TUMORS

in Domestic Animals

I wish to pay tribute to and thank
Dr. Jack Moulton for his years of dedication to
the fields of veterinary oncology and veterinary
pathology, and for entrusting this edition of his
book to me. Dr. Moulton's tireless efforts helped
make *Tumors in Domestic Animals* one of the
landmark textbooks in veterinary pathology.

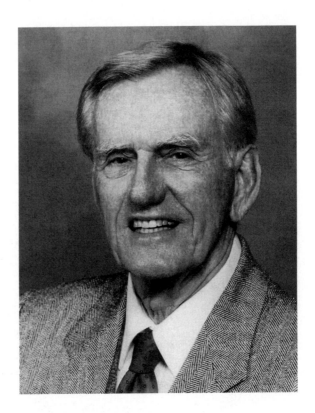

This photograph of Jack was shared with us
by his wife, Idell.

TUMORS
in Domestic Animals

Fourth Edition

Donald J. Meuten, Editor

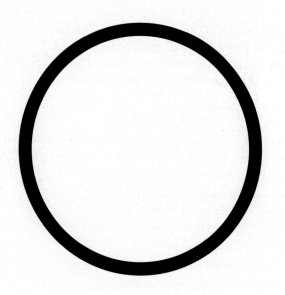

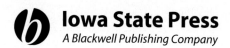

Iowa State Press

A Blackwell Publishing Company

To Mom, the rock in my life.
I will give Travis and Janelle
what you gave to me.

Donald J. Meuten, DVM, PhD, is a professor of pathology in the Department of Microbiology, Pathology, and Parasitology at the College of Veterinary Medicine, North Carolina State University, Raleigh.

© 2002 Iowa State Press
A Blackwell Publishing Company
All rights reserved

Iowa State Press
2121 State Avenue, Ames, Iowa 50014

Orders: 1-800-862-6657
Office: 1-515-292-0140
Fax: 1-515-292-3348
Web site: www.iowastatepress.com

♾ Printed on acid-free paper in the United States of America

Every effort has been made to obtain the necessary permissions for copyrighted material. In the event of any question arising as to the use of any material, the editor and the publisher, while expressing regret for any inadvertent error or oversight, will make the necessary correction in the future printings.

First edition, 1961 © The Regents of the University of California
Second edition, 1978 © The Regents of the University of California
Third edition, revised and expanded, 1990 © The Regents of the University of California
Fourth edition, 2002 © Iowa State Press

Library of Congress Cataloging-in-Publication Data

Tumors in domestic animals / edited by Donald J. Meuten.—4th ed.
    p.; cm.
Includes bibliographical references and index.
    ISBN 0-8138-2652-7 (alk. paper)
    1. Tumors in animals. 2. Veterinary oncology.
    [DNLM: 1. Neoplasms—veterinary. 2. Animals, Domestic. SF 910.T8
    T295 2002] I. Meuten, Donald J.
    SF910.T8 M6 2002
    636.089′6992—dc21   2001005200

The last digit is the print number: 9 8 7 6 5 4 3 2 1

Contents

Preface to the Fourth Edition

Same name, new edition, new authors, new text, new publisher, new and old photos, and a lot more information. In the 12 years since the third edition of *Tumors in Domestic Animals* there has been an enormous expansion of our knowledge about the molecular mechanisms of tumor development and the ancillary aids used to diagnose neoplasms. The information about molecular events in oncology, application of diagnostic techniques, recognition of new tumors, creation of subtypes, new acronyms, new epidemiologic data, paraneoplastic syndromes, treatment regimens, and classification schemes is overwhelming and is a credit to the researchers who generated this information. It was our task to condense this new body of information and present it in a way that is useful to diagnostic pathologists, residents, veterinarians, and oncologists.

In the first three editions of *Tumors in Domestic Animals,* Dr. Moulton and his authors produced one of the landmark textbooks for veterinary pathology. I believe we can maintain that subjective ranking and gather some new readers as well. In deference to all of us, I will not sum our total years of experience with diagnostic material and research; suffice it to say that the blend of these two characteristics in the authors is outstanding, and this is reflected in the quality of each of the chapters.

The format of the previous editions has been maintained, but the text and illustrations are substantially changed or entirely different. Each chapter has a section on relevant clinical pathology, and the black-and-white illustrations in the book are supplemented by color images that are available on CD-ROM. Readers will be able to find salient clinical information, prevalence data, biological behavior, and most importantly, accurate information about gross and microscopic lesions to help diagnostic pathologists establish an accurate morphological diagnosis.

Histopathologic diagnoses are now often supplemented by ancillary diagnostic tests such as immunohistochemistry. This information is provided in an applicable fashion and with the knowledge that it is only one step in the process of establishing a diagnosis—a step that is constantly evolving as more cases and newer techniques are evaluated. For most veterinarians and in most of our diagnostic settings, the morphological diagnosis from H&E stained material is still the gold standard. The clear need for accurate morphological diagnoses in veterinary patient care is even more apparent today with the numerous treatment modalities that are available to oncologists and owners. It is our responsibility to provide as accurate a diagnosis as our capabilities permit and to provide the type of information that clinicians need to make decisions. An excellent example of this is the grading schemes used in the evaluation of connective tissue tumors of the subcutis. It is apparent that the morphological diagnosis is not as predictive of survival or as useful in the selection of treatments as are specific microscopic assessments such as a mitotic index. This has made our job easier and more fulfilling in that we do not have to struggle over the separation of hemangiopericytoma, Schwannoma, neurofibroma, and peripheral nerve sheath tumors to establish a prognosis. Yet we provide applicable information (e.g., grade of connective tissue tumor) that clinical veterinarians need and want to make their decisions. Research projects correlating morphological features of cancer, which a pathologist can provide, with outcome analyses of survival, metastasis, and treatments that clinicians can provide, require a team approach to a much needed area of veterinary oncology. The algorithms that flow from this approach need to be accurate, reproducible, predictive, and simple.

I was delighted when Dr. Moulton asked me to be the next editor of his book. The delight waned about 3 years ago as the enormity of this undertaking became fully apparent, but my enthusiasm is high again as the completion of this project nears. I developed a love-hate relationship with the authors. They loved me when I said their contribution was terrific, and they hated the suggestion of a change. We are a dangerously well informed and opinionated group who need little input from various types of editors. The quality of the authors of this text is such that input was rarely needed; however, to keep us on course and to keep the book a manageable size I asked for modifications. I thank the authors for considering different ideas.

I am deeply indebted to the contributors for their hard work with few rewards, and I take full responsibility for any errors in the text. I thank Dr. Moulton for trusting me with the care of this project and hope he is pleased that his book continues to be a cornerstone of veterinary pathology.

—Don Meuten

Contributing Authors

The number in parentheses following each name is the chapter number.

Capen, Charles C. DVM, PhD (13)
The Ohio State University
Department of Veterinary Biosciences
Columbus, OH

Cooper, Barry J. BVSc, PhD (6)
Cornell University
College of Veterinary Medicine
Ithaca, NY

Cullen, John M. VMD, PhD (1, 9)
North Carolina State University
College of Veterinary Medicine
Raleigh, NC

Dubielzig, Richard R. DVM (8, 15)
University of Wisconsin
School of Veterinary Medicine
Madison, WI

Dungworth, Donald L. BVSc, PhD, MRCVS (7)
University of California
School of Veterinary Medicine
Davis, CA

Else, Rod W. BVSc, PhD, MRCVS (8)
Royal (Dick) School of Veterinary Studies
University of Edinburgh
Edinburgh, Scotland

Goldschmidt, Michael H. BVMS, MRCVS, MSc (2)
University of Pennsylvania
School of Veterinary Medicine
Philadelphia, PA

Head, Kenneth W. BSc, MRCVS (8)
Royal (Dick) School of Veterinary Studies
University of Edinburgh
Edinburgh, Scotland

Hendrick, Mattie J. VMD (2)
University of Pennsylvania
School of Veterinary Medicine
Philadelphia, PA

Higgins, Robert J. BVSc, MSc, PhD (14)
University of California
School of Veterinary Medicine
Davis, CA

Jacobs, Robert M. BSc, DVM, PhD (3)
University of Guelph
Department of Pathology
Guelph, Ontario

Kennedy, Peter C. DVM, PhD (11)
University of California
School of Veterinary Medicine
Davis, CA

Koestner, Adalbert DVM, PhD (14)
The Ohio State University
Department of Veterinary Biosciences
Columbus, OH

MacLachlan, N. James BVSc, MS, PhD (11)
University of California
School of Veterinary Medicine
Davis, CA

Messick, Joanne B. VMD, PhD (3)
University of Illinois
College of Veterinary Medicine
Urbana, IL

Meuten, Donald J. DVM, PhD (10)
North Carolina State University
College of Veterinary Medicine
Raleigh, NC

Misdorp, Wim DVM, PhD (1, 12)
Stadionkade 75III
Amsterdam, The Netherlands

Page, Rodney DVM, MS (1)
Cornell University
College of Veterinary Medicine
Ithaca, NY

Pool, Roy R. DVM, PhD (4, 5)
Mississippi State University
College of Veterinary Medicine
Mississippi State, MS

Popp, James A. DVM, PhD (9)
DuPont Pharmaceutical Company
Stine-Haskell Center
Newark, DE

Thompson, Keith G. BVSc, PhD (4, 5)
Institute of Veterinary, Animal and Biomedical Sciences
Massey University
Palmerston North, New Zealand

Valentine, Beth A. DVM, PhD (6)
Oregon State University
College of Veterinary Medicine
Corvallis, OR

Valli, Victor E. DVM, MSc, PhD (3)
University of Illinois
College of Veterinary Medicine
Urbana, IL

Wilson, Dennis W. DVM, MS, PhD (7)
University of California
School of Veterinary Medicine
Davis, CA

TUMORS

in Domestic Animals

1 An Overview of Cancer Pathogenesis, Diagnosis, and Management

J. M. Cullen, R. Page, and W. Misdorp

CANCER PATHOGENESIS

The Molecular Basis of Cancer

Cancer is a genetic disease. Damage to the cellular genome is a common feature for virtually all neoplasms, despite the facts that neoplasms arise in a broad variety of tissues and that diverse agents such as viruses, mutagenic chemicals, and radiation induce their outgrowth. The genetic damage produced by carcinogens is believed to be random, and many mutations may be inconsequential. Cancer can develop, however, when nonlethal mutations occur in a small subset of the genome, perhaps a few hundred of the 10 thousand genes thought to comprise the mammalian genome. This subset of critical genes can be divided further into two subclasses, oncogenes and tumor suppressor genes, based on their functional attributes. Each of these gene subclasses is discussed below.

Oncogenes

The concept that genes can cause cancer arose from experiments in which animals infected with certain viruses (i.e., retroviruses) rapidly developed tumors. Such viruses were predicted to carry genes, termed *oncogenes*, that transformed normal cells into tumor cells.[1] Years of research into the molecular characteristics of chicken and mouse retroviruses confirmed this prediction, and a wide variety of oncogenes have been isolated and characterized. Surprisingly, the origin of the oncogenic genes was found to be cellular, not viral. That is, the oncogenic retroviruses had acquired (or transduced) certain cellular genes and incorporated them into their genomes. The normal cellular counterparts of the retroviral oncogenes are termed *protooncogenes*. They encode proteins that participate in one or more signal transduction pathways. Such signaling pathways regulate cell proliferation and maturation.[2] Because of their central role in the life cycle of the cell,

protooncogenes have been conserved throughout evolution and vary little from yeast to humans. Once usurped by viruses, the activities of protooncogenes are deregulated via mutation or inappropriate expression and thus perturb mechanisms that strictly regulate the proliferation of mammalian cells.

More than 100 oncogenes have been identified, and their number is expected to increase with continued genetic analyses of neoplasms. Often, the genes are referred to using a three-letter nomenclature that is related to the virus from which they were originally identified. For example, the protooncogene *myc* was originally isolated from the avian *my*elocytomatosis virus, and *erbA* and *erbB* were isolated from avian *erythrob*lastosis virus. The viral oncogene is usually preceded by a v, as in v-*myc* to distinguish it from the related protooncogene (often preceded by a c for cellular, as in c-*myc*). It is important to remember that it is not the gene, but the encoded protein that leads to cell transformation. The proteins encoded by oncogenes are referred to as *oncoproteins*.

A brief review of signal transduction is required to clarify the role of oncogenes in tumor development. Signal transduction pathways convey extracellular stimuli to the nucleus via a cascade of messengers (fig. 1.1 A). Most of the extracellular molecular messengers (usually growth factors) are soluble proteins or polypeptides, although other classes of molecules, such as ions and lipids, can play an important role in signaling. In addition to the soluble factors, the constituents of the extracellular matrix play an important, although generally less well recognized, role in cellular signaling. The extracellular molecules bind to cell receptors that bridge the cell membrane and conduct signals from the outer aspect of the cell into the cytoplasm. Intracellular components of the signaling cascade include cytoplasmic enzymes termed *kinases* (enzymes that attach phosphate atoms onto other proteins) and transcription factors (proteins that regulate gene expression). Such protein messengers are normally in an inactive state or in an active, but regulated, state. Many of

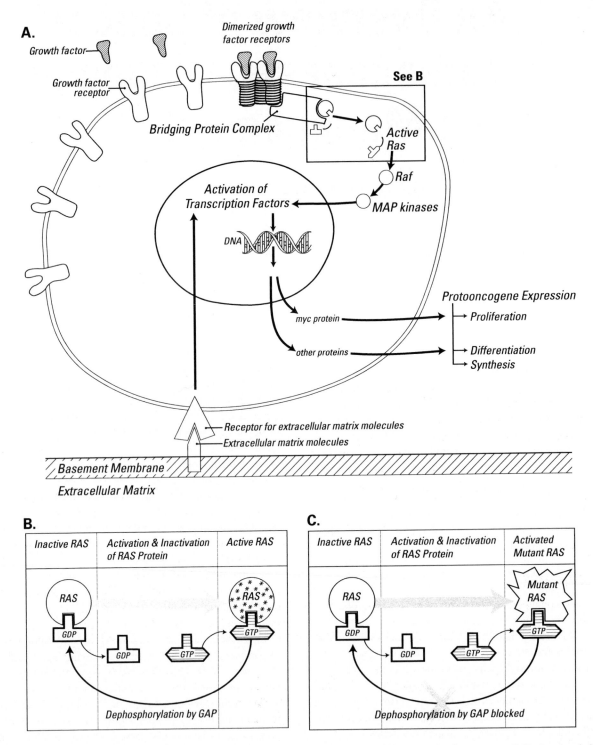

Fig. 1.1.   Signal transduction via RAS protein. **A.** Extracellular stimuli to the nucleus conveyed via a cascade of messengers. **B.** Dephosphorylation by GAP. **C.** Dephosphorylation by GAP blocked.

the messengers can be activated by phosphorylation, and once activated they interact with the next messenger in the cascade, passing on the activation until the message reaches the nucleus. Two groups of kinases that are important in neoplastic transformation phosphorylate the amino acids tyrosine (tyrosine kinases) or serine/threonine (serine/threonine kinases) where they occur in proteins. Swift dephosphorylation returns the proteins to an inactive state, and in normal cells signal transduction is carefully regulated by a matrix of overlapping regulatory pathways.

One of the better characterized signal transduction pathways involves ras protein (fig. 1.1 A,B). Signaling via ras begins when growth factors bind to specific cell surface receptors. This induces the receptors to dimerize, and the dimerized receptors autophosphorylate and undergo a conformational change. As a result of the conformational change, the receptors can interact with an associated bridging protein complex that in turn transfers activation to the ras protein located on the cytoplasmic surface of the cell membrane. Normally, the ras protein is inactive and is bound to guanine diphosphate (GDP). When the ras protein is stimulated it exchanges GDP for guanine triphosphate (GTP) and becomes activated (fig 1.1 B). Ras protein is negatively regulated by GAP (GTPase activating protein), a protein that enhances the hydrolysis of ras-bound GTP to GDP. Activated ras attracts a serine/threonine kinase, termed raf, to the inner aspect of the cell membrane where raf is phosphorylated by membrane associated kinases. Activated raf in turn phosphorylates mitogen activated protein (MAP) kinases, and these kinases migrate to the nucleus, where they stimulate the synthesis of nuclear transcription factors, such as myc. These transcription factors stimulate the expression of genes that cause resting cells either to enter the cell cycle and divide or to alter their differentiation or synthesis patterns.

Conversion of Protooncogenes to Oncogenes

Protooncogenes are converted into oncogenes by one of two means: alteration of gene expression or alteration of gene structure.

Alterations of Gene Expression

Gene expression can be altered via gene amplification, promoter insertion, and/or gene translocation. Each of these genetic mechanisms can lead to the deregulated synthesis of normal (i.e., wild type) protooncogene proteins. Given that proteins, such as ras and erbB, function to stimulate cell proliferation, it is obvious that their overexpression would have dire consequences for homeostasis.

For reasons that are not well understood, tumor cells often sustain excessive rounds of localized DNA replication that can result in the formation of multiple copies (hence the term *gene amplification*) of the same gene or genes. The duplicated genes (or amplicon) may be found in small chromosome-like structures termed *double minutes* or may form concatenated structures within a chromosome that can be identified as homogeneously staining regions (HSRs). HSRs are portions of chromosomes that lack the characteristic banding pattern found in normal chromosomes. In general, gene amplification leads to the overproduction of the products encoded by the genes within the amplicon.

When certain retroviruses insert their genome into cellular DNA, the regulatory elements that normally control viral gene expression can also affect the expression of nearby cellular genes. Viruses and cells have two types of these regulatory elements, enhancers and promoters. Both elements stimulate gene expression, but differ in their functional attributes. Promoters stimulate adjacent genes but must be properly oriented (upstream of the gene) to facilitate expression. Enhancers stimulate promoter activity, but unlike promoters, their capacity to stimulate transcription is orientation independent. Since, in general, viral promoters and enhancers are more potent than their cellular counterparts, they can significantly increase and thus deregulate cellular gene expression. Should a retrovirus integrate within a region of genomic DNA that flanks a protooncogene, transcription of the protooncogene can be deregulated, leading to cell transformation. In most circumstances, viral insertion events affect the regulation of gene expression, not the function of the gene or genes affected.

Gene expression can be altered by spontaneous or carcinogen-induced structural changes in chromosomes, such as insertions, deletions, or translocations. Chromosome translocation results in the movement of portions of one chromosome to another chromosome, or portions may be exchanged between chromosomes in reciprocal translocation events. This process can deregulate transcription by bringing in close juxtaposition active cellular promoters and protooncogenes. One example occurs in both humans and mice: the protooncogene c-*myc* is overexpressed in lymphomas of B cell lineage due to translocation of an active cellular promoter from the immunoglobulin gene to another chromosome that contains c-*myc*.

Alterations of Gene Structure (Function)

Protooncogenes can be transformed into oncogenes following damage to their structure. Structural alterations can occur by mutation of individual nucleotides or alterations that may occur during more global genetic events, such as the translocation of chromosomes. Damage to individual nucleotides (i.e., point mutations) is the most common structural change sustained by protooncogenes. Chemical carcinogens and some forms of radiation exert their influence this way. Mutation of a single nucleotide can lead to the incorporation of a novel amino acid into a protein, and if appropriately localized, the activity of the protein can be profoundly altered. For example, a point mutation in the *ras* gene is often detected in certain mouse tumors. Normally, hydrolysis of GTP to GDP inactivates ras, but point mutations can alter ras protein so that it is unable to interact with GAP and remains constitutively activated (fig 1.1 C). As a consequence, the proliferative signals that emanate from ras proceed unchecked.

In some circumstances the functions of protooncogenes are altered by chromosome translocation. A well-characterized example of this process occurs in the distinctive translocation that produces the Philadelphia chromosome found in many instances of human chronic myelogenous leukemia and some forms of acute myelogenous leukemia (fig. 1.2). During this reciprocal translocation a fragment of a protooncogene (c-*abl*) is moved to a

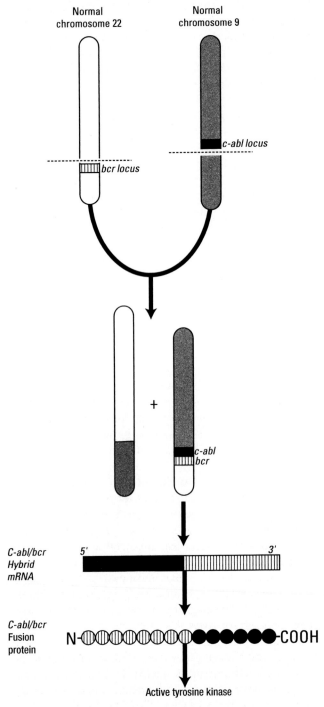

Fig. 1.2. Chromosomal translocation producing an oncogenic fusion protein in chronic myelogenous leukemia in humans.

Classification of Oncogenes

Oncogenes can be grouped into five categories based on the types of oncoproteins they encode. These categories include growth factors, growth factor receptors, intracellular signal transducers, nuclear regulatory proteins (transcription factors), and cyclins (table 1.1). An example of a growth factor, the *sis* protooncogene, encodes the beta chain of platelet derived growth factor. Simian sarcoma virus is a retrovirus that contains the oncogene v-*sis* and can cause transformation of infected fibroblasts by stimulating platelet derived growth factor receptors on their cell surface in an autocrine fashion. In this circumstance the oncoprotein has a normal amino acid sequence but is produced in an abnormal, deregulated amount. Mutant forms of growth factors also occur, and they may inappropriately stimulate receptors by binding to them in an abnormal fashion.

Oncogenes may encode growth factor receptors. A typical growth factor receptor has three components: an extracellular growth factor binding domain, a transmembranous segment, and a cytoplasmic domain with kinase activity. Oncogene encoded growth factor receptors, such as erbB, are often truncated into a form that no longer has the extracellular receptor portion of the normal protein. These abnormal receptors do not require growth factor binding to be stimulated and are constitutively activated.

The intracellular signal transducers are located in the cytosol (e.g., abl, raf) or are membrane associated (e.g., ras, src). Typically, these molecules are protein kinases. Point mutations or more gross structural alterations can constitutively activate these proteins, producing a level of activity that in turn leads to uncontrolled cell proliferation.

Transcription factors are nuclear proteins that regulate gene expression. They bind to selected sites on DNA, alone or in a complex with other proteins to facilitate gene expression. The oncoproteins encoded by *myc, jun,* and *fos* are transcription factors that stimulate expression of genes that are necessary for cell division. Abnormal levels of expression or mutations that alter the function of these proteins can compromise growth control.

Cyclins are a series of proteins that precisely regulate movement through the cell cycle. Individual cyclins are expressed for brief intervals at appropriate points in the cell cycle.[3] The cyclins interact with and activate enzymes termed *cyclin dependant kinases* (cdk). The cdks, in turn, activate proteins that are essential for progression through the cell cycle. Disruption in the function of cyclins leads to dysregulated control of cell replication. Several types of tumors in humans have been described with mutations in the genes that encode cyclins or cyclin dependant kinases.[4,5]

Although mutation and altered expression of oncogenes have been recognized in rodent and human neoplasms for many years, tumors of domestic animals have only recently been examined. Most studies in domestic animals have been conducted on lung, mammary, and lymphoid neoplasms. Mutations in K-*ras* were detected in

site within a gene on another chromosome, termed the *break point cluster region* (bcr). This fusion of genes yields an abnormal hybrid gene that encodes messenger RNA that contains information from both genes. When the message is translated, a hybrid protein, termed a *fusion protein,* results. In this circumstance the fusion protein is an active oncoprotein.

TABLE 1.1. Oncogene categories

	Category	Protooncogene
Growth factors	Platelet derived growth factor (β-chain)	*sis*
	Fibroblast growth factor	*int2*
Growth factor receptors	EGF receptor	*erbB*
	EGF-like receptor	*erbB2*
	CSF-1 receptor	*fms*
	Angiotensin receptor	*mas*
Intracellular signal transducers	GTP-binding protein	*ras*
	Membrane-associated	*src*
	Cytosolic	*abl*
	Cytosolic	*raf*
	Cytosolic	*mos*
Nuclear regulatory proteins	Transcription factor	*myc*
	Transcription factor	*myb*
	Transcription factor	*fos*
	Transcription factor	*jun*
Cell cycle regulators	Cyclins	*cyclin D*
	Cyclin-dependent kinase	*CDK4*

about 25 percent of canine non–small cell pulmonary neoplasms in one study, but no mutations in K-*ras* were found in another study.[6] Lung tumors from dogs exposed to plutonium-239 were characterized by overexpression of c-erbB-2 protein in 18 percent of irradiated dogs, and an increase in epidermal growth factor receptor and its ligand transforming growth factor alpha were found in approximately half of the neoplasms.[7] The c-erbB-2 protein was overexpressed in 74 percent of spontaneous canine mammary cancers and tumor derived cell lines, while no increase was seen in histologically benign mammary tumors.[8] N-*ras* mutations were not found in 10 dogs with mammary carcinoma.[9] Expression of c-*myc* is increased in most malignant plasmacytomas compared to benign plasmacytoma in dogs.[10] Mutated N-*ras* was uncommon in canine lymphoma, occurring in only one of 28 cases.[9] Overexpression of c-*erbB*-2 and c-*myc* was associated with the metastatic potential of canine malignant melanoma cells when transplanted into nude mice.[8] Structural abnormalities and overexpression of the *myc* gene were found in 30 percent of feline leukemias.[11]

Tumor Suppressor Genes

Tumor suppressor genes play a critical role in the control of normal cell growth.[12] They serve as the "brakes" to cell replication. When tumor suppressor genes are inactivated, cells lose regulatory control of cell proliferation. A single intact copy of a tumor suppressor gene is sufficient to maintain control of cell proliferation. When both alleles are lost or damaged the affected cell has a high risk of neoplastic transformation.

To understand the relevance of tumor suppressor gene inactivation in tumorigenesis, a brief review of the normal cell cycle and how it differs from that in neoplastic

cells is warranted (fig. 1.3 A). A review on cell cycle is available.[3] The cell cycle consists of a series of biochemically distinct temporal periods that prepare the cell for division.[13] Following mitosis, a cell may either withdraw from the cell cycle and enter a quiescent stage (G_0 phase) or continue to proliferate. In most instances, cells in G_0 can be recruited into the cell cycle when necessary by interactions with one or more growth factors. The first growth phase of the cell cycle is termed G_1, for the gap in time between mitosis and the next round of DNA synthesis. The duration of this phase of the cell cycle is more variable than the duration of the others, ranging from 6 to 12 hours. During this cell cycle phase, RNA and proteins are synthesized but no DNA is formed. Synthesis of DNA occurs in the S phase during which the DNA content of the cell increases from diploid to tetraploid. The duration of the S phase is similar in all cells and takes from 3 to 8 hours. The S phase is followed by the G_2 phase, a pause of about 3 to 4 hours that precedes mitosis. During the G_2 phase the cell has two complete sets of diploid chromosomes. Mitosis, or the M phase, takes no more than an hour to complete in normal cells.

The ability of cells to restrict or slow their movement through the cell cycle is regulated. This can be observed when normal cells in tissue culture sustain irradiation induced genetic damage.[3,14] Irradiated cells in the early stages of the cell cycle respond by halting their progress prior to the S phase; this pause in the cell cycle has been termed the G_1/S checkpoint. During the pause, DNA that has been damaged by irradiation can be repaired before mutations are passed on to the genomes of daughter cells. In cells in which tumor suppressor genes are absent or not functioning properly, genetic damage is left unrepaired and often leads to genetic instability and additional oncogenic events. A similar checkpoint is present at the transition between the G_2 and the M phase of the cell cycle.

The best characterized of the tumor suppressor genes are *p53* and the retinoblastoma (*Rb*) gene.[15-17] Both of these genes encode nuclear phosphoproteins that regulate cell cycle progression. When the Rb protein is in its nonphosphorylated form it inhibits entry of the cell into the S phase of the cell cycle by binding a transcription factor that stimulates growth promoting genes (fig. 1.3 B).[18] When a cell is stimulated to divide, the Rb protein is phosphorylated, causing it to release sequestered transcription factors that enable cells to enter the S phase. Following the S phase, the Rb protein is dephosphorylated and is, once again, able to bind transcription factors and inhibit entry into the S phase. In tumor cells, the ability of Rb to bind transcription factors is disrupted and the checkpoint is eliminated. For example, oncogenic DNA viruses (discussed later) can disrupt cell cycle control by synthesizing viral proteins that block the uptake of transcription factors by Rb protein.[3]

The *p53* gene encodes a nuclear phosphoprotein that can regulate movement of the cell through the cell cycle.[19,20] Although this phosphoprotein is not involved in regulation of the normal cell cycle, it plays an important

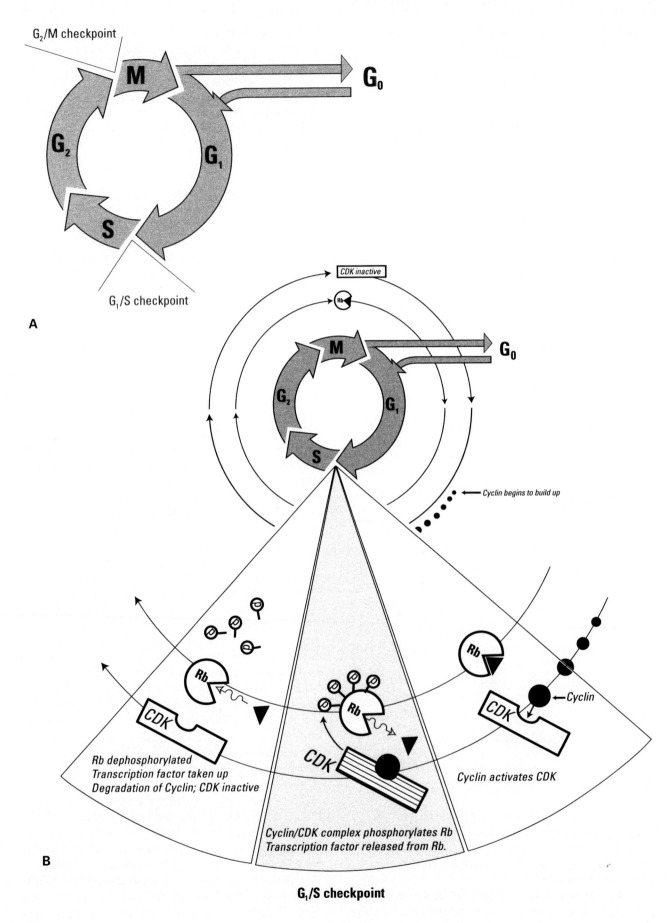

Fig. 1.3. **A.** The normal cell cycle. **B.** The role of Rb, cyclins, and cyclin dependent kinases (CDK) in the normal cell cycle. Note: ▶ = transcription factor; p = phosphorylation.

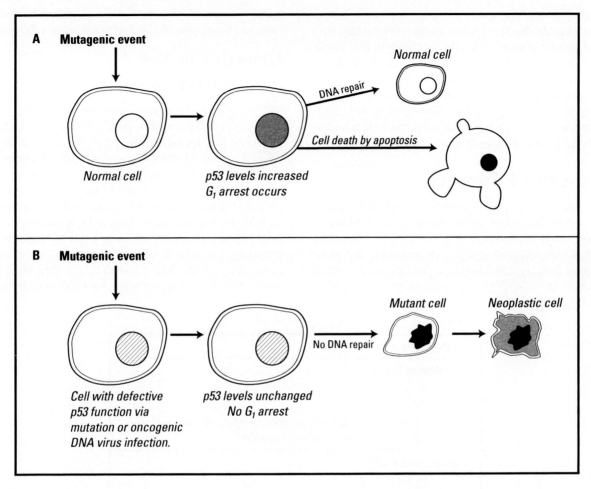

Fig. 1.4.   Effect of p53 function on cellular response to mutagenic events. **A.** Normal p53 function. **B.** Abnormal p53 function.

role in cells that have sustained genetic damage. Through mechanisms that are not well understood, p53 can detect when a cell sustains genetic damage by U.V. light, irradiation, or carcinogenic chemicals and then arrests the entry of the cell into the S phase from the G1 phase of the cell cycle to allow time for the repair of cellular DNA damage. It also induces DNA repair enzymes to aid in elimination of mutations. If the extent of DNA damage is too excessive, p53 can promote cellular apoptosis. Although normally a short-lived protein, after genetic damage, p53 is modified in a way that causes it to have a significantly longer half-life, accumulate in the nucleus, and activate transcription of genes that inhibit specific cyclin-dependent kinases and prevent the phosphorylation of the Rb protein leading to cell cycle arrest (fig. 1.4A). Other effects include expression of genes involved in DNA repair or apoptosis. Cells carrying mutated *p53* genes or cells infected with oncogenic DNA viruses that alter the function of p53, do not arrest before entering the S phase of the cell cycle and are less likely to undergo apoptosis (fig. 1.4B). Affected cells can continue to replicate with damaged DNA, and those that do not develop lethal genetic changes are at risk for acquiring additional genetic damage leading to neoplastic transformation.

The DNA sequence for *p53* is very similar in dogs, cats, and humans.[21] Because mutations in *p53* occur in a high proportion of some types of human neoplasms, the frequency of *p53* mutations in animals has been examined. Mutations in *p53* have been detected in canine neoplasms including thyroid carcinomas,[22] osteosarcomas,[23] and mammary tumors.[24] Equine squamous cell carcinomas have been identified with *p53* mutations, but the significance of these mutations is not clear.[25] Abnormal cellular distribution of p53, indicative of mutant *p53*, has been shown in canine colorectal tumors.[26] The number of neoplasms from domestic species that have been studied is small, and it is not possible to determine the relative frequency of *p53* mutations in different tumor types.

Regulators of Apoptosis

Genes that control programmed cell death can play a significant role in tumor development when they fail to function normally. Certain types of lymphoid tumors serve as an example of the importance of the genes that control apoptosis.[27] These tumors are characterized by an increased expression of a gene, *bcl*-2, that blocks apoptosis. *Bcl*-2 is only one of a family of genes that participate in the regulation of apoptosis. The ability of oncoproteins such as bcl2 to block cell death pathways may enable cells that have sustained genetic damage to escape mechanisms that would stimulate normal cells to undergo programmed cell death. Whereas normal lymphoid cells have a finite life span, the neoplastic lymphocytes that overexpress *bcl-2* persist and slowly form lymphoid masses.[28] Consequently, cells eluding apoptosis could multiply and are at risk to accumulate additional genetic damage that can heighten malignancy.

Growth of Tumors

The biology of cell growth and differentiation is quite similar for normal and neoplastic cells.[3,14] What distinguishes transformed cells from normal cells is deficient regulation of cell proliferation, differentiation, and chromosomal integrity. This aberrant regulation affects several aspects of the natural history of tumor growth including tumor cell growth and differentiation, malignant conversion, and tumor progression and tumor stroma formation.

Growth Kinetics and Differentiation

It is generally agreed upon that most tumors arise from clonal expansion of a single cell that has undergone malignant transformation (fig. 1.5)[29]. To form a clinically detectable mass of about 1 g, a single 10 μ diameter cell would have to increase to a mass of 10^9 cells, taking about 30 population doublings. Only 10 more doublings would yield a 1 kg mass, which is the maximum size compatible with life for humans and is likely to be in excess of a fatal tumor burden for small animal species, although benign neoplasms can grow to larger sizes without such a deleterious effect on the host. Clearly, by the time most neoplasms have been detected, the greater part of their growth

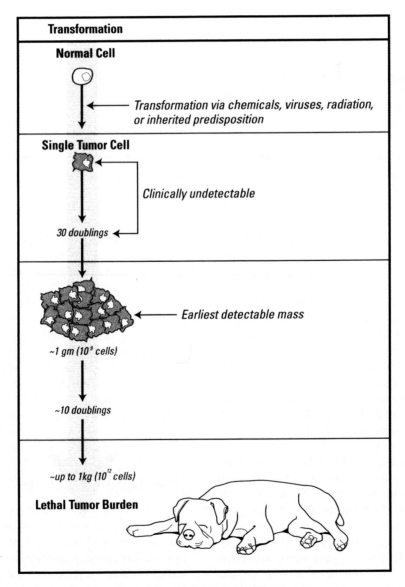

Fig. 1.5.   Tumor cell growth kinetics. Modified from *Hospital Practice* (1983) 18:81, with permission.

is complete. In this example it was assumed that all progeny cells survive and continue to replicate, which as will be discussed below, is an unlikely assumption. If all the tumor cells were to continue to divide and if a 24 hour period to complete the cell cycle were assumed, a 1 g mass would take 30 days to develop, and only 10 additional days would be required for the mass to become lethal.

One goal of tumor biology is to understand the factors that govern the growth of transformed cells and to use this information to assist in earlier detection of neoplasms or to arrest the growth of tumors before they become clinically evident.

The rate at which any tumor increases in size is dependant on three factors: (1) the rate of mitosis of individual cells, (2) the proportion of cells in the replicating pool (growth fraction), and (3) the rate of cell death or differentiation into a postmitotic stage.

Not all neoplasms have a high rate of cell replication. The rate of mitosis does not necessarily separate neoplasms from normal tissue or even benign neoplasms from malignant neoplasms. It is well recognized that the rate of cellular replication in normal tissues, such as the intestinal crypt epithelium, or inflamed tissues can exceed the rate of cell replication in many neoplasms by more than 10-fold.[30-32] Mitotic figures are constant microscopic features of intestinal epithelium and are often seen in areas of neovascularization and fibroplasia. Benign tumors and some tumors that spontaneously regress (e.g., transmissible venereal tumors and histiocytomas) are characterized by a high mitotic index.

The initial growth rate of neoplasms is often exponential, each cell giving rise to two viable daughter cells that enter the cell cycle. Later, constraints on tumor growth develop. These restraints include a lower proportion of cells in the replicative pool and an increase in cell death. Both of these events can be partly attributed to diminished vascular perfusion due to insufficient vascular ingrowth or the dysfunctional vasculature that is characteristic of neoplasms. Cells that lack sufficient nutritive support often leave the replicative pool and remain in the G_0 phase of the cell cycle until adequate nutrient support, including oxygen supply, is available. By the time most tumors are clinically detectable, the majority of the tumor cells are resting in G_0 or a prolonged G_1, not in the replicative pool. Other constraints on tumor growth include the differentiation of some cells into a postmitotic stage in which they are lost from the replicative pool as well as the shedding of other cells from the original mass. In some neoplasms fewer than 10 percent of cells may survive following mitosis due to the loss of genetic integrity. In neoplasms for which the rate of cell death approaches the rate of cell proliferation, the growth of the neoplasm will appear slow despite a high number of mitotic figures. In the end, the rate of growth of a mass is determined by the difference between the rate of cell replication and the rate of cell loss. It should be remembered, however, that the rate of growth of neoplasms is not always consistent. Sudden spurts of growth after long periods of apparent dormancy can occur. This may occur when subclones of cells with greater replicative ability emerge from the population of neoplastic cells through the process of tumor progression.

Tumor growth can be enhanced by the failure of tumor cells to respond to stimuli that would lead to apoptosis. In some tumor cells, the apoptosis pathways are disrupted and these tumor cells fail to die. As a result, tumor growth is facilitated by the accumulation of cells that do not undergo apoptosis.

The clinically relevant aspect of tumor cell growth kinetics centers on its impact on therapy.[33] Classical treatment approaches (chemotherapy and radiation therapy) involve killing cells that are rapidly synthesizing DNA. Tumors with only a small proportion of cells in the replicating pool may not respond well to these types of treatment. The more histologically aggressive appearing masses with high rates of mitosis may be much more responsive to therapy despite their more anaplastic and invasive characteristics.

Malignant Transformation, Progression, and Tumor Heterogeneity

Malignant transformation (or malignant conversion) is the process by which a normal cell acquires the phenotype of a malignant cell. The emergence of the malignant phenotype is dependent on the sequential acquisition of genetic damage until, in a rare event, one cell accumulates sufficient numbers and types of genetic changes to become malignant. There are likely to be many pathways that lead a cell to the malignant phenotype, but they all involve multiple genetic alterations.

Tumor progression is a process by which cells that have developed the malignant phenotype acquire more characteristics that are deleterious to the host (fig. 1.6). Tumor growth starts with a single cell that has undergone neoplastic transformation, and the incipient tumor develops by clonal expansion of this one cell. Initially, all cells in the mass are identical, but due to the lack of regulation of chromosomal integrity the tumor cells acquire genetic changes that give rise to *tumor heterogeneity*. Some genetic changes are lethal to the affected cells, but some changes confer new phenotypes that may have inherent growth advantages. Over time, the tumor mass becomes composed of a heterogeneous cell population, and neoplasms accumulate characteristics that make them more dangerous. As a neoplastic cell replicates, subclones emerge that are more locally aggressive, more likely to metastasize, and less responsive to therapy. This process has been attributed to a greater genetic instability in affected cells. It is because of tumor progression that early detection is associated with improved prognosis. By the time most tumors are detected, however, they are most likely composed of a heterogeneous cell population, because by this time most neoplasms have completed the greater part of their growth.

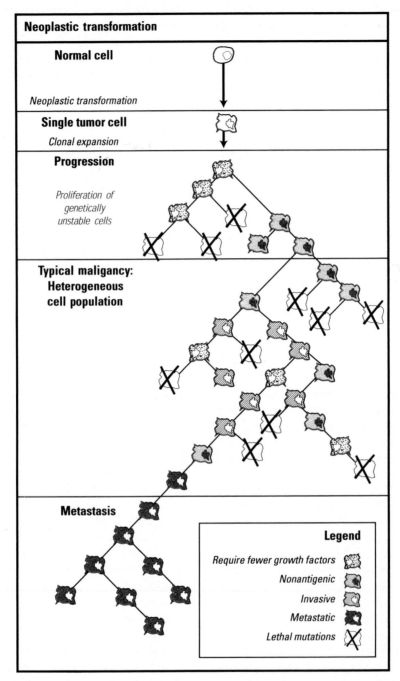

Fig. 1.6.   Tumor heterogeneity. Modified from *Hospital Practice* (1983) 18:81, with permission.

Tumor Angiogenesis and Stroma Formation

Solid neoplasms depend on the blood vessels and supporting stroma that they recruit from adjacent tissue for their survival and growth.[34] Tumor cells that secrete growth factors or stimulate other cells to release angiogenic factors stimulate the vessels and supporting stroma in tumors. Without angiogenesis tumors have to rely on diffusion to provide needed nutrients and eliminate waste products. Tumors lacking the ability to stimulate vascular ingrowth are limited to a diameter of 1–2 mm.[34,35] Moreover, angiogenesis plays an essential role in sustained tumor growth, as well as metastasis.[36] Angiogenesis, measured as the density of the microvasculature within a tumor, has been shown to be a significant prognostic indicator for some human neoplasms such as those of the breast and prostate.[37,38] Because of this powerful effect on tumor growth, angiogenesis is an area of particular interest in tumor biology. Angiogenesis by itself, however, is not an indication of malignancy as even benign neoplasms have the ability to stimulate vascular growth.[39]

The mechanisms of angiogenesis and stroma formation are similar in tumors and in wound healing, although there are some distinct differences in the structure and function of the vessels that are formed during each process.[40] In tumors, the blood vessels are poorly differentiated and are not distributed uniformly through the tumor.[41] Tumor blood vessels tend to be more tortuous and dilated than normal vessels. Blood vessels in tumors often have gaps in the endothelium and are persistently permeable, unlike vessels in healing wounds that have a transient phase of permeability. Increased interstitial pressure due to the permeable vessels and the lack of lymphatics to carry away the leaked fluid lead to edema formation. This edema and the resultant interstitial fluid pressure tend to collapse the vessels within the tumor, thus obstructing local blood flow. The density of vascular supply to tumors is frequently minimally adequate and is deficient in arteriolar supply, in particular. As a result, irregular blood flow and perfusion cause localized areas of hypoxia and anoxia, leading to apoptosis or necrosis.[42]

Tumor stromata are composed of nonneoplastic connective tissue, blood vessels, and inflammatory cells. While the vasculature is an essential component of stroma formation because of its nutrient support of the neoplasm, the greatest proportion of the tumor stroma is nonvascular. The noncellular components of the stroma include collagen types I, III, and V, glycosaminoglycans, proteoglycans, fibronectin, fibrin, and plasma proteins.[43] Fibroblasts, endothelial cells, and inflammatory cells are the principal cellular constituents. Initially, the tumor stroma resembles granulation tissue with a high density of blood vessels and smaller numbers of fibroblasts. The persistent permeability of tumor vessels allows a continued leakage of macromolecules that engenders a perivascular deposition of fibrin that serves as scaffolding for migration of host stromal cells and tumor stroma formation. As this tissue matures, collagenous stroma predominates and vascularity diminishes, creating a desmoplastic or scirrhous response. For reasons that are unclear, the amount of stroma produced by different neoplasms varies considerably. Certain carcinomas such as gastric, transitional cell, and mammary carcinomas are more prone to develop desmoplasia than other neoplasms. The resultant masses are very firm to the touch, and the stroma can comprise a larger proportion of the mass than the tumor cells do.

A newly emerging understanding of epithelial-mesenchymal interactions is clarifying the role of fibroblasts and other stromal elements in tumor growth. Fibroblasts adjacent to carcinomas have a fetal-like phenotype that differs from fibroblasts in other parts of the body.[44,45] Tumor associated fibroblasts release growth factors and proteases in response to cytokines released by neoplastic epithelial cells. The factors released by the fibroblasts can accelerate the process of cancer progression and facilitate tumor cell mobility. For example, scirrhous gastric carcinoma cells can be stimulated to proliferate by normal fibroblasts that are adjacent to tumor cells.[46]

Tumor Growth Characteristics and Clinical Observations

As the mechanisms of tumor growth are clarified, some of the long recognized growth characteristics of tumors can be better understood. For example, umbilication of the surface of a mass commonly results from central necrosis. Central necrosis occurs more often in epithelial than in mesenchymal neoplasms and more often in malignant than in benign neoplasia.[47] This has been attributed to the fact that epithelial neoplasms have a greater dependency on recruited stroma to support tumor cell growth than mesenchymal neoplasms do. Several causes for central necrosis in neoplasms have been proposed; all of them involve disruption of blood flow that supports the growth of the neoplasm, and they may act independently or in conjunction to lead to necrosis within a neoplasm. Although the vessels are composed of normal cells, they do not function as well as normal vessels. They tend to leak plasma constituents in a fashion similar to inflamed vessels. Ischemia may result from inadequate patency or perfusion through the abnormally permeable vasculature or increased tissue pressure at the center of a mass that restricts perfusion of small caliber vessels. Thrombosis within the tumor mass is another possible cause for tumor necrosis. For example, hemangiosarcomas may, due to altered neoplastic endothelial cell–lined vascular spaces, stimulate platelet aggregation or stimulate the coagulation cascade by other mechanisms. Studies in canine neoplasms have shown tissue hypoxia in tumors beginning no more than 1 mm away from capillaries.[48]

Benign and malignant neoplasms can often be distinguished by their pattern of growth during physical examination. A capsule (a circumferential rim of compressed connective tissue) often surrounds benign neoplasms. The capsule is produced primarily by the surrounding normal tissue, possibly in response to tumor derived growth factors, although the tumor may contribute to the capsule in some tumor types. Since the capsule separates the neoplasm from adjoining tissue, benign neoplasms are usually freely moveable when palpated. The term *cancer,* from the Greek for crab, is derived from the early observation that malignant neoplasms tended to attach firmly to adjacent tissues in a "crab-like" fashion. This characteristic is a consequence of invasive behavior that is typical of malignancies. The inability to move overlying skin fully or to discern the margins of a neoplasm by palpation is suggestive of the invasive behavior characteristic of malignancy. Malignant neoplasms may also be surrounded by compressed normal tissue, termed a *pseudocapsule,* that does not restrict tumor invasion but may be misinterpreted at the time of surgery as a true capsule.

Invasion and Metastasis

Metastasis is an inefficient multistep process, and only a very small proportion of cells is able to complete the process.[49] Once a malignancy develops, a metastatic sub-clone may arise within the tumor through the process of tumor progression. Loss of epithelial adhesion by impaired activity of cell adhesion factors such as E cadherins precedes invasion by epithelial tumors. During the transition from noninvasive (in situ) carcinoma to infiltrating carcinoma, malignant cells penetrate the basement membrane. First, tumor cells attach to the basement membrane; subsequently, they secrete hydrolytic enzymes (proteases) that degrade the membrane. The next step is locomotion. Tumor cells migrate into the extracellular matrix and create a pathway through it by the release of various enzymes secreted by the tumor cells and host macrophages. Connective tissues are unequally susceptible to invasive processes. Hyaline cartilage, for example, contains inhibitors of matrix degrading enzymes and is highly resistant to invasion.[50]

Intravasation, entry of tumor cells into the vascular spaces of the blood stream or lymphatics, is facilitated by increased permeability of tumor vessels and increased tumor cell motility. Intravasation via blood vessels is only possible after attachment of tumor cells to the basement membrane of the vessel and degradation of this barrier. Tumor cells can then pass through the junctions between adjacent endothelial cells or pass directly through the intact endothelium. Lymphatic vessels pose less of a barrier to entry than blood vessels because lymphatic vessels lack a basement membrane.

The mere presence of tumor cells in vessels does not ensure that those cells will eventually give rise to metastatic populations. Once tumor cells enter the vasculature, they encounter the array of host cells involved in immune-mediated killing of tumor cells. To survive, the tumor cells must evade intense scrutiny by the host immune response. One way tumor cells evade host defenses is by interacting with blood components, such as platelets and fibrin, to form thrombi. When the tumor cells are enclosed by fibrin, they may be protected from recognition by the immune system and have a better chance to survive in the hostile environment of the blood. Extravasation of surviving tumor cells may occur in a directed, nonrandom fashion. Recent studies help explain the predilection for certain tumors to metastasize to particular organs. Some tumor cells are guided to particular organs because they bind to tissue-specific endothelial cell surface markers. In other tumor types, the cells bear receptors to specific chemokines, home to organs that release the chemokines, and are less likely to be found in organs that do not release these chemokines.[152] Tumor cells then penetrate the endothelium, reversing the process of intravasation.

The newly extravasated tumor clone must next acquire a blood supply. A new vascular network is needed not only to provide nutrients to the growing tumor, but also to carry away waste products. Once a metastatic tumor has established a proper vascular supply, its growth may be limited by inhibitory growth factors, by a restrictive growth environment, or by a cytotoxic response by the host.

There are three principal pathways of metastasis: (1) lymphatic, (2) hematogenous, and (3) transcoelomic.[51]

Lymphatic Metastasis

Lymphatic invasion occurs primarily at the periphery of the tumor. Lymphatic vessels offer little resistance to penetration by tumor cells because they lack a basement membrane. Clumps or single cell tumor emboli may be trapped in the first lymph node encountered, or they may traverse or bypass lymph nodes to form a more distant metastasis, a condition termed *skip metastasis*. Tumor cells are usually first detected histologically in the subcapsular region of the lymph nodes. Based on extensive studies in humans and limited data from animals, carcinomas have a predilection for metastasis by the lymphatic route compared to sarcomas.[52-54]

In dogs with mammary cancer, regional lymph nodes appeared to function as good filters since bypassing the node was found to be extremely uncommon.[55] An enlarged local lymph node does not necessarily mean metastasis has occurred because at this stage the node may be enlarged and palpable due to lymphoid hyperplasia and/or metastasis. In most cases, an enlarged lymph node draining a region with malignancy is probably no longer immunologically effective, but there is no consensus regarding the value of the removal of such an enlarged node.[56] Fine needle aspiration by an experienced cytologist or biopsy for histologic examination may be necessary to distinguish lymphoid hyperplasia from metastasis and to allow appropriate clinical staging and treatment planning.

Hematogenous Metastasis

Tumor cells can enter the blood directly by invasion of blood vessels or indirectly via the lymphatic system that connects with venous tributaries at sites such as the thoracic duct and subsequently enter into the vena cava. Distribution of hematogenous metastases can be explained by the hemodynamic theory based on circulatory anatomy. Briefly, primary tumors spread along the vena cava route (mammary, skin, soft tissue, bone, thyroid tumors) or along the portal vein route (gastrointestinal and pancreatic tumors). The vast majority of tumor cells are arrested in the first capillary bed they encounter. The first capillary filter of the vena caval drainage is the lung, and the liver is the first microvascular field draining the portal vein system. From those sites, tumors can spread to secondary microvascular filters like bone marrow. However, in the human, and to a lesser extent also in domestic animals, preferential metastatic sites can also be explained by organ tropism or the seed and soil hypothesis. Since extravasation requires adhesion to endothelial cells or underlying basement membrane, tumor cell attachment may be directed to specific sites by receptor and ligand interactions. The release of chemokines can also direct some types of tumor cells to specific organs. Organ tropism seems to play a role in metastasis of melanomas in dog and man (brain) and prostatic carcinoma in dog and man (bone). For these tumors occult micrometastases are frequently present at the time of primary tumor diagnosis.

Pulmonary metastases can be nodular, diffuse, or radiating in a linear fashion (lymphangitic type). Nodular pulmonary metastases can be used for determination of growth rate by repeated radiological examination. In dogs, doubling time of pulmonary metastases ranged from 8 to 31 days, shorter than in most human metastases. Nourishment of primary and metastatic lung tumors in dogs is provided by new vessels from the bronchial artery and by non-proliferating branches of pulmonary arteries.[57]

Most osseous metastases have intertrabecular growth. Only in advanced stages are there osteolysis or endosteal and periosteal bone formation.[58] The frequency of osseous metastasis may be underestimated when the bones are not carefully checked radiographically or during the postmortem examination. In a detailed postmortem study, examination of transected bones revealed that 17 percent of dogs with visceral metastasis from a variety of neoplasms also had skeletal metastasis.[58] Sites of predilection are flat bones, including the ribs, the vertebrae, and the metaphyseal region of the long bones. Frequently, multiple sites in the bones are affected, and metastatic involvement of bone is almost always accompanied by concurrent soft tissue metastasis. Most primary tumors responsible for bone metastases in the dog are carcinomas, including mammary gland,[59,60] lungs,[58,59,61] and prostate.[58,59] Metastasis to bone from mammary carcinomas has been reported in cats.[59]

Transcoelomic Metastasis

The coelomic surfaces, covered with a film of fluid, are an ideal site for metastatic seeding. Neoplastic cells shed from a primary tumor may not need to be able to invade the basement membrane if they can survive implanted onto the serosal surface of the body cavity or organs. Implantation of tumor cells in serous cavities is often accompanied by an accumulation of fluid. Peritoneal or pleural carcinomatosis in dogs is associated either with a primary tumor within a coelomic cavity (ovarian, pulmonary carcinoma) or with metastases from carcinoma elsewhere in the body (e.g., mammary carcinoma). Pleuritic carcinomatosis in dogs and cats with mammary carcinoma was found to be invariably associated with the presence of pulmonary metastasis.[55,62] The spread of mesotheliomas is often restricted to the coelomic cavity, the site of origin.

Etiologies of Cancer

Chemical Carcinogenesis

Chemicals are reported to be responsible for the largest proportion of human cancer. The major categories of chemical carcinogens include (1) polycyclic aromatic hydrocarbons such as benzpyrene, which are encountered in tobacco smoke, combusted fossil fuels, and cooked meats, (2) nitrosamines, which may be formed de novo in the stomach from dietary sources, (3) aromatic amines and azo dyes used in industrial applications and once used in food dyes, and (4) a variety of naturally occurring carcinogens, such as the mycotoxin aflatoxin B1, a common contaminant of corn and peanuts. Much of human exposure to carcinogenic chemicals occurs in the workplace or through behaviors such as cigarette smoking. Obviously, direct exposure of domestic animals to potentially carcinogenic chemicals occurs in different ways. However, chemical exposure is not nearly as well documented for domestic animals as it is for humans, and the importance of environmental chemical exposure as a cause of cancer for domestic animals is largely unknown.

A few studies have demonstrated that environmental exposure to carcinogenic chemicals can pose a risk for cancer in domestic animals. An increased risk of bladder cancer in dogs has been associated with topical application of insecticide.[63] The risk was greatest in dogs that were treated more than twice yearly. Obesity was an additional risk factor, possibly because most insecticides are lipid soluble and are stored in body fat. Dogs exposed to household cigarette smoke or other household chemicals had no associated tumor risk,[63] but when the filtering effect of the nose was bypassed in an experimental setting, direct inhalation of cigarette smoke did produce pulmonary adenocarcinomas in laboratory dogs.[64] Exposure to a lawn herbicide, 2,4-dichlorophenoxyacetic acid, was reported to increase the risk of lymphoma in dogs.[65] However, a review of the study design cast doubt on the validity of the design and conclusions of this study.[66] Environmental carcinogens can also affect ruminants. Ingestion of bracken fern was, at least, a cofactor with papillomavirus infection, and the combination led to neoplasms of the digestive and urinary tract.[67,68]

In addition to these environmental carcinogens, many other chemicals have been established as experimental carcinogens for dogs. A few examples include nitrosamines and polycyclic aromatic hydrocarbons. Nitrosamines are potent carcinogens in the canine stomach,[69] lung,[70,71] and liver.[72] Pulmonary neoplasms can be produced by exposure to nitrosamines and several polycyclic aromatic hydrocarbons.[71] Carcinomas in the canine urinary bladder have been induced by 3, 3′-dichlorobenzidine.[73]

The process of carcinogenesis can been divided into two major phases: *initiation* and *promotion*. Initiated cells have a greater likelihood of becoming malignant than normal cells, although initiation alone is insufficient for tumor development. Initiation occurs when cells are exposed to a chemical that can permanently and irreversibly alter their cellular DNA. Usually a single brief exposure to an initiator is sufficient to produce a mutation through formation of covalent bonds between the chemical and a nucleotide in the DNA. Initiation is a two step process. Following the initial genetic damage, a round of replication is required to fix the mutation into the genome as a permanent change.

Chemicals that serve as initiators are highly reactive electrophiles—molecules that form covalent bonds with electron rich targets (nucleophiles) such as DNA, RNA, and proteins to form adducts. Whereas adducts formed

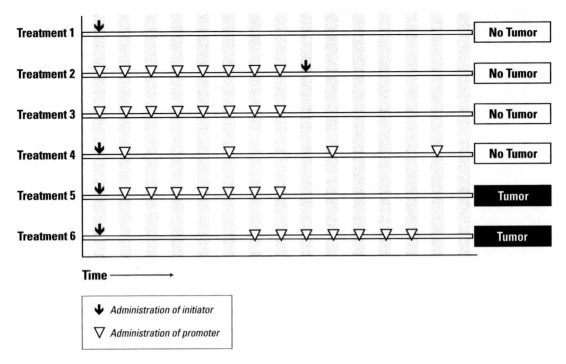

Fig. 1.7. Initiators and promoters in chemical carcinogenesis.

with proteins and RNA can lead to cell death, DNA adducts can cause mutations and are more significant in cancer production. This view is supported by the observation of a general correlation between the amount of DNA adduct formation and tumor yield.[74-76] Thus, most initiators also are mutagens. A few chemicals (direct acting carcinogens) are capable of forming adducts directly with DNA without metabolic activation. However, most initiators require metabolic activation in order to form adducts. They are termed *procarcinogens* or *indirect acting carcinogens.*

Most promoters are nongenotoxic chemicals that do not require metabolic activation and whose effects are reversible. They are not capable of transforming cells by their action alone, but sufficient exposure to promoters after initiation will lead to tumor formation.[77] Promotion only occurs following initiation. Because the effects of promotion are reversible, they must be administered with sufficient frequency and for sufficient duration to produce tumors (fig. 1.7). An important common feature of the diverse array of compounds that can serve as promoters is that most of them alter signal transduction within cells and stimulate clonal replication of initiated cells. Since mutations accumulate more rapidly in dividing cells, clonal expansion of initiated cells increases the risk of additional genetic changes and transformation of the cells to a malignant phenotype. Promoters have the ability to diminish the latency period and increase the number of tumors produced in animals treated with initiators. Chemicals that can initiate and promote neoplasms are termed *complete carcinogens.* An overview of the process of chemical carcinogenesis is shown in figure 1.8.

Viral Carcinogenesis

Viruses have long been recognized as agents of neoplasia in domestic animals. As early as the first decade of the twentieth century, two oncogenic viral infections, an avian leukosis virus and Rous sarcoma virus, were identified in poultry.[78,79] Oncogenic viruses represent a diverse group, including RNA and DNA viruses, and there are a variety of mechanisms involved in neoplastic transformation of infected cells. Despite these differences, there are some consistent features in virus induced cancer. Common factors in virus induced neoplastic transformation include the following: (1) only a single virus particle is needed to infect a cell, and multiple rounds of infection are unnecessary; (2) all or part of the viral genome persists in the transformed cell, but there are often no infectious progeny produced; (3) at least part of the viral genome is expressed; (4) transformation results from corruption of normal cellular growth control signals; and (5) reversion of transformation can be achieved by specific interference with the function of viral effector molecules.[80]

All of the RNA viruses that cause neoplasia are retroviruses, but only some members of the family Retroviridae are oncogenic. Most of the oncogenic retroviruses are classified as mammalian type C retroviruses. These include feline leukemia virus, feline sarcoma viruses, simian sarcoma virus, and a variety of rodent viruses. Bovine leukemia virus is in the HTLV-BLV group. Other retroviruses such as the lentiviruses, including equine infectious anemia virus and the spumaviruses, are not considered to be oncogenic.

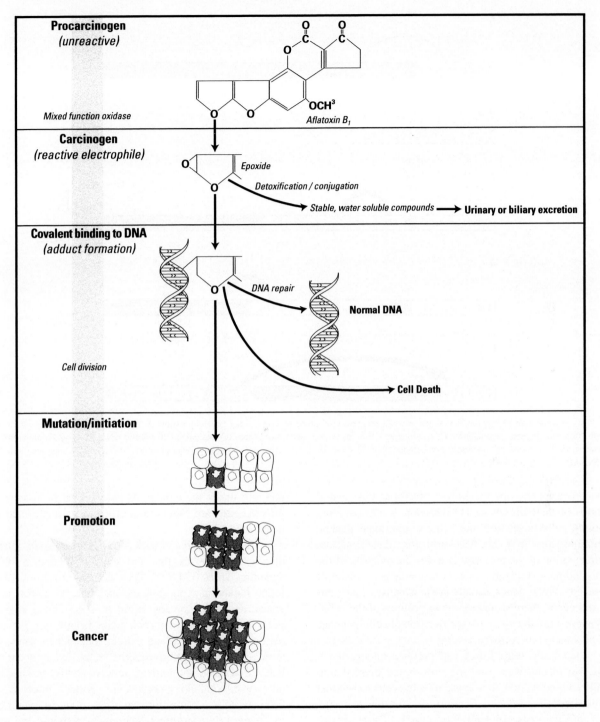

Fig. 1.8. An overview of the process of chemical carcinogenesis.

Retroviruses have a common life cycle. All retroviruses have an RNA genome that is reverse transcribed via an endogenous enzyme, reverse transcriptase, into a double stranded DNA provirus. As an obligatory part of the normal life cycle of retroviruses, the DNA provirus is integrated, usually at random, into the genome of the infected cell. The three major retroviral genes are *gag, pol,* and *env.* The *gag* gene encodes for the capsid (internal) proteins. The *pol* gene encodes the reverse transcrip-

tase enzyme, and the *env* gene encodes the viral envelope proteins. Viral genes, like cellular genes, are expressed under the control of specific promoters (fig. 1.9 A). Retroviral gene expression is under the control of potent viral transcription regulators, termed *long terminal repeats* (LTRs), that flank the ends of the genome [upstream (5′) and downstream (3′)] (fig. 1.9 B). These regulatory regions determine the tissues in which the virus replicates and affect the pathogenicity of different viral strains. The

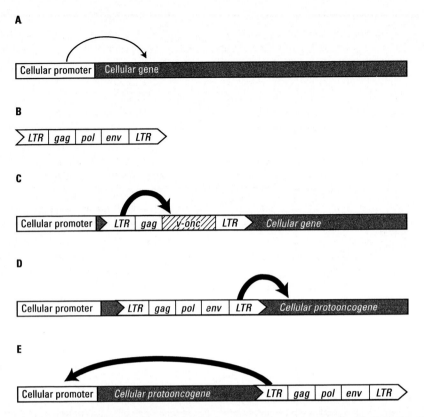

Fig. 1.9. Normal gene expression and effects of oncogenic retroviral promoters on cellular gene expression. **A.** Normal promotion of gene expression in cells. **B.** Retroviral gene organization. **C.** Transducing retrovirus (v-*onc* encodes oncoprotein) integrated into cellular DNA. **D.** *Cis*-activating retrovirus (activation via viral promoter) integrated into cellular DNA. **E.** *Cis*-activating retrovirus (action on cellular promoter via enhancer) integrated into cellular DNA.

oncogenic capacity of retroviruses is facilitated by several features of their life cycle: (1) infection is not cytolytic, enabling cells to survive and acquire additional genetic alterations that may be necessary for transformation; (2) integration of the provirus damages the integrity of the host genome; (3) integrated provirus can acquire intact or damaged cellular genes, usually at the expense of portions of viral genes, thereby incorporating portions of the cellular genome into the virus; (4) the function of cellular genes can be affected by retroviruses.[80]

Oncogenic retroviruses can produce tumors by at least two mechanisms, and the viruses are divided into families based on how they cause infected cells to become neoplastic.[80] *Transducing retroviruses* are able to transform infected cells efficiently and rapidly. These viruses arise from the rare recombination of proviral DNA and host genetic material (fig. 1.9 C). They have a hybrid genome composed of portions of the original viral genome with the addition of a transduced cellular oncogene (v-*onc*). Most of these viruses have lost some part of the viral genome during the incorporation of the oncogene, and as a result, the majority of these viruses can not replicate on their own. A strain of chicken sarcoma virus, Rous sarcoma virus, is an exception to this rule; it contains all the viral genes needed for replication as well as an oncogene. The oncogenes are expressed at high levels since

they are under the control of potent viral promoters and infected cells are rapidly and efficiently transformed into neoplastic cells.

Feline sarcoma viruses (FeSVs) are a group of transducing retroviruses that are closely related to feline leukemia virus (FeLV).[81] They contain a portion of the feline leukemia virus genome and one of several oncogenes, depending on the strain of FeSV. Each strain of FeSV is unique because each arises from a rare recombination between FeLV and cellular oncogenes. Thus, cats with FeSV induced fibrosarcoma are always infected with FeLV. FeSV can not replicate independently, and horizontal transmission does not occur.[80] Kittens injected with FeSV rapidly develop fibrosarcomas, often in a multicentric pattern, but an effective immune response by adults may eliminate the tumors.[82] Other tumor types, such as malignant melanomas, can be induced by some strains of FeSV.[83]

A second group of oncogenic retroviruses are designated *cis-activating retroviruses*. These viruses do not contain an oncogene. During proviral integration these viruses may insert their powerful viral transcription regulatory elements of the LTR region near cellular oncogenes and activate them in a process termed *insertion* or *cis-activation* (Fig. 1.9 D,E). The importance of the regulatory elements in the LTR is substantiated by the observation that in most tumors produced by these viruses only a fragment of the original provirus persists, and the remaining portion usually contains an LTR. Tumors produced by *cis*-activating retroviruses develop over a considerable period of time compared to those that develop from transducing viruses. Given that integration is a relatively random event and that these viruses must integrate into or near the relatively small proportion of the genome that contains protooncogenes, many integration events must occur before one leads to protooncogene activation. FeLV is a *cis*-activating retrovirus. Approximately 20 percent of cats persistently infected with FeLV develop neoplasia and die.[84,85] Tumor development is considerably slower in FeLV infected cats than in cats infected with FeSV. Following experimental infection, there is a 1 to 23 month lag time (5.3 month average) before tumors develop.[86,87] Bovine leukemia virus, which causes B lymphocyte transformation, may function this way also, although it is also possible that a transactivating viral protein (one that activates genes on different chromosomes) may play a role in lymphocyte transformation.[80]

There are several families of oncogenic DNA viruses, including herpesviruses, papovaviruses (including papillomaviruses and polyomaviruses), adenoviruses, hepadnaviruses, and poxviruses.[80] There are several features in common among this diverse group of oncogenic DNA viruses. DNA viruses, unlike retroviruses, transform infected cells by expressing genes of viral origin, and the genes of DNA viruses involved in oncogenesis are essential for the normal viral life cycle.

In the normal life cycle of a DNA virus that has infected a permissive cell (one that supports complete viral replication), early and late viral genes are expressed. Early genes generally are responsible for subverting control of the cell to support viral replication. Some early genes encode multifunctional proteins that interact with cellular genes and are responsible for blocking apoptosis pathways or affecting regulation of cellular replication.[3] Once viral progeny have matured, the infected cells are lysed, and viral particles are released as a result of expression of late genes. Because the infected cells are destroyed as part of the viral life cycle, the possibility of cell transformation is averted (fig. 1.10). In the uncommon situation of aberrant infections of permissive cells or infections of nonpermissive or semipermissive cells, usually only a part of the viral life cycle is completed and no viral progeny are produced. In these circumstances a portion of the viral genome can become integrated into the cellular DNA. If the portion that is integrated contains the early genes, the encoded proteins can dysregulate cellular growth controls. Several DNA virus early genes encode proteins that bind critical cellular proteins such as Rb and p53 that are involved in the regulation of the cell cycle or apoptosis.[88] Because the viral late genes are not expressed, these cells are not lysed, and they survive with a high risk of developing into neoplastic cells.

DNA viruses are responsible for a variety of neoplasms in rodents, avian species, and to a lesser extent, nonhuman primates, but only papillomaviruses are a significant cause of neoplasia in domestic animals. The ubiquitous virus induced wart or viral papilloma is found in virtually all domestic and wild animal species, including the cat.[89] Most virus-induced papillomas are self-limiting and are usually found in young animals.

In humans, malignant transformation of epithelial cells is associated with certain strains of papillomavirus. The oncogenicity of specific strains of papillomaviruses increases with the affinity of the viral proteins for Rb and p53. Like human papillomaviruses, certain strains of bovine papillomavirus (BPV) are more likely to be linked to neoplasms than are others.[67] Infection with BPV-2 and BPV-4 has been associated with malignant neoplasms in cattle. Urinary tract carcinomas develop in BPV-2–infected cattle, and BPV-4 is associated with neoplasms of the digestive tract. The tumor producing effects of BPV in cattle are significantly augmented by concurrent ingestion of quercetin, a chemical found in bracken fern. Several types of neoplasms are more frequent in BPV-4–infected cattle that ingest bracken fern or that are treated with quercetin than in cattle only infected with BPV.[67] Bracken fern ingestion by Scottish cattle increases the number of papillomas and the malignant transformation of papillomas to carcinomas in the digestive tract.[68]

Herpesviruses cause cancer in humans and several nondomestic mammals. Epstein-Barr virus, a human herpesvirus, is linked to Burkitt's lymphoma, oropharyngeal carcinoma, a B cell malignant lymphoma in immunosuppressed humans, and some forms of Hodgkin's disease. Herpes simplex is putatively linked to some human carcinomas as well.[90] *Herpesvirus saimiri* is a virus of squirrel monkeys that produces oropharyngeal ulcerative lesions in the normal host, but infection of owl monkeys and New Zealand white rabbits with this virus can produce T cell malignant lymphoma or lymphoid leukemia.[90] Perhaps the classic oncogenic herpesvirus infection of veterinary interest is Marek's disease. Marek's disease virus is a herpesvirus that infects chickens and produces malignant lymphoma. This was once responsible for very serious economic losses in the avian industry prior to the advent of effective vaccination programs.

Hepadnaviruses, which include hepatitis B virus, woodchuck hepatitis virus, and ground squirrel hepatitis virus, are responsible for an increased risk of liver cancer in their respective hosts.[91] Hepadnavirus infections differ from many other oncogenic DNA virus infections because tumors are produced in the typical host and in cells that are normally infected. However, it appears that, like other DNA viruses, integration of viral genome into the cellular genome is necessary for tumor production. Despite the high risk of liver cancer, approaching 100 percent in chronically infected woodchucks, no oncogene has been identified for this family of viruses.[92] Another group of DNA viruses, the

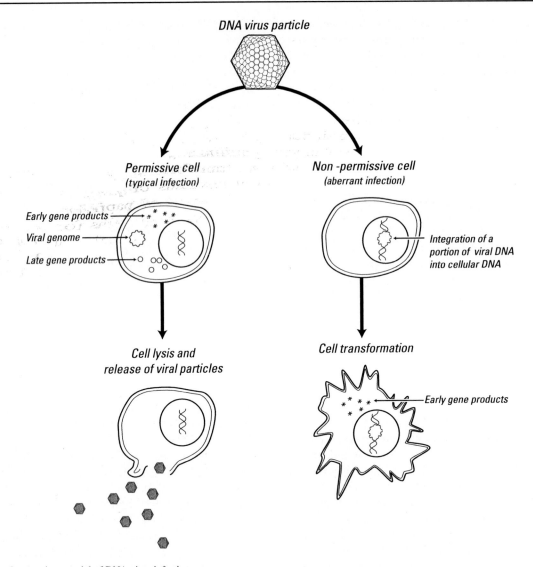

Fig. 1.10.   Oncogenic potential of DNA virus infection.

poxviruses, such as Shope fibroma virus of rabbits, can cause myxomas and fibromas in their typical hosts.[80]

Radiation Induced Carcinogenesis

Radiation can be divided into two major categories.[93] The first is ionizing radiation, produced by various isotopes that emit either gamma rays or particulate radiation (e.g., alpha and beta particles), and the second category is ultraviolet (UV) radiation. Ionizing radiation can damage DNA in two ways. Direct DNA damage occurs when ionizing radiation interacts with DNA molecules and alters individual bases or induces breaks in the DNA strands. Indirect damage to DNA results from ionization of cellular water and subsequent transfer of energy from the water to DNA. Ionizing radiation has a long history as a human carcinogen, starting with skin cancers and leukemia in a number of the earliest radiation workers, including Marie Curie. A more recent demonstration of the dangers of radiation exposure is found in the survivors of the atomic bombings in Japan in the Second World War. Epidemiological studies revealed an increase in leukemias in survivors in the first 10 or so years following radiation exposure and in other neoplasms involving the thyroid, lung, breast, and colon after a greater period of latency.

Ionizing radiation has been shown to produce a variety of neoplasms in dogs. For example, gamma irradiation in young dogs has been proven to increase the risk of mesenchymal and epithelial neoplasms later in life.[94,95] Inhalation of plutonium 239, a source of alpha particles, is linked to induction of pulmonary neoplasia in dogs.[96] There is also a risk of tumor production in dogs by therapeutic radiation exposure. Osteosarcomas are more frequent in dogs that have received intraoperative radiotherapy and external beam radiation.[97–99]

Ultraviolet radiation is divided into three spectra: UV-A, which has recently been shown to be carcinogenic in laboratory animals[100,101]; UV-B, which is a well-known cause of cutaneous neoplasia; and UV-C, a potent mutagen that is efficiently filtered out by the earth's ozone layer before it reaches the surface.[102] UV-B radiation is the portion of the spectrum that is most involved in cutaneous neoplasia. It produces a characteristic mutation at sites in DNA where two pyrimidine bases (i.e., cytosine and thymine) are found together. The radiation produces a dimer of these molecules that can lead to mutation when they are repaired incorrectly. The importance of this type of genetic injury in the pathogenesis of cancer is supported by the presence of mutations in the dipyrimidine regions of the *ras* oncogene and *p53* tumor suppressor gene in both humans and mice following UV-B exposure. The oncogenicity of UV-B radiation may be augmented by its deleterious effect on immunity, which may interfere with the recognition and destruction of tumor cells by the immune system. In contrast to UV-B radiation, UV-A radiation is not efficiently absorbed by DNA and protein. UV-A may cause DNA damage indirectly through the formation of free radicals and active oxygen species.[103,104]

The majority of neoplasms that are induced by UV irradiation arise in the epidermis, site of maximal exposure. In humans, UV exposure increases the risk of squamous cell carcinoma and basal cell carcinomas.[102] Malignant melanomas may also be linked to UV exposure, but the evidence is less persuasive. Squamous cell carcinoma is associated with UV exposure in animals, but more data is needed to determine if other types of skin neoplasia are induced by UV radiation in animals. Most neoplasms arise in white or less pigmented skin and areas of the skin that have a thin hair coat, such as periocular mucocutaneous areas in cattle and the tips of the pinnae in white cats.[105] The moderating effect of cutaneous melanin, which absorbs the UV light, has been proposed as an important protection against UV light-induced damage. However, recent data suggests that melanin may also have deleterious effects. When melanin is exposed to UV light, photodynamic products that are harmful to DNA and other proteins can result.[106]

Hormonal Carcinogenesis

It is now apparent from experimental and clinical evidence that hormones can play a major role in tumor development in organs of the male and female reproductive tract and related secondary sex glands.[107] A common feature underlying the pathogenesis of hormone induced neoplasia is excessive hormonal stimulation of a particular target organ that normally has its growth and function controlled by polypeptide or steroid hormones. Hormonal carcinogenesis appears to be independent of chemical or ionizing radiation–induced initiation. Another feature of hormonal carcinogenesis in humans, and one that may be important in domestic animals, is the association with an inherited genetic predisposition to tumor formation.

There is compelling evidence from studies on the effect of ovariohysterectomy in dogs that the action of hormones can increase the risk of mammary carcinoma.[108] The incidence of mammary neoplasia is 1 in 100 in dogs that had an ovariohysterectomy (OHE) before their first estrus. The protective effect of OHE diminishes as the dogs age. Dogs neutered after the first estrus have a 1 in 12 incidence of mammary tumors. After the second estrus the protective effect of OHE is significantly reduced, and tumor incidence becomes 1 in 4.

Exogenous estrogens and progesterone can also produce hyperplastic and neoplastic lesions. Progesterone can produce mammary hyperplasia (fibroadenoma) in female cats. Administration of estrogens such as diethylystilbestrol induces ovarian carcinomas in female dogs.[109,110] Progesterone and estrogen given in combination produced mammary adenomas and carcinomas when given to intact or neutered female dogs.[111] Toxicological studies and epidemiological studies indicate that progestational compounds have an independent dose related tumorigenic effect in the development of mammary tumors in dogs and cats.[112] The possible role of another endocrine factor, growth hormone, in canine mammary carcinoma has been reported. Treatment of bitches with progesterone can induce overproduction of growth hormone (GH) in the mammary gland, and this may play a role in mammary carcinogenesis in dogs.[113] Immunoreactive GH and GH messenger RNA are found in hyperplastic mammary epithelium, indicating a possible autocrine or paracrine action for this hormone.[114]

Bacterial and Parasite-Induced Carcinogenesis

Neoplasms can arise as a consequence of chronic parasitic infection. The mechanism by which long-term infection results in tumors is not known, but the chronic inflammation and stimulation of cell proliferation are suspected to play a role. Sarcomas of the esophagus have been reported in dogs with long-term infection with *Spirocerca lupi*.[115] Biliary carcinomas in cats and dogs have been linked to infection with the liver fluke *Clonorchis sinensis*.[116]

Humans and mice can develop cancer as a result of chronic infection with *Helicobacter* spp.[117,118] Gastric neoplasms (gastric carcinoma and lymphoma) arise in affected humans, and hepatocellular carcinomas arise in mice.

Tumor Immunity

Tumor immunity is a result of interactions among various cells of the immune system and tumor cells.[119] The occurrence of spontaneous regression, although extremely rare, and the presence of lymphoid infiltrates in and around tumors indicate that immunological defense mechanisms may interfere with the development and growth of tumors. Tumor cells can be recognized by the immune system because they often bear unique tumor specific antigens. These tumor specific antigens arise from mutations of cellular genes that give rise to abnormal proteins that are expressed on the cell surface or to abnormal expression of genes that would not otherwise be expressed. Tumor cells may also bear nonunique tumor associated antigens that are found in tumor cells as well as in other cells in the body. Some of these are oncofetal antigens.

Several types of cells in the immune system can effect tumor cell killing. The regional lymph nodes are the first filters where antigens released by the growing tumor may be presented to immunocompetent cells. Cytotoxic T lymphocytes (CTLs) are a major component of the host immune response against tumor cells. CTLs recognize tumor antigens on the surface of cells that are presented by the major histocompatibility complex I (MHC I). In some cases the CTLs can kill the antigen bearing tumor cells. Natural killer (NK) cells provide a first line of defense, since they can kill tumor cells without prior sensitization. They also participate in antibody dependant cellular cytotoxicity. Natural killer cells may also play a role in the attack on cells that are not recognized by CTLs. Unlike CTLs, which require antigen presentation via MHC I, NK cells are most active against cells with reduced MHC I display. Macrophages are also efficient tumor cell killers, once they are activated by interferon gamma produced by T lymphocytes and NK cells. Humoral factors such as complement and antibodies also play a role. The host immune system is active against tumors in tissue and in the vasculature. The initial response is inhibitory to tumor growth. Later, suppressor T cell activity and blocking factors may become dominant, allowing tumor cells to proliferate.[120]

In nonneoplastic mammary lesions, lymphocytic infiltrates were associated with a greater risk of tumor development, since infiltration was more frequent in lesions that were most likely to be precancerous.[121] In this study, however, there was no significant difference in biologic behavior between mammary tumors with or without lymphocytic infiltration. The prognosis of dogs with lymphoid infiltrates around mammary tumors was relatively favorable in another study,[33] but not so in cats, where lymphoid accumulation was associated with tumor necrosis, an unfavorable prognostic variable.[62] Lymphoid infiltrates occur in other tumor types. Lymphoid infiltrates are associated with regression of histiocytomas in dogs. Other neoplasms that may have lymphoid infiltrates include malignant melanomas, transmissible venereal tumors, dysgerminomas and transitional cell carcinomas in dogs, and postvaccinal sarcomas in cats. With the advent of new markers to identify lymphocyte subsets in domestic animals, lymphoid infiltrates can be better characterized and their activities better understood. This may facilitate use of the immune response as an effective treatment.

Age and Heredity-Related Effects on Tumor Incidence

There is a significant increase in the frequency of neoplasms as animals age.[122] Accumulation of genetic damage over time, diminished immune function, and the long lag time between malignant transformation of a single cell and the emergence of a clinically detectable neoplasm may each be independent or interdependent explanations for increased tumor incidence in the latter third of an animal's life span. However, it should not be overlooked that there is also a small peak of tumor incidence in young animals.[123] The most common neoplasms found in dogs under 6 months of age arise in the hematopoietic system, brain, and skin.[124] In fact, the incidence of tumors in two of these sites, the brain and hematopoietic system, exceeds the tumor incidence in mature dogs for the same sites. Mast cell tumors are also relatively common in young dogs. In young cats and cattle, lymphoid neoplasia is the most frequent type of neoplasia.[123] Mesotheliomas are reported to have a relatively high incidence in neonatal calves.[125] Cutaneous neoplasms (including mastocytosis or mast cell tumors and papillomas) and connective tissue neoplasms are common tumors in young horses.[123]

An inherited predisposition to develop various types of neoplasia has been described in many human families. Similarly, a breed related predisposition to develop certain neoplasms has been recognized in dogs for many years (table 1.2). The Boxer dog stands out as a breed particularly susceptible to the development of a variety of tumors. Osteosarcomas in large breed dogs and central nervous system neoplasms and aortic body tumors in brachycephalic breeds are other examples. Susceptibility to tumors has been traced to the family level in life-long studies of laboratory beagles in a pattern that is similar to those in some human families.[126] There are inherited tendencies to develop melanomas in Sinclair and Hormel miniature pigs and Duroc-Jersey swine.[127,128] Although the specific genetic damage associated with the increased risk for tumors has been identified for some human families, none of the genetic abnormalities responsible for increased tumor susceptibilities in domestic animals has been identified.

Paraneoplastic Syndromes

Paraneoplastic syndromes are defined as systemic complications of neoplasia that are remote from the primary tumor.[129] Frequently, the effects of the paraneoplastic syndrome can be more injurious than the associated malignancy. Paraneoplastic syndromes may serve as diagnostic aids or as specific tumor markers for treatment response and failure. These effects are generally unrelated to the size of the tumor, the presence of metastasis, or the physiologic activity of the tissue of primary origin. Most of the examples in veterinary medicine are associated with the production of native (true) hormone from cells that normally produce that hormone or from the "ectopic" production of a hormone-like peptide by tumor cells that normally do not produce this hormone. Excessive insulin production by neoplastic islet cells and production of a parathormone-like peptide by neoplastic lymphocytes or apocrine cells of the canine anal sac are examples of each category, respectively. In order to definitively establish that a paraneoplastic condition is a result of a specific neoplasm, one or more criteria have to be met. These criteria include the following: (1) concentration of the product

TABLE 1.2. Predilection of dog breeds for tumors

Location and Type of Tumor	High Risk	Low Risk	References
Hematopoietic system (lymphoma)	Boxer	Crossbreeds	132
Hematopoietic system (malignant histiocytosis)	Bernese mountain dog		133
Brain (several types)	Bulldog, Boxer, Boston terrier		134
Skin (mastocytoma, vascular tumors)	Boxer, Bulldog, Retriever		135
	Boxer		136
Skin/other (hemangiosarcoma)	German shepherd		137,138,139
Mammary glands (several types)	Boxer, Spaniel, Pointer, Dachshund, Labrador retriever	German shepherd	140
	English setter, Brittany/springer spaniels	Crossbreeds	141
		Boxer	136
Nose and sinuses (several types)	Airedale, Collie, Scottish terrier		142
Oropharynx (several types)	Boxer, Golden retriever, Cocker spaniel	Beagle, Dachshund	143
Ovary (carcinoma)	Pointer		144
Pancreas (carcinoma, insulinoma)	Airedale terrier		145
	Poodle		146
Thyroid (carcinoma)	Beagle, Boxer, Retriever	Poodle	147
Skeleton (osteosarcoma)	Giant breeds	Small breeds	148
	Boxer, Danish dog, German shepherd, Rottweiler	Crossbreeds	149
Testis	Boxer, Collie, German shepherd		150
Urinary bladder (carcinoma)	Beagle, Collie, Scottish terrier		151

(e.g., calcium) decreases after removal or treatment of the neoplasm (e.g., a malignant lymphoma that was secreting the trophic hormone); (2) product concentrations are maintained after removal of the normal gland that controls the concentration of that product (e.g., calcium concentration remains increased following removal of a parathyroid gland); (3) a positive arteriovenous concentration gradient of the hormone exists across the tumor; and (4) synthesis and secretion of the product by the tumor *in vitro* occurs. In veterinary medicine, the first criterion, decreased concentration of product after tumor ablation, is most commonly used to diagnose a paraneoplastic syndrome.

The pathogenesis of paraneoplastic syndromes has been theorized to result from several processes. Derepression of a gene may result in production of a substance with biologic activity. In fact there may be many products from a given tumor, but only the active substances are detectable. One example would be the production of hormone precursors that do not exhibit activity unless metabolized (i.e., prohormone production). Ectopic receptor production by a tumor has also been reported and accounts for displaced activity of a humoral substance (e.g., thymoma and acetylcholine receptor production). The third theory is termed *forbidden contact* and implies that there is exposure to substances that are normally sequestered from the body (i.e., antigens of normal or neoplastic origin) and therefore are recognized by the immune system as foreign. Immune complex formation from antigenic exposure to these normally sequestered antigens may result in a physiologic or pathologic event leading to clinical signs. Examples include anaphylaxis, coagulopathies, vasculitis, glomerulonephritis, and hemolytic anemia.

The common paraneoplastic syndromes in veterinary medicine are listed in table 1.3. The therapeutic man-

TABLE 1.3. Paraneoplastic syndromes in veterinary oncology

Hematopoietic	Endocrinopathy
Leucocytosis	Hypercalcemia
Leucopenia	Hypoglycemia
Thrombocytosis	Hyperestrogenism
Thrombocytopenia	Hypergastrinemia
Erythrocytosis	Thyrotoxicosis
Anemia	Hyperhistaminosis
Eosinophilia	Hypercatecholaminemia
Coagulopathies	Dysproteinemias
Miscellaneous	
Anorexia/cachexia	
Fever of unknown origin	
Myasthenia gravis	
Hypertrophic osteopathy	
Alopecia	
Neurologic disorders	

agement of paraneoplastic syndromes can be generalized into a stepwise process. The initial goal of managing a patient with a paraneoplastic disease involves controlling clinical signs or processes that may impede further diagnostic evaluation or treating an emergency situation. Disseminated intravascular coagulopathy (DIC), hemolytic anemia, hypoglycemia, serum hyperviscosity, and hypercalcemia are examples of paraneoplastic syndromes that require immediate clinical attention. Following stabilization of the patient and initial management of the clinical signs related to the paraneoplastic syndrome, consideration is then given to treatment of the tumor. The cardinal rule of therapy for the management of paraneoplastic syndromes is that the primary causes must be controlled to expect long-term resolution of the signs. In some cases, the paraneoplastic signs (hyperestrogenism, hypoglycemia, eosinophilia, and hypercalcemia) are controllable with the surgical resection of the tumor. In nonresectable or disseminated neoplasia treatment, radiation therapy or chemotherapy can also cause resolution of the paraneoplastic condition (multiple myeloma, lymphoma). If definitive therapy for the tumor is not expected to be successful, long-term symptomatic therapy of the associated paraneoplastic condition should be considered for palliative purposes. Some of the syndromes are occasionally amenable to long-term control (hyperhistaminosis due to mast cell tumors, hypoglycemia due to insulinoma), while others are not (DIC, hypertrophic osteopathy). For additional discussion of specific paraneoplastic conditions the reader is referred to several reviews.[130,131]

Endocrine syndromes are a frequent manifestation of paraneoplastic disease. Protein hormones, hormone precursors, or cytokines can be produced or metabolized by tumors. Some types of hormones such as steroid hormones and thyroid hormone derivatives and catecholamines are produced exclusively by tumors that have originated from glands that normally produced these substances. The frequency of biologically active peptide producing neoplasms can be explained by the fact that most cells secrete peptide hormones that function in paracrine signaling. These peptide hormones may be expressed in excess when cells become malignant and their numbers increase by clonal expansion.

Cancer cachexia is one of the more common paraneoplastic syndromes encountered in veterinary medicine. Affected animals are anemic, weak, easily fatigued, lose weight, and have diminished immune function. There are characteristic metabolic changes associated with this syndrome that affect carbohydrates, proteins, and lipids. Growth of the tumor occurs at the expense of the host. Increased serum lactate levels and insulin levels characterize abnormal carbohydrate metabolism. There is a loss of muscle mass and hypoalbuminemia in affected animals because protein catabolism exceeds protein synthesis. Wound healing and immunity are also affected by altered protein metabolism. The loss of protein develops because amino acids are redirected from protein synthesis into gluconeogenesis in cancer patients. Although tumor cells are less capable of using lipids for energy than normal cells, cancer cachexia also promotes fat utilization. Cancer cachexia has been attributed to the effects of tumor necrosis factor, interleukins 1 and 6, and interferons gamma and alpha.[132–151]

REFERENCES

1. Lewin, B. (1997) *Genes VI.* Oxford University Press, Inc., Oxford, pp. 1131–1172.

2. Druker, B.J., Mamon, G.J. and Roberts, T.M. (1989) Oncogenes, growth factors, and signal transduction. *N Engl J Med* 321:1383–1391.

3. Schafer, K.A. (1998) The cell cycle: A review. *Vet Pathol* 35:461–478.

4. Xu, L., Davidson, B.J., Murty, V.V.V.S., Li, R.G., Sacks, P.G., Garinchesa, P., Schantz, S.P., and Chaganti, R.S.K. (1994) *TP53* gene mutations and *CCND1* gene amplification in head and neck squamous cell carcinoma cell lines. *Intl J Cancer* 59:383–387.

5. Zhang, S.Y., Caamano, J., Cooper, F., Guo, X., and Klein-Szanto, A.J.P. (1994) Immunohistochemistry of cyclin D1 in human breast cancer. *Amer J Clin Pathol* 102:695–698.

6. Kraegel, S.A., Gumerlock, P.H., Dungworth, D.L., Oreffo, V.I. and Madewell, B.R. (1992) K-ras activation in non-small cell lung cancer in the dog. *Cancer Res* 52:4724–4727.

7. Tierney, L.A., Hahn, F.F., and Lechner, J.F. (1996) erbB-2 and K-*ras* gene alterations are rare in spontaneous and plutonium-239-induced canine lung neoplasia. *Radiat Res* 145:181–187.

8. Ahern, T.E., Bird, R.C., and Bird, A.E. (1993) Overexpression of c-erb b2 and c-myc but not c-ras in canine melanoma cell lines is associated with metastatic potential in nude mice. *Anticancer Res* 13:1365–1372.

9. Mayr, B., Dressler, A., Reifinger, M., and Feil, C. (1998) Cytogenetic alterations in eight mammary tumors and tumor-suppressor gene *p53* mutation in one mammary tumor from dogs. *Amer J Vet Res* 59:69–78.

10. Frazier, K.S., Hines, M.E., Hurvitz, A.I., Robinson, P.G.c and Herron, A.J. (1993) Analysis of DNA aneuploidy and c-myc oncoprotein content of canine plasma cell tumors using flow cytometry. *Vet Pathol* 30:505–511.

11. Miura, T., Tsugitomi, H., Fukasawa, M., Kedoma, T., Shibuya, M., Hasegawa, H., and Hayami, M. (1987) Structural abnormality and over-expression of the myc gene in feline leukemias. *Intl J Cancer* 40:564–569.

12. Fearon, E.R., and Vogelstein, B. (1997) Tumor suppressor and DNA repair gene defects in human cancer. In Holland, J.F., Bast, R.C.J., Morton, D.L., Frei, E.I., Kufe, D.W., and Weichselbaum,R.R. (eds.), *Cancer Medicine.* Williams and Wilkins, Baltimore, pp. 97–117.

13. Lewin, B. (1997) *Genes VI.* Oxford University Press, Inc., Oxford, pp. 1090–1129.

14. Sherr, C.J. (1996) Cancer cell cycle. *Science,* 274: 1672–1677.

15. Levine, A.J. (1997) *P53,* the cellular gatekeeper for growth and division. *Cell* 88:323–331.

16. Whyte, P., Buchkovich, K.J., Horowitz, J.M., Friend, S.H., Raybuck, J., Weinberg, R.A., and Harlow, E. (1988) Association between an oncogene and an anti-oncogene: The adenovirus E1A protein binds to the retinoblastoma gene product. *Nature* 334:124–129.

17. Horowitz, J.M., Yandell, D.W., Park, S.H., Canning, S., Whyte, P., Buchkovich, K.J., Harlow, E., Weinberg, R.A., and Dryja, T.P. (1989) Point mutational inactivation of the retinoblastoma antioncogene. *Science* 243:937–940.

18. Pardee, A.B. (1989) G1 events and regulation of cell proliferation. *Science* 246:603–608.

19. Greenblatt, M.S., Bennett, W.P., Hollstein, M., and Harris, C.C. (1994) Mutations in the *p53* tumor suppressor gene: Clues to cancer etiology and molecular pathogenesis. *Cancer Res* 54:4855–4878.

20. Sinicrope, F.A., Ruan, S.B., Cleary, K.R., Stephens, C., Lee, J.J., and Levin, B. (1995) bcl-2 and p53 oncoprotein expression during colorectal tumorigenesis. *Cancer Res* 55:237–241.

21. Kraegel, S.A., Pazzi, K.A., and Madewell, B.R. (1995) Sequence analysis of canine *p53* in the region of exons 3–8. *Cancer Lett* 92:181–186.

22. Devilee, P., Van Leeuwen, I.S., Vaesten, A., Rutteman, G.R., Vos, J.H., and Cornelisse, C.J. (1994) The canine *p53* gene is subject to somatic mutations in thryoid carcinoma. *Anticancer Res* 14:2039–2046.

23. Van-Leeuwen, I.S., Cornelisse, C.J., Misdorp, W., Goedegebuure, S.A., Kisseberth, W.C., and Rutteman, G.R. (1997) *P53* gene mutations in osteosarcomas in the dog. *Cancer Lett* 111:173–178.

24. Van-Leeuwen, I.S., Hellmen, E., Cornelisse, C.J., and Rutteman, G.R. (1996) *P53* mutations in mammary tumor cell lines and

corresponding tumor tissues in the dog. *Anticancer Res* 16:3737–3744.

25. Pazzi, K.A., Kraegel, S.A., Griffey, S.M., Theon, A.P., and Madewell, B.R. (1996) Analysis of the equine tumor suppressor gene *p53* in the normal horse and in eight cutaneous squamous cell carcinomas. *Cancer Lett* 107:125–130.

26. Wolf, J.C., Ginn, P.E., Homer, B., Fox, L.E., and Kurzman, I.D. (1997) Immunohistochemical detection of *p53* tumor suppressor gene protein in canine epithelial colorectal tumors. *Vet Pathol* 34:394–404.

27. Kroemer, G. (1997) The protooncogene bcl-2 and its role in regulating apoptosis. *Nature Med* 3:614–620.

28. Thompson, C. (1995) Apoptosis in the pathogenesis and treatment of disease. *Science* 267:1456–1462.

29. Vogelstein, B., Fearon, E.R., Hamilton, S.R., Preisinger, A.C., Willard, H.F., Michelson, A.M., Riggs, A.D., and Orkin, S.H. (1987) Clonal analysis using recombinant DNA probes from the X chromosome. *Cancer Res* 46:4806–4813.

30. Fabrikant, J.I., and Cherry, J. (1969) The kinetics of cellular proliferation in normal and malignant tissues. *J Surg Oncol* 1:23–47.

31. Fukuda, K., Iwasaka, T., Hachisuga, T., Sugimori, H.K., Tsugitomi, H., and Mutoh, F. (1990) Immunocytochemical detection of S-phase cells in normal and neoplastic cervical epithelium by anti-BrdU monoclonal antibody. *Anal Quant Cytol Histol* 12:135–138.

32. Teodori, L., Trinca, M.L., Goehdek, W., Hemmer, J., Salvatt, F., Storniello, G., and Mauro, F. (1990) Cytokinetic investigation of lung tumors using the anti-bromodeoyuridine (BUdR) monoclonal antibody method: Comparison with DNA flow cytometric data. *Int J Cancer* 45:995–1001.

33. MacEwen, E.G. (1986) Current concepts in cancer therapy: Biologic therapy and chemotherapy. In Withrow, S.J.M., and MacEwen E.G. (eds.), *Sem Vet Med Surg,* 1:5–16.

34. Folkman, J. (1997) Tumor Angiogenesis. In J.F. Holland, R.C.J. Bast, D.L. Morton, E. Frei, III, D.W. Kufe, and R.R. Weichselbaum (eds.), *Cancer Medicine.* Williams and Wilkins, Baltimore, pp. 181–206.

35. Folkman, J. (1995) Clinical application of research on angiogenesis. *N Engl J Med* 333:1757–1763.

36. Pluda, J.M. (1997) Tumor associated angiogenesis: Mechanisms, clinical implications and therapeutic strategies. *Sem Oncol* 24: 203–218.

37. Weidner, N., Carroll, P.R., Flax, J., Blumenfeld, W., and Folkman, J. (1993) Tumor angiogenesis correlates with metastases in invasive prostate carcinoma. *Amer J Pathol* 143:401–409.

38. Weidner, N., Semple, J.P., Welch, W.R., and Folkman, J. (1991) Tumor angiogenesis and metastasis correlation in invasive breast carcinoma. *N Engl J Med* 324:1–8.

39. Ribatti, D., Vacca, A., Bertossi, M., DeBenedictis, G., Roncali, L., and Dammacco, F. (1990) Angiogenesis induced by B-cell non-Hodgkins lymphomas: Lack of correlation with tumor malignancy and immunologic phenotype. *Anticancer Res* 10:401–406.

40. Dvorak, H.F. (1986) Tumors: Wounds that do not heal: Similarities between tumor stroma generation and wound healing. *N Engl J Med* 315:1650–1659.

41. Konno, H., Tanaka, T., Matsuda, I., Kannai, T., Maruo, Y., Nishino, N., Nakamura, S., and Baba, S. (1995) Comparison of the inhibitory effect of the angiogenesis inhibitor, TNP-470, and mitomycin C on growth and liver metastasis of human colon cancer. *Intl J Cancer* 61:268–271.

42. Tannock, I., and Rotin, D. (1989) Acid pH in tumors and its potential for therapeutic exploitation. *Cancer Res* 49:4373–4384.

43. Yeo, T.K., and Dvorak, H.F. (1995) Tumor Stroma. In Colvin, R.B., Bahn, A.K., and McCluskey, R.T. (eds.), *Diagnostic Immunopathology.* Raven Press, New York, pp. 685–700.

44. Hornby, A.E., and Cullen, K.J. (1998) Mammary tumor fibroblasts are phenotypically distinct from non-tumor fibroblasts. In Goldberg, I.D., and Rosen, E.M. (eds.), *Epithelial-Mesenchymal Interactions in Cancer.* Birkhauser Verlag, Basel, pp. 249–272.

45. Van der Hooff, A. (1988) Stromal involvement in malignant growth. *Adv Cancer Res* 50:159–196.

46. Inoue, T., Chung, Y.S., Yashiro, M., Nishimura, S., Hasuma, T., Otani, S., and Sowa, M. (1997) Transforming growth factor-beta and hepatocyte growth factor produced by gastric fibroblasts stimulate the invasiveness of scirrhous gastric cancer cells. *Jpn J Cancer Res* 88:152–159.

47. Kuntz, C.A., Dernell, W.S., Powers, B.E., Devitt, C., Straw, R.C., and Withrow, S.J. (1997) Prognostic factors for surgical treatment of soft-tissue sarcomas in dogs: 75 cases (1986–1996). *J Amer Vet Med Assoc* 211:1147–1151.

48. Cline, J.M., Thrall, D.E., Rosner, G.I., and Raleigh, J.A. (1994) Distribution of the hypoxia marker CCI-103F in canine tumors. *Int J Radiat Oncol Biol Phys* 4:921–933.

49. Fidler, I.J., and Kripke, M.L. (1977) Metastasis results from pre-existing variant cells within a malignant tumor. *Science* 197:893–895.

50. Pauli, B.U., and Kuettner, K.K. (1982) The regulation of invasion by cartilage-derived antivasion factor. In Liotta, L.A., and Hart, I.R. (eds.), *Tumor Invasion and Metastasis.* M. Nijhoff, Boston, pp. 267–291.

51. Liotta, L.A., and Kohn, E.C. (1997) Invasion and metastasis. In Holland, J.F., Bast, R.C.J., Morton, D.L., Frei, E., III, Kufe, D.W., and Weichselbaum, R.R. (eds.), *Cancer Medicine.* Williams and Wilkins, Baltimore, pp. 165–180.

52. Connolly, J.L., Schnitt, S.J., Wang, H.H., Dvorak, A.M., and Dvorack, H.F. (1997) Principles of cancer pathology. In Holland, J.F., Bast, R.C.J., Morton, D.L., Frei, E., III, Kufe, D.W., and Weichselbaum, R.R. (eds.), *Cancer Medicine.* Williams and Wilkins, Baltimore, pp. 533–555.

53. Fidler, I.J., and Brodey, R.S. (1967) A necropsy study of canine malignant mammary neoplasms. *J Amer Vet Med Assoc* 151:710–715.

54. Brodey, R.S. (1960) A clinical and pathological study of 130 neoplasms of the mouth and pharynx in the dog. *Amer J Vet Res* 21:787–790.

55. Misdorp, W., and Hart, A.A.M. (1979) Canine mammary cancer II: Therapy and causes of death. *J Small Anim Pract* 20:395–404.

56. Rosenthal, R.C. (1998) Mechanism of invasion and metastasis. In Withrow, S.J., and McEwen, E.G. (eds.), *Clinical Veterinary Oncology.* J.B. Lippincott, Philadelphia, pp. 23–28.

57. Jonas, A.M., and Carrington, C.B. (1969) Vascular patterns in primary and secondary pulmonary tumors in the dog. *Amer J Pathol* 56:79–95.

58. Goedegebuure, S.A. (1979) Secondary bone tumors in the dog. *Vet Pathol* 16:520–529.

59. Kas, N.P., Van der Heul, R.O., and Misdorp, W. (1970) Metastatic bone neoplasms in dogs, cats and a lion (with some comparative remarks on the situation in man). *Zentralbl-Veterinarmed A* 17:909–919.

60. Misdorp, W., and Den Herder, B.A. (1966) Bone metastasis in mammary cancer. *Brit J Cancer* 20:496–499.

61. Brodey, R.S., Reid, C.F., and Sauer, R.M. (1966) Metastatic bone neoplasms in the dog. *J Amer Vet Med Assoc* 148:129–142.

62. Weijer, K., and Hart, A.A. (1983) Prognostic factors in feline mammary carcinoma. *J Natl Cancer Inst* 70:709–716.

63. Glickman, L.T., Schofer, F.S., McKee, L.J., Reif, J.S., and Goldschmidt, M.H. (1989) Epidemiologic study of insecticide exposures, obesity, and risk of bladder cancer in household dogs. *J Toxicol Environ Health* 28:407–414.

64. Auerbach, O., Hammond, E.C., Korman, D., and Garfinkel, L. (1970) Effects of cigarette smoking on dogs II. Pulmonary Neoplasms. *Arch Envir Health* 21:754–768.

65. Hayes, H.M., Tarone, R.E., Cantor, K.P., Jessen, C.R., McCurnin, D.M., and Richardson, R.C. (1991) Case-control study of canine malignant lymphoma: Positive association with dog owner's use of 2,4-dichlorophenoxyacetic acid herbicides. *J Natl Cancer Inst* 83:1226–1231.

66. Carlo, G.L., Cole, P., Miller, A.B., Munro, I.C., Solomon, K.R., and Squire, R.A. (1992) Review of a study reporting an association between 2,4-dichlorophenoxyacetic acid and canine malignant lymphoma: Report of an expert panel. *Reg Toxicol Pharmacol* 16:245–252.

67. Jackson, M.E., and Campo, M.S. (1995) Cooperation between bovine papillomaviruses and dietary carcinogens in cancers of cattle. In Barbanti-Brodano, G., Bendinelli, M., and Friedman, H. (eds.), *DNA Tumor Viruses: Oncogenic Mechanisms.* Plenum Press, New York, pp. 111–122.

68. Campo, M.S., O'Shea, J.D., Baron, R.J., and Jarrett, W.F.H. (1994) Experimental reproductions of the papilloma/carcinoma complex of the alimentary tract in cattle. *Carcinogenesis* 15:1597–1601.

69. Amano, Y., and Fukumoto, S. (1987) A study on the cell kinetics of the canine gastric mucosa by the cytofluorometric method: An evaluation of chemically induced gastric cancer. *Gastroenterol Jpn* 22:292–302.

70. Benfield, J.R., Hammond, W.G., Paladugu, R.R., Pak, H.Y., Azumi, N., and Teplitz, R.L. (1986) Endobronchial carcinogenesis in dogs. *J Thorac Cardiovasc Surg* 92:880–889.

71. Benfield, J.R., Shors, E.C., Hammond, W.G., Paladugu, R.R., Cohen, A.H., Jensen, T., Fu, P.C., Pak, H.Y., and Teplitz, R.L. (1981) A clinically relevant canine lung cancer model. *Ann Thorac Surg* 32:592–601.

72. Hirao, K., Matsumura, K., Imagawa, A., Enomoto, Y., Hosogi, Y., Kani, T., Fujikawa, K., and Ito, N. (1974) Primary neoplasms in dog liver induced by diethylnitrosamine. *Cancer Res* 34:1870–1882.

73. Stula, E.F., Barnes, J.R., Sherman, H., Reinhardt, C.F., and Zapp, J.A., Jr. (1978) Liver and urinary bladder tumors in dogs from 3,3′-dichlorobenzidine. *J Environ Pathol Toxicol* 1:475–490.

74. Okey, P., Harper, A.B., Grant, A., and Hill, D.M, (1998) Chemical and radiation carcinogenesis. In Tannock, I.H.R.P. (ed.), *The Basic Science of Oncology.* McGraw-Hill, New York, pp. 166–196.

75. Poirier, M.C., and Weston, A. (1992) DNA adduct measurements and tumor incidence during chronic carcinogen exposure in animal models: Implications for DNA adduct-based human cancer risk assessment. *Chem Res Toxicol* 5:749–755.

76. Wogan, G.N., and Gorelick, N.J. (1985) Chemical and biochemical dosimetry of exposure to genotoxic chemicals. *Environ Health Perspect* 62:5–18.

77. Pitot, H.C., and Cambell, H.A. (1987) An approach to the determination of the relative potencies of chemical agents during the stages of initiation and promotion in multistage hepatocarcinogenesis in the rat. *Environ Health Perspect* 76:49–56.

78. Rous, P. (1910) A transmissible avian neoplasm: Sarcoma of the common fowl. *J Exp Med,* 696–705.

79. Ellermann, B., and Bang, O. (1908) Experimentelle leukamie bei huhnern. *Zentralb Bakteriol* 46:595–609.

80. Nevins, J.R., and Vogt, P.K. (1996) Cell transformation by viruses. In B.N. Fields, D.M. Knipe, and P.M. Howley (eds.), Fields Virology, Lippincott-Raven, Philadelphia, pp. 301–343.

81. Hardy, R.M. (1981) The feline sarcoma viruses. *J Amer Anim Hosp Assoc* 17:981–987.

82. Essex, M., Klein, G., Snyder, S.P., and Harrold, J.B. (1971) Feline sarcoma virus-induced tumors: Correlation between humoral antibody and tumor regression. *Nature* 233:195–196.

83. Shadduck, J.A., Albert, D.M., and Niederkorn, J.Y. (1982) Feline uveal melanomas induced by feline sarcoma virus: Potential model of the human counterpart. *J Natl Cancer Inst* 67:619–627.

84. Dorn, C.R., Taylor, D.O.N., Schneider, R., Hibbard, H.H., and Klauber, M.R. (1968) Survey of animal neoplasms in Alameda and Contra Costa Counties, California, II. Cancer morbidity in dogs and cats from Alameda County. *J Natl Cancer Inst* 40:307–318.

85. Schneider, R. (1983) Comparison and age- and sex-specific incidence rate patterns of the leukemia complex in the cat and the dog. *J Natl Cancer Inst* 70:971–977.

86. Francis, D.P., Cotter, S.M., Hardy, R.M., and Essex, M. (1979) Comparison of virus-positive and virus-negative cases of feline leukemia and lymphoma. *Cancer Res* 39:3866–3870.

87. McClelland, A.J., and Hardy, W.D., Jr. (1980) Prognosis of healthy feline leukemia virus infected cats. *Dev Cancer Res* 4:121–124.

88. Ludlow, J.W., DeCaprio, J.A., Haung, C.M., Lee, W.H., Paucha, E., and Livingston, D.M. (1989) SV40 large T antigen binds preferentially to an underphosphorylated member of the retinoblastoma susceptibility gene product family. *Cell* 56:57–65.

89. Sundberg, J.P., Van Ranst, M., Montali, R., Homer, B.L., Miller, W.H., Rowland, P.H., Scott, D.W., England, J.J., Dunstan, R.W., Mikaelian, I., and Jenson, A.B. (2000) Feline papillomas and papillomaviruses. *Vet Pathol* 37:1–10.

90. Medveczky, P. (1995) Oncogenic transformation of T cells by *Herpesvirus saimiri.* In Barbanti-Brodano, G., Bendinelli, M., and Friedman, H. (eds.), *DNA Tumor Viruses: Oncogenic Mechanisms.* Plenum Press, New York, pp. 239–252.

91. Marion, P.L. (1988) Use of animal models to study hepatitis B virus. *Prog Med Virol* 35:43–75.

92. Popper, H., Shih, J.W.K., Gerin, J.L., Wong, D.C., Hoyer, B.H., London, W.T., Sly, D.L., and Purcell, R.H. (1981) Woodchuck hepatitis and hepatocellular carcinoma: Correlation of histologic with virologic observations. *Hepatology* 1:91–98.

93. Little, J.B. (1997) Ionizing radiation. In Holland, J.F., Bast, R.C.J., Morton, D.L., Frei, E., III, Kufe, D.W., and Weichselbaum, R.R. (eds.), *Cancer Medicine.* Williams and Wilkins, Baltimore, pp. 293–306.

94. Benjamin, S.A., Lee, A.C., Angleton, G.M., Saunders, W.J., Miller, G.K., Williams, J.S., and Brewster, R.D. (1986) Neoplasms in young dogs after perinatal irradiation. *J Natl Cancer Inst* 77:563–571.

95. Benjamin, S.A., Hahn, F.F., Chiffelle, T.L., Boecker, B.B., Hobbs, C.H., Jones, R.K., McClellan, R.O., and Snipes, M.B. (1975) Occurrence of hemangiosarcomas in beagles with internally deposited radionuclides. *Cancer Res* 35:1745–1755.

96. Gillett, N.A., Stegelmeier, B.L., Kelly, G., Haley, P.J., and Hahn, F.F. (1992) Expression of epidermal growth factor receptor in plutonium-239-induced lung neoplasms in dogs. *Vet Pathol* 29:46–52.

97. Barnes, M., Duray, P., DeLuca, A., Anderson, W., Sindelar, W., and Kinsella, T. (1990) Tumor induction following intraoperative radiotherapy: Late results of the National Cancer Institute canine trials. *Int J Radiat Oncol Biol Phys* 19:651–660.

98. Thrall, D.E., Goldschmidt, M.H., Evans, S.M., Dubielzig, R.R., and Jeglum, K.A. (1983) Bone sarcoma following orthovoltage radiotherapy in two dogs. *Vet Radiol* 24:169–173.

99. Gillette, S.M., Gillette, E.L., Powers, B.E., and Withrow, S.J. (1990) Radiation-induced osteosarcoma in dogs after external beam or intraoperative radiation therapy. *Cancer Res* 50:54–57.

100. Berg, R.J., de Latt, A., Roza, L., van der Leun, J.C., and de Gruijl, F.R. (1995) Substitution of equally carcinogenic UV-A for UV-B irradiations lowers epidermal thymine dimer levels during skin cancer induction in hairless mice. *Carcinogenesis* 16:2455–2459.

101. Berg, R.J., de Gruijil, F.R., and van der Leun, J.C. (1993) Interaction between ultraviolet A and ultraviolet B radiation in skin cancer induction in hairless mice. *Cancer Res* 53:4212–4217.

102. Cleaver, J.E., and Mitchell, D.L. (1997) Ultraviolet radiation carcinogenesis. In Holland, J.F., Bast, R.C.J., Morton, D.L., Frei, E., III, Kufe, D.W., and Weichselbaum, R.R. (eds.), *Cancer Medicine.* Williams and Wilkins, Baltimore, pp. 307–318.

103. Tyrrell, R.M., and Keyse, S.M. (1990) New trends in photobiology: The interaction of UVA radiation with cultured cells. *J Photochem Photobiol* 84:349–361.

104. Tyrrell, R.M., and Pidoux, M. (1986) Endogenous glutathione protects human skin fibroblasts against the cytotoxic action of UVB, UVA and near-visible radiations. *J Photochem Photobiol,* 561–564.

105. Hargis, A.M. (1981) A review of solar induced lesions in domestic animals. *Comp Cont Educ Pract Vet* 3:287–296.

106. Menter, J.M., Tounsel, M.E., Moore, C.L., Williamson, G.D., Soteres, B.J., and Willis, I. (1990) Melanin accelerates the tyrosinase-catalyzed oxygenation of p-hydroxyanisole (MMEH). *Pigment Cell Res* 3:90–97.

107. Henderson, B.E., Bernstein, L., and Ross, R.K. (1997) Hormones and the etiology of cancer. In Holland, J.F., Bast, R.C.J., Morton, D.L., Frei, E., III, Kufe, D.W., and Weichselbaum, R.R. (eds.), *Cancer Medicine.* Williams and Wilkins, Philadelphia, pp. 277–292.

108. Schneider, R., Dorn, R.C., and Taylor, D. (1969) Factors influencing canine mammary cancer development and postsurgical survival. *J Natl Cancer Inst* 43:1249–1261.

109. Jabara, A.G. (1962) Induction of canine ovarian tumours by diethylstilbestrol and progesterone. *Aust J Exp Biol Med Sci* 40:139–143.

110. O'Shea, J.D., and Jabara, A.G. (1967) The histogenesis of canine ovarian tumours induced by stilboestrol administration. *Vet Pathol* 4:137–148.

111. Giles, R.C., Giles, R.P., Kwapien, R.P., Geil, R.G., and Casey, H.W. (1978) Mammary nodules in Beagle dogs administered investigational oral contraceptive steroids. *J Natl Cancer Inst* 60:1351–1364.

112. Misdorp, W. (1991) Progestagens and mammary tumours in dogs and cats. *Acta End(Copenh)* 125:27–31.

113. Selman, P.J., Mol, J.A., Rutteman, G.R., Van Peperzeel, H.A., and Rijnberk, A. (1997) Progestin-induced growth excess in the dog originates in the mammary gland. *Endocrinology* 134:287–292.

114. Van Garderen, E., De Wit, M., Voorhout, W.F., Rutteman, G.R., Mol, J.A., Nederbragt, H., and Misdorp, W. (1997) Expression of growth hormone in canine mammary tissue and mammary tumors. *Amer J Pathol* 150:1037–1047.

115. Wandera, J.G. (1976) Further observations on canine spirocercosis in Kenya. *Vet Rec* 99:348–351.

116. Hou, P.C. (1964) Primary carcinoma of bile duct of the liver of the cat infested with *Clonorchis sinensis. J Pathol Bact* 87:239–244.

117. Ward, J.M. (1997) Helicobacter infections of rodents in carcinogenesis bioassays. *Toxicol Pathol* 25: 590

118. Forman, D., Newell, D.G., Fullerton, F., Yarnell, J.W., Stacey, A.R., Wald, N., and Sitas, F. (1991) Association between infection with *Helicobacter pylori* and risk of gastric cancer: Evidence from a prospective investigation. *Brit Med J* 302:1302–1305.

119. MacEwen, E.G. (1989) Immunology and biologic therapy of cancer. In MacEwen, E.G. and Withrow, S.J. (eds.), *Clinical Veterinary Oncology.* Lippincott Co., Philadelphia, pp. 92–105.

120. Rogers, K.S. (1990) The role of regional lymph node in metastasis. *VCS Newsletter* 14:1–3.

121. Gilbertson, S.R., Kurzman, I.D., Zachrau, R.E., Hurvitz, A.I., and Black, M.N. (1983) Canine mammary epithelial neoplasms: biological implications of morphologic characteristics. *Vet Pathol* 20:127–142.

122. Priester, W.A., and McKay, F.W. (1980) The occurrence of tumors in domestic animals. *J Natl Cancer Inst Monog* 54:210–216.

123. Mulvihill, J.J., and Priester, W.A. (1978) Tumours in young domestic animals: Epidemiologic comparisions with man. In Severi, L. (ed.), *Tumors of Early Life in Man and Animals.* Perugia University, Division of Cancer Research, Monteluce.

124. Keller, E.T., and Madewell, B.R. (1992) Location and types of neoplasms in immature dogs: 69 cases (1964–1989). *J Amer Vet Med Assoc* 200:1530–1532.

125. Cotchin, E. (1975) Spontaneous tumours in young animals. *Proc Roy Soc Med* 68:653–655.

126. Schafer, K.A., Schrader, K.R., Griffith, W.C., Muggenburg, B.A., Tierney, L.A., Lechner, J.F., Janovitz, E.B., and Hahn, F.F. (1998) A canine model of familial mammary gland neoplasia. *Vet Pathol* 35:168–177.

127. Flatt, R.E., Middleton, C.C., Tumbleson, M.E., and Mesa-Prez, C. (1968) Pathogenesis of benign cutaneous melanomas in miniature swine. *J Amer Vet Med Assoc* 153:936–941.

128. Oxenhandler, R.W., Adelstein, E.H., Haigh, J.P., Hook, R.R., Jr., and Clark, W.H., Jr. (1979) Malignant melanoma in the Sinclair miniature swine: An autopsy study of 60 cases. *Amer J Pathol* 96:707–720.

129. Morrison, W.B. (1998) Paraneoplastic syndromes and the tumors that cause them. In Morison, W.B. (ed.), *Cancer in Dogs and Cats: Medical and Surgical Management.* Williams and Wilkins, Baltimore, pp. 763–777.

130. Ogilvie, G.K., and Vail, D.M. (1990) Nutrition and cancer. Recent developments. *Vet Clin North Amer Small Anim Pract* 4:969–985.

131. Ruslander, D.A., and Page, R.L. (1995) Perioperative management of paraneoplastic syndromes. *Vet Clin North Amer Small Anim Pract* 1:47–62.

132. Priester, W.A. (1967) Canine lymphoma: Relative risk in the boxer breed. *J Natl Cancer Inst* 39:833–845.

133. Moore, P.F., and Rosin, A. (1986) Malignant histiocytosis of Bernese mountain dogs. *Vet Pathol* 23:1–10.

134. Hayes, H.M., Priester, W.A., and Pendergrass, T.W. (1975) Occurrence of nervous-tissue tumors in cattle, horses, cats, and dogs. *Intl J Cancer* 15:39–47.

135. Priester, W.A. (1973) Skin tumors in domestic animals: Data from 12 United States and Canadian colleges of veterinary Medicine. *J Natl Cancer Inst* 50:457–466.

136. Cohen, D., Reif, J.S., Brodey, R.S., and Keiser, H. (1974) Epidemiological analysis of the most prevalent sites and types of canine neoplasia observed in a veterinary hospital. *Cancer Res* 34:2859–2868.

137. Prymak, C., McKee, L.J., Goldschmidt, M.H., and Glickman, L.T. (1988) Epidemiologic, clinical, pathologic, and prognostic characteristics of splenic hemangiosarcoma and splenic hematoma in dogs: 217 cases (1985). *J Amer Vet Med Assoc* 193:706–712.

138. Waller, T., and Rubarth, S. (1967) Haemangioendothelioma in domestic animals. *Acta Vet Scand* 8:234–261.

139. Pearson, G.R., and Head, K.W. (1976) Malignant hemagioendothelioma in the dog. *J Small Anim Pract* 17:737–745.

140. von Bomhard, D., and Dreiack, J. (1977) Statistische erhebungen uber mammatumoren bei hundinnen. *Kleintier-Praxis* 22:205–209.

141. Priester, W.A. (1979) Epidemiology. In Theilen, G.H., and Madewell, B.R. (eds.), *Veterinary Cancer Medicine.* Lea and Febiger, Philadelphia, pp. 14–32.

142. Madewell, B.R., Priester, W.A., Gillett, E.L., and Sotaniemi, E.A. (1976) Neoplasms of the nasal passages and paranasal sinuses in domesticated animals as reported by 13 veterinary colleges. *Amer J Vet Res* 37:851–856.

143. Dorn, C.R., and Priester, W.A. (1976) Epidemiologic analysis of oral and pharyngeal cancer in dogs, cats, horses, and cattle. *J Amer Vet Med Assoc* 169:1202–1206.

144. Hayes, H.M., Jr., and Young, J.L. (1978) Epidemiologic features of canine ovarian neoplasms. *Gynecol Oncol* 6:348–351.

145. Priester, W.A. (1974) Data from eleven United States and Canadian colleges of veterinary medicine on pancreatic carcinoma in domestic animals. *Cancer Res* 34:1372–1375.

146. Priester, W.A. (1974) Pancreatic islet cell tumors in domestic animals: Data from 11 colleges of veterinary medicine in the United States and Canada. *J Natl Cancer Inst* 53:227–229.

147. Hayes, H.M., Jr., and Fraumeni, J.F., Jr. (1975) Canine thyroid neoplasms: Epidemiologic features. *J Natl Cancer Inst* 55:931–934.

148. Tjalma, R.A. (1966) Canine bone sarcoma: Estimation of relative risk as a function of body size. *J Natl Cancer Inst* 36:1137–1150.

149. Misdorp, W., and Hart, A.A.M. (1979) Some prognostic and epidemiologic factors in canine osteosarcoma. *J Natl Cancer Inst* 62:537–545.

150. Hayes, H.M., Jr., and Pendergrass, T.W. (1976) Canine testicular tumors: Epidemiologic features of 410 dogs. *Intl J Cancer* 18:482–487.

151. Hayes, H.M., Jr., (1976) Canine bladder cancer: Epidemiologic features. *Amer J Epidemiol* 104:673–677.

152. Liotta, L.A. (2001) An attractive force in metastasis. *Nature* 410:24-25.

TUMOR DIAGNOSIS

Classification of Proliferative Lesions

Nonneoplastic Proliferative or Mass-Forming Lesions

Although we now associate the word tumor with a neoplasm, the original meaning of the word tumor is derived from the Greek word for swelling. It is important to remember that not all processes that produce swelling or masses are neoplastic. As part of the initial assessment of a mass, nonneoplastic lesions have to be distinguished from neoplastic lesions because there are several processes that cause tissue enlargement or an abnormal histological appearance that bear some resemblance to neoplasia, but are not neoplastic.

Hyperplasia is an increase in the size of an organ or tissue due to an increase in cell number. The process can be divided into physiologic hyperplasia and pathologic hyperplasia.[1]

Physiologic hyperplasia occurs in response to a known stimulus, serves a purpose, and ceases when the stimulus is removed. Criteria that distinguish physiologic hyperplasia from neoplasia are well characterized (table 1.4). Mammary gland hyperplasia in response to pregnancy and parturition is an example. Hyperplasia can also be compensatory. Following partial hepatectomy, there is a wave of hyperplasia by hepatocytes, endothelial cells, and biliary epithelium that replaces lost tissue and restores hepatic mass to its original amount.

Pathologic hyperplasia involves an increase in tissue size due to an increase in cell replication, but while the process may not be harmful, it is not helpful to the individual. The stimulus for pathologic hyperplasia is frequently attributed to an excess of growth factors, but the precise cause in specific cases is often unknown. Pathologic hyperplasia can be nodular, as seen in the exocrine pancreas, adrenal cortex, and liver of older dogs, or it can be diffuse, as in the prostate of older intact dogs or in the mammary glands of female cats given progestational compounds. Proliferative lesions of the endocrine glands are a particular diagnostic challenge because hyperplastic and benign neoplastic lesions have a similar histological appearance and require careful observation to distinguish focal hyperplastic lesions from neoplasms.

Neoplasms can develop in areas of pathologic hyperplasia. For example, progression from foci of hyperplasia to benign and eventually to malignant neoplasms has been demonstrated in several tissues, including the colon, skin, and liver.[2,3] It is prudent to alert the clinician to carefully observe or monitor tissues that have evidence of this change.

Hypertrophy is an increase in tissue or organ size due to an increase in cell size. Cell types that are incapable

TABLE 1.4.   Comparison of characteristics of physiologic hyperplasia, pathologic hyperplasia, and neoplasia

Physiologic Hyperplasia	Pathologic Hyperplasia	Neoplasia
Example: Callus formation, endocrine	Example: nodular hyperplasia, liver and pancreas	Example: squamous cell carcinoma
Appropriate to needs	Inappropriate	Excessive
Ceases when stimulus ceases	Uncertain	Persistent
Serves a purpose	Purposeless	Purposeless
Reversible	Uncertain	Irreversible
Regulated	Possibly	Autonomous

of cell proliferation (such as neurons) or have scant replicative ability (such as mature cardiac and skeletal muscle) undergo hypertrophy in response to trophic stimuli. This process can also be divided into physiological and pathological categories. The physiological demands of increased exercise will produce hypertrophy of healthy skeletal and cardiac muscle. Cell enlargement can also occur in disease states. Enlarged cardiac myocytes in feline hypertrophic cardiomyopathy, megalocytes, and enlarged hepatocytes in pyrrolizidine exposed cattle are examples of pathological hypertrophy. Cells with the ability to divide may undergo hypertrophy as well as hyperplasia in response to increased demands. Thus, in many tissues, endocrine especially, an increase in organ size may occur as a result of hypertrophy and hyperplasia.

Dysplasia is a nonadaptive change in cell appearance due to a loss of uniformity of individual cells and a loss of their architectural orientation.[1] It is recognized at the light microscopic level by cytological atypia that is still confined to its normal microanatomic sites. Epithelial surfaces, such as the conjunctiva of cattle and cats or the ear tips of white cats, are common sites for dysplastic changes. Dysplasia is generally regarded as a premalignant lesion, but not all dysplastic lesions will result in a neoplasm. Differentiation between dysplasia and *carcinoma* in situ, a noninvasive epithelial neoplasm that has not broken through the basement membrane, can be difficult and usually rests on the degree of cytological atypia.

Quasi-neoplastic lesions are those having some characteristics of neoplasia, but not a sufficient number. *Hamartomas* are an overabundance of normal tissue in a normal location.[4] Vascular hamartomas of the subcutis can produce dark red pigmented "birthmarks." *Choristomas* are normal tissue in an abnormal position. Examples of choristomas include pancreatic exocrine tissue found in the intestinal submucosa or haired skin present on the surface of the cornea. They probably arise from errors in embryogenesis. These abnormalities can be readily distinguished from metastatic lesions by the well-differentiated histological appearance of the cells in question. These lesions are not considered premalignant lesions, and there is no data to suggest they are more prone to develop into neoplasms.

Terminology of Neoplasms

Although pathologists would likely agree that they have a clear concept of what a neoplasm is, a universally acceptable definition that includes all known types of neoplasms is difficult to derive. In the 1950's Willis offered this definition: "A neoplasm is an abnormal mass of tissue. The growth of which exceeds and is uncoordinated with that of the normal tissues and persists in the same excessive manner after cessation of the stimuli which evoked the change."[5] An updated definition, taking into account new knowledge of the etiology of neoplasms, is the following: "A neoplasm is a mass of tissue generated by cells capable of division which have acquired either permanent expressible heritable change or stable epigenetic change so that the same or other cells no longer respond appropriately to one or more normal tissue organizing stimuli, chemical or physical, intracellular or extracellular, in the organism in which it occurs."[6] Once a lesion has been identified as a neoplasm, classification proceeds using a binomial system. In this system neoplasms are categorized on the basis of two elements, their predicted behavior (benign or malignant) and the tissue of origin (mesenchymal or epithelial).

Predicted Behavior: Benign or Malignant

It is a general rule that a benign neoplasm will have less of an impact on the health of an animal than a malignant neoplasm, but this is not always the case. Benign neoplasms that occlude the flow of blood or cerebrospinal fluid can cause life threatening disturbances. Ulcerated benign lesions can hemorrhage or provide portals of entry for systemic bacterial infections. Benign endocrine neoplasms that are functional may be capable of causing systemic disturbances such as hyperadrenocorticism. In contrast to the general rule, not all malignancies are swiftly fatal. Dogs with some malignancies, such as B cell malignant lymphoma, can be predicted to survive one to several years and maintain a good quality of life with appropriate medical management. Beta cell neoplasms of the pancreas in dogs invariably metastasize, but these patients can also be managed for several years with medical therapy. In order to provide accurate prognoses for our patients, we must recognize the inherent variations in the behavior of different types of malignancies and stay abreast of newer anticancer therapies and recent studies that elucidate specific features of neoplasms, such as mitotic index or local invasion, that are most predictive of their behavior.

Characteristics that distinguish benign from malignant lesions are summarized in table 1.5. In different tumor types, exceptions to these guidelines occur. However, the presence of metastasis is irrefutable evidence of malignancy.

Malignant neoplasms span a range of morphological appearances from well differentiated to anaplastic (those with a total lack of differentiation). Identification of the

TABLE 1.5. General characteristics of benign and malignant neoplasms

Characteristic	Benign	Malignant
Metastasis	Does **not** occur.	Often present.
Local invasion	Usually a uniformly expanding mass without evidence of invasion.	Local invasion of surrounding tissue is common.
Growth rate	Typically progressive, but slow. Mitotic figures have normal appearance.	Slow to rapid. May be unpredictable Mitotic figures may be abundant and appear abnormal.
Differentiation	Well-differentiated histologic appearance; resembles tissue of origin.	Usually poorly differentiated; may be anaplastic.
Encapsulation	Frequently present; well delineated.	Usually absent, or if present, invasion may be evident; poorly delineated.

cell of origin in anaplastic tumors can be difficult and may require special techniques (i.e., immunohistochemistry). Characteristic changes in malignant cells include variation in cell size (anisocytosis), variation in nuclear size (anisonucleosis), and an increased nuclear to cytoplasmic ratio approaching 1:1 instead of the more normal 1:4 to 1:6, depending on the cell type. Nuclei may be hyperchromatic, reflecting increased abnormal DNA content (aneuploidy), or they may have open vesicular nuclei indicative of active gene transcription. Nucleoli are often prominent or multiple, indicative of active production of the ribosomal RNA needed for protein synthesis. Mitotic figures tend to be increased and are often bizarre. The increase in mitotic figures can be attributed to a high proportion of cells in the cell cycle and possibly to the presence of abnormal mitotic figures that can not complete cytokinesis normally and therefore remain arrested in this state. Poorly differentiated neoplasms usually are pleomorphic, characterized by unrecognizable histological architecture and marked variations in the size and shape of cells and nuclei. Abnormally sized cells, including multinucleate giant cells, may be seen. Multinucleate giant cells can form by cell fusion (more common in inflammatory conditions) or by nuclear division without cytokinesis (more typical of malignant cells). Multinucleate giant cells seen in malignancy are characterized by a disorganized array of nuclei in contrast to normal multinucleate cells such as osteoclasts in which the nuclei are arranged in an orderly fashion, often with a polar distribution.

The functional capacity of neoplasms usually varies with their degree of differentiation. Benign neoplasms are more likely to have metabolic patterns and synthetic pathways similar to the cell of origin than are carcinomas, and well-differentiated carcinomas are more likely to be functional than poorly differentiated carcinomas. Thus, many endocrine adenomas can produce systemic effects by the secretion of hormones, while generally fewer carcinomas are capable of secreting biologically active hormones or detectable amounts of the native hormone. In domestic animals, neoplasms of the beta cells of the pancreatic islets are an exception to this rule. Most beta cell neoplasms are malignant and functional, secreting insulin.

Tissue of Origin: Mesenchymal or Epithelial

Tissues and the tumors derived from them are divided into mesenchymal or epithelial origin. Mesenchymal elements include connective tissue, striated and smooth muscle, blood cells, and endothelial cells and related tissues (synovium, mesothelium, and meninges). Epithelial cells include squamous epithelia of the skin, cells that line the respiratory, digestive, urinary, and reproductive tracts, all glands, exocrine and endocrine, and cells of neuroectoderm origin such as melanocytes. The tissue of origin and the suffix -*oma* designate benign mesenchymal neoplasms. Thus a benign neoplasm of fibroblasts is a fibroma. Malignant neoplasms of mesenchymal origin use the tissue designation and the suffix -*sarcoma.* A malignant neoplasm of fibroblast origin is a fibrosarcoma. Benign epithelial neoplasms of glandular origin are named by the tissue of origin with the suffix -*adenoma,* as in mammary adenoma. Benign epithelial neoplasms that arise from lining epithelium are usually termed *papillomas.* The tissue of origin and the suffix -*carcinoma* is used for malignant epithelial neoplasms. Those that make histologically evident glands within the neoplasm are termed *adenocarcinomas.* A few exceptions to this scheme that are well established in common usage and are unlikely to change include melanoma and hepatoma, which refer to malignant neoplasms. The alternative terms *malignant melanoma* and *hepatocellular carcinoma* are more accurate. *Lymphoma,* despite the above objections, is the preferred term.

Although most neoplasms are composed of only one tissue type, there are exceptions. A teratoma is a neoplasm that contains tissues that arise from at least two, and usually three, different embryonic germ layers. Representatives of the endodermal, mesodermal, and ectodermal layers such as the digestive tract, muscle, and skin, respectively, are frequently found in these neoplasms. They arise most often in the gonads, but extragonadal sites are recognized. Mixed neoplasms contain two neoplastic tissues. They arise most often in glands such as the mammary gland or the salivary gland. Neoplastic glandular or ductular epithelium and periglandular myoepithelial cells are usually involved.

Tumor Cell Identification

When the histological appearance of a hematoxylin and eosin stained neoplasm is insufficient to provide a diagnosis, several techniques including histochemistry, electron microscopy, immunohistochemistry, and flow cytometry can be used. These techniques may yield a definitive diagnosis, but more often contribute additional information that can be used in context with histological appearance and clinical judgment to make a diagnosis. The basic distinction between epithelial and mesenchymal origin can influence the welfare of the patient, because this information can affect the prognosis and treatment decisions.

Histochemistry

Histochemical stains have been used for many years to identify cells and their products. A list of frequently used histochemical stains and the cells identified by them is presented in table 1.6. Because these stains employ relatively nonspecific chemical reactions that detect substances on the basis of certain chemical properties, such as the ability to reduce silver, more specific immunohistochemical stains have progressively replaced them. That notwithstanding, many histochemical stains continue to be valuable and are used regularly.

TABLE 1.6.   Histochemical stains frequently used in tumor diagnosis

Histochemical Stain	Feature Stained	Cell Type
Fontana-Masson	Melanosomes	Melanocytes
Dopa-oxidase (*frozen tissue*)	Melanosomes	Melanocytes
Masson trichrome	Connective tissue/smooth muscle/osteoid	Fibrocytes/smooth muscle/osteoblasts
PTAH	Z-bands	Skeletal/cardiac muscle (*cross striations*)
Argentaffin	Secretory granules	Endocrine/neuroendocrine cells
Argyrophil/grimelius	Secretory granules	Neuroendocrine cells
Methyl green-pyronin	Ribosomal protein	Plasma cells (*cells with large amounts of RNA*)
Toluidine blue	Mast cell granules*	Mast cells
Giemsa/acid fast	Mast cell granules	Mast cells
Alcian blue (*with/without hyaluronidase*)	Acid mucopolysaccharides	Chondrocytes/matrix- producing cells/mesothelial cells
Reticulin stain	Reticulin fibers	Distinguishes mesenchymal cells from epithelial cells
PAS	Neutral mucopolysaccharides (glycogen)	Mucus-producing carcinomas

*Immature mast cell granules may require treatment with a sulfation technique at an altered pH to be detected.

Electron Microscopy

Transmission electron microscopy can be a useful procedure for tumor identification in selected cases. In all cases, the diagnostician should have a specific feature or features in mind when undertaking ultrastructural examination, since increased magnification alone is unlikely to assist in making a diagnosis of a neoplasm that can not be identified by light microscopy. Prompt collection and proper fixation of tissue are important because many significant details of ultrastructural anatomy are obscured by autolysis. However, depending on the object of the ultrastructural examination, formaldehyde fixed postmortem samples can still be useful. There are only a few general ultrastructural features that distinguish neoplastic cells from normal cells. These features include (1) altered size and the acquisition of odd, often segmented shapes of the nuclei, (2) increased numbers, increased size, and variations in the shape of nucleoli, and (3) small and/or variably sized and shaped mitochondria.[7]

Ultrastructural examination can be used to determine the epithelial or mesenchymal origin of poorly differentiated malignancies. At least two ultrastructural features are retained in anaplastic neoplasms and can be used to distinguish carcinomas from sarcomas; these include the relationship of the cells with their extracellular environment and the presence of cell junctions. Typically, epithelial cells are aligned on a basement membrane, while certain types of mesenchymal cells are separated from each other by their extracellular matrix. Cell junctions (desmosomes, hemidesmosomes, and tight junctions) are other distinguishing features that are characteristic of epithelial cells. The number of cell junctions is usually reduced in malignant cells, so careful review of the tissue may be required.

Electron microscopy can be used to confirm a diagnosis of malignant melanoma when the histological samples appear amelanotic.[7] Neoplastic melanocytes, like normal melanocytes, can be identified by the presence of solitary melanosomes at different stages of development. Melanosomes may acquire odd appearances in neoplastic cells, but the distinctive internal structure is usually retained. Single membrane bound structures containing transversely banded material or striated filaments arranged in spirals or a zigzag pattern are readily recognized and distinguished from lysosomes or other cytoplasmic granules. Compound melanosomes are uncommon in neoplastic melanocytes. In comparison, melanophages usually contain compound melanosomes or a few melanosomes in the later stages of development. This observation is also useful to determine if pigmented cells in local lymph nodes are metastatic melanoma cells or melanophages.

Cytoplasmic granules are particularly useful for transmission electron microscopic identification of neoplasms because the granules are resilient and can be identified when other, more fragile organelles are obscured by autolysis or inadequate fixation. For example, the characteristic appearances and sizes of cytoplasmic granules can identify tumors arising from endocrine cells and leukocytes. Large granular lymphocytes also have distinctive features such as a small number of cytoplasmic granules that are electron dense and have a distinctive electron dense cap. When histochemical stains fail to reveal typical granules in mast cells, they can be identified on the basis of the characteristic ultrastructural appearance of their immature granules. Tumors of skeletal muscle origin can be readily diagnosed by electron microscopy also, since they are characterized by abundant mitochondria and Z bands.

Immunohistochemistry

Immunohistochemistry is an important ancillary diagnostic aid for tumor identification. The advent of a broad variety of antibodies has facilitated the identification of tumors through the use of antibodies that bind to cell-specific proteins. Several detailed reviews on the subject are available.[8-11]

The ubiquitous intermediate filaments, structural cytoplasmic proteins, are the most frequently used targets for immunohistochemical identification of tumors that can not be categorized in H&E stained sections. Cytokeratin and vimentin are the intermediate filaments used most often, because all epithelial cells contain cytokeratins and most mesenchymal cells contain vimentin. Thus the basic distinction between epithelial and mesenchymal origin of an anaplastic malignancy can often be made by detecting either of these proteins in the cytoplasm of the cells in question. Some tumor types, such as mesotheliomas and synovial cell sarcomas, can express both cytokeratin and vimentin. There are many types of cytokeratins, usually divided into high weight and low weight forms that appear in different cell types and at different stages of maturation in particular cell types. Consequently, mixtures of anticytokeratin antibodies are used initially when dealing with poorly differentiated neoplasms. More precise identification of a particular epithelial cell type may be made with individual monoclonal antibodies to distinct types of cytokeratin that are characteristic of certain cell types or different stages of maturation.

Vimentin has a more uniform molecular structure than the cytokeratins, and usually only one antibody is needed to detect this intermediate filament. Different types of mesenchymal tumors can be recognized by their staining reactions using other markers. Tumors arising from striated or smooth muscle can be identified by the presence of the intermediate filament desmin. Proteins other than intermediate filaments can also be used as cell markers. For example, smooth muscle actin can be used to distinguish leiomyosarcomas from other spindle cell neoplasms. Factor VIII–related antigen is found in vascular endothelial cells and can be used to distinguish hemangiosarcomas from lymphangiosarcomas. Neoplastic endocrine cells can be identified by using antibodies to detect specific hormones in their cytoplasm. The immunophenotype of lymphoid and hematopoietic neoplasms can be precisely determined using a panel of monoclonal antibodies that recognize B and T lymphocytes or other differentiation markers. An example of how some neoplasms can be identified using the appropriate commercially available antibodies is shown in figure 1.11. The immunohistochemical method will support, if not supplant, the histological classifications as more antibodies become commercially available. A recent study has revealed the relative inaccuracy of some histological classifications compared to immunophenotyping of canine lymphoid neoplasms.[12]

While the theory of immunohistochemical staining is straightforward, in practice interpretation of histochemical staining results can be challenging. Although normal tissues stain quite consistently, neoplastic cells are less uniform in their staining patterns. Despite the clonal origin of most neoplasms, by the time they are recognized clinically, most are composed of a heterogeneous population of cells with different patterns of gene expression due to tumor progression. Tumor heterogeneity yields inconsistent protein expression (antigen presence) and, therefore, inconsistent staining patterns. Poorly differentiated neoplasms are less likely to express typical proteins of the cell of origin for the tumor. Technical factors such as the concentration of primary antibody and incubation conditions can also affect the proportion of tumor cells that are stained. Often there is considerable variation in the proportion of stained cells in different sites of the same neoplasm. Results are usually interpreted as positive when at least a proportion of cells that are clearly of neoplastic origin, not trapped normal stromal cells or infiltrating inflammatory cells, are stained with appropriate antibodies.

In some malignancies, such as malignant mesotheliomas and synovial cell sarcomas, both cytokeratin and vimentin staining occur. Other malignancies may, in some cases, express both intermediate filaments as well. The majority of studies of immunohistochemical staining patterns of neoplasms fails to demonstrate complete concordance of immunohistochemical staining pattern and histological diagnosis.[13] Errors in interpretation can easily result when only a single antibody is used. A panel of antibodies is more likely to provide accurate and useful information. Therefore staining results should be used as a guide, not a definitive indicator of cell type in neoplastic tissue.

Appropriate fixation, use of controls, and consistent staining technique are essential for proper interpretation of immunohistochemical stains. Different types and duration of fixation can significantly affect antibody binding. Some antibodies will work only on frozen sections, while others require formaldehyde or alcohol fixation. Most commercial antibodies indicate the appropriate fixatives for best results. The duration of fixation is important because antigenic epitopes can be lost during prolonged fixation. Tissue that has spent more than 48 hours in formaldehyde will often be unsatisfactory for immunohistochemistry. Aldehyde fixatives continue to cross-link proteins during fixation and impede access of antibodies to antigenic epitopes or alter the epitopes. Antigen retrieval methods that use cycles of heating and cooling of tissue sections in a buffer solution have been developed to improve antibody binding in overfixed tissues.

Suitable positive and negative controls are essential for accurate interpretation of staining results. It is preferable to have the control and stained sections of the tissue of interest on the same slide rather than on separate slides to ensure consistency in the stain technique. Each section is handled identically, except that primary antibody is added to the section under study, while nonimmune sera at the same concentration as the primary antibody is applied to the control section. No tissue staining should be seen in the negative control section. The optimal control for specificity requires that the primary antibody be incubated with the target antigen and that this mixture then be applied to the tissue of interest. All staining should be eliminated by this procedure, otherwise nonspecific staining is occurring. This is seldom practical for diagnostic situations. Nonspecific staining or lack of appropriate staining requires reassessment of the staining protocol and technique. Antibody concentrations, source of antibody, and incubation times are frequently changed until results are improved.

Flow Cytometry

The flow cytometer is a particularly useful tool for analysis of large populations of cells. With this device, individual cells are examined at a very rapid rate, permitting analysis of tens of thousands of cells in a brief period. Typically cells are stained with antibodies that are tagged with fluorescent dyes. Mixtures of different antibodies, each with different fluorescent tags, can distinguish heterogeneous cell populations into subgroups. Usually, antibodies are used to identify cell surface antigens, but internal proteins can also be studied. Individual cells in suspension, such as blood leukocytes (B and T lymphocytes), are studied most often, but solid tumors can be enzymatically digested into single-cell suspensions and analyzed. The advent of numerous antibodies directed against leukocyte cell membrane antigens that are specific for domestic species has made precise identification of lymphocyte subsets and other leukocyte subtypes by this method possible.[14-16] Typically, malignant cells in blood samples can be distinguished from normal cells and identified as a monoclonal cell population based on the presence of a uniform display of cell surface markers. These markers also identify the cell lineage and degree of differentiation of the affected cells. These data have proven to be clinically relevant in dogs and are likely to become more important as more data are gathered.

Tumor Markers

The presence of certain substances in blood, known collectively as tumor markers, can be correlated with the

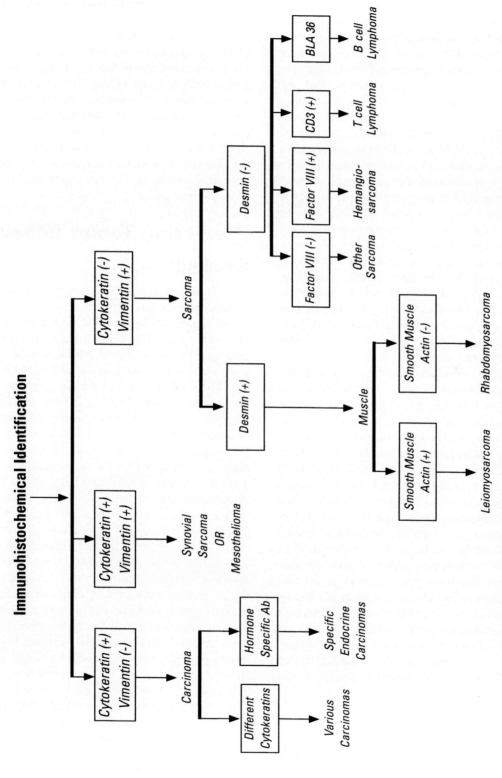

Fig. 1.11. A flowchart for immunohistochemical identification of poorly differentiated neoplasms.

33

appearance of tumors. There is a great deal of interest in tumor markers because they can be used as a relatively noninvasive indication of the presence of tumors and of tumor regrowth following therapy. Oncofetal proteins are one group of tumor cell markers. They are normally expressed in the fetus but are present at very low levels or undetectable in healthy adults. They reappear in the serum of individuals with certain types of neoplasia. An example is alpha-fetoprotein (AFP), which is the predominant serum protein in the fetus but disappears from circulation in the early neonatal period. It is produced by fetal and neoplastic hepatocytes, but not normal adult hepatocytes. In dogs with primary hepatocellular carcinoma and sometimes other neoplasms, including cholangiocarcinomas, serum increases of AFP occur. Immunohistochemical staining of tissue for AFP has been used in dogs to identify hepatocellular carcinoma and biliary carcinoma.[17,18] However, care must be used in interpretation of results since AFP can increase following hepatocellular injury and in regeneration.[19] Another oncofetal marker, carcinoembryonic antigen (CEA) has been identified in dogs with hepatocellular and exocrine pancreatic carcinoma.[17]

A newly identified oncofetal protein, designated oncofetal protein 55, is involved in mRNA transport in serum and may have broad applicability. It is increased in the serum of dogs with a variety of malignancies of mesenchymal or epithelial origin compared to those with benign lesions or no neoplastic disease.[20]

Several other substances can be detected in the serum of tumor bearing animals. Inhibin levels are increased in dogs with Sertoli cell neoplasms.[21] Serum lipid associated sialic acid levels and serum alpha 1-acid glycoprotein are increased in dogs with a variety of malignancies.[22] Some serum tumor markers that are useful to detect prostatic cancer in men, such as acid phosphatase and prostate specific antigen, are not useful as serum markers in dogs with these tumors.[23] Although canine prostate specific esterase is increased in the serum of dogs with benign prostatic hyperplasia compared to normal dogs, enzyme levels can not be used to discriminate dogs with prostatic cancer from those with hyperplasia. In addition to serum, it is also possible to analyze urine and cells collected by urinalysis for substances such as fibroblastic growth factor, which is increased in the urine of dogs with transitional cell carcinoma compared to normal dogs and those with inflammatory lesions of the bladder.[24] Monoclonal antibodies, developed against a substance termed *glycoprotein 72* can distinguish neoplastic urothelial cells from normal and inflamed cells.[25]

Ploidy

Ploidy, the nuclear DNA content of cells, can aid in distinguishing malignant tumors from benign tumors or nonneoplastic lesions.[26] Most somatic cells in the body are diploid, containing one set of chromosomes from each par-

ent. This status is also termed *euploid*. In neoplastic cells, abnormal regulation of chromosomal integrity can lead to abnormal DNA content, termed *aneuploidy*. Aneuploidy has been detected in a variety of canine tumors.[27-38] Significantly higher proportions of malignant neoplasms than of benign tumors or normal cells are aneuploid. The majority of canine malignant melanomas, osteosarcomas, thyroid carcinomas, and transitional cell carcinomas are aneuploid, and most metastatic lesions have a similar or identical ploidy. Thus ploidy can be an aid in distinguishing benign from malignant lesions. About half of canine mammary carcinomas, prostate carcinomas, and plasma cell tumors are aneuploid. In malignant mast cells and lymphocytes only about 20–30 percent of tumors are aneuploid. Only a minority of feline mammary carcinomas were aneuploid. In the tumor types studied so far, there has been little correlation between ploidy and histological or clinical characteristics.

Predicting Tumor Behavior

Grading

In general, cellular morphology is the most accurate predictor of the behavior of a neoplasm.[29,39] However, individual tumor types have specific associations between their prognosis and morphology. These relationships are addressed by morphological grading schemes for several malignant tumors in veterinary medicine.[40-44] Grading is the subdivision of a neoplasm type into categories, or grades, based on those histological features that may be correlated with patient prognosis. Tumor grading schemes should not be confused with histological classification schemes or clinical staging. Tumor grade is based on assessment of morphological criteria such as the degree of cellular differentiation, invasiveness, overall cellularity, mitotic index, and necrosis that are examined alone or in combination. The simplest schemes use a single criterion, such as mitotic index or invasiveness, to establish an appropriate grade. Using these criteria, a given malignant tumor can be assigned to one of several grades from well differentiated (low grade) to poorly differentiated (high grade), depending on the grading convention. Validation of predictive values for tumor grading schemes or algorithms requires that some outcome measure (disease free interval, rate of recurrence, survival) be statistically dependent on grade. In order to validate a grading scheme or to assess the validity of a grading scheme, several concerns must be kept in mind: (1) the outcome measure should be as unambiguous and as unbiased as possible (e.g., tumor recurrence is preferable to overall survival due to the effects of elective euthanasia), (2) treatment should be uniform, including surgical procedures, and (3) retrospective study data is often inaccurate due to infrequent follow-up analysis of the patients and loss of information. Despite these limitations, grading schemes have been proposed for various canine tumors.

Numerous grading schemes have been proposed for dogs and cats, and they have been reviewed recently.[45,46] Some of the grading schemes include the following tumors in dogs: (1) cutaneous mast cell tumor,[40] (2) mammary gland neoplasia,[41] (3) fibrosarcoma, neurofibrosarcoma, and hemangiopericytoma[42] (also designated soft tissue sarcomas or spindle cell sarcomas), (4) cutaneous and ocular melanoma,[47,48] (5) cutaneous and splenic hemangiosarcoma,[43,49] (6) synovial sarcoma,[44] (7) transitional cell carcinoma,[50] (8) lung carcinoma,[51] and (9) bone neoplasms of the skull and mandible.[52,53] Attempts have also been made to grade lymphoma in dogs according to several different and complex grading schemes for non-Hodgkin's lymphoma in humans, with conflicting prognostic results.[25,54,55]

The number of nucleolar organizing regions (AgNORs) is one feature of cells that has been studied as a prognostic indicator. These are proteins associated with DNA loops in the nucleolus that can be distinctly stained with silver stains. The nucleolus is the site of ribosomal RNA synthesis, and ribosomal RNA is needed for protein synthesis. Cells that are rapidly replicating require abundant protein synthesis, and the increase in number and area of AgNORs is correlated with cell proliferation. This relationship has been studied to determine if AgNOR scores can be correlated with tumor identification and behavior. Results have differed among investigators and tissues that have been studied, but in general AgNOR studies offer insight into tumor behavior and detection of malignancy.[56]

Studies that evaluate multiple criteria and preferably analyze them in a multifactoral way will likely prove to be the best at establishing accurate prognoses. It is crucial that diagnostic pathologists know what criteria need to be evaluated and plan accordingly. The simpler these criteria are to determine, the more likely they will be evaluated. For example, it may not be possible to evaluate certain parameters that require frozen sections, special fixatives, or storage media for evaluation when most samples are submitted in formalin.

A common feature used in many of these grading schemes is an estimate of cell replication. Elevated S phase was found to be a prognostic factor of canine mammary carcinoma.[27] Determination of the mitotic index by counting the number of mitotic figures in 10, 40x fields and establishing an average or total number is the most common method. For some tumors, melanomas and connective tissue sarcomas, this criterion has been determined to be the best predictor of survival and/or response to treatment and is as useful as more sophisticated and cumbersome techniques, such as flow cytometry to determine ploidy.[48,49] Although it is tempting to extrapolate these results to all tumors, this is not valid. Histiocytomas and transmissible venereal tumors of dogs are examples of neoplasms with high mitotic indices that can spontaneously regress. When a grading scheme has not been validated for a specific tumor or group of tumors, it may be helpful to report such criteria as mitotic index, invasiveness, and anaplasia, but the pathologist should be aware that these features may or may not be informative predictors of survival or treatment response. Future clinical studies will no doubt correlate basic evaluations such as mitotic index and invasion with newer methods such as flow cytometric characterization of ploidy, replication fraction, tumor doubling times, and cell marker analysis with patient outcome.

In addition to morphological grading schemes, a pathologist also needs to know the literature in order to recognize which tumors have a histological classification correlated with survival. For some neoplasms the identification of the cell type and the species affected are critical components for assessing prognosis because of the established behaviors of some tumors. Malignant smooth muscle tumors and beta cell neoplasms of the pancreatic islets are examples of neoplasms that offer little evidence of their malignant behavior based on histological examination, because they often lack the histological criteria of malignancy. Neoplasms of the apocrine glands of the anal sac in dogs have a uniformly malignant behavior despite a typical well-differentiated appearance. Species of origin can significantly influence prognosis also. Thyroid neoplasms that are large enough to be palpated in dogs are virtually always malignant, but in cats most are benign. Neoplasms of the appendicular skeleton in dogs are most often malignant, but in cats they are more likely to be benign.

Grading Algorithms

Simplified tumor grading algorithms derived from published data on grading of various neoplasms in veterinary medicine can be found in the appendix. The tumor grading schemes are based on relatively objective end points, with descriptions of surgical procedures used and adequate statistical rigor to warrant including them here. The existing grading schemes were modified into algorithms for the sake of simplicity and to enhance uniformity among different users when grading these neoplasms at North Carolina State University College of Veterinary Medicine. Below each algorithm are summaries of the prognostic data taken from the original reference from which the algorithm was derived. Depending on the reference, the prognostic information may be provided in terms of mean posttreatment survival time, percent survival at a given time posttreatment, disease free interval, or metastatic rate. With more clinical experience and new data, such as molecular phenotyping, it is anticipated that modifications to the algorithms will be appropriate. Detailed information on the grading of specific neoplasms can be found in their respective chapters.

Staging

In addition to grading schemes, systems for staging neoplasms have been developed. They are intended to aid in planning treatment and to give some indication of

TABLE 1.7.   TNM Classification scheme for tumors in animals

Primary Tumor

T_0	No evidence of neoplasia
T_1	Tumor <1 cm diameter, not invasive
T_2	Tumor 1–3 cm diameter, locally invasive
T_3	Tumor >3 cm diameter or evidence of ulceration or local invasion

Node

N_0	No evidence of nodal involvement
N_1	Node firm, enlarged
N_2	Node firm, enlarged, and fixed to surrounding tissues
N_3	Nodal involvement beyond the first station

Metastasis

M_0	No evidence of metastasis
M_1	Metastasis to one organ system (e.g., pulmonary metastasis)
M_2	Metastasis to more than one organ system (e.g., pulmonary and hepatic metastases)

prognosis. In addition, they generate uniformity between pathologists and standardize comparisons of the response of tumors to therapy. A staging system used by some veterinary oncologists is based on a system developed by the World Health Organization[57] (table 1.7). Staging is based on the size of the primary tumor, the spread to lymph nodes, and the presence or absence of distant metastases. It employs three main categories to classify tumor stages: local (T), regional (N), and metastatic (M) characteristics. Each tumor has specific criteria for categorization, but there are general rules. Tumor size is graded from T_0 for in situ lesions and T_1 to T_4 for increasing sized tumors. When there is no involvement of the lymph nodes, the designation is N_0. Progressive nodal involvement is reported as N_1 to N_3. Hematogenous metastasis is reported on a scale from M_1 to M_2. The absence of metastasis is reported as M_0. With this system, tumors can be staged by the pattern and extent of spread, which can affect prognosis and treatment decisions. Additional prognostic factors may be used for specific types of tumors. For example, a squamous cell carcinoma on the ear tip has a different prognosis than one on the tonsil. Staging of mast cell tumors in dogs may also include the histological grade.[58]

REFERENCES

1. Cotran, R.S., Kumar, V., and Collins, T. (1999) Neoplasia. In Cotran, R.S., Kumar, V., and Collins, T. (eds.), *Pathologic Basis of Disease*. W.B. Saunders, Philadelphia, pp. 260–327.
2. Farber, E., and Sauer, R.M. (1987) Hepatocarcinogenesis: A dynamic cellular perspective. *Lab Invest* 56:4–42.
3. Slaga, T.J. (1983) *Mechanisms of Tumor-promotion: Tumor Promotion in Internal Organs*. CRC Press, Boca Raton, FL.
4. Willis, R.A. (1962) *The Borderland of Embryology and Pathology*. Butterworths, London.
5. Willis, R.A. (1952) *The Spread of Tumors in the Human Body*. Butterworths, London.
6. Rowlatt, C. (1982) Tissue organization and neoplasms. In Rowlatt, C. (ed.), *The Functional Integration of Cells into Animal Tissues*. Cambridge University Press, Cambridge, pp. 319
7. Ghadially, F.N. (1985) *Diagnostic Electron Microscopy of Tumours*, 2nd ed. Butterworths, London.
8. Moore, A.S., Madewell, B.R., and Lund, J.K. (1989) Immunohistochemical evaluation of intermediate filament expression in canine and feline neoplasms. *Am J Vet Res* 50:88-92.
9. Day, M.J. (1995) Immunophenotypic characterization of cutaneous lymphoid neoplasia in the dog and cat. *J Comp Pathol* 112:79–96.
10. Elias, J.M. (1990) *Immunohistopathology: A Practical Approach to Diagnosis*. ASCP Press, Chicago.
11. True, L.D. (1990) *Atlas of Diagnostic Immunohistopathology*. Lippincott, Philadelphia.
12. Teske, E., Wisman, P., Moore, P.F., and van Heerde, P. (1994) Histologic classification and immunophenotyping of canine non-Hodgkins lymphomas: Unexpected high frequency of T cell lymphomas with B cell morphology. *J Exp Hematol*, 22: 1179–1187.
13. Moore, A.S., Madewell, B.R., and Lund, J.K. (1989) Immunohistochemical evaluation of intermediate filament expression in canine and feline neoplasms. *Amer J Vet Res* 50:88–92.
14. Moore, P.F., Schrenzel, M.D., Affolter, V.K., Olivry, T., and Naydan, D. (1996) Canine cutaneous histiocytoma is an epidermotropic Langerhans cell histiocytosis that expresses CD1 and specific beta 2-integrin molecules. *Amer J Pathol* 148:1699–1708.
15. Moore, P.F., and Olivry, T. (1994) Cutaneous lymphomas in companion animals. *Clin Dermatol*, 12: 499–505.
16. Day, M.J. (1995) Immunophenotypic characterization of cutaneous lymphoid neoplasia in the dog and cat. *J Comp Pathol* 1:79–96.
17. Martin de las Mulas, J., Gomez-Villamandos, J.C., Perez, J., Mozos, E., Estrado, M., and Mendez, A. (1995) Immunohistochemical evaluation of canine primary liver carcinomas: Distribution of alpha-fetoprotein, carcinoembryonic antigen, keratins and vimentin. *Res Vet Sci* 59:124–127.
18. Lowseth, L.A., Gillett, N.A., Chang, I.Y., Muggenburg, B.A., and Boecker, B.B. (1991) Detection of serum alpha-fetoprotein in dogs with hepatic tumors. *J Amer Vet Med Assoc* 199:735–741.
19. Madsen, A.C., and Rikkers, L.F. (1984) Alpha-fetoprotein secretion by injured and regenerating hepatocytes in the dog. *J Surg Res* 37:402–408.
20. Stromberg, P.C., Schumm, D.E., Webb, T.E., Ward, H., and Couto, C.G. (1995) Evaluation of oncofetal protein-related mRNA transport activity as a potential early cancer marker in dogs with malignant neoplasms. *Amer J Vet Res* 56:1559–1563.
21. Hahn, K.A. (1993) Prognostic tumor markers. 11th Am Coll Vet Intern Med Forum 8:573–587. (Abstract)
22. Ogilvie, G.K., Walters, L.M., Greeley, S.G., Henkel, S.E., and Salaman, M.D. (1993) Concentration of alpha-1-acid glycoprotein in dogs with malignant neoplasia. *J Amer Vet Med Assoc* 203:1144–1146.
23. Bell, F.W., Klausner, J.S., Hayden, D.W., Lund, E.M., Liebenstein, B.B., Feeney, D.A., Johnston, S.D., Shivers, J.L., Ewing, C.M., and Isaacs, W.B. (1995) Evaluation of serum and seminal plasma markers in the diagnosis of canine prostatic disorders. *J Vet Int Med* 9:149–153.
24. Allen, D.K., Waters, D.J., Knapp, D.W., and Kuczek, T. (1996) High urine concentrations of basic fibroblast growth factor in dogs with bladder cancer. *J Vet Int Med* 4:231–234.
25. Clemo, F.A., DeNicola, D.B., Morrison, W.B., and Carlton, W.W. (1995) Immunoreactivity of canine epithelial and nonepithelial neoplasms with monoclonal antibody B72.3. *Vet Pathol* 32:147–154.
26. Merkel, D.E., and McGuire, W.L. (1990) Ploidy, proliferative activity and prognosis. *Cancer* 86:1194–1205.
27. Hellmen, E., Bergstrom, R., Holmberg, L., Spangberg, I.B., Hannson, K., and Lindgren, A. (1993) Prognostic factors in canine mammary tumors: A multivariate study of 202 consecutive cases. *Vet Pathol* 30:20–27.
28. Ayl, R.D., Couto, C.G., Hammer, A.S., Weisbrode, S., Ericson, J.G., and Mathes, L. (1992) Correlation of DNA ploidy to tumor histo-

logic grade, clinical variables, and survival in dogs with mast cell tumors. *Vet Pathol* 5:386–390.

29. Teske, E., vanHeerde, P., Rutteman, G.R., Kurzman, I.D., Moore, P.F., and MacEwen, E.G. (1994) Prognostic factors for treatment of malignant lymphoma in dogs. *J Amer Vet Med Assoc* 205:1722–1728.

30. Rutteman, G.R., Cornelisse, C.J., Dijkshoorn, N.J., Poortman, J., and Misdorp, W. (1988) Flow cytometric analysis of DNA ploidy in canine mammary tumors. *Cancer Res* 48:3411–3417.

31. Fox, M.H., Armstrong, L.W., Withrow, S.J., Powers, B.E., LaRue, S.M., Straw, R.C., and Gillette, E.L. (1990) Comparison of DNA aneuploidy of primary and metastatic spontaneous canine osteosarcomas. *Cancer Res* 50:6176–6178.

32. Minke, J.M., Cornelisse, C.J., Stolwijk, J.A., Kuipers-Dijkshoorn, N.J., Rutteman, G.R., and Misdorp, W. (1990) Flow cytometric DNA ploidy analysis of feline mammary tumors. *Cancer Res* 50:4003–4007.

33. Bolon, B., Calderwood-Mays, M.B., and Hall, B.J. (1991) Characteristics of canine melanomas and comparison of histology and DNA ploidy to their biologic behavior. *Vet Pathol* 27:96–102.

34. Clemo, F.A., DeNicola, D.B., Carlton, W.W., Morrison, W.B., and Walker, E. (1994) Flow cytometric DNA ploidy analysis in canine transitional cell carcinoma of urinary bladders. *Vet Pathol* 31:207–215.

35. Teske, E., Rutteman, G.R., Kuipers-Dijkshoorn, N.J., VanDierendonck, J.H., vanHeerde, P., and Cornelisse, C.J. (1993) DNA ploidy and cell kinetic characteristic in canine non-Hodgkin's lymphoma. *Exp Hematol* 21:579–584.

36. Madewell, B.R., Deitch, A.D., Higgins, R.J., Marks, S.L., and deVere-White, R.W. (1991) DNA flow cytometric study of the hyperplastic and neoplastic canine prostate. *Prostate* 18:173–179.

37. Scanziani, E., Caniatti, M., Sen, S., Erba, E., Cairoli, F., and Battocchio, M. (1991) Flow cytometric analysis of cellular DNA content in paraffin wax-embedded specimens of canine mammary tumours. *J Comp Pathol* 105:75–82.

38. Perez-Alenza, M.D., Rutteman, G.R., Kuipers-Dijkshoorn, N.J., Pena, L., Montoya, A., Misdorp, W., and Cornelisse, C.J. (1995) DNA flow cytometry of canine mammary tumours: The relationship of DNA ploidy and S-phase fraction to clinical and histological features. *Res Vet Sci* 58:238–243.

39. Koestner, A. (1985) Prognostic role of cell morphology of animal tumors. *Toxicol Pathol,* 13: 90–94.

40. Patnaik, A.K., Ehler, W.J., and MacEwen, E.G. (1984) Canine cutaneous mast cell tumor: Morphologic grading and survival time in 83 dogs. *Vet Pathol* 21:469–474.

41. Gilbertson, S.R., Kurzman, I.D., Zachrau, R.E., Hurvitz, A.I., and Black, M.N. (1983) Canine mammary epithelial neoplasms: Biological implications of morphologic characteristics. *Vet Pathol* 20:127–142.

42. Bostock, D.E., and Dye, M.T. (1980) Prognosis after surgical excision of canine fibrous connective tissue sarcomas. *Vet Pathol* 17:581–588.

43. Ward, H., Fox, L.E., Calderwood-Mays, M.B., Hammer, A.S., and Couto, C.G. (1994) Cutaneous hemangiosarcoma in 25 dogs: A retrospective study. *J Vet Int Med* 8:345–348.

44. Vail, D.M., Powers, B.E., Getzy, D.M., Morrison, W.B., McEntee, M.C., O'Keefe, D.A., Norris, A.M., and Withrow, S.J. (1994) Evaluation of prognostic factors for dogs with synovial sarcoma: 36 cases. *J Amer Vet Med Assoc* 205:1300–1307.

45. Powers, B.E., Hoopes, P.J., and Ehrhart, E.J. (1995) Tumor diagnosis, grading and staging. *Semin Vet Med,* 10:158–167.

46. Powers, B.E. and Dernell, W.S. (1998) Tumor biology and pathology. *Clin Tech Small Anim Pract* 13:4–9.

47. Bostock-Wilcock, B.P. and Peiffer, R.L. (1986) Morphology and behavior of primary ocular melanomas in 91 dogs. *Vet Pathol* 23:418–424.

48. Bostock, D.E. (1979) Prognosis after surgical excision of canine melanomas. *Vet Pathol* 16:32–40.

49. Spangler, W.L., Culbertson, R., and Kass, P.H. (1994) Primary mesenchymal (nonangiomatous/nonlymphomatous) neoplasms occurring in the canine spleen: Anatomic classification, immunohistochemical, and mitotic activity correlated with patient survival. *Vet Pathol* 31:37–47.

50. Valli, V.E., Norris, A.M., Jacobs, R.M., Laing, E., Withrow, S., Macy, D., Tomlinson, J., McCaw, D., Ogilvie, G.K., and Pidgeon, G. (1995) Pathology of canine bladder and urethral cancer and correlation with tumor progression and survival. *J Comp Pathol* 113:113–130.

51. McNiel E.A., Ogilvie, G.K., Powers, B.E., et al. (1997) Evaluation of prognostic factors for dogs with primary lung tumors: 67 cases (1985-1992). *J Am Vet Med Assoc* 211:1422–1427.

52. Dernell, W.S., Straw, R.C., Cooper, M.F., Powers, B.E., LaRue, S.M., and Withrow, S.J. (1998) Multilobular osteochondrosarcoma in 39 dogs: 1979–1993. *J Amer Anim Hosp Assoc* 34:11–18.

53. Straw, R.C., Powers, B.E., Klausner, J.S., Henderson, R.A., Morrison, W.B., McCaw-D.L., Harvey, H.J., Jacobs, R.M., and Berg, R.J. (1996) Canine mandibular osteosarcoma: 51 cases (1980–1992). *J Amer Anim Hosp Assoc* 32:257–262.

54. Vail, D.M., Kisseberth, W.C., Obradovich, J.E., Moore, F.M., London, C.A., MacEwen, E.G., and Ritter, M.A. (1996) Assessment of potential doubling time (Tpot), argyrophilic nucleolar organizer regions (AgNOR), and proliferating cell nuclear antigen (PCNA) as predictors of therapy response in canine non-Hodgkin's lymphoma. *Exp Hematol* 24:807–815.

55. Weller, R.E., Holmberg, C.A., Theilen, G.H., and Madewell, B.R. (1980) Histologic classification as a prognostic criterion for canine lymphosarcoma. *Amer J Vet Res* 41:1310–1314.

56. Lohr, C.V., Teifke, J.P., Failing, K., and Weiss, E. (1997) Characterization of the proliferation state in canine mammary tumors by the standardized AgNOR method with postfixation and immunohistologic detection of Ki-67 and PCNA. *Vet Pathol* 34:212–221.

57. Owen, L.N. (1980) *TNM Classification of Tumors in Domestic Animals.* World Health Organization, Geneva.

58. Gilson, S.D., and Stone, E.A. (1990) Principles of oncologic surgery. *Comp Cont Educ Pract Vet* 12:827–838.

TUMOR MANAGEMENT

Introduction

The development of a neoplasm represents a continuum of discrete, independent genetic events that confer novel characteristics to cells, such as increased growth rate, metastatic potential, and resistance to immune mediated or drug induced death. Cells with particular constellations of genetic characteristics can develop into malignant neoplasms that threaten the life of the affected individual. The complete extent of this continuum, from preclinical events to overt clinical signs, has been described for few spontaneous neoplasms in animals. Alterations in the structure or function of the organ are most often the first clinical evidence of a neoplasm and represent one extreme of this continuum. Even the best scenario, associated with the identification of a small incidental tumor, fixes the first point of clinical intervention at a late stage in the evolution of that neoplasm. Although gross and microscopic manifestations of malignancy are derived from these late events, such data form the basis of current staging schemes, as well as diagnostic and therapeutic recommendations. Methods to detect genetic and biologic dysregulation have started to emerge as descriptors of the neoplastic condition, and assessment of these early changes may supplant demographic and morphological characteristics as better determinants of outcome. For example, immunological derivation of canine lymphoma (B vs. T cell derived neoplasia) has been determined to be a stronger predictor of response to chemotherapy than other clinical or histological prognostic factors.[1,3,4] Identification of susceptible or affected individuals by molecular testing or by serum analysis will likely transform the diagnosis and management of neoplastic disease in domestic animals in the next several decades.

The purpose of this introductory chapter is to register the current level of expertise on the pathogenesis and management of neoplastic diseases of domestic animals as a means to measure future improvements in this field. In order to accomplish this, we will identify state-of-the-art diagnostic tools and discuss how they have resulted in improved classification schema for several tumor categories. In addition, it will be useful to the reader of this text to review some background on the etiology, genetics, biology, and clinical management of cancer in domestic animals. Table 1.8 describes the relative importance, at the time of this writing, of prognostic factors for neoplasms along the preclinical to clinical continuum within the canine species. It is hopeful and, we believe, probable that many of the categories, which currently are of unknown importance, will be identified and will improve the management of cancer.

Basic Concepts in Cancer Management

Cancer management in companion animals has evolved considerably during the last 15–20 years as a result of several significant factors. Clients are increasingly aware of cancer treatment options for their pets and are often willing to make the emotional and financial commitment to pursue sophisticated diagnostic and therapeutic regimens. Increased information regarding treatment results has enabled clinicians to make better recommendations regarding curative or palliative treatment, and technological advances have made treatment more sophisticated. For instance, new surgical procedures result in prolonged survival for many patients presenting with orofacial tumors and permit limb-sparing for dogs with primary bone tumors; in addition, the development of vascular pedicle grafts and tissue expanders facilitates the reconstruction of normal tissue following tumor resection in situations where this was not previously possible. Radiation therapy has been refined both technologically and in clinical application so that it is now an essential tool for management of incompletely resected solid tumors, nasal tumors, and oral melanoma and for pain relief in patients with bone cancer. The use of chemotherapy in combination with surgery or radiation therapy has resulted in better management of canine hemangiosarcoma and osteosarcoma and of mammary carcinoma in cats. Veterinarians engaged in any type of companion animal practice now manage pets with cancer on a weekly or daily basis and must be familiar with current trends in diagnosis and treatment. A flow chart of the principles of cancer management from a clinician's perspective is shown in figure 1.12. Treatment decisions are based on numerous factors, several of which require transfer of information between clinicians and pathologists during the biopsy process and following removal of normal and tumor tissue at surgery. It is important for clinicians to properly process tissue specimens and provide accurate data regarding clinical management issues such as identification of normal tissue margins of particular concern. It is equally important for pathologists to understand the context of clinical decision making in order to transfer accurate and useful information about the tumor and surrounding normal tissue.

Biopsy Process

Figure 1.13 illustrates a scheme for an approach to the diagnosis of any superficial tumor. Preliminary assessment of the mass should consist of measurements, evaluation of local invasion and attachment of the mass to surrounding tissues, and evaluation of possible regional lymph node involvement. A topographic map of masses located on the patient helps document new lesions and changes in previously identified benign masses. A fine needle aspiration (FNA) should be conducted following the physical examination in most instances. A rapid and final diagnosis is possible for benign processes such as an inclusion cyst or abscess and for neoplastic masses such as mast cell tumors and other round cell tumors (e.g., lymphoma, plasmacytoma, histiocytoma); or a presumptive diagnosis may be made for epithelial/mesenchymal neo-

TABLE 1.8.   Relative importance of prognostic indicators in various categories for canine solid tumors* and lymphoproliferative tumors

Prognostic Category	Solid	Lymphoproliferative
Genetic (mutations, translocations, etc.)	Unknown	Unknown
Biologic (phenotype)	Unknown	++++
Morphologic (mitotic figures, invasion, etc.)	++	+
Physiologic/microenvironmental (hypoxia, cell kinetics, interstitial press)	Unknown	Unknown
Physical (size, site, adherence, invasion)	++	++
Regional metastasis (LN, adj normal tissue)	+++	Not used
Systemic metastasis	++++	Not used
Clinical signs/symptoms	++++	+++

*Solid tumors include sarcomas, mast cell tumors, and mammary gland tumors.

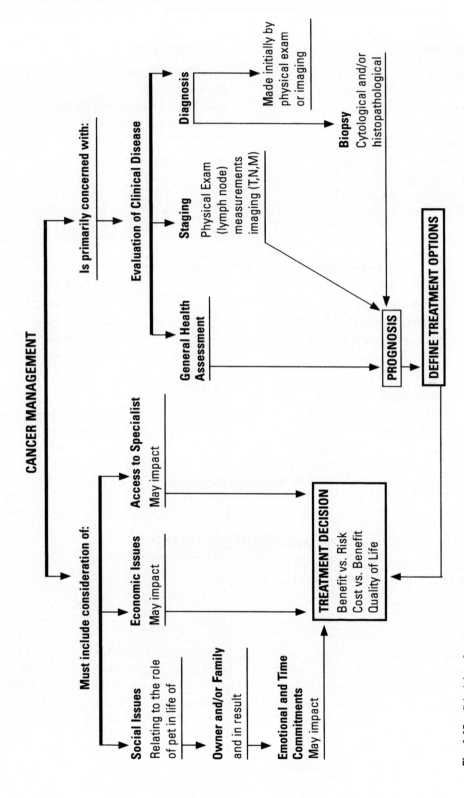

Fig. 1.12. Principles of cancer management.

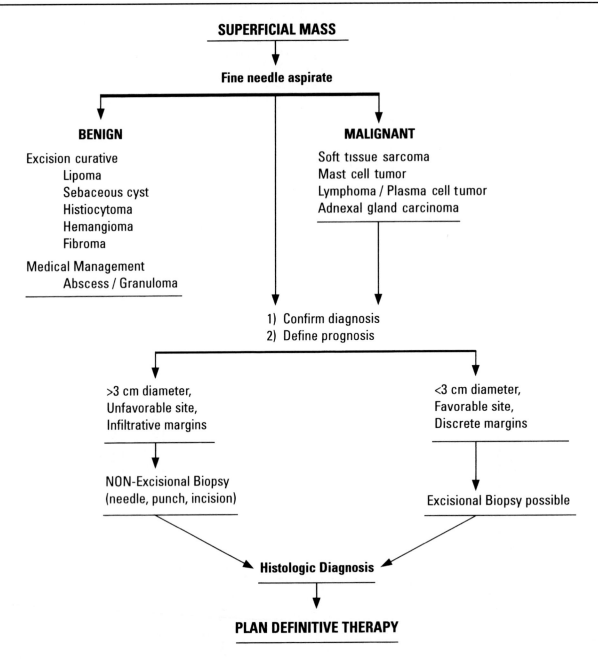

Fig. 1.13. Approach to histological diagnosis of a superficial mass.

plasia. Fine needle aspiration biopsies are often not conducted when a definitive biopsy procedure is preferred based on location of the tumor (e.g., oral/nasal tumor) or when a high potential for an inconclusive result exists (e.g., suspected mesenchymal tumor or mammary neoplasia). Impression smears of biopsy specimens, however, may be useful as a screening tool to consider preliminary treatment options. In many instances, a nondiagnostic aspirate may result from a FNA of a superficial mass. In this situation or when prognostic information from a sample of tissue may be helpful in planning the best treatment,

a biopsy is recommended even if a preliminary diagnosis is made by FNA technique. The decision to perform an excisional biopsy must be made by considering the size of the mass, the site of the mass, and the degree of normal tissue that can be removed with the procedure. When an excisional biopsy is not possible, it is critical to select the biopsy site wisely. The site of a punch or core biopsy must be in an area that will be completely treated once the treatment plan has been determined. This means that the biopsy track should be completely excised or should be in the radiation treatment field. Likewise, the biopsy site and pro-

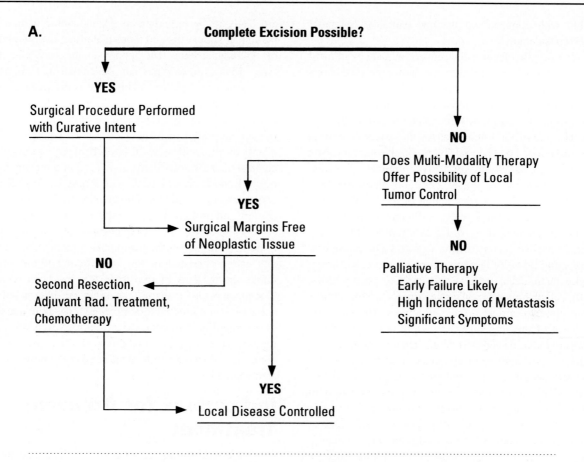

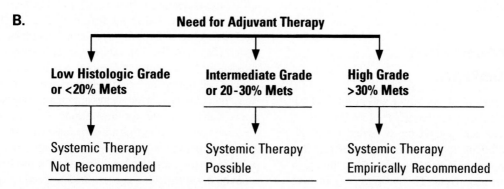

Fig. 1.14. Treatment decision algorithms for solid tumor and adjuvant therapy. **A.** Treatment decision algorithm. **B.** Adjuvant therapy algorithm.

cedure selected should not compromise the future treatment of the tumor by being overly aggressive or likely to dehisce during irradiation. Obtaining adequate tissue for evaluation is essential. If a cutting needle is used, several cores of tumor tissue should be obtained by redirecting the needle through the same surface puncture if possible. From a clinician's perspective, a biopsy should first determine whether a mass is neoplastic or nonneoplastic, then determine the tumor morphological type (e.g., round cell, epithelial, mesenchymal), and lastly, provide any prognostic information helpful for guiding treatment decisions.

The treatment decision algorithm illustrates the process of determining the treatment options for a solid tumor (fig.1.14 A). The ability to achieve a curative outcome is based on assessment of the natural history of the specific tumor type as defined by clinically relevant predictive indicators (i.e., grade) and the available treatment options. A working definition of *curative* often used in veterinary medicine is a likelihood of greater than 50 percent that a given tumor type will be controlled (no detectable recurrence or metastasis) for at least 1 year posttreatment. If available information suggests such control is not possible with conventional therapy, palliative treatment may be considered.

The first therapeutic determination made by clinical veterinarians involves whether the tumor may be completely excised. This is determined by the size of the surgical field necessary to remove all known and probable tumor extent, the site of the tumor, and the skill of the surgeon. The site of the tumor dictates the extent of normal tissue resection. For instance, interscapular injection-site sarcomas in cats require extensive removal of tissue, including portions of dorsal vertebral processes and scapulae, due to the complex nature of the fascial planes within that site. Regions where sufficient normal tissue can not be removed (e.g., distal extremities, skull) may require extensive reconstruction (grafting) or consideration of multimodality therapy. More sophisticated tumor imaging techniques, such as CT or MR, greatly assist presurgical planning for invasive tumors or for tumors located close to critical normal structures. The skill and experience of the surgeon is extremely important. Some tumors are radiation sensitive (e.g., acanthomatous epulis, plasmacytomas, mast cell tumors) and may be considered potentially curable if they are located within a site that is not amenable to complete resection. A combination of radiation and surgery improves outcome in situations when neither treatment modality alone is sufficient to accomplish that goal. Well planned, combined modality therapy is being used more frequently for tumors that are located in difficult sites.

Tissue Processing and Evaluation

Following removal of the tumor and normal tissue, determination of the completeness of resection is extremely important and should be evaluated histologically. It is the clinician's responsibility to ensure that excised tissue is properly marked to orient the pathologist after the tissue has been fixed. This process may involve marking the cut surface with India ink or other dyes or using a labeling system with different suture patterns to indicate areas of special concern such as the deep margin, potential close margins, etc. If the tissue is too large to submit whole, samples of each margin are excised and clearly labeled. Samples from several internal sites on the mass are also submitted. Substantial additional time and cost is necessary to thoroughly examine the margins for neoplastic cells, but this information is vital to the successful management of cancer.

The pathologist's report should be concise and descriptive of the tissue submitted. The report should be free of abbreviations or jargon and use terminology that is clear and readily understood by clinicians reading the report. Careful attention should be paid to the issues that are likely to be important in distinguishing benign from malignant neoplasms and those that affect the morphological grading scheme that applies to the particular tumor type.[2] Many tumor types can be graded to facilitate the prognosis for the patient. (This issue is discussed above in the tumor diagnosis section of this chapter.) It is the pathologist's responsibility to stay abreast of the literature regarding current grading schemes. The report should include the results of all ancillary tests, histochemistry, immunohistochemistry, or electron microscopy used in achieving a diagnosis. Reports should be issued promptly. Any delay in communication with the clinician can delay appropriate therapy and prolong anxiety in the animal's owner.

Frequently, the completeness of excision is an important element of the pathologist's report. The pathologist can be assisted in this undertaking if the surgeon marks the margins of the tissue that has been removed. Completeness of excision can often be determined with assurance for epithelial tumors of the lung, skin, mammary gland, and digestive tract. Determining if excision is complete for mesenchymal malignancies, in particular those composed of spindle cells, is more likely to pose a significant challenge.

Indications for Adjuvant Treatment

The need for adjuvant therapy (radiation, chemotherapy, immunotherapy) is based on a high likelihood of local tumor recurrence following resection or a high rate of metastasis even if the primary tumor is permanently controlled (fig. 1.14 B). Adjuvant radiation therapy is recommended for local control of incompletely resected sarcomas or mast cell tumors and results in long-term control. Adjuvant chemotherapy or adjuvant immunotherapy would be theoretically valuable for any tumor with a substantial metastatic rate. Tumors that are associated with an incidence of distant metastasis exceeding 20 percent may warrant a recommendation for adjuvant treatment if a survival benefit could be documented for that chemotherapeutic protocol. In veterinary medicine, few studies have documented that adjuvant therapy with chemotherapy/immunotherapy prolongs survival. Survival of dogs with osteosarcoma, and perhaps hemangiosarcoma, is significantly prolonged after chemotherapy or immunotherapy use. Cats with mammary carcinoma are believed to benefit from adjuvant chemotherapy. A general recommendation for adjuvant therapy in other types of cancer where metastasis is a life-limiting event is difficult to make given the available data. However, some tumors (e.g., high grade sarcomas in dogs, malignant melanoma) are associated with a high risk of metastasis, and clinical trials are currently being conducted to determine the efficacy of adjuvant therapy in these tumor categories. Prognostic factors that relate to the prognosis following treatment are presented in table 1.9.

TABLE 1.9. **Clinical and histologic prognostic features of canine tumors that relate to prognosis following current treatment recommendations**

| Tumor Category | Prognostic Category | | Treatment Decision[a,b] |
	Clinical Stage	Histological Grade	
Soft tissue sarcoma[c]	Lymph node (+)	Grade 1 or 2 v. 3	Aggressive local tx (surgery +/- radiation therapy alone vs. adjuvant/systematic chemotherapy)[5,6]
Synovial cell sarcoma	Bone invasion	Grade 1 v. 2 v. 3	Aggressive local tx alone (amputation or radiation therapy vs. adjuvant chemotherapy)[7]
Mast cell tumor	Multiple cutaneous nodules, LN(+), or systemic disease	Grade 1 v. 2 v. 3	Local/regional tx (surgery +/- radiation therapy) vs. palliative systemic treatment[8]
Hemangiosarcoma			
Cutaneous	LN(+), systemic disease	Grade 1 v. 2/3	Surgery alone vs. adjuvant chemotherapy[9]
Splenic	Splenic v. extrasplenic	Grade 1 v. 2/3	Palliative surgery v. adjuvant chemotherapy[10]
Osteosarcoma			
Appendicular	LN(+), ploidy, proliferation	None identified	Amputation + chemotherapy v. palliative radiation therapy[11]
Mandibular	As above	Grade 1 v. 2 or 3	Surgery + adjuvant chemotherapy[12]
Multilobular osteochondroma	Mandibular v. other site	Grade 1 v. 2 v. 3	Surgery +/- radiation therapy plus adjuvant chemotherapy[13]
Pulmonary carcinoma	+/- symptoms, LN(+)	Grade 1 v. 2 v. 3	Aggressive surgery v. adjuvant chemotherapy[14]
Mammary carcinoma	>3 cm diameter	Grade 0 or 1 v. 2	Surgery vs. adjuvant systemic treatment[15]
Transitional cell carcinoma	Apical v. trigonal, LN(+)	Grade 1 v. 2 or 3 +/- desmoplasia, +/- lymphoid rxn	Treatment is palliative (piroxicam + chemotherapy)[16]
Nasopharyngeal cavity tumors	Theon stage 1 v. 2	None identified	Radiation therapy +/- chemotherapy for all histologic types[17]
Lymphoma	WHO I-III v. IV/V, a v. b substage, mediastinal mass	B v. T cell phenotype	Aggressive v. palliative chemotherapy/ radiation therapy[1,2,3,18]

Note: rxn = reaction; tx = treatment.

[a]Treatment decisions are based on individual tumor types and prognostic categories. Histologic grade is derived from mitotic index, percentage of the tumor area that is necrotic, and features such as nuclear atypia and cellular pleomorphism.

[b]Superscript numbers following treatment descriptions are references.

[c]Includes fibrosarcoma, hemangiopericytoma, liposarcoma, neurofibrosarcoma, myxosarcoma, malignant fibrous histiocytoma, and undifferentiated sarcoma.

Conclusions

In recent years, there has been remarkable progress made in the understanding of the complex pathogenesis of neoplasia. A schematic overview of the current view of the pathogenesis of cancer is shown in figure 1.15. The molecular mechanisms involved in the neoplastic transformation and regulation of cells have been identified for numerous tumor types. This understanding is beginning to be applied to risk assessment, tumor diagnostics, and anticancer therapy. It is hoped that this new understanding will permit more precise identification of the early stages of neoplasia when, it is presumed, therapy can be more effective.

Therapies that can be developed to specifically target abnormal properties of cancer cells may spare normal cells and may avoid the side effects of many contemporary treatments. Moreover, as the genetic lesions responsible for cancer development and progression are identified, conventional diagnostic techniques and grading algorithms will, it is hoped, become obsolete and be replaced by stronger predictors of outcome.

As a result of collaborative interactions among clinicians, oncologists, and pathologists, new grading schemes have been developed that assist in identifying the important histological features that provide prognostic information for various tumors. It is incumbent upon pathologists to remain well informed about recent developments in classification and grading of neoplasms in order to provide the most useful information to clinicians. However, one should not lose sight of the fact that the ultimate predictor of tumor behavior and patient prognosis remains the morphological assessment of the tissue by the pathologist.

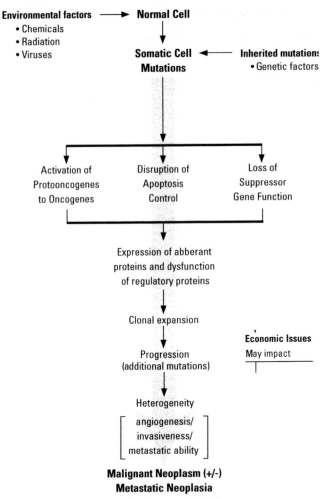

Fig. 1.15. Overview of the process of carcinogenesis [Modified from Cotran et al. (1998) *Pathologic Basis of Disease*; with permission].

REFERENCES

1. Greenlee, P.G., Filippa, D.A., Quimby, F.W., Patnaik, A.K., Calvano, S.E., Matus, R.E., Kimmel, M., Hurvitz, A.I., and Lieberman, P.H. (1990) Lymphomas in dogs: A morphologic, immmunological and clinical study. *Cancer* 66:480–490.

2. Powers, B.E., and Dernell, W.S. (1998) Tumor biology and pathology. *Clin Tech Small Anim Pract* 13:4–9.

3. Ruslander, D.A., Gebhard, D.H., Tompkins, M.B., Grindem, C.B., and Page, R.L. (1997) Immunophenotypic characterization of canine lymphoproliferative disorders. *In Vivo* 11:169–172.

4. Vail, D.M., Kisseberth, W.C., Obradovich, J.E., Moore, F.M., London, C.A., MacEwen, E.G., and Ritter, M.A. (1996) Assessment of potential doubling time (Tpot), argyrophilic nucleolar organizer regions (AgNOR), and proliferating cell nuclear antigen (PCNA) as predictors of therapy response in canine non-Hodgkin's lymphoma. *Exp Hematol* 24:807–815.

5. Bostock, D.E., and Dye, M.T. (1980) Prognosis after surgical excision of canine fibrous connective tissue sarcomas. *Vet Pathol* 17:581-588.

6. Vail, D.M., Powers, B.E., Getzy, D.M., et al. (1994) Evaluation of prognostic factors for dogs with synovial sarcoma: 36 cases. *J Am Vet Med Assoc* 205:1300-1307.

7. Patnaik, A.K., Ehler, W.J., and MacEwen, E.G. (1984) Canine cutaneous mast cell tumor: Morphologic grading and survival time in 83 dogs. *Vet Pathol* 21:469-474.

8. Ward, H., Fox, L.E., Calderwood-Mays, M.B., et al. (1994 Cutaneous hemangiosarcoma in 25 dogs: A retrospective study. *J Vet Int Med* 8:345-348.

9. Prymak, C., McKee, L.J., Goldschmidt, M.H., and Glickman, L.T.

(1988) Epidemiologic, clinical, pathologic, and prognostic characteristics of splenic hemangiosarcoma and splenic hematoma in dogs: 217 cases (1985). *J Am Vet Med Assoc* 193:706-712.

10. Misdorp, W., and Har, A.A.M. (1979) Some prognostic and epidemiologic factors in canine osteosarcoma. *J Nat'l Cancer Inst* 62:537-545.

11. Straw, R.C., Powers, B.E., Klausner, J.S., et al. (1996) Canine mandibular osteosarcoma: 51 cases (1980-1992). *J Am Anim Hosp Assoc* 32:257-262.

12. Dernell, W.S., Straw, R.C., Cooper, M.F., et al. (1998) Multilobular osteochondrosarcoma in 39 dogs: 1979-1993. *J Am Anim Hosp Assoc* 34:11-18.

13. McNiel, E.A., Olgilvie, G.K., Powers, B.E., et al. (1997) Evaluation of prognostic factors for dogs with primary lung tumors: 67 cases (1985-1992). *J Am Vet Med Assoc* 211:1422-1427.

14. Bostock, D.E., Moriarty, J., and Cooper, J. (1992) Correlation between histologic diagnosis, mean nucleolar organizer region count, and prognosis in canine mammary tumors. *Vet Pathol* 29:381-385.

15. Valli, V.E., Norris, A.M., Laing, E., et al. (1995) Pathology of canine bladder and urethral cancer and correlation with tumor progression and survival. *J Comp Pathol* 113:113-130.

16. Theon, A.P., Madwell, B.R., Harb, M.F., and Dungworth, D.L. (1993) Megavoltage irradiation of neoplasms of the nasal and paranasal cavities in 77 dogs. *J Am Vet Med Assoc* 202:1469-1475.

17. Teske, E., vanHeerde, P., Rutteman, G.R., et al. (1994) Prognostic factors for treatment of malignant lymphoma in dogs. *J Am Vet Med Assoc* 205:1722-1728.

18. Rutteman, G.R., Cornelisse, C.J., Dijkshoorn, N.J., et al. (1988) Flow cytometric analysis of DNA ploidy in canine mammary tumors. *Cancer Res* 48:3411-3417.

2 Tumors of the Skin and Soft Tissues

M. H. Goldschmidt and M. J. Hendrick

The category *skin and soft tissues* covers a wide range of tumors among which are many of the most common neoplasms in veterinary medicine. Because lesions and masses involving the skin are easily seen by the owner and brought to the attention of the veterinarian, these lesions frequently will be removed and submitted for histopathologic evaluation.

These tumors have been classified using the revised International Histological Classification of Skin Tumors and Tumor-like Lesions of Domestic Animals.[1,2] This classification system is similar to that found in several recent texts that deal with skin tumors.[3,4,5,6] These references will not be further cited in the text, but they provide extensive information on the clinical aspects and histopathology of skin tumors.

The skin consists of the epidermis and associated appendaged structures, the hair, the sebaceous glands and modified sebaceous glands, the apocrine glands and modified apocrine glands, and the eccrine glands, all supported by a dermis and panniculus. Melanocytes are present between the basal cells of the epidermis and between the germinative cells of the hair follicle bulb. The chapter is divided into two major sections: the first covers epithelial tumors, and the second covers mesenchymal tumors. The section on epithelial tumors includes tumors without squamous and adnexal differentiation, tumors of the epidermis, tumors with adnexal differentiation, and the melanocytic tumors. The section on mesenchymal tumors includes those tumors arising from the supporting mesenchymal tissues of the dermis and subcutis (fibrous connective tissue, blood vessels, lymphatics, nerves, adipose tissue, and smooth muscle) and those round cell tumors of mesenchymal origin that present as cutaneous masses.

Much of the information on incidence, age, sex predilection, and site of occurrence of these tumors in the dog and cat is based on a database of 130,000 surgical pathology accessions (1986–1995) in the Laboratory of Pathology, University of Pennsylvania, School of Veterinary Medicine. Where sufficient numbers of cases were available, the odds ratios were calculated for all canine and feline breeds at increased and decreased risk for each specific tumor. Statistical significance was defined as $p < 0.01$ and was determined by the chi-square test. In the text, the odds ratio is noted in parentheses (OR) after the breed.

GENERAL REFERENCES

1. Goldschmidt, M.H., Dunstan, R.W., Stannard, A.A., von Tscharner, C., Walder, E.J., and Yager, J.A. (1998) *World Health Organization International Histologic Classification of Tumors of Domestic Animals. Histological Classification of Tumors of the Skin of Domestic Animals.* 2nd series, vol. III. Armed Forces Institute of Pathology, Washington, D.C.
2. Hendrick, M.J., Mahaffey, E.A., Moore, F.M., Vos, J.H., and Walder, E.J. (1998) *World Health Organization International Histologic Classification of Tumors of Domestic Animals. Histological Classification of the Mesenchymal Tumors of Skin and Soft Tissues of Domestic Animals.* 2nd series, vol. II. Armed Forces Institute of Pathology, Washington, D.C.
3. Goldschmidt, M.H., and Shofer, F.S. (1998) *Skin Tumors of the Dog and Cat.* Butterworth Heinemann, Oxford, pp. 1–301.
4. Walder, E.J. (1992) In T.L. Gross, P.E. Ihrke, and E.J. Walder. Veterinary *Dermatopathology: A Macroscopic and Microscopic Evaluation of Canine and Feline Skin Disease.* Mosby Yearbook, St. Louis, pp. 330–484.
5. Scott, D.W., Miller, W.H., and Griffin, C.E. (1995) *Small Animal Dermatology.* W.B. Saunders Co., Philadelphia, pp. 990–1126.
6. Yager, J.A., and Wilcock, B.P. (1994) *Color Atlas and Text of Surgical Pathology of the Dog and Cat.* Mosby Yearbook, London, pp. 243–303.

EPITHELIAL TUMORS

M. H. Goldschmidt

EPITHELIAL TUMORS WITHOUT SQUAMOUS AND ADNEXAL DIFFERENTIATION

Epithelial tumors without squamous and adnexal differentiation include basal cell tumors and basal cell carcinoma (infiltrative type and clear cell type).

Basal Cell Tumor

This is an epithelial tumor which shows no epidermal or adnexal differentiation. The tumor cells morphologically resemble the normal basal cells of the epidermis. The tumor, previously classified as a basal cell tumor in the dog, horse, and sheep and as the spindle cell form of a basal cell tumor in the cat, has been reclassified as a trichoblastoma.

Incidence, Age, Breed, and Sex

Basal cell tumors are common in the cat, uncommon in the dog and horse, and rare in other species.[1] Cats as young as 1 year of age may be affected, with a peak incidence between 6 and 13 years of age. Himalayan (2.8), Persian (1.7), and domestic longhair cats (1.5) are at increased risk, and domestic shorthair cats (0.7) are at decreased risk for developing basal cell tumors. There is no sex predilection.

Sites and Gross Morphology

In the cat basal cell tumors are most commonly found on the neck and head. Multicentric basal cell tumors have been reported to occur,[2] but account for only 1 percent of cases.

Most tumors are presented clinically as well circumscribed intradermal and subcutaneous masses. The overlying epidermis may show loss of hairs, and ulceration of the epidermis may also be present. On cut section, many of the tumors are pigmented brown/black. Central cystic degeneration with the accumulation of amorphous dark brown material within the center of the tumor may be found. The mass is frequently well demarcated from the surrounding dermal and subcutaneous tissue.

Histological Features

Many basal cell tumors are well circumscribed intradermal masses, which may extend into the subcutaneous adipose tissue as the tumor enlarges. There is often an association with the overlying epidermis, even in tumors that are ulcerated. The tumor is often multilobulated, with the individual lobules separated by a fibrous stroma. Central cystic degeneration of the tumor lobules is common, with an accumulation of brown/black necrotic debris in the center of the cysts and a zone of viable tumor cells at the periphery (fig. 2.1 A).

The individual tumor cells are small and round to polyhedral in morphology. The nuclei are ovoid, nucleoli are inconspicuous, and few mitotic figures are found. A small amount of cytoplasm is present. Melanocytes may be found interspersed between the basal cells, with transfer of melanin to the neoplastic cells. However, melanophages are often present in the interlobular connective tissue stroma.

Growth and Metastasis

Basal cell tumors do not metastasize. They are usually slow growing intradermal masses. The treatment of choice is surgical excision. Incomplete excision may result in tumor recurrence.

Basal Cell Carcinoma

This is a low grade malignant epithelial tumor which shows no epidermal or adnexal differentiation. The tumor cells morphologically resemble the normal basal cells of the epidermis.

Incidence, Age, Breed, and Sex

Basal cell carcinomas are common in the cat, uncommon in the dog, and rare or not described in other species. Cats and dogs between 3 and 14 years old are affected. No breed predilection has been noted. There is a higher incidence in females then males.

Sites and Gross Morphology

The head and neck are often affected, but some cases present with multiple masses. The tumor, which often shows epidermal ulceration and extensive infiltration of the dermis and subcutaneous tissue, feels firm on palpation.

Histological Features

Two variants of basal cell carcinoma are found, an infiltrative type and a clear cell type. The *infiltrative type* often can be found extending from the basal cells of the epidermis into the dermis and subcutis, as cords and sheets of small, basophilic cells with hyperchromatic nuclei and little cytoplasm (fig. 2.1 B). The nuclei show little pleomorphism, but mitoses are often extremely numerous. Necrosis may be found in the center of the invading cords and islands of tumor cells. Tumor cells show no differentiation to squamous epithelium or adnexal structures. There is often a marked dermal fibroblast proliferation in response to the infiltrating tumor cells. The *clear cell type* of basal cell carcinoma is also invasive, but it often lacks the intimate association with the epidermis seen with the infiltrative type. The cells are larger and have a clear or finely granular cytoplasm. The nuclei are ovoid with inconspicuous nucleoli, and the number of mitoses found is quite variable.

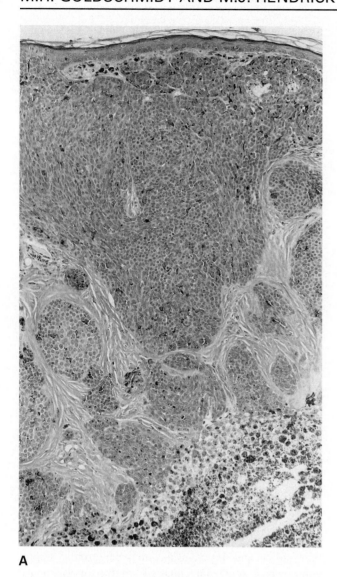

A

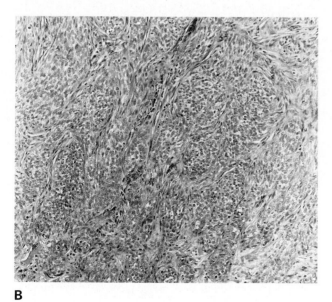

B

Fig. 2.1. **A.** Basal cell tumor, feline. **B.** Basal cell carcinoma, infiltrative type, feline.

Growth and Metastasis

This tumor is locally invasive, but few cases with proven metastases have been reported.[3] Thus, surgical excision is the treatment of choice. Basal cell carcinomas can be differentiated from basal cell tumors by the invasive nature of the tumor, particularly at the base of the mass, often accompanied by dermal fibroplasia.

REFERENCES

1. Diters, R.W., and Walsh, K.M. (1984) Feline basal cell tumors: A review of 124 cases. *Vet Pathol* 21:51–56.
2. Fehrer, S.L., and Lin, S.H. (1986) Multicentric basal cell tumors in a cat. *J Amer Vet Med Assoc* 189:1469–1470.
3. Day, D.G., Couto, C.G., Weisbrode, S.E., and Smeak, D.D. Basal cell carcinoma in two cats. *J Amer Anim Hosp Assoc* 30:265–269.

TUMORS OF THE EPIDERMIS

Tumors of the epidermis include papilloma and inverted papilloma, multicentric squamous cell carcinoma in situ (Bowen's disease), squamous cell carcinoma, and basosquamous carcinoma.

Papilloma (Cutaneous Papillomatosis)

General Considerations

This is a benign, exophytic proliferation of the epidermis. It is caused by infection with a papillomavirus.[1] The lesion should be distinguished from a squamous papilloma (see table 2.1), which is a nonviral proliferation of the epidermis that has many features in common with viral papillomas, both clinically and histopathologically. Canine oral papillomavirus (COPV) infection is discussed in chapter 8, bovine fibropapillomas in chapter 11, and equine sarcoids later in this chapter.

TABLE 2.1. Points of differentiation between viral and squamous papillomas

Viral Papilloma	Squamous Papilloma
Epidermal differentiation may show orthokeratosis or parakeratosis	Epidermal differentiation is normal
Enlarged keratohyaline granules	Normal size to keratohyaline granules
Koilocytes present	Koilocytes absent
Keratinocytes show viral cytopathic effect	Keratinocytes normal
Intranuclear inclusions may be present	No intranuclear inclusions
Elongated rete slant inward	Elongated rete slant outward

A large number of different papillomaviruses have been identified. Each species may be infected by several papillomaviruses, with each virus subtype often associated with a specific tissue.

Incidence, Age, Breed, and Sex

Cutaneous papillomas are common in the horse and in cattle, uncommon in the dog, cat, sheep, and goat, and rare in the pig. In most species, except the goat, young animals are preferentially affected; in goats, adult females are most commonly affected. There are several reports of congenital papillomas in foals,[2,3,4,5] a calf,[6] and a piglet.[7]

There is no known breed predilection for papillomas in horses or cattle. In the goat, Saanen goats are primarily affected.[8] Dogs at increased risk are the Great Dane (4.3), Irish setter (2.9), and beagle (2.3), while mixed breed dogs (0.56) are at decreased risk.

There is no known sex predilection in any species that develops cutaneous papillomas, except the goats, where white lactating animals are primarily affected.[8]

Sites and Gross Morphology

In cattle papillomas occur most commonly at sites of abrasion where the virus can enter the epidermis and produce the cutaneous lesions, including the ears following tattooing.[9] Thus the sites where the papillomas may be found are greatly dependent on the husbandry practices of the agricultural community. Lesions in cattle are most often multicentric and frequently tend to involve the head and neck (fig. 2.2 A). In horses lesions are found primarily around the nose and lips, in goats the udder, in sheep the head and ears, and in dogs the head and multiple body sites. Cutaneous papillomas may also present as multiple plaques in dogs.[10]

Histological Features

Histopathologic features of cutaneous papillomas were studied in the horse by Hamada et al.,[11] who subdivided the naturally developing lesions into three phases: a growing phase, a developing phase, and a regressing phase. The growing phase was characterized by basal cell hyperplasia, mild to moderate acanthosis, hyperkeratosis and parakeratosis, and a few intranuclear inclusion bodies. The developing phase was characterized by marked acanthosis with cell swelling and marked hyperkeratosis and parakeratosis. Many intranuclear inclusion bodies were present in swollen or degenerating cells of the upper spinous and granular cell layer. The regressing phase was characterized by slight epidermal hyperplasia, accentuation of the rete, moderate proliferation of fibroblasts, and collagen deposition along with an infiltrate of T lymphocytes at the epidermal-dermal interface. Papillomas in horses show hypopigmentation of the affected skin, which is due to decreased numbers of melanocytes in the basal layer, abnormal melanosome

formation during melanin synthesis (some of which are transferred to keratinocytes), and abnormal interactions between melanocytes and keratinocytes.[12] Langerhans cells in the epidermis are decreased in number and size during the developing phase, but are increased in number and are hyperfunctional in the regressing phase.[13] There are also abnormalities in the expression of cytokeratins in the papillomavirus infected cells, with expression of a 54kD keratin by the suprabasilar keratinocytes in the infected epidermis. Electron microscopy showed decreased intracytoplasmic tonofilaments and desmosome-tonofilament complexes due to an abnormality in the proliferation and terminal differentiation of keratinocytes in the papilloma.[14]

Papillomas have a core of dermal stroma that supports the proliferating epithelium (fig. 2.2 B). Capillaries within the dermis are often dilated and congested, and when there is secondary bacterial infection, they will show neutrophil margination and exocytosis into the dermis and epidermis. Many cells within the stratum spinosum have a basophilic cytoplasm, which corresponds to the decreased intracytoplasmic tonofilaments noted on electron microscopy and is a viral cytopathic effect. Also seen in the upper spinous layer are cells with eccentric pyknotic nuclei and a perinuclear halo, referred to as koilocytes. In the granular cell layer the keratohyaline granules are often larger than normal and may be round or angular (fig. 2.2 C).

The number of intranuclear inclusion bodies varies from species to species, and in some cases none will be found. In the dog, a variant to the above findings associated with a novel papillomavirus has been found.[10] The lesions are endophytic; intranuclear inclusion bodies are basophilic; and intracytoplasmic eosinophilic aggregates, which represent clumped keratin tonofilaments, are seen.

Etiology

In cattle six different types of bovine papillomavirus have been identified (BPV-1 to BPV-6) and classified into two subgroups, A and B. Subgroup A (BPV-1, BPV-2, BPV-5) will induce fibropapillomas with involvement of dermal fibroblasts and keratinocytes, and subgroup B will induce epithelial papillomas (BPV-3, BPV-6) with only keratinocyte involvement. BPV-4 infects the mucosal epithelium of the upper alimentary canal and induces pure epithelial papillomas.[15] There are other still unidentified bovine papillomaviruses. Other species also have several papillomaviruses but there is less information available on these.

Immunity and Regression

Spontaneous regression of papillomavirus infection in cattle due to a cell-mediated immune response has been noted, with protection from subsequent infection by neu-

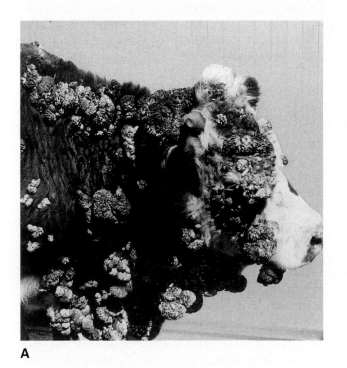

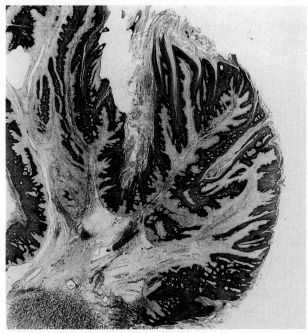

A

B

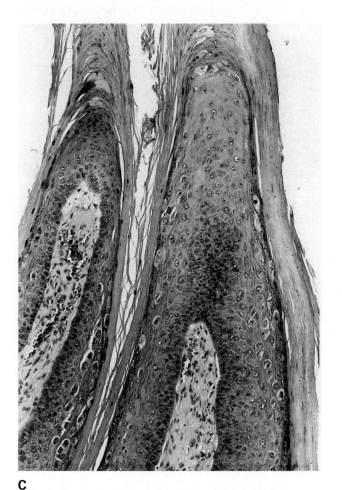

C

Fig. 2.2. Papilloma (cutaneous papillomatosis). **A.** Papillomas in a steer showing cauliflower-like growths. **B.** Papilloma with thickened, irregular epidermis covered by a layer of keratin and supported by proliferative connective tissue. **C.** Proliferating epidermis and vacuolated cytoplasm in the prickle cell layer over the tops of the dermal papillae.

tralizing antibodies and the relapse of animals with persistent papillomavirus infection. Cell-mediated immunity is of greater importance in causing regression of papillomas. Therefore, several prophylactic vaccines have been developed. For many years crude vaccines using viral particles from macerated papillomas, injected intramuscularly, caused regression of lesions in infected cattle and prevented infection of naive animals. However, the use of the viral capsid proteins L1 and L2 in bacteria, yeasts, insect cells, and mammalian cells has achieved protection against BPV-2 and BPV-4 infection.[15] In the dog a formalin-inactivated vaccine provides protection against oral papillomavirus infection.[16]

In regressing papillomas there is a lymphocytic infiltrate at the epidermal-dermal interface. In naturally regressing BPV-4 papillomas, the dermal infiltrate consists predominantly of CD4+ lymphocytes, with fewer gamma-delta T cells and CD8+ lymphocytes. Within the epidermis, gamma-delta T cells and CD8+ lymphocytes predominate.[15] These lymphoid cells are associated with upregulation of ICAM-1 on keratinocytes and E-selectin and VCAM-1 on endothelial cells at the site of infection.

REFERENCES

1. Goldschmidt, M.H., Dunstan, R.W., Stannard, A.A., von Tscharner, C., Walder, E.J., and Yager, J.A. (1998) *World Health Organization. International Histologic Classification of Tumors of Domestic Animals. Histological Classification of Tumors of the Skin of Domestic Animals.* 2nd series, vol. III. Armed Forces Institute of Pathology, Washington, D.C.
2. Njoku, C.O., and Barwash, W.A. (1972) Congenital cutaneous papilloma in a foal. *Cornell Vet* 62:54–57.
3. Scheuler, R.L. (1972) Congenital equine papillomatosis. *J Amer Vet Med Assoc* 162:640.
4. Atwell, R.B., and Summers, P.M. (1977) Congenital papilloma in a foal. *Aust Vet J* 53:299.
5. Garma-Avina, A., Valli, V.E., and Lumsden, J.H. (1981) Equine congenital cutaneous papillomatosis: A report of 5 cases. *Equine Vet J* 13:59–61.
6. Desrocher, A. St.-Jean, G., and Kennedy, G.A. (1994) Congenital cutaneous papillomatosis in a one-year-old Holstein. *Canadian Vet J* 10:646–647.
7. Rieke, H. (1980) An extreme congenital papillomatosis of a piglet. *Dtsch Tierartzl Wochenschr* 87:412–413.
8. Thielen, G., Wheeldon, E.B. East, N., Madewell, B., Lancaster W.D., and Munn, R. (1985) Goat papillomatosis. *Amer J Vet Res* 46:2519–2526.
9. Studdert, M.J., McCoy, K., Allworth, M.B., and Staples, P. (1988) Papilloma of the ears of calves following tattooing. *Aust Vet J* 65:399.
10. Le Net, J.L., Orth, G., Sundberg, J.P., Cassonnet, P., Poisson, L., Masson, M.T., George, C., and Longeart, L. (1997) Multiple pigmented cutaneous papules associated with a novel canine papillomavirus in an immunosuppressed dog. *Vet Pathol* 34:8–14.
11. Hamada, M. Omayada, T., Yoshikawa, H., Yoshikawa, T., and Itakura C. (1990) Histopathologic development of equine cutaneous papillomas. *J Comp Path* 102:393–403.
12. Hamada, M., and Itakura, C. (1990) Ultrastructural morphology of hypomelanosis in equine cutaneous papilloma. *J Comp Path* 103:199–213.
13. Hamada, M. Takechi, M., and Itakura, C. (1992) Langerhan's cells in equine cutaneous papillomas and normal skin. *Vet Pathol* 29:152–160.
14. Hamada, M., Oyamada, T., Yoshikawa, H., Yoshikawa, T., and Itakura, C. (1990) Keratin expression in equine normal epidermis and cutaneous papillomas using monoclonal antibodies. *J Comp Path* 102:405–420.
15. Campo, M.S. (1997) Vaccination against papillomavirus in cattle. *Clin Dermatol* 15:275–283.
16. Bell, J.A., Sundberg, J.P., Ghim, S.J., Newsome, J., Jenson, A.B., and Schlegel, R. (1994) A formalin-inactivated vaccine protects against mucosal papillomavirus infection: A canine model. *Pathobiology* 62:194–198.

Inverted Papilloma

This is a benign, endophytic proliferation of the epidermis that is caused by infection with a papillomavirus.

Incidence, Age, Breed, and Sex

This tumor has only been reported in the dog.[1] The tumor is uncommon. There are insufficient cases reported to identify any age, breed, or sex predilections.

Sites and Gross Morphology

No site predilection has been noted. The lesions are 1–2 cm in diameter and are located within the dermis, extending into the subcutaneous tissue as the lesions increase in size. There is a small pore that opens onto the skin surface. On cut section the invaginated flask mass shows proliferation of thin filiform projections into the center of the mass, where keratin accumulates. There is a well-demarcated border.

Histological Features, Growth, and Metastasis

The histological features are the same as those described for papillomas, with a supporting stroma of connective tissue covered by a hyperplastic epidermis with koilocytosis and enlarged keratohyaline granules. The masses are slow growing and amenable to surgical excision.

Multicentric Squamous Cell Carcinoma in Situ (Bowen's Disease)

This is a malignant tumor of epidermal cells that does not, at the time of histopathologic evaluation, show evidence of invasion through the basement membrane. The tumor has not been associated with extended exposure to ultraviolet light, but in the cat an association with papillomaviruses has been noted.

Incidence, Age, Breed, and Sex

The tumor is most often seen in the cat.[2] A single case has been described in the dog.[3]

In cats the disease is being diagnosed with increasing frequency, possibly due to a papillomavirus infection.[4] Middle-aged to old cats are primarily affected. Although no breed predilection has been noted, most cases have been described in domestic shorthaired cats with a variety of hair-coat colors. No sex predilection has been found, although neutered animals appear to be more commonly affected.[2]

Sites and Gross Morphology

Areas of haired, pigmented skin, including the trunk, limbs, feet, head, and neck, are the primary sites of occurrence, although the lesions are found at multiple sites in most cats. The sites of the tumors and the color coats of affected cats indicate that development of the tumor, in contrast to cases of invasive squamous cell carcinoma, is not related to exposure to ultraviolet light.

Lesions are either irregular, slightly raised, hyperpigmented, and plaque-like or papillated and alopecic, and they vary in size from 0.5 to 3.0 cm in diameter. Several cases with a cutaneous horn overlying the skin tumor have been seen by the author.

Histological Features

The lesions consist of sharply demarcated regions of neoplastic keratinocytes affecting the epidermis and follicular infundibular epithelium without invasion through the basal lamina into the dermis. Two histological subclasses of multicentric squamous cell carcinoma in situ are described, an irregular nonhyperkeratotic type and a verrucous hyperkeratotic type.[2] The irregular nonhyperkeratotic lesions have moderate to severe acanthosis of the epidermis and follicular infundibulum and a mildly undulating surface to the epidermis. The verrucous hyperkeratotic lesions, as the name implies, show the formation of elongated spires of orthokeratin arising from the follicular ostium in addition to hyperkeratosis and dilation of the follicular infundibulum.

The neoplastic cells give the epidermis a disorganized appearance, with loss of polarity of the keratinocytes. The neoplastic cells have large hyperchromatic nuclei, prominent nucleoli, and a clear or vacuolated cytoplasm. Mitotic figures may be found in the suprabasal cells and are usually quite numerous (1–3/200x field) (fig. 2.3 A). Increased melanin may be present within the cells in a few cases. Hyperkeratosis, parakeratosis, and hyperpigmentation of the stratum corneum may be found.

Growth and Metastasis

The lesions continue to enlarge slowly. Local recurrence has not been reported following surgical excision of the masses, but similar lesions may develop at new sites in these cats. Because these are in situ lesions, metastases do not occur.

REFERENCES

1. Campbell, K.L., Sundberg, J.P., Goldschmidt, M.H., Knupp, C., and Reichmann, M.E. (1988) Cutaneous inverted papillomas in dogs. Vet Pathol 25:67–71.
2. Baer, K.E., and Helton, K. (1993) Multicentric squamous cell carcinoma in situ resembling Bowen's disease in cats. *Vet Pathol* 30:535–543.
3. Gross, T.L., and Brimacomb, B.H. (1986) Multifocal intraepidermal carcinoma in a dog histologically resembling Bowen's disease. *Am J Dermatopath* 8:509–515.
4. Scott, D.W., Miller, W.H., and Griffin, C.E. (1995) *Small Animal Dermatology*. W.B. Saunders Co., Philadelphia, pp. 1005–1006.

Squamous Cell Carcinoma

General Considerations

This is a malignant tumor of epidermal cells in which the cells show differentiation to keratinocytes.[1] There are several factors that are associated with the development of a squamous cell carcinoma, including prolonged exposure to ultraviolet light, lack of pigment within the epidermis at the sites of tumor development, and lack of hair or a very sparse hair coat at the affected sites.

Incidence, Age, Breed, and Sex

The tumor is common in the horse, cow, cat, and dog, relatively uncommon in the sheep, and rare in the goat and pig. In all species squamous cell carcinomas may occur in young animals, but the incidence increases with age.

The peak incidence of squamous cell carcinomas in the cat is between 9 and 14 years of age and in the dog between 6 and 10 years of age.

When exposed to solar radiation and higher altitude, cattle breeds at increased risk are those that lack circumocular pigmentation, including the Hereford and Simmenthal; horse breeds at increased risk are the Belgian, Clydesdale, shire, and Appaloosa. The domestic shorthaired cat has an increased risk (1.9), while the Himalayan (0.4), Siamese (0.3), and Persian (0.2) breeds have a decreased risk. The dog breeds at increased risk are the keeshond (3.6), standard schnauzer (2.5), basset hound (2.2), and collie (1.9); the boxer (0.33) is at decreased risk. Short-coated dogs with a white or piebald coat color that pass an extended period of time outdoors also have a higher incidence of cutaneous squamous cell carcinomas.[3,4,5,7] No sex predilection has been noted.

Sites and Gross Morphology

In horses and cattle squamous cell carcinoma occurs primarily at mucocutaneous junctions, particularly the eyelids. In the cat the most common sites are the pinna, eyelids, and planum nasale; in the dog the tumor most frequently occurs on the head, abdomen, forelimbs, rearlimbs, and perineum and digits (see subungual squamous cell carcinoma in the section on nailbed tumors). In sheep the ears are affected. However, in any species this tumor may arise from any site.

Solar dermatosis (actinic keratosis) is the first recognizable change at mucocutaneous junctions or on skin that is sparsely haired and lacks pigment. Erythema, edema, and scaling are followed by crusting, scaling, and thickening of the epidermis with subsequent ulceration. As the tumor becomes invasive of the dermis, the lesion feels more indurated. With time the ulcerated lesion increases in size and depth, and secondary bacterial infection results in a purulent exudate on the surface of the mass.[4]

Squamous cell carcinoma of the eyelid often is associated with a purulent conjunctivitis, while epistaxis, sneezing, ulceration, or swelling are the clinical signs associated with tumors arising from the planum nasale.

In the dog occasional cases of invasive squamous cell carcinomas have been identified in Beagles at the site of prior vaccination with an autogenous papillomavirus vaccine. The latency period reported in these unique cases is 11–34 months. On examination the tumor exhibits no unique features that allow it to be differentiated from other cases of squamous cell carcinoma, other than a rather uncommon tumor location.[8]

Histological Features

Actinic keratosis (squamous cell carcinoma[1,2]) shows epidermal hyperplasia, hyperkeratosis, parakeratosis, acanthosis, accentuation of the epidermal rete, and keratinocyte dysplasia. The affected keratinocytes, which are mostly found in the basal and spinous layer, show loss of polarity, karyomegaly, nuclear hyperchromatism, enlarged and prominent nucleoli, and mitotic figures of basal and suprabasal keratinocytes. Because this lesion is induced by prolonged ultraviolet light exposure, some cases may show solar elastosis,[6] with degeneration and fragmentation of elastic and collagen fibers in the superficial dermis and deposition of thickened, basophilic fibrillar material that stains positive with the van Gieson elastin stain. At this stage there is no invasion through the basement membrane by the dysplastic keratinocytes, such as occurs with squamous cell carcinoma, described below.

Extending into the dermis, with or without an association to the overlying epidermis, are islands, cords, and trabeculae of neoplastic epithelial cells showing a variable degree of squamous differentiation. The amount of keratin, seen as intracytoplasmic, eosinophilic fibrillar material (keratin tonofibers), produced by the neoplastic cells is quite variable; there is extensive keratinization, and in well-differentiated tumors there is formation of distinct keratin "pearls" (fig. 2.3 B,C,D). In poorly differentiated tumors only a few cells have intracytoplasmic eosinophilic keratin tonofibers. Individual tumor cells have large, ovoid, often vesicular nuclei with a single, central, prominent nucleolus, abundant cytoplasm that varies from pale to brightly eosinophilic, and distinct cell borders. In more differentiated tumors it is also possible to recognize intercellular desmosomes, especially in areas where intercellular edema allows them to be more readily identified. The number of mitotic figures is variable, but they are more frequent in less well differentiated tumors. Invasion of the dermis and subcutaneous tissue may evoke a desmoplastic response. Ulceration is accompanied by an infiltrate of neutrophils into the superficial part of the tumor, while plasma cells and lymphocytes are found in the deeper parts of the tumor. The invasive margins of the tumor may show neurotropism as well as invasion of dermal and subcutaneous lymphatics.

Several uncommon variants of squamous cell carcinoma have been described. The spindle cell variant of squamous cell carcinoma is often difficult to differentiate from the surrounding stromal cells. However, the tumor cells stain positive with antikeratin antibodies on immunohistochemical evaluation. Acantholytic squamous cell carcinomas are characterized by marked dyshesion of the neoplastic cells, which results in a pseudoglandular pattern (the basal neoplastic cells having remained attached to the basal lamina), but there is individualization of the neoplastic keratinocytes that make up the centers of the islands of neoplastic squamous cells.

Invasive squamous cell carcinomas in Beagles at the site of prior vaccination with an autogenous papillomavirus vaccine will show positive staining of nuclei in the granular cell layer on immunohistochemical examination for the canine papillomavirus[8].

Growth and Metastasis

Squamous cell carcinomas are mainly slow growing. Most tumors, although invasive, do not show metastatic spread to regional lymph nodes; regional lymph node metastasis is most often found with poorly differentiated tumors or tumors that have been present for a considerable time before they are diagnosed or excised.

Treatment

This is one of the few skin tumors for which several treatment options, other than surgery, are available to the clinician. Cases treated with these methods are usually those that arise at sites that are not amenable to surgical excision with wide margins of normal tissue or those that involve either multicentric tumors or tumors that have been incompletely excised at the time of initial removal.

In dogs these treatments are used for solar induced squamous cell carcinomas and preneoplastic lesions (solar dermatosis). Etretinate for 90 days produces complete regression of preneoplastic lesions but only partial response to invasive tumors.[9] (Acitretin is the main metabolite of etretinate, and it is a substitute for etretinate, which is no longer available.) A somewhat better response was achieved when controlled localized radiofrequency heat was applied in conjunction with isotretinoin, another synthetic retinoid.[10] A second chemotherapeutic approach is the use of intralesional sustained-release gel implants. Using either 5-fluorouracil and/or cisplatin for a minimum of 3 weeks produces partial or total regression of the tumors.[11]

In cats, lesions on the planum nasale, which are the most difficult to adequately excise by surgery alone, are those most often treated with adjuvant therapy. Alternative forms of surgery are cryosurgery, which produced complete remission of tumors of the ears and eyelids and 70 percent of nasal lesions following a single treatment,[12] or laser surgery.[13] Adjunct therapies include intratumoral administration of carboplatin (100 mg/m²) with or without sesame oil as a buffer,[14] photodynamic therapy using aluminum phthalocyanine tetrasulfonate as the photosensitizer,[15] or radiation therapy (10 fractions of 4 Gy over 3.5 weeks).[16]

In horses topical administration of 5-fluorouracil (5-FU) in conjunction with surgical debulking has been used as a treatment for penile and vulvar squamous cell carcinoma[17] or intratumoral chemotherapy with cisplatin (+/- 1 mg/cm³ of tumor tissue/session) in sesame oil has been used to treat skin tumors.[18]

Basosquamous Carcinoma

This is a lowgrade malignancy composed primarily of basal cells with foci of squamous differentiation.[1]

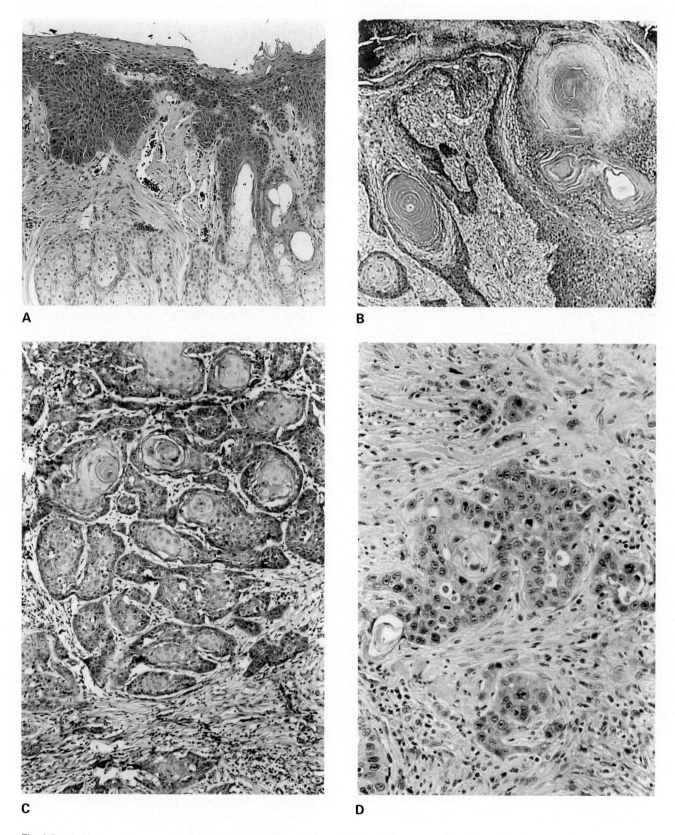

Fig. 2.3. **A.** Multicentric squamous cell carcinoma in situ (Bowen's disease), feline. **B.** Squamous cell carcinoma of the skin. Irregular masses and cords of epidermal cells invading the dermis, feline. **C.** Variably sized masses of concentrically arranged squamous epithelial cells with "horn pearl" formation, feline. **D.** Invasive tumor cells stimulating stromal fibrosis, feline.

Incidence, Age, Breed, and Sex

The tumor is uncommon and is diagnosed most often in the dog. The peak incidence of this tumor is between 6 and 12 years of age. Breeds at increased risk are the Scottish terrier (3.8), English springer spaniel (2.1), cocker spaniel (1.9), and golden retriever (1.6). No sex predilection has been noted.

Sites and Gross Morphology

Basosquamous carcinoma occurs most often on the head, neck and hindlimbs. The tumor is intradermal, often with foci of epidermal ulceration and hair loss. On cut section the tumor extends into the subcutis, may be pigmented brown/black, and is subdivided by connective tissue trabeculae into variably sized lobules, which may show central cyst formation. It may not always be possible to identify the borders of the tumor on gross examination.

Histological Features

At the periphery of the tumor lobules are undifferentiated basaloid cells, as described above (see basal cell tumor). In the center of the lobules the cells show abrupt differentiation and the formation of keratinocytes, which exhibit modest nuclear pleomorphism, mitotic activity, and dyskeratosis (fig. 2.4). Melanin is often present within the peripheral basaloid cells.

Growth and Metastasis

Although relatively slow growing, these tumors may recur at the surgical site if inadequately excised, but metastasis has not been reported. Surgical excision is the recommended treatment.

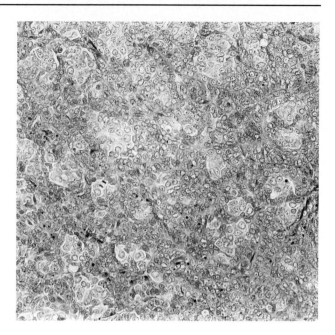

Fig. 2.4.   Basosquamous carcinoma, canine.

REFERENCES

1. Goldschmidt, M.H., Dunstan, R.W., Stannard, A.A., von Tscharner, C., Walder, E.J., and Yager, J.A. (1998) *World Health Organization. International Histologic Classification of Tumors of Domestic Animals. Histological Classification of Tumors of the Skin of Domestic Animals.* 2nd series, vol. III. Armed Forces Institute of Pathology, Washington, D.C.
2. Goldschmidt, M.H., and Shofer, F.S. (1998) *Skin Tumors of the Dog and Cat.* Butterworth Heinemann, Oxford, pp. 37–49.
3. Walder, E.J. (1992) In Gross, T.L., Ihrke, P.E., and Walder, E.J., *Veterinary Dermatopathology: A Macroscopic and Microscopic Evaluation of Canine and Feline Skin Disease.* Mosby Yearbook, St. Louis, pp. 336–340.
4. Hargis, A.M., Thomassen, R.W., and Phemister, R.D. (1977) Chronic dermatosis and cutaneous squamous cell carcinoma in the beagle dog. *Vet Pathol* 14:218–228.
5. Madewell, B.R., Conroy, J.D., and Hodgkins, E.M. (1981) Sunlight-skin cancer association in the dog: A report of three cases. *J Cut Path* 8:434–443.
6. Campbell, G.A., Gross, T.L., and Adams, R. (1987) Solar elastosis with squamous cell carcinoma in two horses. *Vet Pathol* 24:463–464.
7. Nikula, K.J., Benjamin, S.A., Angleton, G.M., Saunders, W.J., and Lee, A.C. (1992) Ultraviolet radiation, solar dermatosis, and cutaneous neoplasia in beagle dogs. *Radiation Res* 129:11–18.
8. Bregman, C.L., Hirth, R.S., et al. (1987) Cutaneous neoplasms in dogs associated with canine oral papillomavirus vaccine. *Vet Pathol* 24:477–487.
9. Marks, S.L., Song, M.D., Stannard, A.A., and Power, H.T. (1992) Clinical evaluation of etretinate for the treatment of canine solar-induced squamous cell carcinoma and preneoplastic lesions. *J Amer Acad Derm* 27:11–16.
10. Levine, N., Earle, M., and Wilson, S. (1990) Controlled localized heating and isotretinoin effects in canine squamous cell carcinoma. *J Amer Acad Derm* 23:68–72.
11. Kitchell, B.K., Orenberg, E.K., Brown, D.M., Hutson, C., Ray, K., Woods, L., and Luck, E. (1995) Intralesional sustained-release chemotherapy with therapeutic implants for treatment of canine sun-induced squamous cell carcinoma. *Eur J Cancer* 31:2093–2098.
12. Clarke, R.E. (1991) Cryosurgical treatment of feline cutaneous squamous cell carcinoma. *Aust Vet Pract* 21:148–153.
13. Shelley, B.A., Bartels, K.E., Ely, R.W., and Clark, D.M. (1992) Use of the neodymium:yttrium-aluminum garnet laser for treatment of squamous cell carcinoma of the nasal planum in a cat. *J Amer Vet Med Assoc* 201:756–758.
14. Theon, A.P., Madewell, B.R., and Van Vechten, M.K. (1996) Intratumoral administration of carboplatin for treatment of squamous cell carcinomas of the nasal plane in cats. *Amer J Vet Res* 57:205–210.
15. Peaston, A.E., Leach, M.W., and Higgins, R.J. (1993) Photodynamic therapy for nasal and aural squamous cell carcinoma in cats. *J Amer Vet Med Assoc* 202:1261–1265.
16. Theon, A.P., Madewell, B.R., Shearn, V.I., and Moulton, J.E. (1995) Prognostic factors associated with radiotherapy of squamous cell carcinoma of the nasal plane in cats. *J Amer Vet Med Assoc* 206:991–996.
17. Fortier, L.A., and Harg, M.A.M. (1994) Topical use of 5-fluorouracil for treatment of squamous cell carcinoma of the external genitalia of horses: 11 cases (1988–1992). *J Amer Vet Med Assoc* 205:1183–1185.
18. Theon, P., Pascoe, J.R., Carlson, G.P., and Krag, D.N. (1993) Intratumoral chemotherapy with cisplatin in oily emulsion in horses. *J Amer Vet Med Assoc* 202:261–267.

TUMORS WITH ADNEXAL DIFFERENTIATION

Follicular Tumors

Follicular tumors with adnexal differentiation include infundibular keratinizing acanthoma, tricholemmoma (bulb type and isthmus type), trichoblastoma (ribbon type, trabecular type, granular type, and spindle type), trichoepithelioma and malignant trichoepithelioma, and pilomatricoma and malignant pilomatricoma.

Infundibular Keratinizing Acanthoma (IKA)

This is a benign tumor showing differentiation to the squamous epithelium of the follicular isthmus. This tumor has been previously referred to as an intracutaneous cornifying epithelioma, intracutaneous keratinizing epithelioma, keratoacanthoma, and squamous papilloma.[1] The dog is the only species affected.

Incidence, Age, Breed, and Sex

The tumor is common in the dog, with a peak incidence between 4 and 9 years of age. However, a relatively large number of these tumors (21 percent of cases) can be found in dogs less than 4 years old. The breeds at increased risk are the Norwegian elkhound (28.9), Yorkshire terrier (4.6), Pekingese (4.1), Lhasa apso (3.5), bichon frise (3.4), German shepherd (3.3), standard poodle (2.4), keeshond (2.3), Samoyed (2.2), and Shetland sheepdog (1.7), while those breeds at decreased risk are the golden retriever (0.5), Siberian husky (0.4), cocker spaniel (0.4), Labrador retriever (0.3), standard schnauzer (0.3), dalmatian (0.2), Great Dane (0.1), rottweiler (0.1), Scottish terrier (0.1), basset hound (0.1), and doberman pinscher (0.1). No sex predilection has been noted.

Sites and Gross Morphology

Infundibular keratinizing acanthoma occurs most commonly on the back, tail, and neck. Multiple tumors on the same dog are common, especially in the Norwegian elkhound, Keeshond, German shepherd, and Lhasa apso (fig. 2.5 A). The tumors are located in the dermis and subcutis and vary in size from 0.3 to 5 cm in diameter. Many tumors have a central pore, which extends to the skin surface and represents the preexisting follicular infundibulum, from the base of which the tumor arises and grows. The pore may be filled with an inspissated keratinous material. Applying gentle digital pressure to the mass often results in expulsion of a grey-white keratinous material through the pore onto the skin surface. Those tumors having no epidermal communication arise as encapsulated intradermal masses.[1]

On cut section there is accumulation of keratin in the center of the mass, with the neoplastic cells at the periphery forming a red-brown zone of viable cells that varies in thickness. The mass is well demarcated from the surrounding dermis and subcutaneous tissue. Any breach in the wall of the tumor will allow keratin to extend into the adjacent dermis and subcutaneous tissue, where it will evoke a severe inflammatory response.

Histological Features

The pore is lined by a stratified squamous keratinizing epithelium with intracytoplasmic keratohyalin granules. From the base of the pore the tumor extends into the dermis and subcutis. There is central aggregation of keratin, which often forms concentric lamellae (fig. 2.5 B). Beneath the keratin, the wall of the tumor consists of large, pale-staining keratinocytes that may contain small basophilic keratohyaline granules. These cells have normochromic nuclei, cell borders are very distinct, and no desmosomes can be seen. Extending outward from the lining cells of the central cavity are cords of epithelial cells, which are only two cells thick (fig. 2.5 C). These cords of cells, which also form the peripheral zone of tumor cells, will anastomose and form small horn cysts with concentric lamellar aggregates of keratin within the cyst lumina (fig. 2.5 D). The cells have central nuclei that are more hyperchromatic than those of the luminal cells, a moderate amount of eosinophilic cytoplasm, and distinct cell borders. Cellular and nuclear pleomorphism and mitotic activity is minimal. A fibrovascular stroma surrounds the tumor and also extends into the tumor between the anastomosing cords of epithelial cells. The stroma may be mucinous and in some cases will show chondroid or osseous metaplasia, a feature also noted with mixed apocrine gland tumors, from which IKA must be differentiated by the morphology of the keratinocytes with their abundant eosinophilic cytoplasm and the lack of glandular tissue within the IKA. Occasional lymphocytes and plasma cells may be present within the stroma. Compression of the surrounding dermal collagen produces a pseudocapsule.

Rupture of the wall of the tumor with release of keratin into the surrounding dermal and subcutaneous tissue will evoke a pyogranulomatous and granulomatous inflammatory response.

Growth and Metastasis

These tumors are benign and do not recur following adequate surgical removal. Thus surgical removal is recommended for solitary tumors or in cases where only a few tumors are present. In those dogs with multiple tumors, treatment with synthetic retinoids has been helpful. One report suggests using isotretinoin (1.7–4 mg/kg/day) or etretinate (1.1–1.5 mg/kg/day).[2]

Tricholemmoma

This is a benign tumor showing differentiation to either the inferior segment or the isthmic segment of the external root sheath of the hair follicle.[3,4]

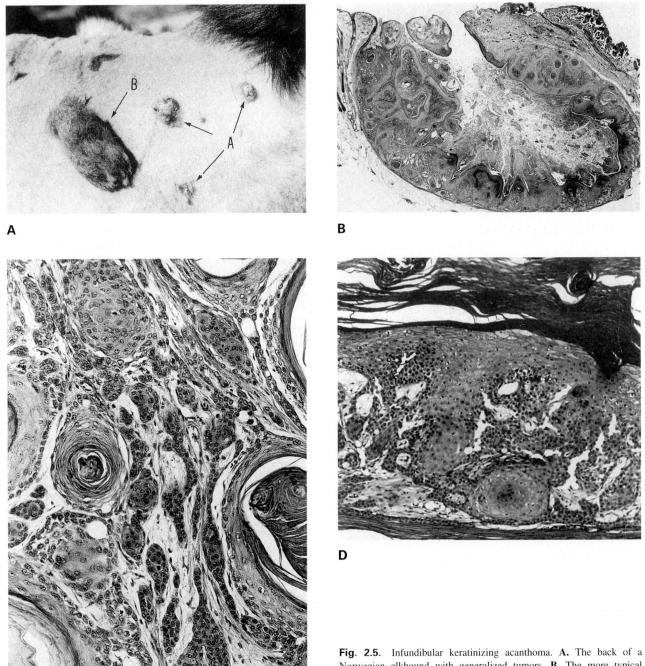

Fig. 2.5. Infundibular keratinizing acanthoma. **A.** The back of a Norwegian elkhound with generalized tumors. **B.** The more typical growths are characterized by a pore that opens to the skin surface and contains a prominent keratin plug. **C.** Anastomosing cords and nests of squamous epithelial cells. **D.** A portion of the wall of a cystic tumor.

Incidence, Age, Breed, and Sex

This tumor is uncommon in the dog and rare or not described in other species. Too few cases have been described to determine any age, breed, or sex predilection.

Sites and Gross Morphology

No site predilection has been established for tricholemmomas. The tumors appear as well-encapsulated intradermal and subcutaneous masses, with hair loss from the overlying skin.

Histological Features

Bulb Type

Two variants of tricholemmomas are described. The *bulb type* shows differentiation to the inferior segment of the hair follicle with islands of epithelial cells surrounded by a fine fibrillar collagenous stroma. The central epithelial cells have a central nucleus and a moderate amount of eosinophilic cytoplasm, while the peripheral cells are arranged in a palisaded fashion on a thickened, eosinophilic basal lamina and have an abundant, pale, vacuolated cytoplasm (fig. 2.6 A).[3,4]

Isthmus Type

The *isthmus type,* as its name implies, shows differentiation to the isthmus segment of the hair follicle. There is often an association with the epidermis. The tumor consists of cords and trabeculae of epithelial cells extending between islands of epithelial cells that exhibit central trichilemmal (no keratohyaline or trichohyaline granules are formed) keratinization (fig. 2.6 B). The neoplastic cells are small and have a moderate amount of pale eosinophilic cytoplasm and small euchromatic nuclei. Melanin may be found within the neoplastic cells. There is some interstitial stroma, which may contain a small amount of mucin. The isthmus type of tricholemmoma must be differentiated from an infundibular keratinizing acanthoma, with which it shares many features. However, the isthmus tricholemmoma has an association with the epidermis, shows no central cyst formation, and exhibits trichilemmal keratinization, whereas the infundibular keratinizing acanthoma shows infundibular keratinization with occasional keratohyaline granules within the cytoplasm of the cells which line the central cyst.

Growth and Metastasis

These are benign skin tumors, which are best treated by wide surgical excision.

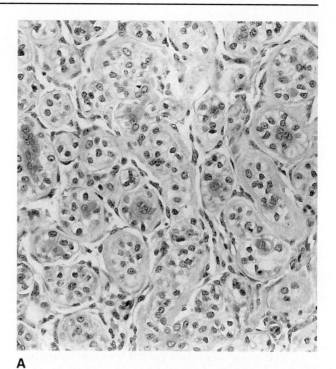

A

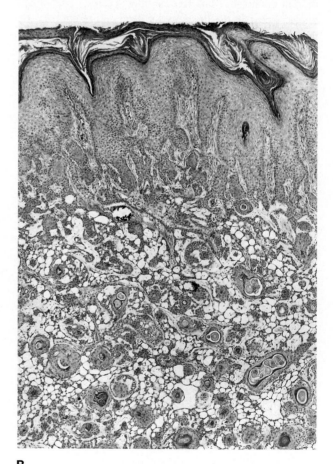

B

Fig. 2.6. Tricholemmoma, canine. **A.** Bulb type. **B.** Isthmus type.

REFERENCES

1. Stannard, A.A., and Pulley, L.T. (1975) Intracutaneous cornifying epithelioma (keratoacanthoma) in the dog: A retrospective study of 25 cases. *J Amer Vet Med Assoc* 167:385–8.
2. White, S.D., Rosychuck, R.A., Scott, K.V., Trettien, A.L., Jonas, L., and Denerolle, P. (1993) Use of isotretinoin and etretinate for the treatment of cutaneous neoplasia and cutaneous lymphoma in dogs. *J Amer Vet Med Assoc* 202:387–391.
3. Diters, R.W., and Goldschmidt, M.H. (1983) Hair follicle tumors resembling tricholemmomas in six dogs. *Vet Pathol* 20:123–5.
4. Walsh, K.M., and Corapi W.V. (1986) Tricholemmomas in three dogs. *J Comp Pathol* 96:115–7.

Trichoblastoma

This is a benign tumor, which is either derived from or shows differentiation to the hair germ of the developing follicle. This tumor was previously classified as a basal cell tumor.

Incidence, Age, Breed, and Sex

This tumor is common in the dog and cat,[1,2,3] uncommon in the horse,[1,2] and rare in other species.[3] Trichoblastomas appear in the literature as basal cell tumors. In the dog the tumor occurs predominantly in animals between 4 and 9 years of age. Breeds at increased risk are Kerry blue terrier (12.3), soft coated Wheaton terrier (3.9), bichon frise (3.7), cock-a-poo (3.0), Shetland sheepdog (2.9), husky (2.5), cocker spaniel (2.1), miniature poodle (2.1), Airedale terrier (2.0), English springer spaniel (1.7), collie (1.6), and Yorkshire terrier (1.5). Breeds at decreased risk are Irish setter (0.4), dachshund (0.4), Scottish terrier (0.4), dalmatian (0.3), Labrador retriever (0.3), doberman pinscher (0.3), basset hound (0.3), standard schnauzer (0.3), miniature schnauzer (0.2), rottweiler (0.2), beagle (0.2), German short haired pointer (0.1), Chihuahua (0.1), shar-pei (0.1), and boxer (0.1). No sex predilection has been noted.

Sites and Gross Morphology

The head and neck are the primary sites of occurrence of trichoblastomas in the dog and cat. The tumors, which are often exophytic masses, may vary in size from 0.5 to 18 cm in diameter. Most extend from the epidermal-dermal interface into the dermis and subcutis. They are well demarcated from the surrounding tissue by a pseudo-capsule of compressed dermal collagen. The overlying epidermis is devoid of hair and may be secondarily ulcerated.

On cut section the tumor is often subdivided into multiple lobules of varying size by connective tissue trabeculae. Some tumors are melanized, and others may show focal or multifocal cystic degeneration.

Histological Features

There are several histological subtypes of trichoblastoma, including the ribbon, medusoid, trabecular, spindle, and granular cell types. However, the considerable vari-ability of these tumors on histological evaluation in no way affects their prognosis, since they are all benign.

Ribbon Type

Ribbon type trichoblastoma consists of long cords of branching and anastomosing cells (fig. 2.7 A). These cords are two or sometimes three cells thick. The cells often have a palisaded appearance and have prominent nuclei and little cytoplasm. The nuclei may appear normochromatic or hyperchromatic, and the nucleoli are inconspicuous. The small amount of cytoplasm is pale eosinophilic, and cell borders are indistinct. The number of mitotic figures seen may be quite variable, with some tumors showing marked mitotic activity. The adjacent stoma can vary from mucinous to collagenous, and the amount of stroma found between the cords of cells is also quite variable. This subtype is most frequently seen in the dog.

Medusoid Type

Medusoid type trichoblastoma is similar to the ribbon type. However, the cords of cells stream outward from a central aggregation of cells, which have a more extensive amount of eosinophilic cytoplasm, mimicking the snakes streaming from the head of the medusa of Greek mythology (fig. 2.7 B). This subtype is most frequently seen in the dog.

Trabecular Type

Trabecular type trichoblastoma consists of multiple lobules of neoplastic cells surrounded by thin bands of interlobular collagenous stroma. The cells at the periphery of the lobules are distinctly palisades, while the cells in the center of the lobules have ovoid to elongated nuclei and a more abundant eosinophilic cytoplasm (fig. 2.7 C). This subtype is most frequently seen in the cat.

Spindle Type

Spindle type trichoblastoma may have an association with the overlying epidermis. The tumor is multilobulated with little interlobular stroma. The morphology of the tumor cell varies depending on whether the cells are cut longitudinally, when they have a spindle-cell morphology, or transversely, when they appear more ovoid (fig. 2.7 D). The fusiform cells often have an interwoven pattern. The tumor may have melanin within the neoplastic cells and within melanophages. This subtype is most frequently seen in cats.

Granular Cell Type

Granular cell type trichoblastoma consists of islands and sheets of neoplastic cells that have an abundant, eosinophilic, granular cytoplasm with distinct cell borders (fig. 2.7 E). The nuclei are small and hyperchromatic, and few mitoses are found. The amount of interstitial collagenous stroma is variable. This subtype is most frequently seen in the dog.[4]

Growth and Metastasis

Most trichoblastomas are slow growing. They recur only after incomplete surgical excision, which is the

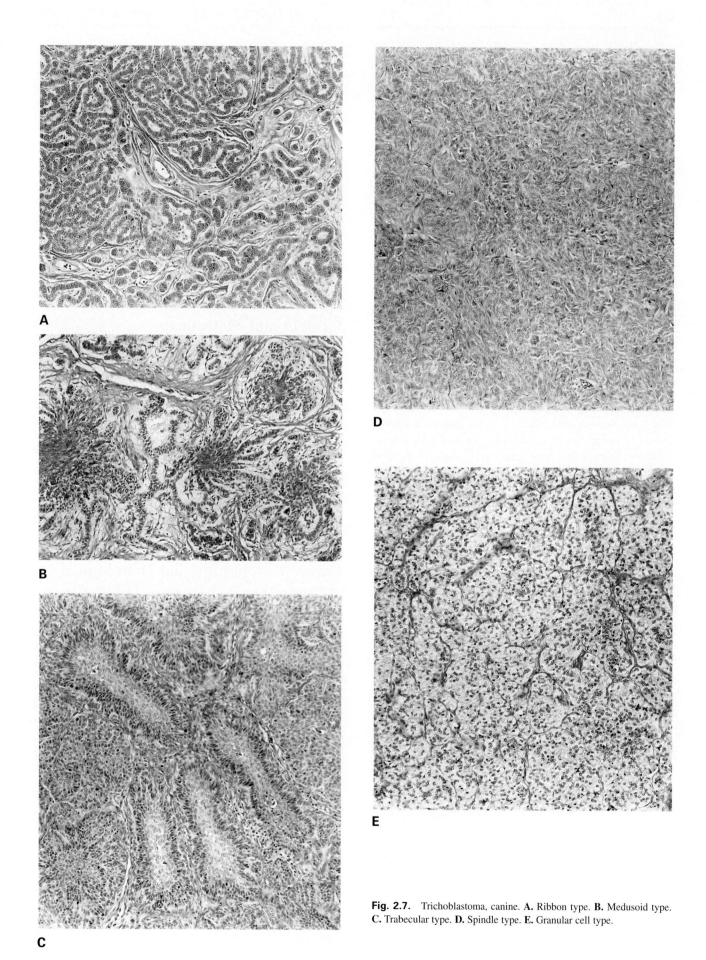

Fig. 2.7. Trichoblastoma, canine. **A.** Ribbon type. **B.** Medusoid type.
C. Trabecular type. **D.** Spindle type. **E.** Granular cell type.

treatment of choice. The tumors are benign and do not metastasize.

Trichoepithelioma

This is a benign tumor showing differentiation to all three segments of the hair follicle; incomplete or abortive trichogenesis is present.

Incidence, Age, Breed, and Sex

Trichoepitheliomas are common in the dog, uncommon in the cat, and rare or not recognized in other species. In dogs they may occur in animals between 1 and 15 years of age, but most cases arise between 5 and 9 years of age. Dog breeds at increased risk are basset hound (14.7), bull mastiff (4.7), Gordon setter (3.4), standard poodle (3.0), Irish setter (3.0), soft coated Wheaton terrier (2.7), English springer spaniel (2.6), golden retriever (2.5), standard schnauzer (2.0), and miniature schnauzer (1.5), whereas breeds at decreased risk are mixed breed (0.9), Labrador retriever (0.5), dachshund (0.5), cocker spaniel (0.5), husky (0.4), Brittany spaniel (0.3), rottweiler (0.3), Yorkshire terrier (0.3), Lhasa apso (0.2), shih tzu (0.2), chow (0.1), doberman pinscher (0.1), shar-pei (0.1), Shetland sheepdog (0.1), and Scottish terrier (0.1). Cats develop trichoepitheliomas primarily between 4 and 11 years of age, and no breed predilection has been noted in this species. Spayed female dogs, but not cats, are at increased risk.

Sites and Gross Morphology

Trichoepitheliomas have a predilection for the back, neck, thorax, and tail, but about 6 percent of cases are multicentric. The tumor is located within the dermis with extension into the subcutaneous tissue. Most tumors are removed when between 0.5 and 5 cm in diameter. Epidermal ulceration, alopecia of the skin overlying the mass, and secondary infection may be present. On cut section there are multiple 1 to 2 mm in diameter grey-white foci with intervening bands of fibrovascular connective tissue. Most tumors have a distinct border, although some trichoepitheliomas can be invasive of the deeper tissues.

Histological Features

The histological appearance will vary depending on the degree of differentiation to the three segments of the hair follicle. Most tumors consist of islands of neoplastic cells surrounded by a stroma, which may be collagenous or somewhat mucinous. In the center of these islands there is an accumulation of keratin and shadow (ghost) cells, whose presence is indicative of matrical differentiation. The outer epithelial cells are often a heterogeneous population, including small cells with hyperchromatic nuclei and little cytoplasm (resembling the undifferentiated cells of the hair bulb), cells that have a lightly eosinophilic cytoplasm and vesicular nuclei (resembling the lower portion of the external root

sheath), or cells with intracytoplasmic trichohyaline granules (as in the inner root sheath of the hair follicle) (fig. 2.8 A).

A cystic variant of trichoepitheliomas may also be found, with one large cyst or several somewhat smaller cysts filled with keratinous debris. At the periphery there is often a very thickened eosinophilic basal lamina, with a single layer of palisaded cells with hyperchromatic nuclei and little cytoplasm on its inner aspect. These cells become more haphazardly arranged toward the center of the cyst, and their nuclei are less hyperchromatic, and the cells have a moderate amount of eosinophilic cytoplasm. Within the lumen of the cyst are shadow (ghost) cells, keratinous material, and cholesterol clefts. Smaller cysts may be found extending into the surrounding tissue from the larger central cyst (fig. 2.8 B).

Growth and Metastasis

Trichoepitheliomas are relatively slow growing. Most respond well to wide surgical excision, and recurrence is only noted with incompletely excised tumors. However, several breeds, especially the basset hound, are predisposed to developing multicentric tumors.

Malignant Trichoepithelioma

This is a malignant tumor with matrical and inner root sheath differentiation, which may metastasize. This uncommon skin tumor has been described only in dogs. No age, breed or sex predilections have been noted in the few cases seen.

Gross Morphology and Histological Features

The tumor is seen as a nodular infiltrative mass involving the dermis and subcutaneous tissue and is indistinguishable grossly from other invasive skin tumors. The tumor cells often have an association with the overlying epidermis or follicular infundibulum and extend as cords and islands of basophilic cells into the dermis (fig. 2.8 C). The center of the larger islands of tumor cells is necrotic, with aggregates of shadow cells, indicative of matrical keratinization. The tumor cells have hyperchromatic nuclei and little eosinophilic cytoplasm. Many mitoses may be present. Occasional cells contain brightly eosinophilic intracytoplasmic trichohyaline granules. Invasion of the deeper tissues often evokes a desmoplastic response. Lymphatic invasion may be seen at the periphery of the tumor.

Growth and Metastasis

The tumor grows rapidly and will show metastatic spread to regional lymph nodes and lungs. However, too few cases are seen to determine whether these tumors would respond to any form of therapy.

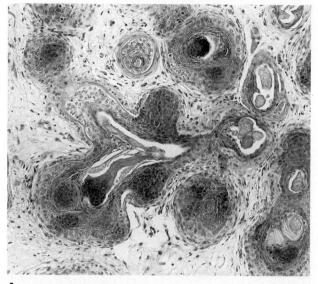

A

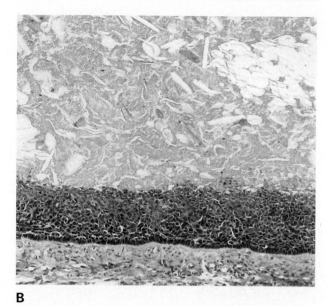

B

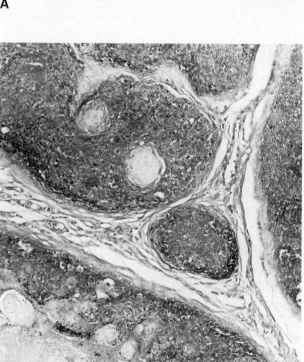

C

Fig. 2.8. Trichoepithelioma. **A.** Canine. **B.** Cystic, canine. **C.** Malignant, canine.

Pilomatricoma

This is a benign follicular tumor showing only matrical differentiation. This tumor was previously referred to as the necrotizing and calcifying epithelioma of Malherbe or pilomatrixoma.

Incidence, Age, Breed, and Sex

Pilomatricomas are most frequently diagnosed in the dog and are rare in the cat and other domestic animals. In dogs most tumors arise between 2 and 7 years of age, and breeds at increased risk are Kerry blue terrier (57.6), soft coated Wheaton terrier (16.3), standard poodle (12.9), Old English sheepdog (8.9), bichon frise (8.1), Airedale terrier (7.1), West Highland white terrier (4.0), standard schnauzer (3.4), basset hound (3.2), miniature poodle (3.2), Lhasa apso (2.1), and miniature schnauzer (1.9). Breeds at decreased risk are mixed breed (0.5), golden retriever (0.5), German shepherd (0.3), beagle (0.3), Labrador retriever (0.3), dachshund (0.1), rottweiler (0.1), husky (0.1), and cocker spaniel (0.1). No sex predilection has been noted.

Sites and Gross Morphology

Most pilomatricomas arise on the back, neck, thorax, and tail. The tumors are firm intradermal masses with alopecia of the overlying skin. The tumors may be difficult to transect due to the presence of bone within the tumor. On cut section the tumor consists of one or several larger lobules of grey-white chalky tissue, but areas of melanization may be found. A distinct border to the tumor is often seen.

Histological Features

At the periphery of the lobules is a zone of basophilic cells with small hyperchromatic nuclei and little cytoplasm (fig. 2.9 A). These basophilic cells may exhibit considerable mitotic activity. As the basophilic cells differentiate toward the center of the lobule, the cells enlarge due to an increase in the amount of eosinophilic cytoplasm associated with each cell. Further differentiation results in loss of the basophilic appearance of the

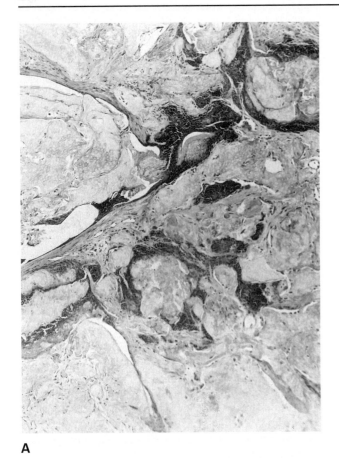

A

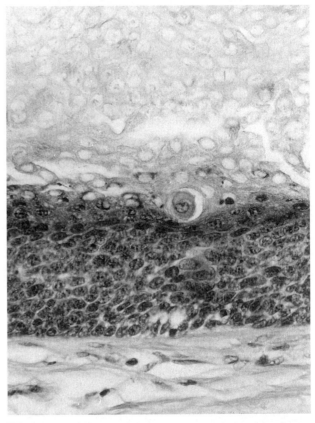

B

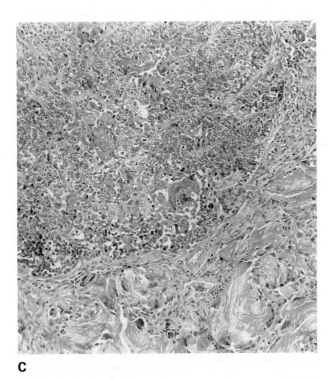

C

Fig. 2.9. Pilomatricoma—canine. **A.** Typical pilomatricoma consisting of variably shaped masses of epithelial cells. **B.** An area of transition from *basal cells* to *shadow cells*. **C.** Malignant pilomatricoma.

nucleus, which can still be recognized as a round empty space surrounded by an abundant eosinophilic cytoplasm and distinct cell borders (fig. 2.9 B). These cells are referred to as *ghost cells* or shadow cells and represent matrical differentiation.

In the center of the lobules the shadow cells accumulate and degenerate. Within the degenerating cells foci of dystrophic calcification and lamellar bone formation may be found. There is an accompanying infiltrate of multinucleated giant cells and fibroblasts. It is unclear if the infiltration of the fibroblasts into the mass evokes the dystrophic mineralization or if the fibroblasts and giant cell infiltration is secondary. Amyloid, which appears as a fine amorphous brightly eosinophilic material, may also be found in the center of the lobules; it stains positive with Congo red and shows an apple green birefringence on polaroscopy. Melanin may be found within the cytoplasm of the tumor cells or within macrophages in the perilobular stroma.

Pilomatricomas that have been present for a long time before being excised will have only a thin rim of basophilic cells at the periphery and marked accumulation of shadow cells in the center of the lobules. The interlobular stroma consists of mature fibrous connective tissue with few inflammatory cells evident.

Growth and Metastasis

Pilomatricomas are benign tumors that are readily removed surgically. Recurrence is uncommon.

Malignant Pilomatricoma

This is a malignant follicular tumor showing only matrical differentiation. (fig. 2.9 C) This is a rare tumor reported only in the dog.[5,6,7,8] Too few cases have been described to determine if there is any breed or sex predilection. However, older dogs appear to be affected.

Sites and Gross Morphology

The cases seen have shown no site predilection. The tumor may, however, show the development of smaller satellite tumors in the adjacent dermis. On cut section the tumor is often multilobulated and invasive and can not be differentiated from an infiltrative trichoepithelioma.

Histological Features, Growth, and Metastasis

The microscopic features are the same as those described above for pilomatricomas, but lymphatic invasion may be found at the periphery of the tumor. These tumors tend to grow quite rapidly and invade the deep dermis and subcutaneous tissues. Metastasis occurs via the lymphatics to regional lymph nodes and lungs. Cases of neural involvement have been reported.[8] Too few cases are seen for any ongoing study of the response of these tumors to therapy, but in the experience of the author those cases that have been treated with radiation therapy and chemotherapy failed to respond to these treatments.

REFERENCES

1. Schuh, J.C., and Valentine, B.A. (1987) Equine basal cell tumors. *Vet Pathol* 24:44–49.
2. Baril, C. (1973) Basal cell tumour of third eyelid in a horse. *Can Vet J* 14:66–67.
3. Gorham, S.L., Penney, B.E., and Bradley, L.D. (1990) Basal cell tumor in a sheep. *Vet Pathol* 27:466–467.
4. Seiler, R.J. (1982) Granular basal cell tumors in the skin of three dogs: A distinct histopathologic entity. *Vet Pathol* 19:23–29.
5. von Sandersleben, J. (1964) Gutartige epitheliale Neubildungen der Haut des Hundes. *Zbl Vet Med* 11:702–728.
6. Sells, D.M., and Conroy, J.D. (1976) Malignant epithelial neoplasia with hair follicle differentiation in dogs. Malignant pilomatrixoma. *J Comp Pathol* 86:121–129.
7. Goldschmidt, M.H., Thrall, D.E., Jeglum, K.A., Everett, J.I., and Wood, M.G. (1981) Malignant pilomatricoma in a dog. *J Cut Pathol* 8:375–381.
8. Rodriguez, F., Herraez, P., Rodriguez, E., and Gomez-Villamandos, J.C. (1995) Espinosa de los Monteros A. Metastatic pilomatrixoma associated with neurological signs in a dog. *Vet Rec* 137:247–248.

Nailbed Tumors

Nailbed tumors with adnexal differentiation include subungual keratoacanthoma (nailbed keratoacanthoma) and subungual squamous cell carcinoma.

Subungual Keratoacanthoma (Nailbed Keratoacanthoma)

This is a benign tumor of the nailbed epithelium. This uncommon tumor has only been described in the dog and cat. Animals 3 to 14 years old are affected, with no breed or sex predilection noted in the cases reported.

Sites and Gross Morphology

The nailbed epithelium of the forelimbs or hindlimbs is the site of origin of the tumor. The nail is often enlarged and may be twisted. Ulceration of the adjacent epidermis, loss of the nail, and secondary bacterial infection are infrequently found. On cut section there is loss of a portion of P3, due to lysis by the expansile mass of the nail bed.

Histological Features

The tumor consists of a symmetric, circumscribed mass of pale eosinophilic keratinocytes with a relatively smooth base. Beneath the basal lamina, the fibrovascular stroma contains some inflammatory cells, especially plasma cells. The basal cells have a more hyperchromatic nucleus and amphophilic cytoplasm. No breach of the basal lamina by neoplastic cells, as may occur with well-differentiated squamous cell carcinomas, is seen. The keratinocytes differentiate without the formation of a granular cell layer and with the formation of broad zones of parakeratin (fig. 2.10).

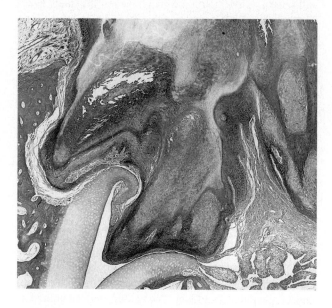

Fig. 2.10.   Canine subungual keratoacanthoma.

Growth and Metastasis

The tumors are slow growing and are cured by amputation of the affected digit.

Subungual Squamous Cell Carcinoma

Incidence, Age, Breed, and Sex

This is a malignant tumor of nailbed epithelium. The tumor is most commonly seen in dogs between 7 and 11 years of age.[1,2] Breeds at increased risk are giant schnauzer (15.0), Gordon setter (13.3), standard poodle (5.9), standard schnauzer (4.9), Scottish terrier (3.7), Labrador retriever (2.4), rottweiler (2.3), dachshund (2.2), miniature schnauzer (1.7), and miniature poodle (1.5). Breeds at decreased risk are golden retriever (0.4), boxer (0.3), Lhasa apso (0.2), collie (0.2), basset hound (0.1), beagle (0.1), and Shetland sheepdog (0.1). No sex predilection has been noted.

Sites and Gross Morphology

This tumor arises from the nailbed epithelium and is the malignant counterpart of the subungual keratoacanthoma. A single digit or multiple digits on the same animal may be involved. Involvement of more than one digit on the same dog may be seen at the time of initial presentation, or these tumors may involve other digits at separate times. There is often loss of the nail with secondary infection of the nail bed. On cut section there is destruction of the bone of P3 by the infiltrating islands of tumor cells, which often appear grey-white. More aggressive tumors show loss of the articular cartilage; alternatively, the articular cartilage may remain intact, while the bone at the periphery of the articular surface has been destroyed by the infiltrating tumor tissue, which invades the joint space between P3 and P2 and may also extend along the bursae of the digital flexor and extensor tendons.

Histological Features

The pertinent histological features of squamous cell carcinoma have been described previously. The infiltrating islands of neoplastic squamous epithelium extend through the basal lamina of the nailbed epithelium with invasion into and destruction of the medullary and cortical bone of P3. There is often lysis of the remaining small pieces of bone by osteoclasts. Superimposed infiltration by neutrophils, plasma cells, and lymphocytes and moderate fibroplasia may be seen.

Growth and Metastasis

The rate of growth of these tumors is variable as is the extent of involvement of the underlying tissues. The entire specimen should be decalcified and examined to determine the extent of involvement of the digital bones and to ensure that clean surgical margins are present.

Metastases are occasionally encountered with cases of subungual squamous cell carcinoma. Metastasis occurs via lymphatics to regional lymph nodes and lungs. In one study, 3 (13 percent) of 24 dogs with subungual squamous cell carcinoma had radiographic evidence of pulmonary metastasis at the time of diagnosis,[1] while in a second study 1 (5 percent) of 21 dogs developed documented pulmonary metastases.[2]

As noted previously, the tumor may involve the bursa of the digital flexor or extensor tendons so that recurrence of the tumor may be noted within the subcutaneous tissue at the amputation site.

REFERENCES

1. Marino, D.J., Matthiesen, D.T., Stefanacci, J.D., and Moroff. S.D. (1995) Evaluation of dogs with digit masses: 117 cases (1981–1991). *J Amer Vet Med Assoc* 207:726–728.
2. O'Brien, M.G., Berg, J., and Engler S.J. (1992) Treatment by digital amputation of subungual squamous cell carcinoma in dogs. *J Amer Vet Med Assoc* 201:759–761.

Sebaceous and Modified Sebaceous Gland Tumors

Sebaceous and modified sebaceous gland tumors with adnexal differentiation include sebaceous adenoma, sebaceous ductal adenoma, sebaceous epithelioma, sebaceous carcinoma, meibomian adenoma, meibomian ductal adenoma, meibomian epithelioma, meibomian carcinoma, hepatoid gland adenoma, hepatoid gland epithelioma, hepatoid gland carcinoma.

Table 2.2 summarizes the histological features of the sebaceous gland neoplasms.

Sebaceous Adenoma, Sebaceous Ductal Adenoma, and Sebaceous Epithelioma

General Considerations

These are tumors showing sebaceous differentiation. Sebaceous adenomas have a preponderance of sebocytes with few basaloid reserve cells and ducts, while sebaceous ductal adenomas have a preponderance of ducts with fewer sebocytes and basaloid reserve cells. Sebaceous epithelioma is of low grade malignancy, and there is a preponderance of basaloid reserve cells with fewer sebocytes and ducts. The dividing line between these tumors may be very arbitrary.

Incidence, Age, Breed, and Sex

These tumors are very common in the dog,[1] uncommon in the cat,[2] and rare in other domestic species. In dogs

TABLE 2.2. Histological features of sebaceous neoplasms

Neoplasm	Histological Features
Hyperplasia	Lobules of glands around a central duct; superficial dermis
Adenoma	Multilobulated; majority of cells are sebocytes; few reserve cells and ducts
Ductal adenoma	Majority of tissue consists of ducts; few sebocytes and reserve cells
Epithelioma	Majority of cells are reserve cells which may show many mitoses but little pleomorphism; few sebocytes and ducts
Carcinoma	Multilobulated; majority of cells are pleomorphic sebocytes; few reserve cells and ducts

the peak incidence is between 8 and 13 years of age. Breeds at increased risk are English cocker spaniel (4.2), cocker spaniel (3.9), Samoyed (2.8), Siberian husky (2.8), cock-a-poo (2.6), Alaskan malamute (2.2), West Highland white terrier (2.0), cairn terrier (1.9), dachshund (1.9), miniature poodle (1.7), toy poodle (1.6), and shih tzu (1.5); breeds at decreased risk are Shetland sheepdog (0.6), golden retriever (0.6), English springer spaniel (0.4), collie (0.3), Irish setter (0.3), doberman (0.2), Great Dane (0.2), German shepherd (0.2), boxer (0.2), weimaraner (0.2), and rottweiler (0.1). There is no sex predilection.

In cats the peak incidence is between 7 and 13 years of age, and Persian cats (2.1) are predisposed to developing the tumors.

Sites and Gross Morphology

In the dog there is a predilection for the tumors to develop on the head; in the cat there is a predilection for tumors on the back, tail, and head, or the tumors may be multicentric. Many of these tumors are exophytic, but there is also an invasive component, which extends into the dermis and may involve the subcutaneous tissue. The elevated, nodular skin masses may exhibit alopecia, hyperpigmentation, and ulceration with secondary infection. Sebaceous tumors are pale yellow to white on cut section and are often divided by fine connective tissue trabeculae into small lobules. Sebaceous ducts may be dilated and filled with keratin. Some tumors, particularly sebaceous epitheliomas, may appear brown/black due to the presence of melanocytes within the tumor.

Histological Features

Sebaceous adenomas extend from the epidermal-dermal interface into the dermis and may involve the subcutis. There are multiple lobules separated by connective tissue trabeculae and remnants of preexisting dermal collagen bundles. At the periphery of the lobules is a rim of small, basophilic reserve cells, which have hyperchromatic nuclei and little cytoplasm. These cells show little or no pleomorphism, but moderate numbers of mitoses may be observed. The reserve cells may be one to several cell layers in thick-

ness. The reserve cells differentiate into mature sebocytes, which have an abundant pale eosinophilic, vacuolated cytoplasm and a small central hyperchromatic nucleus (fig. 2.11 A). The sebocytes do not exhibit mitotic activity. Haphazardly arranged within the tumor are ducts, the outer cells of which have ovoid, vesicular nuclei, a moderate amount of eosinophilic cytoplasm, and distinct cell borders, but lack intercellular desmosomes. These cells become more flattened toward the luminal aspect of the ducts, which are lined by a corrugated, brightly eosinophilic squamous epithelium. Sebocytes are the predominant cell type within sebaceous adenomas.

It is important to differentiate sebaceous adenoma from sebaceous hyperplasia, which is often a multicentric tumor-like lesion of the dog and cat and often represents a senile change. Lesions of sebaceous hyperplasia consist of hyperplastic lobules of mature sebaceous glands arranged around a large sebaceous duct, which often communicates with the follicular infundibulum.

Sebaceous ductal adenomas are characterized by large numbers of variably sized ducts, which contain keratin and some sebum. Fewer reserve cells and sebocytes are seen with this tumor (fig. 2.11 B).

Sebaceous epitheliomas have a preponderance of small, basophilic reserve cells with fewer sebocytes and ducts (fig. 2.11 C). The reserve cells may show considerable mitotic activity. To distinguish this mass from a basal cell carcinoma, it is necessary in some cases to search for individual cells showing evidence of sebaceous differentiation within the tumor. Melanocytes, whose dendritic processes may be found interdigitated between the tumor cells may be present, and melanin granules are seen within the cytoplasm of the reserve cells and within macrophages in the interlobular stroma.

Growth and Metastasis

Sebaceous adenomas and sebaceous ductal adenomas are benign tumors that are cured by wide surgical excision. Sebaceous epitheliomas may recur at the excision site. A small proportion of cases, especially those arising on the head, may show metastasis to regional lymph nodes, but more widespread metastasis has not been noted. These metastatic tumors, primarily those found in the mandibular lymph nodes, often show extensive differentiation to sebocytes and ducts and little mitotic activity of the reserve cells.

Sebaceous Carcinoma

This is a malignant tumor with cells showing sebaceous differentiation.

Incidence, Age, Breed, and Sex

Sebaceous carcinomas are uncommon in the dog and cat and rare in other species.[3] In dogs the peak incidence is between 9 and 13 years of age. Breeds at increased risk are cocker spaniel (4.1), West Highland white terrier (3.2),

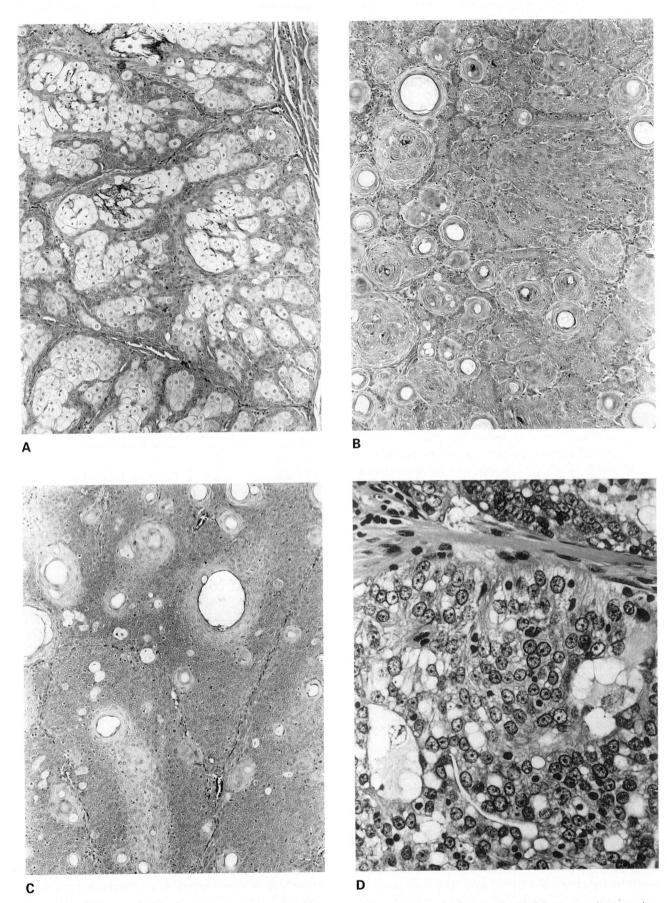

Fig. 2.11.   **A.** Sebaceous adenoma, canine. **B.** Sebaceous ductal adenoma, canine. **C.** Sebaceous epithelioma, canine. **D.** Sebaceous carcinoma, canine.

Scottish terrier (3.1), and Siberian husky (2.9), while breeds at decreased risk are doberman pinscher (0.3) and boxer (0.1). No sex predilection has been noted.

In cats the peak incidence is between 8 and 15 years of age. No breed or sex predilection has been noted.

Sites and Gross Morphology

Sebaceous carcinomas arise primarily on the head and neck in dogs and on the head, thorax, and perineum in cats. The tumors are similar on gross examination and cut section to sebaceous adenoma and epithelioma. A multilobulated intradermal mass is the most common finding.

Histological Features

The tumor is subdivided by fibrovascular connective tissue trabeculae into lobules of varying size. The tumor cells have intracytoplasmic lipid vacuoles, but the degree of lipidization varies from cell to cell within the tumor (fig. 2.11 D). The nuclei are large and hyperchromatic, with prominent nucleoli, and display moderate pleomorphism. The number of mitotic figures found is variable, but atypical mitoses may be found.

The multilobulated appearance of the tumor allows it to be differentiated from a liposarcoma.

Growth and Metastasis

Local infiltration is most often found with sebaceous carcinomas. Metastases are rarely found, but when they do occur it is via lymphatics to regional lymph nodes. More widespread metastases are rarely reported.[4] The treatment of choice is wide surgical excision of the mass.

REFERENCES

1. Scott, D.W., and Anderson, W.I. (1990) Canine sebaceous gland tumors: A retrospective analysis of 172 cases. *Canine Pract* 15:19–21, 24–27.
2. Scott, D.W., and Anderson, W.I. (1991) Feline sebaceous gland tumors: A retrospective analysis of nine cases. *Feline Pract* 19:16–18, 20–21.
3. McMartin, D.N., and Gruhn, R.F. (1977) Sebaceous carcinoma in a horse. *Vet Pathol* 14:532–534.
4. Case, M.T., Bartz, A.R., Bernstein, M., and Rosen, R.A. (1969) Metastasis of a sebaceous gland carcinoma in the dog. *J Amer Vet Med Assoc* 154:661–664.

Meibomian Adenoma, Meibomian Ductal Adenoma, and Meibomian Epithelioma

These tumors arise from the Meibomian glands (tarsal glands) on the inner aspect of the eyelid. They are modified sebaceous glands. Those criteria applied to the classification of sebaceous tumors above also apply to meibomian gland tumors.

Incidence, Age, Breed, and Sex

Meibomian tumors are common in dogs and rare in other species. Dogs between 3 and 15 years old are affected, with the peak incidence between 6 and 11 years of age. Breeds at increased risk are Gordon setter (3.1), Samoyed (2.4), standard poodle (1.7), shih tzu (1.7), Siberian husky (1.6), West Highland white terrier (1.5), and Labrador retriever (1.4). Breeds at decreased risk are rottweiler (0.6), dachshund (0.6), doberman pinscher (0.6), German shepherd (0.6), boxer (0.5), and Yorkshire terrier (0.2). There is no known sex predilection.

Gross Morphology and Histological Features

The tumors, found on the inner aspect of the eyelid, may be brown/black or pale red in appearance and are well demarcated from the surrounding tissue. There may be a small papillomatous exophytic component on the surface of the tumor, but most of the tumor mass is found in the deeper tissues. Histologic features are as described above for sebaceous tumors. However, many meibomian tumors may contain an extensive amount of melanin, but the cell morphology on bleached sections allows them to be readily differentiated from the melanocytomas that also commonly arise on the eyelid.

Growth and Metastasis

The tumors are normally slow growing, and because of their location they are often recognized early in their development and removed. Wide surgical excision is curative, but incomplete excision, especially of larger tumors, will allow the tumor to recur at the surgical site. Further excisions may be more difficult.

Meibomian Carcinoma

This is a malignant tumor of the meibomian glands. This is a rare tumor in all species. Few cases have been reported.[1]

Sites, Gross Morphology, and Histological Features

The tumor can not be distinguished grossly from its benign counterpart on the eyelid. The histology of meibomian carcinoma is as described for sebaceous carcinomas. Location in the meibomian glands of the eyelid is the key to this diagnosis.

Growth and Metastasis

The tumor is locally infiltrative and destructive. Metastases, when found, are via lymphatics to regional lymph nodes.

Hepatoid Gland Adenoma and Hepatoid Gland Epithelioma

General Considerations

These tumors arise from the hepatoid glands (perianal glands, circumanal glands), which are modified sebaceous glands. These glands occur only in Canidae and are referred to as hepatoid glands because the cells morphologically resemble hepatocytes. The glands are located primarily in the perianal region, on the dorsal and ventral aspect of the tail, in the parapreputial area in males, in the abdominal mammary region in females, on the posterior region of the hindlimbs, and on the midline of the back and thorax. Occasionally, they may be found in other locations. Hepatoid gland adenomas are benign tumors that have a preponderance of hepatoid cells with few basaloid reserve cells; hepatoid gland epitheliomas are of low grade malignancy with a preponderance of basaloid reserve cells and fewer hepatoid cells.

Incidence, Age, Breed, and Sex

The peak incidence of the tumor is between 8 and 13 years of age, although both younger dogs (occasionally as young as 2 years old) and older dogs may develop the tumor. Breeds at increased risk are Siberian husky (4.0), Samoyed (2.9), Pekinese (2.8), cock-a-poo (2.3), cocker spaniel (2.1), Brittany spaniel (1.8), Lhasa apso (1.7), shih tzu (1.7), mixed breed (1.5), and beagle (1.5); breeds at decreased risk are German shepherd (0.7), English springer spaniel (0.6), standard poodle (0.6), Labrador retriever (0.5), miniature schnauzer (0.5), Shetland sheepdog (0.5), Great Dane (0.5), golden retriever (0.5), doberman pinscher (0.4), Scottish terrier (0.3), English setter (0.3), boxer (0.1), shar-pei (0.1), and rottweiler (0.1). There is a marked sex predilection, with intact males at increased risk (57 percent of cases) and intact females at decreased risk (9 percent of cases).

Sites and Gross Morphology

The majority of tumors arise in the perianal area, where they may be found as solitary or multiple intradermal masses.[2] The tumors vary from 0.5 to 5 cm in diameter and are frequently ulcerated. The epidermis over nonulcerated tumors is often thin, and hair loss may be noted when the tumor extends into the surrounding haired skin. Tumors arising at other sites may be exophytic or endophytic but are less frequently ulcerated. The most common sites other than the perianal area are the dorsal and ventral aspects of the tail and the parapreputial area.

On cut section hepatoid gland tumors are pale brown and frequently have a distinct multilobulated appearance. Areas of hemorrhage, which may be focal or multifocal and involve large areas of the tumor, are frequently found. Hepatoid gland adenomas may be better encapsulated than hepatoid gland epitheliomas.

Histological Features

Hepatoid gland (circumanal) adenomas are well encapsulated, multilobulated, intradermal and subcutaneous masses. Within the tumor the cells may be arranged as cords, islands, and anastomosing trabeculae of large cells resembling hepatocytes. The cells are polyhedral and have centrally located, large, ovoid, vesicular normochromatic nuclei with a central small nucleolus, abundant eosinophilic cytoplasm, and distinct cell borders. At the periphery of the lobules are the basaloid reserve cells, usually only one cell layer thick, which have small hyperchromatic nuclei and little cytoplasm (fig. 2.12 A). An interlobular stroma, which is rich in blood vessels and may contain inflammatory cells, is found throughout the tumor and at the periphery, where it forms a capsule. In some cases the vessels within the interlobular stroma are extremely ectatic, and there may be hemorrhage into the surrounding tumor tissue. Few mitotic figures will be seen, and these are confined to the reserve cells. Small, round, laminated structures, which represent foci of ductal differentiation, may be scattered throughout the tumor. In some tumors there is the formation of intracytoplasmic vacuoles, evidence of sebaceous differentiation. Hepatoid gland adenomas in male dogs are arranged as anastomosing trabeculae, while in the female there are multiple small islands of tumor cells with a surrounding interlobular stroma.

Hepatoid gland epitheliomas are a low grade malignancy. They are characterized by the majority of cells being reserve cells, with fewer hepatoid cells (fig. 2.12 B). These tumors generally show disorderly growth and usually do not form distinct lobules. The basaloid cells may show marked mitotic activity but little nuclear pleomorphism. The tumor cells may invade the capsule but rarely extend beyond the capsule into the adjacent tissue.

Growth and Metastasis

Hepatoid gland adenomas are slow growing and develop under the influence of androgens[3]. Castration at the time of surgical removal of the tumor is recommended in intact male dogs.[4] Recurrence is uncommon following surgical excision of the tumors; some of the cases thought to be recurrent tumors are de novo tumors arising in the adjacent tissue. It is often possible to find very hyperplastic hepatoid glands adjacent to the tumor; these hyperplastic glands probably progress to form the new tumors in the area of prior surgery.

Hepatoid Gland Carcinoma

This is an uncommon malignant tumor showing differentiation to hepatoid gland epithelium.

Incidence, Age, Breed, and Sex

Dogs between 4 and 15 years of age are affected, with the peak incidence between 8 and 12 years of age. Breeds at

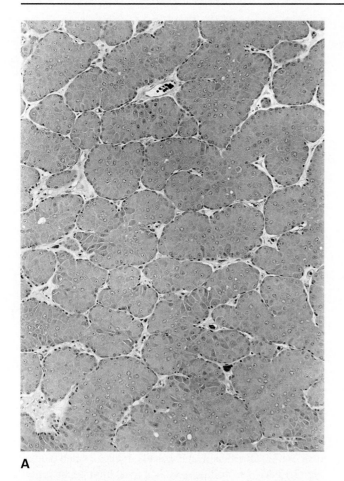

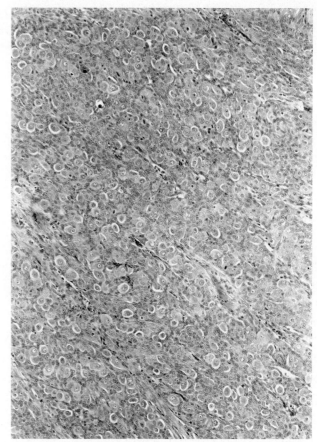

Fig. 2.12. Hepatoid gland, canine. **A.** Adenoma. **B.** Epithelioma. **C.** Carcinoma.

C

increased risk are Siberian husky (8.4), shih tzu (2.6), and mixed breed (1.6). Intact males (69 percent of cases) are at increased risk, but intact females (5 percent of cases) and spayed females (9 percent of cases) are at decreased risk. This is in contrast to previous reports of increased risk for hepatoid gland carcinomas in females.[2]

Sites and Gross Morphology

The primary sites of occurrence of hepatoid gland carcinomas are the perianal, parapreputial, and tail skin. The tumors can not be differentiated from their benign counterpart based on site or gross examination.

Histological Features

Most malignant tumors are less well organized into distinct lobules and trabeculae. The tumor may consist of only one cell type; these cells are undifferentiated, with hyperchromatic nuclei, prominent nucleoli, and little cytoplasm. Only individual cells within the sheets and lobules of tumor cells will show differentiation to hepatoid cells. Other tumors may consist of reserve cells and hepatoid cells: the reserve cells show pleomorphism of their nuclei and abundant mitotic figures, but distinction from the tumor's benign counterpart on cytological features of the cells is difficult; the hepatoid cells have a vacuolated cytoplasm and large nuclei with several prominent nucleoli (fig. 2.12 C).

The most important feature noted on histology that is an indicator of malignancy is invasion of tumor cells into the connective tissue around the tumor and into lymphatics. Care must be exercised in distinguishing true lymphatic invasion from shrinkage artifacts due to retraction of the tumor tissue from the surrounding stroma.

Growth and Metastasis

The rate of growth of hepatoid gland carcinomas is variable. Metastasis occurs via the lymphatic route to the sacral and internal iliac lymph nodes, with subsequent spread to lung and other organs. Criteria to predict metastasis of hepatoid tumors are lacking.

REFERENCES

1. Buyukmihci, N., and Karpinski, L.G. (1975) Cosmetic removal of a sebaceous adenocarcinoma of the eyelid. *Vet Med, Small Anim Clin* 70:1091–1093.
2. Berrocal, A., Vos, J.H., van den Ingh, T.S., Molenbeek, R.F., and van Sluijs, F.J. (1989) Canine perineal tumours. *Zbl Vet Med* 36:739–749.
3. Hayes, H.M., Jr., and Wilson, G.P. (1977) Hormone-dependent neoplasms of the canine perianal gland. *Cancer Res* 37:2068–2071.
4. Wilson, G.P., and Hayes, H.M., Jr. (1979) Castration for treatment of perianal gland neoplasms in the dog. *J Amer Vet Med Assoc* 174:1301–1303.

Apocrine and Modified Apocrine Gland Tumors

Apocrine and modified apocrine gland tumors with adnexal differentiation include apocrine adenoma (complex and mixed), apocrine carcinoma (complex and mixed), apocrine ductal adenoma, apocrine ductal carcinoma, ceruminous adenoma (complex and mixed), ceruminous carcinoma (complex and mixed), anal sac gland adenoma, anal sac gland carcinoma.

Apocrine Adenoma

General Considerations

This is a benign tumor showing differentiation to an apocrine secretory epithelium. Complex apocrine adenoma shows proliferation of glandular and myoepithelial cells; and mixed apocrine adenomas show, in addition to the above, foci of chondroid or osseous metaplasia.[1]

Incidence, Age, Breed, and Sex

Apocrine adenomas are common in the dog, less common in the cat, and rare in other species.[2,3] In dogs the peak incidence is between 8 and 11 years of age. Breeds at increased risk are Lhasa apso (2.4), Old English sheepdog (2.3), collie (2.0), shih tzu (1.8), and Irish setter (1.7), while breeds at decreased risk are miniature schnauzer (0.3), doberman (0.2), boxer (0.2), German short haired pointer (0.2), and great Dane (0.1). No sex predilection has been noted. In cats the peak incidence is between 6 and 13 years of age, and no breed or sex predilection has been noted.

Sites and Gross Morphology

Apocrine adenomas arise more frequently on the head and neck in the dog and on the head in the cat. The tumor is located within the dermis and subcutis, feels soft, and often bulges above the surrounding skin. On cut section some tumors are multilobulated and cystic, the lobules are filled with clear fluid, and there are fine interlobular septa of connective tissue. In other tumors the cysts are smaller, and the connective tissue trabeculae are more conspicuous.

Histological Features

Apocrine adenomas are lined by a single layer of a cuboidal epithelium, with an abundant granular eosinophilic cytoplasm and basally located small nuclei (fig. 2.13 A). The epithelial cells may exhibit decapitation secretion and an accumulation of the secretory product in the glandular lumina, often mixed with macrophages, erythrocytes, and cholesterol crystals. The supporting stroma consists of a fibrovascular connective tissue that is infiltrated by variable numbers of plasma cells and pigment-laden macrophages (ceroidphages). The accumulation of secretions within the lumina of the tumor lobules may result in marked attenuation of the lining epithelial cells. Papillary tumors show invagination of the epithelium and stroma into the lumina of the tumor. Rarely will the flattened myoepithelial cells be seen between the luminal epithelium and the basal lamina.

Complex apocrine adenomas show proliferation of small islands of a glandular epithelium with focal or multifocal proliferation of myoepithelial cells. The myoepithelial cells have a fusiform to stellate shape, euchromatic nuclei, and lightly eosinophilic cytoplasm, and there is a pale basophilic mucinous matrix between the cells. None of these cells shows pleomorphism, and there is little mitotic activity.

Mixed apocrine tumors show metaplasia of the myoepithelial cells, primarily to chondrocytes that blend with the myoepithelial cells described above. The chondrocytes have a central hyperchromatic nucleus and a space between the nucleus and the deeply basophilic chondroid matrix. A few cases also show osseous metaplasia (fig. 2.13 B).

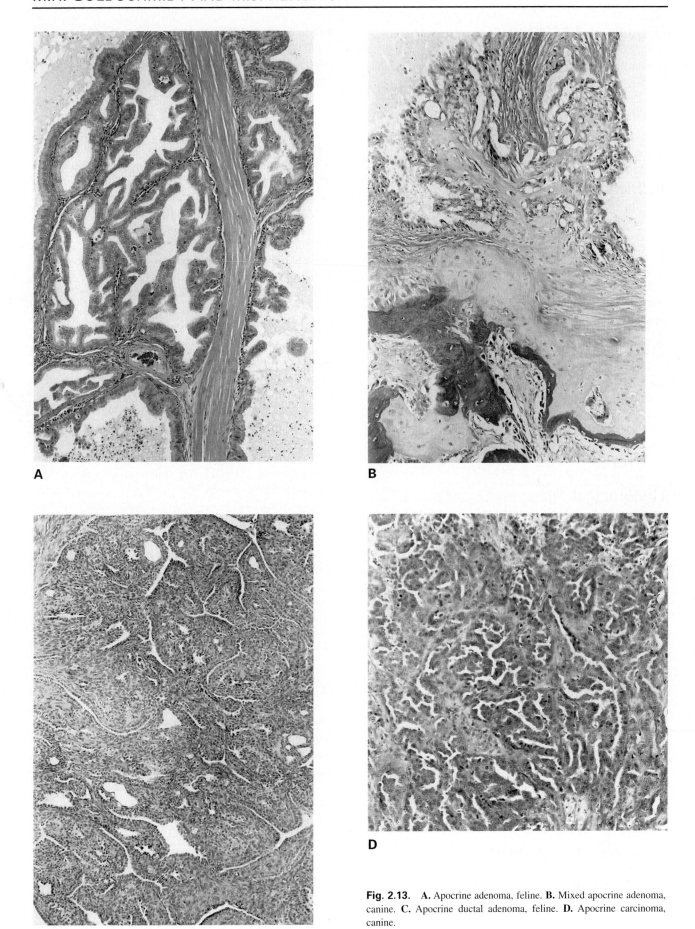

Fig. 2.13. **A.** Apocrine adenoma, feline. **B.** Mixed apocrine adenoma, canine. **C.** Apocrine ductal adenoma, feline. **D.** Apocrine carcinoma, canine.

Growth and Metastasis

Apocrine adenomas are slow growing and do not recur following surgical excision with adequate surgical margins.

Apocrine Ductal Adenoma

This is a benign tumor showing differentiation to an apocrine ductal epithelium.[1]

Incidence, Age, Breed, and Sex

In dogs and cats apocrine ductal adenomas are relatively common.[2,3] The peak incidence in the dog is between 6 and 11 years of age, and in the cat between 5 and 14 years of age. Breeds at increased risk are Old English sheepdog (4.7), golden retriever (2.6), and English springer spaniel (2.4); breeds at decreased risk are miniature poodle (0.2) and doberman pinscher (0.1). No sex predilection has been noted.

Sites and Gross Morphology

In the dog the head, thorax, abdomen, and back are the sites where most tumors occur, while most tumors arise on the head in cats. Apocrine ductal adenomas are located within the deep dermis and subcutis and are well circumscribed but poorly encapsulated. The tumor is multilobulated, and cysts of varying size may be found within the tumor.

Histological Features, Growth, and Metastasis

The hallmark of the apocrine ductal adenoma is the proliferation of a double layer of epithelial cells lining a lumen, which varies in diameter and shape but will often, especially in cats, have the appearance of oriental letters (fig. 2.13 C). The luminal epithelial cells have small, hyperchromatic nuclei and a small amount of pale eosinophilic cytoplasm; the basal cells are more fusiform and have little cytoplasm and a euchromatic nucleus. There is little nuclear or cellular pleomorphism or mitotic activity. Foci of squamous differentiation, such as may normally be seen at the junction of the apocrine duct and the infundibular epithelium, may be found, particularly in dogs. The cells showing squamous differentiation have a granular cell layer with accumulation of small mounds of keratin on the luminal surface. The interlobular stroma is variable in amount and may be infiltrated by a few inflammatory cells. These tumors are slow growing and, although not well encapsulated, are amenable to wide excision.

Apocrine Carcinoma

General Considerations

This is a malignant tumor with differentiation to apocrine secretory epithelium.[1] Complex apocrine carcinomas show proliferation of the glandular epithelium, which is malignant, and myoepithelial cells. In mixed apocrine carcinomas the myoepithelial cells show chondroid or osseous metaplasia.[1]

Incidence, Age, Breed, and Sex

Apocrine carcinomas are relatively common in dogs,[2,3,4] less common in cats,[2,3,4] and infrequently described in other species.[5,6] Dogs between 2 and 15 years old may be affected, with the peak incidence between 8 and 12 years of age. Breeds at increased risk are Old English sheepdog (4.2), shih tzu (2.1), German shepherd (2.0), and cocker spaniel (1.7), while the breed at decreased risk is the doberman pinscher (0.3). In cats the peak incidence is between 5 and 15 years of age, with Siamese cats (2.5) at increased risk and domestic shorthaired cats (0.6) at decreased risk. No sex predilection has been noted.

Sites and Gross Morphology

In both dogs and cats the inguinal and axillary areas are sites where apocrine carcinomas frequently occur, and in cats the perioral region is another favored site. The tumor has various clinical presentations, including nodular intradermal and subcutaneous masses of variable size or a diffuse erosive/ulcerative dermatitis that is referred to as an inflammatory carcinoma.

The nodules vary in size from less than 1 cm to many centimeters in diameter. The inflammatory form is an expansile skin lesion that spreads in a centrifugal manner from a central focus of ulceration. Infiltration of dermal lymphatics and extension to the regional lymph nodes, with blockage of the afferent and efferent lymphatics, may produce severe dermal and subcutaneous edema in the involved area.

On cut section the nodular masses may show central degeneration and necrosis. The tumor is often subdivided by connective tissue trabeculae into multiple lobules. Cyst formation is infrequently found. Fibrosis at the periphery of the mass is often seen with invasive tumors.

Histological Features

Apocrine carcinomas may appear histologically as solid, tubular or cystic tumors, and the cystic tumor may show invagination of the lining epithelial cells to form papillae. The tumor is subdivided into lobules by fibrous trabeculae. The tumor cells have an extensive amount of eosinophilic cytoplasm, which rarely shows the apical blebbing so characteristic of apocrine epithelial cells (fig. 2.13 D). The nuclei are round to ovoid, normochromatic to hyperchromatic, with prominent nucleoli. Cell borders are distinct. There is a variable mitotic rate, usually from one to four mitoses per 400x field. The more anaplastic tumors usually have an abundant amount of eosinophilic cytoplasm, but nuclei are more hyperchromatic and pleomorphic, and mitotic figures are very commonly seen. These tumors, particularly when they infil-trate the deep dermis and subcutaneous tissue, evoke a desmoplastic host response. Great care should be taken to search for evidence of lymphatic invasion by tumor cells, which may be readily found in some cases but is difficult to find in others.

Tumors of apocrine origin stain positively with anti-body to carcinoembryonic antigen. This can be a useful marker to determine apocrine differentiation in a poorly differentiated tumor.[7]

In compound apocrine carcinomas the neoplastic apocrine cells show moderate pleomorphism and mitotic activity, and there is an accompanying periglandular pro-liferation of the myoepithelial cells, as described previ-ously for benign apocrine tumors. The mixed apocrine car-cinomas will show chondroid and occasionally osseous metaplasia of the myoepithelial cells.

Growth and Metastasis

The growth rate of these tumors is quite variable. Inflammatory carcinomas are often rapid growing and metastasize to regional lymph nodes and lungs. Nodular tumors, particularly those located in the perioral region in cats, may be slow growing and slow to metastasize. Inflammatory apocrine carcinomas, like their mammary counterpart, may produce an interstitial pattern on radio-graphic evaluation of the lungs, rather than the nodular pat-tern seen with the nodular form of apocrine carcinomas.

Complex and mixed apocrine carcinomas tend to be slower growing and are usually less malignant with metas-tasis to regional lymph nodes an uncommon event.

Apocrine Ductal Carcinoma

This is a malignant tumor that shows differentiation to apocrine ductal epithelium.[1] This tumor is uncommon and has been reported only in the dog and cat.[2] In these species the peak incidence is between 8 and 13 years of age. No breed or sex predilection has been noted.

Sites and Gross Morphology

The tumor has many features in common with the apocrine ductal adenoma but is more invasive, is poorly circumscribed, and lacks the distinct multilobular appear-ance of its benign counterpart. The tumor is often ulcerated and infiltrative at the margins.[2]

Histological Features

The tubules that make up the tumor are lined by a dou-ble layer of epithelial cells and may contain an eosinophilic secretion. The cells show nuclear and cellular pleomor-phism, nuclear hyperchromasia, and moderate mitotic activ-ity. These tumors seldom exhibit the extensive pleomor-phism seen with apocrine carcinomas. Foci of squamous differentiation are scattered throughout the tumor. Invasion

of the tissue at the periphery of the tumor is a common fea-ture, but lymphatic invasion is infrequently observed.

Growth and Metastasis

These tumors are relatively slow growing, and most are amenable to surgical excision with wide margins. Metastases are uncommon.

Ceruminous Adenoma

General Considerations

This is a benign tumor showing differentiation to ceruminous secretory epithelium.[1] The complex ceremi-nous adenoma shows proliferation of glandular and myoepithelial cells; in addition, the mixed ceruminous adenoma shows foci of chondroid or osseous metaplasia.[1]

Incidence, Age, Breed, and Sex

Benign ceruminous tumors are relatively common in the dog and cat.[2] The tumors are found in dogs and cats between 4 and 13 years of age, with the peak incidence between 7 and 10 years of age. Dog breeds at increased risk are cocker spaniel (7.3) and shih tzu (5.1), while breeds at decreased risk are Labrador retriever (0.3), golden retriever (0.2), and doberman pinscher (0.1). No sex predilection has been noted.

Sites and Gross Morphology

The tumors present as masses within the ear canal, including the vertical ear canal. Ulceration and secondary infection are common. Benign tumors tend be exophytic, especially in dogs. It is often difficult to differentiate benign neoplasms from severe hyperplastic polypoid otitis externa, especially in the Cocker spaniel, a breed predis-posed to developing ceruminous adenomas. Some of the tumors have a dark brown appearance, probably secondary to retention of inspissated cerumen within the lumina of neoplastic glands. In cats these tumors need to be differen-tiated from inflammatory polyps of the external ear, which arise from the middle ear and extend through the tympanic membrane into the external ear; these inflammatory polyps, however, usually occur in younger cats.

Histological Features

Ceruminous adenomas are similar on histology to their cutaneous counterpart, the apocrine adenoma (fig. 2.14 A). However, there is often retention of a brown mate-rial within the glandular lumina, as well as small brown globules within the cytoplasm of the neoplastic glandular epithelium. Many tumors also show aggregation of pigment-laden macrophages within the interstitium, neutrophils within the glandular lumina, and plasma cells in the periglandular stroma. Occasional cases show invasion of neoplastic cells into the intraepidermal ductal portion of the gland (acrosyringium), with small nests of tumor cells in this site .

Superimposed inflammation often makes it difficult to differentiate benign from malignant ceruminous tumors, with the tumor cells appearing more pleomorphic and the nuclei more hyperchromatic. However, the presence of large, hyperchromatic nuclei and invasion through the basal lamina zone are not seen in these cases.

Complex ceruminous tumors (fig 2.14 B) and mixed ceruminous tumors are as described for their apocrine counterparts. Complex ceruminous tumors are not uncommon in dogs.

Growth and Metastasis

The rate of growth of these tumors is usually slow. However, complete surgical excision of the tumor may be difficult to achieve, so that ablation of the ear may be necessary.

Ceruminous Gland Carcinoma

General Considerations

This is a malignant tumor showing differentiation to ceruminous epithelium.[1] The complex ceruminous carcinoma shows malignant proliferation of glandular epithelium and a proliferation of myoepithelial cells; mixed ceruminous carcinomas also show foci of chondroid or osseous metaplasia of the myoepithelial cells.[1]

Incidence, Age, Breed, and Sex

Ceruminous carcinomas are relatively common in the cat and dog. They are more common in cats, with the peak incidence between 7 and 13 years of age. Domestic shorthaired cats (1.6) are predisposed to developing the tumor, while Siamese cats (0.2) are at decreased risk. Dogs between 5 and 14 years of age are mainly affected, with the peak incidence between 9 and 11 years of age. The cocker spaniel (4.8) is at increased risk. Castrated male dogs appear to be predisposed to developing ceruminous carcinomas.

Sites, Gross Morphology, and Histological Features

Carcinomas tend to be infiltrative, erosive, or ulcerated growths. Secondary infection is again common. Carcinomas share many of the features of ceruminous adenomas. However, the tumor cell nuclei are larger and more pleomorphic, often with a single large nucleolus. Mitoses are common. Most cells have an abundant amount of eosinophilic cytoplasm. Intraepidermal infiltration of tumor cells into the acrosyringium may be found (fig. 2.14 C).

Complex ceruminous carcinomas and mixed ceruminous carcinomas have histological features as described previously for their apocrine counterparts.

Growth and Metastasis

The tumors are infiltrative but rarely invade or destroy the cartilage of the ear canal. There is invasion within the dermis and lymphatics, with spread to the parotid lymph node. Surgical excision usually results in total ear ablation.

Anal Sac Gland Adenoma

This is a benign tumor, arising from the apocrine secretory epithelium found in the wall of the anal sac.[1] This tumor is very rare in both the dog and the cat.

Sites and Gross Morphology

The tumor arises from the apocrine glands of the anal sac. These tumors can not be differentiated from their malignant counterpart, which is described below.

Histological Features

There is proliferation of multiple large islands of glandular epithelium. The cells lining the individual glands are cuboidal to columnar with basally located normochromatic nuclei. There is minimal nuclear pleomorphism and mitotic activity (fig. 2.15 A). Cells have an abundant amount of eosinophilic cytoplasm and may exhibit decapitation secretion. Surrounding the glands is a fine fibrovascular connective tissue stroma.

Growth and Metastasis

These are rare tumors. Little is known about their rate of growth.

Anal Sac Gland Carcinoma

This is a malignant tumor, arising from the apocrine secretory epithelium found in the wall of the anal sac.[8,9,10]

Incidence, Age, Breed, and Sex

This tumor is common in dogs and rare in cats.[2,3,4] Dogs between 5 and 15 years of age are primarily affected, with the peak incidence between 7 and 12 years of age. It is the most common malignant tumor in the perineum of dogs. Breeds at increased risk are English cocker spaniel (11.5), German shepherd (2.3), English springer spaniel (2.2), and mixed breed (1.9). Breeds at decreased risk are golden retriever (0.3) and boxer (0.3). A sex predilection is thought to exist, but the data is confusing. The initial reports on this tumor identified an increased risk to females.[8,9,10] The male to female ratio was shown to vary depending on the breed affected, but overall an increased incidence in neutered males and females was noted.[2] However, subsequent evaluation of a larger database has shown that only male castrates are at increased risk.

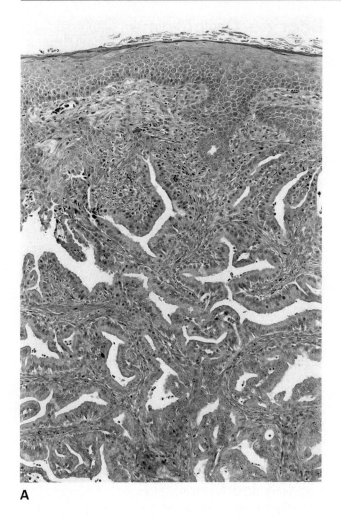

A

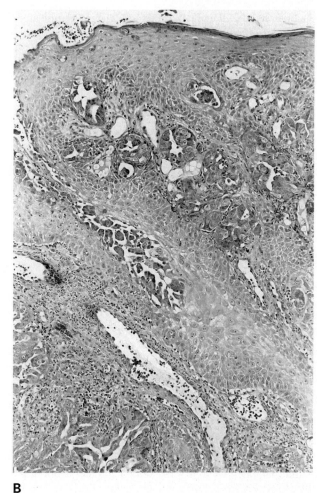

B

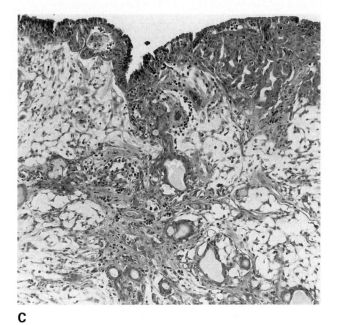

C

Fig. 2.14. **A.** Ceruminous adenoma, canine. **B.** Ceruminous gland carcinoma, canine. **C.** Complex ceruminous adenoma, canine.

Sites and Gross Morphology

The tumors arise from the anal sac glands and are located on the ventrolateral aspect of the anus as intradermal and subcutaneous masses, which often invade deep into the underlying perirectal tissue. Some cases will appear as a perianal mass, impossible to differentiate on gross inspection from hepatoid gland tumors, when they arise in this site. Ulceration is uncommon. The tumors may first be noted by the clinician as a mass when expressing the anal sacs. Large tumors may impinge on the rectum, resulting in straining and difficulty in defecation. Digital examination localizes the tumor to the wall of the anal sac.

A large proportion of cases will develop polyuria, polydipsia, weakness, and hypercalcemia due to the production by the neoplastic cells of a parathyroid hormone–related protein.[10,11]

On gross examination the tumor can often be found in the wall of the anal sac. The stratified squamous lining of the anal sac is often highly melanized, while the surrounding tumor is white; the tumor may appear multilobulated, and occasionally small cysts may be seen.

Histological Features

Three distinct patterns may be found, and one or more of these patterns may be present in a single tumor. The tumor cells may form *solid* sheets of tumor cells, or foci of *rosette* formation may be seen, which may enlarge to form *tubules* of varying diameter that may have an eosinophilic secretion within their lumina.

The cells that make up the *solid* type of anal sac gland carcinoma (fig. 2.15 B) have round to oval normochromatic to hyperchromatic nuclei, a prominent nucleolus, and little eosinophilic cytoplasm. In the *rosette* type (fig. 2.15 C), the nuclei become basally located within the cell, with a small amount of apical eosinophilic cytoplasm radially arranged around a small amount of eosinophilic secretion. The *tubular* type (fig 2.15 D) has a large lumen lined by cuboidal cells with an extensive amount of cytoplasm and hyperchromatic nuclei. The mitotic rate is quite variable. Invasion of the surrounding tissue evokes a desmoplastic response, and invasion of the perirectal muscles is common. Lymphatics may have tumor emboli within their luminae, but true vascular invasion should be differentiated from retraction artifacts, which are commonly encountered when evaluating this tumor.

Growth and Metastasis

The rate of growth is variable, but metastasis is common. The sacral and sublumbar lymph nodes are the most common sites of metastasis, with subsequent spread to lungs and other internal organs, including the spleen. Surgical excision of the tumor may be difficult due to the invasive nature of the tumor and the accompanying desmoplastic host response. Occasionally this tumor is cured by surgery alone, but in cases with lymph node metastasis the prognosis is often poor.

Eccrine Adenoma

This is a benign tumor in the footpad area showing differentiation to an eccrine secretory epithelium.[1] This tumor is rare in all species of domestic animals but common in humans.

Histological Features

The tumor cells have basally located nuclei and very lightly staining eosinophilic cytoplasm. There is little nuclear pleomorphism or mitotic activity.

Eccrine Carcinoma

This is a malignant tumor showing differentiation to eccrine secretory epithelium.[1] This tumor is rare but has been reported in the footpads of the cat and dog, where these glands are normally located. Too few cases have been reported to know whether there is any predisposition to this tumor.

Sites and Gross Morphology

As stated above, most tumors arise from the footpad of the cat and dog. Affected areas are swollen, and often the overlying epidermis is ulcerated. There may be invasion of the adjacent bones of the digit, a feature also found with subungual squamous cell carcinoma and keratoacanthoma.

Histological Features

The neoplastic cells form tubuloacinar structures lined by a single layer or a multilayered epithelium, with a dense collagenous stroma surrounding the epithelial component. The tumor cells are cuboidal to polygonal and have an amphophilic or eosinophilic cytoplasm and large hyperchromatic nuclei with prominent nucleoli (fig. 2.16). Small foci of keratinization may be found. Intraluminal necrotic cells and an eosinophilic secretion may be found. Immunohistochemical staining for carcinoembryonic antigen, normally present in the eccrine duct, will differentiate eccrine carcinomas from squamous cell carcinoma.[7]

Growth and Metastasis

The rate of growth is variable. Metastases are infrequently reported with eccrine carcinomas. Most cases are treated by excision of the tumor with wide margins.

REFERENCES

1. Goldschmidt, M.H., Dunstan, R.W., Stannard, A.A., von Tscharner, C., Walder, E.J., and Yager, J.A. (1998) *World Health Organization International Histologic Classification of Tumors of Domestic Animals. Histological Classification of Tumors of the Skin of Domestic Animals.* 2nd series, vol. III. Armed Forces Institute of Pathology, Washington, D.C.
2. Goldschmidt, M.H., and Shofer, F.S. (1998) *Skin Tumors of the Dog and Cat.* Butterworth Heinemann, Oxford, pp. 1–301.
3. Walder, E.J. (1992) In Gross, T.L., Ihrke, P.E., and Walder, E.J. *Veterinary Dermatopathology: A Macroscopic and Microscopic Evaluation of Canine and Feline Skin Disease.* Mosby Yearbook, St. Louis, pp. 330–476.
4. Kalaher, K.M., Anderson, W.I., Scott, D.W. (1990) Neoplasms of the apocrine sweat glands in 44 dogs and 10 cats. *Vet Rec* 127:400–403.
5. Anderson, W.I., Scott, D.W., and Crameri, F.M. (1990) Two rare cutaneous neoplasms in horses: Apocrine gland adenocarcinoma and carcinosarcoma. *Cornell Vet* 80:339–345.
6. Piercy, D.W.T., Cranwell, M.P., and Collins, A.J. Mixed apocrine (sweat gland) adenocarcinoma in the tail of a cow. *Vet Rec* 134:473–474.

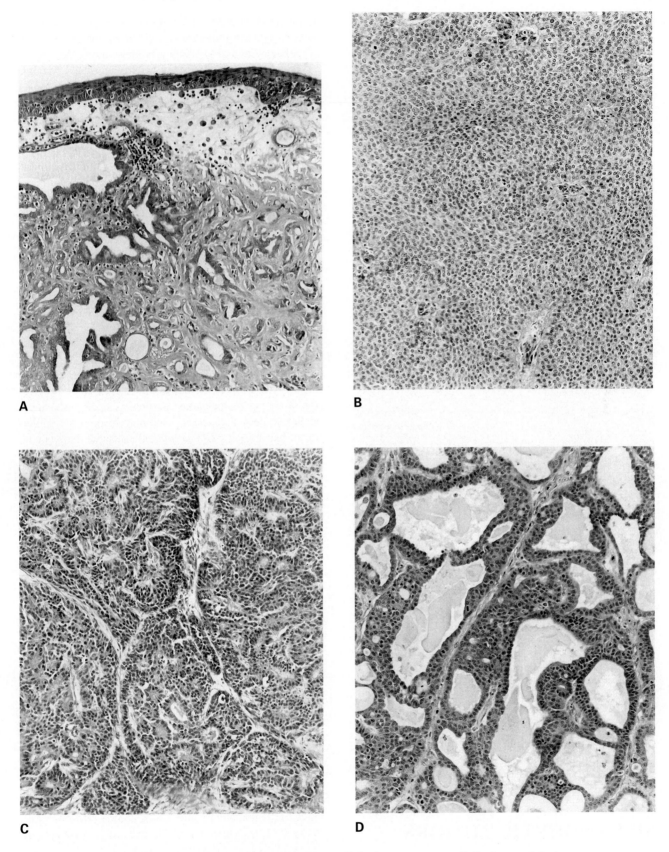

Fig. 2.15. Anal sac gland, canine. **A.** Adenoma. **B.** Carcinoma, solid type. **C.** Carcinoma, rosette type. **D.** Carcinoma, tubular type.

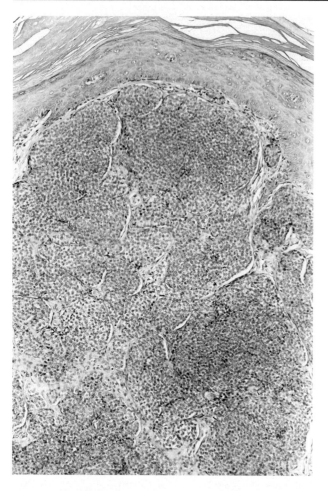

Fig. 2.16.   Eccrine carcinoma, feline.

7. Ferrer, L., Rabanal, R.M., Fondevila, D. and Prats, N. (1990) Immunocytochemical demonstration of intermediate filament proteins, S-100 protein and CEA in apocrine sweat glands and apocrine gland derived lesions of the dog. *J Vet Med* 37:569–576.
8. Goldschmidt, M.H., and Zoltowski, C. (1981) Anal sac adenocarcinoma in the dog: 14 cases. *J Small Anim Pract* 22:119–128.
9. Ross, J.T., Scavelli, T.S., and Mathiesen, D.T. (1991) Adenocarcinoma of the apocrine glands of the anal sac: A review of 32 cases. *J Amer Anim Hosp Assoc* 27:349–355.
10. Meuten, D.J., Cooper, B.J., Capen, C.C., Chew, D.J., and Kociba, G.J. (1981) Hypercalcemia associated with an adenocarcinoma derived from the apocrine glands of the anal sac. *Vet Pathol* 18:454–471.
11. Rosol, T.J., Capen, C.C., Danks, J.A., Suva, L.J., Steinmeyer, C.L., Hayman, J., Ebeling, P.R., and Martin, T.J. (1990) Identification of parathyroid hormone-related protein in canine apocrine adenocarcinoma of the anal sac. *Vet Pathol* 27:89–95.

MELANOCYTIC TUMORS

Melanoblasts are neuroectodermal in origin, and during fetal development they migrate to the skin and hair bulbs. Mature pigment producing cells are referred to as melanocytes. These dendritic cells are found interspersed between the basal keratinocytes of the epidermis and hair bulb. E-cadherin molecules are found on the cell surfaces of melanocytes and keratinocytes; these molecules are the adhesion mechanism between the two cell types. Melanin produced by melanocytes, is stored within melanosomes, and is transferred to keratinocytes by a process known as cytocrinia. Melanosomes accumulate within the cytoplasm of keratinocytes, where they serve to protect the skin from the harmful effects of ultraviolet radiation. Melanoblasts that fail to reach the epidermis will develop into intradermal melanocytes. In the dermis, a second population of melanin-containing cells, melanophages, may be found; these cells have phagocytosed melanin that enters the dermis secondary to leakage from or destruction of epidermal or follicular melanocytes.

A nevus cell is an altered melanocyte. This term is used extensively in conjunction with the description of pigmented lesions in human dermatology and dermatopathology. We have chosen not to use this term in order to avoid any confusion or suggestion that the lesions seen in domestic animals are analogous to their human counterpart.

Three terms used extensively in descriptions of melanocytic neoplasms: *Junctional* refers to the proliferation of neoplastic melanocytes, often as small nests, at the epidermal-dermal junction. This may involve the epidermis or hair follicle.[1] *Compound* indicates that there is both an epidermal and a dermal component to the tumor.[1] *Dermal* indicates that the tumor is only intradermal, with no epidermal component.[1]

Melanocytoma

This is a benign tumor arising from the melanocytes in the epidermis, dermis, or adnexa, but primarily from the external root sheath of the hair follicle.[1]

Incidence, Age, Breed, and Sex

Melanocytomas are common in dogs,[2,3] horses, and certain breeds of swine, less common in cats and cattle, and rare in sheep and goats.

Dogs

Dogs less than a year of age occasionally develop melanocytomas, but it is difficult to establish if these are congenital lesions. The peak incidence is found between the ages of 5 and 11 years. The breeds at increased risk are vizsla (6.8), miniature schnauzer (6.4), standard schnauzer (4.9), Chesapeake Bay retriever (4.0), giant schnauzer (3.5), doberman pinscher (3.4), Airedale terrier (3.0), Irish setter (3.0), Brittany spaniel (2.6), golden retriever (2.2), shar-pei (1.9), rottweiler (1.9), and cairn terrier (1.8). Breeds at decreased risk are Labrador retriever (0.6), mixed breed (0.6), Lhasa apso (0.5), cocker spaniel (0.4), English springer spaniel (0.4), German short haired pointer (0.4), miniature poodle (0.4), beagle (0.3), collie (0.3), Shetland sheepdog (0.2), shih tzu (0.2), weimaraner (0.2), West

Highland white terrier (0.2), basset hound (0.1), toy poodle (0.1), bichon frise (0.1), Old English sheepdog (0.1), and Siberian husky (0.1). No sex predilection has been noted.

Horses

Horses may occasionally develop congenital melanocytomas.[4] Congenital and acquired melanocytomas in horses less than 2 years of age are relatively common, occurring in a variety of breeds and in horses of varied coat color. Females are more commonly affected.[5] Gray horses are predisposed to developing melanocytomas, particularly the Arab and Lipizzaner breeds. These tumors increase in number as the horses age.[6] Horses with other coat colors may occasionally develop melanocytomas as they age.

Swine

Swine have a high incidence of melanocytomas, which may often be found in slaughtered animals.[7] Certain breeds, including the Sinclair, Hormel, and duroc swine, have a high incidence because the tumor is congenital in these breeds. Melanocytomas in these swine breeds are being used as animals models for melanoma in humans. However, it remains unclear how these tumors should be classified, because in some cases they regress spontaneously, while in others they have a malignant biologic behavior, fail to regress, and show metastasis to regional lymph nodes.

Cats

Cats have a low incidence of melanocytomas. Animals between 4 and 13 years old have a greater incidence, and domestic shorthaired cats (2.2) are at greatest risk.[2,8,9]

Cattle

Cattle develop melanocytomas infrequently, but congenital tumors and tumors in young animals have been reported.[10] Angus cattle may be at greater risk than other breeds.

Sites and Gross Morphology

Predilection sites for melanocytomas are the eyelids in dogs, the legs and trunk in young horses, the perineum and tail in older gray horses, and the head in cats. The congenital tumors in swine may be multicentric or may arise in the flank area in the Duroc breed.

Melanocytomas vary considerably in their appearance, which may be related to the length of time they have been present in the skin. The smallest lesions are small, pigmented macules, while the largest lesions are tumors which may be 5 cm or more in diameter. The color of the tumor depends on the amount of melanin within the cells and varies from black through various shades of brown to gray and red. On cut section the epidermis is usually intact, and there is often hair loss. Hyperpigmentation of the epidermis may be present, with much of the dermis often replaced by the tumor, which in larger masses also extends into the subcutaneous tissue. The tumors may have a var-iegated appearance, with areas of pigmentation intermingled with nonpigmented regions.

Of critical importance, particularly in the dog, is the location of the tumor. As a general rule tumors arising from the haired skin are benign, whereas those arising from mucocutaneous junctions are malignant, the only exception being those arising on the eyelids. To determine whether a cutaneous melanocytic neoplasm is benign or malignant requires histological examination. Heavily pigmented tumors require bleaching to remove the melanin and allow the cellular and nuclear morphology to be more easily evaluated.

Histological Features

The intraepidermal component of melanocytomas, seen in junctional and compound melanocytomas, consists of atypical melanocytes that occur either as single cells or small nests of tumor cells in the lower epidermis or the external root sheath of the hair follicle (fig. 2.17 A). Most of these tumor cells are round and have a large amount of intracytoplasmic melanin, which tends to obscure the nuclear morphology. In bleached sections the nuclei are somewhat hyperchromatic and show little pleomorphism (fig. 2.17 C,D). Mitotic figures are infrequently observed.

The dermal component, seen in compound and dermal melanomas, shows a marked variability in the morphology of the neoplastic melanocytes (fig. 2.17 B). Often, the tumor cells in the upper dermis of compound melanocytomas are similar to those found in the epidermis (fig. 2.18 A). However, the tumor cells may also appear epithelioid, with prominent nucleoli, and the cells may be arranged in small groups, subdivided by a fine fibrovascular stroma (fig. 2.18 B).

Dermal melanocytomas may be less cellular. The neoplastic cells are often small spindle cells with intracytoplasmic melanin granules. A variable amount of collagenous stroma often is present between the neoplastic cells. Unless these tumor cells retain the ability to synthesize melanin, it is difficult to distinguish them from dermal fibromas. Some tumors have a more distinct neuroidal morphology so that they are more readily identified as melanocytomas by their neuroepithelial origin (fig. 2.18 C).

An unusual variant of melanocytoma that consists of large round cells with an abundant pale eosinophilic granular cytoplasm is referred to as the balloon-cell melanocytoma.[11] Melanin granules are often difficult to identify within the cytoplasm of these cells but will stain positive with the Fontana–Masson stain for melanin. Nuclei are small and hyperchromatic, and cell borders are quite distinct.

The majority of these tumors show little nuclear or cellular pleomorphism. The number of mitoses is usually low. In the dog those tumors arising from the haired skin that have fewer than three mitotic figures per 10 high power (HP) fields should be considered benign, while those with more than three mitotic figures per 10 high power fields should be considered malignant.

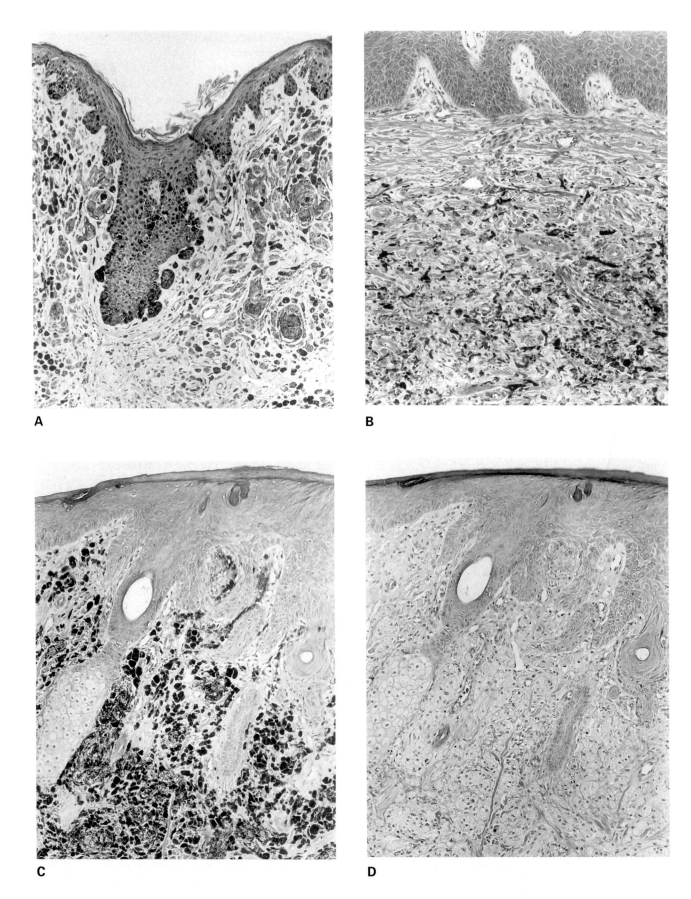

Fig. 2.17. Melanocytoma. **A.** With junctional activity, canine. **B.** Congenital, dermal, bovine. **C.** Dermal, equine. **D.** Dermal, equine, bleached.

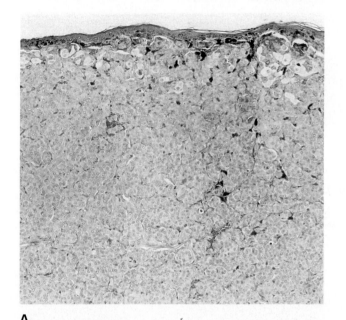

A

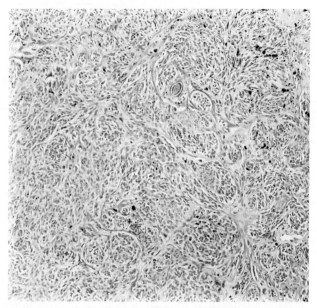

B

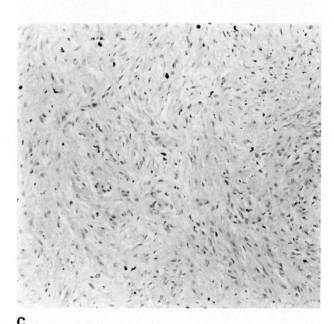

C

Fig. 2.18. Melanocytoma, canine. **A.** Round cell. **B.** Epithelioid. **C.** With neurotization.

Growth and Metastasis

The majority of melanocytomas are slow growing and amenable to surgical excision, which is the treatment of choice.

Cimetidine, an H2 histamine antagonist (2.5 mg/kg of body weight, PO, q 8 h), has been used in the clinical management of progressive, multifocal melanomas in three adult gray horses that were treated for 2 months to 1 year.[12] The number and size of the melanomas decreased substantially.

Malignant Melanoma

This is a malignant tumor of melanocytes.[1]

Incidence, Age, Breed, and Sex

Malignant melanoma is common in the dog[2,3] and uncommon in other domestic species. However, in swine, a proportion of cases, as high as 10–15 percent of selectively bred Sinclair miniature swine with congenital melanoma, behave in a malignant fashion and will show progression and metastasis to regional lymph nodes and lungs. The other 85–90 percent spontaneously regress with no recurrence of the tumor, secondary to a cell-mediated immune response to the tumor.[14]

Dogs between 3 and 15 years old are primarily affected, with the peak incidence between 9 and 13 years of age. Breeds at increased risk are Scottish terrier (3.8), standard schnauzer (3.5), miniature schnauzer (3.5), Irish setter (2.8), golden retriever (2.1), and doberman pinscher (2.1); the breed at decreased risk is the Siberian husky (0.1). No sex predilection has been noted in the dog.

Malignant melanoma is uncommon in the cat, occurring mainly in older cats and showing no sex predilection.

Sites and Gross Morphology

The majority of cases of malignant melanoma in dogs involve the oral cavity and mucocutaneous junction of the lips, with approximately 10 percent of cases arising from the haired skin, with a predilection for the head and scrotum. Cats have a greater proportion of malignant melanomas arising from the skin, primarily the head (lips and nose) and back. Malignant melanoma can not be differentiated from melanocytoma on gross examination. The tumors may be highly pigmented or lack pigment and may invade deeply into the subcutaneous tissue and along fascial planes. Size and degree of pigmentation are not reliable indicators of the malignant potential of melanocytic tumors.

Histological Features

Malignant melanomas arising in the skin often show marked junctional activity. The neoplastic melanocytes are present as small nests or as single cells within the basal portion of the epidermis (fig. 2.19 A). However, the tumor cells may be found in the upper layers of the epidermis, a feature not seen with melanocytomas. The cells within the epidermis have larger nuclei and more conspicuous nucleoli than those found in melanocytomas, and mitoses are more frequently observed. Epidermal ulceration may also be more common with malignant melanoma.

The dermal component often consists of more anaplastic and pleomorphic melanocytes which may be fusiform or epithelioid in shape and contain much or little intracytoplasmic melanin. The tumor may display an interwoven or whorled pattern of fusiform cells (fig. 2.19 B), or nests of epithelioid cells with an interstitial, fine, fibrovascular stroma may be found. Mitoses are usually common (> 3/10 HP fields). Occasionally, foci of chondroid or osseous metaplasia may be seen within the tumor.

The cell type found on histology is of no prognostic significance when evaluating malignant melanomas in the dog. However, the epithelioid type of malignant melanoma in the cat may behave in a more aggressive and malignant fashion.

Growth and Metastasis

Malignant melanomas are often rapidly growing and can be fatal.[13] There is local invasion into the subcutaneous tissue, but intraepidermal spread (analogous to the horizontal growth phase of melanomas in humans) may also be seen; thus surgical margins, particularly the epidermal edges, should be carefully evaluated for the presence of neoplastic melanocytes. Metastasis occurs commonly, with spread via lymphatics to regional lymph nodes and lungs. It is not uncommon for malignant melanoma to spread to other body sites, including unusual locations such as the brain, heart, and spleen.

In cytological and histological evaluation of lymph nodes (particularly mandibular lymph nodes) for evidence of metastasis, care must be taken to differentiate melanophages (which are common in the medullary sinuses due to drainage of melanin pigment from the oral cavity to this node) from neoplastic melanocytes. Bleached sections should be evaluated for evidence of nuclear pleomorphism and prominent nucleoli within the tumor cells, which also tend to be arranged in small nests, both in the cortex and medulla, rather than as single cells within the medulla.

Little progress has been made in the successful treatment of malignant melanoma in humans and in animals.

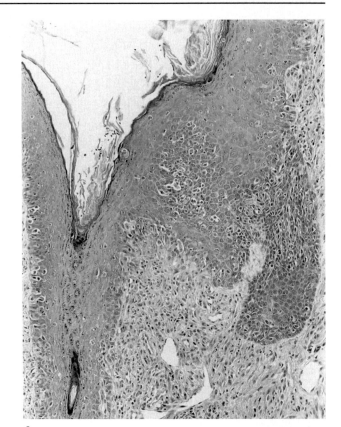

A

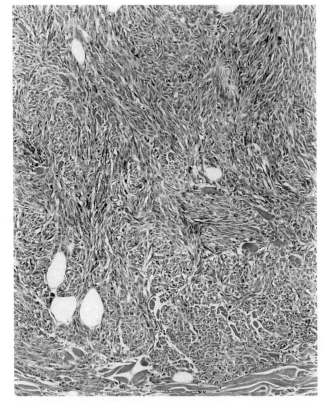

B

Fig. 2.19. Malignant melanoma, canine. **A.** Intraepidermal and dermal. **B.** Malignant melanoma, dermal, spindle cell, canine. (continued)

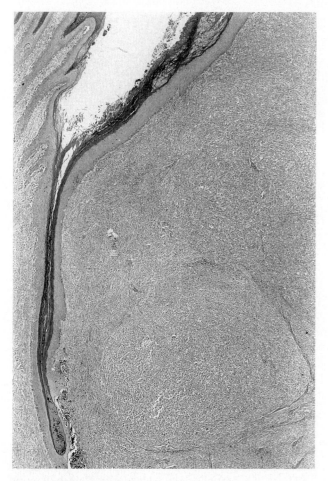

C

Fig. 2.19. (continued) C. Subungual.

Subungual Malignant Melanoma

This is a malignant tumor of melanocytes of the nailbed epithelium (fig. 2.19C).

Incidence, Age, Breed, and Sex

This tumor is common only in the dog and accounts for approximately 8 percent of cases of malignant melanoma.[2] The peak incidence is between 8 and 13 years of age. Breeds at increased risk are Scottish terrier (12.1), standard schnauzer (7.4), Irish setter (4.2), miniature schnauzer (4.2), rottweiler (3.1), and Golden retriever (1.9), while mixed breed dogs (0.5) are at decreased risk. No sex predilection has been noted.

Sites and Gross Morphology

The tumor, which arises in the epithelium of the nail bed, may not be visible on external evaluation, but it may present clinically with paronychia, nail deformity, or nail loss and lameness. Radiographic examination of the affected digit shows lysis of P3. The gross and radio-graphic findings are very similar to those seen with cases of subungual squamous cell carcinoma.

On cut section the tumor may appear variably pigmented brown/black, with invasion and destruction of P3, which correlates with the radiographic findings.

Histological Features

There is often an intraepithelial component of neoplastic melanocytes, either as single cells or as nests in the basal layer. The subepithelial cells are as described above for malignant melanoma. Invasion and destruction of the phalangeal bones, as noted with subungual squamous cell carcinoma, is common.

Growth and Metastasis

Subungual malignant melanoma is usually slow growing, and many will show invasion and destruction of the underlying bone at the time of initial examination. As with other malignant melanomas, these tumors metastasize via lymphatics to regional lymph nodes and lungs. However, those tumors removed at an early stage in their development, prior to subepithelial and bone invasion, tend to have a better prognosis following digital amputation.

REFERENCES

1. Goldschmidt, M.H., Dunstan, R.W., Stannard, A.A., von Tscharner, C., Walder, E.J., and Yager, J.A. (1998) *World Health Organization. International Histologic Classification of Tumors of Domestic Animals. Histological Classification of Tumors of the Skin of Domestic Animals.* 2nd Series. Vol. III. Armed Forces Institute of Pathology, Washington, D.C.
2. Goldschmidt, M.H., and Shofer, F.S. (1998) *Skin Tumors of the Dog and Cat.* Butterworth Heinemann, Oxford, pp. 131–141.
3. Walder, E.J. (1992) In Gross, T.L., Ihrke, P.E., and Walder, E.J. *Veterinary Dermatopathology: A Macroscopic and Microscopic Evaluation of Canine and Feline Skin Disease.* Mosby Yearbook, St. Louis, pp. 451–459.
4. Calderwood Mays, M.B., Mayhew, I.G., Woodard, J.C. (1984) A giant congenital pigmented nevus in a horse. *Amer J Dermatopathol* 6:325–330.
5. Foley, G.L., Valentine, B.A., and Kincaid, A.L. (1991) Congenital and acquired melanocytomas (benign melanomas) in eighteen young horses. *Vet Pathol* 28:363–369.
6. Gebhart, W., and Niebauer, G.W. (1997) Comparative investigations of depigmented and melanomatous lesions in gray horses of the Lipizzaner breed. *Arch Dermatol Res* 259:29–42.
7. Bundza, A., Feltmate, T.E. (1990) Melanocytic cutaneous lesions and melanotic regional lymph nodes in slaughter swine. *Can J Vet Res* 54:301–304.
8. Goldschmidt, M.H., Liu, S.M.S., and Shofer, F.S. (1993) Feline dermal melanoma: A retrospective study. In Ihrke, P.J., Mason, I.S., and White, S.D. (eds.) *Advances in Veterinary Dermatology II.* Pergamon Press, New York pp. 285–291.
9. Miller, W.H., Jr., Scott, D.W., and Anderson, W.I. (1993) Feline cutaneous melanocytic neoplasms: A retrospective analysis of 43 cases (1979–1991). *Vet Dermatol* 4:19–25.
10. Miller, M.A., Weaver, A.D., et al. (1995) Cutaneous melanocytomas in 10 young cattle. *Vet Pathol* 32:479–484.

11. Diters, R.W., Walsh, K.M. (1984) Canine cutaneous clear cell melanomas: A report of three cases. *Vet Pathol* 21:355–356.

12. Goetz, T.E., Ogilvie, G.K., Keegan, K.G., and Johnson, P.J. (1990) Cimetidine for treatment of melanomas in three horses. *J Amer Vet Med Assoc* 196:449–452.

13. Ramos-Vara, J.A., Beissenherz, M.E., Miller, M.A., Johnson, G.C., Pace, L.W., Fard, A., and Kottler, S.J. (2000) Retrospective study of 338 canine oral melanomas with clinical, histological, and immunohistochemical review of 129 cases. *Vet Pathol* 37:597–608.

14. Morgan, C.D., Measel, J.W., Jr., Amoss, M.S., Jr., Rao, A., and Greene, J.F., Jr. (1996) Immunophenotypic characterization of tumor infiltrating lymphocytes and peripheral blood lymphocytes isolated from melanomatous and non-melanomatous Sinclair miniature swine. *Vet Immunol Immunopathol* 55:189–203.

MESENCHYMAL TUMORS

M. J. Hendrick

Mesenchymal tumors of the skin and soft tissues comprise a wide range of entities, some of which are of uncertain classification. Various spindle cell and round cell neoplasms are described below, but the term *tumor* is used broadly, and includes nonneoplastic lesions of clinical importance or interest.

FIBROMA

Fibromas are benign neoplasms of fibrocytes with abundant collagenous stroma.

Incidence, Age, Breed, and Sex

Fibromas are uncommon, but they are most often seen in the dog. They have been reported in cats, but some investigators believe that feline tumors that have the histological appearance of fibromas are actually well-differentiated fibrosarcomas.[1] Canine breeds that are predisposed to the formation of these tumors include Rhodesian ridgebacks, doberman pinschers, and boxers.[1] Fibromas are rare in large animals.[2]

Site and Gross Morphology

Fibromas occur most commonly on the limbs and heads of dogs. The majority of tumors are round to oval intradermal or subcutaneous masses. They are firm, rubbery, and gray/white on cut surface.

Histological Features

This benign tumor is well circumscribed but unencapsulated. It is composed of mature fibrocytes producing abundant collagen (fig. 2.20). The collagenous fibers are repetitive and are usually arranged in interwoven fascicles, more rarely in whorls. The neoplastic fibrocytes are uniform, with oval normochromatic nuclei and an indistinct cytoplasm that blends into the extracellular collagenous stroma. Mitotic figures are rarely observed. Occasionally,

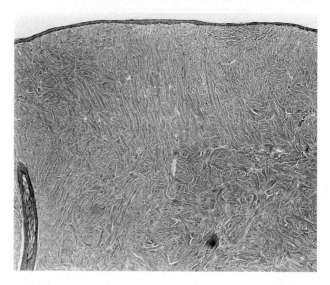

Fig. 2.20. Fibroma, skin, dog. Note the dense pattern of repetitive collagen.

the collagen may be brightly eosinophilic and hyaline, resembling keloids in humans.

Additional Diagnostic Criteria

Collagenous hamartomas (see below) can be distinguished from fibromas by the haphazard arrangement of the collagen fibers, which is similar to normal collagen, and by their superficial dermal location, which often raises the epidermis.

Growth, Metastasis, Treatment

Fibromas are slow growing, and complete excision is curative.

FIBROSARCOMA

This malignant neoplasm has variable presentations depending on species, age, site, and etiopathogenesis. Many other neoplasms (e.g., hemangiopericytoma, malignant melanoma, and leiomyosarcoma) can have regions that are consistent with fibrosarcoma, but careful examination of several sections will usually identify areas characteristic of these other tumors.

Incidence, Age, Breed, Sex, and Site

Although fibrosarcomas occur in all domestic species, they are most commonly seen in adult and aged cats and dogs (mean age of 9 years). Fibrosarcoma is the most common tumor of the cat and has increased in incidence over the last decade, most likely because of its association with vaccination (see below). No breed or sex predisposition has been reported in the cat, but one reference states that golden retrievers and doberman pinschers are at increased risk.[1] Most tumors are focal and can develop anywhere on the body, although head and limbs are most often involved. One exception is the fibrosarcoma of cats that is induced by feline sarcomavirus (FeSV). FeSV is a defective mutant of FeLV; in the presence of FeLV, it can replicate, resulting in oncogenesis. FeSV-associated tumors can occur in individuals as young as a few months of age, with a mean age of 3 years. Tumors in pet cats are rare, but they are often multicentric and can metastasize.[3]

Gross Morphology

The tumor can be circumscribed or infiltrative. Capsules are usually not seen. The cut surface is gray/white and glistening, often with an obvious interwoven fascicular pattern.

Histological Features

Tumors can be well differentiated, with spindle shaped tumor cells arranged in interwoven or *herringbone* patterns (fig. 2.21). Cytoplasm is scant, and nuclei are elongate to oval with inconspicuous nucleoli. More anaplastic tumors can have marked cellular pleomorphism. Ovoid, polygonal, and multinucleated giant cells are seen, often with large round to oval nuclei and prominent nucleoli. The number of mitotic figures varies widely. Peripheral aggregates of lymphocytes are occasionally seen.

Additional Diagnostic Criteria

The diagnosis of fibrosarcoma is usually not difficult; however, in rare instances differentiation from peripheral nerve sheath tumors (PNSTs) and leiomyosarcomas can be problematic. PNSTs usually have finer more delicate cells arranged in shorter interwoven fascicles, palisades, or whorls. The collagenous stroma can be more pronounced in fibrosarcomas than in PNSTs or leiomyosarcomas, and a Masson's trichrome stain will distinguish between collagen and smooth muscle. There has

been much ado about the more rounded shape of nuclei in leiomyosarcomas as opposed to fibrosarcomas, but this feature is not reliable. The cytoplasm of leiomyosarcoma cells tends to be more eosinophilic and abundant and can have a bubbly or vacuolar appearance. Immunohistochemistry is not particularly useful as all these tumors are vimentin positive, and actin positivity is notoriously nonspecific.

Growth, Metastasis, and Treatment

Tumors are infiltrative and recurrent, but metastasis is uncommon. Surgical excision remains the treatment of choice. Radiation can be a successful adjunct therapy, especially when complete excision is difficult. Surgery with follow-up radiotherapy can result in increased tumor-free intervals and overall improved long-term control.[4]

FELINE VACCINE–ASSOCIATED FIBROSARCOMA

General Considerations

This relatively new entity was first described in 1991. Since then it has been shown to be an especially aggressive, recurrent variant of fibrosarcoma with high mortality.[5,6] Other vaccine associated sarcomas occur in the cat (malignant fibrous histiocytomas, osteosarcomas, chondrosarcomas, and rhabdomyosarcomas), but these are seen at decreased incidence.[7,8] The histological features of these other sarcomas are described below and in other chapters, but the information listed here concerning signalment, incidence, site, gross morphology, growth, metastasis, and treatment pertain to all vaccine-associated sarcomas.

Incidence, Age, Breed, and Sex

The tumor is seen in cats as young as 3 years of age, but the mean age is 8.1 years, which is slightly younger than that seen in cats (mean = 9.2 years) with fibrosarcomas that are not vaccine associated.[9] There is no sex predilection. True incidence is difficult to determine, but estimates range from 1:1000 to 1:10,000 tumors per vaccinated cat.[10]

Site and Gross Morphology

Vaccine-associated sarcomas arise at vaccination sites on the neck, thorax, lumbar region, flank, and limbs. The most typical presentation is a well-circumscribed, firm white mass in the subcutis or skeletal muscle, with a cystic center containing thin watery or mucinous fluid.

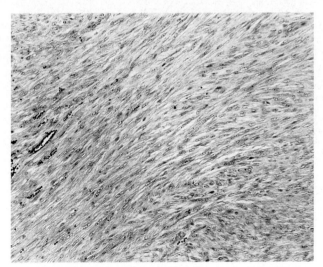

Fig. 2.21.   Fibrosarcoma, subcutis, canine.

Histological Features

At low magnification, the tumor is circular. When in the subcutis, it is usually associated with and extends downward from the panniculus carnosus muscle. There is often a partial fibrous capsule. Despite the circumscribed gross appearance of the tumor, histological "tongues" of tumor are often seen extending away from the mass along fascial planes. Vaccine-associated fibrosarcomas may be well differentiated, with plump spindle cells arranged in interwoven bundles; however, they tend to be more anaplastic, with cells of variable size and shape, pleomorphic nuclei, and increased numbers of multinucleated cells (fig. 2.22 A,B). Peripheral inflammation, consisting predominantly of lymphocytes and macrophages, is common.[11]

Additional Diagnostic Criteria

The presence of peripheral aggregates of macrophages containing globular gray/brown intracytoplasmic material (shown to be aluminum, a common vaccine adjuvant) supports the diagnosis of vaccine associated sarcoma.[6]

The cytological distinction between vaccine associated fibrosarcoma and postvaccinal inflammation is extremely difficult because fibroblasts arising in granulation tissue are often pleomorphic and anaplastic, mimicking neoplastic cells. Excisional biopsy is more reliable and is the method of choice for a definitive diagnosis; however, since there appears to be a continuum from inflammation and fibroplasia to neoplasia, even some histological preparations can be problematic.

Growth and Metastasis

These tumors are highly recurrent, requiring surgical excision one, two, or three times within a 1- or 2-year period.[9] The majority of cats end up being euthanized after repeated surgeries, with or without adjuvant therapy. The metastatic potential of these neoplasms appears to be low initially, but appears to increase with prolonged survival. Metastasis has been reported to occur in regional lymph nodes, mediastinum, and lungs.[9,12,13]

Treatment

Wide surgical margins in all directions should be obtained, which in some cases may include either partial scapulectomy or excision of epaxial muscles and dorsal cervical vertebral processes. Amputation of an involved limb should also be considered. Aggressive surgical excision with wide margins appears to contribute to extended tumor-free interval and survival times in cats.[14,15] Various combinations of immunostimulatory agents and radiotherapy have been used to treat vaccine-associated sarcomas in cats.[19] Preliminary reports suggest that they can extend tumor-free interval and survival times.[16,17]

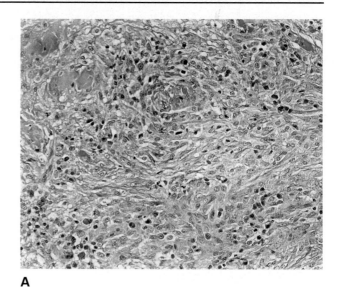

A

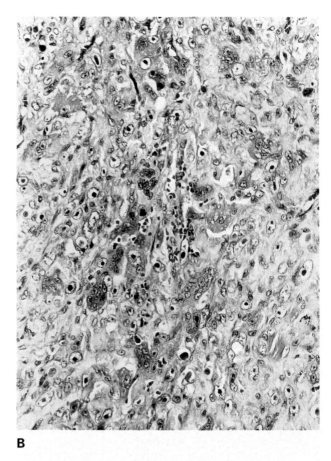

B

Fig. 2.22. **A.** Vaccine-associated fibrosarcoma. **B.** Vaccine-associated sarcoma, anaplastic with giant cells, and an absence of any vaccine-associated products, subcutis, feline.

CANINE MAXILLARY WELL-DIFFERENTIATED FIBROSARCOMA

General Considerations, Age, Sex, Incidence, and Site

This is an uncommon but distinctive variant of fibrosarcoma seen in the muzzle region of adult golden retrievers and other large breed dogs.[18]

Gross Morphology

This tumor usually manifests itself as a lumpy enlargement of the maxillary or, less commonly, the mandibular region. On cut surface, there is a poorly defined firm gray-white mass involving the dermal and subcutaneous tissues.

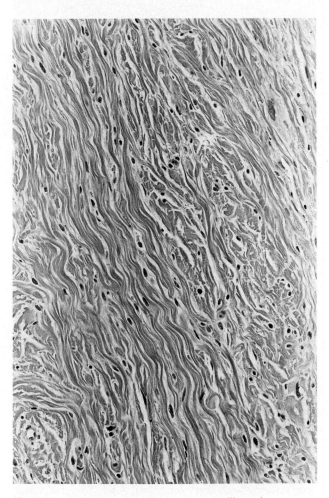

Fig. 2.23. Well-differentiated fibrosarcoma, maxilla, canine.

Histological Features

The neoplasm is composed of well-differentiated fibrocytes and fibroblasts in an extensive connective tissue stroma (fig. 2.23). Nuclear pleomorphism and mitotic figures are rare. The collagen bundles are often haphazard as in the surrounding normal connective tissue, but often there is a repetitive fascicular pattern that sets the tumor apart. Rarely, there is an obvious border with compression, but more often the edge infiltrates the surrounding tissue, making complete excision difficult. There can be a superimposed inflammatory infiltrate, further obscuring the true nature of the neoplastic proliferation.

Additional Diagnostic Criteria

Because of the bland histological appearance of this neoplasm, it could be misdiagnosed as a fibroma or not recognized as abnormal tissue. However, the constellation of breed, site, and histology should lead one to the correct diagnosis.

Growth, Metastasis, and Treatment

Despite the bland appearance of the cells, the neoplasm is progressively infiltrative, with eventual disfigurement and loss of function.

As mentioned above, complete surgical excision is difficult, and other adjuvant therapies have not proven successful.

REFERENCES

1. Goldschmidt, M.H., and Shofer, F.S. (1998) *Skin Tumors of the Dog and Cat.* Butterworth Heinemann, Oxford.
2. Scott, D.W. (1988) *Large Animal Dermatology.* W.B. Saunders Co. Philadelphia, pp. 432–446.
3. Snyder, S.P., and Thielen, G.H. (1969) Transmissible feline fibrosarcoma. *Nature* 221:1074–1075.
4. Withrow, S.J., and MacEwen, EG. (1996) *Small Animal Clinical Oncology.* W.B. Saunders, Philadelphia.
5. Hendrick, M.J., Goldschmidt, M.H. (1991) Do injection site reactions induce fibrosarcomas in cats (lett)? *J Amer Vet Med Assoc* 199:968.
6. Hendrick, M.J., Goldschmidt, M.H., Shofer, F.S., Wang, Y.Y., and Somlyo, A.P. (1992) Postvaccinal sarcomas in the cat: Epidemiology and electron probe microanalytical identification of aluminum. *Cancer Res* 52:19, 5391–5394.
7. Hendrick, M.J., Brooks, J.J. (1994) Postvaccinal sarcomas in the cat: Histology and immunohistochemistry. *Vet Pathol* 31:126–129.
8. Dubielzig, R.R., Hawkins, K.L., and Miller, P.E. (1993) Myofibroblastic sarcoma originating at the site of rabies vaccination in a cat. *J Vet Diagn Invest* 5:637–638.
9. Hendrick, M.J., Shofer, F.S., Goldschmidt, M.H., Haviland, J., et al. (1994) Comparison of fibrosarcomas that developed at vaccination sites and at nonvaccination sites in cats: 239 cases (1991–1992). *J Amer Vet Med Assoc* 205:1425–1429.

10. Kass, P.H., Barnes, W.G., Jr., Spangler, W.L., Chome, B.B., et al. (1993) Epidemiologic evidence for a causal relation between vaccination and fibrosarcoma tumorigenesis in cats. *J Amer Vet Med Assoc* 203:396–405.

11. Doddy, F.D., Glickman, L.T., Glickman, N.W., and Janovitz, E.B. (1996) Feline fibrosarcomas at vaccination sites and non-vaccination sites. *J Comp Pathol* 114:165–174.

12. Rudmann, D.G., Van Alstine, W.G., Doddy, F., Sandsky, G.E., Barkdull, T., and Janovitz, E.B. (1996) Pulmonary and mediastinal metastasis of a vaccination-site sarcoma in a cat. *Vet Pathol* 33:466–469.

13. Esplin, D.G., Jaffe, M.H., (1996) McGill, L.D. Metastasizing liposarcoma associated with a vaccination site in a cat. *Feline Pract* 24:20–23.

14. Davidson, E.B., Gregory, C.R., and Kass, P.H. (1997) Surgical excision of soft tissue fibrosarcomas in cats. *Vet Surg* 26:265–269.

15. Hershey, A.E., Sorenmo, K.U., Hendrick, M.J., Shofer, F.S., and Vail, D.M. (2000) Prognosis for presumed feline vaccine-associated sarcoma after excision: 61 cases (1986–1996). *J Amer Vet Med Assoc* 216:58–61.

16. King, G.K., Yates, K.M., Greenlee, P.G., Pierce, K.R. et al. (1995) The effect of acemannan immunostimulant in combination with surgery and radiation therapy on spontaneous canine and feline fibrosarcomas. *J Amer Anim Hosp Assoc* 31:439–447.

17. Cronin, K.L., Page, R.L., Spodnick, G., et al. (1998) Radiation and surgery for fibrosarcoma in 33 cats. *Vet Radiol and Ultrasound* 39:51–56.

18. Ciekot, P.A., Powers, B.E., Withrow, S.J., Straw, R.C. et al. (1994) Histologically low grade, yet biologically high-grade, fibrosarcomas of the mandible and maxilla in dogs: 25 cases (1982–1991). *J Amer Vet Med Assoc* 204:610–615.

19. Barber, L.G., Sorenmo, K.U., Cronin, K.L., Shofer, F.S. (2000) Combined doxorubicin and cyclophosphamide chemotherapy for nonresectable feline fibrosarcomas. *J Amer Anim Hosp Assoc* 36: 416–421.

EQUINE SARCOID

This unique equine lesion is the result of a nonproductive infection with bovine papillomavirus.[1,2] It is worldwide in distribution and is not related to human sarcoidosis.

Incidence, Age, Breed, and Sex

This most common equine skin tumor can be seen in any age horse, but the majority of cases are seen in individuals younger than 4 years of age.

Site and Gross Morphology

Sarcoids can occur anywhere on the body, but especially the head, lips, legs, and ventral trunk (fig. 2.24 A,B). About 40 percent of affected horses have multiple sarcoids.[3] There are four gross morphological types: verrucous, fibroblastic, mixed, and flat.

Histological Features

Histologically, most lesions are composed of a thickened epidermis with prominent epithelial pegs that extend into a dermal proliferation of fibroblasts that are arranged

in whorls, tangles, or herringbone patterns and contain small amounts of collagen (fig. 2.24 C). Nuclear pleomorphism and mitoses vary, but can be pronounced in rapidly growing or recurrent tumors. There can be difficulty differentiating some sarcoids from fibrosarcomas or nerve sheath

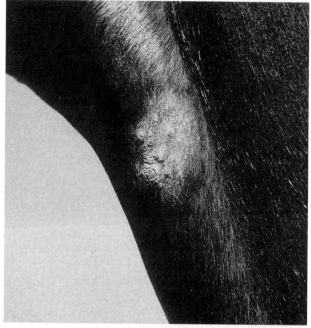

A

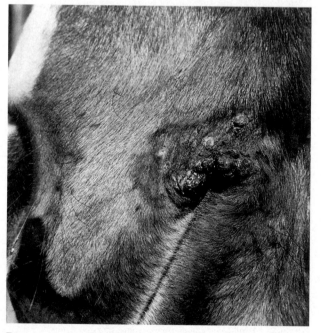

B

Fig. 2.24. Equine sarcoid. **A.** Clinical example on the ventral neck. **B.** Clinical example on commissure of the lip. **(continued)**

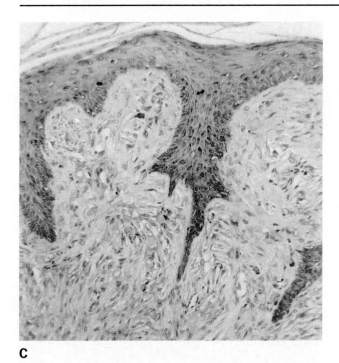

C

Fig. 2.24. (continued) **C.** Proliferation of interwoven fibroblasts and pseudoepitheliomatous hyperplasia.

tumors, especially if there has been ulceration with loss of the distinctive epidermal component. However, these latter tumors are thought to be rare in the horse.

Additional Diagnostic Criteria

Identification of bovine papillomavirus DNA in the nuclei of proliferating fibroblasts by in situ hybridization is diagnostic of sarcoid, but it is seldom necessary due to the unique gross and histological characteristics of this lesion.

Growth, Metastasis, and Treatment

Rare tumors spontaneously regress, but the majority are cured by cryosurgery with clean margins.[4] Recurrence of inadequately excised masses is expected, but metastasis has not been reported.

REFERENCES

1. Otten, N., VonTscharner, C., Lazary, S., Antczak, D.F., et al. (1993) DNA of bovine papillomavirus type 1 and 2 in equine sarcoids: PCR detection and direct sequencing. *Arch Virol* 132:121–131.
2. Angelos, J.A., Marti, E., Lazary, S., Carmichael, L.E. (1991) Characterization of BPV-like DNA in equine sarcoids. *Arch Virol* 119:95–109.
3. Scott, D.W. (1988) *Large Animal Dermatology.* W.B. Saunders Co. Philadelphia, pp. 432–446.
4. Knottenbelt, D.C., and Walker, J.A. (1994) Topical treatment of the equine sarcoid. *Equine Vet Educ* 6:72–75.

MALIGNANT FIBROUS HISTIOCYTOMA

Although still controversial, this uncommon tumor is slowly gaining acceptance in the veterinary literature as a distinct, though histologically diverse, entity.

Human malignant fibrous histiocytoma (MFH) has been divided into subtypes based on the pattern and predominance of the cell types: storiform-pleomorphic, giant cell, inflammatory, and myxoid.[1] Only the first three types have been found with any consistency in domestic animals.[2-5]

Incidence, Age, Breed, Sex, and Site

This tumor occurs in most domestic animal species, but is most frequently seen in the dog; it arises in the skin or spleen as a single, expansile tumor, or it may appear as part of a multiorgan disease that often involves lungs, lymph nodes, spleen, liver, bones, and kidneys.[3,6] Golden retrievers and rottweilers are overrepresented.[3] The relative incidence of focal vs multiorgan MFH in dogs is difficult to determine because most diagnoses are made on biopsy specimens with incomplete follow-up. However, necropsy files at the University of Pennsylvania contain 40 cases of multiorgan MFH in dogs. Two of these animals had skin masses. In the cat, MFH is one of the histological variants of vaccine associated sarcomas,[8] and can also occasionally be seen in the dermis or subcutis in nonvaccine sites. There is no sex predilection. Middle-aged or older individuals are usually affected.

Gross Morphology

The tumor is usually gray/white but can also have red mottling, depending on the amount of hemorrhage and necrosis. Margins are often distinct, but without encapsulation.

Histological Features
Storiform-Pleomorphic

In this variant, fibroblast-like cells are arranged in cartwheel (storiform) patterns, mixed with histiocytoid cells and an infiltrate of lymphocytes, plasma cells, neutrophils, and occasional eosinophils (fig. 2.25 A). Histiocytoid cells are frequently karyomegalic or multinucleate, with nuclear atypia. Some tumors have patchy zones of sclerotic collagenous stroma. This is the most common variant in the skin and organs of dogs.

Inflammatory

As the name implies, an extensive inflammatory cell infiltrate of lymphocytes, plasma cells, eosinophils, and rare neutrophils predominate, with a background of occasionally bizarre histiocytoid cells (fig. 2.25 B). The karyomegaly and nuclear atypia of the histiocytoid cells distinguishes this proliferation from a purely inflammatory process. This variant is rare, and it occurs most often in the spleen of dogs.

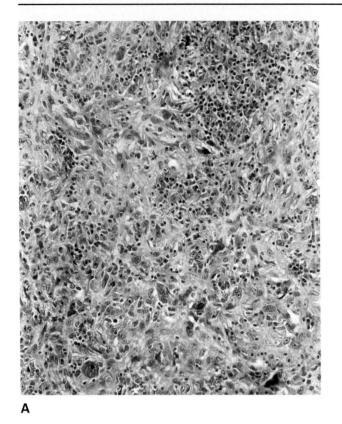

A

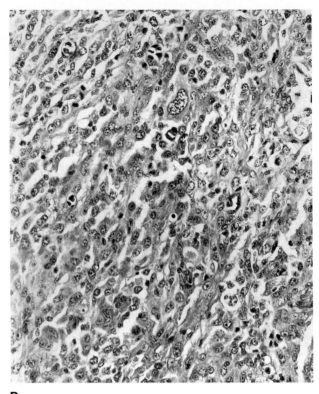

B

C

Fig. 2.25. Malignant fibrous histiocytoma. **A.** Storiform-pleomorphic variant, subcutis, canine. **B.** Inflammatory variant, spleen, canine. **C.** Giant cell variant, skin, canine.

Giant Cell (fig. 2.25 C)

These tumors have numerous multinucleated giant cells mixed with spindle cells and mononuclear histiocytic cells. Although occasionally present, inflammatory cells are not a consistent feature of this variant. The most common subtype in the cat, this tumor has also been called *giant cell tumor of soft parts.*

Additional Diagnostic Criteria

The histological features of the storiform-pleomorphic variant of MFH are unique and are usually diagnostic. However, anaplastic carcinomas with large bizarre karyomegalic cells, desmoplasia, and inflammation can resemble this variant of MFH. Immunopositivity for keratins should distinguish carcinomas from MFH. As mentioned above, the inflammatory variant of MFH is almost always in the spleen and is usually distinguished from inflammation or a nodule of hyperplasia by the nuclear atypia of the histiocytoid cells. The giant cell variant could be confused with either fibrosarcoma with giant cells or osteosarcoma. In fibrosarcoma and osteosarcoma, the giant cell component is not the predominant cell type. Also, the diagnosis of osteosarcoma is contingent upon finding neoplastic osteoid or bone, neither of which is found in giant cell

MFH. Ultrastructural studies reveal the tumor cells in MFH to be characteristic of fibroblasts with or without cytoplasmic filaments consistent with actin.[1,7]

Immunohistochemical analysis is compatible with a fibroblastic/myofibroblastic phenotype, with variable positivity for vimentin, actin, and rarely, desmin.[6,8,9]

Cytology of MFH is often diagnostic as the cell population is a unique mixture of poorly cohesive spindle cells and rounder mononuclear or multinucleated histiocytic cells.

Growth, Metastasis, and Treatment

Dermal or subcutaneous MFH tends to be locally expansile. Reports vary as to the metastatic potential of this neoplasm. This may be due to its multicentric nature and whether or not tumors in other organs represent true metastasis. Any individual with MFH should be given a very guarded prognosis.

Complete excision can be curative for solitary dermal or subcutaneous masses. There is no recognized successful treatment for multicentric MFH.

REFERENCES

1. Enzinger, F.M., and Weiss, S.E. (1995) *Soft Tissue Tumors,* 3rd ed. Mosby, St. Louis, pp. 355–380.
2. Waters, C.B., Morrison, W.B., DeNicola, D.B., Widmer, W.R., et al. (1994) Giant cell variant of malignant fibrous histiocytoma in dogs: 10 cases (1986–1993). *J Amer Vet Med Assoc* 205:1420–1424.
3. Kerlin, R.L., and Hendrick, M.J. (1996) Malignant fibrous histiocytoma and malignant histiocytosis in the dog—convergent or divergent phenotypic differentiation? *Vet Pathol* 33:713–716.
4. Gibson, K.L., Blass, C.E., Simpson, M., and Gaunt, S.D. (1989) Malignant fibrous histiocytoma in a cat. *J Amer Vet Med Assoc* 194:1443–1445.
5. Sartin, E.A., Hudson, J.A., Herrera, G.A., Dickson, A.M., et al. (1996) Invasive malignant fibrous histiocytoma in a cow. *J Am Vet Med Assoc* 208:1709–1710.
6. Hendrick, M.J., Brooks, J.J., and Bruce, E. (1992) Six cases of malignant fibrous histiocytoma of the canine spleen. *Vet Pathol* 29:351–354.
7. Confer, A.W., Enright, F.M., and Beard, G.B. (1981) Ultrastructure of a feline extraskeletal giant cell tumor (malignant fibrous histiocytoma) *Vet Pathol* 18:738–744.
8. Hendrick, M.J., and Brooks, J.J. (1994) Postvaccinal sarcomas in the cat: Histology and immunohistochemistry. *Vet Pathol* 31:126–129.
9. Pace, L.W., Kreeger, J.M., Miller, M.A., Turk, J.R., et al. (1994) Immunohistochemical staining of feline malignant fibrous histiocytomas. *Vet Pathol* 31:168–172.

MYXOMA AND MYXOSARCOMA

These are tumors of fibroblast origin distinguished by their abundant myxoid matrix rich in mucopolysaccharides. Myxomas/myxosarcomas are rare, occurring in middle-aged or older dogs and cats.

Gross Morphology

The majority arise in the subcutis of the trunk or limbs. The gross appearance varies little between myxomas and myxosarcomas. They are soft, gray-white, poorly defined masses which exude a stringy clear mucoid fluid.

Histological Features

Both tumors are composed of an unencapsulated proliferation of stellate to spindle shaped fibroblasts loosely arranged in an abundant myxoid matrix (fig. 2.26). This matrix, rich in acid mucopolysaccharides, stains light blue with routine hematoxylin and eosin (H&E) stains. Cellularity is low, mitoses are rare, and there is little or no cytological atypia in myxomas. Nuclei tend to be small and hyperchromatic. Increases in cellular density, nuclear pleomorphism, and mitoses warrant the diagnosis of myxosarcoma, but the distinction is often subtle.

Growth, Metastasis, and Treatment

Surgical excision is the treatment of choice. Myxomas and myxosarcomas are infiltrative, with poorly defined margins. Recurrence is likely in either case; metastasis is rare, however.

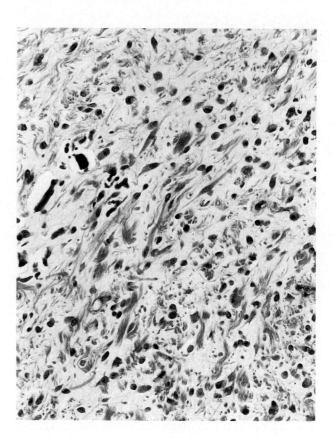

Fig. 2.26. Myxosarcoma, subcutis, canine.

Additional Diagnostic Criteria

Cytological smears of these tumors are often difficult to prepare because of the slimy consistency of the tumor and the paucity of cells that adhere to slides.

TUMOR-LIKE LESIONS

Collagenous Hamartoma

This common nonneoplastic lesion of dogs is a nodular, poorly circumscribed focus of redundant collagen in the superficial dermis. Although this lesion is also called *collagenous nevus,*[1,2] the term *hamartoma,* which precludes confusion of this lesion with pigmented (melanocytic) tumors or tumors present at birth, is preferred. The pathogenesis of collagenous hamartomas is unknown.

It is one of the many common dermal proliferations in aged dogs, and there is no recognized breed or sex predilection.

Site and Gross Morphology

Hamartomas can occur anywhere, but there appears to be a predilection for the digits. These masses are usually small nodular elevations of the epidermis. There can be mild alopecia but no evidence of erosion, ulceration, or other signs of self-trauma.

Histological Features

In contrast to fibromas, the collagen fiber pattern is not repetitive; it is similar to that seen in adjacent normal collagen (fig. 2.27). The proliferation is limited to the superficial dermis and usually results in slight elevation of the epidermis and loss, separation, or distortion of adnexal structures.

Additional Diagnostic Criteria

The differentiation between skin tags and collagenous hamartomas is subtle in some instances and not clinically important. Unlike collagenous hamartomas, which usually show some loss or distortion of adnexa, skin tags are usually pedunculated pieces of excess skin that contain all of the skin's normal constituents. Because of their nipple-like growth, skin tags are subject to external trauma with secondary ulceration and inflammation.

Growth and Treatment

These masses are slow growing and usually are excised to rule out other more clinically significant lesions. Excision is curative.

Nodular Dermatofibrosis of the German Shepherd

This is a rare syndrome of multiple fibrous nodules in the dermis and subcutis. Female German shepherds are preferentially affected, but the disease can occasionally

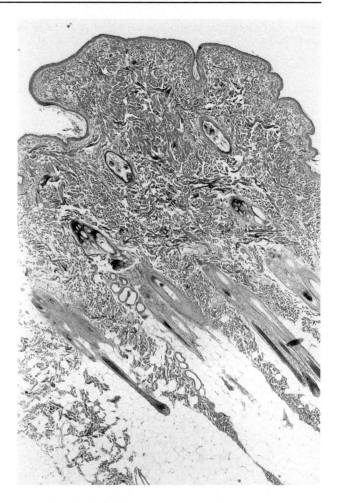

Fig. 2.27. Collagenous hamartoma, skin, canine. Note the haphazard arrangement of collagen that is similar to the adjacent normal collagen.

occur in other breeds. The skin lesions may precede or coincide with unilateral or bilateral renal adenomas or carcinomas.[3,4,5,6,7]

Site and Gross Morphology

The nodules, which can number in the hundreds, are generally found on the limbs, ears, and back. They range from a few millimeters to 4 cm in diameter.[1,2] They are well circumscribed, but when large they can result in alopecia and ulceration of the overlying skin.

Histological Features

There is a focal proliferation of collagen covered by a mildly hyperplastic epidermis. Collagen bundles can be normal or slightly thickened, but are arranged in the haphazard pattern seen in normal dermis. Adnexal structures are normal or hyperplastic. The collagenous proliferation is poorly demarcated from adjacent normal collagen bundles in the dermis, but the subcutaneous portion is well circumscribed and can push or separate normal structures in this location. Inflammation is usually minimal.

Additional Diagnostic Criteria

In contrast to collagenous hamartomas, these lesions are not limited to the superficial dermis, and adnexal structures are normal or hyperplastic. However, these differences can be subtle. It is the multiplicity of these lesions that is unique. When these lesions are found in female German shepherds, clinicians should run additional tests to evaluate the kidneys.

Growth and Treatment

Because of the multicentricity of these lesions, there is no effective treatment. The nodules are benign, but some will be surgically removed for cosmetic reasons or if they interfere with function.

Nodular Fasciitis

The term *nodular fasciitis* has been borrowed from the human literature[8] and refers to a nonneoplastic, enigmatic inflammatory lesion with many clinical and histological features suggestive of a locally invasive fibrosarcoma.

Incidence, Age, Breed, Sex, and Site

This lesion has been reported almost exclusively in the dog (collies, most notably) as a deep dermal or subcutaneous mass, most often found in the corneal and scleral regions of the eye.[9] It is called *nodular granulomatous episcleritis* in this site, but virtually identical lesions can be found on the trunk and limbs of dogs.

Gross and Histological Features

The lesion tends to be firm, nodular, and poorly demarcated. The cut surface is usually gray/white with varying degrees of red mottling. Nodular fasciitis is a mixture of fibroblasts and fibrocytes arranged in short bundles or whorls and mixed with variable amounts of lymphocytes, plasma cells, and macrophages (fig. 2.28). Sometimes the inflammatory infiltrate is marked, obscuring the proliferating spindle cells, but these areas can alternate with zones of acellular sclerotic collagen. Fibroblasts, particularly in the center of the lesion, are immature in appearance, with numerous mitotic figures, sometimes leading to a misdiagnosis of fibrosarcoma. The edges of the lesion often merge with surrounding connective tissue and muscle, resulting in spiky or feathery margins.

Additional Diagnostic Criteria

In lesions of nodular fasciitis where the fibroblast proliferation is minimal or is obscured by inflammatory cells, the lesion can be difficult to distinguish from cutaneous histiocytosis (see below). Nodular fasciitis is usually focal and deep dermal or subcutaneous, as opposed to cutaneous histiocytosis, which tends to be multifocal and more superficial. Also, cutaneous histiocytosis has not been described in the sclera.

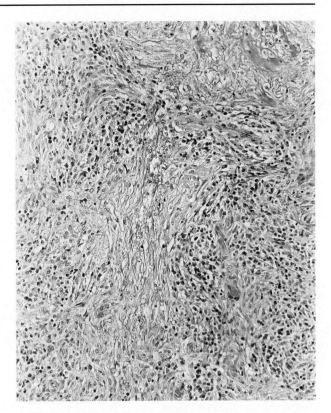

Fig. 2.28. Nodular fasciitis, sclera, canine.

Growth and Treatment

Lesions in the scleral region may show partial regression following corticosteroid therapy, but they tend to recur. Those elsewhere on the body are usually cured by complete excision.

REFERENCES

1. Goldschmidt, M.H., and Shofer, F.S. (1998) *Skin Tumors of the Dog and Cat.* Butterworth Heinemann, Oxford, p. 152.
2. Gross, T.L., Ihrke, P.E., and Walder, E.J. (1992) *Veterinary Dermatopathology: A Macroscopic and Microscopic Evaluation of Canine and Feline Skin Disease.* Mosby Yearbook, St. Louis, pp. 407–408.
3. Perry. W. (1995) Generalised nodular dermatofibrosis and renal cystadenoma in a series of 10 closely related German shepherd dogs. *Aust Vet Pract* 25:90–93.
4. Marks, S.L., Farman, C.A., and Peaston, A. (1993) Nodular dermatofibrosis and renal cystadenomas in a golden retriever. *Vet Dermatol* 4:133–137.
5. Atlee, B.A., DeBoer, D.J., Ihrke, P.J., Stannard, A.A., et al. (1991) Nodular dermatofibrosis in German shepherd dogs as a marker for renal cystadenocarcinoma. *J Amer Anim Hosp Assoc* 27:481–487.
6. Lium, B., and Moe, L. (1985) Hereditary multifocal renal adenocarcinomas and nodular dermatofibrosis in the German shepherd dog: Macroscopic and histopathologic changes. *Vet Pathol* 22:447–455.
7. Suter, M., Lott-Stolz, G., and Wild, P. (1983) Generalized nodular dermatofibrosis in six Alsatians. *Vet Pathol* 20:632–634.

8. Enzinger, F.M., and Weiss, S.E. (1995) *Soft Tissue Tumors,* 3rd ed. Mosby, St. Louis, pp. 167–172.
9. Gwin, R.M., Gelatt, K.N., and Peiffer, R.L. (1977) Ophthalmic nodular fasciitis in the dog. *J Amer Vet Med Assoc* 170:611–614.

CANINE HEMANGIOPERICYTOMA

Although the name of this common mesenchymal neoplasm suggests pericyte origin, the actual histogenesis is uncertain. The name was bestowed because of some minor histological similarities to the tumor in humans, but the actual gross and histological characterisitics of the human tumor are quite different from the canine tumor.[1] Still, the original nomenclature has been retained in veterinary pathology.

Incidence, Age, Breed, and Sex

Hemangiopericytomas are very common in middle-aged or older dogs. Large breed dogs appear overrepresented, but there is no sex predilection. Tumors with a similar morphology occur rarely in cats and are most likely of peripheral nerve sheath origin.

Site and Gross Morphology

Tumors are usually solitary, arise in the subcutis around joints of limbs, and are multilobulated and infiltrative. They have variable gross appearances: white/gray to red, soft to firm, rubbery to "fatty." In fact, many lesions are thought by submitting veterinarians to be lipomas. When cut, these latter tumors may exude a slimy mucoid material.

Histological Features, Growth, and Metastasis

Histologically, the hallmark of this neoplasm is the presence of perivascular whorls of fusiform cells (fig. 2.29). Although this feature may be present in other sarcomas, it is usually dominant in hemangiopericytomas. Cells may also be arranged in interlacing bundles or storiform patterns. The neoplastic cells can range, sometimes within the same tumor, from thick to thin, spindle shaped to almost pyriform, and they are separated by variable amounts of collagenous stroma. In some tumors there is patchy, though abundant, mucinous matrix, which can lead to a misdiagnosis of myxosarcoma. The neoplasm may be well demarcated from the surrounding tissue, but it often invades along fascial planes, leading to frequent recurrences. Cellular pleomorphism and mitotic activity are usually low in primary tumors, but cellular atypia, number of mitoses, and multinucleated forms increase with each recurrence. Reports suggest that mitotic index is the key prognostic feature of hemangiopericytomas and that the usually low metastatic potential of hemangiopericytomas increases with each recurrence.[2,3]

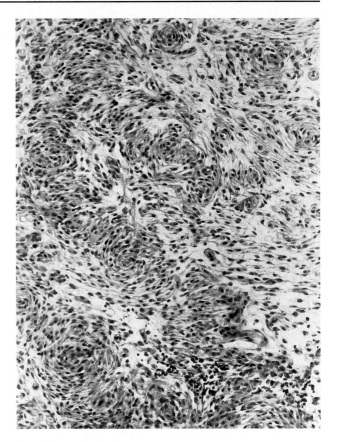

Fig. 2.29. Canine hemangiopericytoma, subcutis, canine.

Additional Diagnostic Criteria

It continues to be difficult to distinguish hemangiopericytomas from peripheral nerve sheath tumors (PNSTs). Histologically, PNSTs are characterized by interwoven bundles of small wavy spindle cells with occasional palisading and whorls. In contrast to hemangiopericytomas, whorls in PNSTs are less prominent, and most whorls encircle sclerotic collagen rather than capillaries. The spindle cells are more delicate and often have more intercellular fibrillar or mucinous matrix than in hemangiopericytoma. Still, there is enough histological crossover to make the differentiation between these two neoplasms difficult. Most diagnoses of these two neoplasms are based on tradition rather than auxiliary tests such as electron microscopy or immunohistochemistry. Reports employing these techniques often have conflicting or ambiguous results. Light and electron microscopic features which have been ascribed to hemangiopericytoma cells include incomplete poorly developed basal laminae, rudimentary intercellular junctions, pinocytotic vesicles, and intracytoplasmic filaments.[4] Pericytes are rather nondescript cells ultrastructurally, and although the features ascribed to hemangiopericytoma cells are compatible with pericytes, they do not preclude the possibility of perineural fibroblast origin, because cells of such origin have identical ultrastructural characteristics. Pericytes are only immunopositive for vimentin; perineural fibroblasts, despite their mesenchymal origin, are reported to be S-100 negative and epithelial membrane antigen (EMA) positive.[1] Theoretically, this latter marker could prove valuable in immunohistochemical differentiation of these two neoplasms, since pericytes should be negative. However, the lack of EMA positivity is most likely irrelevant because work at this laboratory and elsewhere suggests that commercially available antibodies to human EMA do not cross-react with the dog.

Treatment

Aggressive initial surgery is considered the best treatment for hemangiopericytoma. Radiation therapy can result in some tumor control and longer survival times.[5] Chemotherapy has proven unsuccessful.

BENIGN PERIPHERAL NERVE SHEATH TUMOR (NEUROFIBROMA, SCHWANNOMA)

Classically, the term *Schwannoma* is used when the tumor cells are solely of Schwann cell origin. Neurofibroma/sarcoma is used when the tumor is composed of Schwann cells and perineural cells. This distinction can occasionally be made by immunostaining with S-100, GFAP, other neural markers, or leu 7; however, we choose to combine these entities under the title "peripheral nerve sheath tumors" (PNSTs) because most diagnoses are made without these ancillary tests and because the markers, when they are used, are nonspecific. Some pathologists would prefer to restrict the term *peripheral nerve sheath tumor* to those neoplasms that arise and spread within peripheral nerves. Others contend that there is a subset of PNSTs that arise in the skin and subcutis, presumably from small peripheral nerves. Most would agree that there are differences in the histology and biological behavior of these two entities; however, the diagnosis of soft tissue PNSTs is well established in veterinary medicine and pathology.

Incidence, Age, Breed, Sex, and Site

In cats, benign PNSTs are uncommon and are found predominantly on the head.[6,7] The tumor is rare in the dog. In cattle, multiple tumors may be seen in the subcutis, heart, and brachial plexus, resembling von Recklinghausen's disease in humans. Horse PNSTs are most common on the eyelids.[8] Middle-aged or older animals of all species are preferentially affected, but PNSTs can occur in calves and in horses as young as 3 years of age.[8]

Gross Morphology

Tumors are firm to soft, well circumscribed, unencapsulated masses in the dermis (most common in the cat) or subcutis. They are usually white to gray and sometimes bulge slightly on cut surface.

Histological Features

Benign PNSTs are composed of wavy spindle cells arranged in bundles, palisades, and whorls. They have low cellularity, with spindle or polygonal cells loosely distributed in a fibrillar or mucinous matrix. Nuclei are small and normochromatic. The classic Antoni A configuration with Verocay bodies has been considered the hallmark of benign PNSTs (Schwannomas) in humans,[1] but it is rare in tumors of domestic animals. Small nerves are occasionally seen in or adjacent to the tumor, but their presence does not preclude another cell of origin.

Additional Diagnostic Criteria

The various markers that might be used to identify cells of nerve sheath origin (S-100, GFAP, myelin basic protein, neuron specific enolase) are notoriously nonspecific or at present not readily cross-reactive in domestic animal species. The specificity and ease of use of these immunomarkers will undoubtedly improve with time and experience and should, in the future, aid in our ability to diagnose these tumors.

Growth, Metastasis, and Treatment

Complete excision is usually curative, but a few tumors will recur. Recurrence is especially common in horses, often requiring multiple surgeries.[8]

MALIGNANT PERIPHERAL NERVE SHEATH TUMOR

In the dog, malignant PNSTs (neurofibrosarcoma, malignant Schwannoma) and hemangiopericytomas have similar histomorphologic features, and depending on the bias of the educational facility, the two tumors may be "lumped" or "split."

Incidence, Age, Breed, Sex, and Site

Because of the similarities between PNSTs and canine hemangiopericytoma, the true incidence of this tumor is unknown. Most reports describe the site distribution, gross appearance, and biological behavior of this neoplasm as similar to that of hemangiopericytoma, which is not surprising. Malignant PNSTs are uncommon in cats and extremely rare in large domestic animals. Those arising in cats tend to be on the head.[6,7]

Histological Features

The histological features of malignant PNSTs and their similarities to canine hemangiopericytoma are described above. In general, the majority of the cells of malignant PNSTs are arranged in small interwoven bundles with varying amounts of intervening collagenous or mucinous stroma (fig. 2.30). Whorls are seen, but are usually around collagen bundles rather than blood vessels. The classic palisading seen in benign PNSTs is usually absent, and the cells are more densely grouped. Nuclei are oval

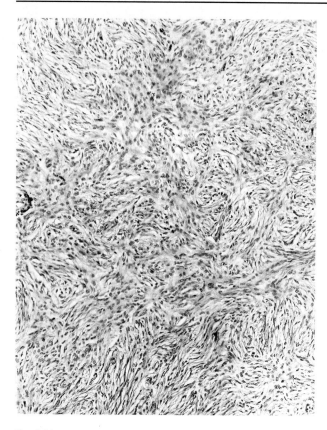

Fig. 2.30. Malignant peripheral nerve sheath tumor, skin, canine.

with mild pleomorphism. The mitotic index varies, but it is usually low to moderate. Scattered lymphocytes and mast cells are commonly seen.

Additional Diagnostic Criteria

Our ability to distinguish these two tumors histologically and biologically will no doubt improve as immunohistochemical evaluation becomes more routine at diagnostic facilities, and as our antibodies become more specific.

Growth, Metastasis, and Treatment

These tumors commonly recur after excision, but metastasis is rare. The therapeutic effects of radiation have not been determined.

REFERENCES

1. Enzinger, F.M., and Weiss, S.E. (1995) *Soft Tissue Tumors,* 3rd ed. Mosby, St. Louis.
2. Bostock, D.E., and Dye, M.T. (1980) Prognosis after surgical excision of canine fibrous connective tissue sarcomas. *Vet Pathol* 17:581–588.
3. Postorino, N.C., Berg, R.J., Powers, B.E., et al. (1988) Prognostic variables for canine hemangiopericytoma: 50 cases (1979–1984). *J Amer Anim Hosp Assoc* 24:501–509.
4. Xu, F.N. (1986) Ultrastructure of canine hemangiopericytoma. *Vet Pathol* 23:643–645.
5. Evans, S.M. (1987) Canine hemangiopericytoma. A retrospective analysis of response to surgery and orthovoltage radiation. *Vet Radiol* 28:13–16.
6. Goldschmidt, M.H., and Shofer, F.S. (1998) *Skin Tumors of the Dog and Cat.* Butterworth Heinemann, Oxford.
7. Gross, T.L., Ihrke, P.E., and Walder, E.J. (1992) *Veterinary Dermatopathology: A Macroscopic and Microscopic Evaluation of Canine and Feline Skin Disease.* Mosby Yearbook, St. Louis, pp. 438–443.
8. Scott, D.W. (1988) *Large Animal Dermatology.* W.B. Saunders Co., Philadelphia, pp. 432–446.

LIPOMA

This is a common benign tumor of well-differentiated adipocytes (fig. 2.31 A) seen in most domestic animals. Rare tumors will contain collagen (fibrolipomas) or clusters of small blood vessels (angiolipomas) (fig. 2.31 B).

Incidence, Age, Breed, and Sex

Lipomas are most common in the dog and uncommon in other species. Female dogs and castrated male cats appear predisposed to the formation of these tumors, and some animals will have multiple tumors at presentation.

Site and Gross Morphology

Predominantly subcutaneous, lipomas occur most commonly in the trunk, gluteal region, and proximal limbs.

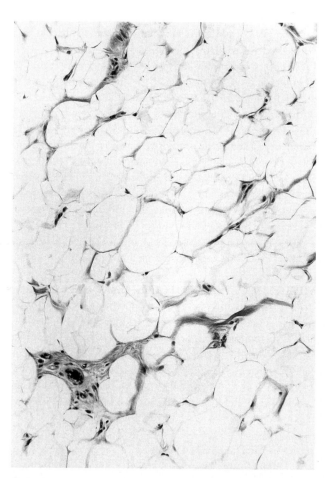

A

Fig. 2.31. Lipoma, subcutis, canine. **A.** Lipoma. (continued)

The tumors are well-circumscribed, unencapsulated, soft white to yellow masses, indistinguishable from normal fat. Most are freely moveable over the underlying deeper tissues and can be easily shelled out. They have a distinctive greasy feel and float in water or formalin. A small percentage of lipomas are infiltrative.[1] These look and feel like their counterparts but invade adjacent connective tissue and skeletal muscle, giving the area a *marbled* appearance (fig. 2.31 C). In the horse, lipomas can arise as pedunculated tumors in the mesentery that often strangulate the bowel. In cats, and rarely in dogs, lipomas containing myeloid cells are seen in the spleen, adrenal, and liver. Called *myelolipomas,* they are discrete, unencapsulated, white fatty masses embedded within the parenchyma.

Histological Features

The cells of lipomas are identical to those in normal adipose tissue. Large clear vacuoles replace the cytoplasm, with peripheralization and compression of nuclei. Some tumors have regions of necrosis, inflammation, and/or fibrosis. The predominant infiltrating cells are foamy macrophages, which occasionally are epithelioid and so numerous that they mimic the pleomorphic

lipoblasts seen in liposarcoma. However, the overall pattern and general bland appearance of the macrophages precludes this diagnosis.

Growth and Treatment

The majority of lipomas are slow growing expansile masses that are cured by excision. Infiltrative lipomas, although benign, are more difficult to completely excise and may require multiple excisions (fig. 2.31 C).

LIPOSARCOMA

This malignant counterpart to the lipoma is rare in domestic animals but can be divided into subtypes based on cellular morphology. There is not an accepted classification for these subtypes, and most authors have simply applied nomenclature from the human literature.[2] In this author's experience, liposarcomas in animals can be divided into well-differentiated and anaplastic tumors, the latter called *pleomorphic* by other authors.[3,4] Another variant, *myxoid,* is the least common and most distinctive of the subvariants.[5]

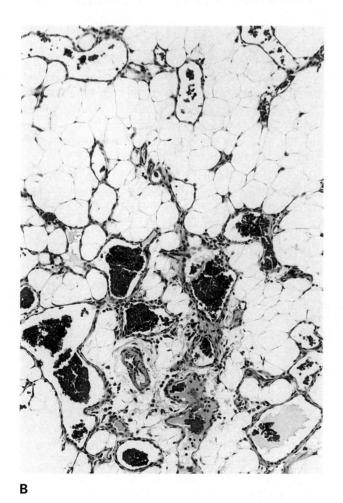

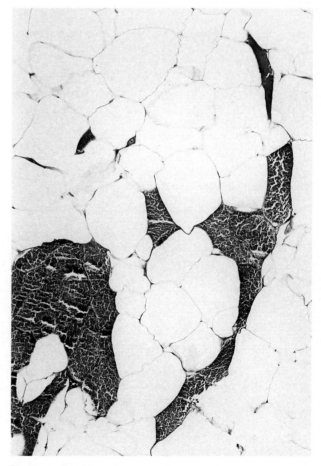

B

C

Fig. 2.31. (continued) **B.** Angiolipoma. **C.** Infiltrative lipoma, flank, canine.

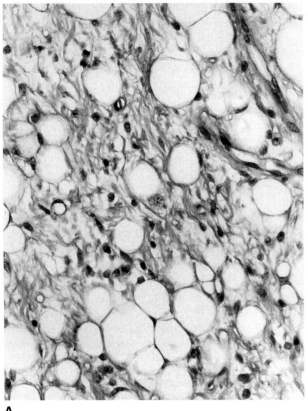

A

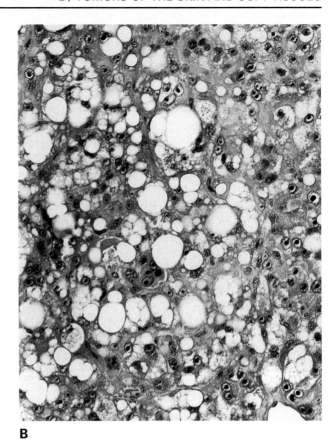

B

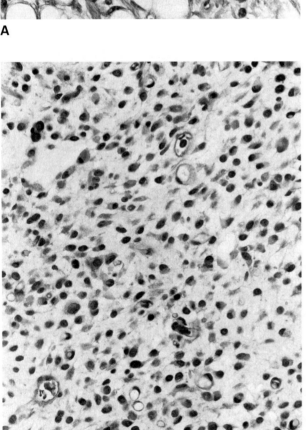

C

Fig. 2.32. Liposarcoma, subcutis, canine. **A.** Well differentiated. **B.** Pleomorphic. **C.** Myxoid. Rare lipid-containing cells distinguish this tumor from a myxosarcoma.

Incidence, Age, Breed, and Sex

Liposarcomas occur in all domestic species but are rare. They are probably most common in the canine; Shetland sheepdogs are preferentially affected.[3] There is no sex predisposition, but the incidence increases with age.

Site and Gross Morphology

The gross appearance of these tumors varies depending on the amount of lipid they produce. Some mimic lipomas, but others are firm, gray-white subcutaneous masses infiltrating adjacent soft tissues and muscle.

Histological Features

Most tumors are composed of round to polygonal cells arranged in sheets, with little or no collagenous stroma. In the well-differentiated variant (fig. 2.32 A), the majority of cells resemble normal adipocytes, with a single clear fat vacuole and a peripheral nucleus. Other cells have variably sized round to oval nuclei and abundant cytoplasm that contains variably sized lipid droplets. The diagnosis in these cases is clear.

The anaplastic or *pleomorphic* variant (fig. 2.32 B) has cells of highly variable morphology mixed with large bizarre multinucleated cells. Diagnostic intracytoplasmic fat vacuoles are usually present, but only in a small percentage of cells. This rare tumor mimics the pleomorphic variant of malignant fibrous histiocytoma. However, the lack of a significant collagenous stroma or a spindle-cell population in a storiform pattern precludes the diagnosis of MFH.

The myxoid variant (fig. 2.32 C) is identified by the presence of scattered spindle cells, lipocytes, and lipoblasts loosely arranged in a "bubbly" mucoid stroma that is alcian blue positive. Resembling myxosarcoma, this tumor is differentiated by the presence of lipid filled vacuoles within the cytoplasm of some of the neoplastic cells. Demonstration of lipid may require histochemistry or ultrastructural study.

Growth and Metastasis

Despite histological distinctions, there appears to be no difference in the biologic behavior of these variants of liposarcoma. Recurrence is common, but reports of metastasis, usually to lung, liver, or bone, are rare.[6]

Treatment

Radiation therapy and chemotherapy have not been shown to have any efficacy against liposarcoma. Complete surgical excision is the best approach.

REFERENCES

1. Bergman, P.J., Withrow, S.J., Straw, R.C., and Powers, B.E. (1994) Infiltrative lipoma in dogs: 16 cases (1981–1992). *J Amer Vet Med Assoc* 205:322–324.
2. Enzinger, F.M., and Weiss, S.E. (1995) *Soft Tissue Tumors,* 3rd ed. Mosby, St. Louis, pp. 438–453.
3. Goldschmidt, M.H., and Shofer, F.S. (1998) *Skin Tumors of the Dog and Cat.* Butterworth Heinemann, Oxford, p. 199.
4. Gross, T.L., Ihrke, P.E., and Walder, E.J. (1992) *Veterinary Dermatopathology: A Macroscopic and Microscopic Evaluation of Canine and Feline Skin Disease.* Mosby Yearbook, St. Louis, pp. 435–436.
5. Messick, J.B., and Radin, M.J. (1989) Cytologic, histological and ultrastructural characteristics of a canine myxoid liposarcoma. *Vet Pathol* 26:520–522.
6. Theilen, G.H., and Madewell, B.R., eds. (1987) *Veterinary Cancer Medicine,* 2nd ed. Lea and Febiger, Philadelphia, p. 292.

HEMANGIOMA

Incidence, Age, Breed, Sex, and Site

Common in dogs, but rare in other domestic animals, hemangiomas are benign tumors of vascular endothelium. They are dermal or subcutaneous tumors occurring anywhere on the body. There is evidence that in some light skinned, short haired dog breeds, hemangiomas may be caused by prolonged exposure to sunlight.[1] Hemangiomas can occur in very young horses, usually on the distal limbs. Hemangiomas in swine are rare, and when present they are usually seen in the scrotum of Yorkshire and Berkshire boars.[2] In the horse and pig, hemangiomas can be congenital.[2]

Gross Morphology

The tumors are well-demarcated, encapsulated masses which range from bright red to dark brown. The darker colored specimens are often mistaken for melanomas. In larger specimens, the cut surface reveals a honeycomb pattern of fibrous trabeculae separating blood filled cavities. In the horse and pig, there is a verrucous variant of hemangioma that is less well demarcated, multinodular, and associated with epidermal hyperkeratosis.[2]

Histological Features

Most tumors are well circumscribed and are composed of variably sized vascular spaces filled with erythrocytes and lined by a single layer of uniform endothelial cells (fig. 2.33 A,B). Organized thrombi are often found in tumors, with foci of hemosiderosis. Variants of these tumors have been called *cavernous* or *capillary,* based on the size of the vascular channels. In the cavernous type, the large channels are separated by a fibrous connective tissue stroma, which can contain lymphocytes and other inflammatory cells. Capillary variants have little stroma, a more cellular appearance, and larger, sometimes pleomorphic, nuclei. Mitotic figures are rare.

Growth, Metastasis, and Treatment

Hemangiomas are generally slow growing and are cured by complete excision. Cryosurgery may be necessary in some of the verrucous variants in large animals.[2]

HEMANGIOSARCOMA

Incidence, Age, Breed, Sex, and Site

Hemangiosarcoma most commonly presents as a multicentric disease involving the spleen, liver, lungs, and right auricle of dogs, especially the German shepherd and golden retriever breeds. The tumor is less frequently seen in the cat, and rarely in large domestic animals.[2,3] The incidence in cats appears to be on the rise, and it is seen on the head (eyelids, especially), distal limbs, and paws.[3,4] Unusual solitary sites of hemangiosarcoma in the dog include the urinary bladder serosa and the capsule of the kidney. Cutaneous involvement can be solitary or, rarely, part of the multicentric syndrome. Some canine dermal hemangiosarcomas appear to be the result of chronic solar irradiation.[1] Short haired, light skinned breeds such as greyhounds, whippets, and American pit bulls are at increased risk, and a small percentage of canine tumors may represent malignant transformation of hemangiomas.[1,3,5]

There is continued controversy over whether multicentric hemangiosarcoma in the dog represents true multicentric origin rather than one primary tumor with metastasis. Based on the knowledge of common metastatic patterns of sarcomas in general, it seems unlikely that there is one primary tumor. The right auricle and spleen could be considered as possible primary sites, but these two sites are commonly involved in the same animal, and neither would be considered as a likely metastatic site. Also, one histo-

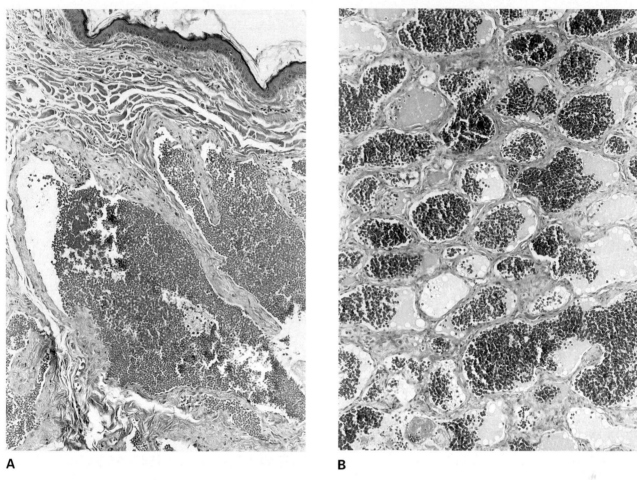

Fig. 2.33. Hemangioma. **A.** Skin, canine. **B.** Canine skin with uniformly sized vessels containing red blood cells and lined by inconspicuous endothelial cells.

logical pattern seen in hepatic hemangiosarcoma demonstrates a scattered "multihit" type of early neoplastic transformation of sinusoidal endothelial cells that would be difficult to explain as metastasis.

Gross Morphology

Dermal or subcutaneous hemangiosarcoma is usually a single well-defined mass which is red/brown to black, soft to firm, and exudes blood when cut.

Histological Features

Histologically, the neoplastic cells are highly variable, ranging from spindle shaped to polygonal to ovoid, and usually form recognizable vascular clefts or channels somewhere in the tumor (fig. 2.34 A). The cells lining the clefts often have prominent, bulging nuclei that are pleomorphic and hyperchromatic. Mitotic figures are frequent. In some areas, the stroma between the clefts is acellular, hyaline, and brightly eosinophilic. There can be large solid areas, indistinguishable from fibrosarcoma or other poorly

differentiated sarcomas. Conversely, there can be large areas of hemorrhage with few cells that mimic hematomas.

Additional Diagnostic Criteria

Traditionally, factor VIII immunopositivity has been considered diagnostic of hemangiosarcoma. Unfortunately, experience has shown that many hemangiosarcomas will *not* stain with this antibody and that some tumors with the histological appearance of lymphangiomas or lymphangiosarcomas *will* stain for factor VIII.

Cytological diagnosis of hemangiosarcoma can be difficult because of the large amount of hemorrhage in the sample. Pleomorphic spindle cells may be seen, but the proportion of these cells may be small.

Growth and Metastasis

Visceral hemangiosarcomas are highly aggressive tumors with a poor prognosis. Death is often associated with rupture of nodules or masses and resultant hemoabdomen or hemopericardium. Cutaneous hemangiosarcomas are less aggressive than their visceral counterparts, with lower metastatic potential and longer survival times.[1,3]

Treatment

Surgical excision is the preferred choice for dermal or subcutaneous hemangiosarcomas. Various chemotherapeutic regimes have been attempted on dogs with multicentric visceral disease with little success.[6,7]

LYMPHANGIOMA AND LYMPHANGIOSARCOMA

General Considerations and Classification

These are tumors of lymphatic endothelium. As with myxomas and myxosarcomas, the distinction between benign and malignant tumors can be minimal.

Incidence, Age, Breed, and Sex

These are rare tumors in all species. Many are congenital or occur within the first few months of life, lead-

ing some to interpret these lesions as nevi rather than neoplasms.[3]

Site and Gross Morphology

ÏLymphangiomas and lymphangiosarcomas tend to be found in the subcutis along the ventral midline and limbs as poorly demarcated dermal masses that are soft and spongy to the touch. They are often wet on cut surface and exude a clear serous fluid.

Histological Features

Histologically, the neoplastic cells resemble normal endothelial cells; however, the cells grow directly on bundles of dermal collagen, dissecting them and forming numerous clefts and channels (fig. 2.34 B). The majority of clefts are devoid of cells, but occasional erythrocytes may be seen, presumably due to trauma or extravasation from nearby blood vessels. Most of the neoplastic cells in lymphangiomas are bland, and mitoses are not evident. The malignant tumor differs little from its benign counterpart except for its increased cellular pleomorphism. Cells lining the clefts and channels have more rounded nuclei with hyperchromatism and a few mitotic figures.

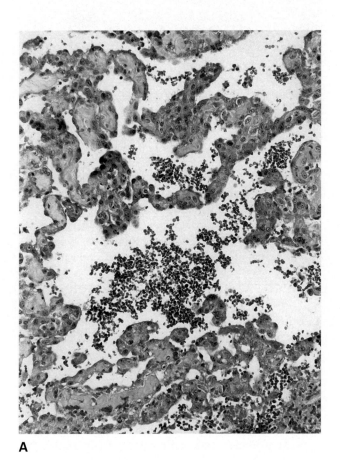

A

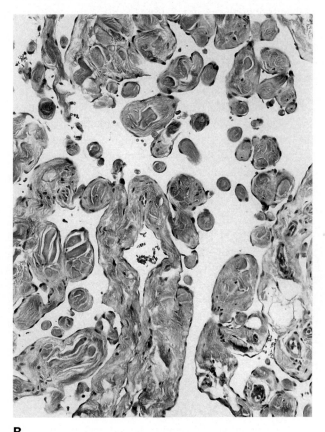

B

Fig. 2.34. Hemangiosarcoma and lymphangiosarcoma, çanine, skin. **A.** Hemangiosarcoma, irregularly shaped and sized vessels with plump endothelial cells lining and filling trabeculae between lumens. **B.** Lymphangiosarcoma, thin, flat endothelium, collagen filled trabeculae, and lumens devoid of red blood cells.

Additional Diagnostic Criteria

The distinction between hemangioma/hemangiosarcoma and lymphangioma/lymphangiosarcoma is based on the apparent close apposition of the cells on the collagen bundles and the relative lack of blood cells in the channels in the latter. Ultrastructurally, lymphangiosarcomas are reported to lack a basal lamina and have discontinuous endothelial cells as opposed to hemangiosarcomas, which have a basal lamina and continuous endothelial cells.[8]

Growth, Metastasis, and Treatment

The infiltrative growth of these tumors makes borders difficult to assess. Recurrence is common. Metastasis is rare. Early surgical excision can be curative. There is little published data on the success of any other modalities. One reported case of lymphangioma was cured by radiation therapy.[9]

FELINE VENTRAL ABDOMINAL ANGIOSARCOMA

There is controversy over whether this tumor is of blood vessel or lymphatic origin. The term *angiosarcoma* is therefore preferred (fig. 2.35).

Incidence, Age, Breed, Sex, and Site

This rare tumor is seen only in the cat, where it presents as a distinctive lesion on the caudoventral abdominal wall.

Gross Morphology

The caudoventral abdominal wall and mammary region has a diffuse "bruised" appearance, as if there were dermal and subcutaneous hemorrhage. When cut, the region is discolored red/black and oozes a serosanguineous fluid. A distinct mass is usually not discernible, but the area can vary in texture from soft and gelatinous to firm.

Histological Features

Histologically, the subcutis in this area is diffusely edematous, hemorrhagic, and infiltrated by neoplastic endothelial cells that form clefts and channels. Most neoplastic cells hug the collagen and show moderate to marked nuclear pleomorphism. Although there is extensive hemorrhage throughout the area, the vascular channels of the neoplasm usually contain only a few erythrocytes. Scattered throughout the tumor and the adjacent soft tissues are lymphocytes, plasma cells, and hemosiderophages.

Additional Diagnostic Criteria

It is controversial whether the endothelial cell proliferation in this syndrome is of blood or lymphatic vessel origin.[3,8,10,11] Therefore, the diagnosis of lymphangiosarcoma is favored by some authors, based on light micro-

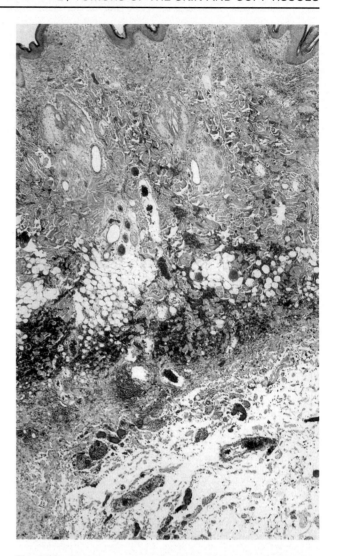

Fig. 2.35.   Angiosarcoma, ventral abdominal skin and subcutis, feline.

scopic evidence of the close association of the neoplastic cells with collagen bundles and on the lack of a continuous basal lamina ultrastructurally.[8] Factor VIII immunostaining is positive in some tumors, negative in others. The use of the term *angiosarcoma* avoids this controversy and may be a more appropriate name for this entity at this time.

Growth, Metastasis, and Treatment

The extensive infiltrative growth of this neoplasm leads to frequent recurrences. Metastasis is rare. Repeated surgical excision has been the only recognized treatment.

KAPOSI-LIKE VASCULAR TUMOR

An extremely rare and controversial diagnosis, this entity has been recognized solely in the dog.[12] Of the few cases seen, all have been in middle-aged to old female dogs.

Site and Gross Morphology

Tumors are single or multiple, usually involving tongue and/or skin. In one case, multiple dermal lesions were present on the limbs, and submucosal masses were found in the tongue and rectum. Tumors are nodular, usually less than a centimeter in diameter. They are raised, red-brown to black, soft, and covered by alopecic skin.

Histological Features

The masses are composed of a well-demarcated collection of bland nonvacuolated spindle cells that form small angular slit spaces, often containing extravasated erythrocytes, in the dermis or submucosa (fig. 2.36 A). Within the spindle cell population, most cases have some open irregular vascular spaces resembling lymphatics (fig. 2.36 B). The nuclei are small and oval, with rare atypia. Peripherally, cavernous vascular channels are seen, accompanied by hemosiderin deposits and infiltrates of lymphocytes and plasma cells. Morphologically, the tumors have features of Kaposi's sarcoma and kaposiform hemangioendothelioma of humans.[13]

Additional Diagnostic Criteria

The nodular appearance with central slits and more peripheral, blood filled, cavernous spaces edged by hemosiderin give this lesion a unique appearance dissimilar to any other vascular or spindle cell tumor in the dog. Intracellular PAS-positive hyaline globules, a distinguishing feature of Kaposi's sarcoma in humans, are seen in some canine tumors.[13] In contrast to hemangiosarcoma, only rare neoplastic spindle cells are immunohistochemically positive for factor VIII. One dog tested positive for p24 HIV protein via Western blot analysis. The significance of this finding is unknown.

Growth, Metastasis, and Treatment

Single tumors are usually cured by excision. Dogs with multiple tumors can have an indolent course, with remissions and recurrences. Because of the rarity of this lesion, information regarding treatment is lacking.

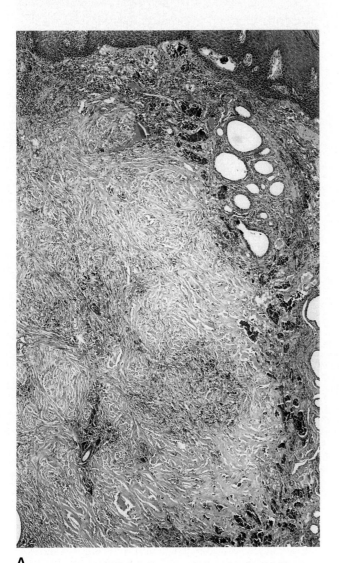

A

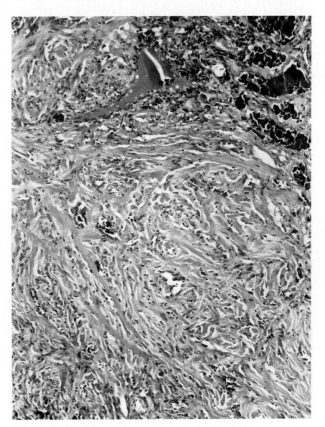

B

Fig. 2.36.   Kaposi-like vascular tumor, canine. **A.** Tongue. **B.** Skin, with bland spindle cells and irregular vascular slits.

SCROTAL VASCULAR HAMARTOMA

This is a proliferative vascular hamartoma rather than a true neoplasm. It is occasionally misdiagnosed as hemangiosarcoma by individuals unaware of the true nature and behavior of this lesion.

Incidence, Age, Breed, Sex, and Site

This rare lesion is seen in dog breeds with pigmented scrotal skin. It first appears in middle-aged individuals and progresses and enlarges with time.[3]

Gross Morphology and Histological Features

Initially, the lesion is a region of brown/black discoloration on the scrotal skin. It develops into a firm plaque in the superficial dermis.

Histologically, there is a poorly circumscribed proliferation of vessels in the dermis (fig. 2.37). The redundant vessels range from large hyperplastic arteries with thick muscular walls to capillary buds and are lined by endothelial cells with rounded nuclei. Atypia and mitoses are rare, but the proliferative capillary areas can resemble hemangioma or hemangiosarcoma.

Additional Diagnostic Criteria

The recognition of variably sized, disorganized, but relatively normal vessels with the characteristics of veins, arterioles, and capillaries marks this as a hamartomatous lesion and distinguishes it from hemangioma or hemangiosarcoma.

Treatment

Complete surgical excision is curative.

BOVINE CUTANEOUS ANGIOMATOSIS

This is a benign vasoproliferative lesion that is thought to be either an abnormal repair response to injury or an idiopathic hamartoma.

Incidence, Age, Breed, Sex, and Site

Reports of this rare lesion are few and indicate that the lesion occurs in young adult cattle in Great Britain, France, and the United States.[14,15] Mean age is 5.5 years. Most masses are on the back, but they can be seen anywhere on the skin.

Gross Morphology

These occur as single or multiple, poorly circumscribed, soft, fleshy, sessile to pedunculated masses. They range from pink to gray to red. Some lesions can bleed profusely and uncontrollably.

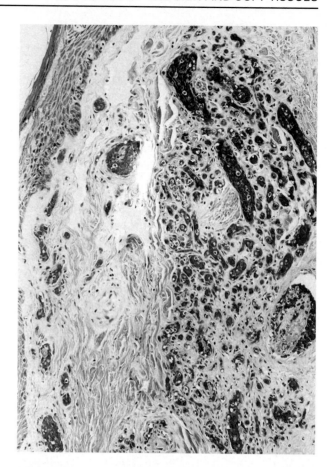

Fig. 2.37. Vascular hamartoma, scrotum, canine.

Histological Features

There is a nonencapsulated mixture of arteries, veins, and capillaries that is associated with an often intense inflammatory infiltrate. The proliferating vessels are of various calibers, and in some areas the lumina are indistinct. Separating the vessels are scattered fibroblasts and variable amounts of collagen. Authors liken the lesion to exuberant granulation tissue, but the classic perpendicular orientation of vessels to collagen seen in granulation tissue is lacking.

Growth and Treatment

These are benign lesions that can be cured by complete excision. Rare tumors can be associated with extensive hemorrhage and blood loss.

REFERENCES

1. Hargis, A.M., Ihrke, P.J., Spangler, W.L., and Stannard, A.A. (1992) A retrospective clinicopathologic study of 212 dogs with cutaneous hemangiomas and hemangiosarcomas. *Vet Pathol* 29(4):316–328.
2. Scott, D.W. (1988) *Large Animal Dermatology.* W.B. Saunders Co., Philadelphia, pp. 432–446.

3. Gross, T.L., Ihrke, P.E., and Walder, E.J. (1992) *Veterinary Dermatopathology: A Macroscopic and Microscopic Evaluation of Canine and Feline Skin Disease.* Mosby Yearbook, St. Louis, pp. 422–426.

4. Miller, M.A., Ramos, J.A., and Kreeger, J.M. (1992) Cutaneous vascular neoplasia in 15 cats: Clinical, morphologic, and immunohistochemical studies. *Vet Pathol* 29:329–336.

5. Goldschmidt, M.H., and Shofer, F.S. (1998) *Skin Tumors of the Dog and Cat.* Butterworth Heinemann, Oxford, pp. 210–216.

6. Hammer, A.S., Couto, C.G., Filppi, J., Getzy, D., et al. (1991) Efficacy and toxicity of VAC chemotherapy (vincristine, doxorubicin, and cyclophosphamide) in dogs with hemangiosarcoma. *J Vet Int Med* 5:160–166.

7. Withrow, S.J., and MacEwen, E.G. (1996) *Small Animal Clinical Oncology.* W.B. Saunders, Philadelphia, pp. 524–526.

8. Swayne, D.E., Mahaffey, E.A., and Haynes, S.G. (1989) Lymphangiosarcoma and haemangiosarcoma in a cat. *J Comp Pathol* 100:91–96.

9. Turrel, J.M., Lowenstine, L.J., and Cowgill, L.D. (1988) Response to radiation therapy of recurrent lymphangioma in a dog. *J Amer Vet Med Assoc* 193:1432–1434.

10. Carpenter, J.L., Andrews, L.K., and Holzworth, J. (1987) Tumors and tumor-like lesions. In Holzworth, J. (ed.), *Diseases of the Cat.* W.B. Saunders, Philadelphia, pp. 483–486.

11. Mughannam A. (1991) Subcutaneous hemangiosarcoma in the cat. *Calif Vet* 45:28–29.

12. Hendrick, M.J., Goldschmidt, M.H., Helfand, S.C., and Senior, M.B. (1986) Kaposi's sarcoma in a dog. Proceedings of the 37th Annual Meeting of the American College of Veterinary Pathologists, p.117.

13. Enzinger, F.M., and Weiss, S.E. (1995) *Soft Tissue Tumors,* 3rd ed. Mosby, St. Louis, pp. 658–669.

14. Cotchin, E., and Swarbrick, O. (1963) Bovine cutaneous angiomatosis: A lesion resembling human pyogenic granuloma (granuloma telangiectaticum). *Vet Rec* 75:437–444.

15. Lombard, C., and Levesque, L. (1964) A new disease in France; Hemangiomatosis of the skin and nasal mucosa in Normandy cows. *C R Acad Sci (Paris)* 258:3137–3138.

MAST CELL TUMOR

Mast cell tumors are ubiquitous in domestic animal species. The neoplasms can be focal or multicentric in the skin and may occasionally involve internal viscera such as spleen, liver, and intestine. There is species variation in location and biological behavior, but the similarities outweigh the differences.

Canine Mast Cell Tumors

Incidence, Age, Breed, and Sex

Boxers, pugs, Boston terriers, bull terriers, weimaraners, and Labrador retrievers are predisposed to the development of these cutaneous tumors, which can be single or multicentric.[1,2] Most tumors occur in middle-aged dogs. There is no sex predilection.

Site and Gross Morphology

In the dog, the skin is the most common site of involvement, but mast cell tumors can develop in the intestine, liver, spleen, or elsewhere. Mast cell tumors have a highly variable gross appearance, but many are erythematous, alopecic, and edematous masses or plaques. Most tumors are white to light yellow, but much of the color and consistency of the neoplasm is dependent on the degree of degranulation and secondary inflammation occurring in the tumors. Ulceration is common in larger tumors.

Histological Features

Luckily, most neoplastic mast cells in the dog resemble their normal counterparts, making diagnosis relatively easy. The cells are round to polygonal with round central to slightly eccentric nuclei and moderate, pale pink cytoplasm containing granules which stain light gray/blue with hematoxylin and eosin (H&E) or purple with metachromatic stains. Eosinophils are almost always found in canine mast cell tumors and can sometimes be the predominant cell type. Many tumors will have wide peripheral aggregates of eosinophils that should not be interpreted as part of the tumor when evaluating margins. *Collagenolysis,* sclerosis, edema, necrosis, and secondary inflammation are often seen in mast cell tumors, and when severe, they can mask neoplastic cells and make assessment of surgical margins difficult. Many reports have suggested a correlation between degree of cellular differentiation and biologic behavior.[3,4] Thus, *grading systems* have developed in the hopes of prognosticating these tumors. The most widely used system provides three grades: grade one tumors are confined to the dermis, and grade two and three tumors extend into the subcutis but differ in their degree of differentiation.[4] In this system, *Grade I* (fig. 2.38 A) tumors are well-differentiated superficial dermal tumors with few to no mitoses. *Grade II* (fig. 2.38 B) tumors are larger tumors that are less well circumscribed and extend into the deeper dermis and subcutis. There is mild nuclear pleomorphism, and the mitotic index is higher than in Grade I tumors but usually less than two per 40x field. *Grade III* (fig. 2.38 C) tumors extend into the subcutis and are composed of anaplastic cells with variably sized, sometimes large, nuclei and prominent nucleoli. Cytoplasmic granules are less numerous and are sometimes unidentifiable without the use of special histochemical stains (Giemsa, toluidine blue, astral blue) especially in Grade III neoplasms. Mitotic figures are frequent, and many are atypical in less well differentiated mast cell tumors. In those tumors with marked anaplasia and little or no granule staining, other features such as eosinophil infiltrates, multifocal collagenolysis, and dilated apocrine glands will aid in the diagnosis. Ectasia of apocrine glands is a common, yet unexplained, feature of many canine mast cell tumors.

Additional Diagnostic Criteria

In recent years, investigators have evaluated the benefit and efficacy of using means other than histological grading for prognosis. Specifically, the presence of agyrophilic nucleolar organizer regions (AgNORs) and DNA ploidy were evaluated as indicators of prognosis.[5,6] AgNORs are indirect measurements of cell proliferation, and counts can be made on paraffin embedded tissue or on

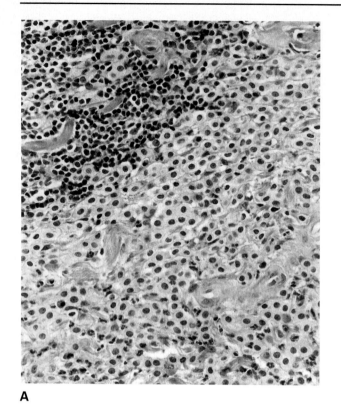

A

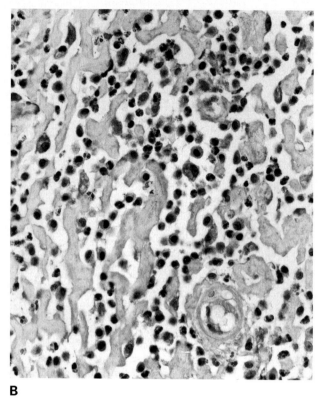

B

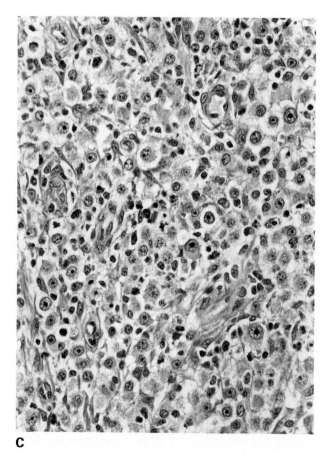

C

Fig. 2.38. Mast cell tumors in canine skin. **A.** Grade I. **B.** Grade II. **C.** Grade III.

cytological specimens. Studies showed that higher AgNOR counts correlated well with poorer prognosis and that this technique was less subjective than histological grading and as predictive of biological behavior.[5,6] Evaluation of DNA ploidy was not as predictive, although it did suggest that dogs with aneuploid tumors tended to have shorter survival times.[7]

The cytological diagnosis of mast cell tumor is fairly straightforward in the majority of cases due to the presence of numerous cytoplasmic granules. Many suspected mast cell tumors that do not stain metachromatically with "quick-type" stains will exhibit metachromasia if stained with Giemsa or Wright-Giemsa stains. However, histological evaluation is necessary for grading and assessment of surgical margins. Infrequent mast cell tumors also do not stain metachromatically in histological preparations. In these situations shifting the pH of the stain to a more acidic solution, employing a battery of stains (Giemsa, acid fast stains, Luna's, etc.), or using triethylenemelamine (TEM) is sometimes required to identify the cytoplasmic granules. The presence of collagenolysis, eosinophils, and dilated apocrine glands makes it likely that a poorly differentiated round cell tumor is of mast cell origin.

Gastroduodenal ulceration is sometimes seen in association with cutaneous or visceral mast cell tumors in the dog. The excess histamine produced by the tumor causes receptor-mediated hypersecretion of HCl by the parietal cells. Most ulcers tend to be in the pylorus or anterior duodenum because of a decreased production in these areas of the mucus that acts as a barrier to excess acid in the rest of the stomach. When present, these ulcers could be an indication of mast cell tumor in the dog.

Growth and Metastasis

As mentioned above, the biological behavior of canine mast cell tumors correlates with histological grade. Well-differentiated tumors (Grade I) have little evidence of recurrence after surgical excision and a 3 year survival rate of approximately 90 percent.[3] Moderately differentiated tumors (Grade II) have low to moderate metastatic potential and a 3 year survival rate of approximately 55 percent.[3,4,5] As expected, poorly differentiated tumors (Grade III) have the highest metastatic rates and a 3 year survival rate of only 10–15 percent. Recurrence after surgical excision is fairly common in Grade II and III tumors, most likely because these tumors are deeper, are less well circumscribed, and often have more necrosis, edema, and hemorrhage, which obscures tumor margins. Metastasis in all cases is first to regional lymph nodes, then later, rarely, to spleen and liver.

Treatment

The optimal treatment of mast cell tumor is wide surgical excision and adjuvant radiation therapy for tumors where complete excision is impossible.[8,9] Although systemic and/or intralesional steroids are commonly used by many veterinarians, the support for this is anecdotal.[9]

Feline Mast Cell Tumors

Incidence, Age, Breed, and Sex

Mast cell tumors are less common in cats than in dogs. The majority of cats are over 4 years of age, and there is no sex predilection. Siamese cats are at high risk for developing mast cell tumors,[1,10] including the rare *histiocytic* variant. Multicentricity of tumors is much more common in cats than dogs.

Gross Morphology

Feline mast cell tumors usually present as firm, tan papules, plaques, or nodules in the skin. The overlying epidermis is usually alopecic and pink. When multiple tumors are present, they may be clustered together or dispersed widely over the body. Ulceration can be seen in larger lesions.

Histological Features

Most cutaneous mast cell tumors in cats are benign, superficial dermal, well-demarcated lesions composed of sheets of uniform cells resembling normal feline mast cells (fig. 2.39 A). The neoplastic cells have little to no pleo-

morphism, and mitoses are absent. Eosinophil infiltrate is rare, but scattered clusters of small lymphocytes are commonly seen. Poorly differentiated mast cell tumors (fig. 2.39 B) are occasionally seen in which the neoplastic cells are moderately to markedly pleomorphic with large, often eccentric, nuclei and frequent mitoses. These tumors tend to infiltrate more deeply into the dermis and subcutis and are accompanied by increased numbers of eosinophils.

A rare variant, called *histiocytic* (fig. 2.39 C), occurs in juvenile to middle-aged Siamese cats.[11] In these tumors the neoplastic cells are large, polygonal to round, with abundant light pink cytoplasm and round hypochromatic nuclei. Mitoses are infrequent. These tumors often have moderate numbers of eosinophils and lymphoid aggregates. The overall appearance is that of granulomatous inflammation, and it is sometimes diagnosed as such by those unfamiliar with the histological appearance of this form of mast cell tumor.

Additional Diagnostic Criteria

Well-differentiated mast cell tumors in the cat present no diagnostic challenge, but poorly differentiated and histiocytic variants may require special metachromatic stains (Giemsa, toluidine blue, astral blue), which are almost always positive on a percentage of the cells in these tumors.

Growth and Metastasis

Complete excision of the well-differentiated form is usually curative, although as mentioned above some cats will develop multiple tumors simultaneously or sequentially. The biological behavior of the other two variants is not as clear. One group of investigators reported increased recurrence and suspected visceral metastasis in cats with the histiocytic variant,[11] but another study found no correlation between cell differentiation and prognosis.[12]

Mast Cell Tumors in Other Species

Mast cell tumors occasionally arise in horses, cattle, and pigs. The histological appearance of the neoplastic cells varies from well differentiated (typical in the horse) to pleomorphic.

Horses

Most tumors in the horse are in males, occur as focal masses on the head or legs, and respond to complete excision. Tumors are invariably benign. Some of these tumors appear in very young animals and spontaneously regress, leading some to argue that at least some mast cell lesions in the horse are not neoplastic. Mast cells are well differentiated and are accompanied by numerous eosinophils. Eosinophils may be prominent in some tumors, and coupled with the presence of collagenolysis and mineraliza-

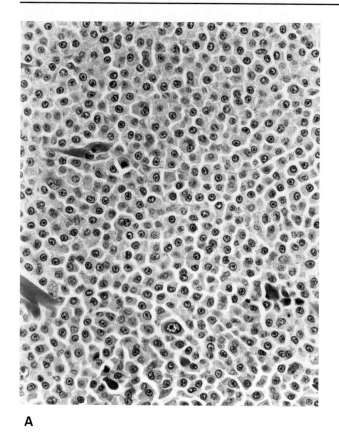

A

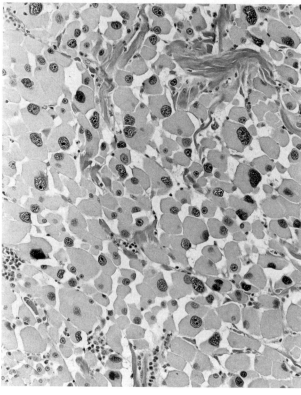

B

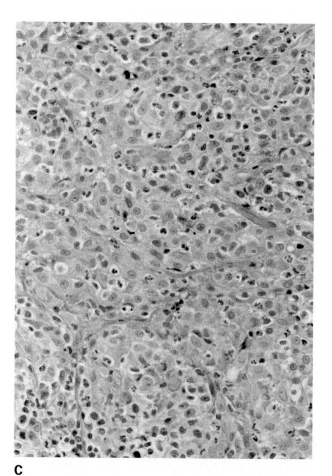

C

Fig. 2.39. Mast cell tumors, skin, feline. **A.** Well differentiated. **B.** Poorly differentiated variant. **C.** Histiocytic variant, skin, feline.

tion, may lead to a misdiagnosis of equine collagenolytic granuloma. Collagenolytic granulomas may be mast cell–rich, but they are generally confined to the dorsum of the neck, withers, and saddle area and have areas of collagenolysis (often with mineralization), foci of inflammation and giant cells, and disseminated and sometimes large aggregates of eosinophils; they are also steroid responsive.

Cattle

In contrast to horses, the majority of bovine mast cell tumors are malignant and have high metastatic potential.[13,14]

Rare reports of porcine mast cell tumors state that they can be cutaneous or visceral.[14]

REFERENCES

1. Goldschmidt, M.H., and Shofer, F.S. (1998) *Skin Tumors of the Dog and Cat.* Butterworth Heinemann, Oxford.
2. Gross, T.L., Ihrke, P.E., and Walder, E.J. (1992) *Veterinary Dermatopathology: A Macroscopic and Microscopic Evaluation of Canine and Feline Skin Disease.* Mosby Yearbook, St. Louis.
3. Patnaik, A.K., Ehler, W.J., and MacEwen, E.G. (1984) Canine cutaneous mast cell tumor: Morphologic grading and survival time in 83 dogs. *Vet Pathol* 21:469–474.
4. Bostock, D.E. (1973) The prognosis following surgical removal of mastocytomas in dogs. *J Small Anim Pract* 14:27–40.

5. Bostock, D.E., Crocker, J., Harris, K., Smith, P. (1989) Nuclear organiser regions as indicators of postsurgical prognosis in canine spontaneous mast cell tumors. *Brit J Cancer* 59:915–918.

6. Kravis, L.D., Vail, D.M., Kisseberth, W.C., Ogilvie, G.K., et al. (1996) Frequency of argyrophilic nuclear organizer regions in fine-needle aspirates and biopsy specimens from mast cell tumors in dogs. *J Amer Vet Med Assoc* 209:1418–1420.

7. Ayl, R.D., Couto, C.G., Hammer, A.S., Weisbrode, S., et al. (1992) Correlation of DNA ploidy to tumor histologic grade, clinical variables, and survival in dogs with mast cell tumors. *Vet Pathol* 29:386–390.

8. al-Sarraf, R., Mauldin, G.N., Patnaik, A.K., Meleo, K.A. (1996) A prospective study of radiation therapy for the treatment of grade 2 mast cell tumors in 32 dogs. *J Vet Int Med* 10:376–378.

9. Vail, D.M. (1996) Mast cell tumors. In Withrow, S.J., and MacEwen, E.G. (eds.), *Small Animal Clinial Oncology*. W.B. Saunders, Philadelphia, pp. 192–210.

10. Miller, M.A., Nelson, S.L., Turk, J.R., Pace, L.W., et al. (1991) Cutaneous neoplasia in 340 cats. *Vet Pathol* 28:389–395.

11. Wilcock, B.P., Yager, J.A., and Zink, M.C. (1986) The morphology and behavior of feline cutaneous mastocytomas. *Vet Pathol* 23:320–324.

12. Buerger, R.G., and Scott, D.W. (1987) Cutaneous mast cell neoplasia in cats: 14 cases (1975–1985). *J Amer Vet Med Assoc* 190:1440–1444.

13. Shaw, D.P., Buoen, L.C., and Weiss, D.J. (1991) Multicentric mast cell tumor in a cow. *Vet Pathol* 28:450–452.

14. Scott, D.W. (1988) *Large Animal Dermatology*. W.B. Saunders Co., Philadelphia, pp. 432–446.

CANINE CUTANEOUS HISTIOCYTOMA

Recent immunohistochemical and ultrastructural studies of canine cutaneous histiocytoma indicate that this round cell tumor is a localized form of self-limiting Langerhans cell histiocytosis.[1,2]

Incidence, Age, Breed, and Sex

This benign tumor is extremely common and is unique to dogs. The majority occur in dogs less than 4 years of age, but dogs of any age can be affected. Purebred dogs are predisposed toward development of histiocytomas, including Scottish terriers, bull terriers, boxers, English cocker spaniels, flat coated retrievers, doberman pinschers, and Shetland sheepdogs.[3]

Site and Gross Morphology

This is the classic *button tumor,* a smooth, pink, raised mass usually covered by alopecic skin. Ulceration is common, leading to central umbilication. Head and pinnae are preferential sites. A small percentage of dogs will have multiple cutaneous histiocytomas either synchronously or sequentially.[3,4] This is presumably due to an alteration in host immunity but does not reflect any change in the benign behavior of the tumor(s).

Histological Features

The histological appearance varies greatly, depending on the age of the lesion and the degree of necrosis and secondary inflammation. Typically, there is a dermal infiltrate of densely packed, mildly pleomorphic, round cells arranged in cords and sheets. There is little or no stroma, and adnexal structures are obliterated. The cells extend from the *dermoepidermal junction* (where the parallel, cord arrangement is most prominent) to the deep dermis and panniculus (fig. 2.40 A). Deeper portions of the neoplasm tend to be narrower than those near the epidermis, giving the tumor a wedge shaped appearance at low magnification. The neoplastic cells look histiocytic, with bean shaped to ovoid nuclei and moderate, lightly eosinophilic cytoplasm (fig. 2.40 B). Mitotic figures are numerous, but nuclear atypia and multinucleated forms are rare. In some tumors, clusters of neoplastic cells infiltrate the epidermis, mimicking the so-called Pautrier abscesses of cutaneous lymphosarcoma. Dense aggregates of mature lymphocytes and plasma cells are commonly seen at the base of the tumor and are presumed to be part of the host's immune response and to be partially responsible for tumor regression. In some cases these inflammatory cells predominate, obscuring the residual histiocytic tumor cells. However, the overall wedge shaped appearance of the lesion at low magnification, coupled with the typical clinical presentation (e.g., button tumor on the head of a young dog), should aid the diagnosis. Older tumors are often ulcerated, and areas of necrosis, which can be extensive, are present in some regressing tumors, usually at the deep and lateral margins.

Additional Diagnostic Criteria

Recent studies have shown the tumor cells in canine histiocytoma to have an immunophenotype of Langerhans cells.[1,2] Langerhans cells (LCs) in humans and dogs express major histocompatibility complex class II molecules and a variety of leukocyte antigens characteristic of dendritic cells. These include CD1a, CD1b, CD1c, and CD11c. Canine histiocytoma cells express CD1 molecules (CD1a, -b, and -c), CD11c, and major histocompatibility complex class II. They do not express Thy-1 or CD4, which are positive in other non-Langerhans cell dendritic cells in humans. Ultrastructurally, the cells have coated vesicles, regularly laminated bodies, paracrystalline structures, and deep invaginations of the plasma membrane, structures seen in a human Langerhans cell tumor.[1] Birbeck's granules, characteristic rod shaped granules found in the cytoplasm of human Langerhans cells by electron microscopy, are not present in canine Langerhans cells. In approximately 35% of tumors, the majority of cells stain strongly positive for lysozyme; in another 25%, there is regional positivity.[16]

Growth and Treatment

Histiocytomas have been referred to, humorously, as "surgical emergencies." One must remove them quickly before they regress. Complete excision is curative. Occasional tumors will recur, but it is unclear whether these are true recurrences or de novo tumors.

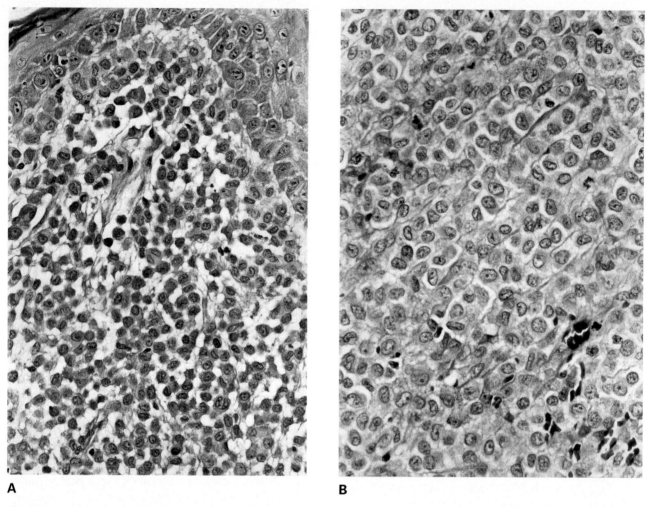

Fig. 2.40. Cutaneous histiocytoma. **A.** Neoplastic cells immediately subjacent to the epidermis or infiltrating the epidermis are features of canine histiocytoma. **B.** Higher magnification of neoplastic cells.

CUTANEOUS HISTIOCYTOSIS

This is an uncommon multifocal nodular cutaneous proliferation of histiocytes, recently shown to be of dermal dendritic immunophenotype.[15] The lesion is not thought to be neoplastic, but is similar to the proliferative histiocytoses of humans (Letterer-Siwe syndrome, Hand-Schüller-Christian disease).

Incidence, Age, Breed, and Sex

Cutaneous histiocytosis has only been described in the dog, most often in collies, border collies, Shetland sheepdogs, briards, Bernese mountain dogs, and golden retrievers.[3] There is no age or sex predilection.

Site and Gross Morphology

Lesions can occur anywhere on the skin, but especially on the face and planum nasale. Single and coalescing nodules are seen, covered by epidermis that is sometimes alopecic or ulcerated. There can be bulbous

enlargement of the planum nasale with swelling of the underlying nasal mucosa. This leads to difficulty in breathing and characteristic "bubble blowing."[5]

Histological Features

Sheets of large histiocytic cells with pale eosinophilic, often vacuolated, cytoplasm are present in the dermis, accompanied by diffusely scattered mature lymphocytes and neutrophils (fig. 2.41 A). A distinctive feature of this lesion is the lack of granuloma formation. There is no organization to this mixed cellular proliferation. The histiocytes are mildly pleomorphic, and mitotic figures are sometimes present, but the lesion as a whole resembles disorganized, undirected inflammation. Special stains and cultures are invariably negative for microorganisms.

Additional Diagnostic Criteria

There is considerable clinical and histological overlap of this syndrome with systemic histiocytosis, an extremely rare disease reported to occur in Bernese mountain dogs.[6] The cells in cutaneous and systemic histiocytosis have been shown to be of dermal dendritic cell lineage,[15] and they both can form similar nodular proliferations in the muzzle, planum nasale, and other areas of the skin. Both stain positively for lysozyme. Some solitary lesions wax and wane, but what distinguishes systemic histiocytosis from cutaneous histiocytosis is that in the former there is progression to widespread involvement of lymph nodes and viscera. Systemic histiocytosis is considered by most authors to be nonneoplastic, but its behavior can not be considered benign since most dogs with this disease are euthanized. These two syndromes have been called "reactive histiocytoses"[15] and are part of a spectrum of proliferative histiocytic lesions in the dog, much like the histiocytosis X complex in humans. The more aggressive nature of systemic histiocytosis may be a manifestation of the genetically determined inability of the Bernese mountain dog to control these cell proliferations.

Growth and Treatment

Cutaneous histiocytosis lesions can be slow or fast growing. There can be spontaneous regression of some lesions, and others are responsive, at least temporarily, to steroid therapy.

MALIGNANT HISTIOCYTOSIS

This is the most aggressive syndrome in the spectrum of histiocytic diseases and the most obscure in origin. Most recent investigations suggest that the cells of malignant histiocytosis are of variable immunophenotypes, some expressing antigens consistent with dendritic cells, while others express antigens consistent with bone marrow monocyte origin.[7] Malignant histiocytosis is quite distinctive from the other histiocytic disorders in its lightmicroscopic appearance and biological behavior.

Incidence, Age, Breed, and Sex

First described in the Bernese mountain dog, this uncommon but highly malignant round cell neoplasm has since been reported in various dog and cat breeds, as well as other domestic species.[8,9,10] In the dog, there is a predilection for rottweilers, golden retrievers, and Bernese mountain dogs.[11]

Site and Gross Morphology

Classically, malignant histiocytosis involves viscera, most notably spleen, liver, lung, kidney, lymph nodes, and bones, but skin tumors can occur, either alone or as part of the multiorgan disease.[11,12,13] The skin lesions can be single or multiple, solitary or clustered. They are usually purple/red nodules or plaques, covered by alopecic, thickened epidermis. Lesions in viscera may be diffuse or nodular and are usually white to pink/purple, soft and bulging.

Histological Features

There is a multifocal to diffuse infiltrate of large round to polygonal cells with ovoid to reniform nuclei and abundant eosinophilic cytoplasm, sometimes containing phagocytosed erythrocytes, hemosiderin, or cellular debris (fig. 2.41 B; see also fig. 3.28). The discrete cells form loose sheets with little or no stroma. Some cells resemble normal macrophages, but others will show marked variation in size and shape, with a range of 15 to 60 μm in diameter. Nuclei also vary in size and shape, are hyperchromatic, and often contain multiple prominent nucleoli. There is marked atypia, and numerous mitoses are seen, many of which are bizarre. Multinucleate forms are often present in large numbers and show the same marked atypia. Inflammatory cells (e.g., neutrophils, lymphocytes, and plasma cells) can be seen scattered among the neoplastic cells but do not usually constitute a significant percentage of the total population.

Additional Diagnostic Criteria

Cytological diagnosis of malignant histiocytosis is fairly straightforward. The cells are recognizable as macrophages, but their marked atypia precludes a diagnosis of inflammation. Immunohistochemical analysis of frozen sections should reveal positive staining for lysozyme and, to a lesser degree, alpha-1-antitrypsin. Cells express CD45, CD18/11a, CD11c, CD1 (a, b, and c) MHC class II, ICAM-1 (intercellular adhesion molecule), CD44, and CD49d.

Some animals with extensive erythrophagocytosis can become anemic due to sequestration of red blood cells within tumor cells.

Growth, Metastasis, and Treatment

The disease is uniformly fatal after a progressive course that usually involves the many organs listed above. Attempts at chemotherapy have been unsuccessful. There is no known treatment.

XANTHOMA

Xanthomas are nonneoplastic masses composed of large foamy macrophages. Seen frequently in birds, they also occur in domestic animals. The appearance of these lesions is usually associated with abnormal plasma levels of cholesterol or triglycerides, but solitary, idiopathic xanthomas have also been reported.[5,14]

Incidence, Age, Breed, and Sex

Seen rarely in the cat and less so in the dog, xanthomas can be focal or multifocal in the skin. In the cat, the lesions have been seen secondary to spontaneous or megestrol acetate–induced diabetes mellitus.

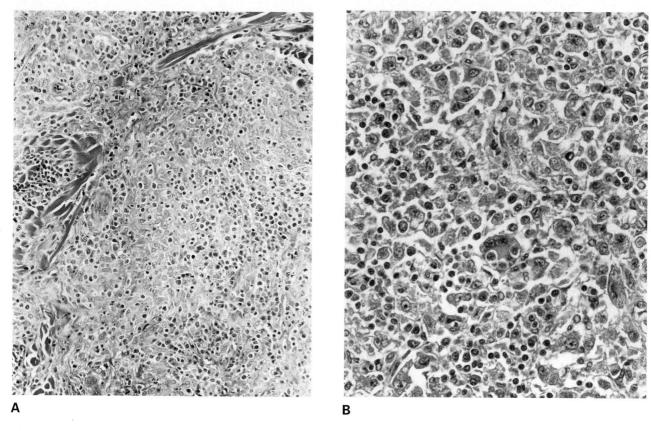

Fig. 2.41. Histiocytosis. **A.** Cutaneous, skin, canine. **B.** Malignant, skin, canine. Note the phagocytosis by the tumor cells.

Gross Morphology and Histological Features

The lesion usually presents as smooth white to pale yellow raised nodules or plaques in the skin. Lipid filled macrophages (fig. 2.42) are seen diffusely throughout the dermis, forming granulomas, often associated with cholesterol clefts. Between the cells are lakes of finely granular to amorphous acellular material.

Additional Diagnostic Criteria

Xanthomas must be differentiated from granulomatous inflammation secondary to infectious agents such as fungi or mycobacteria. These latter lesions do not have cholesterol clefts, and special stains will be positive for organisms. This author has seen a few lesions in Siamese cats that resembled xanthomas but were, in fact, mast cell tumors. The cells in these lesions were large, often multinucleated, with markedly foamy to vacuolated cytoplasm. Despite the lipoid appearance to the cytoplasm, the cells stained strongly with metachromatic stains for mast cells. This suggests that one variant within the histiocytic type of mast cell tumor in cats can mimic xanthoma. Features that may help to distinguish this variant of mast cell tumor from xanthoma are the infiltrating eosinophils and scattered lymphocytic aggregates present in the former.

Growth and Treatment

Single lesions respond to surgical excision. Multiple lesions can also be surgically excised if necessary for cosmetic reasons, but if the predisposing abnormal lipid levels persist, new lesions could appear.

REFERENCES

1. Marchal, T., Dezutter-Dambuyant, C., Fournel, C., Magnol, J.P., et al. (1995) Immunophenotypic and ultrastructural evidence of the Langerhans cell origin of the canine cutaneous histiocytoma. *Acta Anatom* 153:189–202.
2. Moore, P.F., Schrenzel, M.D., Affolter, V.K., Olivry, T., and Naydan, D. (1996) Canine cutaneous histiocytoma is an epidermotropic Langerhans cell histiocytosis that expresses CD1 and specific beta 2-integrin molecules. *Amer J Pathol* 148:1699–1708.
3. Goldschmidt, M.H., and Shofer, F.S. (1998) *Skin Tumors of the Dog and Cat.* Butterworth Heinemann, Oxford.
4. Bender, W.M., and Muller, G.H. (1989) Multiple, resolving, cutaneous histiocytoma in a dog. *J Amer Vet Med Assoc* 194:535–537.
5. Gross, T.L., Ihrke, P.E., and Walder, E.J. (1992) *Veterinary Dermatopathology: A Macroscopic and Microscopic Evaluation of Canine and Feline Skin Disease.* Mosby Yearbook, St. Louis, pp. 198–201.
6. Moore, P.F. (1984) Systemic histiocytosis of Bernese mountain dogs. *Vet Pathol* 21:554–563.

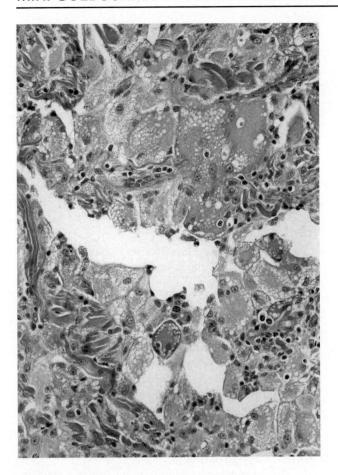

Fig. 2.42.   Xanthoma, skin, feline.

PLASMA CELL TUMOR

This tumor has had many incarnations; it has previously been called *atypical histiocytoma* and *reticulum cell sarcoma,* and it has been misclassified for a few years as a neuroendocrine (Merkel cell) tumor.[1,2] In 1989, investigators identified immunoglobulin in the cytoplasm of the neoplastic cells,[3,4] and since then the diagnosis of Merkel cell tumor has been essentially abandoned. It is important to note that although some cases of multiple myeloma can have skin involvement, most cutaneous plasma cell tumors are de novo proliferations unassociated with primary bone marrow neoplasia.

Incidence, Age, Breed, Sex, and Site

The majority of plasma cell tumors occur in older dogs; rare tumors occur in the cat. Dog breeds preferentially affected include cocker spaniels, Airedale terriers, Kerry blue terriers, standard poodles, and Scottish terriers.[5]

Gross Morphology

Most plasma cell tumors are single, small, slightly raised dermal nodules covered by alopecic, occasionally ulcerated, skin. Some animals will have multiple plasma cell tumors at presentation. The pinnae and digits are preferentially affected. Other sites are oral cavity and rectum. On cut surface, the tumor is well demarcated but unencapsulated, and the color varies from white to red.

Histological Features

Although the gross appearance and site predilection of plasmacytomas resemble those of histiocytomas, the histological differences are apparent at low magnification. Sheets of round cells with pleomorphic nuclei are seen in poorly defined cords and nests (fig. 2.43). Scattered throughout this population are distinctive cells with large hyperchromatic nuclei. These cells can be mononuclear, multilobulated, or multinucleated, and at low magnification these cells serve as a useful diagnostic marker for this neoplasm. Despite this nuclear pleomorphism, the cells are generally round with scant to moderate eosinophilic to amphophilic cytoplasm. Most neoplastic cells do not have the typical plasma cell *clock-face* nuclear chromatin pattern; however, toward the periphery of the tumor, where the cells are not as densely packed, the cells more closely resemble normal plasma cells, with rare cells showing perinuclear clear zones or circular cytoplasmic packets. The mitotic index varies, but is usually low.

Amyloid can be found in a small percentage of cutaneous or oral plasma cell tumors. It is immunoglobulin derived (primary) amyloid composed of lambda light chains; it can be found in large lakes or in small deposits scattered throughout the tumor between cells and, occasionally, in blood vessel walls.

7. Moore, P.F. (2000) Canine histiocytic diseases: Proliferation of dendritic cells is key. Proceedings of the 55th Annual Meeting of the American College of Veterinary Pathologists, Amelia Island, FL, December 2000.

8. Moore, P.F., and Rosin, A. (1986) Malignant histiocytosis of Bernese mountain dogs. *Vet Pathol* 23:1–10.

9. Freeman, L., Stevens, J., Loughman, C., and Tompkins, M. (1995) Malignant histiocytosis in a cat. *J Vet Int Med* 9:171–173.

10. Lester, G.D., Alleman, A.R., Raskin, R.E., and Calderwood Mays, M.B. (1993) Malignant histiocytosis in an Arabian filly. *Equine Vet J* 25:471–473.

11. Kerlin, R.L., and Hendrick, M.J. (1996) Malignant fibrous histiocytoma and malignant histiocytosis in the dog—Convergent or divergent phenotypic differentiation? *Vet Pathol* 33:713–716.

12. Hayden, D.W., Waters, D.J., Burke, B.A., and Manivel, J.C. (1993) Disseminated malignant histiocytosis in a golden retriever: Clinicopathologic, ultrastructural, and immunohistochemical findings. *Vet Pathol* 30:256–264.

13. Schmidt, M.L., Rutteman, G.R., Wolvekamp, P.T.C., and Van Niel, M.H.F. (1993) Clinical and radiographic manifestations of canine malignant histiocytosis. *Vet Quarterly* 15:117–120.

14. Fawcett, J.F., Demaray, S.Y., Altman, N. (1977) Multiple xanthomatosis in a cat. *Feline Pract* 5:31–33.

15. Affolter, V.K., and Moore, P.F. (2000) Canine cutaneous and systemic histiocytosis: Reactive histiocytosis of dermal dendritic cells. *Amer J Dermatopathol* 22:40–48

16. Moore, P.F. (1986) Utilizaton of cytoplasmic lysozyme immunoreactivity as a histocytic marker in canine histocytic disorders. *Vet Pathol* 23:757–762.

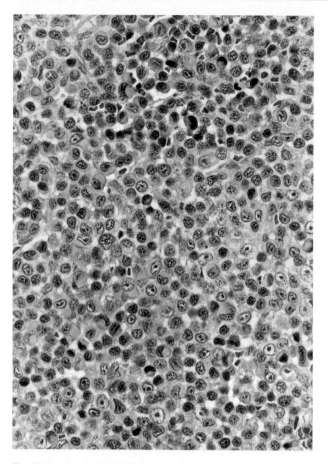

Fig. 2.43. Plasma cell tumor, skin, canine.

Additional Diagnostic Criteria

The histological features of plasma cell tumors are distinctive, and diagnosis is usually not difficult, especially in the more differentiated variants. However, markedly anaplastic tumors can be misdiagnosed as malignant histiocytosis (see fig. 3.20). Some of the cells in plasma cell tumors will stain positively with methyl green pyronine because of their high concentration of RNA; however, this stain is not specific. Positive thioflavine T cytoplasmic fluorescence can distinguish plasma cell tumors from other round cell neoplasms.[6] The identification of monoclonal immunoglobulin (usually IgG) or immunoglobulin light chains (usually lambda) by immunofluorescence or immunoperoxidase will confirm the diagnosis in less differentiated tumors.

Growth, Metastasis, and Treatment

The majority of cutaneous plasma cell tumors in the dog are benign. Most are cured by complete excision, though a few will recur. In one study, tumors with amyloid appeared to have a higher recurrence rate, but the overall numbers were too low to make any definitive statements about the prognostic significance of amyloid in plasma cell tumors.[7] Metastasis to distant skin sites has been reported rarely and probably reflects cases of multiple myeloma

with skin involvement. Unlike in multiple myeloma, monoclonal gammopathy has not been reported in cases of single or multiple cutaneous or oral plasma cell tumors. The behavior of canine plasma cell tumors does not seem to have any relationship to the degree of pleomorphism or atypia. The behavior of feline plasma cell tumors is difficult to assess because of the rarity of the lesion.

LYMPHOMA

General Considerations and Classification

Lymphoma is an important and common tumor in dogs and cats; this brief discussion centers on the cutaneous form of lymphoma.

Incidence, Age, Breed, Sex, and Site

Lymphoma of the skin is rare in all species, but is more commonly seen in dogs and cats. The mean age in dogs and cats is 10 years. There is no breed predilection in cats, but briards, English cocker spaniels, bulldogs, Scottish terriers, and golden retrievers are predisposed to cutaneous lympoma.[5] Most of the tumors are on the trunk, but lesions can appear anywhere on the body.

Gross Morphology

There is marked variability to the gross appearance of cutaneous lymphoma, which appears to correlate with the cell type (T or B) that is involved. As in humans, the lesions may manifest as patches, plaques, or tumors. *Patches* are uncommon in animals, but these erythematous scaly macules can wax and wane over many years. *Plaques* can develop from patches or arise de novo. As the name implies, these are areas of thickened, plaque skin, often covered by scaly and partially alopecic skin. Pruritis is common and often leads to ulceration. The color ranges from pink to brown. *Tumors* are variably sized, intradermal masses that can show ulceration, crusting, and alopecia. All of these forms can be single or multifocal in the skin.

Histological Features

Cutaneous lymphoma in humans has traditionally been divided into the *epitheliotropic* and *nonepitheliotropic* forms. Cases in dogs and cats seem to fall quite well into these categories, and the veterinary profession has adopted this nomenclature.

Epitheliotropic Tumors

In epitheliotropic tumors, the neoplastic cells are T cells and have an affinity for epidermis and adnexal epithelium. The descriptive, but misleading name *mycosis fungoides,* has been applied to this form of lymphoma because of its gross appearance. Neoplastic lymphocytes, which can range from small well-differentiated cells to large histiocytoid cells, invade the epidermis either diffusely or in small clusters (Pautrier microabscesses). Similar infiltrates are seen in hair follicular and apocrine gland epithelial cells. Sometimes the infiltrate is so even that at first low magnification inspection the only change is a slight basophilia and hyperplasia of the basal cell layers of the epidermis and adnexa. Closer examination will reveal the lymphocytic population. Neoplastic cells are also seen in the dermis, but it is the epitheliotropism that distinguishes this form. Mitotic activity in this form is usually low.

Nonepitheliotropic Tumors

Nonepitheliotropic tumors are of B or T cell origin and are characterized by sheets and clusters of neoplastic lymphocytes. Again, cells can vary tremendously in morphology, even in tumors in the same animal. Neoplastic lymphocytes are often intermingled with normal lymphocytes, plasma cells, and histiocytes, and the true neoplastic nature of the lesion can be hidden. When the neoplastic cells are small and well differentiated, diagnosis can be difficult. Lymphoblastic, immunoblastic, or histiocytic forms can usually be recognized by their characteristic nuclear and cytoplasmic features. Mitotic indices vary from moderate to high.

Additional Diagnostic Criteria

The identification of lymphocyte lineage can usually be accomplished by the use of a panel of anitibodies directed at canine and feline leukocyte antigens; however, interpretation of these should be made in conjunction with thorough histological evaluation of H&E sections.

Growth, Metastasis, and Treatment

Cutaneous lymphoma tends to be a progressive disease, beginning with the development of multicentric skin tumors and ultimately involving the regional lymph nodes and viscera. Treatment, which has consisted of various combinations of chemotherapeutic drugs, retinoids, and topical mechlorethamine has proven unrewarding.[8] Most treatment is aimed at palliation.

CANINE TRANSMISSIBLE VENEREAL TUMOR

This tumor is unusual in many regards. It is of unknown cell origin and is transmitted by physical transplantation rather than infectious means, and the chromosome count of the cells of the neoplasm is 59 rather than the normal 78 found in other cells of the dog. As the name implies, it is primarily located on the genitalia or, less commonly, on the lips or other portions of the skin or mucosa that come in contact with the genitalia. Transmission is usually during coitus.

Incidence, Age, Breed, and Sex

Dogs of both sexes and all ages are affected, but the tumor is more commonly seen in female dogs that have reached sexual maturity. The distribution of transmissible venereal tumor (TVT) throughout the world is patchy and unexplained. The disease is enzootic in some regions of the Caribbean (e.g., Puerto Rico), but it has never been reported in the British Isles. TVTs are seen frequently in portions of the midwestern United States, but are uncommon in the mid-Atlantic and relatively common in the southeastern states. It occurs in pockets in Europe, Africa, and Asia.

Gross Morphology

TVTs vary in their gross appearance, but most are proliferative verrucous, papillary, or nodular masses protruding from the surface of the penis or vulva (fig. 2.44 A,B). The tumors can be small single nodules or multilobulated masses (fig. 2.44 C) as large as 15 cm in diameter. The surface is usually ulcerated and friable, with a smooth or granular appearance.

Histological Features

The neoplasm is composed of loose sheets, rows and cords of relatively uniform round to ovoid cells. Cell margins are generally indistinct. Nuclei are large, round, with a single centrally placed nucleolus surrounded by marginated chromatin. There is a moderate amount of light pink to clear cytoplasm. The mitotic index is high. Variable numbers of lymphocytes, plasma cells and macrophages infiltrate the tumor. In regressing tumors, increased inflammation and zones of necrosis and fibrosis are often present.

Additional Diagnostic Criteria

The primary differentials for TVTs are other round cell tumors of the skin: histiocytoma, lymphoma, and mast cell tumor. The location of the tumor should play an important role in diagnosis; genital round-cell lesions should be considered TVTs until proven otherwise by special stains, electron microscopy, or immunohistochemistry. TVTs were shown to have immunoreactivity with lysozyme, alpha-1-antitrypsin, and vimentin.[9,10] They were negative for keratins, S-100 protein, lambda light-chain immunoglobulins, IgG, IgM, and CD3 antigen. Although these implied a histiocytic immunophenotype, more recent studies indicate that TVT is composed of immature leukocytes, likely myeloid in origin (see chapter 11). Ultrastructurally, TVT cells are nondescript, but their unique karyotype is diagnostic.

On routine H&E stained slides, the nuclear and cytoplasmic differences between TVTs and histiocytomas can be subtle. Cytological preparations have better nuclear preservation and should be used to help confirm the diagnosis. Lymphocytic and plasma cell infiltration is not a feature of lymphomas.

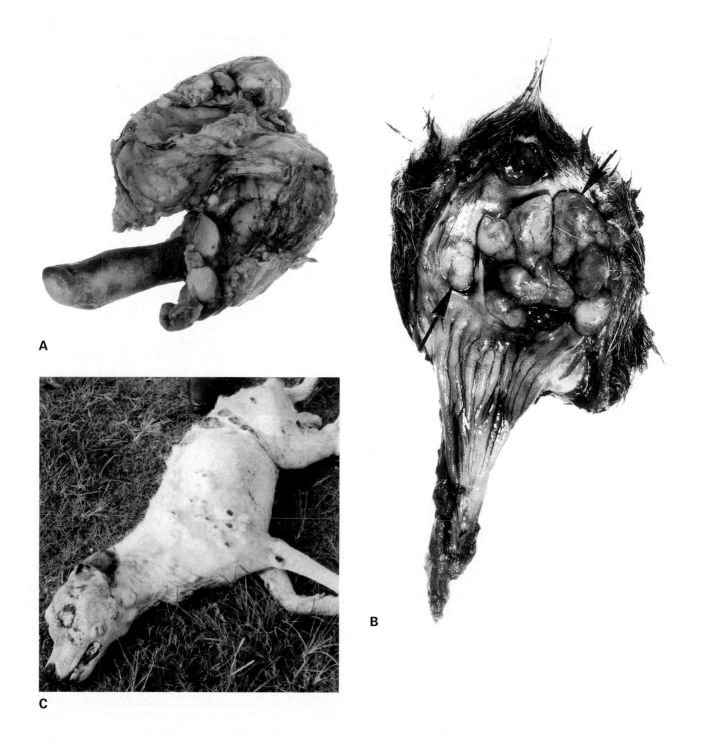

A

B

C

Fig. 2.44. Canine transmissible venereal cell tumor. **A.** Lateral view of the penis of a dog, showing a large tumor involving caudal parts of the penis. The dorsoventral measurement of this tumor is 10 × 12 cm. Approximately 6 cm of the normal penis is visible. **B.** Multiple polypoid growths (arrows) in the vagina of a bitch. **C.** Mongrel stray dog with advanced tumor involvement of the skin and subcutaneous, periorbital, and buccal tissues. Many of the lesions are ulcerated and hemorrhagic.

Growth, Metastasis, and Treatment

Tumors grow rapidly at first and then remain static for a time, with eventual spontaneous regression after several months. Regression is the result of a humoral immune response (IgG) that makes the dog highly resistent to subsequent tumor implantation. There is infrequent metastasis to regional lymph nodes and, rarely, to viscera.

REFERENCES

1. Nikoloff, B.J., Hill, J., and Weiss, L.M. (1985) Canine neuroendocrine carcinoma. A tumor resembling histiocytoma. *Amer J Dermatopathol* 7:579–586.
2. Whiteley, L.O., and Leininger, J.R. (1987) Neuroendocrine (Merkel) cell tumors of the canine oral cavity. *Vet Pathol* 24:570–572.
3. Baer, K.E., Patnaik, A.K., Gilbertson, S.R., et al. (1989) Cutaneous plasmacytomas in dogs: A morphologic and immunohistochemical study. *Vet Pathol* 26:216–221.
4. Rakich, P.M., Latimer, K.S., Weiss, R., et al. (1989) Mucocutaneous plasmacytomas in dogs: 75 cases (1980–1987). *J Amer Vet Med Assoc* 194:803–810.
5. Goldschmidt, M.H., and Shofer, F.S. (1998) *Skin Tumors of the Dog and Cat.* Butterworth Heinemann, Oxford, pp. 252–270.
6. Brunnert, S.R., Altman, N,H. (1991) Identification of immunoglobulin light chains in canine extramedullary plasmacytomas by thioflavine T and immunohistochemistry. *J Vet Diag Invest* 3:245–251.
7. Rowland, P.H., Valentine, B.A., Stebbins, K.E., et al. (1991) Cutaneous plasmacytomas with amyloid in six dogs. *Vet Pathol* 28:125–130.
8. Withrow, S.J., and MacEwen, E.G. (1996) *Small Animal Clinial Oncology.* W.B. Saunders, Philadelphia, p. 467.
9. Mozos, E., Mendez, A., Gomez-Villamandos, J.C., Martin De Las Mulas, J., et al. (1996) Immuno-histochemical characterization of canine transmissible venereal tumor. *Vet Pathol* 33:257–263.
10. Marchal, T., Chabanne, L., et al. (1997) Immunophenotype of the canine transmissible venereal tumour. *Vet Immunol Immunopathol* 57:1–11.

3 Tumors of the Hemolymphatic System

R.M. Jacobs, J.B. Messick, and V.E. Valli

LYMPHOID TUMORS

Introduction

Biological Implications of Tumor Classification

The purpose of all disease classification systems is to define disease entities based on their biological behavior. In the process of defining criteria for various disease entities, we may err by lumping together similar lesions that have different biological behaviors or, alternatively, by creating subtypes of diseases that do not have unique progression and, therefore, do not deserve to be separately identified. In veterinary hematopathology, major inference is drawn from experience in human medicine where it is presumed that diseases with a similar presentation and morphology will mimic the biology of the human counterpart and will respond in a similar manner to various therapies. For the dog, sufficient experience has been gained in the therapy of hematopoietic tumors to confidently state that hematopoietic tumors diagnosed using human classification systems will, if reliably identified, behave and respond in a manner similar to their human counterparts. We are less certain of these correlations in other species.

Some general statements can be made which will assist diagnosticians and therapists in applying the information gained from a careful identification of hematopoietic neoplasms. Firstly, those hematopoietic tumors with a high mitotic rate, whether of myeloid or lymphoid histogenesis, can be expected to be tumors which will progress rapidly, causing death of the animal. Since most of our chemotherapeutic modalities are cell-cycle dependent, it is also true that tumors with a high mitotic rate are most likely to enter remission as a result of aggressive therapy. In contrast, hematopoietic tumors with a very low mitotic and death rate, which are therefore largely tumors of accumulation, tend to progress slowly, perhaps with survival of a year or more in the absence of treatment. These tumors may be amenable to treatment with drugs that are membrane dependent and active or to radiation; however, since very few of the cells are in an active phase of growth and division, they will be less injured by aggressive chemotherapy than benign cells of marrow and intestine that normally have a high proliferation rate. In this chapter, the lymphoid tumors are classified according to the National Cancer Institute Working Formulation, which identifies lymphoma subtypes based on their histomorphology into low, intermediate, and high grade groups. Subsequently, the International Lymphoma Study Group has produced the Revised European American Lymphoma (REAL) system, which has the advantage of separating lymphomas with similar morphology but different biological behavior on the basis of their B or T cell subtype. While this is a useful advance for those who already have a specialist's knowledge of lymphomas and their behavior, the REAL system is a *list* of B and T derived tumors that, in general, indicate biological behavior without division into low, intermediate, and high grade lesions. The updated WHO classification of tumors of hematopoietic and lymphoid tissues is a more complete list than the REAL system and includes acute and chronic myeloproliferative diseases as well as myelodysplastic syndromes, the histiocytoses, and mast cell tumors. In animals, as in humans, the T cell lymphomas are generally more aggressive than B cell types and respond less well to therapy. In addition, with 18 years of experience in use of the Working Formulation, not only have new entities been identified, but some of the original categories have been shown to not be biologically different and therefore can be effectively combined.

Myeloid tumors in this chapter are classified on the basis of the French/American/British system for acute leukemias that identifies the subtypes from M0 for an undifferentiated or stem cell tumor to M7 for acute tumors of the megakaryocytic system. In this case, the numbers indicate the direction of maturation of the myeloid cell line rather than the characteristic rate of progression. In contrast, the chronic myeloid tumors are classified simply on the basis of their cell type as either neutrophil, eosinophil, monocytic, or platelet, with the chronic leukemia of the erythroid system known as polycythemia vera. The acute lymphoid leukemias are classified as L1 to L3 based on morphology; all are large cells with a high proliferative rate and a short course in the untreated state. In contrast, the chronic lymphocytic leukemias tend to be of smaller cells with a very low proliferative rate but much higher peripheral blood lymphocyte counts.

Diagnostic Strategies

The approach to the diagnosis of hematopoietic neoplasms should proceed with particular attention to cell size and mitotic rate. In the case of true leukemias with bone marrow involvement, it is important to determine whether the tumor is of myeloid or lymphoid origin; in poorly differentiated tumors of either type, this may require special stains for a definitive answer. The distinction between these two types of tumors is important in terms of the rate of tumor progress. Primitive myeloid tumors preferentially invade subendosteal areas and drive benign hematopoietic cells centripetally in the marrow cavity, where they tend to undergo terminal differentiation rather than self-renewal. Acute or primitive lymphoid leukemias, on the other hand, colonize the bone marrow in a random fashion that tends to displace the myeloid progenitors much more slowly and allows more time for benign cells to convert fatty to hematopoietic marrow in the face of the advancing tumor. For these reasons, acute myeloid tumors tend to cause marrow failure much more rapidly than acute lymphoid tumors. Thus, acute myeloid tumors are characterized by early marrow failure with neutropenia, thrombocytopenia, anemia, and death due to septicemia and hemorrhage. Untreated cases may progress from diagnosis to termination in 3 weeks or less. The acute leukemias of monoblastic or myelomonocytic type tend to progress more slowly than myeloblastic or promyelocytic leukemias because of the array of interleukins that are produced by the monocytic progenitors and that tend to stimulate benign myelopoiesis and delay marrow failure. The acute tumors of the erythroid system, erythremic myelosis and erythroleukemia, are rapidly progressive diseases for which there is no effective therapy. The megakaryoblastic leukemias tend to have a short course because of the production of associated cytokines; one of these, platelet derived growth factor, is suspected of involvment with the early onset of myelofibrosis and marrow failure. Both chronic myeloid and chronic lymphoid leukemia tend to be diseases diagnosed by accident with the recognition of high numbers of mature-appearing blood cells, often during routine examinations of animals that appear otherwise to be in good health. As a basic rule of thumb, all leukemias are accompanied by blast cells in the peripheral blood, albeit at very low numbers in the chronic leukemias. Finally, the myelodysplasias are diseases characterized by a hyperplastic marrow with cytopenias of one or more of the cell lines in the peripheral blood. Depending on the type of dysplasia and the stage at which it is diagnosed, the animals may live a year or more with supportive therapy, including transfusions of whole blood, but will ultimately die due to marrow failure or acute leukemia.[94]

In the diagnosis of lymphomas, it is necessary to provide the clinician with both a morphological and an immunohistochemical determination of B or T cell type. Thus, the lesion should be characterized as low, intermediate, or high grade (similar to the categories of the Working Formulation), and the histogenetic derivation must be provided (figs. 3.2 and 3.3). In general, the small cell lymphomas such as small cell lymphocytic lymphoma, small cleaved cell lymphoma, and intermediate small cell lymphoma all tend to be lesions more characterized by accumulation than by proliferation; they are therefore likely to be less responsive to aggressive chemotherapy than the acute leukemias (see figs. 3.30–3.33). In the intermediate grade lymphomas, the true follicular lymphomas are unusual lesions in animals and are primarily seen in the cat and dog (figs. 3.4–3.8). In the REAL classification, the follicular lymphomas are not identified by cell type (small cleaved cell, mixed cell, and large cell) but by grade (Grade I to III), based on the proportions of small cleaved lymphocytes (centrocytes) and larger, more vesicular cells (centroblasts) present. Follicular lymphomas with 0–5 centroblasts per high power (HP) field will be classed as Grade I, those with 6–15 centroblasts per HP field as Grade II, and those with 15 or more centroblasts per HP field as Grade III. All follicular lymphomas tend to be relatively indolent and are characterized by slow expansion of lymph nodes with thinning of the capsule; but colonization of perinodal structures does not occur until late in the disease process. Included in the intermediate grade lymphomas are the mixed small cleaved and large cell types now known as T-cell-rich B cell lymphomas (fig. 3.9). Also included are the large cell lymphomas, including the cleaved cell variant (fig. 3.10) and immunoblastic lymphomas (fig. 3.11), which according to human experience, do not differ in behavior from large cell lymphomas and do not deserve to be included in the high grade category. This grouping of categories is pragmatic, since it is somewhat arbitrary in deciding whether to call a lesion diffuse large or immunoblastic, based on whether the predominant cell type has central or peripheral nucleoli. The T-cell-rich B cell lymphoma (fig. 3.9) is the characteristic subcutaneous tumor of the horse, where the lesions may be multiple; it is also seen in the dog and cat (fig. 3.1). These lesions tend to be slowly progressive and do not respond well to chemotherapy, at least insofar as shrinkage of tumors is concerned, because of the large component of stromal tissue characteristic of these lesions. Since the malignant B cells may constitute as few as 5 percent or less of the tumor mass, with the rest being benign reactive T cells, one should not be discouraged when a marked reduction in lymph node size is not achieved on the initiation of aggressive chemotherapy. Horses will live a year or more with this type of tumor without treatment and are usually destroyed because of multiple subcutaneous tumors. In contrast, the large cell, large cleaved cell, and

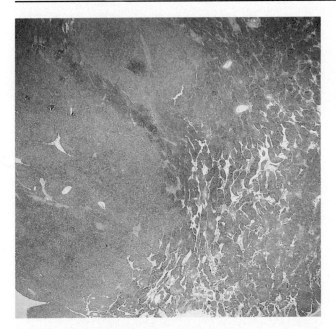

Fig. 3.1. In situ lymphoma. Mesenteric lymph node from a 5-year-old male cat. A diffuse tumor of the mixed cell type (T-cell-rich B cell) has involved the outer cortex and is compressing the residual benign medullary cords and sinuses. H&E ×10.

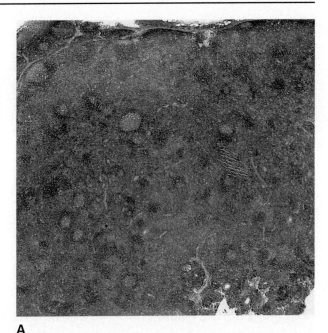

A

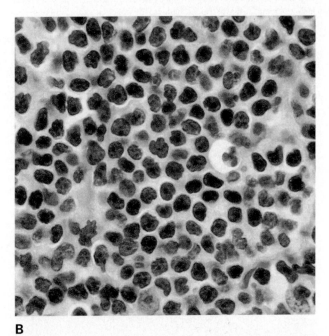

B

immunoblastic lymphomas tend to have high mitotic rates; and those that are of the B cell type, at least, tend to enter into complete remission with an aggressive combination therapy, which typically lasts several months. Further remissions may be obtained by using the initial or different therapeutic protocols.

Finally, the high grade lymphomas, consisting of small noncleaved cell (fig. 3.12) and lymphoblastic (fig. 3.13) lymphomas, require careful examination and identification. Lymphoblastic lymphomas are frequently of T cell type and are the type of lymphoma in the dog most often associated with hypercalcemia. It is essential to recognize that both lymphoblastic and small noncleaved cell lymphomas are small cell tumors with high mitotic rates, which differentiates them from the low grade small cell lymphomas. Dogs with lymphoblastic lymphomas may not survive more than 90 days, even with aggressive treatment. In contrast, the small noncleaved cell lymphomas, which are by definition of the B type, tend to undergo an early and complete remission on appropriate therapy and are potentially curable diseases, at least in children and possibly also in animals.

Focal lesions such as plasmacytoma (see fig. 3.19) or granulocytic sarcoma (see fig. 3.44) tend to be diagnosed based on cell type; they tend to be relatively indolent and, where appropriate, responsive to surgical removal. In contrast, multiple myeloma (see fig. 3.18) must be approached with considerable caution if there is marked hypergammaglobulinemia. In animals with 8 g/dl or more of protein,

Fig. 3.2. Diffuse small lymphocytic lymphoma (DSL). **A.** Popliteal lymph node from a 7-year-old spayed female Siamese cat that suffered a tibial fracture 5 years earlier that was treated with a bone implant. On architectural examination, the node capsule is thinned and the capsule and peripheral sinus are bridged in multiple areas, with colonization of perinodal tissues. There is loss of cortex and medullary differentiation, and there are fading germinal centers throughout the tissue. H&E ×10. **B.** Detail of A. The nuclei are 1-1.5 red cells in diameter and retain a round appearance with occasional shallow indentations. The chromatin is characteristically deeply stained. The nuclear membranes are irregularly thickened, there is retention of small chromocenters, and there are some focal areas of parachromatin clearing. There are occasional medium and large cells present that contain nucleoli, and mitoses are rare. H&E ×1600.

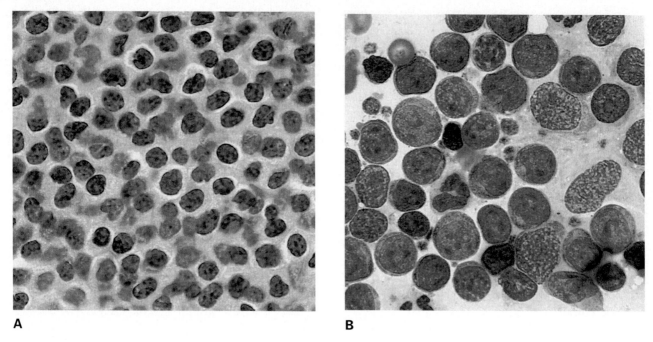

A

B

Fig. 3.3. **A.** Diffuse small lymphocytic intermediate lymphoma (DSLI), lymphoplasmacytoid type. Submandibular node from a 10-year-old neutered male golden retriever presented with greatly enlarged submandibular nodes and mildly enlarged prescapular nodes. The histology is similar to figure 3.1; there is effacement of architecture in a node and thickened medullary trabeculae. The nuclei are generally round, slightly larger, and more vesicular than in DSL, and occasional nuclei have shallow, sharp indentations. There is thickening of nuclear membranes and retention of small chromocenters, but some cells have focal areas of parachromatin clearing. Mitoses are absent, and there is an increased amount of quite deeply stained cytoplasm. H&E ×1600. **B.** DSLI imprint. Fine needle aspirate from the prescapular lymph node of a 9-year-old male dog with mild, shifting lymphadenopathy over the past year. Shows more typical cytology; nuclei are generally round and up to 1.5 red cells in diameter, have more prominent chromocenters, and have infrequent small nucleoli. Plasma cells (center) have abundant cytoplasm and larger, more prominent chromocenters. Wright's ×1600.

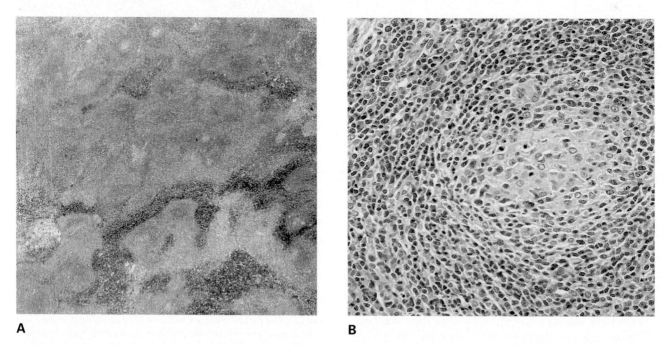

A

B

Fig. 3.4. Mantle cell lymphoma. **A.** Mandibular lymph node from an 11-year-old male Siberian husky. At the architectural level, there is complete replacement of normal architecture with "back-to-back" nodular proliferations of relatively pale cells surrounding a small cluster of dark (benign) cells at their center. The capsule is thin and taut with an intact peripheral sinus and without colonization of perinodal structures. H&E ×10. **B.** Detail of A. Characteristic histological features of this tumor are the arrangement of the malignant cells around fading germinal centers and the relatively abundant cytoplasm that renders these cells less dense in appearance on architectural examination. H&E ×140.

122

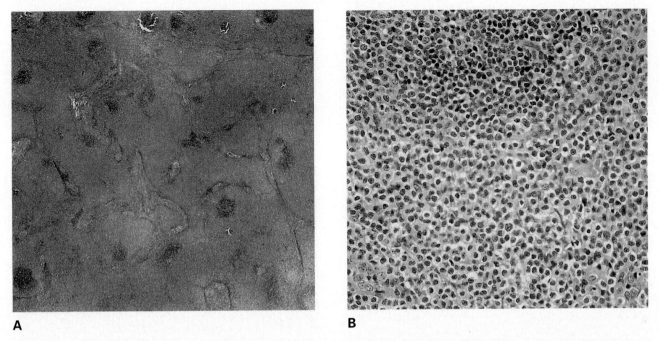

A

B

Fig. 3.5. Marginal zone lymphoma. **A.** Prescapular lymph node from a 5.5-year-old female rottweiler that subsequently developed generalized lymphadenopathy. Marginal zone cells occupy the area immediately outside of the mantle cells surrounding the germinal centers. At the architectural level, this tumor is characterized by evidence of previous chronic follicular hyperplasia, with fading germinal centers throughout the node and increased thickness of the collagenous trabeculae. The marginal zone cells have larger and less dense nuclei than the mantle cells and more abundant pale-stained cytoplasm, which contributes to the lighter staining cuffs of proliferating cells around residual germinal centers. H&E ×20. **B.** Detail of A. Mantle cells of a fading germinal center (top center) are surrounded by a band of slightly larger cells with more abundant pale-staining cytoplasm. H&E ×320.

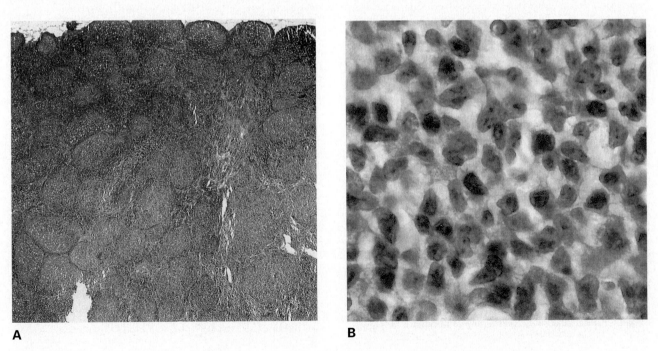

A

B

Fig. 3.6. Follicular small cleaved cell lymphoma (FSC). **A.** Popliteal lymph node from a 22-year-old cat with generalized lymphadenopathy. The capsule is thin and distended, the peripheral sinus is intact, and colonization of perinodal structures is not present. Normal architecture is effaced by closely packed nodular proliferations, with a lighter center and narrow darker mantle zones. The specific criteria for diagnosis of follicular lymphomas are that the postcapillary venules must be *between,* not within, the follicular proliferations and that the cellularity of the nodules must be *homogeneous* without evidence of the deep and superficial pole "polarity" characteristic of benign germinal centers. H&E ×10. **B.** Detail of A. The tissue consists of small cells up to 1.5 red cells in diameter that are densely stained, have irregular margins, and have angular and indented nuclei with thickened nuclear membranes and prominent chromocenters. There are nucleoli in an occasional larger cell, and mitoses are rare. H&E ×1600.

123

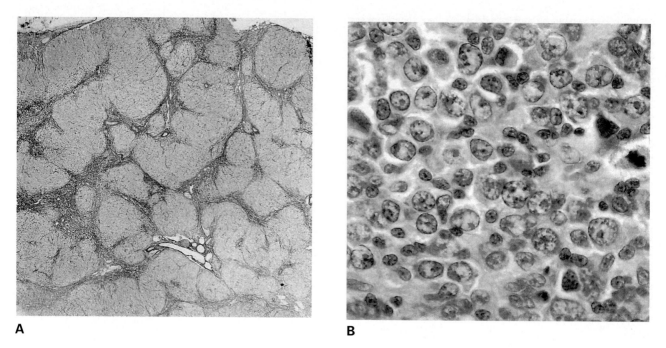

Fig. 3.7. Follicular mixed cell lymphoma (FM). **A.** Peripheral lymph node from a 7-year-old male cat with a mediastinal mass. The node is enclosed by an intact but greatly thinned peripheral capsule with a focally compressed but largely intact peripheral sinus. There is complete effacement of normal node architecture; it is replaced with tightly compressed "back-to-back" nodular proliferations that lack mantle zones. Reticulin ×10. **B.** Detail of A. The cells within the nodular structures consist in all areas of roughly equal numbers of small, medium, and large lymphocytes. The small cleaved lymphocytes have hyperchromatic nuclei and multiple chromocenters and lack nucleoli; the intermediate population of lymphocytes has relatively round nuclei, approximately 1.5 red cells in diameter; and the large cells have generally round nuclei that are more typically 3 red cells in diameter. These larger cells have vesicular nuclei with irregular thickening of the nuclear membranes and a finely branched chromatin pattern; both intermediate and large cell types have moderately prominent, typically single nucleoli. There is an abundant background matrix in which the lymphocytes are irregularly distributed without apparent cellular boundaries. There are numerous eosinophils and neutrophils in the compressed stromal areas between the nodular structures. H&E ×800.

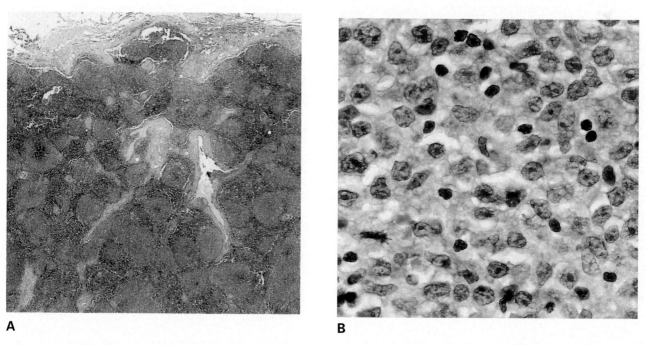

Fig. 3.8. Follicular large cell lymphoma (FL). **A.** Enlarged lymph node from a dog. At the architectural level, there is moderate thinning of the capsule, with an open and focally distended peripheral sinus. The outer cortex is remarkable in that there is complete paracortical atrophy and isolation of nodular proliferations, some of which have a central area of darker staining cells. In the body of the node, these nodular structures are tightly faceted and are delineated by a thin rim of compressed paracortical structures without normal mantle zones. H&E ×10. **B.** Detailed A. The darker cells in the centers of the nodular proliferations are small benign lymphocytes that are mildly vesiculated and resemble intermediate small cell lymphoma (DSLI). The predominant cells in the focal proliferations are a homogeneous population of large cells with nuclei 3 red cells in diameter; these are generally round but occasionally have irregularly indented nuclear membranes. The nuclei are vesicular, and have irregularly thickened nuclear membranes, a coarsely branched chromatin pattern with prominent parachromatin clearing, and either one prominent central nucleolus or two to three moderate sized nucleoli, some of which typically impinge on the nuclear membrane. There are one to three mitoses in most of the nodular areas that lack the polarity of benign germinal centers. H&E ×800.

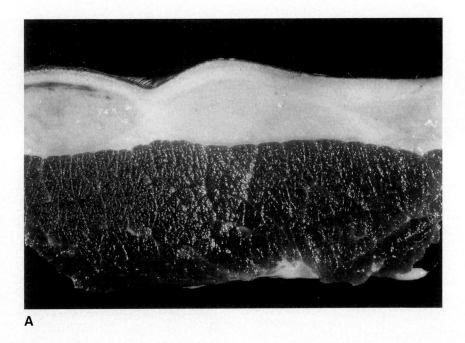

A

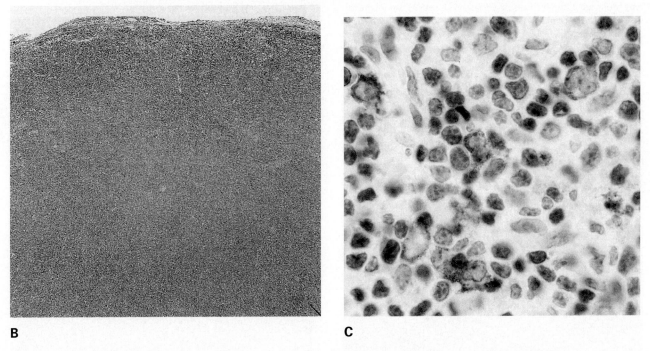

B

C

Fig. 3.9. **A.** Equine multifocal subcutaneous lymphoma. Cross section of subcutaneous lesions from a 7-year-old standardbred mare. Note that the skin is intact above the tumor masses, which are enlarging locally without invasion of the skin or underlying muscle. **B.** Diffuse mixed cell lymphoma (DM or T-cell-rich B cell lymphoma). A 1.5 cm subcutaneous mass from a 6-year-old male castrated quarter horse with multiple lesions. The lesion is typically solidly cellular and loosely encapsulated from compression of surrounding tissues. The heavy connective tissue background contributes to the uniformity of the architectural examination. H&E ×30. **C.** Detail of B. There is a constant mixed small and large cell population. Note that the small cells are likely benign small cleaved lymphocytes. The large cells are marked with a CD-79a (Pan B cell) reagent, and the small cells reacted positively with CD-3 (Pan T cell; not shown). The large lymphocytes with vesicular nuclei have one to three prominent nucleoli and constitute 5–10 percent of the cells present. The pale-staining oblong nuclei represent benign connective tissue proliferation. ×1000.

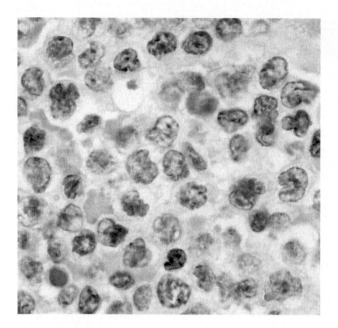

Fig. 3.10. Diffuse large cleaved cell lymphoma (DLC). Lymph node from an 11-year-old male dog with generalized lymphadenopathy. The tumor cells are 2 to 3 red cells in diameter with sharply and irregularly indented nuclear membranes. The nuclei are vesicular, with a branched chromatin pattern, and nucleoli frequently impinge on the nuclear membranes. H&E ×1280.

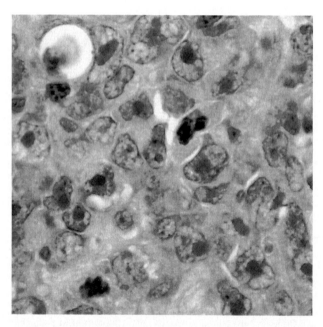

Fig. 3.11. Immunoblastic polymorphous lymphoma (IBP). Pyloric submucosa from an 8-year-old male domestic shorthair cat. The tumor consists of cells with large nuclei that vary markedly in size and shape, with many nuclei 3 or more red cells in longest dimension. The nuclei have both shallow and sharp indentations and irregular multiple infoldings, and nuclear membranes are sharply delimited with irregular thickening. The chromatin pattern is finely branched, larger chromocenters largely absent, and there is prominent parachromatin clearing. There are characteristically one or two large central nucleoli. Cells have abundant cytoplasm, and cell boundaries are indistinct. There are both high apoptotic and high mitotic rates, with a mean of 8.6 mitoses per 1000 × field. H&E ×1600.

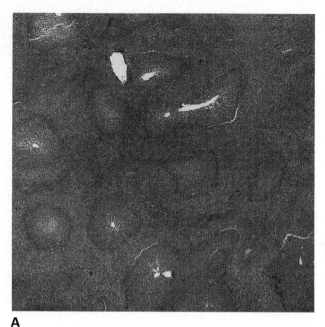

A

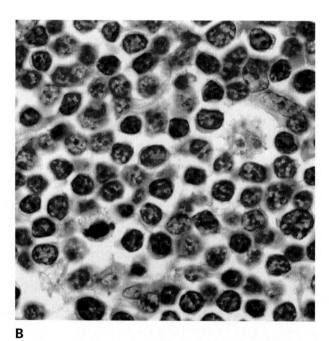

B

Fig. 3.12. Small noncleaved cell lymphoma (SNC). **A.** Liver from a 6-month-old Yorkshire pig. Marked infiltration of hepatic tissue, with tumor arising in the portal areas and forming a "bridging" confluence to surround central veins. H&E ×10. **B.** Detail of A. The tumor consists of a relatively uniform population of lymphocytes, predominantly 1.5 red cells in diameter. There is quite marked irregular thickening of the nuclear membranes, prominent parachromatin clearing, and a coarsely branched hyperchromatic chromatin pattern. There are characteristically *one to three small nucleoli* and a moderate amount of quite densely stained cytoplasm. There is an average of four mitoses per 100 × field. SNC lymphomas with this degree of uniformity of cell type are referred to as *Burkitt type* in human pathology. While the cell type is similar in size to the small intermediate cell lymphomas, the irregular parachromatin clearing, multiple nucleoli, and high mitotic rate are indications that this is a high grade lymphoma. H&E ×1280.

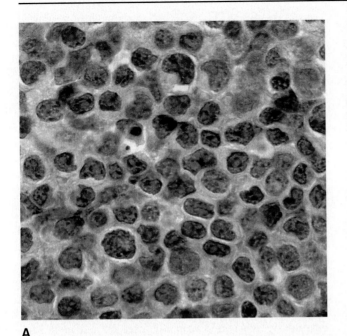

A

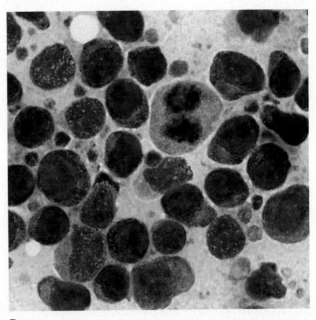

B

Fig. 3.13. **A.** Lymphoblastic convoluted lymphoma (LBC). Submandibular lymph node from a 6-year-old spayed female cocker spaniel. The tumor consists of cells with nuclei approximately 1.5 red cells in diameter that are characterized by multiple sharp, shallow indentations. The major characteristic of this tumor is the *chromatin,* which has a *finely dispersed pattern* with a few small chromocenters; *nucleoli are absent or obscured.* There are frequent apoptotic cells, and the chromatin of mitotic cells is less distinct than in other high grade lymphomas, making the relatively high proliferative rate less easily recognized. H&E ×1280. **B.** Fine needle aspirate from the lymph node in A. The tumor cells are 1.5 to 2 red cells in diameter, with the nuclei appearing round and the membrane indentations being much less apparent than in the histological preparation. The chromatin pattern is hyperchromatic and finely granular with a few large chromocenters. Nucleoli tend to be obscured in intact cells but are apparent in bare nuclei. Wright's ×1280.

there is serious danger of sludging of red cells in the peripheral circulation and the development of shock with even light anesthesia. This is particularly true in those cases with a uniformly enlarged spleen that may have focal areas of infarction and harbor occult sepsis. The extranodal lymphomas of peripheral T cell type (fig. 3.14) present a diagnostic dilemma because of their cytological heterogeneity, which mimics infectious granuloma formation. While a variety of extranodal lymphomas exist in human medicine, the mixed small cleaved and large cell type appears to be most common in animals; it resembles the T-cell-rich B cell lymphoma, with the difference that there is greater cytological heterogeneity than in T- and B-cell-rich T cell lymphomas. All peripheral T cell lymphomas are characterized by a vibrant fine vascular proliferation, and the malignant cells have vesicular nuclei with water-clear cytoplasm. These lesions tend to be relatively indolent; they may respond well for a matter of months to low-grade therapy, such as steroids, and ultimately progress to generalized lymphoma of the large T cell type.

In summary, for all hematopoietic neoplasms, it is highly desirable to undertake whatever histochemical or immunohistochemical assistance is required to provide the clinician with the correct morphological and histogenetic characterization. These characteristics do correlate with biological behavior, and as more data are accumulated, further associations will undoubtedly become evident.

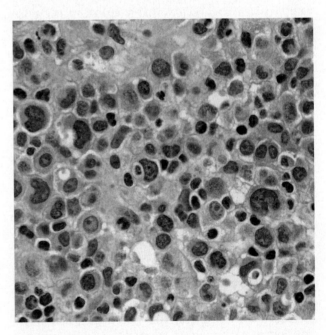

Fig. 3.14. Peripheral T cell lymphoma. A distinctive lymphoid neoplasm that characteristically appears as a single nodal or extranodal lesion that may be mistaken for granulomatous inflammation. A 15-year-old castrated male mixed breed cat presented with an 1.5 cm subcutaneous mass on the left hock. On architectural examination, the mass was solidly cellular with multifocal areas of ischemic necrosis. Cytologically, the lesion is heterogenous, with a background population of small cleaved lymphocytes and a smaller population of large cells with nuclei 2 to 3 red cells in diameter that have peripheralized hyperchromatic chromatin and a single prominent nucleolus. There is abundant cytoplasm, and cellular boundaries are often distinct, presenting an epithelioid appearance. The atypical cells marked strongly with CD-3 reagent. H&E ×720.

The Lymphomas

General Considerations

Classification Schemes

With time and advances in the understanding of the pathogenesis of hemolymphatic cancer there has been a slow evolution of classification schemes. It has become clear that some tumor types respond to a treatment protocol while other tumors do not. Therefore, response to treatment and, hence, prognosis, may be predicted by the tumor type. These associations have been well established in people, and there is good comparative evidence that lymphoma classification and response to therapy are associated in the dog.[1-5] Classification schemes have been applied in the other domestic animals,[6] which aids greatly in facilitating communication between pathologists and clinicians and in the prospective collection of data regarding treatment protocol evaluation. Some classification schemes have been more successful than others; these schemes have survived, and with other modalities of cell characterization, they form the basis for typing tumor cells.

Since the beginning of the last decade, the National Cancer Institute—Working Formulation (NCI-WF)[7] has become the standard for classification of human lymphomas in the United States, while the Kiel system[8,9] is used in much of Europe. Both systems are based on standard histological techniques readily applicable to animal tumors. Recently, revisions have been proposed which add phenotypic and genotypic procedures to routine histology.

Age and Tumor Topography

In some species it is clear that the distribution of lymphoid tumors differs characteristically between young (juvenile) and old (adult) animals. Interestingly, in cattle and cats, this relationship between age and distribution of lesions also has etiological implications. Lymphomas in adult cattle and young to middle-aged cats are associated with oncornaviral infection. In contrast, lymphomas in cattle less than 1 year of age[10] and gastrointestinal lymphoma[11] in older cats are largely unassociated with (productive) oncornaviral infection.

The classification according to the anatomic distribution of lesions is based on the observation that there are, generally, repeatable patterns of organ involvement characteristic of lymphoma in a species and at particular ages. The distribution of lesions will dictate the nature of the symptoms and sometimes the biological behavior. For example, hypercalcemia, one of the most common paraneoplastic disorders, may accompany canine T cell lymphomas in the anterior mediastinum.

The most common descriptive terms are alimentary, cutaneous or subcutaneous, multicentric or generalized, thymic or mediastinal, and solitary, regional, or extranodal lymphomas. Multicentric lymphomas are most commonly seen in animals. With some important species differences, the following tissues most often affected are the peripheral lymph nodes (often in a symmetrical manner), liver, spleen, kidneys, heart, gastrointestinal tract, and bone. In thymic lymphomas there is involvement of the anterior mediastinum, sometimes with invasion into adjacent structures. Those cases described as alimentary have involvement of the intestinal wall, mesenteric lymph nodes, and occasionally, other abdominal organs. At least early in the disease there is no spread anterior to the diaphragm. Solitary, regional, or extranodal lymphomas are classified by their unique location (e.g., renal, ocular, central nervous system, nasopharyngeal); these terms should only be used to describe the early disease process.[12-15] Rarely is the lymphoma confined to one site, but when clinical signs are predictive of a system, that anatomic system is usually appended to the name (e.g., ocular lymphoma, CNS lymphoma, etc.). Interestingly, in people some solitary lymphomas have unique ethnogeographic characteristics.[16] Proving the existence of a solitary lymphoma will depend on how vigorously tumors are searched for and on the sensitivity of various modalities used to assess the extent of the disease. Localization of lymphomas is, at least in part, dependent on "homing" characteristics based on cell surface adhesion molecules.[17]

Cutaneous lymphomas are subdivided into epitheliotrophic and nonepitheliotrophic varieties. The former originates in the skin and does not spread to other tissues until late in the disease. The latter form may be an expression of multicentric lymphoma or, if present in isolation, may be considered a variety of solitary or extranodal lymphoma. The subcutaneous lymphomas may present with multiple lesions, particularly in the horse (see fig. 3.9).

Cytology and Histology

Lymphoma will initially distort and eventually totally efface the normal lymph node architecture (see figs. 3.1 and 3.2). With lymphoid hyperplasia there may be colonization of the lymph node capsule, but the peripheral sinus usually remains intact. In contrast, with neoplasia the peripheral sinus is often destroyed, particularly with high grade lymphoma. Tissue and cellular characteristics helpful in distinguishing lymphoid hyperplasia from neoplasia are summarized in table 3.1.

Extensive experience in humans has shown that the biological behavior of lymphoid tumors can be predicted as low, intermediate, or high grade based on the estimation of mitotic index and characterization of tissue architecture and cellular details. Mitotic figures are counted as the number per field at 1000x magnification so that low, intermediate, and high grade categories correspond to 1 or less per field, 2–4 per field, and 5 or more per field, respectively. Usually 10 fields are assessed. At lower magnifications mitotic figures and pyknotic cells can not be reliably distinguished. At least in the dog, there is a strong positive correlation between proliferative index and the low and high grade categories.[18]

TABLE 3.1.   Histological characteristics helpful in distinguishing lymphoproliferative disorders

Characteristics	Hyperplasia	Neoplasia
Tissue architecture such as follicles, parafollicular areas, corticomedullary demarcation, and peripheral sinus	Normal architecture retained; follicles, paracortex, and medullary cords may be singly or collectively prominent	Compression and/or destruction of normal architecture; postcapillary venules are excluded from follicular lesions and become atrophic in diffuse arrangements of cells
Cell populations	Often increased numbers of granulocytes, mast cells, macrophages, and plasma cells	Monotypic
Cell size and nuclear shape	Variable	Monomorphic but occasionally dimorphic (i.e., mixed type); there are no lymphomas with three or more malignant cell types
Chromatin pattern	Large, coarse, and dense chromocenters with little detail	Fewer large chromocenters, more branching chromatin strands and other finely detailed structures
Nucleoli	Uniform size and shape and usually a uniform deposition of chromatin around the rim	More frequent, variable size and shape, irregular and discontinuous condensation of chromatin
Nature of follicular cells and parafollicular integrity	Marked variation in cell type across the diameter of the follicle; even with marked hyperplasia some paracortex remains to separate follicles	Parafollicular atrophy, uniformity in cell type across the diameter of the follicle but some changes in the density of cells

Tumors are described in terms of tissue architecture (follicular or diffuse), nuclear size (small or large), and nuclear shape (cleaved or noncleaved). Cell size is determined relative to the diameter of red cells. Small nuclei have diameters of 1 to 1.5 red cell diameters (see figs. 3.2, 3.3–3.5) while large nuclei have diameters equal to or greater than 2 red cell diameters (see figs. 3.7, 3.9–3.11). These tissue and cellular characteristics were assembled into a scheme [known as the National Cancer Institute Working Formulation for Non-Hodgkin's Lymphomas (NCI-WF)] that has been proven to correlate with biological behavior, response to treatment, and prognosis in humans with lymphoma.[7] As mentioned above, this scheme is also useful for the description of lymphomas in all of the domestic animals and has been shown to correlate with outcome in dogs.[1,3,4] The anatomical distribution of lesions, histological type, and immunophenotype should all be considered when designing treatment protocols since in various circumstances each has utility in predicting response to therapy in animals. Prognostic factors important in canine and feline lymphomas are summarized in table 3.2.

The tumor type based on a single biopsy generally reflects the nature of all tumors within an individual at that point in time. However, over time there may be a focal or general transformation of smaller cell types into larger and more aggressive forms. Treatment tends to shift the transformation in the opposite direction so that larger cell types are replaced by smaller cells.[3]

Previous histocytological schemes included the terms lymphoblastic (least differentiated), prolymphocytic, and lymphocytic (most differentiated). Lymphoblastic was used to describe a large cell with medium to high nuclear to cytoplasmic ratio (N/C), fine chromatin pattern, and prominent nucleoli. The prolymphocytic cells have large nuclei with a low N/C ratio, and the mature lymphocytic cell types have small nuclei with a high N/C ratio and increasingly aggregated chromatin. The disappearance of nucleoli and decreased nuclear size indicate progression toward a well-differentiated cell type.

Veterinary pathologists have tended to apply *blastic* uniformly across all large cell types. In the NCI-WF, REAL, and WHO classifications, *lymphoblastic* refers to an aggressive small cell lymphoma having nuclei with dense uniform chromatin and inapparent nucleoli (see fig. 3.13). The logic for this terminology lies in lymphocyte biology taken in the context of hematopoiesis. Here the progenitor or memory cell is a small potentially long-lived resting cell that when stimulated may undergo blast transformation and then terminal differentiation. Blast cells give rise to differentiated progeny; hence, the term *lymphoblast* was used to describe a small lymphocyte. Cells previously termed *lymphoblasts* by veterinary pathologists should be correctly described as *large lymphocytes*.

The term *histiocytic* is still used occasionally to describe large cell lymphomas. Its usage in lymphoproliferative diseases should be curtailed since it implies a histiocytic origin. Use of the term *histiocytic* should be restricted to those cases where the cell type is proven to be derived from the mononuclear phagocyte cell lineage.

Nuclear size alone is not a criterion of clinical progression in human or animal lymphomas. Thus, both lymphoblastic and small noncleaved cell lymphomas (see figs. 3.12, 3.13), as defined in the NCI-WF, are small cell tumors with nuclei less than 2 red cells in diameter that have a high mitotic rate and are clinically aggressive.

Recognition of mitotic rate as a branch point (algorithm 3.1) in distinguishing indolent from aggressive small cell lymphomas is an important diagnostic criterion.[1]

Other classification schemes (table 3.3), based on similar architectural and cellular characteristics, have been applied in dogs.[5,35,45,46] Like the NCI-WF, these schemes demonstrate that some tumor types do respond better to specific treatment protocols. Not surprisingly, different classification schemes seem to be associated with various aspects of outcome. For example, the Kiel classification applied in dogs appeared helpful in prognosticating relapse.[35] Most studies show that high grade tumors respond better to chemotherapy than low grade tumors.[3,35,45] Dogs with low grade tumors may have slowly progressive disease and live a relatively long time without intensive treatment; however, low grade tumors are less common in animals. Most lymphomas in animals are intermediate to high grade and are composed of large cells (table 3.4).[47]

Hodgkin's-like lymphomas with the characteristic Reed-Sternberg or lacunar cells are rarely recognized in animals.[47,48] Lymphocytes in the lymphocyte predominant type of Hodgkin's disease would be similar to diffuse small cell lymphoma seen in animals (see fig. 3.25).

Two unusual subtypes of lymphoma in people, the mantle cell and marginal zone lymphomas, have recently been recognized in animals. The mantle cell lymphoma (see fig. 3.4) is composed of small to medium-size lymphocytes with irregular cleaved nuclei, absent to small nucleoli, and little cytoplasm. These neoplastic cells form an expanded mantle cuff surrounding residual germinal centers, thus creating a subtle follicular pattern. In the spleen, the follicles in mantle cell lymphoma coalesce and replace the red pulp. The cells of marginal zone lymphoma (see fig. 3.5) have more cytoplasm and less nuclear irregularity. Architecturally, marginal zone lymphomas form an expanding layer of cells surrounding atrophic follicles, and in the spleen, they are less invasive of the red pulp than mantle cell lymphoma.

There are some remarkable differences between animal studies utilizing lymphoma classification schemes. The most prominent is the high prevalence of follicular lymphomas in the European cases of canine lymphomas (table 3.3).[35] This could be due to differences in diagnostic criteria, to the stage in the disease when a diagnosis is made, or to unique geographical, etiological, and genetic circumstances.

Other Phenotypic Characteristics

Some of the alternative approaches for characterizing tumor cells, such as immunohistochemistry and cytochemistry, may not optimally preserve morphology. This is not a problem if the tumor is quite homogeneous in nature, but tumors may contain large numbers of nonneoplastic cells. For example, a heterogenous picture is seen in some B cell lymphomas containing large numbers of T cells, termed *T-cell-rich B cell lymphoma.*[49] Presumably, the T cells are reacting against tumor associated antigens on the transformed B cells (see fig. 3.9). If one is looking for the expression of specific surface or cytoplasmic constituents but cannot distinguish various normal and abnormal cell types, then it is impossible to make any valid conclusions. As few as 5 percent of the cells in a lesion may stain for a particular marker; when there is this paucity of staining one must be satisfied that there is marked homogeneity of tumor cells and few inflammatory cells and that the staining is attributable to the tumor cells.

Cytochemical staining has proven to be useful in characterizing hemolymphatic neoplasias. Reagents for these stains are easily obtained, protocols are well established, and staining characteristics are known for most animals.[50,51] With few exceptions, lymphocytes do not stain with Sudan black B or for peroxidase activity, but cells of granulocytic/monocytic origin stain positively (see fig. 3.38 B). Other commonly utilized stains are for nonspecific and specific esterases, acid and alkaline phosphatase, and lysozyme. A summary of cytochemical staining for various cell types is presented in table 3.5. Most enzyme cytochemical reactions are performed on rapidly air dried blood smears, bone marrow smears, or imprints of tumors although some reactions have been performed on plastic embedded tissue sections.[52]

Prior to obtaining a biopsy for immunostaining, one should plan carefully to have the proper reagents and protocol to get the correctly processed sample to the laboratory in a timely manner. Many antigens are not preserved well in formalin. Even those antigens that are detectable in formalin-fixed tissues may be destroyed if tissues are stored in formalin longer than 24 hours. In table 3.5 CD markers and other antigens printed in boldface type denote those that can be demonstrated in formalin-fixed, paraffin-embedded tissues, usually with the aid of antigen retrieval protocols including enzyme digestion or microwave treatment. Sources of monoclonal and polyclonal antibodies used to detect CD antigens are listed elsewhere.[54] Blood or bone marrow samples on which flow cytometry will be performed are anticoagulated using ACD or EDTA. Immunohistochemistry is routinely done on snap frozen tissue which is then processed for frozen sectioning.[53]

Characterization of tumors beyond routine histology is important since nonmorphological attributes have been shown to be significantly associated with response to therapy and survival times. For example, dogs with T cell lymphomas have a lower complete response to chemotherapy as well as shorter remission and survival times than dogs with B cell tumors.[5,28] Dogs with lymphomas that have more rapid growth characteristics, such as short doubling times, and increased numbers of nuclear organizing regions, overall, have a better prognosis.[23] Prognostic features are summarized in table 3.2, above.

TABLE 3.2. Prognostic factors for canine and feline lymphomas

Species	Variable	Comments	References
Canine	Breed and gender	More favorable prognosis in small dogs and female dogs; males may have a higher incidence of T-cell lymphoma	19, 23
	Hypercalcemia	Mean survival time shorter in hypercalcemic dogs and, consequently, those with anterior mediastinal mass of T cell origin and with renal failure; hypercalcemic dogs without anterior mediastinal mass had longer remission and survival times	5, 24, 25
	Corticosteroid treatment prior to combination chemotherapy	Shorter remissions were associated with prior steroid treatment	26
	Response to therapy	Survival time longer in dogs with lymphoma that achieves complete remission	21, 27
	Anatomic site	A poor prognosis may be associated with primary cutaneous, diffuse gastrointestinal, and primary central nervous system lymphomas; solitary lesions in the skin and intestine may be amenable to surgery and radiation	28
	Clinical stage and substage within the modified World Health Organization staging system	More favorable prognosis when involvement is limited to a single lymph node or lymphoid tissue in a single organ, excluding bone marrow (i.e., stage I/II); dogs in stage I/II may achieve complete remission, have longer remissions, or have longer survival; bone marrow and blood involvement (i.e., stage V) and the presence of systemic signs (i.e., substage b) herald an unfavorable prognosis	5, 19-21, 27-32
	Histomorphology	Conflicting data: Kiel classification was found to be prognostic for time to relapse and for survival time between treated and untreated dogs; Working Formulation predicted survival time. In a recent study both classification systems were found to be unreliable prognosticators. Dogs with high and intermediate grade lymphomas more often achieve complete remission and may have longer remission times and survival, but early relapse may occur; low grade lymphomas respond less well to chemotherapy but may have longer survival times than high grade lymphomas	5, 29, 33-36
	Immunophenotype	Decreased survival time with T cell lymphomas; decreased expression of B5 and expression of P-glycoprotein prior to treatment are associated with shorter survival; relapse may be seen in association with P-glycoprotein expression	5, 34, 35, 37-39
	Proliferative index	Survival is prolonged in lymphomas having a larger mean AgNOR area, larger total AgNOR area, shorter distance between two AgNORs, and a smaller AgNOR area to nucleus ratio; longer disease-free period associated with a smaller number of AgNORs per nucleus and greater mean AgNOR area, maximal AgNOR area, and total AgNOR area; AgNOR better than PCNA in predicting response to therapy; Ki67 staining had no prognostic value; high mitotic rate associated with poor prognosis; positive correlation between proliferative index and low and high grade tumors	18, 23, 33, 34
	Karyotype	Dogs with lymphoma that had trisomy 13 have longer survival	40
Feline	Response to therapy	Cats with lymphoma that have complete remission survive longer than those with partial remission	41, 42
	FeLV status	Antigenemia is associated with poorer survival, although there is no association with response to therapy; FeLV negative cats with stage I/II lymphoma had longer survival than similarly affected FeLV negative cats; cats with renal lymphoma may have a better prognosis if FeLV negative	13, 41, 42
	Anatomic site	Some controversy: may or may not be longer complete remission in cases of mediastinal lymphoma; peripheral lymphadenopathy (atypical lymphoid hyperplasia?) without other organ involvement may be associated with longer complete remission; cats treated for renal lymphoma may relapse with CNS lymphoma	13, 41, 43, 44
	Clinical stage	Cats with stage I/II lymphoma (single nodal or extranodal tumor, including anterior mediastinum, but without lesions in liver, spleen, CNS, blood, or bone marrow) more often achieve complete remission and longer survival than those with stages III/IV/V	13, 42

131

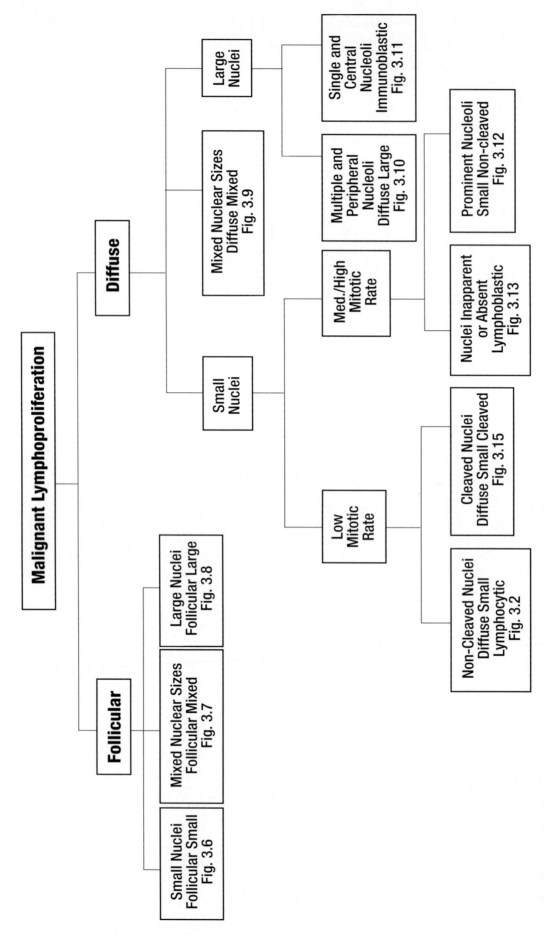

Algorithm 3.1. Algorithm for classification of canine lymphomas using the NIH working formulation.

TABLE 3.3.   Modification of the human non-Hodgkin's lymphoma working formulation for use in animals, percentages of major cell types[7,47]

Grade	Tissue Architecture, Nuclear Size, and Nuclear Shape	Cat (n=506)	Cattle (n=1195)	Dog (n=285)	Horse (n=81)	Pig (n=136)	Human (n=1014)
Low	Diffuse small lymphocytic (DSL)	2.4	1.8	4.9	1.2	0.5	4.1
	DSL—plasmacytoid	2.4	1.0	—	9.9	0.5	—
	DSL—intermediate	5.5	4.3	—	13.6	1.0	—
	Follicular small cleaved	0.2	0.3	0.0	0.0	0.0	25.5
	Follicular mixed	0.6	0.0	0.4	0.0	0.0	8.8
Intermediate	Follicular large	0.2	0.1	0.4	0.0	0.0	4.3
	Diffuse small cleaved	6.7	1.1	5.9	1.2	0.0	7.8
	Diffuse mixed	7.5	2.2	2.1	38.3	3.0	7.6
	Diffuse large cleaved	13.4	35.5	0.0	2.5	0.0	—
	Diffuse large noncleaved	8.5	30.6	20.0	23.5	60.0	22.4
High	Immunoblastic	37.2	2.3	24.9	6.2	8.0	9.0
	Lymphoblastic	2.6	1.6	17.2	3.7	3.0	4.8
	Small noncleaved	14.6	18.6	24.2	2.5	24.0	5.7
	Small noncleaved—Burkitt type	—	0.8	—	1.2	0.0	—

TABLE 3.4.   Frequencies (%) of cell types in two classification schemes for canine lymphomas

Working Formulation	Kiel Formulation	Carter[1] n = 285 (%)	Greenlee[5] n = 176 (%)	Teske[35] n = 116 (%)
Low Grade				
	Lymphocytic			
	Lymphoplasmacytic			
Diffuse, small lymphocytic	Lymphoplasmacytoid	4.9	10.2	—
Follicular, predominately small cleaved cells	Centrocytic, follicular	0.0	—	12.1
Follicular, mixed	Centroblastic/centrocytic, follicular, small cells	0.4	1.1	4.3
Intermediate Grade				
Follicular, predominately large	Centroblastic/centrocytic, follicular, large cells	0.4	3.4	31
Diffuse, small cleaved	Centrocytic, diffuse	5.9	3.4	8.6
Diffuse, mixed	Centroblastic/centrocytic, diffuse, small cells	2.1	5.1	5.2
Diffuse, large cleaved	Centrocytic, diffuse, large cells	—	—	—
Diffuse, large noncleaved	Centroblastic monomorphous	20	48.3	30.2
	Centroblastic polymorphous			
High Grade				
Immunoblastic	Immunoblastic	24.9	25.6	6
Lymphoblastic	Lymphoblastic	17.2	0.6	—
Small noncleaved	Lymphoblastic	24.2	3.2	—

Genotypic Characteristics

Karyotypic and molecular genetic changes have played exceedingly important roles in the understanding and diagnostics of human hemolymphatic neoplasias. To a limited extent, these powerful technologies have been exploited in the study of animal lymphomas.[83-85] Chromosomal changes, such as translocations, are characterized by traditional cytogenetic analysis and fluorescence in situ hybridization. Immunoglobulin and T cell receptor gene rearrangements are detected by Southern hybridization and the polymerase chain reaction. Many of these changes are acquired following the transforming event and increase in number and complexity with tumor progression. However, there are instances in people [86,87] and animals [83,84,88] where the changes are probably important etiologically and can be used to establish clonality, detect minimal residual disease, and assist in prognostication. Some specific chromosomal translocations define particular human cancers.[89]

Electron Microscopy and Morphometry

Ultrastructure has been used to study cells in lymphomas of most species of animals. Features unique to a particular species are mentioned in the following sections. The lymphocyte, compared with other cell types, is relatively devoid of cytoplasmic inclusions/organelles and nuclear/nucleolar changes. These characteristics of lymphocytes may be helpful, diagnostically, when attempting

TABLE 3.5. Special stains in hemolymphatic neoplasia (antigens that are bolded can be detected in formalin-fixed tissue)

Tumor Cell Type	Stain	Comments	References
Erythrocytes	Enzyme cytochemistry	May stain positively for specific esterase and acid phosphatase	51
Granulocyte	Enzyme cytochemistry	Positive staining for specific esterase, Sudan Black B, and peroxidase in all of the common species; early myeloblasts are negative for peroxidase	50, 55-57
Histiocyte	Antibodies to CD antigens	Acute granulocytic (and lymphoid) leukemias stain for CD34	54
	Immunoreactive lysozyme	Although most histiocytes are postive some may be negative; monocytes, PMNs, and various epithelial cells may also stain; dendritic antigen presenting cells are negative	58
	Antibodies to CD antigens	Most of the canine histiocytic proliferative diseases involve dendritic antigen presenting cells, and these are positive for CD1/CD18 and negative for **CD3/CD79a**: epidermal Langerhans cells lack Thy-1, while dermal Langerhans cells express abundant Thy-1; dendritic antigen presenting cells in the Langerhans cell histiocyoses (cutaneous and systemic histiocytosis) express CD4 and Thy-1 (CD90), while the neoplastic dendritic antigen presenting cell in the histiocytoma, histiocytic sarcoma, and malignant histiocytosis do not express CD4 and Thy-1 (CD90)	59, 60
Lymphocyte	Specific esterase	Some equine and bovine lymphocytes may stain	50
	Nonspecific esterase	All of the common species have some positive staining lymyphocytes (fluoride resistant), usually localized and granular; usually stains T cells, but some B cells may be positive; positive staining in feline LGLs; lymphocytes in all of the common species are negative for peroxidase and Sudan Black B	50, 61-64
	Antibodies to CD antigens	Most acute lymphoid (and myeloid) leukemias express CD34, which is expressed on lymphohematopoietic stem and progenitor cells. Canine thymocytes, T cells, and some B cell leukemias are Thy-1 positive	60
B	Antibodies to CD antigens, surface immunoglobulins, methyl green pyronin (MGP)	Stain positively for one or more of CD21, **CD79a, anti-IgM, anti-IgD, anti-IgG, anti-IgA**; κ and λ **light chains**; **CD79a** is most useful for demonstrating a B cell origin since it is present at almost all stages of development and is present regardless of surface immunoglobulin isotype; CD21 is present on mature B cells; immature and activated B cells stain positively for **BLA36 (CD20)**, and most B cell CLLs in the dog stain for CD21; about 80% of canine cutaneous plasmacytomas stain for **CD79a**; CD1 is frequently expressed in canine B cell chronic lymphocytic leukemia; lymphocytes in lymphocytosis and leukemia in BLV-infected stain for CD5, a marker for the B-1 subset of B cells; mature plasma cells quite well with MGP, poorly differentiated plasma cells may not stain, and early erythroid and eosinophils may stain with MGP; the usefulness of light chain staining to demonstrate clonality is limited in animals since chickens, dogs, cats, horses, cattle, and sheep express predominately or exclusively λ **light chains; κ light chains** are almost exclusively produced in mice and rabbits; swine and people produce about equal amounts of either light chain	59, 60, 65-71
T	Antibodies to CD antigens, perforin, and enzyme cytochemistry	Stain positively for one or more of **CD3**, CD4, CD8, CD49d, and Thy-1; canine PMNs stain for CD4, while PMNs of other species do not; CD3 is most useful for demonstrating a T cell origin; hypercalcemia often associated with CD4 positive cells; most cases of canine mycosis fungoides are CD8 positive, and most are δγT cells; 85% of nonepitheliotrophic cutaneous lymphomas in the dog are **CD3** positive; about 70% of canine chronic lymphocytic leukemias (CLL) are T cells (most are CD8 positive); about 55% of canine CLLs for αβ2 (**CD11d/CD18**); immunoreactivity for perforin and specific esterase activity present in LGLs	59, 60, 65-67, 69, 72
Non-B, Non-T	Antibodies to CD antigens	Absence of staining for B and T cell markers, activated NK cells, may express cytoplasmic **CD3**; a case of non-B, non-T lymphoma was Thy-1 positive	59, 60, 65
Mast cell	Toluidine blue, enzyme immunocytochemistry, antibody to stem cell factor receptor (KIT)	Degranulated mast cells may have numerous cytoplasmic vacuoles; positive staining for acid phosphatase, specific and nonspecific esterase; normal and neoplastic mast cells express KIT, expression is highest in most poorly differentiated mast cell tumors	51, 73

(continued)

TABLE 3.5. continued

Tumor Cell Type	Stain	Comments	References
Megakaryocytes	Nonspecific esterase, serine sensitive acetylcholinesterase, platelet glycoproteins 1b, IIb, **IIIa, vWF** antigen	Nonspecific esterase shows diffuse cytoplasmic staining (partially fluoride sensitive); in bone marrow sections, megakaryocytic cytoplasm is strongly marked with CD-79α, V.E. Valli, personal communication	52, 74-77
Monocyte	Nonspecific esterase	Considerable variability in intensity, usually diffuse, inhibited by fluoride whereas the activity in granulocytes, lymphocytes, and macrophages is not fluoride sensitive	50, 51, 78, 79
	Specific esterase	Some bovine and equine monocytes stain positively	50
	Peroxidase	Some canine and equine monocytes may contain a few positive granules	50, 55
	Sudan Black B	Occasional granules in all animals except sheep, less intense staining than that seen in neutrophils	55
	Antibodies to CD antigens	Some monocytes express CD1c; granulocytes, monocytes, and some macrophages express **CD11**: monocytes and subsets of macrophages and B cells express CD14; monocytes and eosinophils stain with Thy-1, but canine neutrophils are negative	59, 60
Myelomonocyte	Enzyme cytochemistry	Postivity for nonspecific esterase (fluoride sensitive) and peroxidase	64
	Antibodies to CD antigens	CLAW 27 and 51 (possibly identifying CD15), CLAW 016 identifying **CD11b**	80, 81
Various	Cell proliferation markers	**Ki67, PCNA, AgNOR, P-glycoprotein**	18, 23, 37, 66, 82

to distinguish cancers that possess similar *round cell* morphologies.

Morphometry has been used extensively in human lymphomas to quantitate various cellular characteristics and confirm differences in cell types usually assessed qualitatively by pathologists.[90-92] Technically, morphometry is labor intensive, but automated instrumentation is slowly being introduced. Although many of the various cell types described in lymphomas are reliably distinguished by qualitative assessments, some cell types do require morphometry, the outcome of which influences the diagnosis and prognosis. Morphometric studies of lymphomas in dogs[2] and cattle[93] have shown that most of the cell types described in the various classification schemes are distinct entities with very little overlap in measurements.

REFERENCES

1. Carter, R.F., Valli, V.E.O., and Lumsden, J.H. (1986) The cytology, histology and prevalence of cell types in canine lymphoma classified according to the National Cancer Institute Working Formulation. *Can J Vet Res* 50:154–164.
2. Carter, R.F. (1987) Cell types in canine lymphoma: Morphology, morphometry, phenotypes, and prognostic correlations. Ph.D. Thesis, University of Guelph, pp. 49–86.
3. Carter, R.F., Harris, C.K., Withrow, S.J., Valli, V.E.O., and Susaneck, S.J. (1987) Chemotherapy of canine lymphoma with histopathological correlation: Doxorubicin alone compared to COP as first treatment regimen. *J Amer Anim Hosp Assoc* 23:587–596.
4. Carter, R.F., and Valli, V.E.O. (1988) Advances in the cytologic diagnosis of canine lymphoma. *Sem Vet Med Surg (Small Anim)* 3:167–175.
5. Greenlee, P.G., Filippa, D.A., Quimby, F.W., Patnaik, A.K., Calvano, S.E., Matus, R.E., Kimmel, M., Hurvitz, A.I., and Lieberman, P.H. (1990) Lymphomas in dogs: A morphologic, immunologic, and clinical study. *Cancer* 66:480–490.
6. Valli, V.E., McSherry, B.J., Dunham, B.M., Jacobs, R.M., and Lumsden, J.H. (1981) Histocytology of lymphoid tumors in the dog, cat, and cow. *Vet Pathol* 18:494–512.
7. National Cancer Institute. (1982) The non-Hodgkin's lymphoma pathologic classification project: Summary and description of a working formulation for clinical usage. *Cancer* 49:2112–2135.
8. Lennert, K., Mohri, N., Stein, H., Kaiserling, E., and Müller-Hermelink, H.K. (1978) Malignant lymphomas other than Hodgkin's disease. In *Handbuch der Speziellen Pathologischen Anatomie und Histologie.* Springer Verlag, Berlin, pp. 1–833.
9. Lennert, K., and Feller, A.C. (1990) *Histopathologie der Non-Hodgkin-Lymphome (nach der akturalisierten Kiel-Klassifikation),* 2nd ed. Springer Verlag, Berlin.
10. Miller, J.M., Miller, L.D., Olson, C., and Gillette, K.G. (1969) Virus-like particles in phytohemagglutinin-stimulated lymphocyte cultures with reference to bovine lymphosarcoma. *J. Natl. Cancer Inst* 43:1297–1305.
11. MacEwen, E.G. (1996) Feline Lymphoma and Leukemias. In Withrow, S.J., and MacEwen, E.G. (eds.) *Small Animal Clinical Oncology,* 2nd ed. W.B. Saunders Co., Philadelphia, pp. 479–495.
12. Couto, C.G., Cullen, J., Pedroia, V., and Turrel, J.M. (1984) Central nervous system lymphosarcoma in the dog. *J Amer Vet Med Assoc* 184:809–813.
13. Mooney, S.C., Hayes, A.A., Matus, R.E., and MacEwen, E.G. (1987) Renal lymphoma in cats: 28 cases (1977–1984). *J Amer Vet Med Assoc* 191:1473–1477.
14. Lane, S.B., Kornegay, J.N., Duncan, J.R., and Oliver, J.E., Jr. (1994) Feline spinal lymphosarcoma: A retrospective evaluation of 23 cats. *J Vet Int Med* 8:99–104.
15. Weaver, M.P., Dobson, J.M., and Lane, J.G. (1966) Treatment of intranasal lymphoma in a horse by radiotherapy. *Equine Vet J* 28:245–248.
16. Cheung, M.M.C., Chan, J.K.C., Lau, W.H., Foo, W., Chan, P.T., Ng, C.S., and Ngan, R.K. (1998) Primary non-Hodgkin's lymphoma of the nose and nasopharynx: Clinical features, tumor immunophenotype, and treatment outcome in 113 patients. *J Clin Oncol* 16:70–77.
17. Pals, S.T., Drillenburg, P., Radaszkiewicz, T., and Manten-Horst, E. (1997) Adhesion molecules in the dissemination of non-Hodgkin's lymphomas. *Acta Haematol* 97:73–80.
18. Fournel-Fleury, C., Magnol, J.P., Chabanne, L., Ghernati, I., Marchal, T., Bonnefond, C., Byron, P.A., and Felman, P. (1997) Growth fractions in canine non-Hodgkin's lymphoma as determined *in situ* by the expression of the Ki-67 antigen. *J Comp Pathol* 117:61–72.
19. Keller, E.T., MacEwen, E.G., Rosenthal, R.C., Helfand, S.C., and Fox, L.E. (1993) Evaluation of prognostic factors and sequential combination chemotherapy with doxorubicin for canine lymphoma. *J Vet Int Med* 7:289–295.
20. MacEwen, E., Hayes, A., Matus, R., and Kurzman, I. (1981) Cyclic combination chemotherapy of canine lymphosarcoma. *J Amer Vet Med Assoc* 178:1178–1181.
21. MacEwen, E.G., Hayes, A.A., Matus, R.E., and Kurzman, I. (1987) Evaluation of some prognostic factors for advanced multicentric lymphosarcoma in the dog: 147 cases (1978–1981). *J Amer Vet Med Assoc* 190:564–568.
22. Schneider, R. (1983) Comparison of age- and sex-specific incidence rate patterns of the leukemia complex in the cat and the dog. *J Natl Cancer Inst* 70:971–977.
23. Vail, D.M., Kisseberth, W.C., Obradivich, J.E., Moore, F.M., London, C.A., MacEwen, E.G., and Ritter, M.A. (1996) Assessment of potential doubling time (Tpot), argyrophilic nucleolar organizer regions (AgNOR), and proliferating cell nuclear antigen (PCNA) as predictors of therapy response in canine non-Hodgkin's lymphoma. *Ex Hematol* 24:807–815.
24. Rosenburg, M., Matus, R., and Patnaik, A. (1991) Prognostic factors in dogs with lymphoma and associated hypercalcemia. *J Vet Internal Med* 5:268–271.
25. Weller, R.E., Theilen, G.H., and Madewell, B.R. (1982) Chemotherapeutic responses in dogs with lymphosarcoma and hypercalcemia. *J Amer Vet Med Assoc* 181:891–893.
26. Price, G.S, Page, R.L., Fischer, B.M, Levine, J.F., and Gerig, T.M.. (1991) Efficacy and toxicity of doxorubicin/cyclophosphamide maintenance therapy in dogs with multicentric lymphosarcoma. *J Vet Int Med* 5:259–262.
27. Cotter, S.M. (1983) Treatment of lymphoma and leukemia with cyclophosphamide, vincristine, and prednisone: I. Treatment of dogs. *J Amer Anim Hosp Assoc* 19:159–165.
28. MacEwen, E.G., and Young, K.M. (1996) Canine lymphoma and lymphoid leukemias. In Withrow, S.J., and MacEwen, E.G. (eds.), *Small Animal Clinical Oncology,* 2nd ed. W.B. Saunders Company, Philadelphia, pp. 451–479.
29. Carter, R.F., Harris, C.K., Withrow, S.J., Valli, V.E.O., and Susaneck, S.J. (1987) Chemotherapy of canine lymphoma with histopathological correlations: Doxorubicin alone compared to COP as first treatment regimen. *J Amer Anim Hosp Assoc* 23:587–596.
30. MacEwen, E.G., Brown, N.O., Patnaik, A.K., Hayes, A.A., and Passe, S. (1981) Cyclic combination chemotherapy of canine lymphosarcoma. *J Amer Vet Med Assoc* 178:1178–1181.
31. Owen, L.N. (ed.) (1980) *TNM Classification of Tumors in Domestic Animals.* World Health Organization, Geneva, Switzerland, pp. 46–47.
32. Squire, R.A, Bush, M., Melby, E.C, Neeley, L.M., and Yarbrough, B. (1973) Clinical and pathologic study of canine lymphoma: Clinical staging, cell classification, and therapy. *J Natl Cancer Inst* 51:565–574.

33. Kiupel, M., Bostock, D.E., and Bergmann, V. (1998) The prognostic significance of AgNOR- and PCNA-counts and histopathological grading of canine malignant lymphomas. *J Comp Pathol* 119:407–418.

34. Kiupel, M., Teske, E., and Bostock, D. (1999) Prognostic factors for treated canine malignant lymphoma. *Vet Pathol* 36:292–300.

35. Teske, E., van Heerde, P., Rutteman, G.R., Kurzman, I.D., Moore, P.F., and MacEwen, E.G. (1994) Prognostic factors for treatment of malignant lymphoma in dogs. *J Amer Vet Med Assoc* 205:1722–1728.

36. Hahn, K.A., Richardson, R.C., Teclaw, R.F., Cline, J.M., Carlton, W.W., DeNicola, D.B. and Bonney, P.L. (1992) Is maintenance chemotherapy appropriate for the management of canine malignant lymphoma? *J Vet Int Med* 6:3–10.

37. Lee, J.J., Hughes, C.S., Fine, R.L., and Page, R.L. (1996) P-glycoprotein expression in canine lymphoma. *Cancer* 77:1892–1898.

38. Moore, A.S., Leveille, C.R., Reimann, K.A., Shu, H., and Arais, I.M. (1995) The expression of P-glycoprotein in canine lymphoma and its association with multidrug resistance. *Cancer Invest* 13:475–479.

39. Ruslander, D.A., Gebhard, D.H., Tompkins, M.B., Grindem, C.B., and Page, R.L. (1997) Immunophenotypic characterization of canine lymphoproliferative disorders. *In Vivo* 11:169–172.

40. Hahn, K.A., Richardson, R.C., Hahn, E.A., and Christman, C.L. (1994) Diagnostic and prognostic importance of chromosomal aberrations identified in 61 dogs with lymphosarcoma. *Vet Pathol* 31:528–540.

41. Cotter, S.M. (1983) Treatment of lymphoma and leukemia with cyclophosphamide, vincristine, and prednisone: II. Treatment of cats. *J Amer Anim Hosp Assoc* 19:165–172.

42. Mooney, S.C., Hayes, A.A, MacEwen, E.G., Matus, R.E., Geary, A., and Shurgot, B.A. (1989) Treatment and prognostic factors in lymphoma in cats: 103 cases (1977–1981). *J Amer Vet Med Assoc* 194:696–702.

43. Jeglum, K.A., Whereat, A., and Young, K. (1987) Chemotherapy of lymphoma in 75 cats. *J Amer Vet Med Assoc* 190:174–178.

44. Ogilvie, G.K., and Moore, A.S. (1996) Lymphoma in cats. In *Managing the Veterinary Cancer Patient: A Practice Manual*. Veterinary Learning Systems Co., Inc., Trenton, NJ, pp. 249–259.

45. Gray, K.N., Raulston, G.L., Gleiser, C.A., and Jardine, J.H. (1984) Histologic classification as an indication of therapeutic response in malignant lymphoma of dogs. *J Amer Vet Med Assoc* 184:814–817.

46. Krueger, G.R.F., and Konorza, G. (1979) Classification of animal lymphomas: The implications of applying Rappaport's classification for human lymphomas to experimental tumors. *Exp Hematol* 7:305–314.

47. Valli, V.E.O. (1992) The hematopoietic system. In Jubb, K.V.F., Kennedy, P.C., and Palmer, N. (eds.), *Pathology of Domestic Animals*, 4th ed. Academic Press, San Diego, pp. 113–157.

48. Smith, D.A., and Barker, I.K. (1983) Four cases of Hodgkin's disease in striped skunks (*Mephitis mephitis*). *Vet Pathol* 20:223–229.

49. Steele, K.E., Saunders, G.K., and Coleman, G.D. (1997) T-cell-rich B-cell lymphoma in a cat. *Vet Pathol* 34:47–49.

50. Jain, N.C. (1986) Cytochemistry of normal and leukemic leukocytes. In *Schalm's Veterinary Hematology*, 4th ed. Lea and Febiger, Philadelphia, pp. 909–939.

51. Facklam, N.R., and Kociba, G.J. (1986) Cytochemical characterization of feline leukemic cells. *Vet Pathol* 23:155–161.

52. Colbatzky, F., and Hermanns, W. (1993) Megakaryoblastic leukemia in one cat and two dogs. *Vet Pathol* 30:186–194.

53. Madewell, B.R., and Griffey, S.M. (2000) Modern diagnostic strategies for cancer: Sampling guidelines. In Bonagura, J.D. (ed.), *Kirk's Current Veterinary Therapy XIII, Small Animal Practice*. W.B.Saunders Co., Philadelphia, pp. 452–458.

54. Vernau, W., and Moore, P.F. (1999) An immunophenotypic study of canine leukemias and preliminary assessment of clonality by polymerase chain reaction. *Vet Immunol Immunopathol* 69:145–164.

55. Jain, N.C. 1970. A comparative study of leukocytes of some animal species. *Folia Hematol* 94:49–63.

56. Grindem, C.B., Stevens, J.B., and Perman, V. (1986) Cytochemical reactions in cells from leukemic dogs. *Vet Pathol* 23:103–109.

57. Facklam, N.R., and Kociba, G.J. (1985) Cytochemical characterization of leukemic cells from 20 dogs. *Vet Pathol* 22:363–369.

58. Moore, P.F. (1986) Utilization of cytoplasmic lysozyme immunoreactivity as a histiocytic marker in canine histiocytic disorders. *Vet Pathol* 23:757–762.

59. Moore, P.F., Affolter, V.K., and Vernau, W. (2000) Immunophentyping in the dog. In Bonagura, J.B. (ed.), *Kirk's Current Veterinary Therapy XIII, Small Animal Practice*. W.B. Saunders Co., Philadelphia, pp. 505–509.

60. Moore, P., Affolter, V., Olivry, T., and Schrenzel, M. (1998) The use of immunological reagents in defining the pathogenesis of canine skin diseases involving proliferation of leukocytes. In Kwotcha, K., Willemse, T., and von Tscharner, C. (eds.), *Advances in Veterinary Dermatology*. Vol. 3. Butterworth Heinmann, Oxford, pp. 77–94.

61. Osbaldiston, G.W. Sullivan, R.J., and Fox, A. (1978) Cytochemical demonstration of esterases in peripheral blood leukocytes. *Amer J Vet Res* 39:683–685.

62. Raich, P.C., Takashima, I., and Olson, C. (1983) Cytochemical reactions in bovine and ovine lymphosarcoma. *Vet Pathol* 20:322–329.

63. Grindem, C.B. (1996) Blood cell markers. *Vet Clin N Amer Small Anim Pract* 26:1043–1063.

64. Grindem, C.B., Stevens, J.B., and Perman, V. (1985) Cytochemical reactions in cells from leukemic cats. *Vet Clin Pathol* 14:6–12.

65. Teske, E., Wisman, P., Moore, P.F., and van Heerde, P. (1994) Histologic classification and immunophenotyping of canine non-Hodgkin's lymphomas: Unexpected high frequency of T cell lymphomas with B cell morphology. *Exp Hematol* 22:1179–1187.

66. Kiupel, M., Teske, E., and Bostock, D. (1999) Prognostic factors for treated canine malignant lymphoma. *Vet Pathol* 36:292–300.

67. Caniatti, M., Roccabianca, P., Scanziani, E., Paltrinieri, S., and Moore, P.F. (1996) Canine lymphoma: Immunocytochemical analysis of fine-needle aspiration biopsy. *Vet Pathol* 33:204–212.

68. Day, M.J., Kyaw-Tanner, M., Silkstone, M.A., Lucke, V.M., and Robinson, W.F. (1999) T-cell-rich B-cell lymphoma in the cat. *J Comp Pathol* 120:155–167.

69. Kariya, K., Konno, A., and Ishida, T. (1997) Perforin-like immunoreactivity in four cases of lymphoma of large granular lymphocytes in the cat. *Vet Pathol* 34:156–159.

70. Butler, J.E. (1998) Immunoglobulin diversity, B-cell and antibody repertoire development in large farm animals. *Rev Sci Tech* 17:43–70.

71. Arun, S.S., Breuer, W., and Hermanns, W. (1996) Immunohistochemical examination of light chain expression (λ/κ ratio) in canine, feline, equine, bovine, and porcine plasma cells. *Zentralbl Veterinarmed A* 43:573–576.

72. Darbès, J., Majzoub, M., Breuer, W., and Hermanns, W. (1998) Large granular lymphocyte leukemia/lymphoma in six cats. *Vet Pathol* 35:370–379.

73. Reguera, M.J., Rabanal, R.M., Puidgemont, A., and Ferrer, L. (2000) Canine mast cell tumors express stem cell factor. *Amer J Dermatopathol* 22:49–54.

74. Bolon, B., Burgelt, C.D., Harvey, J.W., Meyer, D.J., and Kaplan-Stein, D. (1989) Megakaryoblastic leukemia in a dog. *Vet Clin Path* 18:69–72.

75. Joshi, B.C., and Jain, N.C. (1977) Experimental immunologic thrombocytopenia in dogs: A study of thrombocytopenia and megakaryocytopoiesis. *Res Vet Sci* 22:11–17.

76. Messick, J., Carothers, M., and Wellman, M. (1990) Identification and characterization of megakaryoblasts in acute megakaryoblastic leukemia in a dog. *Vet Pathol* 27:212–214.

77. Pucheu-Haston, C.M., Camus, A., Taboada, J, Gaunt, S.D., Snider, T.G., and Lopez M.K. (1993) Megakaryoblastic leukemia in a dog. *J Amer Vet Med Assoc* 207:194–196.

78. Jain, N.C., Madewell, B.R., Weller, R.E., and Geissler, M.C. (1981) Clinical-pathological findings and cytochemical characterization of myelomonocytic leukemia. *J Comp Pathol* 91:17–31.

79. Yam, L.T., Li, C.Y., and Crosby, W.H. (1971) Cytochemical indentification of monocytes and granulocytes. *Amer J Clin Pathol* 55:283–290.

80. Cobbold, S., and Metcalfe, S. (1994) Monoclonal antibodies that define canine homologues of human CD antigens: Summary of the First International Canine Leukocytes Antigen Workship (CLAW). *Tissue Antigens* 43:137–154.

81. Jain, N.C., Madewell, B.R., Weller, R.E., and Geissler, M.C. (1981) Clinical-pathological findings and cytochemical characterization of myelomonocytic leukaemia in 5 dogs. *J Comp Pathol* 91: 17–31.

82. Ginn, P.E. (1996) Immunohistochemical detection of P-glycoprotein in formalin-fixed and paraffin-embedded normal and neoplastic canine tissue. *Vet Pathol* 33:533–541.

83. Schnurr, M.W., Carter, R.F., Dubé, I.D., Valli, V.E., and Jacobs, R.M. (1994) Nonrandom chromosomal abnormalities in bovine lymphoma. *Leukemia Res* 18:91–99.

84. Fivenson, D.P., Saed, G.M., Beck, E.R., Dunstan, R.W., and Moore, P.F. (1994) T-cell receptor gene rearrangement in canine mycosis fungoides: Further support for a canine model of cutaneous T-cell lymphoma. *J Invest Dermatol* 102:227–230.

85. Momoi Y., Nagase, M., Okamoto, Y., Okuda, M., Susaki, N., Watari, T., Goitsuka, R., Tsujimoto, H., and Hasegawa, A. (1993) Rearrangement of immunoglobulin and T-cell receptor genes in canine lymphoma/leukemia cells. *J Vet Med Sci* 55:775–780.

86. Gascoyne, R.D. (1997) Pathologic prognostic factors in aggressive non-Hodgkin's lymphoma. *Hematol/Oncol Clin N Amer* 11:847–862.

87. Rezuke, W.N., Abernathy, E.C., and Tsongalis, G.J. (1997). Molecular diagnosis of B- and T-cell lymphomas: Fundamental principles and clinical applications. *Clin Chem* 43:1814–1823.

88. Heeney, J.L., and Valli, V.E.O. (1990) Transformed phenotype of enzootic bovine lymphoma reflects differentiation-linked leukemogenesis. *Lab Invest* 62:339–346 .

89. Gascoyne, R.D., Adomat, S.A., Krajewski, S., Krajewska, M., Horsman, D.E., Tolcher, A.W., O'Reilly, S.E., Hoskins, P., Coldman, A.J., Reed, J.C., and Connors, J.M. (1997) Prognostic significance of Bcl-2 protein expression and Bcl-2 gene rearrangement in diffuse aggressive non-Hodgkin's lymphoma. *Blood* 90:244–251.

90. Dardick, I., Sinnott, N.M., Hall, R., Bajenko-Carr, T.A., and Setterfield, G. (1983) Nuclear morphology and morphometry of B-lymphocyte transformation. Implications for follicular center cell lymphomas. *Amer J Pathol* 111:35–49.

91. Crocker, J. (1984) Morphometric and related quantitative techniques in the study of lymphoid neoplasms: A review. *J Pathol* 143:69–80.

92. Hall, T.L., and Fu, Y.S. (1985) Applications of quantitative microscopy in tumor pathology. *Lab Invest* 53:5–21.

93. Vernau W., Jacobs, R.M., Davies, C., Carter, R.F., and Valli, V.E.O. (1998) Morphometric analysis of bovine lymphomas classified according to the National Cancer Institute Working Formulation. *J Comp Pathol* 118:281–289.

94. Blue, J.T. (2000) Myelodysplastic syndromes and myelofibrosis. In Feldman, B.F., Zinkl, J.G., and Jain, N.C. (Eds.) *Schalms Veterinary Hematology,* 5th ed. Lippincott, Williams, and Wilkins, pp. 682–688.

Canine

Demographics

The prevalence of lymphoma in the dog is second only to that in cats. In the general canine population, the annual incidence rate is 13 to 24 cases of lymphoma per 100,000 dogs at risk.[1,2] Pups as young as 4 months of age may be seen with lymphoma, but 80 percent of cases are seen in 5- to 11-year-old dogs. The relative risk is significantly higher for boxers.[3,4] Other breeds that may have a predisposition are basset hound, St. Bernard, bullmastiff, Scottish terrier, Airedale, and bulldog. Dachsunds and Pomeranians may be underrepresented among dogs with lymphoma. Cases of lymphoma may also appear in families of rottweilers and otter hounds.[5,6] There is no significant sex predilection.

Clinical Characteristics

Untreated dogs with multicentric lymphoma have a life expectancy averaging 10 weeks, but a few may live from 6 to 12 months. Survival in dogs with the alimentary form is about 8 weeks. Older dogs with lymphoma tend to survive longer than younger dogs.[7]

The most common form of lymphoma in the dog is the multicentric type. In one series, the multicentric type accounted for 84 percent of cases of lymphoma.[8] About 80 percent of dogs with the multicentric type present with bilateral and symmetrical peripheral lymphadenopathy. The lymph nodes are smooth and usually freely mobile. There is no pain or fever associated with the lymphadenopathy. Subcutaneous edema may be present, presumably due to interference with lymphatic drainage. Other symptoms can be highly variable and are dependent on which organs are involved and on the presence of paraneoplastic syndromes. Splenomegaly is present in about half of the cases. Liver, tonsils, anterior mediastinum, and other organs may sometimes be involved. Bone marrow invasion may be suspected if there is some combination of anemia, petechiae, fever, and the presence of atypical lymphocytes on the peripheral blood film. Lymphoma is one of the most common canine tumors causing hypercalcemia; this is often associated with polyuria.

Alimentary involvement is the second most common form of canine lymphoma and accounts for 5 to 7 percent of cases.[9] Once there is diffuse involvement, affected dogs will show weight loss and often have diarrhea. In early cases, it is difficult to distinguish lymphocytic plasmacytic enteritis from alimentary lymphoma.[10] The transition of lymphocytic plasmacytic enteritis to gastrointestinal lymphoma in basenjis supports the concept that chronic lymphoid hyperplasia may be a risk factor for the development of lymphoma.[11]

Thymic or mediastinal lymphomas account for about 5 percent of canine lymphomas. Of dogs with lymphoma and hypercalcemia, almost half have the mediastinal form (see fig. 3.24).[11,12]

Solitary and cutaneous lymphomas are rare in the dog. Symptoms associated with the solitary lymphomas depend entirely on the organ distribution and degree of dysfunction. The least common form of canine lymphoma is the cutaneous variety; here there may be multifocal to generalized skin involvement, sometimes with pruritis. The canine epitheliotrophic lymphomas usually consist of

CD8[+] T cells.[12,13] In contrast, similar tumors in people are of the CD4[+] variety. The T cells of one form of cutaneous lymphoma, mycosis fungoides, have unique deeply convoluted or cerebriform nuclei. The Sézary syndrome occurs when these same cells appear in the circulation. Nonepitheliotrophic cutaneous lymphomas may be of B or T cell origin. However, recent evidence indicates that the majority are CD3[+], a T cell phenotype.[14] Solitary lymphoma of the gastrointestinal tract was reported in four dogs, two of which had T cell lymphoma.[14]

Clinical Pathology

The majority of dogs with lymphoma are hematologically normal. A mild normocytic normochromic nonregenerative anemia, attributable to chronic disease, is seen in approximately one-third of dogs with lymphoma.[15,16] Marrow invasion may be accompanied by rubricytosis. Hemolytic anemia is rarely seen. A mild to moderate neutrophilia is seen in 25 to 40 percent of dogs with lymphomas. Lymphocytosis and lymphopenia are seen with about equal frequencies of approximately 20 percent, respectively.[16] The detection of neoplastic lymphocytes in circulation is an uncommon phenomenon, although the chances of such a finding increase as the disease progresses coincident with an increased likelihood of bone marrow metastasis.[17] In one series of 53 dogs with multicentric lymphoma, 28 percent, 34 percent, and 55 percent had neoplastic cells in peripheral blood, bone marrow aspirate smears, and bone marrow core sections, respectively.[18] Thrombocytopenia has been reported in 30 to 50 percent of dogs with lymphoma, but spontaneous hemorrhage is rarely reported.[19] Dogs with lymphoma may have decreased humoral immune responsiveness but appear to have intact cell mediated immune responses.[20-22] A variety of immune mediated diseases, such as immune mediated thrombocytopenia and hemolytic anemia, may be seen in dogs with lymphoma. However, only immune mediated thrombocytopenia was significantly associated with lymphoma and may be considered a risk factor for the development of lymphoma.[23]

Hypercalcemia is seen in approximately 10 percent of canine lymphomas.[24,25] Although any topographic form of canine lymphoma may be associated with hypercalcemia, it occurs in almost half of the cases with mediastinal masses and is associated with cells of T cell origin (see fig. 3.24).[26] This paraneoplastic syndrome results from the secretion of a parathormone-like peptide from the tumor cells.[27-29]

Less common paraneoplastic changes seen in canine lymphomas are monoclonal and polyclonal gammopathies, polyneuropathy, polycythemia, and hypoglycemia. Monoclonal gammopathies may be seen in lymphomas without plasmacytoid differentiation (see fig. 3.18). When present in sufficient concentration, they can result in a hyperviscosity syndrome and occasionally renal disease (myeloma kidney).

Nervous system involvement commonly results in a pleocytosis.[30,31] The brain and cervical spine are most often involved, and the pattern of infiltration is multifocal and leptomeningeal.

Gross Pathology

The majority (more than 80 percent) of dogs with lymphoma have the multicentric type. Peripheral lymph nodes are often bilaterally and symmetrically enlarged. The alimentary, mediastinal, solitary, and cutaneous forms appear less frequently. Virtually all organ systems can be invaded by the neoplastic cells, which accounts for the very broad range of clinical symptoms seen with lymphoma. Affected lymph nodes are soft to rubbery and generally not adherent to adjacent tissues. On cut section, affected lymph nodes bulge and are homogeneous in texture; once there is complete effacement there is loss of the corticomedullary demarcation. The color may range from lightly reddish to gray to light tan to white. Necrotic foci may be present in large masses. Unusually firm nodes or extranodal tumors are characteristic of the diffuse mixed cell type of tumor, which has fine sclerosis (see fig. 3.9).

Infiltration of spleen and liver can result in two general patterns: symmetrical enlargement or nodular proliferations. Even in a spleen that is uniformly enlarged with lymphoma there may be prominent follicular structures on cut section that mimic nodular hyperplasia. Liver involvement can range from an accentuated lobular pattern (see fig. 3.12 A) to large multifocal tumor nodules. In the alimentary form, there are thickened intestinal walls sometimes with large nodules (see fig. 3.17). Enlarged mesenteric lymph nodes may fuse to form large masses. Invasion of other tissues, whether part of the multicentric or solitary forms, appears as whitish gray soft nodular lesions. Nervous system involvement is usually in the brain and cervical spine. It is often difficult to detect grossly since the colors of neural, lymphoid, and fatty tissue are similar. For the same reason, metastasis to the bone marrow may be difficult to detect; however, the absence of a normally reddish marrow should create suspicion. Occasionally, lymphoid tumors undergo central necrosis, and infarction is sometimes found in lymph node, bone marrow (see fig. 3.33), and spleen.

Histologic, Phenotypic, and Genotypic Characteristics

The classification schemes in tables 3.3 and 3.4, above, show that the high grade tumors (immunoblastic, lymphoblastic, small noncleaved) account for about two-thirds of canine lymphoma. Another 20 percent of canine lymphomas are of the intermediate grade diffuse large type.[32] In all the animal lymphomas, follicular and low grade tumors are unusual relative to their prevalence in humans (see figs. 3.4–3.8, 3.15). For example, follicular tumors account for almost 40 percent of lymphomas in people but 1 percent or less of the lymphomas in any animal species (see table 3.4). The importance of histological classification and other phenotypic characteristics with regards to prognosis is summarized in table 3.2.

When dogs are presented for diagnosis, involved lymph nodes have usually lost their normal architecture, which is replaced by diffuse sheets of monomorphic cells. Occasionally, dogs are presented early in the disease process, when it can be a challenge to distinguish hyperplasia from neoplasia; a further level of complexity arises in those few cases of follicular lymphoma and, rarely, with in situ lymphoma (see fig. 3.1). Invasion of the lymph node more often effaces the cortex of the node prior to destroying the medulla. In advanced lesions there is usually capsular and extracapsular proliferation. Perinodal lymphocytes may also be seen in increased numbers in hyperplasia, but the peripheral sinus is generally not destroyed unless hyperplasia is accompanied by sepsis and sclerosis (see table 3.1).

Cytological analysis of fine needle aspirates of lymph nodes are helpful in the diagnosis of lymphoma (see fig. 3.13 B).[32-36] The lack of architecture does not often limit the utility of cytological preparations since follicular lymphomas and other unique anatomical forms are uncommon. The presence of cytoplasmic fragments or lymphoglandular (Söderström) bodies in a tissue aspirate of an extranodal mass supports a lymphoid origin for the neoplastic cell type and, at least in people, has some utility in the diagnosis of lymphoma and in distinguishing lymphoma from other malignant tumors.[37] In dogs, lymphoglandular bodies were significantly more common in B cell and high grade lymphomas than in T cell tumors.[38]

When planning prospective trials to establish the efficacy of a treatment, both cytological and histological specimens should be obtained. An oncologist will commence antineoplastic therapy following a definitive diagnosis of lymphoma by a skilled cytologist. Cytology is a convenient way to monitor progress and response to therapy, and to assist in staging, and to detect recurrence.

Diffuse and follicular patterns may appear in the spleen; with either pattern, extensive involvement is not required for symptoms of hypersplenism to be found. Disregarding the various anatomical forms of lymphoma, splenic involvement is found in about half of dogs with lymphoma.[39] When there is difficulty in distinguishing splenic nodular hyperplasia from lymphoma, it is helpful to apply the concepts outlined in table 3.1 and look for similarities between splenic cell populations and infiltrates in other organs (see fig. 3.50). Additionally, lymphoma will frequently be associated with atrophy of the periarteriolar lymphoid sheaths and with subendothelial lymphocyte colonization of large veins within the thick fibromuscular trabeculae.

Liver involvement is most often multifocal, with the largest masses of neoplastic cells congregating around portal triads (see fig. 3.12 A). Smaller accumulations may be found around central veins; the dog is unique in that lymphatics are found adjacent to the central vein.[39] In contrast, with lymphoid leukemia and myeloproliferative diseases the pattern of neoplastic infiltration in the spleen and liver is sinusoidal and diffuse (see fig. 3.35 A). Extramedullary hematopoiesis may co-exist with hepatic and splenic lymphoma.

Bone marrow invasion generally occurs late in the disease process. Bone marrow core biopsies revealed involvement in 55 percent of dogs with multicentric lymphoma at initial presentation.[18] Patterns of invasion have been described as focal, mixed, interstitial, and packed, although the utility of this classification system has not been established.[40] Over 70 percent of multicentric lymphomas that had reached bone marrow were growing in mixed or interstitial patterns in paratrabecular and perivascular sites.

Renal lymphoma is sometimes found bilaterally. Lesions are usually present surrounding outer cortical blood vessels, and with more advanced disease these lesions will coalesce and extend deeper into the cortex and then the medulla. Paraneoplastic syndromes seen with lymphoma, such as hypercalcemia and myeloma (i.e., myeloma kidney), may result in renal insufficiency.

Cutaneous lymphomas are divided into the epitheliotrophic (fig. 3.16) and nonepitheliotrophic varieties.[41-43] Cutaneous plasmacytoma is considered separately and is described below. The range of cell types in the nonepitheliotrophic form parallels those found in multicentric lym-

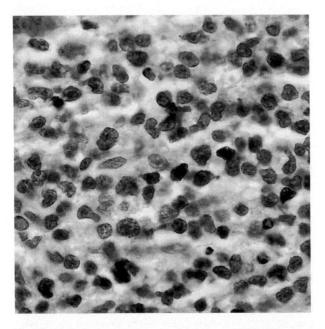

Fig. 3.15. Diffuse small cleaved cell lymphoma (DSC). Mature cat. The cell type is similar to that in figure 3.6 B, follicular small cleaved cell. The nuclei are small and irregular in outline with angular and indented forms. There is little internal nuclear detail, and nucleoli and mitoses are rarely found. H&E ×800.

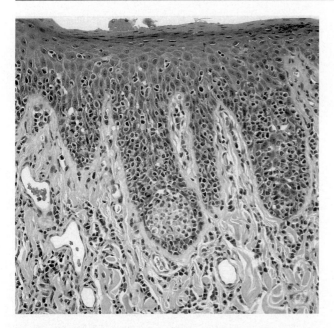

Fig. 3.16. Cutaneous T cell lymphoma, epitheliotrophic type. An 8-year-old male boxer dog was presented for examination of a tumor on the lower left lip margin, which was removed by excisional biopsy. There is a mild and irregular infiltration of tumor cells into the papillary and reticular dermis, a heavy colonization of the epidermal rete pegs, and a focal cystic area of tumor colonization (center). H&E ×200.

phoma. These are most often diffuse uncircumscribed infiltrates growing in the deep dermis or subcutis. Previously these were thought to be B cells, but now they have been shown to be predominately CD3+ T cells.[13] The epitheliotrophic form in dogs results from the infiltration of the epidermis with CD8+ T cells. Presumably, these T cells display an integrin that helps to localize them in the epithelium. There is some controversy whether the subdivisions of epitheliotrophic lymphoma (e.g., mycosis fungoides, pagetoid reticulosis, Woringer-Kolopp disease) are distinct clinicopathological entities or simply reflect temporal changes seen over the prolonged course of the same disease. A pragmatic classification system proposed for human cutaneous lymphomas refers to these lesions collectively as cutaneous T cell lymphomas (CTCL) with various descriptive subdivisions (fig. 3.16).[44] Particularly early in the disease process, the mononuclear cell infiltrate is characteristically pleomorphic, and many plasma cells may be present. Reactive helper and suppressor cells have been identified in canine epitheliotrophic lymphoma[12] but appear less frequent in the nonepitheliotrophic form.[13] Once the lesions of epitheliotrophic lymphoma are fully developed there are distinct histopathological changes. Neoplastic cells are pleomorphic, often having a cerebriform nuclear shape, which may be called the *mycosis cell.* In tumors with an interface pattern, these cells form a linear band within the superficial dermis and within the follicular and sweat gland epithelium. The mycosis cells

will appear in the epithelium as individual cells within a clear halo of spongiosis. With disease progression, clusters of neoplastic cells may appear in small vesicles termed *Pautrier microabscesses.* These latter structures are pathognomonic for mycosis fungoides. Occasionally, the mycosis cells will appear in circulation, heralding a leukemic phase termed the *Sézary syndrome.*[45,46]

Angiotropic lymphoma (malignant angioendotheliomatosis) is a rare form of lymphoma in the dog.[47-49] Gross lesions are variable and include infarcts, nodular masses, symmetrical organ enlargement, and accentuated lobular patterns. Brain, eye, lung, spleen, liver, lymph node, and bone marrow may be affected. Histologically, there is an intravascular proliferation of neoplastic cells within the lumina of lymphatics, sinuses, and blood vessels. The subdendothelium may show invasion. Cells are quite pleomorphic, and mitoses are frequent. Despite the characteristic histological appearance, leukemia is not present. The neoplastic cells have ultrastructural characteristics consistent with lymphocytes. Immunochemical evidence has shown the cells to be negative for factor VIII related antigen and positive for cytoplasmic immunoglobulin.

Reagents and staining protocols for immunophenotyping have been well described.[35,50-53] Various special stains and their utility in diagnosis and prognosis are summarized in tables 3.2 and 3.5. Approximately 70 percent of canine lymphomas are of a B cell phenotype, and depending on the study, T cell tumors accounted for 10 to 40 percent of cases.[26,35,54-56] Null-cell lymphomas occur with a frequency of about 2 percent.[56] Dogs with B cell tumors that have less than normal B5 immunoreactivity have significantly decreased progression-free survival and overall survival times.[56] In one series, the majority of lymphomas with the T cell phenotype were small cell, low grade tumors with occasional high grade pleomorphic types and, rarely, high grade, small noncleaved cell tumors.[35] Thymic or mediastinal tumors tend to have a T cell origin and are more often associated with hypercalcemia. In a study of 175 dogs with lymphoma, hypercalcemia was found only with CD4+ lymphomas.[56] Alimentary lymphomas are more often of B cell origin. Dogs with T cell lymphomas have a significantly greater risk of relapse and early death compared with cases of B cell lymphoma.[56] As mentioned above, the cutaneous lymphomas, whether epitheliotrophic or nonepitheliotrophic, are mostly T cell derived. Tumor cells from dogs with lymphoma appear to more frequently express P-glycoprotein, the product of the multidrug resistance gene, following chemotherapy and relapse, indicating acquired drug resistance.[57,58] Pretreatment expression of P-glycoprotein was a significant negative predictor of overall survival.[58] Reagents and protocols for the immunohistochemical detection of P-glycoprotein in canine tissues have been well described.[59] Potential doubling time and the frequency of argyrophilic nucleolar organizer regions (AgNORs) in tumor cells from dogs with lymphoma were significant predictors of first remission duration.[60]

Etiology and Transmission

Although there are reports of retroviral activity or retroviruses being identified in cultured canine lymphoma cells, it is not clear if these are exogenous or endogenous viruses, and there are no definitive data showing that these retroviruses have an etiological role.[61-64] Like other species, endogenous retroviral sequences have been identified in normal and neoplastic canine lymphoid tissue.[65]

An association between canine lymphomas and exposure to 2,4-D has been suggested but has not been proved conclusively.[66-68] No association was found in a recent study based upon reanalysis of previous case-control data that suggested an association.[69] There is growing evidence that people exposed to 2,4-D have a higher risk of lymphoma,[70-73] providing impetus to design better controlled and larger studies in animals and people. One study showed a significant association between dogs with lymphoma and exposure to electromagnetic radiation; however, further work is needed to decrease the effects of bias and confounding variables.[74]

Karyotypic abnormalities are common in canine lymphomas.[75] However, no consistent changes have been found, suggesting that the detected abnormalities were probably acquired once the transforming event had taken place.[76,77] In a study of 61 dogs with lymphoma in which chromosome banding was done, 25 percent of dogs with trisomy 13 had significantly longer first remission and survival times than dogs with other primary chromosomal changes.[78] About 21 percent of canine lymphomas are aneuploid, and most of these are hyperdiploid. A relationship was not found between DNA ploidy or cell kinetics and cell type or prognosis.[79]

Although there has been some success in transplanting lymphoma cells between dogs,[80-82] canine lymphoma has not been induced in mature recipient dogs receiving cell-free preparations.

REFERENCES

1. Bäckgren, A.W. (1965) Lymphatic leukemia in dogs. An epizootiological, clinical and haematological study. *Acta Vet Scand* 6(Suppl. 1):80.
2. Dorn, C.R., Taylor, D.O., Schneider, R., Hibbard, H.H., and Klauber, M.R. (1968) Survey of animal neoplasms in Alameda Contra Costa counties, California II. Cancer morbidity in dogs and cats from Alameda County. *J Natl Cancer Inst* 40:307–318.
3. Priester, W.A., and McKay, F.W. (1980) The occurrence of tumors in domestic animals. *Natl Cancer Inst, Monograph* 54:1–210.
4. Teske, E. (1994) Canine malignant lymphoma: A review and comparison with human non-Hodgkin's lymphoma. *Vet Quarterly* 16:209–219.
5. Teske, E., Vos J.P. de, Egberink, H.F., and Vos, J.H. (1994) Clustering in canine malignant lymphoma. *Vet Quarterly* 16:134–136.
6. Onions, D.E. (1984) A prospective survey of familial canine lymphosarcoma. *J Natl Cancer Inst* 72:909–912.
7. Squire, R. (1969) Spontaneous Hematopoietic Tumors of Dogs. In Lingemen, C.H., and Garner, F.M., (eds.), *Comparative Morphology of Hematopoietic Neoplasms.* National Cancer Institute Monograph

32. U.S. Government Printing Office, Washington, D.C., pp. 97–116.
8. Madewell, B.R., and Theilen, G.H. (1987) Hematopoietic neoplasms, sarcomas and related conditions. Part IV: Canine. In Theilen, G.H., and Madewell, B.R., (eds.), *Veterinary Cancer Medicine,* 2nd ed. Philadelphia, Lea and Febiger, pp. 392–407.
9. Couto, C.G., Rutgers, H.C., Sherding, R.G., and Rojko, J. (1989) Gastrointestinal lymphoma in 20 dogs: A retrospective study. *J Vet Int Med* 3:73–78.
10. Breitschwerdt, E.B., Waltman, C., Hagastad, H.V., Ochoa, R., McClure, J., and Barta, O. (1982) Clinical and epidemiological characterization of a diarrheal syndrome in basenji dogs. *J Amer Vet Med Assoc* 180:914–920.
11. Rosenberg, M.P., Matus, R.E., and Patnaik, A.K. (1991) Prognostic factors in dogs with lymphoma and associated hypercalcemia. *J Vet Int Med* 5:268–271.
12. Moore, P.F., Olivry, T., and Naydan, D. (1994) Canine cutaneous epitheliotrophic lymphoma (mycosis fungoides) is a proliferative disorder of CD8+ T-cells. *Amer J Pathol* 144:421–429.
13. Day, M.J. (1995) Immunophenotypic characterization of cutaneous lymphoid neoplasia in the dog and cat. *J Comp Pathol* 112:79–96.
14. Steinberg, H., Dubielzig, R.R., Thomson, J., and Dzata, G. (1995) Primary gastrointestinal lymphosarcoma with epitheliotropism in three shar-pei and one boxer dog. *Vet Pathol* 32:423–426.
15. Madewell, B.R., and Feldman, B.F. (1980) Characterization of anemias associated with neoplasia in small animals. *J Amer Vet Med Assoc* 176:419–425.
16. Madewell, B.R. (1986) Hematological and bone marrow cytological abnormalities in 75 dogs with malignant lymphoma. *J Amer Anim Hosp Assoc* 22:235–240.
17. Squire, R.A., Bush, M., Melby, E.C., Neeley, L.M., and Yarbrough, B. (1973) Clinical and pathologic study of canine lymphoma: Clinical staging, cell classification, and therapy. *J Natl Cancer Inst* 56:565–574.
18. Raskin, R.E., and Krehbiel, J.D. (1989) Prevalence of leukemic blood and bone marrow in dogs with multicentric lymphoma. *J Amer Vet Med Assoc* 194:1427–1429.
19. Grindem, C.B., Breitschwerdt, E.B., Corbett, W.T., Page, R.L., and Jans, H.E. (1994) Thrombocytopenia associated with neoplasia in dogs. *J Vet Int Med* 8:400–405.
20. Onions, D.E., Owen, L.N., and Bostock, D.E. (1978) Leukocyte migration inhibition responses in canine lymphosarcoma. *Intl J Cancer* 22:503–507.
21. Weiden, P.L., Storb, R., and Kolb, H.J., Ochs, H.D., Graham, T.C., Tsoi, M.S., Schroeder, M.L., and Thomas, E.D. (1974) Immune reactivity in dogs with spontaneous malignancy. *J Natl Cancer Inst* 53:1049–1056.
22. Owen, L.N., Bostock, D.E., and Halliwell, R.E.W. (1975) Cell-mediated and humoral immunity in dogs with spontaneous lymphosarcoma. *Eur J Cancer* 11:187–191.
23. Keller, E.T. (1992) Immune-mediated disease as a risk factor for canine lymphoma. *Cancer* 70:2334–2337.
24. Weller, R.E., Holmberg, C.A., Theilen, G.H., and Madewell, B.R. (1982) Canine lymphosarcoma and hypercalcemia: Clinical, laboratory and pathologic evaluation of twenty-four cases. *J Small Anim Pract* 23:649–658.
25. Meuten, D.J., Kociba, G.J., Capen, C.C., Chew, D.J., Segre, G.V., Levine, L., Tashjian, A.H., Voelkel, E.F., and Nagode, L.A. (1983) Hypercalcemia in dogs with lymphosarcoma. Biochemical, ultrastructural and histomorphometric investigations. *Lab Invest* 49:553–562
26. Greenlee, P.G., Filippa, D.A., Quimby, F.W., Patnaik, A.K., Calvano, S.E., Matus, R.E., Kimmel M., and Hurvitz, A.I. (1990) Lymphomas in dogs: A morphologic, immunologic, and clinical study. *Cancer* 66:480–490.
27. Weir, E.C., Burtis, W.J., Morris, C.A., Brady, T.G., and Insogna, K.L. (1988a) Isolation of a 16,000 dalton parathyroid hormone-like protein from two animal tumors causing humoral hypercalcemia of malignancy. *Endocrinology* 123:2744–2752.

28. Weir, E.C., Norrdin, R.W., Matus, R.E., Brooks, M.B., Broadus, A.E., Mitnick, M., Johnson, S.D., and Insogna, K.L. (1988b) Humoral hypercalcemia of malignancy in canine lymphosarcoma. *Endocrinology* 122:602–608.

29. Rosol, T.J., and Capen, C.C. (1992) Mechanisms of cancer-induced hypercalcemia. *Lab Invest* 67:680–702.

30. Couto, C.G., Cullen, J., Pedroia, V., and Turrel, J.M. (1984) Central nervous system lymphosarcoma in the dog. *J Amer Vet Med Assoc* 184:809–813.

31. Rosin, A. (1982) Neurologic disease associated with lymphosarcoma in 10 dogs. *J Amer Vet Med Assoc* 181:50–53.

32. Carter, R.F., Valli, V.E.O., and Lumsden, J.H. (1986) The cytology, histology and prevalence of cell types in canine lymphoma classified according to the National Cancer Institute Working Formulation. *Can J Vet Res* 50:154–164.

33. Carter, R.F., and Valli, V.E.O.. (1988) Advances in the cytologic diagnosis of canine lymphoma. *Sem Vet Med Surg (Small Anim)* 3:167–175.

34. Caniatti, M., Roccabianca, P., Scanziani E., Paltinieri, S., and Moore, P.F. (1996). Canine lymphoma: Immunocytochemical analysis of fine-needle aspiration biopsy. *Vet Pathol* 33:204–212.

35. Fournel-Fleury, C., Magnol, J.P., Bricaire, P., Marchal, T., Chabanne, L., Delverdier, A., Bryon, P.A., and Fleman, P. (1997) Cytohistological and immunological classification of canine malignant lymphomas: Comparison with human non-Hodgkin's lymphomas. *J Comp Pathol* 117:35–59.

36. Teske, E., and van Heerde, P.. (1996) Diagnostic value and reproducibility of fine-needle aspiration cytology in canine malignant lymphoma. *Vet Quarterly* 18:112–115.

37. Bangerter, M., Hermann, F., Griesshammer, M., Gruss, H.-J., Hafner, M., Heimpel, H., and Binder, T. (1997) The abundant presence of Soderstrom bodies in cytology smears of fine-needle aspirates contributes to distinguishing high-grade non-Hodgkin's lymphoma from carcinoma and sarcoma. *Ann Hematol* 74:175–178.

38. Teske, E., Wisman, P., Moore, P.F., and van Heerde, P. (1994) Histologic classification and immunophenotyping of canine non-Hodgkin's lymphomas: Unexpected high frequency of T cell lymphomas with B cell morphology. *Exp Hematol* 22:1179–1187.

39. Moulton, J.E., and Harvey, J.W. (1990) Tumors of the lymphoid and hematopoietic tissues. In Moulton, J.E. (ed.), *Tumors in Domestic Animals,* 3rd ed. University of California Press, Berkeley, pp. 231–307.

40. Raskin, R.E., and Krehbiel, J.D. (1988) Histopathology of canine bone marrow in malignant lymphoproliferative disorders. *Vet Pathol* 25:83–88.

41. Wilcock, B.P., and Yager, J.A. (1989) The behavior of epidermotropic lymphoma in twenty-five dogs. *Can Vet J* 30:754–756.

42. Goldschmidt, M.H., and Shofer, F.S. (1992) Cutaneous lymphosarcoma. In *Skin Tumors of the Dog and Cat.* Pergamon Press, Oxford, pp. 252–264.

43. Brown, N.O., Nesbitt, G.H., Patnaik, A.K., and MacEwen, E.G. (1980) Cutaneous lymphosarcoma in the dog: A disease with variable clinical and histologic manifestations. *J Amer Anim Hosp Assoc* 16:565–572.

44. Burg, G., Dummer, R., Dommann, S., Nestle, F., and Nickoloff, B. (1995) Pathology of cutaneous T-cell lymphomas. *Hematol/Oncol Clin N Amera* 9:961–994.

45. Thrall, M.A., Macy, D.W., Snyder, S.P., and Hall, R.L. (1984) Cutaneous lymphosarcoma and leukemia in a dog resembling Sézary syndrome in man. *Vet Pathol* 21:182–186.

46. Foster, A.P., Evans, E., Kerlin, R.L., and Vail, D.M. (1997) Cutaneous T-cell lymphoma with Sézary syndrome in a dog. *Vet Clin Pathol* 26:188–192.

47. Dargent, F.J., Fox, L.E., and Anderson, W.I. (1988) Neoplastic angioendotheliomatosis in a dog: An angiotropic lymphoma. *Cornell Vet* 78:253–262.

48. Kilrain, C.G., Saik, J.E., Jeglum, K.A. (1994) Malignant angioendotheliomatosis with retinal detachment in a dog. *J Amer Vet Med Assoc* 204:918–921.

49. Steinberg, H. (1996) Multisystem angiotropic lymphoma (malignant angioendotheliomatosis) involving the humerus in a dog. *J Vet Diag Invest* 8:502–505.

50. Moore, P.F., Rossitto, P.V., and Danilenko, D.M. (1990) Canine leukocyte integrins: Characterization of a CD18 homologue. *Tissue Antigens* 36:211–220.

51. Moore, P.F., Rossitto, P.V., Danilenko, D.M., Wielenga, J.J., Raff, R.F., and Severns, E. (1992) Monoclonal antibodies specific for canine CD4 and CD8 define functional T-lymphocyte subsets and high-density expression of CD4 by canine neutrophils. *Tissue Antigens* 40:75–85.

52. Cobbold, S.P., and Metcalfe, S. (1994) Monoclonal antibodies that define canine homologues of human CD antigens: Summary of the First International Canine Leukocyte Antigen Workshop (CLAW). *Tissue Antigens* 43:137–154.

53. Grindem, C.B., Page, R.L., Ammerman, B.E., and Breitschwerdt, E.B. (1998) Immunophenotypic comparison of blood and lymph node from dogs with lymphoma. *Vet Clin Pathol* 27:16–20.

54. Teske, E., van Heerde, P., Rutteman, G.R., Kurzman, I., Moore, P.F., and MacEwen, E.G. (1994) Prognostic factors for treatment of malignant lymphoma in dogs. *J Amer Vet Med Assoc* 205:1722–1728.

55. Appelbaum, F.R., Sale, G.E., Storb, R., Charrier, K., Deeg, H.J, Graham, T., and Wulff, J.C. (1984) Phenotyping of canine lymphoma with monoclonal antibodies directed at cell surface antigens. Classification, morphology, clinical presentation, and response to chemotherapy. *Hematol Oncol* 2:151–168.

56. Ruslander, D.A., Gebhard, D.H., Tompkins, M.B., Grindem, C.B., and Page, R.L. (1997) Immunophenotypic characterization of canine lymphoproliferative disorders. *In Vivo* 11:169–172.

57. Moore, A.S., Leveille, C.R., Reimann, K.A., Shu, H., and Arias, I.M. (1995) The expression of P-glycoprotein in canine lymphoma and its association with multidrug resistance. *Cancer Invest* 13:475–479.

58. Lee, J.J., Hughes, C.S., Fine, R.L., and Page, R.L. (1996) P-glycoprotein expression in canine lymphoma. *Cancer* 77:1892–1898.

59. Ginn, P.E. (1996) Immunohistochemical detection of P-glycoprotein in formalin-fixed and paraffin-embedded normal and neoplastic canine tissues. *Vet Pathol* 33:533–541.

60. Vail, D.M., Kisseberth W.C., Obradovich, J.E., Moore, F.M., London, C.A., MacEwen, E.G., and Ritter, M.A. (1996) Assessment of potential doubling times (T_{pot}), argyrophilic nucleolar organizer regions (AgNOR), and proliferating cell nuclear antigen (PCNA) as predictors of therapy response in canine non-Hodgkin's lymphoma. *Exp Hematol* 24:807–815.

61. Ghernati, I., Auger, C., Chabanne, L., Corbin, A., Bonnefort, C., Magnol, J.P., Fournel, C., Rivoire, A., Monier, J.C., and Rigal, D. (1999) Characterization of a canine long-term T cell line (DLC 01) established from a dog with Sézary syndrome and producing retroviral particles. *Leukemia* 13:1281–1290.

62. Onions, D. (1980) RNA dependent DNA polymerase activity in canine lymphosarcoma. *Eur J Cancer* 16:345–350,

63. Tomley, F.M., Armstrong, S.J., Mahy, B.W.J., and Owen, L.N. (1983) Reverse transcriptase activity and particles of retroviral density in cultured canine lymphosarcoma supernatants. *Brit J Cancer* 47:277–284.

64. Safran, N., Perk, K., Eyal, O., and Dahlberg, J.E. (1992) Isolation and preliminary characterization of a novel retrovirus isolated from a leukaemic dog. *Res Vet Sci* 52:250–255.

65. Colbatzky, F., and Jacobs, R.M. (1992) Detection of retroviral-like elements in genomic DNA of dogs with and without lymphoma. 73rd Annual Meeting of the Conference of Research Workers in Animal Diseases, Chicago, p. 57.

66. Carlo, G.L., Cole, P., Miller, A.B., Munro, I.C., Solomon, K.R., and Squire, R.A. (1992) Review of a study reporting an association between 2,4-dichlorophenoxyacetic acid and canine malignant lymphoma: Report of an expert panel. *Regul Toxicol Pharmacol* 16:245–252.

67. Hayes, H.M., Tarone, R.E, and Cantor, K.P. (1995) On the association between canine malignant lymphoma and opportunity for exposure to 2,4-dichlorophenoxyacetic acid. *Environ Res* 70:119–125.

68. Hayes, H.M., Tarone, R.E., Cantor, K.P., Jessen C.R., MacCurnin, D.M., and Richardson, R.C. (1991) Case-control study of canine malignant lymphoma: Positive association with dog owner's use of 2,4-dichlorophenoxyacetic acid herbicides. *J Natl Cancer Inst* 83:1226–1231.

69. Kaneene, J.B., and Miller, R. (1999) Reanalysis of 2,4-D and the occurrence of canine malignant lymphoma. *Vet Hum Toxicol* 41:164–170.

70. Blair, A. (1990) Herbicides and non-Hodgkin's lymphoma: New evidence from a study of Saskatchewan farmers. *J Natl Cancer Inst* 82:544–545.

71. Hardell, L., Erickson, M., Lenner, P., and Lundgre E. (1981) Malignant lymphoma and exposure to chemicals, especially organic solvents, chlorophenols and phenoxy acids: A case-control study. *Brit J Cancer* 43:169–176.

72. Hoar, S.K., Blair, A., Holmes, F.F., Boysen, C.D., Robel, R.J., Hoover, R., and Fraumeni, J.F. (1986) Agricultural herbicide use and risk of lymphoma and soft tissue sarcoma. *J Amer Med Assoc* 256:1141–1147.

73. Zahm, S.H., and Blair, A. (1992) Pesticides and non-Hodgkin's lymphoma. *Cancer Res (Suppl)* 52:5485s-5488s.

74. Reif, J.S., Lower, K.S., and Ogilvie, G.K. (1995) Residential exposure to magnetic fields and risk of canine lymphoma. *Amer J Epidemiol* 141:352–359.

75. Grindem, C.B., and Buoen, L.C. (1986) Cytogenetic analysis of leukemic cells in the dog. A report of 10 cases and a review of literature. *J Comp Pathol* 96:623–635.

76. Idowu, L. (1976) Observations on the chromosomes of a lymphosarcoma in a dog. *Vet Rec* 99:103.

77. Swayne, D.E., Michalski, K., and McCaw, D. (1987) Cutaneous lymphosarcoma with abnormal chromosomes in a dog. *J Comp Pathol* 97:609–614.

78. Hahn, K.A., Richardson, R.C., Hahn, E.A., and Chrisman, C.L. (1994) Diagnostic and prognostic importance of chromosomal aberrations identified in 61 dogs with lymphosarcoma. *Vet Pathol* 31:528–540.

79. Teske, E., Rutteman, G.R., Kuipers-Dijkshoorn, N.J., van Dierendonck, J.H., van Heerde, P., and Cornelisse, C.J. (1993) DNA ploidy and cell kinetic characteristics in canine non-Hodgkin's lymphoma. *Exp Hematol* 21:579–584.

80. Cohen, H., Chapman, A.L., Eberg, J.W., Bopp, W.J., and Gravelle, C.R. (1970) Cellular transmission of canine lymphoma and leukemia in beagles. *J Natl Cancer Inst* 45:1013–1023.

81. Kakuk, T.J., Hinz, R.W., Langham, R.F., and Conner, G.H. (1968) Experimental transmission of canine malignant lymphoma to the beagle neonate. *Cancer Res* 28:716–723.

82. Moldovanu, G., Moore, A.E., Friedman, M., and Miller, D.G. (1966). Cellular transmission of lymphosarcoma in dogs. *Nature* 210:1342–2343.

Feline

Demographics

Lymphoma is the most common neoplasm of cats. Greater than half of all feline hemolymphatic tumors are lymphomas.[1,2] In the San Franciso area, the annual incidence of feline lymphoma was 41.6 per 100,000 cats at risk,[3] while others estimated the rate to be 200 per 100,000 cats at risk.[4] Prevalence rates for lymphomas of 1.6 percent of cats in the general population and 4.7 percent of hospitalized sick cats have been reported.[5] Affected cats show a bimodal age distribution, with peaks appearing in early adulthood at approximately 2 years of age and then in mature cats 6 to 12 years of age.[6,7] Cats as young as 6 months of age may be affected. Purebred cats, in particular the Siamese, may be predisposed.[8] Although there are conflicting data, lymphomas may be more common in male cats, presumably because of behavioral characteristics that make transmission of feline leukemia virus (FeLV) more efficient.[9] Prevalence rates of lymphoma appear to vary with geographic location, which may reflect regional differences in the prevalence rates, strains of FeLV, and genetic backgrounds of the cats.

Clinical Characteristics

Mortality rates of untreated cats with lymphoma are about 40 and 75 percent at 4 and 8 weeks following diagnosis, respectively.[10] As with the dog, clinical signs are referable to the organ systems involved in the disease process. Unlike the dog, most cats with lymphoma present with anterior mediastinal or abdominal masses; peripheral lymphadenopathy is unusual in cats with lymphoma. Therefore, respiratory difficulty, weight loss, diarrhea, vomiting, and constipation are often observed. The mediastinal form is more common in young cats, and the extranodal and alimentary forms are more common in older cats.[2,5,8,11] Anemia may be present as a result of FeLV infection or as a consequence of myelophthisis. The effects of FeLV may be direct (e.g., cytotoxicity) or indirect (through the production of cytosuppressive molecules). Myelophthisis results from a disturbance in the hematopoietic inductive microenvironment (HIM) and is presumably mediated by a combination of physical crowding of marrow elements, competition for nutrients, immune mediated disease, and production of cytokines by proliferating cells. An altered HIM has been demonstrated in association with FeLV infection.[12-14] If myelophthisis is present, there may be fever and petechial hemorrhage, reflecting decreased granulocyte and platelet production, respectively. Immune complex nephritis and bilateral renal lymphoma may result in renal failure.

Clinical Pathology

The pathogenic strains of FeLV and feline immunodeficiency virus (FIV) are often associated with lymphopenia, nonregenerative anemia, pancytopenia, lymphoma, or leukemia. These hematological changes have been reviewed in detail elsewhere.[15] Proliferative and antiproliferative changes are somewhat dependent on viral strain. For example, pure red cell aplasia is strongly associated with subgroup C FeLV. The FeLV associated nonregenerative anemia may be macrocytic.[16]

Approximately two-thirds of cats with lymphoma have some hematological abnormality.[17] About 50 percent of cats with lymphoma are reported to have marrow invasion, and a similar percentage have moderate to marked nonregenerative anemia. Leukopenia and lymphopenia are seen in about one-quarter and one-half of cats with lymphoma, respectively.

With progression of the disease there is increased likelihood of metastasis to the bone marrow, resulting in multiple cytopenias. Once the disease is established in the marrow, there is potential for leukemic lymphoma. Almost two-thirds of cats, irrespective of anatomical distribution, were reported to have neoplastic cells in the peripheral blood.[17] To reliably detect small numbers of neoplastic lymphocytes in blood is difficult. The finding of "atypical" or "potentially malignant" cells on a blood film should not be used in isolation but should stimulate one to obtain a bone marrow sample and, if splenomegaly is present, a splenic biopsy. Current concepts suggest that there are always malignant cells in the blood with lymphoma and that the potential for spread is determined by the homing patterns of the tumor cells, which permit them to attach to endothelium in a preferred site and undergo transmural migration. Since neoplastic lymphoproliferative diseases in all of our domestic animals are most often tumors of solid tissues, a definitive diagnosis is almost always made using fine needle aspiration cytology or excisional biopsy.

The anemia and other cytopenias are usually due to myelophthisis; however, in the alimentary form there is often some hemorrhage. Immune mediated cytopenias are much less common in cats than in dogs with lymphoma. Other rarely reported paraneoplastic syndromes reported in cats with lymphoma are eosinophilia, hypercalcemia, and various gammopathies; the latter two may be associated with renal failure.[18-22] Immune complex nephritis, seen in association with FeLV infection, is another form of paraneoplastic disease. Affected cats will have proteinuria, and immune complex aggregates are seen ultrastructurally in subepithelial, subendothelial, and mesangial locations.[2]

Gross Pathology

Although an anatomic site is often used to "categorize" lymphoma in domestic animals, seldom is the lymphoma confined to that site unless the lesion is localized because of "homing" factors on the tumor cells. Most cases are multicentric or regionally distributed. The alimentary form is most common,[23-25] although in some series of cases mediastinal or thymic tumors are as frequent or slightly more frequent.[26] These forms are followed, in decreasing order, by the multicentric, solitary, and cutaneous forms.

Lesions in the gastrointestinal tract are often regionalized and appear in the form of nodular masses; although they usually occur in the jejunum and ileum, they can be found anywhere from the stomach to the rectum. The nodules may result in stenosis and proximal dilatation. Diffuse laminar thickening of the intestinal wall, although frequent in the dog and occasional in the horse, is less often seen in feline lymphomas. Mesenteric lymph nodes, kidneys, and liver are often involved.

In the thymic form, large masses occupy the anterior mediastinum. These are associated with fluid accumula-tion in the pleural space; the nature of the fluid may range from chylous to hemorrhagic and often contains neoplastic cells. Mediastinal, sternal, and hilar lymph nodes are frequently involved. Lungs are compressed dorsally and are rarely infiltrated with tumor.

Widespread involvement of deep lymph nodes and involvement of the liver, gastrointestinal tract, kidneys, spleen, and bone marrow are seen in the multicentric form. The kidneys are the most common site for the solitary form, and bilateral involvement is usual. Nasopharyngeal lymphoma is more common in the cat than in the dog. Cutaneous lymphomas in the cat are rare; most are of the nonepitheliotrophic variety. The predominately T cell nature of the disease in cats has been confirmed.[27-29] Ocular lymphoma, although rare, is seen more commonly in cats than dogs.

Lymphomas of the peripheral and central nervous systems (CNS) account for about 12 percent of cases of feline lymphoma.[30] The median age of affected cats was 24 months, almost all were FeLV positive, and the vast majority (approximately 90 percent) of lesions were located within the thoracolumbar spine.[30] Neoplastic lymphocytes usually invade along the epidural space and less commonly infiltrate the neuropil. Symptoms are often subtle and variable but may include seizures, anisocoria, Horner's syndrome, rapidly progressive ataxia, paresis, and paralysis. Lymphoma in the central nervous system will commonly cause a marked pleocytosis, with 90 percent or more of the cells being neoplastic lymphocytes, in the dog,[31,32] but neoplastic lymphocytes were found in only 6 of 17 cases of feline CNS lymphoma.[30] Although cerebrospinal fluid (CSF) was obtained from the cerebellomedullary cistern in 12 of the 17 cases, 3 of the 6 cases of CNS lymphoma in which neoplastic lymphocytes were found were detected by examination of CSF obtained from the lumbar cistern, suggesting that this site in the cat may more often reveal lymphoma cells. Dogs more often have multifocal leptomeningeal involvement within the brain and cervical spine, factors which increase the likelihood of finding tumor cells in the cerebellomedullary cistern.

Histologic, Phenotypic, and Genotypic Characteristics

Similar to dogs, cats have predominately intermediate and high grade lymphomas (see table 3.4). However, large cleaved cell lymphomas are more frequent while large noncleaved and lymphoblastic lymphomas are less frequent compared to dogs. The immunoblastic lymphomas account for about 37 percent of all of the feline lymphomas (see table 3.4) (see fig. 3.11).

The development of neoplastic lesions has been studied through the use of experimentally induced lymphomas.[33] Alimentary lymphoid neoplasia commences in the germinal centers of Peyer's patches, later extending to other locations within the lamina propria, and finally invading the muscularis and regional lymph nodes. The lymphoepithelial lesion characteristic of mucosal associated lymphoid tissue (MALT) lymphoma in people[34] has been recognized in animals, including the cat (fig. 3.17). These tumors may be quite localized, permitting effective surgical removal. Neoplasia in mesenteric and other lymph nodes and the spleen also begins in association with follicles. In contrast, the T cell lymphomas begin in paracortical zones. Accordingly, these observations led to the concept that alimentary lymphomas were B cells, while lymphomas of thymic dependent areas, such as node paracortex, were of T cell origin. Immunophenotyping[35,36] and T cell receptor beta gene rearrangement studies support these data and indicate that the majority of FeLV related lymphomas in the mediastinum are of T cell origin. Multicentric tumors often have a non-B non-T phenotype and genotype.[37] There appears to be considerable phenotypic and genotypic heterogeneity, perhaps indicating that the transforming event is directed at lymphoid precursors.[36] Interestingly, in Australia 70 percent of feline lymphomas had a B cell immunophenotype, suggesting that environmental and genetic influences may differ with geography.[38] There are no significant associations between outcome and measures of cell proliferations (AgNOR and PCNA staining) and the CD3 immunophenotype in feline lymphomas.[39,40] However, FeLV positivity is significantly associated with shorter remissions and survival time.[40]

Occasional lymphoid tumors arising from the alimentary tract, chest, and other solitary sites have few to many azurophilic to eosinophilic cytoplasmic granules. At least some of these tumors have been classified as large granular lymphomas (LGLs) and are presumably NK cells or

cytotoxic T cells.[41,42] There is no association with FeLV. One cell line derived from a case of LGL was chronically infected with FeLV,[43] but FeLV could not be demonstrated in another cell line that produced retrovirus particles and reacted with antiendogenous feline retrovirus (RD-114) antiserum.[44] Large granular cells can also be derived from a number of nonlymphoid cell types (e.g., globule leukocyte tumors of intestine, mast cells, eosinophils, and enterochromaffin cells), so that tumors labeled as large granular may in fact be a heterogeneous group of granulated round cell neoplasms. In general, the cytoplasmic granules of globule leukocyte tumors are larger and more numerous than granules in large granular lymphocyte tumors; however, immunohistochemistry or related approaches should be used for definitive identification. Recently, perforin-like immunoreactivity was shown to be a useful marker in a small series of cases of LGLs.[45]

Karyotype

Trisomy of C_2 has been reported in a few cats with thymic lymphoma, suggesting that it may be a nonrandom event; however, additional studies are needed.[46,47] Similarly, further work is needed to assess the significance of karyotypic changes, including translocations, detected in cell lines derived from feline lymphomas.[48,49]

Etiology and Transmission

The primary agent that causes lymphoma in cats is an oncornavirus, the feline leukemia virus (FeLV). Besides causing neoplastic transformation in target cells, FeLV routinely causes a broad variety of non-neoplastic diseases. FeLV is an exogenous oncornavirus that is transmitted horizontally.[50] The genomic organization of all of the oncornaviruses is quite similar. Very simply, one long terminal repeat (LTR) flanks either end of a series of genes, designated *gag, pol,* and *env,* that code for the structural proteins of the virion. The gag protein produces the internal structural proteins associated with the viral core and the nucleocapsid. These internal structural proteins are detected by commercial kits used for the detection of FeLV viremia. Enzymes coded by the *pol* gene allow for the reverse transcription of the viral RNA strand into DNA (reverse transcriptase), duplication of the viral DNA to form a provirus (DNA polymerase), integration of the provirus into the host cell genome (integrase or endonuclease), and proteolytic cleavage of large precursor proteins into their final forms (protease). The *env* gene codes for the envelope glycoprotein (gp70) and the transmembrane protein (p15E), which are important for viral attachment and movement into the cytoplasm of the target cell.

Cats exposed to FeLV make antibodies primarily to the internal structural proteins and the envelope glycoprotein. Antibodies to the internal structural proteins are not protective but are likely important in the development of immune mediated diseases, such as immune complex nephritis, seen in association with chronic FeLV infections. Antibodies made to the envelope glycoprotein

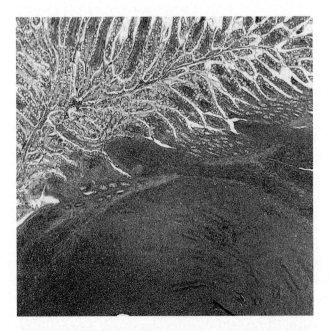

Fig. 3.17. Mucosal associated lymphoid tumor (MALT). Small intestine of a 10-year-old female cat with enteric lymphoma. In addition to a large submucosal tumor mass, the malignant cells are actively invading and destroying mucosal glands. H&E ×30.

(gp70) are neutralizing and are most important in the development of protective immunity, hence the inclusion of gp70 in FeLV vaccines. The transmembrane protein (p15E) is important in mediating the immunosuppressive effects of FeLV and also in the development of nonregenerative anemia. One additional protein displayed on the surface of cells transformed by FeLV is the feline oncornavirus associated cell membrane antigen (FOCMA). FOCMA results from recombination of the FeLV *env* gene with endogenous retroviral sequences; thus, FOCMA is a mutant form of gp70. Anti-FOCMA antibodies provide some protection against the development of FeLV related neoplasias, but have no effect on the nonneoplastic consequences of FeLV infection. The presence of anti-FOCMA antibodies in a FeLV exposed cat with a negative test result for FeLV antigenemia may indicate a subdetectable antigenemia, compartmentalized FeLV infection,[51] or a latent FeLV infection. Such cats are more likely to show signs of immunodeficiency than similar cats without the anti-FOCMA antibodies.[52]

FeLV isolates can be categorized by their ability to infect different cell types in culture.[53,54] Subgroup A replicates exclusively in feline cells; B and C can replicate in a wide variety of cells, even some of human origin. Subgroups B and C arose from mutational or recombinational events with endogenous retroviral sequences in the *env* gene. Subgroup A viruses account for about 90 percent of FeLV infections; it seems to be easily transmitted and causes a rapid viremia. Subgroups B and C are seen as coinfections with subgroup A isolates; about 50 percent of FeLV infected cats also carry subgroups A and B, while only about 1 percent carry subgroups A and C. Subgroup A viruses alone are not highly pathogenic, but persistent infections over a long period can cause lymphoma. In this long prodromal phase, virulent versions of FeLV-A evolve by mutation and recombination. For example, recombinants of FeLV-A and cellular genes *myc* and *fes* will cause thymic lymphoma and fibrosarcoma, respectively.[55-57] Coinfections with subgroups A and B are associated with myeloproliferative disease, myelosuppression, and immunosuppressive disorders. Subgroup C infections are associated with aplastic anemia in kittens. A replication-defective FeLV, termed *FeLV-FAIDS,* causes a rapidly fatal immunodeficiency; a mutation in the *env* gene accounts for the increased virulence.[58]

FeLV positive test results (i.e., FeLV antigenemia) are found in 2 to 3 percent of cats in North America and in about 13 percent of cats in contact with other cats in a hospital, cats in multi-cat household, and known FeLV exposed cats. Cats that are ill are 3 times more likely to have a positive test result than healthy cats. In multi-cat households, in which FeLV infection is endemic, up to 30 percent of cats may be persistently viremic. Male cats are slightly more often infected than females.

The virus may reside in any tissue and is present in bodily secretions and excretions. Major modes of transmission are via respiratory secretions, tears, saliva, and urine. Keeping cats in close contact allows transmission through mutual grooming, fighting, sneezing, and sharing of litter pans or feeding/water bowls. Although not transmitted via the egg/sperm, the fetus can become infected by the transplacental route, exposure to blood and urogenital fluids at birth, or by ingestion of milk. Fetal and neonatal death is seen in about 80 percent of FeLV infected queens. About 20 percent of surviving kittens born to infected queens will be FeLV infected.[59]

The virus enters the body after contacting nasopharyngeal tissues. It replicates in lymphoid tissues in that region and then spreads and multiplies farther in other lymph nodes in the head and neck. Small numbers of infected mononuclear cells carry the virus to all other parts of the body. There is a great deal of virus multiplication in lymphoid tissues of the alimentary tract, spleen, and bone marrow. Later, virus is produced in crypt epithelial cells and in most mucosal and glandular epithelial cells.[53,54] The entire process takes 4 to 6 weeks until persistent viremia is established.

Age at first exposure to FeLV is an important determinant of outcome. Persistent viremia is seen in up to 100 percent of exposed neonates and up to 50 percent of kittens exposed at older than 8 weeks of age. Less than 30 percent of adolescent and mature cats become persistently viremic. Most persistently viremic cats die within 2 to 3 years of FeLV related neoplastic or nonneoplastic diseases, the latter outcome being more frequent. The nonneoplastic consequences are often associated with immunosuppression, which may be mediated by FeLV induced apoptosis of T cells.[60] About 70 percent of exposed adult cats either never show antigenemia or are transiently viremic. It is highly unlikely that latently infected cells will ever be removed since the retroviral life cycle includes incorporation of the provirus in the host cell DNA. FeLV exposed aviremic cats occasionally convert to productive infections; however, the fact that cats with anti-FOCMA antibody have immunodeficiency diseases suggests that latency is not without consequence or is perhaps not truly latent, but rather subdetectable or compartmentalized.[51] FeLV provirus is detected in the tumors of cats with lymphoma more frequently by the polymerase chain reaction than by methods based on the demonstration of antigen, indicating that some infections are indeed subdetectable.[61,62] Cats that are apparently latently infected do not transmit virus.[63] Corticosteroid treatment and stress may cause reactivation.

Overall, approximately 70 percent of cats with lymphoma have FeLV antigenemia. Generally, young cats with lymphoma tend to be FeLV positive, while older cats with lymphoma tend to be negative. The rate of positivity varies with the anatomic form of lymphoma: alimentary, 30 percent; mediastinal, 90 percent; multicentric, 80 percent; and cutaneous, less than 10 percent.[26] About 80 percent of cats with lymphomas of the central nervous system are FeLV positive. Some of the feline lymphomas that appear to be FeLV negative are presumed to be caused by FeLV; the integrated provirus is able to cause neoplastic transformation in the absence of productive infection.[64-66] Most B cell tumors and lymphomas of the alimentary tract in old cats were believed to be FeLV negative; however, in one study the frequency of FeLV positivity was about the same in young and old cats with lymphoma, whether or not the tumors were of B cell or T cell origin.[62]

The exact mechanism by which FeLV causes lymphoid neoplasia is unknown, but the following play direct or indirect roles[67]: (1) Mutations in the *env* gene may increase pathogenicity by altering the display of cell surface epitopes, changing cell membrane signaling, and altering cell growth regulation.[68,69] Altering of cell surface epitopes may facilitate escape from immune surveillance. (2) Direct repeats in the viral LTR may augment enhancer and promoter functions, possibly increasing the expression of protooncogenes located in close proximity.[70,71] (3) The integration of FeLV provirus adjacent to host protooncogenes (insertional mutagenesis) may result in the overexpression of the latter.[72] (4) FeLV proviruses that have recombined with endogenous FeLV sequences or cellular protooncogenes are strongly associated with some forms of lymphoma.[73] The genetic mechanisms involved are distinct for the thymic lymphomas of T cell origin and those of extrathymic, extranodal, non-B non-T cell origin.[74]

There is growing evidence of a role for the feline immunodeficiency virus (FIV) in the development of lymphoma. FIV infected cats have a significantly greater risk of developing lymphoma and other stromal and epithelial tumors.[75,76] The relative risk of developing leukemia/lymphoma in FIV infected cats is 5 times the rate observed in uninfected cats. In the case of FeLV infected cats, the relative risk increases to 62 times normal, while with a dual infection of FeLV and FIV the relative risk is 77 times normal.[75] The lymphomas seen in association with FIV infection are frequently in extranodal sites, such as kidney and liver, occur in older cats, are usually of the high grade immunoblastic or centroblastic type, and tend to be of B cell origin.[77-80] It appears that most often FIV operates indirectly in the development of lymphoma[81,82]; however, FIV was incriminated in causing lymphoma in an experimentally inoculated cat.[83]

Idiopathic Lymphadenopathies

FIV infected cats may have persistent lymphadenopathy due to follicular hyperplasia and expansion of paracortical areas due to an influx of plasma cells. In the terminal stages of the FIV infection lymph nodes undergo involution.[84] Persistent lymphadenopathy has been described in experimental infections with FeLV and in a series of clinical cases of mostly FeLV positive young (range, 5 months to 2 years) cats.[85] Changes included increased frequency of postcapillary venules, lack of follicles and sinuses, and paracortical expansion caused by the infiltration of histiocytes, lymphocytes, immunoblasts, and plasma cells. In most cases, the lymphadenopathy was transient. Histological changes in lymph node biopsies from a small series of

mostly FeLV negative young (range, 1 to 4 years) adult cats with lymphadenopathy were supportive of lymphoma.[86] Four of these six cats had histories of recent upper respiratory and urinary tract infections, and two lived in households with FeLV positive cats but did not have FeLV antigenemia. Despite the evidence supporting lymphoma, the lymph nodes had increased vascularity; primary and secondary follicles with active germinal centers; plasma cells, histiocytes, and granulocytes in subcapsular and medullary sinuses; and lack of capsular invasion. This suggests that the lymph nodes were not totally effaced by the malignancy or that the process was a nonmalignant atypical immune response. Follow-up studies, over 12 to 84 months, revealed resolution of the lymphadenopathy, supporting the latter alternative. In another series of mature cats with solitary lymphadenopathies, proliferation of capillary-sized vascular channels in the interfollicular pulp was reported.[87] These studies suggest caution in diagnosing lymphoma when there are mixtures of cell types, nonuniform lymphocyte morphology, retention of follicles, and proliferation of small blood vessels. In contrast, the peripheral T cell lymphomas (see fig. 3.14), including extranodal types, are characterized by cellular heterogeneity and small vessel proliferation but lack follicles. The small vessel proliferation appears to be a feature of T cell areas in both malignant and benign (paracortical) proliferations.

Transmissible Feline Fibrosarcoma

The feline sarcoma virus (FeSV) evolved from FeLV by mutation and recombination with host cellular genes. FeSV has lost part of *gag,* all of *pol,* and all or part of *env* but has picked up one of many cellular oncogenes.[2] FeSV is termed *replication defective* because the genes coding for proteins important for the formation of new virions are defective. In order to propagate itself it must coexist with a replication-competent FeLV. The acquisition of a cellular oncogene enhances virulence so that FeSV infection, made productive by coinfection with FeLV, can quickly cause the development of fibrosarcomas. Osseous or chondroid differentiation is sometimes found. The time to tumor development after exposure is shorter in kittens than in adult cats; tumors often present as multiple subcutaneous masses, and in about one-third of cases there may be metastasis. FeSV may also cause malignant transformation of other cell types, such as the melanocyte.[88,89] FeSV induced tumor cells express FOCMA; hence, those animals with protective levels of anti-FOCMA antibody either do not develop tumors or show tumor regression. However, in a cat that has had a tumor regress, other fibrosarcomas may develop upon exposure to a different strain of FeSV.[90,91] Overall, about 2 percent of spontaneous feline fibrosarcomas are associated with FeSV.[2] Solitary fibrosarcomas in older cats and those occurring at sites of inflammation, trauma, or vaccination are unassociated with FeLV-FeSV. In these instances, affected cats test negative for FeLV antigen.[92]

REFERENCES

1. Couto C.G. (1989) Oncology. In Sherding, R. (ed.), *The Cat: Diseases and Clinical Management.* Churchill-Livingston, New York, pp. 589–647.

2. Hardy, W.D. (1981) Hematopoietic tumors of cats. *J Amer Anim Hosp Assoc* 17:921–940.

3. Dorn, C.R., Taylor, D.O.N., and Hibbard, H.H. (1967) Epizootiologic characteristics of canine and feline leukemia and lymphoma. *Amer J Vet Res* 28:993–1001.

4. Essex, M., and Francis, D.P. (1976) The risk to humans from malignant diseases of their pets: An unsettling issue. *J Amer Anim Hosp Assoc* 12:386–390.

5. Meincke, J.E., Hobbie, W.V., and Hardy, W.D. (1972) Lymphoreticular malignancies in the cat. *J Amer Vet Med Assoc* 160:1093–1098.

6. Schneider, R. (1972) Feline malignant lymphoma: Environmental factors and the occurrence of this viral cancer in cats. *Intl J Cancer* 10:345–350.

7. Couto, C.G. (1992) Lymphoma in the cat and dog. In Nelson, R.W., and Couto, C.G. (eds.), *Essentials of Small Animal Internal Medicine.* Mosby Year Book, St. Louis, pp. 861– 870.

8. Court, E.A., Watson, A.D.J., and Peaston, A.E. (1997) Retrospective study of 60 cases of feline lymphosarcoma. *Aust Vet J* 75:424–427,

9. Dorn, C.R., Taylor, D.O., Schneider, R., Hibbard, H.H., and Klauber, M.R. (1968) Survey of animal neoplasms in Alameda and Contra Costa Counties, California. II. Cancer morbidity in dogs and cats from Alameda County. *J Natl Cancer Inst* 40:307–318.

10. Jarrett, W.F.H., Crighton, G.W., and Dalton, R.G.. (1966) Leukaemia and lymphosarcoma in animals and man. I. Lymphosarcoma or leukaemia in the domestic animals. *Vet Rec* 79:693–699.

11. Slayter, M.V., Farver, T.B., and Schneider, R. (1984) Feline malignant lymphoma: Log-linear multiway frequency analysis of a population involving the factors of sex and age of animal and tumor cell type and location. *Amer J Vet Res* 45:2178–2181.

12. Wellman, M.L., Kociba, G.J., Mathes, L.E., and Olsen, R.G. (1988) Suppression of feline bone marrow fibroblast colony-forming units by feline leukemia virus. *Amer J Vet Res* 49:227–230.

13. Testa, N.G., Onions, D.E., and Lord, B.I. (1988) A feline model for the myelodysplastic syndrome: Pre-leukemic abnormalities caused in cats by infection with a new isolate of feline leukaemia virus (FeLV), AB/GM1. *Haematologica* 73:317–320.

14. Linenberger, M.L., and Abkowitz, J.L. (1992) Modulation of marrow stromal growth-promoting and inhibitory activities by feline leukemia virus (FeLV). *Blood* 80(Suppl 1): 180a.

15. Linenberger, M.L., and Abkowitz, J.L. (1995) Haematological disorders associated with feline retrovirus infections. *Bailliere's Clin Haematol* 8:73–112.

16. Weiser, M.G., and Kociba, G.J. (1983) Erythrocyte macrocytosis in feline leukemia virus associated anemia. *Vet Pathol* 20:687–697.

17. Theilen, G.H., and Madewell, B.R. (1987) Hematopoietic neoplasms, sarcomas and related conditions. Part II. Feline. In Theilen, G.H., and Madewell, B.R. (eds.), *Veterinary Cancer Medicine.* 2nd ed. Lea and Febiger, Philadelphia, pp. 354–381.

18. Zenoble, R.D., and Rowland, G.N. (1979) Hypercalcemia and proliferative, myelosclerotic bone reaction associated with feline leukovirus infection in a cat. *J Amer Vet Med Assoc* 175:591–595.

19. Chew, D.J., Schaer, M., Liu, S.K., and Owens, J. (1975) Pseudohyperparathyroidism in a cat. *J Amer Anim Hosp Assoc* 11:46–52.

20. McMillan, F.D. (1985) Hypercalcemia associated with lymphoid neoplasia in two cats. *Feline Pract* 15:31–34.

21. Dust, A., Norris, A.M., and Valli, V.E.O. (1982) Cutaneous lymphosarcoma with IgG monoclonal gammopathy, serum hyperviscosity and hypercalcemia in a cat. *Can Vet J* 23:235–239.

22. MacEwen, E.G., and Hurvitz, A.I. (1977) Diagnosis and management of monoclonal gammopathies. *Vet Clin N Amer Small Anim Pract* 7:119–132.

23. Mahony O.M., Moore, A.S., Cotter, S.M., Engler, S.J., Brown, D., and Penninck, D.G. (1995) Alimentary lymphoma in cats: 28 cases (1988–1993). *J Amer Vet Med Assoc* 207:1593–1598.

24. Head, K.W., and Else, R.W. (1981) Neoplasia and allied conditions of the canine and feline intestine. *Vet Ann* 21:190–208.

25. Brodey, R.S. (1966) Alimentary tract neoplasms in the cat: A clinicopathologic survey of 46 cases. *Amer J Vet Res* 27:74–80.

26. MacEwen, E.G. (1996) Feline lymphoma and leukemias. In Withrow, S.J., and MacEwen, E.G. (eds.), *Small Animal Clinical Oncology,* 2nd ed. W.B. Saunders Co., Philadelphia, pp 479–495.

27. Tobey, J.C., Houston, D.M., Breur, G.J., Jackson, M.L., and Stubbington, D.A. (1994) Cutaneous T-cell lymphoma in a cat. *J Amer Vet Med Assoc* 204:606–609.

28. Caciolo, P.L., Nesbitt, G.H., Patnaik, A.K., and Hayes, A.A. (1984) Cutaneous lymphosarcoma in the cat: A report of nine cases. *J Amer Anim Hosp Assoc* 20:491–496.

29. Day, M.J. (1995) Immunophenotypic characterization of cutaneous lymphoid neoplasia in the dog and cat. *J Comp Pathol* 112:79–96.

30. Lane, S.B., Kornegay, J.N., Duncan, J.R., and Oliver, J.E., Jr. (1994) Feline spinal lymphosarcoma: A retrospective evaluation of 23 cats. *J Vet Int Med* 8:99–104.

31. Rosin, A. (1982) Neurologic disease associated with lymphosarcoma in 10 dogs. *J Amer Vet Med Assoc* 181:50–53.

32. Couto, C.G., Cullen, J., Pedroia, V., and Turrel, J.M. (1984) Central nervous system lymphosarcoma in the dog. *J Amer Vet Med Assoc* 184:809–813.

33. Mackey, L.J., and Jarrett, W.F.H. (1972). Pathogenesis of lymphoid neoplasia in cats and its relationship to immunologic cell pathways. I. Morphologic aspects. *J Natl Cancer Inst* 49:853–865.

34. Taal, B.G., Boot, H., van Heerde, P., de Jong, D., Hart, A.A.M., and Burgers, J.M.V. (1996) Primary non-Hodgkin lymphoma of the stomach: Endoscopic pattern and prognosis in low versus high grade malignancy in relation to the MALT concept. *Gut* 39:556–561.

35. Cockerell, G.L., Krakowka, S., Hoover, E.A., Olsen, R.G., and Yohn, D.S. (1976) Characterization of feline T- and B- lymphocytes and identification of an experimentally induced T-cell neoplasm in the cat. *J Natl Cancer Inst* 57:907–913.

36. Rojko, J.L., Kociba, G.J., Abkowitz, J.L., Hamilton, K.L., Hardy, W.D., Ihle, J.N., and O'Brien, S.J. (1989) Feline lymphomas: Immunological and cytochemical characterization. *Cancer Res* 49:345–351.

37. Athas, G.B., Choi, B., Prabhu, S., Lobelle-Rich, P.A., and Levy, L.S. (1995) Genetic determinants of feline leukemia virus-induced multicentric lymphomas. *Virology* 214:431–438.

38. Gabor, L.J., Canfield, P.J., and Malik, R. (1999) Immunophenotypic and histological characterisation of 109 cases of feline lymphosarcoma. *Aust Vet J* 77:436–441.

39. Rassnick, K.M., Mauldin, G.N., Moroff, S.D., Mauldin, G.E., McEntee, M.C., and Mooney, S.C. (1999) Prognostic value of argyrophilic nucleolar organizer region (AgNOR) staining in feline intestinal lymphoma. *J Vet Int Med* 13:187–190.

40. Vail, D.M., Moore, A.S., Ogilvie, G.K., and Volk, L.M. (1998) Feline lymphoma (145 cases): Proliferation indices, CD3 immunoreactivity, and their association with prognosis in 90 cats receiving therapy. *J Vet Int Med* 12: 349–354.

41. Franks, P.T., Harvey, J.W., Calderwood-Mays, M., Senior, D.F., Bowen, D.J., and Hall, B.J. (1986) Feline large granular lymphoma. *Vet Pathol* 23:200–202.

42. Wellman, M.L., Hammer, A.D., Dibartola, S.P., Carothers, M.A., Kociba, G.J., and Rojko, J. (1992) Lymphoma involving large granular lymphocytes in cats, 11 cases (1982–1991). *J Amer Vet Med Assoc* 201:1265–1269.

43. Goitsuka, R., Ohno, K., Matsumoto, Y., Hayashi, N., Momoi, Y., Okamoto, Y., Watari, T., Tsujimoto, H., and Hasegawa, A. (1993) Establishment and characterizaion of a feline large granular lymphoma cell line expressing interleukin 2 receptor α-chain. *J Vet Med Sci* 55:863–865.

44. Cheney, C.M., Rojko, J.L., Kociba, G.J., Wellman, M.L., DiBartola, S.P., Rezanka, L.J., Forman, L., and Mathes, L.E. (1990) A feline large granular lymphoma and its derived cell line. *In Vitro Cell Develop Biol* 26:455–463.

45. Kariya, K., Konno, A., and Ishida, T. (1997) Perforin-like immunoreactivity in four cases of lymphoma of large granular lymphocytes in the cat. *Vet Pathol* 34:156–159.

46. Grindem, C.B., and Buoen, L.C. (1989) Cytogenetic analysis in nine leukaemic cats. *J Comp Pathol* 101:21–30.

47. Hare, W.C.D, Weber, W.T., McFeely, R.A., and Yang T. (1966) Cytogenetics in dog and cat. *J Small Anim Pract* 7:575–592.

48. Wu, F.Y., Iijima, K., Tsujimoto, H., Tamura, Y., and Higurashi, M. 1995. Chromosomal translocations in two feline T-cell lymphomas. *Leukemia Res* 19:857–860.

49. Gulino, S.E. (1992) Chromosome abnormalities and oncogenesis in cat leukemias. *Cancer Genet Cytogenet* 64:149–157.

50. Jarrett, O. (1991) Overview of feline leukemia virus research. *J Amer Vet Med Assoc* 199:1279–1281.

51. Hayes, K.A., Rojko, J.L., and Mathes, L.E. (1992) Incidence of localized feline leukemia virus infection in cats. *Amer J Vet Res* 53:604–607.

52. Swenson, C.L., Kociba, G.J., Mathes, L.E., Hand, P.J., Neer, C.A., Hays, K.A., and Olsen, R.G. (1990) Prevalence of disease in nonviremic cats previously exposed to feline leukemia virus. *J Amer Vet Med Assoc* 196:1049–1052.

53. Hoover, E.A., and Mullins, J.I. (1991) Feline leukemia virus infection and diseases. *J Amer Vet Med Assoc* 199:1287–1297.

54. Rojko, J.L., and Kociba, G.J. (1991) Pathogenesis of infection by the feline leukemia virus. *J Amer Vet Med Assoc* 199:1305–1310.

55. Levy, L.S., Gardner, M.B., and Casey, J.W. (1984) Isolation of a feline leukaemia provirus containing the oncogene *myc* from a feline lymphosarcoma. *Nature* 308:853–856.

56. Mullins, J.I., Brody, D.S., Binari, R.C. Jr., and Cotter, S.M. (1984) Viral transduction of *c-myc* gene in naturally occurring feline leukaemias. *Nature* 308:856–858.

57. Besmer, P. (1983) Acute transforming feline retroviruses. Curr. *Topics Microbiol Immunol* 107:1–27.

58. Mullins J.I., Hoover, E.A., Overbaugh, J., Quakenbush, S.C., Donahue, P.R., and Poss., M.L. (1989) FeLV-FAIDS-induced immunodeficiency syndrome in cats. *Vet Immunol Immunopathol* 21:25–37.

59. Pedersen, N.C. (1988) Feline leukemia virus infection. In Pratt, P.W. (ed.), *Feline Infectious Diseases.* American Veterinary Publications, Goleta, CA, pp. 83–106.

60. Rojko, J.L., Fulton, R.M., Rezanka, L.J., Williams, L.L., Copelan, E., Cheney, C.M., Reichel, G.S., Neil, J.C., Mathes, L.E., Fisher, R.G., and Cloyd, M.W. (1992) Lymphocytotoxic strains of feline leukemia virus induce apoptosis in feline T4-thymic lymphoma cells. *Lab Invest* 66:418–426.

61. Jackson, M.L., Haines, D.M., Meric, S.M., and Misra, V. (1993) Feline leukemia virus detection by immunohistochemistry and polymerase chain reaction in formalin-fixed, paraffin-embedded tumor tissue from cats with lymphosarcoma. *Can J Vet Res* 57:269–276.

62. Jackson, M.L., Wood, S.L., Misra, V., and Haines, D.M. (1996) Immunohistochemical identification of B and T lymphocytes in formalin-fixed, paraffin-embedded feline lymphosarcomas: Relation to feline leukemia virus status, tumor site, and patient age. *Can J Vet Res* 60:199–204.

63. Rojko, J.L., Hoover, E.A., Quakenbush, S.L., and Olsen, R.G. (1982) Reactivation of latent feline leukemia virus infection. *Nature* 198:385–388.

64. Hardy, W.D., McClelland, A.J., Zuckerman, E.E., Snyder, H.W., MacEwen, E.G., Francis, D., and Essex, M. (1980) Development of virus non-producer lymphosarcomas in pet cats exposed to FeLV. *Nature* 288:90–92.

65. Francis, D.P., Cotter, S.M., Hardy, W.D., and Essex, M. (1979) Comparison of virus-positive and virus-negative cases of feline leukemia and lymphoma. *Cancer Res* 39:3866–3870.

66. Hardy, W.D., Zuckerman, E.E., MacEwen, E.G., Hayes, A.A., and

Essex, M. (1977) A feline leukaemia virus and sarcoma virus-induced tumor-specific antigen. *Nature* 270:249–251.

67. Rezanka, L.J., Rojko, J.L., and Neil, J.C. (1992) Feline leukemia virus: Pathogenesis of neoplastic disease. *Cancer Invest* 10:371–389.

68. Rohn, J.L., Linenberger, M.L., Hoover, E.A., and Overbaugh, J. (1994) Evolution of feline leukemia virus variant genomes with insertions, deletions and defective envelope genes in infected cats with tumors. *J Virol* 68:2458–2467.

69. Roy-Burman, P. (1996) Endogenous *env* elements: Partners in generation of pathogenic feline leukemia viruses. *Virus Genes* 11:147–161.

70. Matsumoto, Y., Momoi, Y., Watari, T., Goitswka, R., Tsukimoto, H., and Hasegawa, A. (1992) Detection of enhancer repeats in the long terminal repeats of feline leukemia viruses from cats with spontaneous neoplastic and nonneoplastic diseases. *Virology* 189:745–749.

71. Pantginis, J., Beaty, R.M., Levy, L.S., and Lenz, J. (1997) The feline leukemia virus long terminal repeat contains a potent genetic determinant of T-cell lymphomagenicity. *J Virol* 71:9786–9791.

72. Levy, L.S., Lobelle-Rich, P.A., Overbaugh, J, Abkowitz, J.L., Fulton, R., and Roy-Burman, P. (1993) Coincident involvement of *flvi-2, c-myc,* and novel *env* genes in natural and experimental lymphosarcomas induced by feline leukemia virus. *Virology* 196:892–895.

73. Sheets, R.L., Pandey, R., Jen, W., and Roy-Burman, P. (1993) Recombinant feline leukemia virus genes detected in naturally occurring feline lymphosarcomas. *J Virol* 67:3118–3125.

74. Levy, L.S., Starkey, C.R., Prabhu, S., and Lobelle-Rich, P.A. (1997) Cooperating events in lymphomagenesis mediated by feline leukemia virus. *Leukemia* 11:232–241.

75. Shelton, G.H., Grant, C.K., Cotter, S.M., Gardner, M.B., Hardy, W.D.J., and DiGiacomo, R.F. (1990) Feline immunodeficiency virus and feline leukemia virus infections and their relationship to lymphoid malignancies in cats: A retrospective study (1968–1988). *J Acquir Immune Defic Syn* 3:623–630.

76. Hutson, C.A., Rideout, B.A., and Pedersen, N.C. (1991) Neoplasia associated with feline immunodeficiency virus infection in cats of Southern California. *J Amer Vet Med Assoc* 199:1357–1362.

77. Ishida, T., and Tomoda, I. (1990) Clinical staging of feline immunodeficiency virus infection. *Jpn J Vet Sci* 52:645–648.

78. Poli, A., Abramo, F., Baldinotti, F., Pistello, M., DaPrato, L., and Bendinelli, M. (1994) Malignant lymphoma associated with experimentally induced feline immunodeficiency virus infection. *J Comp Pathol* 110:319–328.

79. Callanan, J.J., McCandlish, I.A.P., O'Neil, B., Lawrence, C.E., Rigby, M., Pacitti, A.M., and Jarrett, O. (1992) Lymphosarcoma in experimentally induced feline immunodeficiency virus infection. *Vet Rec* 130:293–295.

80. Callanan, J.J., Jones, B.A., Irvine, J., Willett, B.J., McCandlish, I.A.P., and Jarrett, O. (1996) Histologic classification and immunophenotype of lymphosarcomas in cats with naturally and experimentally acquired feline immunodeficiency virus infections. *Vet Pathol* 33:264–272.

81. Terry, A., Callanan, J.J., Fulton, R., Jarrett, O., and Neil, J.C. (1995) Molecular analysis of tumors from feline immunodeficiency virus (FIV)-infected cats: An indirect role for FIV? *Intl J Cancer* 61:227–232.

82. Endo, Y., Cho, K., Nishigaki, K., Momoi, Y., Nishimura, Y., Mizuno, T., Goto, Y., Watari, T., Tsujimoto, H., and Hasegawa, A. (1997) Molecular characteristics of malignant lymphomas in cats naturally infected with feline immunodeficiency virus. *Vet Immunol Immunopathol* 57:153–167.

83. Beatty, J.A., Callanan, J.J., Terry, A., Jarrett, O., and Neil, J.C. (1998) Molecular and immunophenotypical characterization of a feline immunodeficiency virus (FIV)-associated lymphoma: A direct role for FIV in B-lymphocyte transformation. *J Virol* 72:767–771.

84. Sparger, E.E. (1993) Current thoughts on feline immunodeficiency

virus infection. *Vet Clin N Amer Small Anim Pract* 23:173–191.

85. Moore, F.M., Emerson, W.E., Cotter, S.M., and DeLellis, R.A. (1986) Distinctive peripheral lymph node hyperplasia of young cats. *Vet Pathol* 23:386–391.

86. Mooney, S.C., Patnaik, A.K., Hayes, A.A., and MacEwen, E.G. (1987) Generalized lymphadenopathy resembling lymphoma in cats: Six cases (1972–1976). *J Amer Vet Med Assoc* 190:897–900.

87. Lucke, V.M., Davies, J.D., Wood, C.M., and Whitebread, T.J. (1987) Plexiform vascularization of lymph nodes: An unusual but distinctive lymphadenopathy in cats. *J Comp Pathol* 97:109–119.

88. McCullough, B., Schaller, J., Shadduck, J.A., and Yohn, D.S. (1972) Induction of malignant melanomas associated with fibrosarcomas in gnotobiotic cats inoculated with Gardner feline fibrosarcoma virus. *J Natl Cancer Inst* 48:1893–1895.

89. Shadduck, J.A., Albert, D.M., and Niederkorn, J.Y. (1982) Feline uveal melanomas induced with feline sarcoma virus: Potential model of the human counterpart. *J Natl Cancer Inst* 67:619–627.

90. Johnson, L., Pedersen, N.C., and Theilen, G.H. (1985) The nature of immunity to Snyder-Theilen fibrosarcoma virus-induced tumors in cats. *Vet Immunol Immunopathol* 9:283–300.

91. Sarma, P.S., Log, T., and Theilen, G.H. (1971) ST feline sarcoma virus: Biological characteristics and *in vitro* propagation. *Proc Soc Exp Biol Med* 137:1444–1448.

92. Rojko, J.L., and Hardy, W.D. Jr. (1994) Feline leukemia virus and other retroviruses. In Sherding, R.G. (ed.), *The Cat: Diseases and Clinical Management,* 2nd ed., Churchill Livingston, NY, pp. 263–432.

Bovine

Demographics

In cattle, lymphoma is the most common neoplasm in predominately dairy producing areas; however, ocular squamous cell carcinoma is more frequent if production type is disregarded. In the United States, the annual incidence rate in slaughtered cattle is 18 per 100,000.[1] There are no breed or sex predispositions. Differences in apparent rates of lymphoma between dairy and beef breeds are attributable to major differences in average age and management factors. Although the risk for lymphoma increases with age, there is a bimodal distribution with one peak under 1 year of age and a larger peak between 5 and 8 years of age. Lymphoid tumors have been found in the fetus. A study in Minnesota showed that the incidence rates were 8.5, 19.7, and 25.6 per 100,000 cattle at 2 to 5 years of age, 6 to 9 years of age, and 10 years of age or greater, respectively.[2,3]

Clinical Characteristics

There is decreased feed consumption and milk production in affected cattle. Symptoms vary with the organ systems involved. Many affected cattle are afebrile and appear with persistent nonpainful peripheral lymphadenopathy. Tumors within the alimentary tract often cause the symptoms of vagus indigestion, interfere with rumen motility, cause abomasal dilatation, melena, and diarrhea. Some adults may suffer from posterior paresis resulting from epidural infiltration of the spinal nerve roots. In advanced cases, exophthalmus, sometimes bilateral, is commonly found. Occasionally animals will die suddenly due to acute hemorrhage from a ruptured spleen or abomasal ulcer. Peritonitis may occur when an abomasal ulcer perforates the serosa. The myocardium is a common site for lymphoma, and if severe, the tumor may interfere with the conduction mechanism resulting in arrhythmias and sudden death. Rarely, a tumor in the myocardium may cause acute hemorrhage resulting in cardiac tamponade. Brisket edema and abdominal effusions are seen when there is congestive heart failure. Fertility is decreased, although pregnant cows with lymphoma can conceive and carry a fetus to term. Marked involvement of the uterus can be mistaken for a fetus.

In adult animals (2 or more years of age), the disease appears to be enzootic, or behaves as an infectious disease, while in juveniles (under 2 years of age) the disease occurs sporadically. The etiological agent of the enzootic form is the bovine leukemia virus (BLV), but sporadic cases have no evidence for a role played by BLV. Rare exceptions have been reported.[4]

There are four clinicopathological forms that are roughly correlated with age: (1) the calf or juvenile form seen in calves usually less than 6 months of age, (2) the thymic form seen more frequently in beef breeds from 6 to 18 months of age, (3) the adult form seen in cattle greater than 2 years of age, and (4) the cutaneous form seen in cattle 2 to 3 years of age.

Calves with lymphoma have symmetrical peripheral lymphadenopathy, sometimes marked organomegaly, and often leukemia. Large masses are present in the ventral neck and anterior mediastinum in the thymic form, and esophageal compression may result in bloat. Occasionally, lymph nodes in head and other sites anterior to the diaphragm are affected, and sometimes there is marked infiltration of the bones of the maxilla and mandible. Dams of affected calves are normal.

Adults have a multicentric appearance of tumors and at least half of affected cattle present with peripheral lymphadenopathy. Infiltration of the retrobulbar fat and nervous system involvement are relatively common late occurrences in the affected adult. Frank leukemia, as distinguished from persistent lymphocytosis (PL), can occur in the latter stages of the adult form. Melena in an adult dairy cow with lymphoma is often associated with abomasal ulceration resulting from diffuse infiltration with tumor. Often calves, yearlings, and adults with lymphoma are presented late in the disease process, at which time the lesions are virtually all multicentric. Apparent, primary involvement of the mandible with extension to regional lymph nodes has been reported.[5]

The cutaneous form is a unique clinical entity.[6-10] The initial lesions appear as urticarial-like and then progress into raised, circular, hairless lesions, mostly concentrated over the neck, shoulders, and perineal areas. Some may be ulcerated and have central necrosis. Typically, these lesions are attributed to ringworm and other inflammatory skin diseases; hence, the time to diagnosis is usually quite long. Lesions appear and then regress for months, and at times the skin may be free of lesions. Lymphadenopathy is absent during this phase. Eventually, the animals develop the multicentric form of lymphoma.

Clinical Pathology

About two-thirds of adult cattle with lymphoma have normal hemograms; the remainder have mild nonregenerative anemias and/or mild to moderate changes in leukocyte numbers. Some of the leukocytotic adult cattle will have neutrophilias. Others have benign reactive lymphocytoses, some of which may be persistent (i.e., persistent lymphocytosis or PL). As with other animals, leukemia is a relatively rare event until late in the disease. Overall, about 10 percent of cattle with lymphoma present with leukemia.[11] Lymphoid leukemia is common in calves with lymphoma, where marrow infarction and myelophthisis are also frequently present (see fig. 3.33).[12] The finding of small numbers of atypical lymphocytes in the peripheral blood of adult cattle should create suspicion and stimulate one to look further for additional evidence of lymphoma in the marrow and spleen. However, even more so than in other species, one should be very cautious about identifying the rare atypical mononuclear cell as a neoplastic cell in cattle, young animals in particular. Cattle often produce reactive lymphocytes and monocytes in response to inflammation. Although posterior paresis is common in the terminal stages, it is unusual to see a pleocytosis since the infiltration along the nerve roots and spinal column is epidural. Neoplastic cells can sometimes be found in pericardial, pleural, or peritoneal cavities. A diagnosis of lymphoma should be made by aspirational cytology or excisional biopsy of the largest and most easily accessible mass.

Earlier in the twentieth century, European researchers realized that an infectious agent was likely involved in causing lymphoma in adult cattle since cases clustered in time and space.[13] Upon further examination they found that cattle with sustained increases in peripheral blood lymphocyte numbers [persistent lymphocytosis (PL)], when compared with the age-matched upper reference limit, had a predisposition to develop lymphoma. On this basis, they designed and carried out large programs aimed at culling cattle with PL, and over time there was a marked decrease in the incidence of lymphoma.[13] Experimental inoculation of cattle and sheep with the BLV causes PL in about one-third of animals.[14] Furthermore, about two-thirds of cattle with lymphoma have a history of PL. Although some investigators have considered PL to be a form of chronic lymphocytic leukemia, it has been shown definitively that PL is a benign polyclonal B cell, CD5+ proliferation[15] and can be considered a paraneoplastic syndrome in an individual with lymphoma. Chronic infections, such as trypanosomiasis, brucellosis, and tuberculosis, may also result in PL. As well, peripheral blood lymphocyte counts are partially under genetic control.[16] Paraneoplastic syndromes common in other species, such as hypercalcemia and gammopathies, have not been reported in cattle with

lymphoma. Most adult cattle with lymphoma have decreased concentrations of all immunoglobulin classes.[17,18]

Gross Pathology

Lesions in calves are in most internal and superficial lymph nodes, spleen, liver, and bone marrow. Infarction in the bone marrow cavity of shafts of long bones is seen frequently although the ends of long bones (see fig. 3.33), vertebral bodies, and ribs may also be affected.[12] Occasionally there is infiltration of the alimentary tract, skeletal muscle, and subperiosteal bone.

In the thymic cases there is usually a single large mass in the ventral neck or in the thoracic inlet. Lymph nodes in the anterior chest and head may also be involved, and in some cases there is infiltration into muscles in the head and extensive infiltration into the bones of maxilla and mandible.

The most common sites of involvement in the adult are deep and superficial lymph nodes, heart (most frequent in right atrium), abomasum, duodenum, kidneys, uterus, liver, spleen, epidural space in the lumbar spinal column and nerve roots, retrobulbar fat, and occasionally hemolymph nodes. Nervous system lesions can easily be overlooked since they grossly appear almost indistinguishable from fat. Often the tubular organs, such as the alimentary tract and uterus, show marked symmetrical thickening of the wall. Organ involvement may be diffuse or focal.

Cattle with cutaneous lymphoma are rarely necropsied early in the disease process when lesions are exclusively skin associated. In the late stages of the disease, lesions are indistinguishable from those of the adult multicentric form.

Histological, Phenotypic, and Genotypic Characteristics

The diffuse large and small noncleaved cell types account for about 60 percent of the sporadic lymphomas (see table 3.4).[19] Mitotic indexes are significantly lower in sporadic lymphomas compared with the enzootic lymphomas.

Almost two-thirds of adult lymphoid tumors are composed of diffuse large cleaved (see fig. 3.10) and diffuse large noncleaved cell types in about equal frequency (see table 3.4). The diffuse large cleaved cell type accounted for 38 percent of adult lymphomas and 14 percent of the sporadic lymphomas. Using the mitotic index as an indicator of tumor grade, these two cell types in bovine lymphomas are considered high grade tumors.[19] Follicular lymphomas in cattle are exceedingly rare and accounted for about 0.3 percent of a series of 1198 cases of bovine lymphoma. This is in marked contrast to people, in whom follicular lymphomas account for more than one-third of lymphomas. Early lesions in adults are found most often in the medullary sinuses of superficial lymph nodes and subepicardially in the right atrium.[20,21] A single case of lymphoma composed of large granular lymphocytes was reported in an 11-year-old Ayrshire.[22] The cow had a multicentric distribution of lesions typical of the adult enzootic form of lymphoma but was BLV negative.

The histological lesions of cutaneous lymphoma are epitheliotrophic and resemble mycosis fungoides. Pautrier microabscesses are present in the early stages of the disease. Typical cerebriform nuclear outlines can be seen when thin paraffin-embedded sections are viewed at oil immersion or when imprints are examined.

Reagents and protocols for the immunophenotyping of bovine lymphocytes have been well described.[23] Lymphomas in adult cattle consist predominately of mature B cells (MHC II$^+$, gamma$_1^+$, gamma$_2^+$, lambda$^+$, and CD5$^+$) based on immunophenotyping and immunoglobulin gene rearrangement studies.[24-29] Since 90 percent of bovine light chains are normally of the lambda variety,[30] light chain studies have limited usefulness for proving clonality in cattle unless the tumor cells produce kappa light chain. The sporadic forms can be of either B cell or T cell lineages.[31-33] Cytoplasmic staining for alpha-naphthylacetate esterase and T cell receptor beta and delta rearrangements were demonstrated in a series of sporadic lymphomas.[34]

Ultrastructural studies of lymphomas in cattle have been reported.[35,36] A unique finding is the presence of *nuclear pockets* that are finger-like projections or loops of nuclear membranes. A small fraction of tumor cells have this morphological characteristic; they appear in association with the presence of C type retroviruses.[37,38]

Chromosomal analysis, utilizing nonbanding approaches, failed to reveal any consistent karyotypic change, although there were frequent random chromosomal changes and diploid or hyperdiploid numbers.[39-43] Subsequently, a banding study identified probable primary karyotypic changes, the most frequent being an isochromosome 26.[44] Trisomy 5 was a common secondary alteration.

Etiology and Transmission

The prevalence of anti-BLV antibodies varies with geographic region. In dairy intensive areas the prevalence ranges between 30 and 50 percent.[43-46] The prevalence in beef cattle is less than 10 percent.

Features of transmission have been reviewed elsewhere.[11] Briefly, transmission is horizontal and normally occurs with close contact over extended periods of time. There must be exchange of blood or other fluids containing infected cells so that whole cells are transferred. Infected cells enter through the skin and the alimentary, reproductive, or respiratory tract. This can occur by ingestion of blood, milk, or saliva or by inhalation of droplets of mucus or saliva. BLV may be transmitted by natural service but is not transmitted by artificial insemination using frozen semen. Blood-contaminated surgical instruments and multidose syringes can be very efficient mechanisms for transmission since only 2500 lymphocytes from a BLV infected cow are required.[14] There is experimental evidence showing that biting insects are capable of transmitting BLV.[47-49] Cattle with PL appear to be more efficient transmitters, hence, the recommendation in control programs to eliminate PL animals early in implementation. Whole cells in milk and colostrum can be transferred to the neonate; however, maternal anti-BLV antibody will neutralize free virus. For this reason, colostrum and milk are thought to be unimportant routes for transmission. Calves getting colostrum from a BLV infected dam will be protected until maternal antibody disappears at about 6 months of age. Transplacental infection and probably exposure to blood and other fluids during parturition can account for up to 20 percent of BLV infections. It seems that most infections occur at about the time heifers are introduced into the adult milking herd. The virus is easily destroyed by pasteurization and does not exist free in the environment for more than a few hours.

After initial infection there is a brief period of viremia followed by a very long incubation period. Once BLV infected cells enter through the skin or the alimentary or respiratory tract the provirus integrates randomly into the host cell genome and then lives a very quiescent existence. Although there is no detectable long-term viremia, latency is evidently incomplete since anti-BLV antibodies persist for life, indicating some limited or compartmentalized viral production. Anti-BLV antibodies are easily detected using an agar gel immunodiffusion test,[50] which remains the official test for import/export in most countries. Chronically BLV infected adult cattle that are persistently seronegative have been found rarely.[4,51] Certain BLV strains may be associated with seronegativity.[52] Uncharacterized plasma factors are potent inhibitors of BLV production in vitro, and they likely play an important role, with nonstructural viral proteins, in limiting expression in vivo, thereby potentially influencing the rate of tumor development.[53] Occasionally, seronegativity may occur in an infected animal during the periparturient period and with concurrent viral infections. Measures of production and reproduction are generally normal during the incubation period,[54] although some deficits have been reported.[55] BLV infected cattle may be culled at a higher rate than uninfected herdmates,[56] may not reach their potential for milk fat production,[57] and may have changes in serum immunoglobulin concentrations, the nature of the immunoglobulins, and production of autoantibodies.[17,18] Despite perturbations of the immune system, BLV infected cattle are not clinically immunosuppressed. The other bovine retroviruses (bovine immunodeficiency virus, bovine syncytial virus) do not appear to work in concert with BLV to produce disease or lymphoma.[58,59]

BLV is the etiological agent of the enzootic form of lymphoma that is seen in adult cattle.[60] There are rare reports of lymphomas in adult cattle unassociated with BLV.[4,61] BLV is an exogenous oncornavirus and shares the same genomic structure and replicative strategy as other members of the retrovirus family. BLV is most closely related phylogenetically to the human T cell leukemia virus. There is no evidence for the existence of subgroups with differing virulences as there is for FeLV. BLV is unlike FeLV, which becomes pathogenic when it recombines with cellular oncogenes. The mechanism of BLV oncogenesis is unknown, but is thought to involve expression of a specialized region of the viral genome that may *trans* activate cellular genes which regulate cell growth. Since only 5 to 10 percent of BLV infected cattle ever develop lymphoma,[62] it is presumed that the incubation period is longer than the lifespan of most infected animals. On an annual basis, it is estimated that 1 in 1000 to 1 in 250 BLV infected cattle develop lymphoma.[63] Undoubtedly, variables that play a role in a multistep process that culminates in neoplastic transformation include all of the following: genetic background, chronic lymphoid hyperplasia, environmental factors, age at exposure, virus dose, acquisition of karyotypic abnormalities, oncogene and tumor suppressor gene expression, and permissiveness for viral transcription by decreasing host factors that downregulate virus production. The complexity of this process and the relatively short lifespan of cattle likely accounts for the low rate of tumor formation. The positive relationship between age and incidence of lymphoma (see above, Demographics) is consistent with the cumulative effects of multiple risk factors.

The sporadic forms (juvenile, thymic, cutaneous) of lymphoma have largely been unassociated, on the basis of epidemiological and virological evidence, with BLV. There are rare reports of monoclonal integration of BLV in sporadic tumors supporting an etiological role for BLV.[4] A familial thymic (T cell) lymphosarcoma unassociated with BLV has been reported.[64,65] Almost all affected calves were sired by the same bull, and cases clustered in an 18-month period. An 11-month-old calf died of a multicentric T cell lymphoma 5 months following experimental inoculation with the bovine immunodeficiency virus (BIV),[66] raising the possibility of an association between the sporadic lymphomas and BIV.

B cells in persistently lymphocytotic cows have upregulated expression of *pim-1* and c-*myc* suggesting that protooncogene dysregulation may be an important step in lymphomagenesis.[67] Cells from most sporadic lymphomas expressed c-*myb,* but there was no expression in B cells from enzootic lymphomas.[68] A series of T cell sporadic lymphomas had the same c-*myb* mutation associated with increased transcription-activating activity.[69] Three of 6[70] and 12 of 18[71] adult cattle with BLV related lymphomas had point mutations in *p53,* suggesting a potential role for this mutated tumor suppressor gene in tumor development. The defect was not detected in BLV infected asymptomatic cattle. Altered expressions of protooncogenes have been detected, but their roles in the development of persistent lymphocytosis and lymphoma have not been established.

REFERENCES

1. Migaki, G. (1969) Hematopoietic neoplasms of slaughter animals. In Lingeman, C.H., and Garner, F.M. (eds.), *Comparative Morphology of Hematopoietic Neoplasms.* National Cancer Institute Monograph 32. U.S. Government Printing Office, Washington, D.C., pp. 121–151.

2. Anderson, R.K., Sorensen, I.K., Perman, V., Dirks, A., Snyder, M.M., and Bearman, J.E. (1971) Selected epizootiologic aspects of bovine leukemia in Minnesota (1961–1965). *Amer J Vet Res* 32:563–577.

3. Sorensen, D.K., Anderson, R.K., Perman, V., and Sautter, J.H. (1964) Studies of bovine leukemia in Minnesota. *Nord Vet Med (Suppl 1)* 16:562–572.

4. Jacobs, R.M., Song, Z., Poon, H., Heeney, J.L., Taylor, J.A., Jefferson, B., Vernau, W., and Valli, V.E.O. (1992) Proviral detection and serology in bovine leukemia virus-exposed normal cattle and cattle with lymphoma. *Can J Vet Res* 56:339–348.

5. Hamir, A.N., Perkins, C., and Jones, C. (1989) Bovine mandibular lymphosarcoma. *Vet Rec* 125:238.

6. Clegg, F.G., and Moss, B. (1965) Skin leucosis in a heifer: An unusual clinical history. *Vet Rec* 77:271–272.

7. Marshak, R.R., Hare, W.C.D., Dutcher, R.M., Schwartzman, R.M., Switzer, J.W., and Hubben, K. (1966) Observations on a heifer with cutaneous lymphosarcoma. *Cancer* 19:724–734.

8. Miller, L.D., and Olson, C. (1971) Regression of bovine lymphosarcoma. *J Amer Vet Med Assoc* 158:1536–1541.

9. Okada, K., Yamaguchi, A., Ohsima, K., Numakunai, S., Itoh, H., Seimiya, Y., and Koyama, H. (1989) Spontaneous regression of bovine cutaneous leukosis. *Vet Pathol* 26:136–143.

10. Zwahlen, R.D., Tontis, A., and Schneider, A. (1987) Cutaneous lymphosarcoma of helper/inducer T-cell origin in a calf. *Vet Pathol* 24:504–508.

11. Jacobs, R.M. (1986) Bovine lymphoma. In Olsen, R., Krakowka, S., and Blakeslee, J. (eds.), *Comparative Pathobiology of Viral Diseases.* CRC Reviews, Baton Rouge, LA, pp. 21–51.

12. Doige, C.E. (1987) Bone and bone marrow necrosis associated with the calf form of sporadic bovine leukosis. *Vet Pathol* 24:186–188.

13. Bendixen, H.J. (1965) Bovine enzootic leukosis. *Adv Vet Sci Comp Med* 10:129–204.

14. VanDerMaaten, M.J., and Miller, J.M. (1978) Susceptibility of cattle to bovine leukemia virus infection by vaious routes of exposure. In Beutvelzen, P., Hilgers, J., and Yohn, D.S. (eds.), *Advances in Comparative Leukemia Research.* Elsevier, North Holland, Amsterdam, pp. 29–32.

15. Depelchin, A., Letesson, J.J., Lostrie-Trussart, N., Mammerickx, M., Portetelle, D., and Burny, A. (1989) Bovine leukemia virus (BLV)-infected B-cells express a marker similar to the CD5 T-cell marker. *Immunol Lett* 20:69–76.

16. Ferrer, J.F. (1980) Bovine lymphosarcoma. *Adv Vet Sci Comp Med* 24:1–68.

17. Jacobs, R.M., Valli, V.E.O., and Wilkie, B.N. (1980) Serum electrophoresis and immunoglobulin concentration in cows with lymphoma. *Amer J Vet Res* 41:1942–1946.

18. Trainen, Z., Ungar-Waron, H., Meiron, R., Barnea, A., and Sela, M. (1976) IgG and IgM antibodies in normal and leukaemic cattle. *J Comp Pathol* 86:571–580.

19. Vernau, W., Valli, V.E.O., Dukes, T.W. Jacobs, R.M., Shoukri, M., and Heeney, J.L. (1992) Classification of 1198 cases of bovine lymphoma using the National Cancer Institute Working Formulation for human non-Hodgkin's lymphomas. *Vet Pathol* 29:183–195.

20. Dungworth, D.L., Theilen, G.H., and Ward, J.M. (1968) Early detection of the lesions of bovine lymphosarcoma. *Bibl Haematol* 30:206–211.

21. Järplid, B. (1964) Studies on the site of leukotic and preleukotic changes in the bovine heart. *Vet Pathol* 1:366–408.

22. Saari, S., and Järvinen, A.-K. (1994) Multicentric lymphoma involv-

ing large granular lymphocytes in a cow. *Zentralbl Veterinarmed A* 41:791–794.

23. Davis, W.C., Marusic, S., Lewin, H.A., Splitter, G.A., Perryman, L.E., McGuire, T.C., and Gorham, J.R., (1987) The development and analysis of species specific and cross reactive monoclonal antibodies to leukocyte differentiation antigens and antigens of the major histocompatibility complex for use in the study of the immune system in cattle and other species. *Vet Immunol Immunopathol* 15:337–376.

24. Aida, Y., Okada, K., and Amanuma, H. (1993) Phenotype and ontogeny of cells carrying a tumor-associated antigen that is expressed on bovine leukemia virus-induced lymphosarcoma. *Cancer Res* 53:429–437.

25. Chiba, T., Hiraga, M., Aida, Y., Ajito, T., Asahina, M., Wu, D., Ohshima, K., Davis, W.C., and Okada, K. (1995) Immunohistologic studies on subpopulations of lymphocytes in cattle with enzootic bovine leukosis. *Vet Pathol* 32:513–520.

26. Heeney, J.L., and Valli, V.E.O. (1990) Transformed phenotype of enzootic bovine lymphoma reflects differentiation-linked leukemogenesis. *Lab Invest* 62:339–346.

27. Onuma, M., Sagata, N., Okada, K., Ogawa, Y., Ikawa, Y., and Ohshima, K. (1982). Integration of bovine leukemia virus DNA in genomes of bovine lymphosarcoma cells. *Microbiol Immunol* 26:813–820.

28. Takashima, I., Olson, C., Driscoll, D.M., and Baumgartener, L.E. (1977) B-lymphocytes and T-lymphocytes in three types of bovine lymphosarcoma. *J Natl Cancer Inst* 59:1205–1209.

29. Vernau, W., Jacobs, R.M., Valli, V.E.O., and Heeney, J.L. (1997) The immunophenotypic characterization of bovine lymphomas. *Vet Pathol* 34:222–225.

30. Hood, L., Gray, W.R., Sanders, B.G., and Dreyer, W.J. (1967) Light chain evolution. In Cold Spring Harbor Symposium on Quantitative Biology—Antibodies 32:133–446.

31. Asahina, M., Kimura, K., Murakami, K., Ajito, T., Wu, D.L., Goryo, M., Aida, Y., Davis, W.C., and Okada, K. (1995) Phenotypic analysis of neoplastic cells from calf, thymic, and intermediate forms of bovine leukosis. *Vet Pathol* 32:683–691.

32. Sasaki, Y., Ishiguro, N., Horiuchi, M., Shinagawa, M., Osame, S., Furuoka, H., Matsui, T., Asahina, M., and Okada, K. (1997) Characterization of differentiation antigens expressed in bovine lymphosarcomas. *J Comp Pathol* 116:13–20.

33. Tani, K., Asahina, M., Wu, D.L., Ajito, T., Murakami, K., Goryo, M., Aida, Y., Davis, W.C., and Okada, K. (1997) Further analysis of the phenotype and distribution of tumor cells in sporadic B-cell and T-cell lymphomas in the lymph node and spleen of cattle. *Vet Immunol Immunopathol* 55:283–290.

34. Ishiguro, N., Matsui, T., and Shinagawa, M. (1994) Differentiation analysis of bovine T-lymphosarcoma. *Vet Immunol Immunopathol* 41:1–17.

35. Fujimoto, Y., Miller, J., and Olson, C. (1969) The fine structure of lymphosarcoma in cattle. *Path Vet* 6:15–29.

36. Ueberschär, S. (1968) Zytologische untersuchungen bei der rinderleukose. *Zentralbl Veterinarmed B* 15:163–173.

37. Weber, A., Andrews, J., Dickinson, B., Larson, V., Hammer, R., Dirks, V., Sorensen, D., and Frommes, S. (1969) Occurrence of nuclear pockets in lymphocytes of normal, persistent lymphocytotic and leukemic adult cattle. *J Natl Cancer Inst* 43:1307–1315.

38. Olson, C., Miller, J.M., Miller, L.D., and Gillette, K.G. (1970) C-type virus and lymphocytic nuclear projections in bovine lymphosarcoma. *J Amer Vet Med Assoc* 156:1880–1883.

39. Grimoldi, M.G., Poli, G., Sartorelli, P., Caldora, C., Oldani, L., and Locatelli, A. (1983) Karyotype analysis of lymphocytes from cattle at different stages of bovine leukemia virus infection. *Brit Vet J* 139:240–246.

40. Hare, W.C.D., McFeely, R.A., Abt, D.A., and Feierman, J.R. (1964) Chromosomal studies in bovine lymphosarcoma. *J Natl Cancer Inst* 33:105–118.

41. Hare, W.C.D., Yang, T.J., and McFeely, R.A. (1967) A survey of chromosome findings in 47 cases of bovine lymphosarcoma (leukemia). *J Natl Cancer Inst* 38:383–392.

42. Weinhold, E., and Müller, A. (1971) Untersuchungen über chromosomenanomalien bei der rinderleukose. *Berl Münch Tierärztle Wschr* 84:146–149.

43. Weipers, W.L., Jarrett, W.F.H., Martin, W.B., Crighton, F.W., and Stewart, M.F. (1964) Lymphosarcoma in domestic animals. *Ann Rep Brit Emp Cancer Campaign* 42:682–685.

44. Schnurr, M.W., Carter, R.F., Dubé, I.D., Valli, V.E., and Jacobs, R.M. (1994) Nonrandom chromosomal abnormalities in bovine lymphoma. *Leukemia Res* 18:91–99.

45. Heald, M.T.S., Waltner-Toews, D., Jacobs, R.M., and McNab, W.B. (1992) The prevalence of anti-bovine leukemia virus antibodies in dairy cows and associations with farm management practices, production and culling in Ontario. *Prev Vet Med* 14:45–55.

46. Miller, J.M., and VanDerMaaten, M.J. (1981) Bovine leukosis—Its importance to the dairy industry in the United States. *J Dairy Sci* 65:2194–2203.

47. Bech-Nielsen, S., Piper, C.E., and Ferrer, J.F. (1978) Natural mode of transmission of the bovine leukemia virus: Role of blood-sucking insects. *Amer J Vet Res* 39:1089–1092.

48. Oshima, K., Okada, K., Numakunai, S., Yoneyama, Y., Sato, S., and Takahashi, K. (1981) Evidence on horizontal transmission of bovine leukemia virus due to blood-sucking Tabanid flies. *Jpn J Vet Sci* 43:79–81.

49. Buxton, B., Schultz, R., and Collins, W.E. (1982) Role of insects in the transmission of bovine leukosis virus: Potential for transmission by mosquitoes. *Amer J Vet Res* 43:1458–1459.

50. Miller, J.M., and Olson, C. (1972) Precipitating antibody to an internal antigen of the C-type virus associated with bovine lymphosarcoma. *J Natl Cancer Inst* 49:1459–1461.

51. Eaves, F.W., Molly, J.B., Dimmock, C.K., and Eaves, L.E. (1994) A field evaluation of the polymerase chain reaction procedure for the detection of bovine leukaemia virus proviral DNA in cattle. *Vet Microbiol* 39:313–321.

52. Fechner, H., Blankenstein, P., Looman, A.C., Elwert, J., Geue, L., Albrecht, C., Kurg, A., Beier, D., Marquardt, O., Ebner, D. (1997) Provirus variants of the bovine leukemia virus and their relation to the serological status of naturally infected cattle. *Virology* 237:261–269.

53. Taylor, J., and Jacobs, R.M. (1993) Effects of plasma and serum on the *in vitro* expression of bovine leukemia. *Lab Invest* 69:340–346.

54. Jacobs, R.M., Heeney, J.L., Godkin, M.A., Leslie, K.E., Taylor, J.A., Davies, C., and Valli, V.E.O. (1991) Production and related variables in bovine leukaemia virus-infected cows. *Vet Res Commun* 15:463–474.

55. Brenner, J., Van-Haam, M., Savir, D., and Trainen, Z. (1989). The implication of BLV infection in the productivity, reproductive capacity and survival rate of a dairy cow. *Vet Immunol Immunopathol* 22:299–305.

56. Thurmond, M.C., Maden, C.B., and Carter, R.L. (1985) Cull rates of dairy cattle with antibodies to bovine leukemia virus. *Cancer Res* 45:1987–1989.

57. Wu, M.-C., Shanks, R.D., and Lewin, H.A. (1989) Milk and fat production in dairy cattle influenced by advanced subclinical bovine leukemia virus infection. *Proc Natl Acad Sci* 86:993–996.

58. Jacobs, R.M., Pollari, F.L., McNab, B., and Jefferson, B. (1995) A serological survey of bovine syncytial virus in Ontario: Associations with bovine leukemia and immunodeficiency-like viruses, production records, and management practices. *Can J Vet Res* 59:271–278.

59. Flaming, K.P., Frank, D.E., Carpenter, S., and Roth, J.A. (1997) Longitudinal studies of immune function in cattle experimentally infected with bovine immunodeficiency-like virus and/or bovine leukemia virus. *Vet Immunol Immunopathol* 56:27–38.

60. Miller, J.M., Miller, L.D., Olson, C., and Gillette, K.G. (1969) Virus-like particles in phytohemagglutinin-stimulated lymphocyte cultures with reference to bovine lymphosarcoma. *J Natl Cancer Inst* 43:1297–1305 .

61. Divers, T.J., Casey, J.N., Finley, M., and Delaney, M. (1995) Sporadic multicentric lymphosarcoma in a three-year-old bull. *J Vet Diag Invest* 7:164–166.

62. Ferrer, J.F., Marshak, R.R., Abt, D.A., and Kenyon, S.J. (1979) Relationship between lymphosarcoma and persistent lymphocytosis in cattle: A review. *J Amer Vet Med Assoc* 175:705–708.

63. Burny, A., Bruck, C., Chantrenne, H., Cleuter, Y., Dekegel, D., Ghysdael, J., Kettman, R., Leclercq, M., Leunen, J., Mammerickx, M., and Portetelle, D. (1980) Bovine leukemia virus: Molecular biology and epidemiology. In Klein, G. (ed.), *Viral Oncology*. Raven Press, NY, p. 231.

64. DaCosta, B., Djilali, S., Kessler, J.L., Sacré, B., Femenia, F., and Parodi, A.-L.(1991) Epidemiological and pathological studies of a familial thymic lymphosarcoma in bovine species. *Leukemia* 5:420–424.

65. Parodi, A.L., DaCosta, B., Djilali, S., Michel, B., Aloginouwa, Th., Femenia, F., Crespeau, F., Fontaine, J.J., and Thibier, M. (1989) Preliminary report of familial thymic lymphosarcoma in holstein calves. *Vet Rec* 125:350–353.

66. Rovid, A.H., Carpenter, S., Miller, L.D., Flaming, K.P., Long, M.J., VanDerMaaten, M.J., Frank, D.E., Roth, J.A. (1996) An atypical T cell lymphoma associated with bovine immunodeficiency-like virus infection. *Vet Pathol* 33:457–459.

67. Stone, D.M., Norton, L.K., Magnuson, N.S, and Davis, W.C. (1996) Elevated *pim*-1 and c-*myc* proto-oncogene induction in B lymphocytes from BLV-infected cows with persistent B lymphocytosis. *Leukemia* 10:1629–1638.

68. Asahina, M., Ishiguro, N., Wu, D., Goryo, M., Davis, W.C., and Okada, K. (1996) The proto-oncogene c-*myb* is expressed in sporadic bovine lymphoma, but not in enzootic bovine leukosis. *J Vet Med Sci* 58:1169–1174.

69. Shinagawa, T., Ishiguro, N., Horiuchi, M., Matsui, T., Okada, K., and Shinagawa, M. (1997) Deletion of c-*myb* exon 9 induced by insertion of repeats. *Oncogene* 14:2775–2783.

70. Ishiguro, N., Furuoka, H., Matsui, T., Horiuchi, M., Shinagawa, M., Asahina, M., and Okada, K. (1997) *p53* mutation as a potential cellular factor for tumor development in enzootic bovine leukosis. *Vet Immunol Immunopathol* 55:351–358.

71. Zhuang, W., Tajima, S., Okada, K., Ikawa, Y., and Aida, Y. (1997) Point mutation of *p53* tumor suppressor gene in bovine leukemia virus-induced lymphosarcoma. *Leukemia* 3:344–346.

Small Ruminants

Demographics

The prevalence of lymphoma per 100,000 slaughtered sheep varies between countries: 0.5 in the United States,[1] 21 in Great Britain,[2] 46 in New Zealand.[3] Lymphoma accounts for 21 to 41 percent of all condemnations of slaughtered sheep in the United States and Great Britain.[4] Most cases are in animals older than 3 years of age, but occasionally cases have been found in animals less than a year of age.[5] There was no gender or breed predisposition. Hepatic, pulmonary, and intestinal tumors are more common in some geographic regions.[6]

Rare cases of lymphoma have been reported in the goat.[7-10] In one study describing 10 goats with lymphoma (age range, 2 to 16 years of age), it was found that these affected goats accounted for 2.4 percent of all goats and 55 percent of all goats with tumors necropsied over a 6-year period.[11] There was no apparent sex or breed predisposition. Thymomas are common in aged dairy goats (see fig. 3.23).[12]

About a third of BLV infected sheep and cattle develop persistent lymphocytosis (PL). Two-thirds of cattle with lymphoma have a history of PL.[13] PL appears to be a rare outcome of BLV infection in goats.[14-17]

Gross Pathology and Histological, Phenotypic, and Genotypic Characteristics

Generally, the distribution of lesions in small ruminants with lymphoma parallels that seen in cattle. The multicentric form is most common in sheep and goats.[18] Most affected animals present with symmetrical lymphadenopathy, although sometimes peripheral lymph nodes may not show gross evidence for involvement. Iliac, cervical, and mediastinal lymph nodes are most often affected in cases of ovine lymphoma. Lymphadenopathy of internal lymph nodes was a consistent finding in the 10 cases of caprine lymphoma; affected peripheral lymph nodes were seen in only 3 cases.[11] Other commonly affected organs in sheep and goats with lymphoma are spleen, liver, kidney, alimentary tract, skeletal muscle, and heart. Mandible and maxillary bone involvement have been reported in goats with lymphoma.[11,19] Occasionally, in sheep gross lesions of lymphoma are found only in the kidney. The alimentary form is next most common in sheep, although there may be regional differences;[3] there appears to be no distinctive alimentary form in goats. Thymic and skin tumors do occur in both species, but the cutaneous involvement is subsequent to a multicentric process. Two cases of C cell hyperplasia and one case of C cell carcinoma were found among 11 sheep with experimentally induced lymphoma.[20]

A traditional classification scheme applied in cases of ovine lymphoma identified the most common histological type as lymphoblastoid, followed in decreasing frequency by lymphoblastoid/prolymphocytic, prolymphocytic, lymphocytic, and reticulum cell sarcoma.[18] However, tumor cell types displayed pleomorphism, particularly when cells were immature. More mature cell types have been reported in some ovine lymphomas.[2]

Immunophenotypes of lymphoid tumors in sheep have been studied; both T and B cell varieties occur, although most alimentary lymphomas were of B cell origin.[21-23] In experimentally induced lymphomas in sheep, tumor cells were of B cell origin, with or without CD5,[24,25] unlike lymphomas in cattle, which more consistently express CD5.[26]

Etiology and Transmission

Epidemiological and virological evidence support a retroviral etiology for spontaneous lymphomas in sheep.[27-29] Viral isolates from sheep with lymphoma cannot be distinguished from the BLV.[30,31] Sheep are exquisitely sensitive to the lymphomagenic properties of BLV; two-thirds of experimentally inoculated sheep develop lymphoma within 3 years.[14] The immunopathology of BLV in sheep has been extensively studied because it is a very useful model of lymphomagenesis.[24,32,33] BLV is not readily transmitted through natural mechanisms between sheep.[34] There are reports of sporadic and enzootic forms of the disease, parallelling the situation in cattle.[18,35]

As well, goats develop lymphoma as a result of experimental inoculation of BLV but are less sensitive to the lymphomagenic effects of BLV than sheep.[36] Anti-BLV antibodies have not been found in goats with spontaneously occurring lymphoma.[8,11]

REFERENCES

1. Migaki, G. (1969). Hematopoietic neoplasms of slaughtered animals. In Lingeman, C.H., and Garner, F.M. (eds.), *Comparative Morphology of Hematopoietic Neoplasms.* National Cancer Institute Monograph 32. U.S. Government Printing Office, Washington, D.C., pp. 121–151.

2. Anderson, L.J., and Jarrett, W.F.H. (1968). Lymphosarcoma (leukemia) in cattle, sheep, and pigs in Great Britain. *Cancer* 22:398–405.

3. Webster, W.M. (1966). Neoplasia in food animals with special reference to high incidence in sheep. *N Z Vet J* 14:203–214.

4. Bostock, D.E., and Owen, L.N. (1973) Porcine and ovine lymphosarcoma: A review. J. Natl. Cancer Inst. 50:933–939.

5. Cordes, D.O., and Shortridge, E.H. (1971) Neoplasms of sheep: A survey of 256 cases recorded at Ruakura Animal Health Laboratory. *N Z Vet J* 19:55–64.

6. Moulton, J.E., and Harvey, J.W. (1990) Tumors of the lymphoid and hematopoietic tissues. In Moulton, J.E. (ed.), *Tumors in Domestic Animals,* 3rd ed. University of California Press, Berkeley, pp. 231–307.

7. Baker, J.C., and Sherman, D.M. (1982) Lymphosarcoma in a Nubian goat. *Vet Med Small Anim Clin* 77:557–559.

8. DiGrassie, W.A., and Wallace, M.A., and Sponenberg, D.P. (1997) Multicentric lymphosarcoma with ovarian involvement in a Nubian goat. *Can Vet J* 38:383–384.

9. Matthews, J.G. (1992) Caprine tumors seen in a mixed practice. *Goat Vet Soc J* 13:52–54.

10. Schalm, O.W., Jain, N.C., and Carrol, E.J. (1975) *Veterinary Hematology,* 3rd ed. Lea and Febiger, Philadelphia, p. 595.

11. Craig, D.R., Roth, L., and Smith, M.C. (1986) Lymphosarcoma in goats. *Comp Cont Educ Pract Vet* 8:S190–S197.

12. Hadlow, W.J. (1978) High prevalence of thymoma in the dairy goat. *Vet Pathol* 15:153–169.

13. Ferrer, J.F. (1980) Bovine lymphosarcoma. *Adv Vet Sci Comp Med* 24:1–68.

14. Olson, C., and Baumgartener, L.E. (1976) Pathology of lymphosarcoma in sheep induced with bovine leukemia virus. *Cancer Res* 36:2365–2373.

15. Mammerickx, M., Portetelle, D., and Burny, A. (1981) Experimental cross-transmission of bovine leukemia virus (BLV) between several animal species. *Zentralbl Veterinarmed B* 28:69–81.

16. Hoss, H.E., and Olson, C. (1974) Infectivity of bovine C-type (leukemia) virus for sheep and goats. *Amer J Vet Res* 35:633–637.

17. Ressang, A.A., Baars, J.C., Calafat, J.,Mastenbrock, N., and Quak, J. (1976) Studies on bovine leukaemia. III. The haematological and serological response of sheep and goats to infection with whole blood from leukaemic cattle. *Zentralbl Veterinarmed B* 23:662–688.

18. Johnstone, A.C., and Manktelow, B.W. (1978) The pathology of spontaneously occurring malignant lymphoma in sheep. *Vet Pathol* 15:301–312.

19. DeSilva, L.N., Winter, M.H., Jackson, P.G.G., and Bostock, D.E. (1985) Lymphosarcoma involving the mandible of two goats. *Vet Rec* 117:276.

20. Okada, H., Fujimoto, Y., Ohshima, K., and Matsukawa, K. (1991) C cell hyperplasia and carcinoma developing in sheep with experimentally-induced lymphosarcoma. *J Comp Pathol* 105:313–322.

21. Németh, P., Horváth, Z., and Kelényi, G. (1979) T-cell lymphoblastoma in sheep. *Acta Vet Acad Sci Hungaricae* 27:303–311.

22. Tagashima, I., and Olson, C. (1980) Bovine leukosis virus in sheep, lymphocyte modification and surface immunoglobulin-bearing cell numbers. *Vet Microbiol* 5:1–12.

23. Dixon, R.J., Moriarty, K.M., and Johnstone A.C. (1984) An immunological classification of ovine lymphomas. *J Comp Pathol* 94:107–113.

24. Murakami, K., Aida, Y., Kageyama R, Numakunia, S., Ohshima, K., Okada, K., and Ikawa, Y. (1994) Immunopathologic study and characterization of the phenotype of transformed cells in sheep with bovine leukemia virus-induced lymphosarcoma. *Amer J Vet Res* 55:72–80.

25. Birkebak, T.A., Palmer, G.H., Davis, W.C., Knowles, D.P., and McElwain, T.F. (1994) Association of GP51 expression and persistent CD5+ B-lymphocytes expansion with lymphomagenesis in bovine leukemia virus infected sheep. *Leukemia* 8:1890–1899.

26. Aida, Y., Okada, K., and Amanuma, H. (1993) Pheontype and ontogeny of cells carrying a tumor-associated antigen that is expressed on bovine leukemia virus-induced lymphosarcoma. *Cancer Res* 53:429–437.

27. Paulsen, J., Best, E., Frese, K., and Rudolph, R. (1971) Enzootische lymphatische leukose bei schafen-lymphozytose, pathologische anatomie une histologie. *Zentralbl Veterinarmed B* 18: 33–43.

28. Paulsen, J., Rudolph, R., Hoffman, R., Weiss, E., and Schliesser, Th. (1972) C-type virus particles in phytohemagglutinin-stimulated lymphocyte cultures with reference to enzootic lymphatic leukosis in sheep. *Med Microbiol Immunol* 158:105–112.

29. Paulsen, J., Rudolph, R., and Miller, J.M. (1974) Antibodies to common ovine and bovine C-type virus specific antigen in serum from sheep with spontaneous leukosis and from inoculated animals. *Med Microbiol Immunol* 159:105–114.

30. Paulsen, J., Rohde, W., Pauli, G., Harms, E., and Bauer, H. (1976a) Comparative studies on ovine and bovine C-type particles. *Bibl Haematol* 43:190–192.

31. Rohde, W. Pauli, G., Paulsen, J., Harms, E. and Bauer, H. (1978) Bovine and ovine leukemia viruses. I. Characterization of viral antigens. *J Virol* 26:159–164.

32. Brandon. B., Gatei, M.H., Naif, H.M, Daniel, R.C., and Lavin, M.F. (1989) Observations on blood leukocytes and lymphocyte subsets in sheep infected with bovine leukemia virus: A progressive study. *Vet. Immunol Immunopathol* 23:15–27.

33. Ohshima, K., Aida, Y., Kim, J., Okada, K., Chiba, T., Murakami, K., and Ikawa, Y. (1991) Histopathology and distribution of cells harboring bovine leukemia virus (BLV) proviral sequences in ovine lymphosarcoma induced by BLV inoculation. *J Vet Med Sci* 53:191–199.

34. Kenyon, S.J., Ferrer, J.F., McFeely, R.A., and Graves, D.C. (1981) Induction of lymphosarcoma in sheep by bovine leukemia virus. *J Natl Cancer Inst* 67:1157–1163.

35. Paulsen, J. (1976b) Comparative studies in bovine and ovine leukosis. *Vet Microbiol* 1:211–218.

36. Olson, C., Kettmann, R., Burny, A., and Kaja, R. (1981) Goat lymphosarcoma from bovine leukemia virus. *J Natl Cancer Inst* 67:671–673.

Equine

Demographics

Case reports of equine lymphomas are relatively common,[1,2] but representative prevalence rates remain unknown. In abattoir surveys, lymphoma accounts for 1.7 to 50.6 per 100,000 horses slaughtered between 1958 and 1967.[3] Necropsy surveys suggest that lymphoma accounts for 0.2 to 3.0 percent of equine tumors.[4-8] At the University of California, Davis, lymphoma was the fifth most common neoplasm in horses after squamous cell carcinoma, dermal fibrosarcoma, melanoma, and ovarian granulosa cell tumor.[9] Half of affected horses are between 4 and 9 years of age; only 10 percent are under 4 years of age. The disease has been reported rarely in newborns and aborted fetuses.[10] There are no apparent gender or breed predispositions.

Clinical Characteristics

Weight loss, lethargy, and fever are commonly reported. Specific symptoms are dependent upon the distribution of lesions, but the diagnosis is often challenging. Most horses with lymphoma have peripheral lymphadenopathy and/or abdominal masses; these may be associated with ventral edema and colic, respectively.[11-13] Respiratory difficulties may be seen with involvement of the upper respiratory tract or with large masses originating in the area of the thymus or mediastinal/hilar lymph nodes. Although epidermal involvement is rare in the horse, subdermal nodules are common. In one series of horses, lymphoid tumors of the skin and subcutis slightly exceeded the frequency of lymphadenopathy.[9] In other studies, the frequency of skin involvement was much lower.[1,11,12,14] The subdermal masses, from 1 to 4 cm in diameter, are often distributed symmetrically over the neck and shoulders and along the perineum and preputium. Although most cases of equine lymphoma have a short clinical course, a small percentage appears to have a prolonged course that may extend over months to years. The latter cases tend to be those with subcutaneous involvement (see fig. 3.9).[9,15]

Clinical Pathology

Nonregenerative anemia is seen in about half of the horses with lymphoma.[11,12] However, hemolytic anemia with regeneration does occur, particularly in association with alimentary, splenic, and hepatic involvement. The regenerative anemias are often Coombs positive, supporting an immune pathogenesis, and can be considered a paraneoplastic syndrome.[16,17] Thrombocytopenia is seen consistently when there is immune hemolytic anemia, but is seen in less than 20 percent of cases overall. Hematological changes are less often seen in association with the skin form.[9] Hypercalcemia has been reported as a paraneoplastic syndrome in horses with lymphoma in which there is no renal infiltration.[11] Malabsorption and hypoproteinemia may be seen with diffuse intestinal involvement.[18,19]

Abnormal immature lymphocytes are reported to appear in the peripheral blood of 25 to 50 percent of horses with lymphoma.[1,2,12] Leukemia occurs once there is bone marrow metastasis and is usually a terminal event. As with other animal species, caution should be the rule when small numbers of "atypical" lymphocytes are detected; their presence should stimulate one to look elsewhere for

further supportive evidence. Confirmation of the diagnosis is usually made by biopsy of the largest accessible mass. Occasionally, diagnostic material may be aspirated from body cavity fluids.

Gross Pathology

Most cases are of the multicentric variety.[11-14] The next most frequent form is alimentary,[9,20,21] and thymic and skin (epitheliotrophic) forms are rare. As described above, subdermal nodules are commonly found as part of the multicentric form. The lymphadenopathy is often regionalized so that groups of lymph nodes (e.g., superficial, mediastinal, or alimentary) are similarly affected. Liver and spleen are commonly infiltrated. Occasionally, there is rupture of a massively enlarged spleen, resulting in sudden death. Other organs affected, in decreasing frequency, are heart, small intestine, kidney, colon, cecum, urinary bladder, peritoneum, and bone marrow.

Histological, Phenotypic, and Genotypic Characteristics

When 81 horses with lymphoma were classified according to the Working Formulation (see table 3.3), 38 percent had diffuse mixed type (see fig. 3.9) and 24 percent had diffuse large cell type. Ninety percent had low or intermediate grades of tumors.[15] One study indicated that most equine lymphomas were high grade,[22] but the criteria for this designation differed from that used previously.[15] The high frequency of the mixed cell type in equine lymphomas accounts for the relative lack of monomorphism compared to lymphomas in other species. In other studies utilizing traditional classification schemes, most lymphomas were classified as lymphocytic, prolymphocytic, or lymphoblastic, and the remainder had various forms of the histiocytic cell type.[14,23] Cells in diffuse mixed tumors stain for B and T cell markers (see fig. 3.9); therefore, using the term *histiocytic* to describe these tumors creates unnecessary confusion and should be avoided. Rare cases of large granular cell lymphoma[24] and Sézary syndrome have been reported.[25] The ultrastructural features of equine (diffuse mixed) lymphomas have been described.[14,26,27] The significance of large crystalline mitochondrial inclusions in equine lymphoma cells is unknown.[26,28]

Reagents and protocols for the immunohistochemical characterization of equine lymphomas have been well described and may be performed in formalin-fixed, paraffin-embedded tissues.[22,29,30] In a retrospective analysis of 31 cases of equine lymphoma, 24 had tumors derived from B cells, 11 of which (33 percent of 31 cases) had frequent nonneoplastic T cells.[22] In these latter cases, large neoplastic B cells were interspersed with small lymphocytes (T cells) and were classified as T-cell-rich (large) B cell tumors. Eight out of 11 T-cell-rich B cell tumors had subcutaneous tumors, suggesting an association between phenotype and topography. The unusually high prevalence of diffuse mixed or T-cell-rich B cell tumors in horses is primarily due to the relatively frequent occurrence of the subcutaneous form of lymphoma. Six of the 31 cases were derived from T cells, and all of the horses with large T cell tumors had mediastinal masses.

Although various infectious agents (retroviruses and coryneform bacteria) have been found in association with equine lymphomas, their etiological significance remains unknown.[26,28,31] The presence of bacterium in tumors may simply represent persistence in an immunosuppressed host. Transmission experiments have been unsuccessful.[32]

REFERENCES

1. Neufeld, J.L. (1973a) Lymphosarcoma in the horse: A review. *Can Vet J* 14:129–135.
2. Neufeld, J.L. (1973b) Lymphosarcoma in a mare and review of cases at the Ontario Veterinary College. *Can Vet J* 14:149–153.
3. Migaki, G. (1969) Hematopoietic neoplasms of slaughter animals. In Lingeman, C.H., and Garner, F.M. (eds.), *Comparative Morphology of Hematopoietic Neoplasms.* National Cancer Institute Monograph 32. U.S. Government Printing Office, Washington, D.C., pp. 121–151.
4. Baker, J.R., and Ellis, C.E. (1981) A survey of postmortem findings in 480 horses 1958–1980. (1) Causes of death. *Equine Vet J* 13:43–46.
5. Bastianello, S.S. (1983) A survey of neoplasia in domestic species over a 40-year period from 1935 to 1974 in the republic of South Africa. IV. Tumors occurring in equidae. *Onderstepoort J Vet Res* 50:91–96.
6. Cotchin, E., and Baker-Smith, J. (1975) Tumors in horses encountered in an abattoir survey. *Vet Rec* 97:339.
7. Kerr, K.M., and Alden, C.L. (1974) Equine neoplasia—A ten year survey. *Proc Ann Assoc Vet Lab Diag* 17:183.
8. Sundberg, J.P., Brunstein, T., Page, E.H., Kirkham, W.W., and Robinson, F.R. (1977) Neoplasms of equidae. *JAVMA* 170:150–152.
9. Madewell, B.R., and Theilen, G.H. (1987) Hematopoietic Neoplasms, Sarcomas and Related Conditions. Part VI. Equine. In Theilen, G.H., and Madewell, B.R. (eds.), *Veterinary Cancer Medicine,* 2nd ed. Lea and Febiger, Philadelphia, pp. 431–437.
10. Haley, R.J., and Spraker, T. (1983) Lymphosarcoma in an aborted equine fetus. *Vet Pathol* 20:647–649.
11. Rebhun, W.C., and Bertone, A. (1984). Equine lymphosarcoma. *J Amer Vet Med Assoc* 184:720–721.
12. VanDenHoven, R., and Franken, P. (1983). Clinical aspects of lymphosarcoma in the horse: A clinical report of 16 cases. *Equine Vet J* 15:49–53.
13. Savage, C.J. (1998) Lymphoproliferative and myeloproliferative disorders. *Vet Clin North Am Equine Practice* 14:563–578.
14. Fujimoto, Y., Kadota, K., Moriguchi, R., Kiryu, J., Matsukawa, K., and Chihaya, Y. (1982) Pathological observations on equine leukemia complex in Japan. *Bull Equine Res Inst Jpn* 19:69–88.
15. Valli, V.E.O. (1992) Equine lymphoma. In Jubb, K.V.F., Kennedy, P.C, and Palmer, N. (eds.), *Pathology of Domestic Animals,* 4th ed. Academic Press, San Diego, pp. 147–149.
16. Reef, V.B., Dyson, S.S., and Beech, J. (1984) Lymphosarcoma and associated immune-mediated hemolytic anemia and thrombocytopenia in horses. *J Amer Vet Med Assoc* 184:313–317.
17. Farrelly, B.T., Collins, J.D., and Collins, S.M. (1966) Autoimmune hemolytic anemia in the horse. *Irish Vet J* 20:42–45.
18. Roberts, M.C., and Pinsent, P.J.N. (1975) Malabsorption in the horse associated with alimentary lymphosarcoma. *Equine Vet J* 7:166–172.
19. Platt, H. (1987) Alimentary lymphomas in the horse. *J Comp Pathol* 97:1–10.
20. Humphrey, M., Watson, D.A., Edwards, H.G., and Wood, C.M. (1984) Lymphosarcoma in a horse. *Equine Vet J* 16:547–548.
21. Wiseman, A., Petrie, L., and Murray, M. (1974) Diarrhoea in the horse as a result of alimentary lymphosarcoma. *Vet Rec* 95:454–457.
22. Kelley, L.C., and Mahaffey, E.A. (1998) Equine malignant lymphomas: Morphologic and immunohistochemical classification. *Vet Pathol* 35:241–252.
23. Platt, H. (1988) Observations on the pathology of non-alimentary lymphomas in the horse. *J Comp Pathol* 98:177–194.
24. Grindem, C.B., Roberts, M.C., McEntee, M.F., and Dillman, R.C. (1989) Large granular lymphocyte leukemia in a horse. *Vet Pathol* 22:86–88.
25. Staempfli, H.R., McAndrew, K.H., Valli, V.E.O., and McEwen, B.J. (1988) An unusual case of lymphoma in a mare. *Equine Vet J* 20:141–143.
26. Sheahan, B.J., Atkins, G.J., Russell, R.J., and O'Connor, J.P. (1980) Histiolymphocytic lymphosarcoma in the subcutis of two horses. *Vet Pathol* 17:123–133.
27. Madewell, B.R., Carlson, G.R., Maclachlan, N.J., and Feldman, B.F. (1982) Lymphosarcoma with leukemia in a horse. *Amer J Vet Res* 43:807–812.
28. Detilleux, P.G., Cheville, N.F., and Sheahan, B.J. (1989) Ultrstructure and lectin histochemistry of equine cutaneous histiolymphocytic lymphosarcomas. *Vet Pathol* 26:409–419.
29. Asahina, M., Murakami, K., Ajito, T., Goryo, M., and Okada, K. (1994) An immunohistochemical study of an equine B-cell lymphoma. *J Comp Pathol* 111:445–451.
30. Collins Kelley, L., Mahaffey, E.A., Bounous, D.I., Antczak, D.F., and Brooks, R.L., Jr. (1997) Detection of equine and bovine T- and B-lymphocytes in formalin-fixed paraffin-embedded tissues. *Vet Immunol Immunopathol* 57:187–200.
31. Tomlinson, M.J., Doster, A.R., and Wright, E.R. (1979) Lymphosarcoma with virus-like particles in a neonatal foal. *Vet Pathol* 16:629–631.
32. McKercher, D.G., Wada, E.M., Straub, O.C., and Theilen, G.H. (1963) Possible viral etiology of bovine and equine leukemia. *Ann NY Acad Sci* 108:1163–1172.

Swine

Demographics

Lymphoma is the most frequently reported cancer of swine based on abattoir surveys in several countries.[1-4] The rates of lymphoma have been estimated at 2, 6.35, and 6.5 per 100,000 slaughtered swine in the United States, Czechoslovakia, and France, respectively.[4-6] In the United States and some European countries lymphoma accounts for 23 to 41 percent of slaughtered swine condemned for neoplasia.[7] There is no observed breed predisposition. One study indicated that females were affected twice as often as males.[8] Affected pigs are often 1 year old or less; the mediastinal form tends to appear in younger pigs than the multicentric variety does.[8,9]

Gross Pathology

The multicentric form of the disease is most frequent and accounts for about two-thirds of pigs with lymphoma. Peripheral lymphadenopathy is less commonly noted than visceral lymph node involvement. In one series, only the multicentric and mediastinal forms were found.[8,9] Commonly affected organs are spleen, liver, kidney, and bone marrow.[10,11]

Histological and Phenotypic Characteristics

Of 136 cases of lymphoma in pigs (table 3.4), 60 percent were of the diffuse, large, noncleaved type, while 24 percent were the small noncleaved type (see fig. 3.12). In another series of 36 pigs with lymphoma, 16 were classified as the Burkitt type, while 15 were of the mixed cell variety. Occasional cases with immunoblastic and medium-sized cell types were found.[8] Interestingly, the organ distribution of cell types classed as Burkitts (uniform type of SNC) more closely resembled the disease in children. Ten of 26 cases of ileal lymphoma in pigs were classed as having the diffuse, large, noncleaved cell type.[12] Membrane reactivity for alkaline phosphatase and diffuse cytoplasmic staining for acid phosphatase and nonspecific esterase were also demonstrated in this series of cases; most cases had cells that stained for IgM. Follicular lymphoma and plasmacytoma have also been described and immunophenotypically defined.[13-15] Antibodies reactive against normal and neoplastic porcine lymphocytes and immunohistochemical staining protocols have been well described.[16] Swine lymphomas, other than those arising in the thymus, are of B cell origin.[17] A case of lymphoma with large epithelioid cells, ostensibly of T cell origin, has been described.[18]

Etiology and Transmission

C type viruses have been associated with naturally occurring cases of lymphoma in swine,[19,20] but transmission studies have not been reported. An endogenous porcine C type virus has been found in a cell line derived from an apparently healthy pig; this virus is not infectious but is vertically transmitted.[21-23]

A genetic predisposition to develop lymphoma is evident in inbred herds.[24,25] In one instance, disease expression appeared in an autosomal recessive fashion.[24,26,27] Pigs with hereditary lymphoma had multicentric tumors (mostly involving visceral lymphoid tissue) and lymphoid leukemia, terminating with anemia and thrombocytopenia. Affected piglets were detected as early as 6 weeks of age. Most lived to 4 to 6 months of age; only rarely did any survive to 18 months of age.

REFERENCES

1. Bastianello, S.S. (1983) A survey of neoplasia in domestic species over a 40-year period from 1935 to 1974 in the Republic of South Africa III. Tumors occurring in pigs and goats. *Onderstepoort J Vet Res* 50:25–28.
2. Cotchin, E. (1960) Tumors of farm animals. A survey of tumors examined at the Royal Veterinary College, London, during 1950–1960. *Vet Rec* 72:816–821.
3. Fisher, L.F., and Olander, H.J. (1978) Spontaneous neoplasms of pigs—A study of 31 cases. *J Comp Pathol* 88:505–517.
4. Vitovec, J. (1977) Statistical data on 120 porcine tumors collected over the years 1964–1973 in South Bohemia. *Zentralbl Veterinarmed A* 24:779–786.
5. Migaki, G. (1969) Hematopoietic neoplasms of slaughter animals. In Lingeman, C.H., and Garner, F.M. (eds.), *Comparative Morphology of Hematopoietic Neoplasms.* National Cancer Institute Monograph 32. U.S. Government Printing Office, Washington, D.C., pp. 121–151.
6. Renier, F., Chevrel, L., Friedmann, J.C., Gaquiere, G., and Guelfi, J. (1966) Some considerations on porcine leukoses. *Nouv Rev Fr Hematol* 6:239–251.
7. Bostock, D.E., and Owen, L.N. (1973) Porcine and ovine lymphosarcoma: A review. *J Natl Cancer Inst* 50:933–939.
8. Hayashi, M., Tsuda, H., Okumura, M., Sakata, T., Ito, N., and Suchi, T. (1988) Histopathological classification of malignant lymphomas in slaughtered swine. *J Comp Pathol* 98:11–21.
9. Anderson, L., and Jarrett, W.F.H. (1969) A classification of lymphoid neoplasms of domestic animals. In Lingeman, C.H., and Garner, F.M. (eds.), *Comparative Morphology of Hematopoietic Neoplasms.* National Cancer Institute Monograph 32. U.S. Government Printing Office, Washington, D.C., pp. 343–353.
10. Chevrel, M.L., Rénier, F., Richier, M.E., Ramée, M.P., and Tréguer, F. (1969). Le lymphosarcome porcin. *Rec Méd Vét* 145:135–147
11. Monlux, A.W., Anderson, W.A., and Davis, C.L. (1956). A survey of tumors occurring in cattle, sheep, and swine. *Amer J Vet Res* 17:646–677.
12. Tanimoto, T., Minami, A., Yano, S., and Ohtsuki, Y. (1994) Ileal lymphoma in swine. *Vet Pathol* 31:629–636.
13. Kadota, K., and Niibori, S. (1985) A case of swine follicular lymphoma with intracytoplasmic immunoglobulin inclusions. *J Comp Pathol* 95:599–608.
14. Kadota, K., Ishino, S., and Nakajima, H. (1986a). Immunological and ultrastructural observations on swine thymic lymphoma. *J Comp Pathol* 96:371–378.
15. Kadota, K., and Nakajima, H. (1988) Histological progression of follicular centre cell lymphomas to immunoglobulin-producing tumors in two pigs. *J Comp Pathol* 99:145–158.
16. Tanimoto, T., and Ohtsuki Y. (1996) Evaluation of antibodies reactive with porcine lymphocytes and lymphoma cells in formalin-fixed, paraffin-embedded, antigen-retrieved tissues sections. *Amer J Vet Res* 57:853–859.
17. Kadota, K., Nemoto, K., Mabara, S., and Shirai, W. (1986b) Three types of swine immunoglobulin-producing tumors: Lymphoplasmacytic lymphosarcoma, immunoblastic lymphosarcoma, and plasmacytoma. *J Comp Pathol* 96:541–550.
18. Kadota, K. A case of swine T-cell lymphoma with Lennert's lesion. (1987) *Jpn J Vet Sci* 49:913–916.
19. Strandström, H., Veijalainen, P., Moennig, V., Hunsmann, G., Schwartz, H., and Schafer, W. (1974). C-type particles produced by a permanent cell line from a leukemic pig. I. Origin and properties of the host-cells and some evidence for the occurrence of C-type like particles. *Virology* 57:175–178.
20. Moennig, V., Frank, H., Hunsmann, G., Ohms, P., Schwarz, H., and Schaper, W. (1974) C-type particles produced by a permanent cell line from a leukemic pig. II. Physical, chemical and serological characterization of the particles. *Virology* 57:179–188.
21. Busse, C., Marschall, H.J., and Moennig, V. (1978) Further investigations on the porcine lymphoma C-type particle (PLCP) and the possible biological significance of the virus in pigs. *Ann Rech Vet* 9:651–658.
22. Busse, C., Marschall, H.J. Frenzel, B., and Moenning, V. (1981) Partial analysis of the polypeptide composition of a porcine lymphoma C-type particle (PLCP). *Zentralbl Veterinarmed B* 28:118–125.
23. Todaro, G.J., Benveniste, R.E., Lieber, M.M., and Sherr, C.J. (1974) Characterization of a type C virus released from porcine cell line PK(15). *Virology* 58:65–74.
24. McTaggart, H.S., Head, K.W., and Laing, A.H.T. (1971) Evidence for a genetic factor in the transmission of spontaneous lymphosarcoma (leukaemia) of young pigs. *Nature* 232:557–558.
25. Saito, Y., Normura, Y., Shirota, K., Yomakoshi, J., Hizawa, H., Kashima, T., Hara, I., Shinoda, M., and Miyashita, I. (1982) Famil-

ial leukemia of swine—A report on two cases in consecutive two generations and one related case. *Bull Azabu Univ* 3:201–202.

26. Head, K.W., Campbell, J.G., Imlah, P., Laing, A.H., Linklater, K.A., and McTaggart, H.S. (1974) Hereditary lymphosarcoma in a herd of pigs. *Vet Rec* 95:523–527.

27. McTaggart, H.S., Laing, A.H., Imlah, P., Head, K.W., and Brownlie, J.E. (1979) The genetics of hereditary lymphosarcoma of pigs. *Vet Rec* 105:36.

Plasma Cell Neoplasia

Tumors of plasma cells result from the monoclonal proliferation of B cells. The cutaneous plasmacytomas are characterized by benign behavior, while multiple myelomas arising in bone marrow (fig. 3.18) and extramedullary plasmacytomas may be malignant (figs. 3.19 and 3.20). Although the cutaneous and extramedullary plasmacytomas have very different behaviors, they are sometimes grouped as solitary plasmacytomas. The solitary osseous plasmacytoma should be regarded as an early event in multiple myeloma.[1]

Cutaneous Plasmacytoma

The cutaneous plasmacytomas are primarily tumors of old dogs (mean, 9–10 years; range, 2–22 years).[2-6] Large breeds are more often affected, but there is no sex predisposition. Lesions occur on the trunk, limbs, head (particularly the external pinnae and ear canals), and the oral cavity including the gingiva and tongue. Rare cases have been reported in the cat.[7-9] In the past, these tumors have been labeled as atypical histiocytomas, reticulum cell sarcomas, or poorly differentiated round cell tumors.[3,4] Some plasmacytomas have been incorrectly identified as cutaneous neuroendocrine tumors.[10]

At presentation, the tumors are usually solitary, raised, pink nodules from 1 to 2 cm in diameter. Much larger and ulcerated lesions may be present. The frequency with which multiple lesions are reported varies with the study but is always less than 20 percent.[2,10,11] The location is primarily dermal but may extend into subcutaneous tissue; there is no infiltration of the epidermis. Tumors are nonencapsulated and are composed of sheets of plasma cells with little to marked heterogeneity. Some may show frequent bi- and multinucleation, multilobation, and karyomegaly. Chromatin is often clumped and peripheralized. If nucleoli are present they are usually single, small, and centrally placed. Variable amounts of amphophilic cytoplasm and prominent Golgi zones are present. Even in very heterogenous tumors, small numbers of more typical plasmacytoid cells are found, supporting the diagnosis. Plasmacytomas were categorized into hyaline, mature, cleaved, asynchronous, and polymorphous-blastic types.[12] Tumors composed of typical plasma cells (mature type) were infrequent, while approximately 70 percent were of the cleaved and asynchronous types. A uniform language for describing these pleomorphic tumors will be a helpful diagnostic aid. There was no association between proliferation rate and category, suggesting limited usefulness as a tumor grading system.

Although nonspecific, cells with plasmacytoid differentiation stain positive with methyl green pyronin. Negative staining with toluidine blue helps to eliminate mast cell tumor. Immunohistochemical staining (see table 3.5) for cytoplasmic IgG (for which most are positive), IgA, and vimentin has been reported.[4,13] Plasmacytoma cells and related tumors do not stain for cytokeratin and S-100.[10] Immunoglobulin-lambda-light chain-associated amyloid was demonstrated in a series of canine cutaneous plasmacytomas[5]; these constitute about 3 percent of canine cutaneous plasmacytomas. The presence of amyloid is frequently associated with local reoccurrence despite wide surgical excision.[5,10] Hypercalcemia and monoclonal gammopathy have been reported rarely.[2]

Cutaneous plasmacytomas are considered benign neoplasms, and complete surgical excision is generally curative in those tumors lacking amyloid. There is a single case report of a cutaneous plasmacytoma metastatic to a regional lymph node.[14] If multiple cutaneous lesions, lymphadenopathy, or other clinicopathological observations supportive of systemic disease are present, then extramedullary plasmacytoma or multiple myeloma should be considered since the prognosis is markedly different.

Other tumors to be distinguished from plasmacytoma are melanoma, histiocytoma, epitheliotropic lymphoma, and transmissible venereal tumor (TVT). The presence of a narrow zone of compressed dermis between the tumor and overlying epithelium is helpful in distinguishing plasmacytoma from histiocytoma, melanoma, and epitheliotropic lymphoma.[15] The histiocytoma is closely associated with the hyperplastic epithelium and is composed of cells with cleaved bean-shaped nuclei. Melanomas are invasive and may show intraepithelial growth, and many will show at least small numbers of melanin granules. Immunohistochemistry (S-100, cytokeratin, neuron specific enolase) can be used to support an epithelial origin. It is important to make this distinction because melanomas of the oral cavity and digit (locations where plasmacytomas are often found) have greater malignant potential than melanomas from other sites. Pautrier microabscesses are characteristic of epitheliotropic lymphoma. The TVT has a characteristic exophytic growth pattern and is composed of relatively uniform cells with a generous amount of clear cytoplasm.

Extramedullary Plasmacytoma

The extramedullary plasmacytomas are largely seen in old dogs (range, 3 to 10 years). There is no sex predisposition. Cocker spaniels represented 24 percent of dogs in one series of cases, relative to 4 percent in the hospital population, which suggests a breed predisposition.[16] Most arise in the gastrointestinal tract, particularly the rectal mucosa.[3,17,18] Less commonly, the tumors have been found

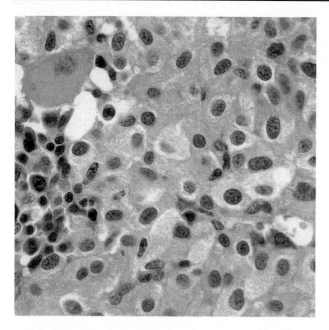

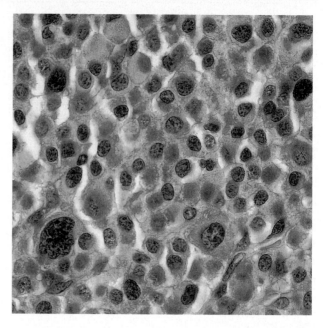

Fig. 3.18. Myeloma. A 6-year-old spayed female rottweiler was presented for examination because of reduced activity and was found to have normocytic, normochromic, nonresponsive anemia. A bone marrow aspirate revealed decreased normal cells plus large undifferentiated cells. A marrow core biopsy was taken. Focal areas of hematopoiesis are present (left), and there is phthisis of normal marrow elements and bone by a solid proliferation of cells that have round to oval hyperchromatic nuclei and a very low mitotic rate. The cells have abundant moderately amphophilic cytoplasm and irregularly distinct cellular boundaries. H&E ×800.

Fig. 3.20. Plasmacytoma, anaplastic. Gastric biopsy from 12.5-year-old female Alaskan malamute with a history of chronic diarrhea. The lamina propria is expanded by cells with nuclei generally 1.5 to 3 red cells in diameter that are round to oval, with hyperchromatic, coarsely granular chromatin and numerous small chromocenters. Nucleoli are irregularly present and not prominent. Significant to the interpretation of malignancy, multinucleation is present in most fields, with as many as four nuclei in a single cell. The cytoplasm is abundant, with moderate staining density, and tends to be eccentrically placed. Mitoses are present in about one-half of the fields, and occasional very large nuclei are present. H&E ×800.

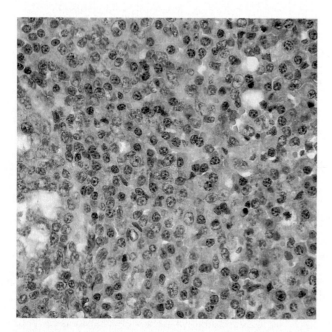

Fig. 3.19. Splenic plasmacytoma. A mature female domestic shorthair cat was examined because of weight loss. At the left, a fading germinal center with almost complete loss of small mature mantle cells is surrounded by a dense population of larger cells with abundant eccentric cytoplasm. Paranuclear lighter areas of Golgi zones are visible in some cells. H&E ×500.

in the esophagus, gastric mucosa (see fig. 3.20), lung, spleen, kidney, vertebral canal, and brain.[6,19-22] Extramedullary plasmacytomas have also been reported in cats[9] and horses.[23,24]

Amyloid of immunoglobulin lambda light chain origin, demonstrated by either thioflavine T or Congo red staining, has been described in association with extramedullary plasmacytomas in dogs, cats, and horses.[24-28] Amyloid detection has some diagnostic usefulness: 60 percent of canine extramedullary plasmacytomas had thioflavine T staining, while other round cell tumors did not stain.[16] Staining for amyloid in the presence of inflammation should be interpreted cautiously since reactive plasma cells will also stain positively.

Tumors may be multinodular or may cause diffuse thickening of the intestinal wall. Metastasis to regional lymph nodes is usual. The plasma cells in tumors may be well differentiated or moderately heterogeneous including multinucleation. An absence of melanin granules and even a small amount of plasmacytoid differentiation will help to distinguish this tumor from melanoma. In difficult cases, immunohistochemistry (see table 3.5) can be used to demonstrate cytoplasmic immunoglobulin (most commonly IgG), although as few as 5 percent of tumor cells may stain positively. Melanomas will stain positively for S-100. Metaplastic bone and cartilage may occasionally be present.[25] Widespread metastasis to other abdominal organs has been reported, and in some there is production of a monoclonal gammopathy (see below) and other characteristics of multiple myeloma.[29,30] However, once there is bone or bone marrow involvement, the disease should be designated as multiple myeloma. Malignant extramedullary plasmacytomas have more aneuploidy and increased c-myc oncoprotein content relative to their benign cutaneous counterparts.[31] There is a single case report of a metastatic plasmacytoma in a cat.[9]

Multiple Myeloma

Multiple myeloma is rare in animals and accounts for less than 1 percent of all malignant neoplasms. Cases have been reported in the cat, cow, dog, horse, and pig. In the dog, 8 percent of hemolymphatic tumors are multiple myelomas (see fig. 3.18).[32] There is no sex predisposition. Depending on the study, the mean age of affected dogs and cats is between 8 and 9 years (canine range, 30 months to 16 years).[33,34]

In one study, German shepherds were overrepresented relative to the hospital population[32] Multiple myeloma is much rarer in the cat than in the dog and is unassociated with FeLV or FIV.[33,35] The etiology of multiple myeloma remains unknown; however, genetic predispositions, viral infections, chronic antigenic stimulation, and exposure to environmental carcinogens are all thought to be contributing factors. Risk factors in people are occupations in the agriculture industry and exposure to petroleum products and radiation.[36,37] It has been suggested that in humans chronic herpes viral infection induces macrophage cytokine production, which drives plasma cell production and ultimately malignant transformation.[38]

The pathological changes associated with multiple myeloma are due to the neoplastic proliferation of B cells in bone marrow and other organs and usually high levels of a myeloma (M) protein in blood. Pathological changes include characteristic osteolytic bone lesions, hypercalcemia, renal disease, hemorrhage, hyperviscosity syndrome, immunodeficiency, cytopenias, and cardiac abnormalities. The bone lesions are seen in 25 to 66 percent of dogs with IgG and IgA types of multiple myeloma.[32,34] Affected bones are usually the vertebrae, ribs, pelvis, skull, and the metaphyses of the long bones. Lameness and pathological fractures are among the most common presenting symptoms of dogs with multiple myeloma. Dogs with IgM multiple myeloma (Waldenstrom's macroglobulinemia) and cats rarely have skeletal lesions. Hypercalcemia is seen in 15 to 20 percent of dogs with multiple myeloma and may result from tumor cells producing osteoclast activating substances. From 33 to 50 percent of canine patients have renal disease (*myeloma kidney*), usually having multiple causations including tumor metastasis, proteinuria resulting in casts, hypercalcemia, amyloidosis, sludging of hyperviscous blood, and upper urinary tract infection. Dogs with multiple myeloma that have

hypercalcemia, lytic bone lesions, or Bence Jones proteinuria have decreased survival.[32]

A diagnosis of multiple myeloma is made when there is bone marrow plasmacytosis, lytic bone lesions, and a serum and/or urine M protein. Bone marrow infiltration may be diffuse or focal. The diagnosis should be considered when plasma cells account for greater than 30 percent of bone marrow cells. Lytic bone lesions will have the highest density of plasma cells. Metastatic sites are most commonly lymph nodes, spleen, liver, and kidneys. Plasma cell leukemia is seen rarely. Cells range from poorly to well-differentiated plasma cells and may have eosinophilic round to crystalline cytoplasmic inclusions.[23] Cells are often larger than normal plasma cells, and anisokaryosis and multinucleation may be prominent and cytoplasm abundant. The more undifferentiated cells may have single nucleoli. The mitotic rate is low and is estimated at 1:20,000 myeloma cells, much lower than the 8:1000 for normal marrow. Thus, therapy based on cell cycle is not indicated.

The M protein is also described as a monoclonal gammopathy or a paraprotein that may be a whole immunoglobulin molecule of any class or a heavy or light chain. Light chains in urine, termed *Bence Jones proteins,* are found in 25 to 40 percent of dogs with multiple myeloma[32,34] and have been reported in about 60 percent of cats.[11,39,40] In dogs with multiple myeloma, the M protein is usually IgG or IgA, with approximately equal frequencies.[32,33] In those cases where the M protein is IgM, the disease may be referred to as Waldenstrom's macroglobulinemia. In contrast to the focal lysis of bone characteristic of multiple myeloma, the Waldenstrom's cases present more like lymphoma with involvement of lymph nodes, liver, spleen, and bone marrow without bone lysis. The cells do not have typical plasmacytoid features and are more similar to the cells of small lymphocytic lymphoma of the intermediate type, usually with a mild and irregular increase in cytoplasmic volume as in lymphoplasmacytoid lymphoma (see fig. 3.3 A). Most multiple myelomas in cats produce IgG.[40] Biclonal gammopathy has been reported in a case of canine multiple myeloma.[41] The frequency with which biclonal gammopathies are detected in animal multiple myelomas will likely increase once immunofixation is used routinely in veterinary laboratories,[42] as has been the experience in human laboratory medicine. About half of all cases of multiple myelomas in people are biclonal.[43] Generally, the concentration of the M protein is proportional to the tumor burden. The effect of treatment can be assessed by sequential monitoring of the serum M protein concentration. Increased concentrations of serum globulins are seen in most cases of multiple myeloma, but it is possible to have a concentration within the reference range because the concentrations of normal immunoglobulins may be markedly decreased. There are rare reports of nonsecretory multiple myeloma in the dog.[1]

It is important to be aware of the nonneoplastic diseases of animals in which a monoclonal gammopathy may be present in serum. These include ehrlichiosis, leishmaniasis, feline infectious peritonitis, chronic pyoderma, and rarely, idiopathic (so-called benign or of unknown significance) disease. [44-47] The M proteins formed in association with these nonneoplastic diseases generally have stable and modest concentrations, are unassociated with Bence Jones proteins, osteolysis, or cytopenias resulting from myelophthisis. In addition, the serum concentrations of other immunoglobulin classes are normal or increased. B cells other than plasma cells may produce large quantities of M proteins. Examples are the cells of the acute and chronic lymphoid leukemias and lymphomas, even of the skin variety. [48,49] These should be described as leukemias or lymphomas with monoclonal gammopathy. Immunohistochemistry may be used to demonstrate that the cytoplasmic immunoglobulin and the M protein are of the same class.

REFERENCES

1. MacEwen, E.G., Patnaik, A.K., Hurvitz, A.I., and Bradley, R. (1984) Nonsecretory multiple myeloma in two dogs. *J Amer Vet Med Assoc* 184:1283–1286.

2. Clark, G.N., Berg, J., Engler, S.J., and Bronson, R.T. (1992) Extramedullary plasmacytomas in dogs: Results of surgical excision in 131 cases. *J Amer Anim Hosp Assoc* 28:105–111.

3. Rakich, P.M., Latimer K.S., Weiss, R., and Steffens, W.L. (1989) Mucocutaneous plasmacytomas in dogs: 75 cases (1980–1987). *J Amer Vet Med Assoc* 194:803– 810.

4. Baer, K.E., Patnaik, A.K., Gilbertson, S.R., and Hurvitz, A.I. (1989) Cutaneous plasmacytomas in dogs: A morphologic and immunohistochemical study. *Vet Pathol* 26:216–221.

5. Rowland, P.H., Valentine, B.A., Stebbins, K.E., and Smith, C.A. (1991) Cutaneous plasmacytomas with amyloid in six dogs. *Vet Pathol* 28:125–130.

6. Kyriazidou, A., Brown, P.J., and Lucke, V.M. (1989) An immunohistochemical study of canine extramedullary plasma cell tumors. *J Comp Pathol* 100:259–166.

7. Lucke, V.M. (1987) Primary cutaneous plasmacytoma in the dog and cat. *J Small Anim Pract* 28:49–55.

8. Kryiazidou, A., Brown, P.J., and Lucke, V.M. (1989) Immunohistochemical staining of neoplastic and inflammatory plasma cell lesions in feline tissues. *J Comp Pathol* 100:337–341.

9. Carothers, M.A., Johnson, G.C., DiBartola, S.P., Liepnicks J., and Benson, M.D. (1989) Extramedullary plasmacytoma and immunoglobulin-associated amyloidosis in a cat. *J Amer Vet Med Assoc* 195:1593–1597.

10. Goldschmidt, M.H., and Shofer, F.S., (1992) *Skin Tumors of the Dog and Cat*. Pergamon Press, Oxford, pp. 25–270.

11. Ogilvie, G.K., and Moore, A.S. (1996) Plasma cell tumors of extramedullary sites. In *Managing the Veterinary Cancer Patient: A Practice Manual*. Veterinary Learning Systems Co., Inc., Trenton, NJ, p. 287.

12. Platz, S.J., Breuer, W., Pfleghaar, S., Minkus, G., and Hermanns, W. (1999) Prognostic value of histopathological grading in canine extramedullary plasmacytomas. *Vet Pathol* 36:23–27.

13. Day, M.J. (1995) Immunophenotypic characterization of cutaneous lymphoid neoplasia in the dog and cat. *J Comp Pathol* 112:79–96.

14. Trigo, F.J, and Hargis, A.M. Canine cutaneous plasmacytoma with regional lymph node metastasis. (1983) *Vet Med Small Anim Clin* 78:1749–1751.

15. Yager, J.A., and Wilcock, B.P. (1994) Round cell tumors. In *Surgical Pathology of the Dog and Cat: Dermatopathology and Skin Tumors*. Mosby, London, pp. 273–286.

16. Brunnert, S.R., and Altman, N.H. (1991) Identification of immunoglobulin light chains in canine extramedullary plasmacytomas by thioflavine T and immunohistochemistry. J. *Vet Diag Invest* 3:245–251.

17. Trevor, P.B., Saunders, G.K., Waldrom, D.R., and Leib, M.S. (1993) Metastatic extramedullary plasmacytoma of the colon and rectum in a dog. *J Amer Vet Med Assoc* 203:406–409.

18. MacEwen, E.G., Patnaik, A.K., Johnson, G.F., and Hurvitz, A.I. (1984) Extramedullary plasmacytoma of the gastrointestinal tract in two dogs. *J Amer Vet Med Assoc* 184:1396–1398

19. Hamilton, T.A., and Carpenter, J.L. (1994) Esophageal plasmacytoma in the dog. *J Amer Vet Med Assoc* 204:1210–1211.

20. Brunnert, S.R., Dee, L.A., Herron, A.J., and Altman, N.H. (1992) Gastric extramedullary plasmacytoma in a dog. *J Amer Vet Med Assoc* 200:1501–1502.

21. Jackson, M.W., Helfand, S.C., Smedes, S.L., Bradley, G.A., and Schultz, R.D. (1994) Primary IgG secreting plasma cell tumor in the gastrointestinal tract of a dog. *J Amer Vet Med Assoc* 204:404–406.

22. Sheppard, B.J., Chrisman, C.L., Newell, S.M., Raskin, R.E., and Homer, B.L. (1997) Primary encephalic plasma cell tumor in a dog. *Vet Pathol* 34:621–627.

23. Jacobs, R.M., Kociba, G.J., and Ruoff, W.W. (1983) Monoclonal gammopathy in a horse with defective hemostasis. *Vet Pathol* 20:643–647.

24. Linke, R.P., Geisel, O., and Mann, K. (1991) Equine cutaneous amyloidosis derived from an immunoglobulin lambda-light chain. Immunohistochemical, immunochemical and chemical results. *Biol Chem Hoppe Seyler* 372:835–843.

25. Ramos-Vara, J.A., Miller, M.A., Pace, L.W., Linke, R.P., Common, R.S., and Watson, G.L. (1998) Intestinal multinodular A lambda-amyloid deposition associated with extramedullary plasmacytoma in three dogs: Clinicopathological and immunohistochemical studies. *J Comp Pathol* 119:239–249.

26. Platz, S.J., Breuer, W., Geisel, O., Linke, R.P., and Hermanns, W. (1997) Identification of lambda light chain amyloid in eight canine and two feline extramedullary plasmacytomas. *J Comp Pathol* 116:45–54.

27. Breuer W., Colbatzky F., Platz, S., and Hermanns, W. (1993) Immunoglobulin-producing tumors in dogs and cats. *J Comp Pathol* 109:203–216.

28. Rowland, P.H., and Linke, R.P. (1994) Immunohistochemical characterization of lambda light-chain-derived amyloid in one feline and five canine plasma cell tumors. *Vet Pathol* 31:390–393.

29. Trevor, P.B., Saunders, G.K., Waldrom, D.R., and Leib, M.S. (1993) Metastatic extramedullary plasmacytoma of the colon and rectum in a dog. *J Amer Vet Med Assoc* 203:406–409.

30. Lester, S.J., and Mesfin, G.M. (1980) A solitary plasmacytoma in a dog with progression to a disseminated myeloma. *Can Vet J* 21:284–286.

31. Frazier, K.S., Hines, M.E., Hurvitz, A.I., Robinson, P.G., and Herron, A.J. (1993) Analysis of DNA aneuploidy and c-myc oncoprotein content of canine plasma cell tumors using flow cytometry. *Vet Pathol* 30:505–511.

32. Matus, R.E., Leifer, C.E., MacEwen, E.G., and Hurvitz, A.I. (1986) Prognostic factors for multiple myeloma in the dog. *J Amer Vet Med Assoc* 188: 1288–1291.

33. MacEwen, E.G., and Hurvitz, A.I. (1977) Diagnosis and management of monoclonal gammopathies. *Vet Clin N Amer Small Anim Pract* 7:119–132.

34. Osborne, C.A., Perman, V., Sautter, J.H., Stevens, J.B., and Hanlon, G.F. (1968) Multiple myeloma in the dog. *J Amer Vet Med Assoc* 153:1300–1319.

35. Engle, G.C., and Brodey, R.S. (1969) A retrospective study of 395 feline neoplasms. *J Amer Anim Hosp Assoc* 5:21–31.

36. Cuzick, J., and DeStavola, B. (1988) Multiple myeloma. A case control study. *Brit J Cancer* 57:516–520.

37. Linet, M.S., Sioban, D.H., and McLaughlin, J.K. (1987) A case-control study of multiple myeloma in whites: Chronic antigenic

stimulation, occupation and drug use. *Cancer Res* 47:2978–2981.

38. Rettig, M.B., Ma, H.J., Vescio, R.A., Pold, M., Schiller, G., Belson, D., Savage, A., Nishikubo, C., Wu, C., Fraser, J., Said, J.W., and Berenson, J.R. (1997) Kaposi's sarcoma-associated herpesvirus infection of bone marrow dendritic cells from multiple myeloma patients. *Science* 276:1851–1854.

39. Drazner, F.H. (1982) Multiple myeloma in the cat. *Comp Cont Educ Pract Vet* 4:206–216.

40. Forrester, S.D., Greco, D.S., and Relford, R.L. (1992) Serum hyperviscosity syndrome associated with multiple myeloma in two cats. *J Amer Vet Med Assoc* 200:79–82.

41. Jacobs, R.M., Couto, C.G., and Wellman, M.L. (1986) Biclonal gammopathy in a dog with myeloma and cutaneous lymphoma. *Vet Pathol* 23:211–213.

42. Jacobs, R.M. (1982) The qualitative analysis of canine immunoglobulins and myeloma proteins by immunofixation. *Vet Clin Pathol* 11:7–10.

43. Kyle, R.A. (1977) Multiple myeloma. Reviw of 869 cases. *Mayo Clin Proc* 50:29–40.

44. Matus, R.E., Leifer, C.E., and Hurvitz, A.I. (1987) Use of plasmapheresis and chemotherapy for treatment of monoclonal gammopathy associated with Ehrlichia canis infection in a dog. *J Amer Vet Med Assoc* 190:1302–1304.

45. Hoenig, M., and O'Brien, J.A. (1988) A benign hypergammaglogulinemia mimicking plasma cell myeloma. *J Amer Anim Hosp Assoc* 24:688–690.

46. Font, A., Closa, J.M., and Mascort, J. (1994) Monoclonal gammopathy in a dog with visceral leishmaniasis. *J Vet Int Med* 8:233–235.

47. Burkhard, M.J., Meyer, D.J., Rosychuk, R.A., O'Neil, S.P., and Schultheiss, P.C. (1995) Monoclonal gammopathy in a dog with chronic pyoderma. *J Vet Int Med* 9:357–360.

48. Dust, A., Norris, A.M., and Valli, V.EO. (1982) Cutaneous lymphosarcoma with IgG monoclonal gammopathy, serum hyperviscosity and hypercalcemia. *Can Vet J* 23:235–239.

49. Williams, D.A., and Goldschmidt, M.H. (1982) Hyperviscosity syndrome with IgM monoclonal gammopathy and hepatic plasmacytoid lymphosarcoma in a cat. *J Small Anim Pract* 23:311–323.

Thymoma

Thymoma is a neoplasm of the anterior mediastinum and is composed of thymic epithelium in which there are various degrees of benign lymphocytic infiltration (figs. 3.21–3.23). It is an uncommon tumor that has been reported in dogs, cattle, cats, horses, pigs, and sheep.[1-6] In these species, thymomas appear in adult to aged animals. The median age of affected dogs is 10 years (minimum age 2.5 years).[7] There are no proven sex or breed predispositions, although medium and large canine breeds may be more often affected[8]; Labrador and German shepherd dogs were overrepresented in one study.[5] An exception is the goat, in which a 25 percent frequency was found in a closed herd of Saanen dairy goats.[9]

Common presenting signs are respiratory distress and edema in the ventral head and neck and, rarely, the forelimbs; however, thymomas may be an incidental finding, particularly in goats. Myasthenia gravis, characterized by muscle weakness and megaesophagus, is seen in up to 40 percent of dogs and rarely in cats with thymoma.[10-12] A diagnosis of myasthenia gravis is confirmed by clinical improvement following the administration of edrophonium chloride (Tensilon test) and by the demonstration of serum autoantibodies to the acetylcholine receptor. For unknown reasons, symptoms of myasthenia gravis and autoantibodies may become apparent following surgical excision.[7] Animals may show hypersalivation and dysphagia. Pleural effusion is often present and may be chylous in nature. Second malignancies (osteosarcoma, mammary cancer), a variety of immune mediated skin diseases, hypercalcemia, polydipsia/polyuria, and polymyositis have also been reported in animals with thymoma (fig. 3.24).[5,8,10,13-15] In cats, there is no association with FeLV.[14,16]

Tumors are mostly found in the anterior mediastinum but may extend from the neck to the posterior mediastinum and are usually nodular and encapsulated, causing compression of adjacent tissues. The normally distinct corticomedullary junction is absent. Multiple biopsies should be obtained since the tumors may be cystic, contain areas of hemorrhagic necrosis, and are generally heterogenous in character. Macro- and microscopic, protein filled cysts are commonly observed. The tumors may be categorized as *lymphocyte* predominant, *epithelial* predominant, or *mixed.* In people, epithelial cells are classified by various criteria, but this distinction may not be a useful prognosticator in animals.[7] Most epithelial cells in animal thymomas have an elongate or spindle shape and stain positively for cytokeratin. Round to oval to polygonal shaped epithelial cells are less frequent. Cytoplasmic margins are ill defined. Nuclei are generally pale staining and vesicular; often a single prominent nucleolus is present. An unusual variant is clear cell thymoma. These are large round cells with abundant clear cytoplasm and distinct cytoplasmic margins.[9,17,18] The pattern arrangement of the epithelial cells may be described as solid, trabecular, cribriform, whorled, or rosette. Occasionally, there may be an angiocentric distribution of epithelial cells. Concentric clusters of epithelial cells with markedly eosinophilic cytoplasm are termed *Hassall's corpuscles.* Classical Hassall's corpuscles were found in 3 of 13 canine and feline thymomas.[6] Lymphocytes are predominately small or are heterogeneous, but about a third of thymomas have predominately large lymphocytes. Lymphoid follicles may be present, particularly in thymomas of the dog and cat. Thymomas often have variable numbers of mast cells, eosinophils, macrophages, melanocytes, plasma cells, and neutrophils.[3] Some or all of these cells admixed with lymphoid cells are characteristic findings in aspirational cytology of thymomas in dogs. The epithelial cells may or may not be present in cytologic preparations. Thymomas of goats (fig. 3.23) may contain myoid cells (containing cross-striations), a normal thymic constituent of this species, small mammals, birds, and reptiles.[9] Myoid cells are often found adjacent to Hassall's corpuscles and are large round cells with a generous amount of eosinophilic and granular cytoplasm. In addition, the cytoplasm may contain concentrically arranged fibrils.[9]

When large numbers of lymphocytes are present, the lesion must be distinguished from thymic lymphoma. Serial sections should be examined for epithelial cells, and immunohistochemical staining for cytokeratin is helpful (figs. 3.23 D, 3.24 C). Furthermore, thymic lymphomas tend to occur in younger animals, they do not have a heterogeneous inflammatory component, the lymphocytes are monomorphous and most often large (fig. 3.24), and very often there is regional lymph node involvement. In lymphocyte predominant thymomas, there is often dilatation of perivascular spaces; this is not a feature of thymic lymphoma. Other neoplasms to be distinguished from thymoma are metastatic carcinoma and tumors of the aortic body.

Thymic hyperplasia is rarely reported and may be difficult to distinguish from lymphocyte predominant thymoma. The presence of rare cytokeratin positive cells in sequential sections denotes thymoma. The normal corticomedullary arrangement is retained in hyperplasia, but this distinction is not always clear in rare thymomas with medullary differentiation.[9,18-20]

Older dogs with thymomas and dogs with lymphocyte predominant thymomas tended to have longer survivals, but upon multivariate analysis only the absence of megaesophagus was significantly associated with longer survival following surgery.[7] Most thymomas have a benign biological behavior. Less than one-third are metastatic or malignant in that they are locally invasive; there are rare reports of distant metastases.[11,13,21,22] Although malignant thymoma and thymic carcinoma are used interchangably, the latter is specifically defined as thymic epithelial neoplasia and is classified into squamous cell carcinoma,[23,24] small cell carcinoma, clear cell carcinoma, and adenosquamous carcinoma. There are single case reports of a dog with a thymic adenocarcinoma and a calf with thymic carcinoma showing neuroendocrine differentiation.[25,26]

Hodgkin's-Like Lymphoma

Hodgkin's disease is a malignant lymphoproliferative disease of people. The disease has an association with Epstein-Barr virus, although virus negative tumors do occur.[27] The pathological diagnosis is based on the detection of the Reed-Sternberg cell in an appropriate cellular and architectural background. The cellular components, and thus the background appearance, define the histological variants of Hodgkin's disease; in order of declining prognosis, these are lymphocytic predominance (< 5 percent of cases) (fig. 3.25), nodular sclerosis (> 60 percent), mixed cellularity (less than 30 percent), and lymphocytic depletion (< 5 percent). The prognosis varies with the predominance of lymphocytes versus Reed-Sternberg cells. The early disease is unique in that lesions spread only between contiguous groups of lymph nodes and the spleen and adjacent organs.

The Reed-Sternberg cell arises by clonal proliferation of a B cell and has a deeply lobulated nucleus, giving the appearance of multinucleation; or they may be truly bi- or multinucleated.[28] Often, the nuclei in Reed-Sternberg cells

that appear binucleate are mirror images of each other. The nuclei have characteristic inclusion-like acidophilic nucleoli. The cytoplasm of the Reed-Sternberg cell is often arti-

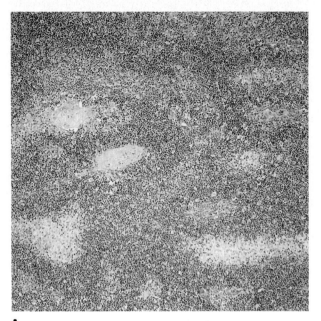

A

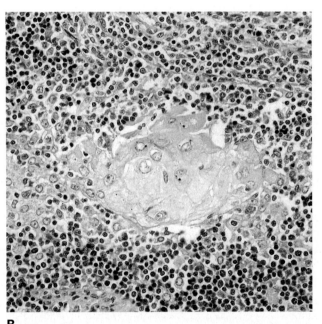

B

Fig. 3.21. Thymoma. **A.** A 2-year-old, large, mixed breed dog presented for vomition after eating, and a large anterior mediastinal mass was removed. At the architectural level, the tissue is composed of an irregular intermixture of epithelial and lymphoid areas. The epithelial areas have widely spaced pale-staining cells; the lymphoid areas are of variable density and consist of irregular aggregations of cortical and medullary cells. H&E ×80. **B.** Detail of A. A lighter area at the center consists of epithelial cells that have enlarged and matured into a Hassall's corpuscle. The surrounding lymphocytes are largely small and mature. H&E ×320.

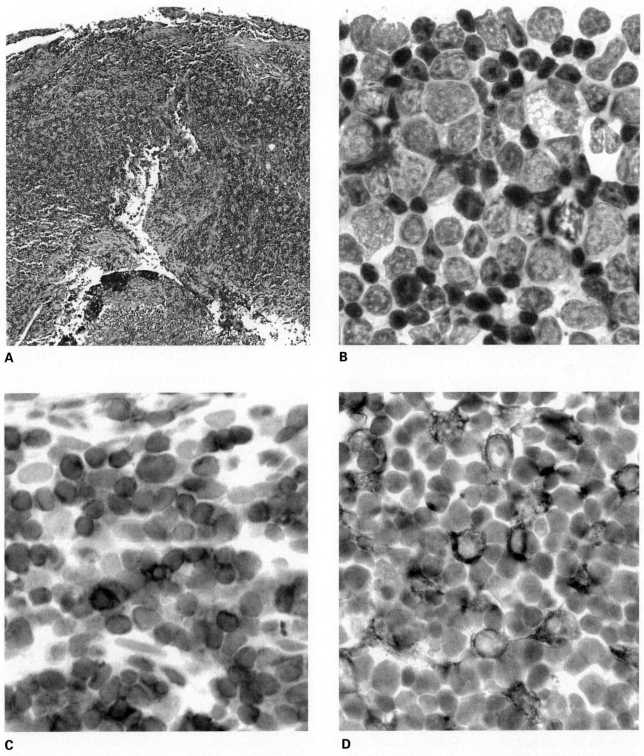

Fig. 3.22. Thymoma. **A.** A 7-year-old male Rodesian Ridgeback dog presented with dyspnea and was found to have extensive pleural effusion and a thoracic mass. After removal of 500 ml of pleural fluid, a fine needle aspirate was made of a mediastinal mass. A highly cellular sample was obtained containing an even distribution of small mature lymphocytes and large lymphocytes with large chromocenters, irregular parachromatin clearing, and only occasional small nucleoli. Wright's ×800. No epithelium was identified, but the regular intermixing of lymphocyte types and the mature chromatin suggested a benign condition, and thymoma was suggested. **B.** A tru-cut biopsy was obtained that had a diffuse nonlobulated architecture with irregular fine bands of collagen and a uniform mixture of large and small lymphocytes and single large pale-staining cells. H&E ×100. **C.** On CD-3 staining, a high proportion of both the large and small lymphocytes stained positively, indicating T cell differentiation. CD-3 ×800. **D.** On staining with cytokeratin, the large cells with lightly stained cytoplasm with H&E were strongly positive, indicating epithelial differentiation. Isolated Hassall's corpuscles were found. On surgery, an 8–11 cm mass was removed with uneventful recovery.

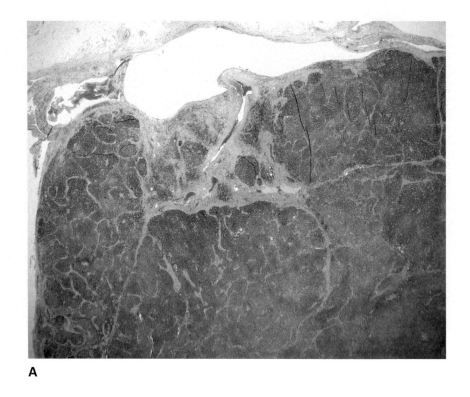

A

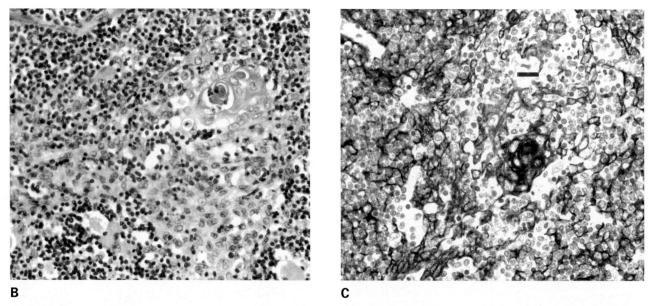

B   C

Fig. 3.23. **A.** A 15-year-old pet female goat died without being observed to be ill. On necropsy, there was massive pleural effusion with lung collapse and a 13 cm diameter mediastinal mass. Histologically, the mass was encapsulated, and a predominant population of small darkly stained lymphocytes was segmented by fine fibrous septation. H&E ×10. **B.** In pale staining areas, Hassall's corpuscles were surrounded by elongated spindle cells with lightly stained vesicular nuclei. H&E ×250. **C.** On staining for cytokeratin, the Hassall's corpuscles and spindle cells were stongly positive, indicating epithelial differentiation. Cytokeratin ×320.

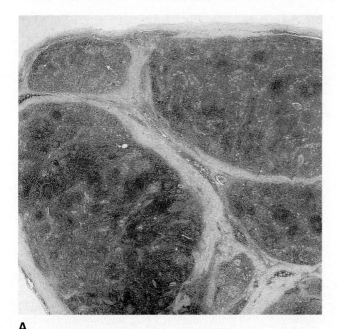

A

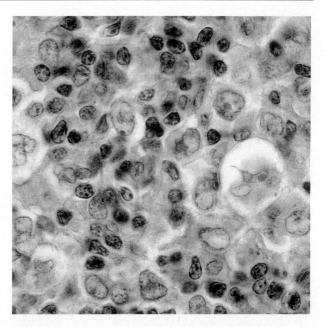

Fig. 3.25. Hodgkin's-like lymphoma, lymphocytic/histiocytic type. Lymph node, mature skunk (from a wildlife farm) that presented with multiple enlarged nodes in the neck area. The animal was in very good body condition and had abundant fat reserves. There is a predominant background of small lymphocytes, numerous elongated pale stromal cells, and a few large lymphocytes with prominent central nucleoli. Two large *lacunar cells* with irregularly convoluted *popcorn type* nuclei are present. H&E ×1000.

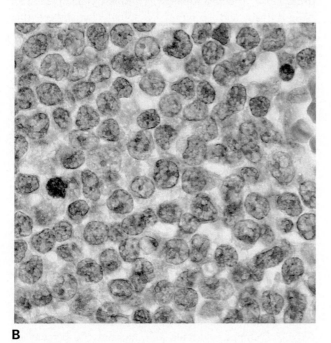

B

Fig. 3.24. Thymic lymphoma. **A.** A 6-year-old castrated male boxer was presented for polydipsia and polyuria of 1 month's duration. On biochemical examination, the dog was found to have hypercalcemia, and radiographs identified a mediastinal mass 7 cm in diameter, which was surgically removed. A small triangular projection on the mass was fibrous and septate and apparently represented residual thymus, while the major part of the mass was a diffuse proliferation of lymphocytes. The mass is heavily encapsulated with irregular collagenous septation. The cortical and medullary distinction has been obliterated by a background population of cells in which there are numerous germinal centers consisting of pale foci surrounded by a dark cuff of mantle cells. H&E ×10. **B.** Detail of A. The major mass consists of a dense proliferation of lymphocytes with nuclei that are 1.5 red cells in diameter and have a branched chromatin pattern and a single small but prominent nucleolus. Cytoplasmic boundaries are indistinct. A mitotic figure is present on the left center. H&E ×1000.

factually shrunken away from the surrounding dense background of lymphocytes or fibrous tissue; the term *lacunar cell* is used to describe this variant cell (fig. 3.25). The *popcorn* or multilobulated (fig. 3.25) variant of the Reed-Sternberg cell is strongly associated with the lymphocyte predominant type of Hodgkin's disease, and the lacunar cell with the nodular sclerosis type.

Hodgkin's-like lesions have been reported in the dog, horse, pig, and skunk.[29-31] Some lesions suspected of being Hodgkin's-like have proven to be atypical mast cell tumors or granulomatous inflammatory lesions.[32]

In dogs reported with Hodgkin's-like disease there is widespread lymph node involvement and lesions in the liver, spleen, lung, and occasionally skin.[30,33] The lymph node involvement in affected dogs is unlike that in people, where a single node or group of lymph nodes is involved at presentation, likely because dogs are examined at a later stage of progression.

REFERENCES

1. Momotani, E., Nakamura, N., and Shoya, S. (1981) Morphologic evidence of the histogenesis of epithelial thymoma in a cow. *Amer J Vet Res* 42:114–121.
2. Parker, G.A., and Casey, H. W. (1976) Thymomas in domestic animals. *Vet Pathol* 13:353–364.

3. Al-Zubaidy, A. J. (1981) Malignant thymoma with metastases in a dog. *Vet Rec* 109:490–492.

4. Sandison, A.T., and Anderson, L.J. (1969) Tumors of the thymus in cattle, sheep, and pigs. *Cancer Res* 29:1146–1150.

5. Day, M.J. (1997) Review of thymic pathology in 30 cats and 36 dogs. *J Small Anim Pract* 38:393–403.

6. Rae, C.A., Jacobs, R.M., and Couto, G.C. (1989) A comparison between the cytological and histological characteristics in thirteen canine and feline thymomas. *Can Vet J* 30:497–500.

7. Atwater, S.W., Powers, B.E., Park, R.D., Straw, R.C., Ogilvie, G.K., and Withrow, S.J. (1994) Canine thymoma: 23 cases (1980–1991). *J Amer Vet Med Assoc* 205:1007–1013.

8. Aronsohn, M. (1985) Canine thymoma. *Vet Clin N Amer Small Anim Pract* 15:755–767.

9. Hadlow, W.J. (1978) High prevalence of thymoma in the dairy goat. Report of seventeen cases. *Vet Pathol* 15:153–169.

10. Aronsohn, M.G., Schunk, K.L., Carpenter, J.L., and King, N.W. (1984) Clinical and pathologic features of thymoma in 15 dogs. *J Amer Vet Med Assoc* 184:1355–1362.

11. Poffenbarger, E., Klausner, J.S., and Caywood, D.D. (1985) Acquired myasthenia gravis in a dog with thymoma: A case report. *J Amer Anim Hosp Assoc* 21:119–124.

12. Scott-Moncrieff, J.C., Cook, J.R, and Lantz, G.C. (1990) acquired myasthenia gravis in a cat with thymoma. *J Amer Vet Med Assoc* 196:1291–1293.

13. Bellah, J.R., Stiff, M.E.,and Russell, R.G. (1983) Thymoma in the dog: Two case reports and review of 20 additonal cases. *J Amer Vet Med Assoc* 183:306–311.

14. Carpenter, J.L., and Holzworth, J. (1982) Thymoma in 11 cats. *J Amer Vet Med Assoc* 181:248–251.

15. Godfrey, D.R. (1999) Dermatosis and associated systemic signs in a cat with thymoma and recently treated with an imidacloprid preparation. *J Small Anim Pract* 40:333–337.

16. Gores, B.R., Berg, J., Carepenter, J.L., Aronsohn, M.G. (1994) Surgical treatment of thymoma in cats: 12 cases (1987–1992). *J Amer Vet Med Assoc* 204:1782–1785.

17. Mettler, F., and Hauser, B. (1984) Clear cell thymoma in a dog. *J Comp Pathol* 94:315–317.

18. Mackey, L. (1975) Clear-cell thymoma and thymic hyperplasia in a cat. *J Comp Pathol* 85:367–371.

19. Rosai, J., and Levine, G.D. (1976) Tumors of the thymus. In Firminger, H.I. (ed.) *Atlas of Tumor Pathology.* 2nd series, fascicle 13. Armed Forces Institute of Pathology, Washington, D.C.

20. Simpson, R.M., Waters, D.J., Gebhard, D.H., and Casey, H.W. (1992) Massive thymoma with medullary differentiation in a dog. *Vet Pathol* 29:416–419.

21. Olchowy, T.W.J., Toal, R.L., Brenneman, K.A., Slauson, D.O., and McEntee, M.F. (1996) Metastatic thymoma in a goat. *Can Vet J* 37:165–167.

22. Robinson, M. (1974) Malignant thymoma with metastasis in a dog. *Vet Pathol* 11:172–180.

23. Carpenter, J.L., and Valentine, B.A. (1992) Squamous cell carcinoma arising in two feline thymomas. *Vet Pathol* 29:541–543.

24. Whiteley, L.O., Leininger, J.R., Wolf, C.B., and Ames, T.R. (1986) Malignant squamous cell carcinoma in a horse. *Vet Pathol* 23:627–629.

25. Abdi, M.M., and Elliott, H. (1994) A thymic carcinoma with glandular differentiation in a dog. *Vet Rec* 134:141–142.

26. Anjiki, T., and Kadota, K. (1999) Thymic carcinoma with neuroendocrine differentiation in a calf. *J Vet Med Sci* 61:853–855.

27. Dolcett, R., and Boiocchi, M. (1998) Epstein Barr virus in the pathogenesis of Hodgkin's disease. *Biomed Pharmacother* 52:13–25.

28. Jox, A., Wolf, J., and Diehl, V. (1997) Hodgkin's disease biology: Recent advances. *Hematol Oncol* 15:165–171.

29. Hoerni, B., Legrand, E., and Chauvergne, J. (1970) Les réticulopathies. Animales de type hodgkinien. *Bull Cancer* 57:37–54.

30. Wells, G.A. (1974) Hodgkin's disease-like lesions in the dog. *J Pathol* 112:5–10.

31. Smith, D.A., and Barker, I.K. (1983) Four cases of Hodgkin's disease in striped skunks *(Mephitis mephitis)*. *Vet Pathol* 20:223–229.

32. Moulton, J.E., and Harvey, J.W. (1990) Tumors of the Lymphoid and Hematopoietic Tissues. In Moulton, J.E. (ed.), *Tumors in Domestic Animals,* 3rd ed. University of California Press, Berkeley, pp. 231–307.

33. Maeda, H., Ozaki, K., Honaga, S., and Narama, I. (1993) Hodgkin's-like lymphoma in a dog. *Zentralbl Veterinarmed A* 40:200–204.

Histiocytic Proliferative Diseases

The histiocytic diseases have come under intense scrutiny in recent years.[1] A better understanding of this seemingly complex set of diseases has come with the development of immunophenotyping reagents.[2]

Histiocytic cells are derived from bone marrow precursor cells that differentiate to either macrophages or dendritic cells. The macrophage is primarily involved with phagocytosis and secretion of soluble substances that influence the inflammatory process. An important role of the dendritic cell is to process and present antigen to T cells, a function shared with other cells classified as *antigen presenting cells.* The benign or reactive histiocytic proliferative diseases in dogs are due to proliferation of antigen presenting cells.[2] Such proliferations in people are termed the *Langerhans cell histiocytoses.*

The benign or reactive canine histiocytic proliferative diseases are cutaneous histiocytoma (fig. 3.26), cutaneous histiocytosis (CH) and systemic histiocytosis (SH) (fig. 3.27). Cutaneous histiocytoma is a benign skin tumor that originates from the epidermal Langerhans cell[3] and is predominately a solitary tumor of young dogs that undergoes spontaneous regression associated with infiltration by CD8 T cells. Multiple histiocytomas are reported, and regression may be prolonged in the shar-pei breed. Histiocytoma cells may migrate to regional lymph nodes; lymphadenopathy will regress along with the primary cutaneous lesion.[1,3] Histiocytoma cells lack CD4 and Thy-1 (CD90) epitopes (see table 3.5), and only 60 percent are positive for lysozyme.

The cutaneous and systemic histiocytoses are seen in middle-aged to old dogs. There is no breed or sex predisposition for CH.[4] Systemic histiocytosis is found in mostly male Bernese mountain dogs and rottweilers, golden and Labrador retrievers, Belgian shepherd, border collie, Irish water spaniel, standard poodles, and mixed breed dogs of either sex.[5,6] Both varieties are characterized by multiple lesions within and beneath the skin that tend to wax and wane. The most common sites are the head, neck, perineum, scrotum, and extremities. Lesions are multifocal to diffuse, often with an angiocentric distribution, and they are composed of large bland histiocytic cells accompanied by frequent lymphocytes and neutrophils. Eosinophils and plasma cells may be present. Thrombosis and necrosis

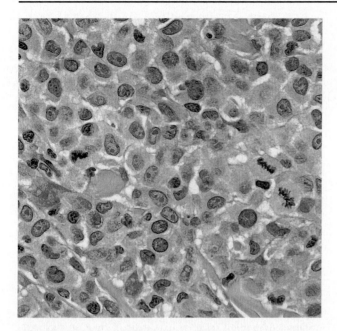

Fig. 3.26. Cutaneous histiocytoma. Focal skin lesion from the ventral lateral thorax of a 1-year-old female Beagle. Bands of reticular collagen are separated by an infiltration of cells with vesicular nuclei approximately 3 red cells in diameter that are round to oval or indented in outline, with peripheralized chromatin and a characteristically single prominent central nucleolus. There are frequent mitoses and an infiltration of a few small cleaved lymphocytes. The tumor cell cytoplasm is abundant and likely amphophilic, and the cellular boundaries are irregularly distinct. H&E ×720.

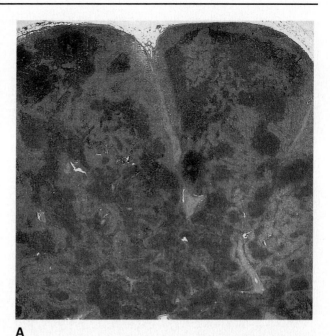

A

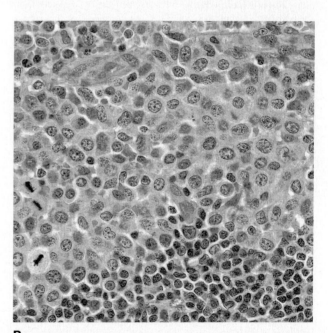

B

Fig. 3.27. Systemic histiocytosis. **A.** Inguinal lymph node from a 1.5-year-old male redbone hound, which had two previous skin tumors removed, diagnosed as cutaneous histiocytoma. Architecturally, the node was markedly enlarged with a thinned capsule and destruction of normal architecture by proliferation of pale-appearing tissue surrounding and compressing residual benign darker areas. H&E ×10. **B.** Detail of A. Foci of small, benign, paracortical lymphocytes (bottom) are surrounded by a cuff of larger cells with round to oval vesicular nuclei and frequent mitoses (left). There is abundant finely granular, mildly eosinophilic cytoplasm with irregularly distinct cellular boundaries. H&E ×720.

occur with angioinvasion. Cell types in CH and SH are indistinguishable in hematoxylin and eosin stained tissue sections. The cells consistently express CD4 and Thy-1, suggesting that they are derived from activated dermal Langerhans cells (see table 3.5). CH and SH may be distinguished by clinical progression; cutaneous histiocytosis may regress spontaneously in association with aggressive T cell infiltration, and about 50 percent of affected dogs respond to immunosuppression with corticosteroids.[1] However, SH is more aggressive than CH and will eventually extend to regional lymph nodes; occasionally there may be generalized lymphadenopathy. Other sites of involvement in SH are the nasal cavity, eyelids, sclera, lung, spleen, liver, and bone marrow. Spontaneous regression is uncommon with SH, and corticosteroids have little effect. Regression of lesions has been achieved with cyclosporin and leflunomide treatment, but reoccurrence may be seen with cessation of therapy.[1]

The malignant forms of the histiocytic proliferative disorders are localized and disseminated varieties of histiocytic sarcoma (HS) (fig. 3.28). The disseminated variety of HS has been termed *malignant histiocytosis* (MH). Cells in the malignant forms do not express CD4 and usually do not express Thy-1, while CH and SH cells are characteristically positive for CD4 and Thy-1. Immunohistochemistry, for the demonstration of either T cell (CD3) or B cell (CD79) markers, is useful in distinguishing the histiocytic

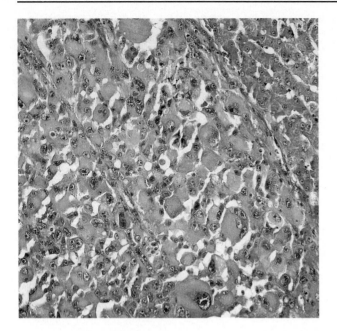

Fig. 3.28. Malignant histiocytosis. Liver from a 7-year-old male cat with a history of rapid weight loss. Lesions are focal and sharply demarcated. Nuclei are vesicular, are variable in size and shape, have occasional multinucleation, and may be larger than adjacent hepatocytes. Nucleoli are very large. The cytoplasm is variable in amount and often voluminous. H&E ×200.

proliferative disorders (which are CD3 and CD79 negative) from large cell lymphomas (see table 3.5); large cell lymphomas will also be much more monomorphic and will be composed of cells with less abundant cytoplasm.

Localized histiocytic sarcomas occur most frequently in middle-aged to old flat-coated retrievers, golden and Labrador retrievers, and rottweilers. Lesions appear as rapidly growing solitary masses in cutaneous and subcutaneous sites, usually on a distal limb adjacent to a joint. Occasional tumors may be found in spleen, liver, gastric wall, and tongue. Cells are large and pleomorphic, ranging from round to polygonal to spindle shape. Multinucleation and unusual mitotic figures may be seen. Inflammatory infiltrates are usually minimal. The tumors are locally invasive and destructive. Metastasis, at least from limb lesions, does not occur until late in the disease process. Procedures such as wide surgical excision and limb amputation may be curative. Tumors to be distinguished from localized histiocytic sarcoma are tumors of the nerve sheath, hemangiopericytoma, hemangiosarcoma, plasma cell tumors, mast cell tumors, and synovial cell sarcoma.

Malignant histiocytosis (MH), or disseminated histiocytic sarcoma, is a rapidly progressive disease seen in middle-aged to old dogs. Bernese mountain dogs, rottweilers, golden and Labrador retrievers, and flat-coated retrievers of either sex are most often affected.[7,8] Malignant histiocytosis has been reported in the cat and horse.[9,10] At least in the Bernese mountain dog, the trait is inherited in a polygenic fashion. There is a higher frequency of the disease in offspring of affected parents, and the heritability of the

trait is 0.298.[11] The disease may present as a rapidly progressive, usually nonresponsive anemia with splenomegaly. Coombs positive anemias have been reported in association with MH. The tumor cells may show extensive erythrophagy.[12] If it is felt that the phagocytic activity of the tumor cells plays an important role in causing the anemia or multiple cytopenias, then the terms *erythrophagocytic syndrome* or *hemophagocytic syndrome* may be utilized. A case report suggested that serum ferritin may have usefulness as a marker for MH.[13] Epidermis and dermis are rarely involved. Viscera involved are usually the spleen, liver, lymph nodes, lung, and bone marrow. Lung lesions may be confused with anaplastic large cell carcinoma, which will stain positively for cytokeratin, and a variety of granulomatous diseases. The latter usually have a significant inflammatory component and an angiocentric distribution. The histological appearance of the tumor is indistinguishable from the localized variety (HS). It is unknown if cells in either of the reactive forms may undergo malignant transformation or if the cells in localized HS may acquire characteristics permitting wider dissemination.

Lymphomatoid Granulomatosis

Lymphomatoid granulomatosis is a rare lymphoproliferative disease, first described in people with pulmonary disease.[14] Although lung lesions predominate, other organs commonly affected are skin, kidneys, and the central nervous system. Histologically there is an angiocentric distribution of large mononuclear cells with variable numbers of other inflammatory cells. Lymphoma eventually appears in 12 to 47 percent of affected human patients.[15] Overall mortality is 38 to 85 percent, and the median survival time is 14 months.[15] The disease may represent a progression from inflammation to lymphoid neoplasia.

A similar disease has been described in the dog.[16-19] In dogs, pulmonary lesions with metastasis to hilar lymph nodes are most frequent. Skin involvement is uncommon, although in one report, multiple granulomatous skin lesions associated with lymphadenopathy were found in two of three affected dogs.[20] Occasionally, myocardium, skeletal muscle, bronchial and mediastinal lymph nodes, liver, and mesenteric fat and blood vessels are affected. Splenic involvement is rare. Two of seven affected dogs had peripheral lymphadenopathy, suggesting a progression to systemic disease and lymphoma.[16] Lesions are difficult to distinguish from various granulomatous and mixed inflammatory diseases. Usually, with lymphomatoid granulomatosis there are solitary to multinodular white or tan masses at the base of the caudodorsal lung lobes. Histologically, the lesions have an angiocentric and peribronchiolar pattern composed of large undifferentiated mononuclear cells accompanied by variable numbers of lymphocytes, plasma cells, eosinophils, neutrophils, macrophages, and multinucleated cells (fig. 3.29). Isch-

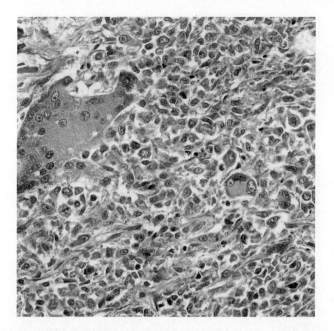

Fig. 3.29. Lymphomatoid granulomatosis. A 9-year-old spayed female basset hound had chest radiographs that demonstrated a right cranial lobe lung mass, which was removed. Histologically, there is solid infiltration of the lung, surrounding airways, and vascular structures. Cytologically, the tumor is variable and consists of small lymphocytes as well as large lymphocytes and multinucleated giant cells. H&E ×320.

emic necrosis occurs due to the angioinvasive and angiodestructive behavior. Pulmonary lesions may be confused *with pulmonary infiltrates with eosinophils,* eosinophil granuloma, heartworm disease, or disseminated histiocytic sarcoma.[16] Negative immunohistochemical staining for CD3 and positive staining for lysozyme and alpha-1-antitrypsin support a histiocytic rather than a lymphoid origin.[20] The anaplastic cells in dogs with lymphomatoid granulomatosis do not stain for lysozyme or alpha-1-antitrypsin immunoreactivity.[16,18] In two of three cases, 10 to 50 percent of the large lymphohistiocytic cells stained for CD3, while none stained for heavy and light chain markers of B cells, suggesting that the canine disease may be an atypical form of T cell lymphoma.[20] Frequent small CD3 positive cells were found throughout and around the tumors. A larger series of canine cases needs to be more fully characterized immunohistochemically. In a review of the disease in people, it was concluded that the lesion is a malignant B cell proliferation with an exuberant and benign T cell reaction (T-cell-rich B cell lymphoma) associated with Epstein-Barr virus infection.[21]

REFERENCES

1. Affolter, V.K., and Moore, P.F. (2000) Canine cutaneous histiocytic diseases. In Bonagura, J.D. (ed.), *Kirk's Current Veterinary Therapy XIII, Small Animal Practice.* W.B. Saunders Co., Philadelphia, pp. 588–591.
2. Moore, P., Affolter, V., Olivry, T., and Schrenzel, M. (1998) The use of immunological reagents in defining the pathogenesis of canine skin diseases involving proliferation of leukocytes. In Kwotcha, K., Willemse, T., and von Tscharner, C. (eds.), *Advances in Veterinary Dermatology,* vol. 3. Butterworth Heinmann, Oxford, pp. 77–94.
3. Moore, P.F., Schrenzel, M.D., Affolter, V.K., Olivry, T., and Naydan, D. (1996) Canine cutaneous histiocytoma is an epidermotrophic Langerhans cell histiocytosis which epxresses CD1 and specific β2 integrin molecules. *Amer J Pathol* 148:1699–1708.
4. Calderwood-Mays, M.B., and Bergeron, J.A. (1986) Cutaneous histiocytosis in dogs. *J Amer Vet Med Assoc* 188:377–381.
5. Moore, P.F. (1984) Systemic histiocytosis of Bernese mountain dogs. *Vet Pathol* 21:554–563.
6. Paterson, S., Boydell, P., and Pike, R. (1995) Systemic histiocytosis in the Bernese mountain dog. *J Small Anim Pract* 36:233–236.
7. Moore, P.F., and Rosin, A..(1986) Malignant histiocytosis in Bernese mountain dogs. *Vet Pathol* 23:1–10.
8. Rosin, A., Moore, P., and Dubielzig, R. (1986) Malignant histiocytosis in Bernese mountain dogs. *J Amer Vet Med Assoc* 188:1041–1045.
9. Court, E.A., Earnest-Koons, K.A., Barr, S.C., and Gould, W.J. (1993) Malignant histiocytosis in a cat. *J Amer Vet Med Assoc* 203:1300–1302.
10. Lester, G.D., Alleman, A.R., Raskin, R.E., and Mays, M.B. (1993) Malignant histiocytosis in an Arabian filly. *Equine Vet J* 25:471–473;
11. Padgett, G.A., Madewell, B.R., Keller, E.T., Jodar, L., and Packard, M. (1995) Inheritance of histiocytosis in Bernese mountain dogs. *J Small Anim Pract* 36:93–98.
12. Wellman, M. L., Davenport, D. J., Morton, D., and Jacobs, R. M. (1985). Malignant histiocytosis in four dogs. *J Amer Vet Med Assoc* 187:919–921.
13. Newlands, C.E., Houston, D.M., and Vasconcelos, D.Y. (1994) Hyperferritinemia associated with malignant histiocytosis in a dog. *J Amer Vet Med Assoc* 205:849–851.
14. Liebow, A.A., Carrington, C.R.B., and Friedman, P.J. (1972) Lymphomatoid granulomatosis. *Human Pathol* 3:457–558.
15. Katzenstein, A.L., Carrington, C.B., and Liebow, A.A. (1979) Lymphomatoid granulomatosis: A clinicopathologic study of 152 cases. *Cancer* 43:360–373.
16. Berry, C.R., Moore, P.F., Thomas, W.P., Sisson, D., and Koblik, P.D. (1990) Pulmonary lymphomatoid granulomatosis in seven dogs. (1976–1987). *J Vet Int Med* 4:157–166.
17. Lucke, V.M., Kelly, D.F., Harrington, G.A., Gibbs, C., and Gaskell, C.J. (1979) A lymphomatoid granulomatosis of the lungs of young dogs. *Vet Pathol* 16:405–412.
18. Leblanc, B., Masson, M.T., Andreu, M., Bonnet, M.C., and Paulus, G. (1990) Lymphomatoid granulomatosis in a beagle dog. *Vet Pathol* 27:287–289.
19. Fitzgerald, S.D., Wolf, D.C., and Carlton, W.W. (1991) Eight cases of canine lymphomatoid granulomatosis. *Vet Pathol* 28:241–245.
20. Smith, K.C., Day, M.J., Shaw, S.C., Littlewood, J.D., and Jeffery, N.D. (1996) Canine lymphomatoid granulomatosis: An immunophenotypic analysis of three cases. *J Comp Pathol* 115:129–138.
21. Jaffe, E.S., and Wilson, W.H. (1997). Lymphomatoid granulomatosis: Pathogenesis, pathology and clinical implications. *Cancer Surv* 30:233–248.

The Lymphoid Leukemias

Leukemia is the presence of malignant cells of hemolymphatic origin in the blood and bone marrow. Leukemias in animals are uncommon relative to their frequency in people, but the true frequency in animals is unknown. In dogs, approximately 30 percent of leukemias are of the lymphoid type.[1-3] In general, leukemias in domestic animals are recognized clinically once there is extensive marrow involvement by tumor cells, when the consequences of cytopenias (anemia, thrombocytopenia, neutropenia) require veterinary assistance.

Lymphoid leukemias almost always arise from the bone marrow and tend to be more common in younger individuals. Occasionally, leukemias may arise in the thymus or spleen, then spread to the bone marrow, and finally colonize other peripheral lymphoid organs. Adults are more often afflicted with lymphoma, initially a disease of peripheral lymphoid organs. Lymphoma is the most common form of malignant lymphoproliferation in animals. Late in the disease process of lymphoma, neoplastic lymphocytes may invade the bone marrow and subsequently appear in the peripheral blood as a leukemic event. This has been described as lymphosarcoma cell leukemia, lymphoma with leukemia, or leukemic lymphoma. Thus, the tissue distributions of malignant lymphocytes in lymphoma and lymphoid leukemia converge late in the disease processes. It is important to distinguish the two diseases in their early stages since therapy and prognosis are different.

The history, physical examination, and sequential complete blood counts are important factors used to support the diagnosis of lymphoid leukemia; however, the ultimate proof is provided by assessment of the bone marrow. Optimally, aspirate smears and a core biopsy of the bone marrow should be obtained. Oncologists will commence treatment on the basis of clinical assessment and a definitive cytological diagnosis.

Cytochemical staining, immunophenotyping, and ultrastructural examination are useful tools for distinguishing immature lymphoid cells from poorly differentiated granulocytic cells (table 3.5).[1,4-9] The presence of primary granules and positive staining for nonspecific esterase activity and Sudan Black B support a nonlymphocytic origin. Lymphoid cells characteristically show a perinuclear clearing, with cytoplasmic basophilia increasing toward the cell membrane; this characteristic is sometimes helpful in distinguishing lymphoid cells from developing erythroid and myeloid cells. It is essential to make the distinction between lymphoid and nonlymphoid neoplasia since the treatment protocols and prognoses are quite different.

Lymphoid leukemias are roughly divisible into acute lymphoblastic (ALL) and chronic lymphocytic (CLL) forms based on history, physical examination, clinicopathological data, and cell type. ALL is more common than CLL in animals.[10]

Acute Lymphoblastic Leukemia (ALL)

ALL may account for 5 to 10 percent of canine lymphoid neoplasias (see figs. 3.30–3.32).[11] In a series of 30 dogs with ALL, the median age was 5.5 years, and the age range was from 1 to 12 years.[12] German shepherds accounted for almost 30 percent of the cases, and slightly more males were affected than females (3:2). The average age of cats with ALL is less than 5 years, with a range from

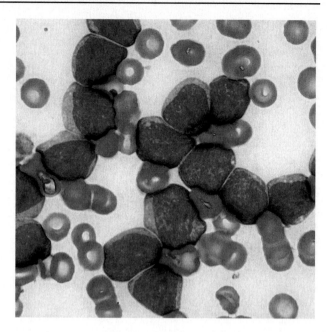

Fig. 3.30. Acute lymphoblastic leukemia (ALL), L1 type. Blood from a 10-year-old spayed female golden retriever, lethargic for 2 weeks. Presented for depression and anorexia. Popliteal nodes were mildly enlarged, and the liver border was palpable. Total leukocyte count was $422 \times 10^3/\mu l$, with 97 percent lymphocytes, 8.9 g/dl hemoglobin, and $67 \times 10^3/\mu l$ platelets. The L1 type ALL has uniform nuclei approximately 2 red cells in diameter with uniformly compact chromatin and residual chromocenters; nucleoli are generally absent. There is a high nuclear cytoplasmic ratio. Wright's ×1000.

6 months to 14 years.[13] ALL is a fulminant disease and often rapidly fatal. Anorexia, weight loss, pale mucous membranes, and hepatosplenogmegaly may be present. About half of the dogs with ALL have lymphadenopathy, but this is mild relative to the prominence of this change in dogs with lymphoma. Lymphadenopathy is more common in cats with ALL than in dogs, but again this change is mild.[13] Calves with ALL often present with marked lymphadenopathy and organomegaly.[14] The disease is rare in the horse.[15,16] Leukocytosis is common in dogs with ALL and is generally less than 50,000 cells per µl, although extreme leukocytoses are occasionally reported.[2,12,17] Marked nonregenerative anemia and thrombocytopenia may be present. Platelet counts may be falsely increased due to the presence of cytoplasmic fragments of leukemic cells. Numbers of neutrophils are often markedly decreased (< 1000 per µl) in canine patients with ALL, except for those having the large granular lymphocyte (LGL) variety of ALL. Dogs in the latter subset often have neutrophilia.[18]

Cats with ALL often present with normal to low leukocyte counts.[19] Such animals may initially have multiple cytopenias or pancytopenia, and malignant cells may be difficult to find even with careful examination of the peripheral blood smear. The diagnosis of leukemia is made only upon bone marrow cytological examination, hence the importance of bone marrow examination in patients

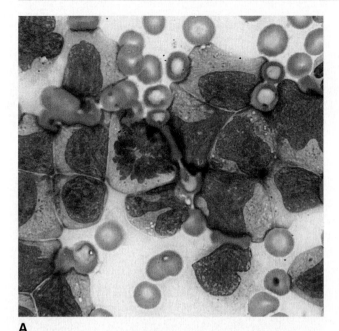

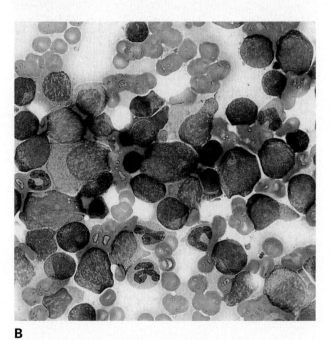

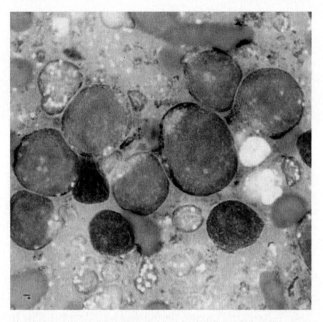

Fig. 3.32. Acute lymphoblastic leukemia, L3 type. Mature dog. The nuclei are round to oval and about 2.5 red cells in diameter, with deeply stained chromatin and *prominent* nucleoli. There is a moderate amount of quite highly basophilic cytoplasm with *sharply delineated peripheral vacuoles*. The vacuoles contain lipid material that readily stains with fat stains (Sudan Black B), and the multifocal reaction needs to be distinguished from the more diffuse reaction typical of early myeloid cells. Wright's ×1600.

Figs.s 3.31. Acute lymphoblastic leukemia, L2 type. **A.** Blood from a 10-year-old spayed female golden retriever with a 1 month history of weakness and anorexia. The dog had hepatomegaly, an enlarged spleen, generalized lymphadenopathy, and moderate jaundice. The blood contained $307 \times 10^3/\mu l$ leukocytes, of which 88 percent were lymphocytes, 4.4 g/dl hemoglobin, and $18 \times 10^3/\mu l$ platelets. The nuclei are 2 to 3 red cells in diameter, often irregularly indented. Small residual chromocenters are present in some nuclei, with the larger cells having one to three small nucleoli. Cells have abundant pale cytoplasm. There is a metaphase in right of center. Wright's ×1280. **B.** Bone marrow aspirate from a dog with ALL L2. There is typically almost complete atrophy of the erythroid system, and the marrow granulocyte reserves are markedly reduced. The variability of size and shape of the tumor cells is more apparent than in the blood. There is irregularly abundant cytoplasm, and nucleoli are more prominent in the residual benign myeloid precursors than in the L2 cells. Wright's ×800.

with nonregenerative anemias and other unexplained cytopenias. Such cases are sometimes referred to as *aleukemic leukemias.* Sequential examination of the peripheral blood will inevitably demonstrate increasing numbers of neoplastic cells, referred to as the *blast cell crisis.* On the presumption that there is no increased peripheral destruction of the normal blood cells, the multiple cytopenias are attributed to myelophthisis, a complex process mediated by proliferating cells physically crowding normal cells and altering the hematopoietic inductive microenvironment, competition for nutrients, autoimmunity, and secretion of suppressor substances by tumor cells.

The pattern of lymphoid colonization of the bone marrow in the lymphoid leukemias tends to be random. In contrast, the acute nonlymphocytic leukemias tend to proliferate from the subendosteum, which is the preferred site for normal hematopoiesis. Thus, myelophthisis tends to arise more quickly in the nonlymphocytic leukemias.

The FAB (France, America, and Great Britain) classification scheme for human ALL[20] can be utilized in animals. The morphological characteristics of ALLs according to the FAB classification are based on nuclear to cytoplasmic ratio, nuclear size and shape, number and size of nucleoli, and cytoplasmic basophilia and vacuolization (table 3.6). ALL is also classified by immunophenotyping and cytogenetics. In people, prognosis tends to decline from L1 to L3. Childhood ALL is predominately of the L1 type, and long-term remissions are achieved with intensive combination chemotherapy therapy in about 80 percent of patients. In contrast, adults with ALL more often have the L2 and L3 varieties, and less than a third of these patients have long-term remissions. Presently, various morphological and immunophenotypic characteristics of ALL cell types do not appear to be associated with longer survival in dogs.[18]

The three ALL cell types described in the FAB classification (table 3.6) do appear in animals and are correspondingly small (L1, see fig. 3.30), large and heterogenous (L2, see fig. 3.31 A,B), or large and homogeneous often with cytoplasmic vacuoles that sometimes stain for lipid (L3, see fig. 3.32). Overall, the L2 variety is most common in animals. There is some overlap in morphology between the smaller ALL cell types and the cell types seen with CLL. In these instances, history, presenting signs, and the presence of other hematological abnormalities may be helpful in distinguishing the two diseases.

Most animal species with ALL usually have only mild loss of condition and mild pallor and lymphadenopathy. In contrast, calves may be cachectic and have marked symmetrical lymphadenopathy. Viscera anterior to the diaphragm are usually normal except for the lymph nodes and thymus in the calf. The liver is markedly enlarged in the calf, with irregular pale areas and an accentuated lobular pattern on cut surface. Hepatomegaly, if present in the cat and dog, is mild. The spleen is often moderately and symmetrically enlarged and is dry and fleshy on cut surface, occasionally with focal pale areas in all species. Bone marrow is usually congested but with some fat stores remaining. Calves sometimes have almost solid infiltration of all marrow cavities and large yellowish areas of necrosis surrounded by hyperemia, resulting from infarction (fig. 3.33).

Microscopically, the bone marrow in terminal cases is virtually 100 percent cellular, with densely packed mononuclear cells (fig. 3.31 B). These are usually of medium to large size but with some heterogeneity (table 3.6). Nucleoli are usually single and centrally located. Cytoplasm is moderate in amount and basophilic. Occasional megakaryocytes and islands of developing erythroid cells are present, but the marrow granulocyte reserves are either markedly decreased or absent. Lymph nodes may have follicular atrophy, and tumor cells are present in paracortical areas and postcapillary venules. Splenic changes include a thin capsule, follicular atrophy, and broad sheets of monomorphic cells occupying the sinus areas. Infarcts

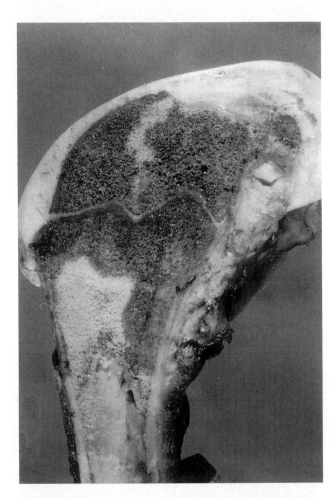

Fig. 3.33. Bone marrow infarction. Hemisection of femur from a 2-week-old calf. The infarcted area (pale) characteristically involves the diaphyseal cavity and focal areas within the cancellous bone of the extremities.

TABLE 3.6.   Classification schemes for acute lymphoid leukemia (modified from Valli, 1992)[21]

World Health Organization (WHO)	Microlymphoblastic	Prolymphocytic	Lymphoblastic
French, American, British (FAB)	L1	L2	L3
Prevalence (%)			
People	80	15	5
Animals	10	60	30
Cytological Features			
Cell size	Predominately small	Large, heterogeneous	Large, homogeneous
Chromatin	Homogeneous	Heterogeneous	Fine, homogeneous
Nucleoli	Absent or small	Absent or small	Prominent
Nuclear shape	Round, rarely cleaved	Irregular, clefting common	Regularly oval to round
Cytoplasmic Features			
Volume	Low	Moderate	Moderate
Basophilia	Slight to moderate	Moderate	Intense
Vacuolization	Absent to variable	Absent to variable	Often numerous

may be present, and there is usually little extramedullary hematopoiesis. The pattern of liver involvement is diffuse and sinusoidal with some portal colonization. The density of tumor cells within sinusoids is usually reflected in the number of tumor cells in the peripheral circulation. There is usually some degree of periacinal ischemic degeneration. Colonies of tumor cells may be very widespread but are most commonly found in the kidneys, testes, meninges, intestine, and pancreas.

In one series of dogs with ALL, tumor cells were characterized as null cell (4/9) or T cell (3/9) phenotype; only two of nine dogs with ALL had tumor cells with a B cell phenotype.[22] In another series of 13 dogs with ALL, six cases were B cell (CD79) and seven were morphologically of the LGL variety.[18] Of the seven LGL ALL cases three were typed as T cell (CD3) and four were considered NK cells. Interestingly, all cases of LGL ALL had marked hepatosplenomegaly and no or minimal bone marrow involvement at presentation, suggesting that acute and chronic LGL leukemia is a primary splenic disease.[18] From 60 to 80 percent of cats with ALL are FeLV positive, and most of the ALLs are of a T cell phenotype.[23] Tumor cells from calves considered to have ALL have been negative for B cell and T cell markers.[24,25]

Chronic Lymphocytic Leukemia (CLL)

CLL is primarily a disease of cattle, cats, and dogs, usually 8–10 years of age or older. The median age of dogs with CLL is 10.5 years, and in one study of 22 dogs, males were slightly more often affected (1.8:1).[26] Affected dogs usually have no prominent symptoms, other than lethargy, and the disease is discovered almost incidentally when the peripheral blood is checked for some other reason.[27-30] The disease is rare in cats (figs. 3.34, 3.35).[31,32] CLL is a slowly progressive disease and there is probably a prodromal period of months to years.[27,30] Mild lymphadenopathy is present in up to 80 percent of dogs with CLL upon physical examination but hepatomegaly and splenomegaly are just as frequent but usually more prominent when the disease is well advanced.[26] Mild nonregenerative anemia (hematocrits greater than 20 percent) and thrombocytopenia (more than 100,000 per µl) are present. Severe cytopenias are more characteristic of ALL than CLL. The leukocyte count usually exceeds 50,000 cells per µl, but cell counts in canine CLL range from 15,000 to 1,600,000 cells per µl.[18] Normal absolute numbers of granulocytes are usually present, but the predominant leukocyte is a small lymphocyte with round nuclei and densely clumped chromatin. Only a small rim of cytoplasm is present. The morphological maturity of these cells belies the fact that they are malignant. Nucleoli are present but are inapparent. At the time of diagnosis, at least 30 percent of the bone marrow cells are of a similar morphology. Rarely, the cells in CLL may be of a larger cell type with more abundant cytoplasm (fig. 3.34 A), making the distinction from ALL

on morphological grounds very difficult. In one series of 73 dogs with CLL, it was found that no CLL cells stained for CD34, whereas ALL cells and acute nonlymphoid leukemia cells stained positively.[18]

Alternatives for lymphocytosis should always be considered, although the degree of lymphocytosis seen with benign reactive diseases seldom attains the levels seen with CLL. The persistent lymphocytosis (PL) associated with bovine leukemia virus infection in cattle is a nonneoplastic polyclonal B cell response and seldom exceeds 20,000 cells per µl. The cells are variable in size and shape, with a homogeneous retiform chromatin pattern. Occasionally, PL in cattle is incorrectly referred to as a form of CLL. Other causes of lymphocytosis are chronic antigenic stimulation including postvaccinal lymphocytosis, epinephrine-induced (excitement) lymphocytosis (particularly in young cats), and adrenocortical insufficiency.

At necropsy of animals with CLL there is usually good body condition. Mild pallor may be present. Hepatomegaly is mild to moderate, and an accentuated lobular pattern is present. Splenomegaly is often marked terminally. Small focal accumulations of tumor cells may be grossly visible in the spleen, liver, and renal cortices. Lymph nodes may be enlarged, but this is never a prominent feature (fig. 3.35 B). The bone marrow cavity is often uniformly reddened.

When CLL is discovered incidentally or when the patient is presented with mild symptoms, the marrow may or may not show involvement, apparently depending upon the B cell or T cell nature of the proliferating cell.[18] It appears that the canine B cell CLLs arise in the bone marrow; alternatively, T cell CLLs apparently originate from the spleen, and as the disease advances, the bone marrow subsequently becomes involved. In terminal cases, the bone marrow is essentially 100 percent cellular regardless of immunophenotype. A small number of fat vacuoles and megakaryocytes may be the only remaining normal elements. There is a monomorphous population of densely packed small mononuclear cells having a diameter slightly larger than red cells. Portal triads in the liver are heavily infiltrated (fig. 3.35 A), but sinusoidal invasion is often less than in ALL despite the greater number of tumor cells seen in the peripheral blood with CLL. The spleen may have a few residual follicles, but the normal features are largely replaced by monomorphous tumor cells filling sinus areas; these cells cytologically resemble the bone marrow. Earlier in the disease process, there may be a considerable amount of extramedullary hematopoiesis coexistent with the tumor. Uninvolved lymph nodes will show atrophy and sinus histiocytosis. Lymph node involvement is usually diffuse and cortical. Postcapillary venules may be prominent. In the medulla, there is invasion of cords but not sinuses (fig. 3.35 B). Tumor colonization may be found in most tissues, including the central nervous system.

CLL can be distinguished from leukemic lymphoma of small cells by the usual mild degree of lymph node involvement in CLL. Additionally, early marrow involvement with

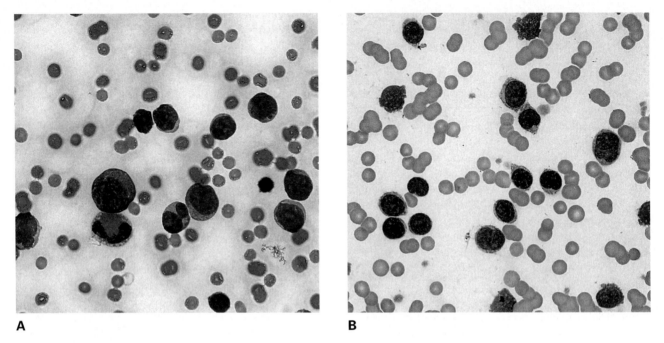

Fig. 3.34. **A.** Chronic lymphocytic leukemia, large cell type. A 4-year-old castrated male domestic shorthair cat presented with lethargy and weight loss of several months duration. The blood leukocytes totaled $228 \times 10^3/\mu l$ with 94 percent lymphocytes, 3.1 g/dl of hemoglobin, and platelets estimated at 10 $\times 10^3/\mu l$. **NOTE:** Anemia is nonresponsive, with lack of anisocytosis and polychromasia. The nuclei are generally 2.0 to 2.5 red cells in diameter, usually round, and occasionally cleft. Chromatin is coarsely granular, and nucleoli are small or absent. There is a moderate amount of quite highly basophilic cytoplasm. The larger cells with nucleoli suggest a shift to an accelerated phase. Wright's ×800. **B.** Chronic lymphocyte leukemia, small cell type. A 14-year-old male cat was presented for examination because of loss of 2.5 pounds over the last 2 years. The leukocytes totaled $110 \times 10^3/\mu l$, primarily lymphocytes, with a packed cell volume of 25 percent. The nuclei are generally 1.5 red cells in diameter, are frequently indented, and have deeply stained chromatin; nucleoli are not apparent. Cytoplasm is scanty and lightly stained. The anemia is of moderate severity and nonresponsive. Wright's ×800.

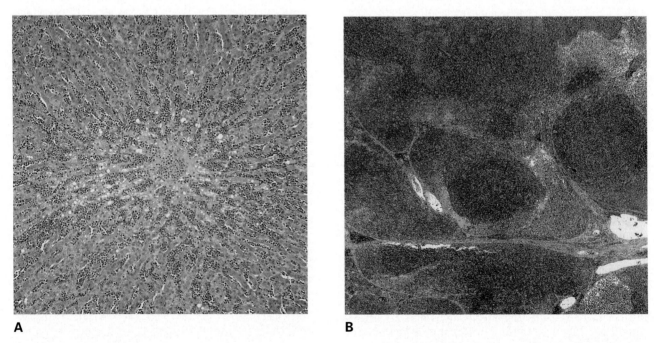

Fig. 3.35. **A.** Sinusoidal pattern of hepatic colonization in CLL. The liver from a 14-year-old standardbred mare. There are narrow but irregular foci of tumor cells in the midzone areas and marked distention of sinusoids in the central vein area (center), where there is loss of normal staining density of hepatocytes due to ischemic degeneration and fatty vacuolization. H&E ×80 **B.** CLL, lymph node "homing" of tumor cells to medullary cords. There is diffuse infiltration of the cortex, with thinning, but not abridgement, of the node capsule. Medullary cords are expanded by tumor cells, and the medullary sinuses are compressed and relatively empty. H&E ×10.

leukemic lymphoma is more often focal. Occasionally, CLL in people may undergo a transformation to a more malignant phenotype. This phenomenon has been reported in dogs that developed lymphoma following a prolonged period of CLL in remission.[26] In people, a small number of CLL cases evolve into ALL, myeloma, or an aggressive large cell lymphoma termed *Richter's syndrome.*

Seventy-five percent of canine CLLs (n = 85) were shown to be a T cell (CD3) disorder with a CD8 phenotype.[18,33] Approximately a quarter of the cases had a B cell phenotype (CD79a, CD21), and a similar proportion had monoclonal gammopathies.[18,33] An earlier series of 22 dogs with CLL reported 70 percent with monoclonal gammopathies.[26] The most frequent paraprotein was IgM. Total serum protein and globulin concentrations may be normal. Occasionally, dogs with CLL may have a hyperviscosity syndrome.[34,35] The tumor cells in people with CLL may have cell surface immunoglobulin but are nonsecretory. Most cats with CLL are FeLV and FIV negative.

CLL of the large granular lymphocyte type (LGL) occurs in a high proportion of aged F344 rats[36] and rarely in Sprague-Dawley rats, cats, horses, and cattle (fig. 3.36). In a series of 73 cases of canine CLL, 54 percent had the morphological characteristics of LGLs.[18] The LGL tumor cells were almost exclusively of the T cytotoxic/suppressor (CD8, CD11d) cell lineage and were thought to be primary splenic tumors similar to those in the rat.[18] Simultaneous positive or negative staining for CD4 and CD8 were occasionally encountered. Positive staining for CD4 is found in canine neutrophils, which may cause false positives if gat-

ing is incorrect. The tumor cells in all CLL cases failed to stain with CD34.

Another T cell type of CLL occurs in the dog,[37] horse, and cow as part of the leukemic syndrome of mycosis fungoides termed *Sézary syndrome.* A retrovirus was isolated from a long-term culture of canine Sézary cells, but the role of this virus in the development of the disease remains unknown.[38] The Sézary cell as it appears in the dermis of the skin and in the blood has a markedly convoluted nuclear membrane that is best demonstrated in ultrathin sections. In people with Sézary syndrome, the prognosis varies inversely with the number of cerebriform cells in circulation.

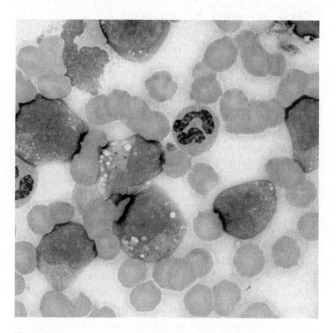

Fig. 3.36. Large granular lymphocytic leukemia. Blood from a 2.5-year-old English setter presented for intense pruritus. Characteristic features of the condition are the presence of prominent azurophilic granules that may be poorly stained and appear as vacuoles. Wright's ×1200.

REFERENCES

1. Grindem, C.B., Stevens, J.B., and Perman, V. (1986) Cytochemical reactions in cells from leukemic dogs. *Vet Pathol* 23:103–109.
2. Couto, C.G. (1985) Clinicopathologic aspects of acute leukemias in the dog. *J Amer Vet Med Assoc* 186:681–685.
3. Grindem, C.B. (1986) Cytogenetic analysis of leukemic cells in the dog: A report of 10 cases and a review of the literature. *J Comp Pathol* 96:623–635.
4. Raskin, R.E., and Nipper, N.M. (1992) Cytochemical staining characteristics of lymph nodes from normal and lymphoma-affected dogs. *Vet Clin Pathol* 21:62–67.
5. Facklam, N.R., and Kociba, G.J. (1985) Cytochemical characterization of leukemic cells from 20 dogs. *Vet Pathol* 22:363–369.
6. Facklam, N.R., and Kociba, G.J. (1986) Cytochemical characterization of feline leukemic cells. *Vet Pathol* 23:155–161.
7. Grindem, C.B., et al. (1985) Cytochemical reactions in cells from leukemic cats. *Vet Clin Pathol* 14:6–12.
8. Grindem, C.B. (1985) Ultrastructural morphology of leukemic cells from 14 dogs. *Vet Pathol* 22:456–462.
9. Grindem, C.B. (1985) Ultrastructural morphology of leukemic cells in the cat. *Vet Pathol* 22:147–155.
10. Cotter, S.M., and Essex, M. (1977) Animal model: Feline acute lymphoblastic leukemia and aplastic anemia. *Amer J Pathol* 87:265–268.
11. MacEwen, E.G., Patnaik, A.K., and Wilkins, R.J. (1977) Diagnosis and treatment of canine hematopoietic neoplasms. *Vet Clin N Amer Small Anim Pract* 7:105–132.
12. Matus, R.E., Leifer, C.E, and MacEwen, E.F. (1983) Acute lymphoblastic leukemia in the dog: A review of 30 cases. *J Amer Vet Med Assoc* 183:859–862.
13. Grindem, C.B., Perman, V., and Stevens, J.B. (1985) Morphological classification and clinical and pathological characteristics of spontaneous leukemia in 10 cats. *J Amer Anim Hosp Assoc* 21:227–236.
14. Muscoplat, C.C., Johnson, D.W., Pomeroy, K.A., Olson, J.M., Larson, V.L., Stevens, J.B., and Sorenson, D.K. (1974) Lymphocyte subpopulations and immunodeficiency in calves with acute lymphocytic leukemia. *Amer J Vet Res* 35:1571–1573.
15. Roberts, M.C. (1977) A case of primary lymphoid leukaemia in a horse. *Equine Vet J* 9:216–219.
16. Green, P.D., and Donovan, L.A. (1977) Lymphosarcoma in a horse. *Can Vet J* 18:257–258.
17. Henry, C.J., Lanevschi, A., Marks, S.L., Beyer, J.C., Nitschelm, S.H., and Barnes, S. (1996) Acute lymphoblastic leukemia, hypercalcemia, and pseudohyperkalemia in a dog. *J Amer Vet Med Assoc* 208:237–239.

18. Vernau, W., and Moore, P.F. (1999) An immunophenotypic study of canine leukemias and preliminary assessment of clonality by polymerase chain reaction. *Vet Immunol Immunopathol* 69:145–164.

19. MacKey, L.J, and Jarrett, W.R.H. (1972) Pathogenesis of lymphoid neoplasia in cats and its relationship to immunological cell pathways. I. Morphologic aspects. *J Natl Cancer Inst* 49:853–865.

20. Bennett, J.M., Catovsky, M., Daniel, M.T., Flandrin, G., Galton, D.A.G., Gralnick, H.R., and Sultan, C. (1976) FAB Cooperative Group (1976) Proposals for the classification of the acute leukemias. *Brit J Haematol* 33:451–458.

21. Valli, V.E.O. (1992) The Hematopoietic System. In Jubb, K.V.F., Kennedy, P.C., and Palmer, N. (eds.), *Pathology of Domestic Animals,* 4th ed. Academic Press, San Diego, pp. 113–157.

22. Ruslander, D.A., Gerhard D.H., Tompkins, M.B., Grindem, C.B., and Page, R.L. (1997) Immunophenotypic characterization of canine lymphoproliferative disorders. *In Vivo* 11:169–172.

23. Essex, M.E. (1982) Feline leukemia: A naturally occurring cancer of infectious origin. *Epidemiol Rev* 4:189–203.

24. Raich, P.C,. Takashima, I., and Olson, C. (1983) Cytochemical reactions in bovine and ovine lymphosarcoma. *Vet Pathol* 20:322–329.

25. Takashima, I., Olson, C., Driscoll, D.M., and Baumgartener, L.E. (1977) B-lymphocytes and T-lymphocytes in three types of bovine lymphosarcoma. J. Natl. *Cancer Inst* 59:1205–1209.

26. Leifer, C.E., and Matus, R.E. (1986) Chronic lymphocytic leukemia in the dog: 22 cases (1974–1984). *J Amer Vet Med Assoc* 189:214–217.

27. Hodgkins, E.M., Zinkl, J.G., and Madewell, B.R. (1980) Chronic lymphocytic leukemia in the dog. *J Amer Vet Med Assoc* 177:704–707.

28. Kristensen, A.T., Klausner, J.S., Weiss, D.J., Schultz, R.D., and Bell, F.W. (1991) Spurious hyperphosphatemia in a dog with chronic lymphocytic leukemia and an IgM monoclonal gammopathy. *Vet Clin Pathol* 20:45–48.

29. Harvey, J.W., Terrell, T.G., Hyde, D.M., and Jackson, R.I. (1981) Well-differentiated lymphocytic leukemia in a dog: Long term survival without therapy. *Vet Pathol* 18:37–47.

30. Couto, C.G., and Sousa, C. (1986) Chronic lymphocytic leukemia with cutaneous involvement in a dog. *J Amer Anim Hosp Assoc* 22:374–379.

31. Cotter, S.M., and Holzworth, J. (1987) disorders of the hematopoietic system. In Holzworth, J. (ed.), *Diseases of the Cat: Medicine and Surgery.* W.B. Saunders Co., Philadelphia, pp. 755–807.

32. Thrall, M.A. (1981) Lymphoproliferative disorders: Lymphocytic leukemia and plasma cell myeloma. *Vet Clin N Amer Small Anim Pract* 11:321–347.

33. Ruslander, D.A., Gerhard D.H., Tompkins, M.B., Grindem, C.B., and Page, R.L. (1997) Immunophenotypic characterization of canine lymphoproliferative disorders. *In Vivo* 11:169–172.

34. Braund, K.G., Everett, R.M., and Albert, R.A. (1978) Neurologic manifestations of monoclonal IgM gammopathy associated with lymphocyte leukemia in a dog. *J Amer Vet Med Assoc* 172:1407–1410.

35. MacEwen, E.G., Hurvitz, A.I., and Hayes, A. (1977) Hyperviscosity syndrome associated with lymphocytic leukemia in three dogs. *J Amer Vet Med Assoc* 170:1309–1312.

36. Stromberg, P.C. (1985) Large granular lymphocyte leukemia in F344 rats. Model for human T gamma lymphoma, malignant histiocytosis, and T-cell chronic lymphocytic leukemia. *Amer J Pathol* 11:517–519.

37. Foster, A.P., Evans, E., Kerlin, R.L., and Vail, D.M. (1997) Cutaneous T-cell lymphoma with Sézary syndrome in a dog. *Vet Clin Pathol* 26:188–192.

38. Ghernati, I., Auger, C., Chabanne, L., Corbin, A., Bonnefont, C., Magnol, J.P., Fournel, C., Rivoire, A., Monier, J.C., and Rigal, D. (1999) Characterization of a canine long-term T-cell line (DLC 01) established from a dog with Sézary syndrome and producing retroviral particles. *Leukemia* 13:1281–1290.

THE MYELOPROLIFERATIVE DISORDERS

Myeloproliferative disorders are a group of conditions of one or more of the myeloid stem cells and their progeny characterized by abnormal bone marrow differentiation and maturation. For the purposes of this chapter, the term *myeloproliferative disease* will be reserved for those conditions characterized as leukemia. The myelodysplastic syndromes are defined to include conditions characterized by ineffective hematopoiesis and peripheral blood cytopenias that may terminate in marrow failure or leukemia (algorithm 3.2 and table 3.7).

The hematopoietic stem cells have the unique property of self-renewal, giving rise to progeny that are ultimately identical in appearance and function. The self-renewal of the stem cells in the bone marrow, the proliferation and differentiation of hematopoietic progenitor cells, and their survival are regulated by hematopoietic growth factors (cytokines). The cytokines known to be most important in the regulation of normal hematopoiesis and that may be involved in malignant hemeatopoiesis are shown in algorithm 3.2.

Myeloid leukemias are autonomous clonal proliferations arising in a single progenitor stem cell in the bone marrow. The leukemic cells have morphologic, immunological, and often functional characteristics of the normal hematopoietic progenitors which correspond to the point at which their differentiation ceased.

The Acute Myeloid Leukemias

Introduction

As a group, the acute myeloid leukemias (AML) are characterized by the presence of blasts and immature cells in the peripheral blood and bone marrow (table 3.8). The aspirated bone marrow specimen from an animal with AML is usually highly cellular, with a lack of fat and nearly complete phthisis of normal marrow cells. The total leukocyte count is usually elevated, but may be normal or even decreased. Thrombocytopenia and anemia are common features of AML. These are generally considered to be due to inadequate production by bone marrow that is heavily infiltrated by the neoplastic population. Recent studies indicate that both altered cell composition and functional abnormalities of stromal/accessory cells and their products (cytokines and extracellular matrix molecules) may contribute to the cytopenias (see algorithm 3.3).[1]

The diagnosis of AML relies heavily on identification of individual blast cells in Wright-stained peripheral blood and bone marrow films (see figs. 3.37–3.42). A core biopsy is usually less helpful in identifying primitive cells. Nevertheless, it provides the best assessment of cellularity, can

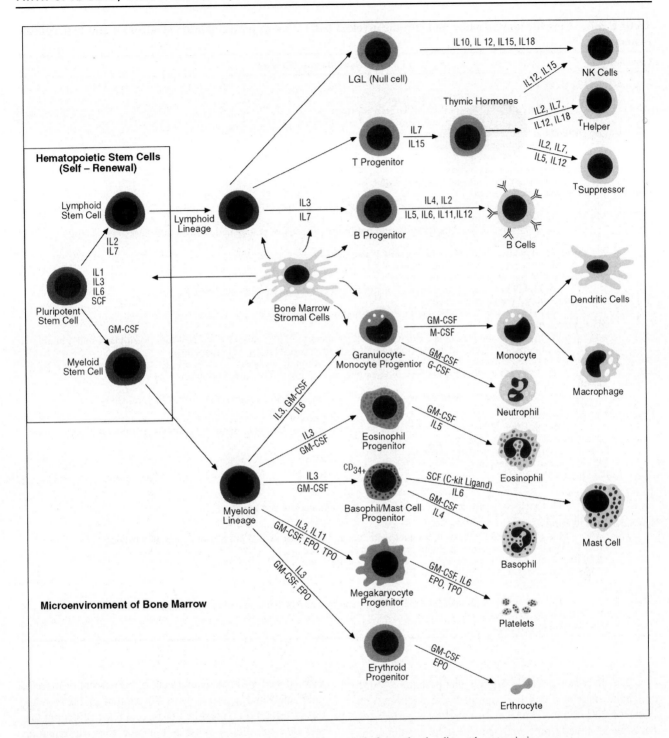

Algorithm 3.2. Algorithm for hematopoietic proliferation and cytokine control of normal and malignant hematopoiesis.

occasionally identify aggregates of leukemic cells not found on a bone marrow aspirate, and is essential for the evaluation of myelofibrosis. The optimal procedure is always to carry out both an aspirate and a core biopsy, with additional slides prepared to permit special stains after an initial examination.

In 1976 hematologists from France, America, and Great Britain (FAB) proposed a system to improve the accuracy of diagnosis and to standardize classification of acute myeloid leukemias in humans.[2] This classification system, which has been modified over the years,[3,4] was subsequently expanded and modified for use in classifying the myeloproliferative disorders of dogs and cats.[5,6] The proposed classification system for AML in dogs and cats, derived from the FAB system, classifies acute myeloid leukemias according to the proportions and identity of the blast cells and the degree of differentiation in the leukemic population (see table 3.7).

TABLE 3.7. Classification of acute and chronic myeloid leukemias with myeloblastic syndromes and hyperplastic responses

Classification	Bone Marrow Findings

Acute Myeloid Leukemia
　　M1 Poorly differentiated myeloblastic leukemia
　　　　　　1. $\geq$30% blasts; >3% blasts MPO/SBB positive;
　　　　　　　　　<10% promyelocytes and more mature granulocytes
　　M2 Differentiated myeloblastic leukemia
　　　　　　2. $\geq$30% blasts; $\geq$3% blasts MPO/SBB positive;
　　　　　　　　　$\geq$10% promyelocytes and more mature granulocytes
　　M2-Eo Differentiated myeloblastic leukemia
　　M2-B Differentiated myeloblastic leukemia with basophilic maturation
　　M3 Promyelocytic leukemia
　　　　　　3. $\geq$30% myeloblasts and abnormal promyelocytes; intense MPO/SBB positivity
　　M4 Myelomonocytic leukemia
　　　　　　4. $\geq$30% myeloblasts, monoblasts, and promonocytes; >20% granulocytic cells; >20% monocytic cells;
　　　　　　　　　monocytosis $\geq$5 $\times$ 10^9/l
　　M4-Eo Myelomonocytic leukemia with abnormal eosinophils
　　M4-B Myelomonocytic leukemia with abnormal basophils
　　M5a Poorly differentiated monoblastic leukemia
　　　　　　5. Monoblasts and promonocytes constitute $\geq$80% of nonerythroid cells (NEC)
　　M5b Differentiated monocytic leukemia
　　　　　　6. $\geq$30% to <80% of NEC are monoblasts and promonocytes
　　M6 Erythroleukemia
　　　　　　7. Erythroid component is $\geq$50% of all nucleated cells (ANC), and $\geq$30% of NEC are myeloblasts and monoblasts
　　　　　　　　　or $\geq$30% of ANC are blasts (including rubriblasts, myeloblasts, and monoblasts)
　　M6-Er/EM Erythroleukemia with erythroid predominance/Erythremic myelosis
　　　　　　8. Erythroid component is $\geq$50% of the ANC, and $\geq$30% of ANC are rubriblasts
　　M7 Megakaryoblastic leukemia
　　　　　　9. $\geq$30% blasts; >50% megakaryocytic cells by immunologic markers and/or ultrastructural study

Chronic Myeloid Leukemia
　　　　　　10. $\geq$6% but <30% blasts of ANC in bone marrow and marked increase in cell counts in peripheral blood
　　CML Chronic myeloid leukemia
　　CMML Chronic myelomonocytic leukemia
　　MM Megakaryocytic myelosis
　　PV Polycythemia vera

Mast Cell Leukemia
　　　　　　11. Extensive proliferation of mast cells in the bone marrow and blood

Myelodysplastic Syndrome
　　　　　　12. $\geq$6% but <30% blasts of all nucleated cells in bone marrow and prominent dysplastic changes
　　MDS-Er Myelodysplastic syndrome with erythroid predominance
　　MDS-RC Myelodysplastic syndrome—refractory cytopenia
　　MDS-EB Myelodysplastic syndrome—excess blasts

Hyperplasia
　　　　　　13. <6% blasts of all nucleated cells in bone marrow and increase in cell counts in peripheral blood
　　EH Erythroid hyperplasia
　　MH Myeloid hyperplasia

The diagnosis of AML requires that peripheral blood and bone marrow films be examined and a differential count of 200 or more bone marrow cells be performed. Knowledge gained from serial hematological examinations may be essential for appropriate classification of the myeloproliferative disorders. To distinguish the various subtypes of AML[5] from the myelodysplastic syndromes, the Animal Leukemia Study Group (ALSG) proposed the modified algorithm 3.3. This scheme has been expanded to include various subtypes of myelodysplastic syndromes, chronic myeloid leukemias (CML), and both myeloid and erythroid hyperplasia.[6,7] Based on the ALSG classification scheme, if the blast cell count constitutes 30 percent or more of all nucleated cells (ANC) in the bone marrow, an acute leukemia may be diagnosed. For diagnosis of acute leukemia in the case of a bone marrow with erythroid pre-dominance (erythroid component of 50 percent or more of total nucleated cells), at least 30 percent of the nonerythroid cells (NEC) must be blasts, or a blast cell count that includes rubriblasts must be greater than or equal to 30 percent of all nucleated cell (ANC).

Histological architectural differences between AML and lymphoma are usually sufficient to identify the former disorder as a primary leukemia.[8] However, cytochemical stains may be needed to aid in subclassification and to distinguish AML from leukemias of lymphoid origin. There are several monoclonal antibodies that are useful in distinguishing surface antigens on myeloid and lymphoid cells. Various cytochemical and immunohistochemical stains are used to identify cell lineage in AML (see table 3.5). The utility of cytochemical markers in animals has been primarily defined in dogs and cats.

TABLE 3.8.   Morphological features of blasts in AML subtypes

Blast Feature	Blast Type and Subtype						
	M1	M2	M3	M4	M5	M6	M7
	Myeloblast				Monoblast	Rubriblast (and Myeloblast)	Megakaryoblast
Cell size	15 to 20 μm				15 to 20 μm	15 to 20 μm, (if megaloblastoid upward to 25 μm)	Highly variable, ranging from small to large (7 to 20 μm) but multinucleate forms are upward to 70 μm
Nuclear chromatin	Finely stippled or smooth and evenly distributed, but stains less purple than rubriblast				Stippled to finely reticular	Stippled and may be slightly clumped; stains more purple than myeloblast	Coarsely to finely reticular with minimal clumping in micromegakaryoblast
Nuclear shape	Round to oval, N:C ratio is high (> 1.5) nuclear outline is regular				Oval or slightly indented or may have slightly irregular nuclear outline (nuclear foldings or undulations)	Round and often eccentric; high N:C ratio; nucleus of cell occupies 3/4 of cell; may be binucleate	Round to oval ; often centrally placed; frequently multinucleated
Nucleolus	One or more distinct or indistinct				One or more, but often indistinct	One or two, prominent with nucleolar rings	One to three prominent nucleoli
Cytoplasm	Scant to moderate amount; may contain few primary granules; in M3 there are numerous prominent azurophilic granules				Moderately abundant and nongranulated	Nongranular, with or without a lightly stained Golgi region	Scant to moderately abundant; cytoplasmic blebs; may contain azurophilic granules
Cytoplasmic basophillia	Moderate blue				Light to moderate blue	Deep blue	Deep blue
Cytoplasmic vacuolation	Infrequent				Occasionally	Infrequent	Frequently

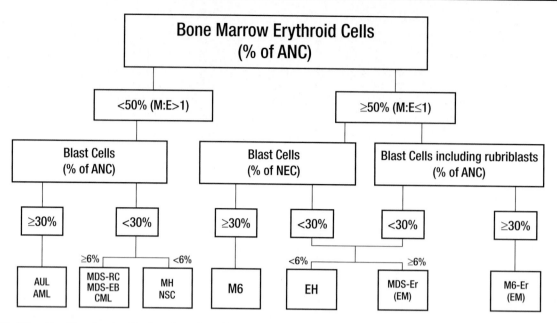

Algorithm 3.3. Algorithm for classification of myeloproliferative disorders. A proposed scheme to classify myeloid and erythroid leukemias, myelodysplastic syndromes, and hyperplastic bone marrow responses. [Modified from Jain N.C., Blue, J.T., Grindem, C.B., et al. (1991) A report of the animal leukemia study group: Proposed criteria for classification of acute myeloid leukemias in dogs and cats. *Vet Clin Pathol* 20:63–82; with permission.] **KEY:** Blast cells include myeloblasts, monoblasts, and megakaryoblasts. Lymphocytes, plasma cells, macrophages, and mast cells were excluded from all nucleated cells (**ANC**). The nonerythroid cells (**NEC**) were ANC minus erythroid cells. **AUL** = acute undifferentiated leukemia; **AML** = acute myeloid leukemias including M1–M5 and M7; **CML** = chronic myeloid leukemias; **MDS-RC** = myelodysplastic syndrome with refractory cytopenia; **MDS-EB** = myelodysplastic syndrome with excess blasts; **MH** = myeloid hyperplasia; **NSC** = no significant changes; **M6** = erythroleukemia; **EH** = erythroid hyperplasia; **MDS-Er** = myelodysplastic syndrome with erythroid predominance; **M6-Er** = erythroleukemia with erythroid predominance; **EM** = erythremic myelosis. [*Vet Clin Pathol* 20(3):63–82; with permission.]

Cytochemical Markers

A panel of cytochemical markers have been developed to aid in the morphological distinction of myeloid leukemias in dogs and cats.[9,10,11] Sudan Black B (SBB) and chloroacetate esterase (CAE) serve as granulocytic markers for leukemic cells in most domestic animals. Myeloperoxidase (MPO) activity is present in the progranulocytes and later stages of granulocytes and monocytes of normal animals, but is not present in the blasts of leukemic dogs and is not a reliable marker.[12] Diffuse cytoplasmic staining for alpha-naphthylbutyrate esterase (ANBE) is a marker for monocyte differentiation. A focal staining pattern with ANBE is seen in canine T cells and feline large granular lymphocytes.[13] Myeloid cells may react positively with nonspecific esterases; the staining is inhibited by fluoride in monocytes but persists in granulocytes, lymphocytes, and macrophages. Positive alkaline phosphatase staining occurs in acute myeloid and myelomonocytic leukemias, and possibly in some lymphocytic leukemias. The markers used to identify acute megakaryoblastic leukemia in dogs and cats include positive cytochemical staining for one or more of the following: serine-sensitive acetylcholinesterase, alpha-naphthylacetate esterase, naphthol AS-D acetate esterase, and positive immunohistochemical staining for either platelet glycoprotein IIIa or Factor VIII related antigen.[14,15]

Myeloid Immunocytochemical Markers

A series of monoclonal antibodies that recognize surface antigens on myeloid and lymphoid cells was characterized and the findings published in 1994 by the first workshop on canine leukocyte antigens (CLAW). Some monoclonal antibodies were identified that are directed against antigen groups, termed *cluster designations* (CD); these antibodies are considered to be restricted to cells committed to a specific lineage.[16] Two such monoclonal antibodies, CLAW 27 and CLAW 51 were found to be specific to a granulocyte/monocyte antigen (possibly CD15). A single monoclonal antibody (CLAW 016) against CD11b, an antigen group commonly considered to be restricted to cells of myeloid differentiation (granulocyte or monocyte lineage), was identified. Blast cells of the megakaryocytic lineage in people can be identified by the presence of surface glycoproteins Ib, IIb/IIIa complex, and IIIa.[3] The CLAW identified four antibodies, 086, 087, 095, and 101, that had strong reactivity with platelets. Although likely candidates for binding the glycoprotein IIb/IIIa complex (CD41/CD61), other platelet adhesion molecules such as CD51 and CD42 could not be ruled out. Antibodies to the von Willebrand factor antigen (Factor VIII related antigen) and platelet glycoprotein IIIa can be used to distinguish the megakaryocytic lineage in dogs and cats[14,15,17] Erythroblastic cells carry glycophorins on their surface and CD71 antigens; however, no monoclonal antibodies were identified that recognized these moieties.[13]

Peripheral Blood and Clinical Manifestations

Patients with AML often present with signs related to a combination of bone marrow and/or organ failure. The typical presentation is an animal with good body condition and hair coat, in collapse and with epistaxis. The most commonly observed clinical signs include weight loss, weakness and malaise, anorexia, infections of variable severity, or hemorrhagic findings such as petechiae, ecchymoses and/or epistaxis. Persistent fever was more common among dogs with AML and was not recognized in the ALL cases described by Couto.[18]

Generally, the findings on physical examination are nonspecific and variable. Examination of the mucous membranes often reveals pallor due to an underlying anemia. Anemia may be the result of reduced erythroid production and myelophthisis, complicated by thrombocytopenic hemorrhage. Lymphadenopathy has been observed more commonly in ALL than in AML cases. Nonetheless, hepatomegaly and splenomegaly were common findings in both leukemic groups. Ocular lesions, which included hyphema, glaucoma, retinal detachment, chorioretinitis, chemosis, and conjunctivitis, were found in 29 percent of dogs with AML reported by Couto.[18]

Most cats and dogs with AML present with anemia and thrombocytopenia, while leukocytosis was reported in only 37 percent and 57.1 percent of the cases in two studies.[5,19] Leukocytosis due to circulating neoplastic cells was more dramatically increased in dogs with acute lymphocytic leukemia (ALL) than in those with AML.[18] Blast cells were present in peripheral blood in 98 percent of cases examined by the ALSG. While circulating blasts were found in 68 percent of feline AML cases, logic would suggest that unless blasts are present in the peripheral blood leukemia should not be diagnosed. Occasionally in AML cases, marked leukopenia at presentation may obscure the diagnosis until a bone marrow examination is performed. Although dyshematopoiesis has been described in all AML subtypes, megaloblastic rubricytes and giant metamyelocytes and bands are among the most common dysplastic changes reported.

Frequency of Myeloproliferative Disorders

Myeloproliferative disorders occur most frequently in dogs and cats, but they are also recognized in other domestic and wild animals.[20,21] In dogs and cats, myeloproliferative disorders represent approximately 5 percent and 10 to 15 percent of hemolymphatic neoplasms, respectively.[8]

Acute myeloblastic leukemia, with and without differentiation, was the most frequently diagnosed myeloproliferative disorder in two studies (see figs. 3.37, 3.38).[5,6] The frequency of this diagnosis approached 30 percent in both studies. Erythroleukemia, (M6-Er) with and without erythroid predominance (M6), was the second most frequent subtype of AML in myeloproliferative disorders of cats, while monoblastic/monocytic leukemia (M5) was the second most commonly diagnosed subtype in the study involving both dogs and cats (see figs. 3.40, 3.41).

Once the diagnosis of acute leukemia has been made, the next distinction is to determine if the lesion is of myeloproliferative or lymphoproliferative origin. Next, the subtype of acute leukemia should be identified, for example, M1–M7, to provide a framework for the development of effective treatment protocols.

Chemotherapy

Unfortunately, current therapies for all subtypes of AML recognized in veterinary medicine are similar, and outcomes are generally poor. Therefore, the advantages to clinical management of this classification are presently limited.

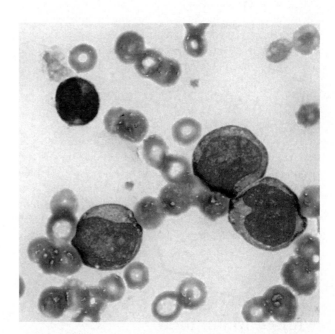

Fig. 3.37. Acute myeloid leukemia without maturation (M1). A 3-year-old springer spaniel was presented because of depression and epistaxis of acute onset. The dog was in excellent body condition with mucosal pallor and petechiae. Hematologically there was a normal leukocyte count with marked left shift, neutropenia, thrombocytopenia, and anemia. The malignant blasts have nuclei 1.5 to 2 red cells in diameter that are round or oval without indentations. The chromatin pattern is generally fine, and there are one to three moderately prominent nucleoli present that are irregularly associated with chromocenters. The cytoplasm is moderate in amount, highly basophilic, without azurophilic granulation, and focally vacuolated. The diagnosis rests on the history of acute onset with undifferentiated blasts in circulation and characteristically no or only mild leukocytosis. Special stains (Sudan Black B) are required to rule out ALL. Wright's ×1280.

Unlike therapeutic approaches to ALL, the agents useful for treatment of AML are largely nonspecific in action and are toxic to the bone marrow, potentially rendering it aplastic. Therefore, meticulous attention to supportive care is essential since death may occur during remission induction as a consequence of treatment induced pancytopenia. Consideration should also be given to the use of either allogeneic or autologous bone marrow transplantation in AML patients, which probably represents their greatest chance for prolonged disease-free survival.[22] The current treatment protocols for AML result in survival times that, from the start of treatment, seldom exceed 5 to 9 months and may be as short as a few weeks.[10,23] Newer therapies used in human medicine may offer more successful future strategies; these include growth factors and interferon therapy, alone or in combination with antimetabolites[24] and oligodeoxynucleotides, which inhibit specific gene expression[25].

Classification

The classification system for AML is based on morphological characteristics of Wright-stained cells in peripheral blood and, preferably, a differential count of 200 or more nucleated cells in bone marrow smears. Cytochemical and immunochemical staining of cells on blood and bone marrow smears facilitate lineage identification (see table 3.5).[5] The acute myeloid leukemias include the following eight categories (AUL and M1 through M7).

AUL—Acute Undifferentiated Leukemia

It is not possible to reliably distinguish between AUL and ALL based simply on morphology. Included in this category are blast cells of uncertain lineage that resemble myeloblasts but are negative at the light microscopic level when stained with SBB. Blast cells of *lymphoid morphology* that stain strongly for alkaline phosphatase activity, as well as blast cells with pseudopodia, fall into the AUL category. The myeloid nature of these leukemias can only be definitively determined by immunological means (see fig. 3.38 A,B).

M1—Myeloblastic Leukemia without Maturation

M1 is characterized by little evidence of granulocytic differentiation and by a predominance of blasts in bone marrow with presence of blasts in the peripheral blood. The predominate cell is a myeloblast, comprising more than 30 percent of all marrow nucleated cells (ANC). In addition, 10 percent or less of the nonerythroid cells (NEC) are maturing granulocytes (promyelocytes to segmented granulocytes) (fig. 3.37). The blast cells from patients with M1 may be distinguished from those in ALL based on cytomorphology. In M1, the blasts are larger than cells in ALL, have more prominent, often multiple, nucleoli, and may have primary granules. To confirm a diagno-

sis of M1, typical blast cells must stain positive for a granulocytic marker such as SBB (see fig. 3.38 B), CAE, or MPO (see table 3.7)). Dyspoiesis of the normal cell lines remaining in the marrow can be expected.

M2—Myeloblastic Leukemia with Maturation

In contrast to M1, the M2 subtype shows obvious maturation which proceeds to and beyond the promyelocyte stage (fig. 3.38). Although myeloblasts constitute equal to or greater than 30 percent of all marrow nucleated cells (ANC), the differentiation along granulocytic lines exceeds 10 percent of the NEC. Cytoplasmic granulation is generally more obvious with a disproportionate number of promyelocytes compared to segmented neutrophils. The

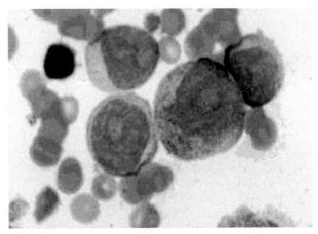

A

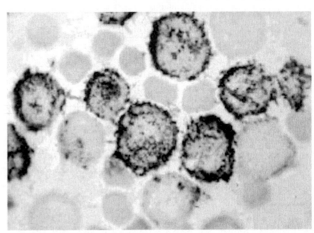

B

Fig. 3.38. Acute myeloid leukemia with maturation, M2. Bone marrow from a cat. **A.** Blast cells similar to M1 (Figure 3.37) are present. Maturation is present to the level of promyelocytes, with more abundant cytoplasm and a few azurophilic granules; some more mature progeny are also seen. Wright's ×1,600. **B.** Marking of primary cytoplasmic granules distinguishes M2 from acute lymphoblastic leukemia. Sudan Black B ×1600.

granules of the promyelocytes are usually uniformly distributed in the cytoplasm, but may be packeted near the Golgi. In most cases of M2, granulocytic maturation is along the neutrophilic pathway, but maturation to eosinophils or basophils has also been reported in animals.[6,26] Such cases are designated M2-Eo and M2-B.

M3—Promyelocytic Leukemia

Acute promyelocytic leukemia is one of the most distinctive subtypes of AML due to the unusually heavily granulated cytoplasm. A hypogranular form, in which the progranulocyte granules fail to stain but may be identified with electron microscopy, occurs in people.[27] In both forms of M3, staining with SBB is strongly positive (fig. 3.38 B). The hypogranular form of the disease in people is associated with disseminated intravascular coagulation subsequent to aggressive cytoreductive therapy. A specific chromosomal translocation (15;17) occurs that results in the up regulation of the myeloperoxidase gene.[28] There are no reports to date of M3 in animals.

M4—Acute Myelomonocytic Leukemia

Myelomonocytic leukemia is characterized by neoplasia of both the granulocytic and monocytic lineages (fig. 3.39). Together, myeloblasts and monoblasts constitute 30 percent or more of all marrow nucleated cells (ANC), with differentiated granulocytes and monocytes each representing more than 20 percent of the NEC. Granulocytic differentiation is usually along the neutrophilic pathway; however, eosinophilic (M4-Eo) or basophilic (M4-B) cell types may occur. The monocytic component is characterized by a lightly granulated and uniformly basophilic cytoplasm, without Golgi zone, but with folded nuclei. Monocytic lineage can be confirmed by demonstrating fluoride-sensitive staining for the nonspecific esterases (NSEs) (alpha-naphthylacetate esterase or alpha-naphthylbutyrate esterase).

M5—Monoblastic/Monocytic Leukemia

Acute monocytic leukemia is characterized by blood and marrow blasts that stain with fluoride-sensitive NSEs. Acute monocytic leukemia can be subdivided on the degree of differentiation into monoblastic (M5a, when more than 80 percent of monocytic cells in the marrow are monoblasts) or monocytic (M5b, when less than 80 percent of the monocytic cells are monoblasts) (fig. 3.40). Monoblasts are usually large cells with abundant, moderately to occasionally deeply basophilic cytoplasm that is sometimes vacuolated and may contain scattered azurophilic granules. The nuclei vary from round to convoluted and have a fine or lacy chromatin pattern and one or more nucleoli. Promonocytes usually contain prominent azurophilic granules, and the cytoplasm is more basophilic than that in the monoblast. The peripheral blood may contain cells of the monocytic lineage that are more differen-

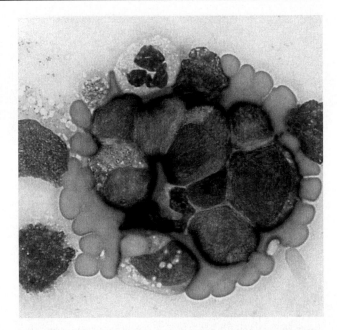

Fig. 3.39. Acute myelomonocytic leukemia, M4. A 10-year-old male neutered domestic shorthair cat was presented for anorexia and depression. Blood contains $96 \times 10^3/\mu l$ leukocytes, of which 98 percent are immature and 44 percent were blasts. Hemoglobin was 3.2 g/dl, with platelets $32 \times 10^3/\mu l$. Two undifferentiated blasts with progeny are present; the blasts have fine chromatin, prominent nucleoli, and minimal highly basophilic cytoplasm; the progeny include a promyelocyte with a few azurophilic granules and a promonocyte with prominent cytoplasmic vacuolization; a bilobed neutrophil, the progeny of a malignant myelocyte is also present. The key to the diagnosis is the presence of blast cells with evidence for maturation into *both* granulocytic and monocytic cell lines. Confirmation of cell lineage is made by the use of alpha-naphthyl acetate (or butyrate) esterase stains (for identification of blasts of the monocytic series) and chloroacetate esterase (for blasts and progranulocytes of the myeloid series). Wright's ×1280.

tiated or mature than those found in the bone marrow. The granulocytic component in M5 is less than 20 percent of NEC. Dyserythropoiesis can be expected to be present. M5 is infrequently diagnosed in cats but may constitute a quarter of myeloproliferative diseases in dogs. Malignant histiocytosis (MH) can be thought of as a more fully differentiated form of malignancy in the monocyte/macrophage system. MH is characterized by solid focal tumors in the spleen, liver, bone marrow, and lymph nodes, often with marked erythrophagocytosis and nonregenerative anemia (see fig. 3.28).

M6—Erythroleukemia

M6 is an acute myeloproliferative disease in which there is concurrent neoplasia in both the granulocytic and erythroid lineages, initially known as DiGuglielmo's syndrome.[29] The marrow contains excess blasts of both series, with the erythroid component predominating. Malignant blasts of both series must be present in peripheral blood to satisfy the diagnosis. The disease is peracute, and anemia and thrombocytopenia are severe. This uncommon syndrome is most frequently recognized in cats. In people, the

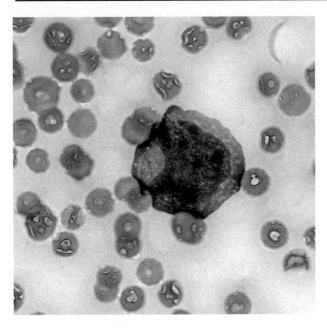

Fig. 3.40. Acute monocytic leukemia, M5b. A 7-year-old holstein cow was presented because of anorexia, diarrhea, and cessation of milk production. The blood contained 17×10^3 leukocytes/μl, of which 10 percent were monoblasts and promonocytes. Hemoglobin was 2.8 g/dl and 25×10^3/μl platelets. Blasts are undifferentiated large cells with fine chromatin, multiple nucleoli, and rather basophilic cytoplasm. Promonocytes have retention of nucleoli plus some chromocenters and increased volume of basophilic cytoplasm that is finely vacuolated. Wright's ×1600.

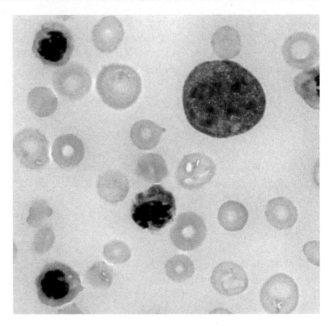

Fig. 3.41. Erythremic myelosis, M6-Er. A 12-year-old holstein cow suffered a progressive loss of weight and milk production. Blood contains 122×10^3 nucleated cells/μl, of which 93 percent are rubricytes at varying stages of maturation. There are 3.8 g/dl of hemoglobin without reticulocytes, and there is an upward shift in the MCV to 59 fl. Platelets are 38×10^3/μl. Prorubricytes with multiple nucleoli and coalescing chromocenters are accompanied by maturing metarubricytes, one of which has an atypical nucleus. The diagnosis is made on the basis of severe anemia with rubricytosis, including blasts but without reticulocytes. Wright's ×1600.

disease may begin as a primary malignancy of the erythroid system that may persist (as is most common in animals) or progress from erythremic myelosis to erythroleukemia and terminate as AML.

M6-Er—Erythremic Myelosis

M6-Er is characterized by neoplasia in the erythroid system only (DiGuglielmo's disease). There is severe nonresponsive anemia, usually with marked rubricytosis that may exceed 100,000 per μl. Primitive cells of benign lineages may appear in the blood, but the M6-Er can be distinguished from M6 by the great preponderance of early and often megaloblastic erythroid precursors in the marrow, with phthisis of other elements. The disease is most often seen in cats but occurs rarely in dogs and cattle (fig. 3.41).[8,30-32] Dyserythropoietic changes are often seen in M6-Er, with erythroid precursors showing features such as nuclear/cytoplasmic asynchrony, nuclear lobulation and binuclearity, karyorrhexis, and cytoplasmic vacuolation. Erythropoiesis may be predominantly megaloblastic, and phagocytosis by abnormal erythroid precursors may be observed. There are several reports of transition from M6-Er to M6 in cats.[32] The transition from one morphological type of leukemia to another has been reported in animals[33] and may be described as *lineage infidelity*.

The numerous circulating nucleated red cells in M6-Er can superficially mimic the finding in acute hemolytic ane-

mias; however, in benign disease, the absence of rubriblasts or very immature erythroid cells in the peripheral blood and an increased reticulocyte count are characteristic of acute hemolysis with regeneration. The marked anemia seen with erythremic myelosis is nonregenerative. Rubricytes in erythremic myelosis are maturation arrested and do not mature normally. *Haemobartonella felis* may be present but should be recognized as an incidental finding because of the lack of polychromasia and presence of blasts in the blood. The megaloblastic changes in erythremic myelosis are unresponsive to treatment with vitamin B_{12} or folate.

M7—Megakaryoblastic Leukemia

This is a disease characterized by neoplasia of the megakaryocytic precursors accompanied by thrombocytopenia and anemia. The diagnosis is suggested by morphological features of blasts that include cytoplasmic protrusions or budding and large bizarre platelets (fig. 3.42). The blasts may be undifferentiated and resemble large lymphoblasts. The diagnosis of M7 can be confirmed by positive immunohistochemical staining reactions of malignant blasts for Factor VIII-related antigen and platelet glycoprotein IIIa.[15,17] Acetylcholinesterase activity can also be demonstrated in megakaryoblasts. M7 leukemia is accompanied by rapidly progressive myelofibrosis and marrow failure.[14]

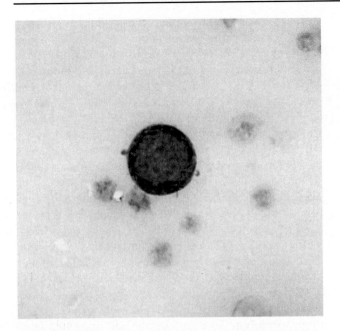

Fig. 3.42 Acute megakaryoblastic leukemia, M7A. Blood from a 6-year-old male collie presented because of dyspnea and lethargy. Upon examination, mucous membranes were found to be very pale. Blood contains 19.8 × 10³ nucleated cells/µl, of which 55 percent were primitive type. There was 1.9 g/dl of hemoglobin, and there were normal numbers of platelets with marked variation in size, granulation, and basophilia. Blastic cells have hyperchromatic chromatin, multiple nucleoli, and a small amount of highly basophilic cytoplasm. The narrow cytoplasmic protrusions are characteristics of this type of tumor. Wright's ×1600.

The Chronic Myeloid Leukemias

Introduction

The term *chronic myelogenous leukemia* (CML) refers to a group of clonal neoplastic disorders characterized by gradually increasing numbers of differentiated hematopoietic cells that result in a marked leukocytosis, erythrocytosis, or thrombocytosis. It has been suggested that the primary defect in chronic leukemias may not be unregulated proliferation of leukemic stem cells but rather *discordant maturation,* such that a slight delay in cell maturation results in the increased myeloid mass.[34]

CML is predominantly a disease of the older dog and cat, but may occur at any age and has been reported in other species (see fig. 3.43).[8] Typically, the onset of CML is insidious, with a gradual increase in peripheral cell numbers, splenomegaly, hepatomegaly, and increasingly severe systemic signs such as anorexia and weight loss. At any time during the course of CML, there may be a relatively abrupt change in the course of the disease to a terminal blastic phase. Transformation into acute leukemia is common in human CML patients and does occur in dogs and cats. Death may be related to organ infiltration and dysfunction or may occur because of hemorrhage and severe infection during chronic or terminal phases. In dogs and cats, the prognosis is very much better for CML (months to years) than for AML (weeks to months).[7]

The chronic myeloid leukemias include all chronic granulocytic leukemias that may be of the neutrophil, eosinophil or basophil type, as well as chronic monocytic leukemia, chronic myelomonocytic leukemia, polycythemia vera, and megakaryocytic myelosis (essential thrombocythemia). Myelodysplastic changes occur in both the myelodysplastic syndrome (MDS) and in CML; however, in MDS the marrow dysplastic changes culminate in ineffective hematopoiesis (marrow hypercellularity and peripheral blood cytopenias). In contrast, cell counts in the peripheral blood of CML patients are markedly increased.[5] Low and normal numbers of bone marrow blast cells, accompanied by a peripheral blood neutrophilia more than twice normal, are more consistent with myeloid hyperplasia than with chronic leukemia or MDS.[6] Features such as neutrophil toxicity, increased inflammatory proteins, and identification of an inflammatory nidus are helpful in distinguishing severe myeloid hyperplasia or leukemoid responses from CML. The rebound hematopoiesis characteristic of dogs and cats following a leukopenia due to increased peripheral consumption or chemical/viral myelotoxicity may be confused with leukemia and can be ruled out by sequential examinations of blood and bone marrow.

Chronic Myeloid Leukemia

Chronic myeloid or granulocytic leukemia (CML) in people is associated with a characteristic chromosome abnormality known as the *Philadelphia chromosome.* In virtually all cases of CML, a translocation of cytogenetic material results in a fused gene; sequences in the breakpoint cluster region (*bcr*) of chromosome 22 are fused with the cellular oncogene, c-*alb,* from chromosome 9 to form a hybrid gene (*bcr-alb*). This reciprocal translocation is thought to be essential in causation of CML because it is associated with elevated tyrosine kinase activity.[34] A striking biochemical abnormality in CML of people, still unexplained, is the reduction of leukocyte alkaline phosphatase activity in the leukemic cells.[35]

CML is a rare myeloproliferative disorder in animals (see fig. 3.43). There is often a history of weight loss that may occur over several months, with depression and weakness associated with myelophthisic anemia. In the peripheral blood, there is a variable degree of a granulocytosis, with a predominance of mature granulocytes; however, some or all other granulocytic precursor stages may also be found.[36] Although in certain inflammatory diseases, one or more of the neutrophil functions may be defective,[37] it has been suggested that in CML the neoplastic granulocytes may have enhanced function. The phagocytic capacity, superoxide generation, and secretion of enzymes have been markedly increased in neoplastic granulocytes.[38] Enhanced GM-CSF (granulocyte macrophage–colony stimulating factor) synthesis was hypothesized to be the

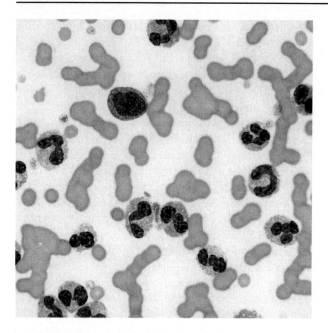

Fig. 3.43. Chronic myeloid leukemia, eosinophil type. A 9-year-old male cat was presented because of weight loss over the last 2 months. Blood contained 120×10^3 leukocytes/µl, of which 75 percent were eosinophils at all stages of maturation, and blast forms were present. There was 8.7 g/dl of hemoglobin and 86×10^3 platelets/µl. The bilobed forms are typical of granulocytes that enter the blood at the myelocyte or earlier stage. Wright's ×800.

cause for the observed cellular hyperresponsiveness. It has also been shown that CML in mice may be induced by retroviral transduction of the gene for GM-CSF, again suggesting that excessive synthesis of this factor may induce leukemia.[39] Gross lesions include pallor with splenomegaly, hepatomegaly, and diffusely reddened marrow. Histological lesions, include pronounced granulocyte proliferation and accumulation in bone marrow and spleen.[38,40]

Chronic Basophilic Leukemia

Basophilic leukemia in seven dogs was diagnosed based on light microscopic evaluation of the neoplastic cells.[41] Cytochemical stains such as omega-exonuclease, a specific marker for basophils, in combination with the granulocyte marker CAE, have been shown to be helpful in establishing a diagnosis.[42] The neoplastic basophilic population may be sensitive to hydroxyurea, however hydroxyurea may also produce severe bone marrow suppression.

Chronic Eosinophilic Leukemia

Chronic eosinophilic leukemia (EL) is rare in the cat (fig. 3.43) and dog, and the diagnosis may be difficult to establish. Typically, the patient has a marked proliferation of mature eosinophils and minimal increase in marrow blast cells. The differential diagnoses must include reactive

eosinophilia and hypereosinophilic syndrome (HES). A reactive eosinophilia is defined as an absolute eosinophil count of 1500 per µl or greater in which an underlying cause for the eosinophilia is recognized. The most common underlying causes of eosinophilia are exo- and endoparasitism, feline asthma, eosinophilic granuloma complex, eosinophilic enteritis, and neoplasia, in particular mast cell tumors.[43] However, the distinction between HES and CML of the eosinophilic type is less clear, and it has been suggested that these two conditions are variants of the same disorder. Both are associated with a prolonged idiopathic peripheral and tissue eosinophilia and organ dysfunction.[44,45] In people, IL-5 produced by activated CD4+ T cells may play a crucial role in the induction of eosinophilia in HES, whereas chromosomal translocations and gene deletions resulting in overproduction of this cytokine are involved in the pathogenesis of eosinophilic CML.[46] The presence of rare blasts in the peripheral blood, morphological abnormalities in eosinophils (intermediate forms containing both eosinophilic and basophilic granules), and immature eosinophilic infiltrates in the tissues have been used to support the diagnosis of EL.[43,47] Although most cats with myeloproliferative disease are FeLV positive, cats with EL are FeLV negative.[48] Cats with EL have a higher average myeloid/erythroid (M:E) ratio, with abnormal and immature eosinophils occurring more frequently and in higher proportions in the peripheral blood that in cats with reactive eosinophilias.[43] The hematocrit of leukemic cats was also significantly lower than in HES cats. A slight female predisposition was noted in the HES population. Malignancy in the granulocytic system that is primary in extramedullary sites is frequently of the eosinophil type and is termed *granulocytic sarcoma* (fig. 3.44).

Chronic Myelomonocytic Leukemia

As in the acute form of this disease, there is concurrent neoplasia of the granulocytic and monocytic lineages (fig. 3.45). The clinical syndrome is one of chronic disease with weight loss and poor appetite. There is characteristically a persistent low white cell count of about 4000 per µl, with a prominent "monocytic" component accompanied by anemia and marrow myeloid hyperplasia. Repeated examinations of blood and marrow are necessary, as are special stains and immunophenotyping, to confirm the diagnosis.

Mast Cell Leukemia

Since the mast cell is derived from a myeloid stem cell, mast cell leukemia (fig. 3.46) should be regarded as a myeloproliferative disorder.[49] Mastocytosis may occur as a de novo leukemia or may be associated with one or more solid tumors in dogs, cats, and horses. Mast cell leukemia and malignant solid tumors are characterized by uncon-

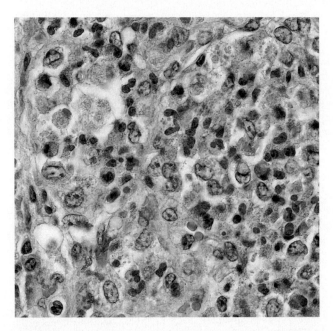

Fig. 3.44. Granulocytic sarcoma. Lung from a mature cat. Primitive mononuclear cells are blasts and promyelocytes of the eosinophil series; these are identified by their progeny, which have typical bilobed nuclei and prominent cytoplasmic granulation. H&E ×800.

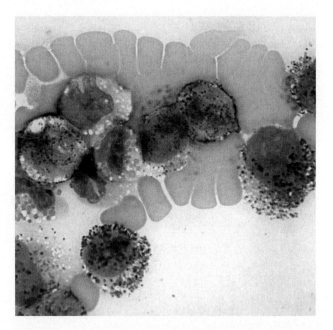

Fig. 3.46. Mast cell leukemia with basophilia. A 4-year-old spayed female saluki presented with severe depression, epistaxis, and icterus. The blood contained 45×10^3 leukocytes/µl, of which 40 percent were mast cells, 24 percent eosinophils, and 5 percent basophils. There was 18 g/dl of hemoglobin and 40×10^3 platelets/µl. A mast cell containing both eosinophilic and basophilic granules is present with a poorly granulated basophil and a mature neutrophil. The presence of increased numbers of basophils in the blood is closely associated with myeloid leukemia. Wright's ×1280.

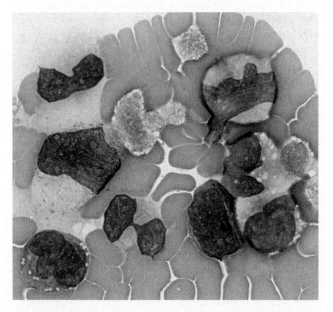

Fig. 3.45. Chronic myelomonocytic leukemia. A 5-year-old male Maltese dog was presented with a history of anorexia, lethargy, and weight loss for the past year. Blood contains 4.3×10^3 leukocytes/µl, of which 43 percent were *monocytoid* and 14 percent were bands and younger, 11.5 g/dl of hemoglobin, and 40×10^3 platelets/µl. Peripheral blood contains bilobed neutrophils, suggesting release from marrow at the myelocyte stage, and a predominant population of cells with irregularly shaped nuclei, some of which have hyperchromatic chromatin and small nucleoli. Cytoplasm is moderate to abundant in amount, with variable basophilia and infrequent cytoplasmic vacuolations. The condition was previously referred to as preleukemic syndrome and is now recognized as a form of myelodysplasia with a high probability of conversion to marrow failure or frank leukemia. Wright's ×1280.

trolled and progressive proliferation and infiltration of mast cells into various organs. In people, a diagnosis of mast cell leukemia is indicated if more than 10 percent atypical mast cells are found in blood.[50] The use of basic dyes such as Giemsa and toluidine blue may be helpful in demonstrating the specific metachromatic granules of the mast cells in tissue sections. Mild transient peripheral blood mastocytosis may be seen in acute inflammatory conditions, particularly those of the skin and gastrointestinal tract. Relative or absolute increases in bone marrow mast cells should be anticipated in hypoplastic and aplastic bone marrows of animals with, for example, estrogen toxicity.[51] The characteristic gross lesion of mastocytosis in the cat is marked splenomegaly (fig. 3.47). Mast cell tumors can be found throughout the alimentary tract.

Mast cells and basophils express certain similarities in mediator content, histochemical characteristics, and function; however, these lineages are distinct. Unlike basophils, the development and secretory function of mast cells are dependent on stem cell factor, the ligand for the receptor encoded by c-*kit*. The events responsible for mast cell proliferation in the leukemic process are largely unknown, but in people and dogs a derangement of the c-*kit* receptor and/or its ligand likely plays a primary role in this disease.[52-54]

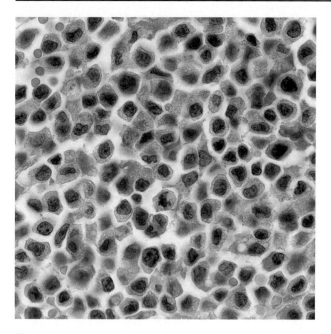

Fig. 3.47. Mast cell tumor. The spleen of a 16-year-old female domestic longhair cat with a history of anorexia, weight loss, and multiple cutaneous tumors that have developed over the last several months. There is atrophy of normal lymphoid tissue and solid filling of the sinus areas with a population of cells of moderate size that have round to irregular nuclei with hyperchromatic chromatin. Nucleoli are occasionally present, and there are frequent mitoses (center). The cytoplasm is abundant and finely granulated with distinct cellular boundaries. H&E ×800.

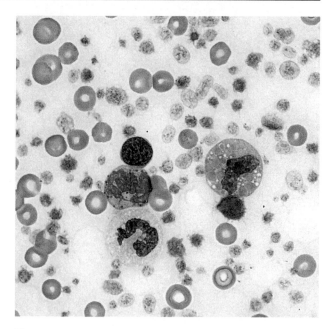

Fig. 3.48. Megakaryocytic myelosis. A 7-year-old Labrador female dog presented because of depression over the last several weeks. Blood contained 10×10^3 leukocytes/μl and increased numbers of basophils with irregular segmentation and immaturity to the promyelocyte stage. There is 2.9 g/dl hemoglobin and as many as 500 platelets per 100 × field, with the total count estimated at 2.4 million/μl. The blood film is representative of severe nonresponsive anemia with a massive increase in numbers of platelets, which vary in size, shape, granulation, and basophilia. Wright's ×1000.

Megakaryocytic Myelosis (Essential Thrombocythemia)

Megakaryocytic myelosis is an uncommon myeloproliferative disorder in dogs (fig. 3.48) and cats and is the chronic form of neoplasia in the megakaryocytic system. It is generally a disease of older animals and may be associated with hemorrhagic or thrombotic tendencies. The disorder is characterized by a persistent increase in numbers of platelets, some of which may be large or have variable, usually reduced, granulation and pale sky-blue basophilia. Typically, the bone marrow has increased numbers of normal or atypical megakaryocytic cells and persistently elevated platelet counts, often in excess of 1,000,000 per μl.[55-58] Plasma thrombopoietin was reported as normal in one dog with probable essential thrombocythemia.[58] Megakaryocytic myelosis may progress to megakaryoblastic leukemia, sometimes making the distinction difficult. Unequivocal diagnosis of megakaryocytic myelosis may require repeated examinations. Reactive thrombocytosis, which may be caused by acute infection, iron deficiency, chronic inflammatory diseases, or other myeloproliferative disorders, must be excluded before a diagnosis of megakaryocytic myelosis can be established.[59]

Polycythemia Vera

Polycythemia vera (PV) is characterized by an autonomous overproduction of normal appearing red cells. In people, the disease is accompanied by leukocytosis, thrombocytosis, and hepatosplenomegaly; myelofibrosis or acute leukemia may eventually develop. Primary erythrocytosis is sometimes used to describe the disease in animals since the hematological abnormalities and hepatosplenomegaly observed in people are unusual in animals. The disease is generally unsuspected, and the clinical course is indolent. Although a rare disease in animals, it has been described in the cat, dog, mice, and cattle.[60-62] Hematocrits in dogs with PV range from 65 to 82 percent.[61]

The diagnosis of PV requires an assessment of both plasma volume and red cell blood mass. Patients with an increased red cell mass are polycythemic; if the plasma volume is decreased (i.e., dehydration, shock) there is relative polycythemia. Absolute polycythemia may be present if the plasma volume is normal or increased. The determination of arterial blood oxygen saturation and serum erythropoietin concentration are necessary for making the distinction between primary and secondary forms of absolute polycythemia. Absolute polycythemia is classified as secondary if the patient is hypoxic or has a tumor and an increased serum concentration of erythropoietin.[63]

Absolute polycythemia is classified as primary (myeloproliferative disease or polycythemia vera) if the patient is not hypoxic, there are no other tumors, and the serum concentration of erythropoietin is normal or decreased.[64,65] In PV, the serum erythropoietin concentration is often undetectable and reticulocyte numbers are within normal limits. Occasionally, microcytic red cells are present in PV patients due to accelerated utilization of iron stores. Bone marrow examination is rarely helpful in making the diagnosis because, most often, there are no morphological abnormalities and the M:E ratios are normal, even if marrow cellularity is increased; occasional mild erythroid hyperplasia may be found.[61]

The Myelodysplastic Syndromes

The FAB classification of acute myeloid leukemias includes a group of conditions designated as myelodysplastic syndromes (MDSs).[5] Prior terminology has included refractory anemia, preleukemia, and smoldering acute leukemia. [66-68] The MDSs are a group of bone marrow disorders characterized by ineffective and dysplastic hematopoiesis that in people progresses to leukemia in 40–60 percent of cases.[69] The hematopoietic abnormalities in MDS include one or more cytopenias in the peripheral blood, while the bone marrow is most often hypercellular or normocellular with features of abnormal cellular maturation or dysplastic hematopoiesis (table 3.9). However, dysplastic changes are not confined to MDS, and reversible changes may occur in hematopoietic precursors secondary to the administration of certain drugs,[70,71] in certain dietary deficiencies, [72-74] following a severe leukopenic episode,[75] or in association with myeloid hyperplasia (MH).[6] Chloramphenicol has been reported to produce sideroblasts and siderocytes, while vincristine may produce nuclear fragmentation in bone marrow erythroid cells.[72,73] Although not associated with anemia, dyserythropoiesis including macrocytosis, megaloblastosis, and nuclear fragmentation has been reported to occur in toy and miniature poodles.[76]

More recently, it was suggested that three subtypes of MDS that occur in people have counterparts in the veterinary context.[7] The use of this scheme to distinguish prognostic subgroups has not yet been evaluated. A subtype was designated the myelodysplastic syndrome–refractory cytopenia (MDS-RC). Cases such as the refractory thrombocytopenias that have been reported in dogs in which there were ineffective thrombopoiesis and dysmegakaryopoiesis preceding the development of AML would fall into the MDS-RC subtype. The proposed veterinary scheme also combined refractory anemias with excess blasts or blasts in transformation into a single subtype, designated myelodysplastic syndrome with excess blasts (MDS-EB) (fig. 3.49). The third subtype, MDS-Er, is unique to the veterinary scheme. These are cases of MDS,

TABLE 3.9.   **Hematologic abnormalities and dysplastic changes in AML and MDS**

Peripheral Blood	Bone Marrow
Erythropoiesis	
Anemia (normocytic, normochromic & non-regenerative)	Hyperplasia (common), normoplasia, or hypoplasia
Anisocytosis & poikilocytosis	Increased blasts*
Normocytic macrocytes	Macronormoblastic erythropoiesis
Megaloblastosis	Megaloblastic or megaloblastoid erythropoiesis
Basophilic stippling	Sideroblastic erythropoiesis
Howell-Jolly bodies and nuclear fragments	Dysplastic erythropoiesis
Sideroblasts	Nuclear fragmentation or karyorrhexis, nuclear budding,
Nucleated red blood cells	unequal nuclear division, bi- or multi-nuclearity, enlarged
Blast cells	nucleoli, ringed sideroblasts, cytoplasmic vacuolation,
	defective hemoglobinization, asynchronous maturation
Granulopoiesis	
Neutropenia (common), neutrophilia (uncommon)	Granulocytic hyperplasia or granulocytic hypoplasia
Neutrophils with hyposegmented nuclei (acquired	Increased blasts*
Pelger-Huet anomaly), hypersegmented nuclei, or ring nuclei	Multinucleation
Persistent cytoplasmic basophilia	Hypo- or hypergranular promyelocytes or myelocytes
Abnormal cytoplasmic granulation	Lack of mature neutrophils
Monocytosis, eosinophilia (uncommon), basophilia (uncommon)	
Blast cells	Increased monocytic, eosinophilic, or basophilic lineage
Thrombopoiesis	
Thrombocytopenia (common) thrombocytosis (uncommon)	Megakaryocytic hyperplasia or hypoplasia
Giant platelets	Increased blasts *
Agranular platelets or platelets with giant granules	Dwarf or micromegakaryocytes
Vacuolated platelets	Multinucleation
Micromegakaryocytes	Megakaryocytes with large nucleus or multiple small nuclei
Blast cells	Abnormal granulation and vacuolation

*AML is defined by the bone marrow having equal to or greater than 30% blasts while the bone marrow in MDS is defined as equal to or greater than 6% but less than 30% blasts.

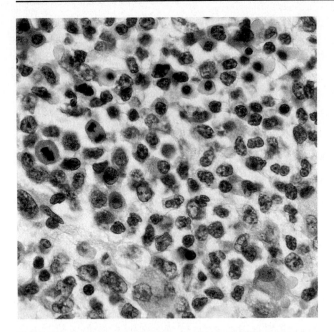

Fig. 3.49. Refractory anemia with excess blasts (RAEB). A mature cat with chronic nonresponsive anemia and recurring infections. Histologically, the marrow has reduced cellular density, an increased number of stromal cells and proliferative (dividing) phase cells, reduced marrow granulocyte reserves, and erythroid phthisis. H&E ×800.

usually in cats, in which erythroid progenitor cells are dominant in the bone marrow.[7]

Myelofibrosis

Fibroblastic proliferation and deposition of reticulin and/or collagen in the bone marrow defines myelofibrosis. Often the disease is suspected in animals that have combinations of cytopenias or pancytopenia and in which difficulty is experienced in obtaining aspirated bone marrow material (*dry tap*). Leukoerythroblastosis and poikilocytosis, including teardrop erythrocytes or dacryocytes, have been described in cats and dogs with myelofibrosis. Increased fibrous tissue may be apparent or may be easily demonstrated using reticulin or trichrome stains on core biopsies of bone marrow. Areas of bone marrow distant from blood vessels should be evaluated since a delicate network of reticulin and specialized fibrocytes is normally present around blood vessels.

In people, the marrow fibrosis that is seen with agnogenic myeloid metaplasia, a form of chronic myeloproliferative disease or trilineage neoplasia, occurs as a result of a reactive process. Both megakaryocytes and monocytes have been implicated in producing cytokines that upregulate fibroblast proliferation, collagen synthesis, angiogenesis, and osteogenesis.[77] Similar cases have been recorded in animals, but proof of an underlying hematological stem cell neoplasia is lacking. Myelofibrosis and/or osteosclerosis have been recognized in cats with myeloproliferative disease and in FeLV infected cats.[78-82] A dog with apparent

megakaryocytic leukemia, myeloid metaplasia, myelofibrosis, and osteosclerosis has been reported.[83] Myelofibrosis was described in dogs with smoldering granulocytic leukemia resulting from radiation exposure.[84] Dogs with hereditary pyruvate kinase deficiency may develop myelofibrosis and osteosclerosis as a terminal event.[85] An inherited form of myelofibrosis was described in pygmy goats.[86] Affected goats died between 6 and 12 weeks of age with anemia and neutropenia. Marrows showed megakaryocytic hyperplasia, and many organs had prominent extramedullary hematopoiesis.

Most cases of myelofibrosis in animals are idiopathic or occur secondarily in association with other diseases such as bone marrow necrosis.[87-89] Sequential bone marrow core biopsies have demonstrated that myelofibrosis is reversible in some cases.[87,89]

Splenic Lymphoid Hyperplasia and Nonlymphoid Splenic Diseases

Splenomegaly, for any reason, may result in increased destruction of peripheral blood cells or hypersplenism. Hematologically, hypersplenism is recognized as various peripheral blood cytopenias and increased bone marrow cellularity. Pancytopenia is an uncommon manifestation. Occasionally, hypersplenism may be seen in the absence of splenomegaly; however, the increased destruction and reticuloendothelial hyerplasia is evident microscopically, and hypersplenism can be demonstrated using radiolabeled blood cells and scintigraphy.

Splenomegaly is associated with a broad variety of illnesses. Congestion causing symmetrical enlargement may arise from heart failure, splenic torsion, and barbital anesthesia. Splenic hematomas are common and are usually single. Although very rare, some storage diseases due to inherited metabolic defects may cause splenomegaly from accumulation of substrate. Amyloidosis may cause symmetrical splenic enlargement. Systemic bacterial, rickettsial, protozoal, fungal, parasitic, and viral infections commonly produce lymphoid hyperplasia and often produce increased demands for the production of blood cells, resulting in extramedullary hematopoiesis or myeloid metaplasia. Hypereosinophilic syndrome may be associated with splenomegaly, particularly in cats, and can be considered a form of myeloid metaplasia. Splenomegaly is common in dogs with immune hemolytic anemia and results from a combination of splenic erythropoiesis and reticuloendothelial hyperplasia associated with the destruction of sensitized erythrocytes. Lymphoid and myeloid proliferations may be nodular or symmetrical, although in the dog nodular splenic enlargements predominate.[90,91] Nodular hyperplasia is seen in old dogs as single or multiple nodules, sometimes bulging from the surface. Nodules are composed of lymphocytes and histiocytes.

Lymphoid follicles are usually a prominent feature. Significant thrombocytopenia may result from altered venous blood flow around a relatively small focal hyperplastic nodule (fig. 3.50 A).

Splenic neoplasia may be primary or metastatic. The splenic tumors include lymphoma, myeloma, hemangioma, hemangiosarcoma, other sarcomas (leiomyosarcoma, fibrosarcoma, osteosarcoma, chondrosarcoma, malignant fibrous histiocytoma),[92,93,94] histiocytic proliferative disease, myelolipoma, and mast cell tumor. In a series of canine splenectomy specimens, fibrohistiocytic nodules appeared to form a continuum between nodular lymphoid hyperplasia and malignant stromal neoplasia (malignant fibrous histiocytoma, fig. 3.51). Interestingly, those lesions with a predominance of lymphoid cells were associated with longer survival whereas lesions with greater numbers of fibrohistiocytic cells and higher mitotic index had higher short-term mortality.

Agnogenic myeloid metaplasia, often with myelofibrosis, is a clonal proliferative disorder recognized in people and is a form of myeloproliferative (hematological malignancy) disease.[77]

Recently, splenectomy specimens from 65 dogs with severe and progressive splenomegaly were reviewed.[95] The clinicopathological syndromes of hemophagocytosis and hypersplenism were associated with microscopic splenic lesions of myeloid metaplasia, histiocytosis, erythrophagocytosis, and thrombosis with segmental infarction. Approximately half of the dogs had malignant histiocytic proliferative disease. The presence of splenic giant cells was significantly associated with an extremely poor prognosis. All dogs with splenic giant cells were dead at the end of the follow-up period, while dogs without this change were all alive at this time.

Splenic involvement is found in 57 percent of dogs, 43 percent of cats, and 30 percent of cattle with lymphoma.[96] The pattern is usually diffuse, with a uniform cell type in sinus areas, and there is at least mild atrophy of germinal centers and periarteriolar lymphoid sheaths. Follicular lymphoma and lymphoid hyperplasia are more difficult to distinguish. A similar follicular pattern of invasion in liver and lymph nodes and subendothelial invasion of large muscular sinuses in the spleen are supportive of lymphoma. Additionally, with follicular lymphoma there is essentially complete loss of the small mantle cuff lymphocytes normally present in the corona of benign splenic germinal centers. There is a uniformity of lymphocyte size as one traverses the follicle from side to side.

REFERENCES

1. Mayani, H. (1996) Composition and function of the hemopoietic microenvironment in human myeloid leukemia. *Leukemia* 10:1041–1047.

2. Bennett, J.M., Catovsky, D., Daniel, M.T., Flandrin, G., Galton, D.A.G., Gralnick, H.R., and Sultan, C. (1976) Proposals for the classification of acute leukemias (FAB cooperative group). *Brit J Haemotol* 33:451–458.

3. Bennett, J.M., Catovsky, D., Daniel, M.T., Flandrin, G., Galton, D.A.G., Gralnick, H.R., and Sultan, C. (1985a) Criteria for the diag-

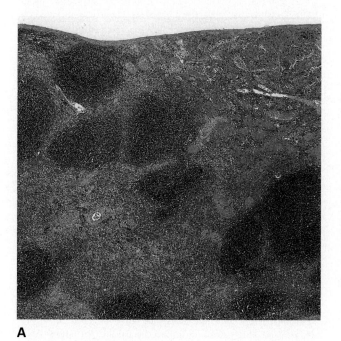

A

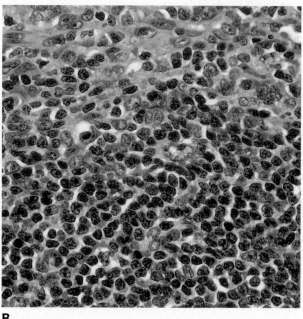

B

Fig. 3.50. Splenic nodular hyperplasia. **A.** A 3-year-old female standard poodle was presented for repeated oral bleeding associated with low platelet counts. Splenectomy was performed, and a 1.5 cm nodule was sectioned. Multifocal areas of lymphoid proliferation and a diffuse involvement of sinus areas had involved a focal area of the spleen and resulted in adjacent sinus distension. H&E ×30. **B.** Detail of A. The focal areas of lymphoid proliferation are composed of small, benign, mature lymphocytes with a few medium and large cells. H&E ×720.

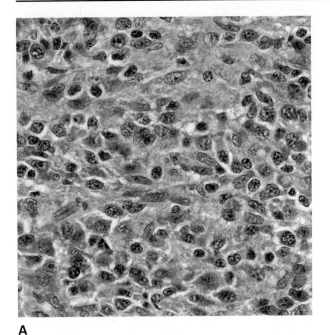

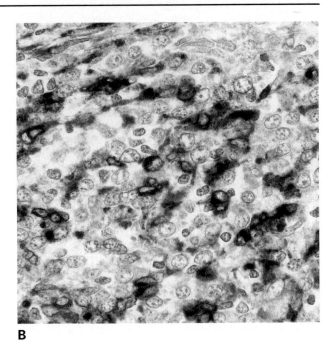

A

B

Fig. 3.51. Malignant fibrous histiocytoma. **A.** A 7-year-old male castrated golden retriever was presented because of an enlarged prescapular lymph node; this, as well as a mass from the axillary area, was removed. The mass is composed of a solid proliferation consisting of stromal cells with oval nuclei intermixed with a population of round cells that appear to be small and medium lymphocytes and larger cells with irregularly indented nuclei. H&E ×720. **B.** Immunohistochemical staining for lysozyme. On staining for macrophages, there are numerous positively staining cells compressed between surrounding stromal cells and lymphocytes. Lysozyme ×720.

nosis of acute leukemia of megakaryocyte lineage (M7) *Ann Int Med* 103:460–462.

4. Bennett, J.M., Catovsky, D., Daniel, M.T., Flandrin, G., Galton, D.A.G., Gralnick, H.R., and Sultan, C. (1985b) Proposed revised criteria for the classification of acute myeloid leukemias. *Ann Int Med* 103:620–629.

5. Jain, N.C., Blue, J.T., Grindem, C.B., Harvey, J.W., Kociba, G.J., Krehbiel, J.D., Latimer, K.S., Raskin, R.E., Thrall, M.A., and Zinkl, J.G. (1991) Proposed criteria for classification of acute myeloid leukemia in dogs and cats. *Vet Clin Pathol* 20:63–82.

6. Jain, N.C. (1993) Classification of myeloproliferative disorders in cats using criteria proposed by the animal leukemia study group: A retrospective study of 181 cases (1969–1992) *Comp Haematol Internat* 3:125–134.

7. Raskin, R. E. (1996) Myelopoiesis and myeloproliferative disorders. *Vet Clin N Amer Small Anim Pract* 26:1023–1042.

8. Valli V.E.O. (1992) The hematopoietic system. In Jubb, K.V.F., Kennedy, P.C., and Palmer, N. (eds.), *Pathology of Domestic Animals,* 4th ed. Academic Press, San Diego, pp. 114–133.

9. Facklam, N.R., and Kociba, G.J. (1985) Cytochemical characterization of leukemic cells from 20 dogs. *Vet Pathol* 22:363–369.

10. Grindem, C.B., Stevens, J.B., and Perman, V. (1986) Cytochemical reactions in cells from leukemic dogs. *Vet Pathol* 23:103–109.

11. Facklam, N.R., and Kociba, G.J. (1986) Cytochemical characterization of feline leukemic cells. *Vet Pathol* 23:155–161.

12. Jain, N.C. (1986) Cytochemistry of normal and leukemic leukocytes. In *Schalm's Veterinary Hematology,* 4th ed. Lea and Febiger, Philadelphia, pp. 909–939.

13. Grindem, C.B. (1996) Blood cell markers. *Vet Clin N. Amer Small Anim Pract* 26(5):1043–1064.

14. Messick, J., Carothers, M., and Wellman, M. (1990) Identification and characterization of megakaryoblasts in acute megakaryoblastic leukemia in a dog. *Vet Pathol* 27:212–214.

15. Colbatzky, F., and Hermanns, W. (1993) Acute megakaryoblastic leukemia in one cat and two dogs. *Vet Pathol* 30:186–194.

16. Cobbold, S., and Metcalfe, S. (1994) Monoclonal antibodies that define canine homologues of human CD antigens: Summary of the First International Canine Leukocyte Antigen Workshop (CLAW). *Tissue Antigens* 43:137–154.

17. Pucheu-Haston, C.M., Camus, A., Taboada, J., Gaunt, S.D., Snider, T.G., and Lopez, M.K. (1995) Megakaryoblastic leukemia in a dog. *J Amer Vet Med Assoc* 207:194–196.

18. Couto, C.G. (1985) Clinicopathologic aspects of acute leukemias in the dog. *J Amer Vet Med Assoc* 186:681–685.

19. Blue, J.T., French, T.W., and Kranz, J.S. (1988) Non-lymphoid hematopoietic neoplasia in cats: A retrospective study of 60 cases. *Cornell Vet* 78:21–42.

20. Monteith, C.N., and Cole, D. (1995) Monocytic leukemia in a horse. *Can Vet J* 36:765–766.

21. Durando, M.M., Allerman, A.R., and Harvey, J.W. (1994) Myelodysplastic syndrome in a quarter horse gelding. *Equine Vet J* 26:83.

22. Gasper, P.W., Rosen, D.K., and Fulton, R. (1996) Allogeneic marrow transplantation in a cat with acute myeloid leukemia. *J Amer Vet Med Assoc* 208:1280–1284.

23. Grindem, C.B., Stevens, J.B., and Perman, V. (1985) Morphological classification and clinical and pathologic characteristics of spontaneous leukemia in 17 dogs. *J Amer Anim Hosp Assoc* 21:219–226.

24. San Miguel, J.F, Sanz, G.F., Vallespi, T., Canizo, M.C., and Sanz, M.A. (1996) Myelodysplastic syndromes. *Critical Rev Oncol Hematol* 23:57–93.

25. Gewirtz, A. M. (1997) Antisense oligonucleotide therapeutics for human leukemia. *Crit Rev Oncog* 8:93–109.

26. Bounous, E.I., Latimer, K.S., and Campagnoli, R.P. (1994) Acute myeloid leukemia with basophilic differentiation (AML, M2-B) in a cat. *Vet Clin Pathol* 23:15.

27. Neame, P.B., Soamboonsrup, P., Leber, B., Carter, R.F., Sunisloe, L., Patterson, W., Orzel, A., Bates, S., and McBride, J.A. (1997)

Morphology of acute promyelocytic leukemia with cytogenetic or molecular evidence of the diagnosis: Characterization of additional microgranular variants. *Amer J Hematol* 56:131–142.

28. de The, H., Chomienne, C., Lanotte, M., Degos, L., and Dejean, A. (1990) The t(15;17) translocation of acute promyelocytic leukemia fuses the retinoic acid receptor α gene to a novel transcribed locus. *Nature* 347, 558–561.

29. Goldberg, S.L., Noel, P., Klumpp, T.R., and Dewald, G.W. (1998) The erythroid leukemias: A comparative study of erythroleukemia (FAB M6) and DiGuglielmo disease. *Amer J Clin Oncol* 21:42–47.

30. Watson, A.D.J., Huxtable, C.R.R., and Hoskins, L.P. (1974) Erythremic myelosis in two cats. *Aust Vet J* 50:29–33.

31. Zawidzka, Z.Z., Janzen, E., and Grice, H.C.(1964) Erythremic myelosis in a cat. A case resembling DiGuglielmo's syndrome in man. *Pathol Vet* 1:530–541.

32. Shimada, T., Matsumoto, Y., Okuda, M., Momoi, Y., Bonkobara, M., Watari, T., Goitsuka, R., Ono, D., Goto, N., and Tsujimoto, H. (1995) Erythroleukemia in two cats naturally infected with feline leukemia virus in the same household. *J Vet Med Sci* 57:199–204.

33. Harvey, J.W., Shields, R.P., and Gaskin, J.M. (1978) Feline myeloproliferative disease: Changing manifestations in the peripheral blood. *Vet Pathol* 15:437–448.

34. Clarkson, B.D., Strife, A., Wisniewski, D., Lambek, C., and Carpino, N. (1997) New understanding of the pathogenesis of CML: A prototype of early neoplasia. *Leukemia* 11:1404–1428.

35. Silver, R.T. (1993) Chronic myeloid leukemia. In Holland, J.F., Frei III, E., Bast, R.C., Jr., Kufe, D.W., Morton, D.L., and Weichselbaum, R.R. (eds.), *Cancer Medicine,* 3rd ed. Lea and Febiger, Philadelphia, pp. 1934–1942.

36. Jain, N.C. (1986). The neutrophils. In Jain, N.C. (ed.), *Schalm's Veterinary Hematology,* 4th ed. Lea and Febiger, Philadelphia, pp. 676–730.

37. Gosset, K.A., McWilliams, P.S., Enright, F.M., and Cleghorn, B. (1983) In vitro function of canine neutrophils during experimental inflammatory disease. *Vet Immunol Immunopathol* 5:151–159.

38. Thomsen, M.K., Jensen, A.L., Skar-Nielsen, T., and Flemming, K. (1991) Enhanced granulocyte function in a case of chronic granulocytic leukemia in a dog. *Vet Immunol Immunopathol* 28:143–156.

39. Daley, G.Q., Van Etten, R.A., and Baltimore, D. (1990) Induction of chronic myelogenous leukemia in mice by P210*bcr/alb* gene of the Philadelphia chromosome. *Science* 247:824–830.

40. Dungworth, D.L., Goldman, M., Switzer, J.W. and McKelvie, D.H. (1969) Development of a myeloproliferative disorder in beagles continuously exposed to ⁹⁰SR. *Blood* 34:610–632.

41. Mears, E.A., Raskin, R.E., and Legendre, A.M. (1997) Basophilic leukemia in a dog. J. Vet. Internal Med. 11:92–94.

42. Mahaffey, E.A., Brown, T.P., Duncan, J.R. Latimer, K.S., and Brown, S.A. (1987) Basophilic leukemia in a dog. *J Comp Pathol* 97:393–399.

43. Huibregtse, B.A., and Turner, J.L. (1994) Hypereosinophilic syndrome and eosinophilic leukemia: A comparison of 22 hypereosinophilic cats. *J Amer Anim Hosp Assoc* 30:591–599.

44. McEwen, S.A., Valli, V.E.O., and Hulland, T.J. (1984) Hypereosinophilic syndrome in cats: A report of three cases. *Can J Comp Med* 49:248–253.

45. Saxon, B., Hendrick, M., and Waddle, J. (1991) Restrictive cardiomyopathy in a cat with hypereosinophilic syndrome. *Can Vet J* 32:367–369.

46. Schrezenmeier, H., Thome, S.D. Tewald, F., Fleischer, B., and Raghavachar, A. (1993) Interleukin-5 is the predominant eosinophilopoietin produced by cloned T lymphocytes in hypereosinophilic syndrome. *Exp Hematol* 21:358–365.

47. Finlay, D. (1985) Eosinophilic leukemia in the cat: A case report. *Brit Vet J* 141:74.

48. Hardy, W.D., Jr. (1981) Hematopoietic tumors of cats. *J Amer Anim Hosp Assoc* 17:941–949.

49. Metcalfe, D.D., Baram, D., and Mekori, Y.A. (1997) Mast cells. *Physiol Rev* 77:1033–1079.

50. Torrey, E., Simpson, K., Wilbur, S., Munoz, P., and Skikne, B. (1990) Malignant mastocytosis with circulating mast cells. *Am J Hematol* 34:283–286.

51. Gaunt, S.D., and Pierce, K.R. (1986) Effects of estradiol on hematopoietic and marrow adherent cells of dogs. *Amer J Vet Res* 47:906–909.

52. Galli,S.J., and Hammel, I.(1994) Mast cell and basophil development. *Curr Opin Hematol* 1:33–39.

53. Reguera, M.J., Rabanal, R.M., Puigdemont, A., and Ferrer, L. (2000) Canine mast cell tumors express stem cell factor receptor. *Amer J Dermatopathol* 22:49–54.

54. London, C.A., Galli, S.J., Yuuki, T., Hu, Z.Q., Helfand, S.C., and Geissler, E.N. (1999) Spontaneous canine mast cell tumors express tandem duplication in the proto-oncogene c-*kit*. *Exp Hematol* 27:689–697.

55. Evans , R.J., Jones, D.R.E., and Gruffydd-Jones, T.J. (1982) Essential thrombocythaemia in the dog and cat: A report of four cases. *J Small Anim Pract* 23:457–467.

56. Harvey, J.W., Henderson, C.W., French, T.W., and Meyer, D.J. (1980) Myeloproliferative disease with megakaryocytic predominance in a dog with occult dirofilariasis. *Vet Clin Pathol* 11:5–11.

57. Dunn, J.K., Heath, M.F., Jefferies, A.R., Blackwood, L., McKay, J.S., and Nicholls, P.K. (1999) Diagnostic and hematologic features of probable essential thrombocythemia in two dogs. *Vet Clin Pathol* 28:131–138.

58. Bass, M.C., and Schultze, A.E. (1998) Essential thrombocythemia in a dog: Case report and a literature review. *J Amer Anim Hosp Assoc* 34:197–203.

59. Jain N.C. (1993) The platelets. In *Essentials of Veterinary Hematology.* Lea and Febiger, Philadelphia, p. 124.

60. Kaneko, J.J. (1968) Iron metabolism in familial polycythemia of Jersey calves. *Amer J Vet Res* 29:949–952.

61. McGrath, C.J. (1974) Polycythemia vera in dogs. *J Amer Vet Med Assoc* 164:1117–1121.

62. Khanna, C., and Bienzle, D. (1994) Polycythemia vera in a cat: Bone marrow culture in erythropoietin-deficient medium. *J Amer Anim Hosp Assoc* 30:45–49.

63. Giger, U. (1991) Serum erythropoietin concentrations in polycythemic and anemic dogs. In *Proceedings 9th Annual College Veterinary Internal Medicine Forum,* New Orleans, LA, pp. 143–145.

64. Cook, S.M., and Lothrop, C.D., Jr. (1994) Serum erythropoietin concentrations measured by radioimmunoassay in normal, polycythemic, and anemic dogs and cats. *J Vet Int Med* 8:18–25.

65. Hasler, A.H., and Giger, U. (1996) Serum erythropoietin values in polycythemia cats. *J Amer Anim Hosp Assoc* 32:294–301.

66. Maggio, L., Hoffman, R., Cotter, S.M., Dainiak, N., Mooney, S., and Maffei, L.A. (1978) Feline Preleukemia: An animal model of human disease. *Yale J Biol Med* 51:469–476.

67. Madewell, B.R., Jain, N.C., and Weller, R.E. (1979) Hematologic abnormalities preceding myeloid leukemia in three cats. *Vet Pathol* 16:510–519.

68. Couto, C.G., and Kallet, A.J. Preleukemic syndrome in a dog. (1984) *J Amer Vet Med Assoc* 184:1389–1392.

69. Masey, J.A. (1997) The myelodysplastic syndromes. *Br J Biomed Sci* 54:65–70.

70. Alleman, A.R., and Harvey, J.W. (1993) The morphologic effects of vincristine sulfate on canine bone marrow cells. *Vet Clin Pathol* 22:36–41.

71. Harvey, J.W., Wokfsheimer, K.J., and Simpson, C.F. (1985) Pathologic sideroblasts and siderocytes associated with chloramphenicol therapy in a dog. *Vet Clin Pathol* 14:36–42.

72. Harvey, J.W., French, T.W., and Meyers, D.J. (1982) Chronic iron deficiency anemia in dogs. *J Amer Anim Hosp Assoc* 18:946–962.

73. Fyfe, J.C., Giger, U., Hall, C.A., Jezyk, P.F., Klumpp, S.A., Levine, J.S., and Patterson, D.G. (1991) Inherited selective intestinal cobalamin malabsorption and cobalamin deficiency in dogs. *Pediatr Res* 29:24–31.

74. Myers, S., Wiks, S., and Giger, U. (1995) Macrocytic anemia caused by naturally occurring folate deficiency in the cat. *Vet Pathol* 32:547.

75. Messick, J.B., McCullough, S.M., Treadwell, N.G., Solter, P.F., and Hoffmann, W.E. (1997) What is your Diagnosis? A 15-year-old domestic shorthair cat. [Dysmyelopoiesis secondary to a severe leukopenic episode] *Vet Clin Pathol* 26:23.

76. Canfield, P.J., and Watson, A.D. (1989) Investigations of bone marrow dyscrasia in a poodle with macrocytosis. *J Comp Pathol* 101:269–278.

77. Tefferi, A. (2000) Myelofibrosis with myeloid metaplasia. *N Eng J Med* 342:1255–1265.

78. Hardy, W.D., Jr. (1981) Hematopoietic tumors of cats. *J Amer Anim Hosp Assoc* 17:921–940.

79. Hoover, E.A., and Kociba, G.J. (1974) Bone lesions in cats with anemia induced by feline leukemia virus. *J Natl Cancer Inst* 53:1277–1284.

80. Flecknell, P.A., Gibbs, C., and Kelly, D.F. (1978) Myelosclerosis in a cat. *J Comp Pathol* 88:627–631.

81. Zenoble, R.D., and Rowland, G.N. (1979) Hypercalcemia and proliferative, myelosclerotic bone reaction associated with feline leukovirus infection in a cat. *J Amer Vet Med Assoc* 175:591–595.

82. Blue, J.T. (1988) Myelofibrosis in cats with myelodysplastic syndrome and acute myelogenous leukemia. *Vet Pathol* 25:154–160.

83. Rudolph, R., and Hubner, C. (1972) Megakaryozytenleukose bein Hund. *Kleintier-Praxis* 17:9–13.

84. Dungworth, D.L., Goldman, M., Switzer, J.W., and McKelvie, D.H. (1969) Development of a myeloproliferative disorder in beagles continuously exposed to ^{90}Sr. *Blood* 34:610–632.

85. Prasse, K.W. (1977) Pyruvate kinase deficiency. In Kirk, R.W. (ed.), *Current Veterinary VII, Small Animal Practice.* W.B. Saunders,

86. Cain, G.R., East, N., and Moore, P.F. (1994) Myelofibrosis in young pygmy goats. *Comp Haematol Int* 4:167–172.

87. Weiss, D.J., and Armstrong, P.J. (1985) Secondary myelofibrosis in three dogs. *J Amer Vet Med Assoc* 187:423–425.

88. Reagan, W.J. (1993) A review of myelofibrosis in dogs. *Toxicol Pathol* 21:164–169.

89. Hoff, B., Lumsden, J.H., and Valli, V.E.O. (1985) An appraisal of bone marrow biopsy in assessment of sick dogs. *Can J Comp Med* 49:34–42.

90. Spangler, W.L., and Culbertson, M.R. (1992) Prevalence, type, and importance of splenic diseases in dogs: 1,480 cases (1985–1989). *J Amer Vet Med Assoc* 200:829–834.

91. Spangler, W.L., and Culbertson, M.R. (1992) Prevalence and type of splenic diseases in cats: 455 cases (1985–1991). *J Amer Vet Med Assoc* 201:773–776.

92. Weinstein, M.J., Carpenter, J.L., and Schunk, J.M. (1989) Nonangiogenic and nonlymphomatous sarcomas of the canine spleen: 57 cases (1975–1987). *J Amer Vet Med Assoc* 195:784–788.

93. Kerlin, R.L., and Hendrick, M.J. (1996) Malignant fibrous histiocytoma and malignant histiocytosis in the dog—convergent or divergent phenotypic differentiation. *Vet Pathol* 33:713–716.

94. Spangler, W.L., and Kass, P.H. (1998) Pathologic and prognostic characteristics of splenomegaly in dogs due to fibrohistiocytic nodules: 98 cases. *Vet Pathol* 35:488–498.

95. Spangler, W.L., and Kass, P.H. (1999) Splenic myeloid metaplasia, histiocytosis, and hypersplenism in the dog (65 cases). *Vet Pathol* 36:583–593.

96. Valli, V.E.O. (1992) The hematopoietic system. In Jubb, K.V.F., Kennedy, P.C., and Palmer, N. (eds.), *Pathology of Domestic Animals*, 4th ed. Academic Press, San Diego, p. 236.

4 Tumors of Joints

R. R. Pool and K. G. Thompson

INTRODUCTION
General Considerations

Several neoplastic and nonneoplastic lesions occur in the region of joints, tendon sheaths, bursae, and fasciae of domestic animals, but most are rare and not well characterized. Such lesions may arise from the synovioblastic mesenchyme or from any of the supporting tissues of the synovium or fascia, including fibrous, adipose, vascular and nervous tissue. The most common and best understood of these lesions is synovial sarcoma, but even this tumor is rare in animals. In dogs and cats, malignant synovial tumors outnumber benign joint lesions, but in horses, most synovial growths are benign.[1] These tumors are seldom reported in other domestic species.

No treatise on neoplasms of joints and related structures in domestic animals currently exists. There are only two published reviews of joint tumors in animals,[2,3] both of which deal primarily with synovial sarcomas of canine joints. The World Health Organization (WHO) bulletin on the histological classification of bone and joint tumors[4] includes only synovial sarcoma and villonodular synovitis as tumors and tumor-like lesions of joints and related tissues. This chapter presents a broader range of lesions, including tumors of tendon sheaths and fascia, and a range of nonneoplastic lesions that occur close to joints. Certain of these lesions also occur at other sites and are therefore mentioned in other chapters.

Diagnostic Considerations

Because of the similarity between synovial tumors and other mesenchymal tumors, the potential for misdiagnosis is high. This problem is compounded by the infrequent occurrence of such tumors in domestic animals and the lack of familiarity among pathologists with the variety of morphological patterns produced. An accurate clinical history combined with knowledge of the radiographic and macroscopic findings will enhance the likelihood of making a correct diagnosis.

Clinical Characteristics

Synovial tumors typically present as solitary lesions in older animals. They may be confused on clinical examination with a resolving infection, an organizing hematoma, synovial osteochondromatosis, tumoral calci-

nosis, or one of the idiopathic proliferative lesions of the synovium affecting a tendon sheath or a joint. Anatomical location of the lesion and the species of the animal affected are important diagnostic considerations. For example, villonodular synovitis affects only the metacarpophalangeal joint of racing thoroughbreds or quarter horses. Benign synovial tumors of tendons and tendon sheaths primarily involve the extensor and flexor tendons of the distal part of the limbs of dogs and cats, whereas malignant synovial tumors of joints occur mainly in the large weight-bearing joints of canine limbs.

Radiographic Evaluation

Radiographic examination using at least two views is helpful in assessing the approximate size and location of the lesion. Radiography will usually indicate whether a tumor is centered on or in the joint or a tendon sheath, whether it contains foci of mineralization, and whether there is any involvement of the adjacent bone. Sequential radiographs are helpful in estimating the rate of growth of the tumor. Benign synovial lesions involving bone organs evoke *nonaggressive* radiographic signs.[5] For example, villonodular synovitis of horses produces a characteristic abruptly bordered depression in the dorsal cortex of the distal end of the cannon bone at the insertion line of the joint capsule of the fetlock joint. Malignant tumors of joints usually produce *aggressive* radiographic signs of bone destruction[5] and are first detected as indistinct areas of osteolysis along the joint capsule insertion lines in the ends of bones on both sides of a diarthrodial joint. Radiographs may not distinguish, however, between primary and metastatic tumors of joints or tendon sheaths.

Pathological Considerations

Knowledge of the exact anatomical location of a synovial tumor may be critical for making a definitive diagnosis because microscopic patterns of synovial tumors may mimic those of other soft tissue neoplasms. Pathologists must rely on the observations of the surgeon who resected the mass or must carefully dissect out the lesion themselves. It should also be remembered that certain members of this group of tumors may arise in unexpected sites. For example, synovial tumors may arise in intermuscular fasciae unassociated with joints and tendon sheaths.[3]

To fully appreciate the range of histological patterns of tumors and tumor-like lesions of joints and related

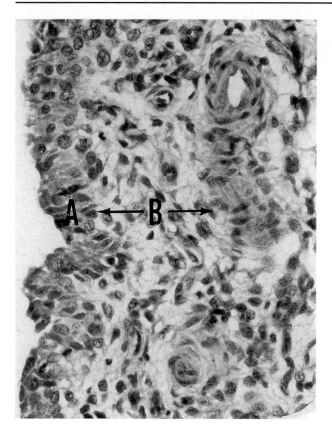

Fig. 4.1. Synovial lining of a normal equine joint. Synoviocytes not only line the intimal layer *(A)* of the synovial membrane, but they are also the most common cell type in the subintimal layer *(B)*.

structures, the pathologist should be familiar with the microscopic appearance of joints, tendons and tendon sheaths, bursae, ligaments, fasciae, and adjacent soft tissues in animals of all age groups. Synoviocytes not only line the surface of synovial membranes, but they are also the most common cell type found in the subsynovial tissue (fig. 4.1). Synovial tissue also lines tendon sheaths and bursae. Cells with light and electron microscopic features of synoviocytes are found in intermuscular fascia and in the interfascicular framework of muscles, tendons, and ligaments, where they produce the proteoglycan that provides the suppleness of these soft tissues. In response to trauma, chronic irritation and other nonspecific influences, this cell population may undergo metaplasia to form fibrous tissue and cartilage. Fibrocytes of tendons and ligaments commonly undergo metaplasia to produce chondroid tissue within tendons and ligaments and in the fibrous layer of joint capsules that have been subjected to chronic trauma or degenerative joint diseases. Synovial chondromas arise from metaplasia of synoviocytes in the synovial lining of joints with chronic degenerative joint disease. Some chondrosarcomas arising in soft tissues possibly originate in nests of metaplastic chondrocytes.

In most cases, histopathology is required in order to make a definitive diagnosis of lesions in the region of joints. Cytological examination of fine needle aspiration biopsies or scrapings prepared from tissue biopsies may

provide useful information on the nature of the tumor cells. However, the number of cells harvested for examination from such lesions is often small, and the architectural details, which are so important in making a diagnosis of synovial sarcoma, are not apparent.

REFERENCES

1. Pool, R.R. (1990) Tumors and tumor-like lesions of joints and adjacent soft tissues. In Moulton J.E. (ed.), *Tumors in Domestic Animals,* 3rd ed. University of California Press, Berkeley.
2. Madewell, B.R., and Pool, R.R. (1978) Neoplasms of joints and related structures. *Vet Clin N Amer* 8:511–521.
3. Lipowitz, A.J., Fetter, Q.W., and Walker, M.A. (1979) Synovial Sarcoma of the Dog. *J Amer Vet Med Assoc* 174:76–81.
4. Slayter, M.V., Boosinger, T.R., Pool, R.R., DÑmmrich, K., Misdorp, W., and Larsen, S. (1994) *Histological Classification of Bone and Joint Tumors of Domestic Animals.* World Health Organization. 2nd series, vol. 1. Armed Forces Institute of Pathology, American Registry of Pathology, Washington, D.C.
5. Morgan, J.P. (1979) Systemic radiographic interpretation of skeletal diseases in small animals. *Vet Clin N Amer* 4:611–626.

BENIGN TUMORS AND TUMOR-LIKE LESIONS IN AND AROUND JOINTS

These lesions are uncommon, and because they are reported so seldom in domestic animals, their clinicopathological features are incompletely characterized. The lesions in animals are generally named after human disorders perceived to be their analogs. This classification procedure has two deficiencies. First, the nomenclature for this group of human lesions has not been standardized,[1,2] and second, appropriate detailed comparative studies of the morphology and biological behavior of these lesions have not been done. In this section the authors have attempted, where applicable, to follow the morphological criteria used for the diagnosis of comparable disease processes in humans and have merged that with information known about lesions in animals. The benign tumors and reactive lesions covered in this chapter are listed in table 4.1.

Benign Synovioma

This term has been used to classify tumor-like nodules found occasionally in the capsule of the human knee joint, but its use is discouraged.[2] Microscopically, these lesions are composed of complex, slit-like cavities lined by hyperplastic, but otherwise normal, synovial cells. Lining cells are supported by well-differentiated fibrous tissue, usually infiltrated with chronic inflammatory cells. Similar lesions have been seen in the synovium of joints and tendon sheaths of horses, dogs, and goats.[3] The infrapatellar pouch of the stifle joint is a common location for such lesions in dogs (fig. 4.2). On histological examination,

TABLE 4.1.   Benign tumors and tumor-like lesions of joints

Benign synovioma
Idiopathic proliferative lesions of the synovium
　　Pigmented villonodular synovitis of joints
　　Localized nodular synovitis of joints
　　Villonodular synovitis of the equine metacarpophalangeal
　　　joint
　　Localized nodular tenosynovitis
　　Benign giant cell tumor of tendons and tendon sheaths
　　Fibroma of tendons and tendon sheaths
　　Metabolic disorders of the synovium
　　"Myxoma" of the synovium
Synovial hemangioma or hamartoma of horses
Synovial chondroma and osteochondroma
Tumoral calcinosis
Ganglia, synovial cysts, and adventitious bursitis
Heterotopic, metaplastic, and reactive bone formation in soft
　　tissues
　　Fibrotic myopathy and ossifying myopathy of horses
　　Localized myositis ossificans of the dog and cat
　　Generalized myositis ossificans of the pig and cat

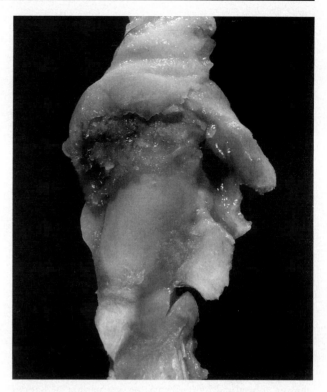

Fig. 4.2.   Tumor-like lesion of chronic synovial hyperplasia in the infra-patellar pouch of a canine stifle joint. The term *benign synovioma* should not be used for these reactive lesions.

these "tumors" include foci of chronic synovitis, villous hyperplasia without a major inflammatory cell response, and hematomas in varying stages of organization. The diagnosis and description should match these histological lesions rather than be classified as a tumor.

Idiopathic Proliferative Lesions of the Synovium

The synovium is a complex tissue composed of synoviocytes arising from synovioblastic mesenchyme and of supporting subsynovial soft tissues such as blood vessels, nerves, fat cells, and fibroblasts. Well-differentiated benign tumors (e.g., hemangiomas, Schwannomas, lipomas, and fibromas) may arise from the supporting cell population. Tumors of supporting tissue have the same morphological appearance and clinical behavior as tumors arising in other soft tissue sites. Although benign tumors of subsynovial soft tissues are apparently rare in animals, their origin in subsynovial tissue most likely goes unrecognized unless the lesion is carefully dissected. By contrast, idiopathic proliferative responses and tumors of the synovium arise only from cells of synovioblastic mesenchyme, and the synovial origin of these lesions is more apparent because of their unique morphology.

Villonodular Synovitis of Joints and Tendon Sheaths

General Considerations

This disorder is characterized by a diffuse pigmented villonodular lesion or a localized nodular lesion in the joint capsule of a knee, ankle, hip, or shoulder joint, or a localized nodular lesion in a tendon sheath (i.e., nodular tenosynovitis) in the hands or feet of young adults or middle-aged persons.[4,5] A lesion of nodular tenosynovitis (also called localized villonodular tenosynovitis, giant cell

tumor of the tendon sheath, benign giant cell tumor of soft tissue, or xanthofibroma) may be attached to a tendon, to a tendon sheath, or to muscle fascia. It may also arise in deep fibrous tissue.[2]

Clinically, there is swelling, pain, and limited motion of the affected part. Erosion of adjacent bony structures may occur. Treatment involves surgical excision, but local recurrence is a frequent problem.[6] Progression to malignancy does not occur.[5]

Grossly, the diffuse lesion is a brown, papillary, spongy mass with nodular areas, and it derives its color from hemosiderin. The solitary lesions are nodular and lobulated and may also have brown pigmentation.

Histologically, the diffuse and solitary lesions are similar except for the prominence of villous structures in the diffuse lesion of joints. Papillary projections and fibrous tissue are intermixed with a pleomorphic population of synoviocytes, foamy cells, and hemosiderin-laden macrophages. Mitotic figures are easily found in the proliferating synoviocytes, and multinucleated giant cells are invariably present.[1]

The etiology of this disorder is unknown, and lack of understanding of its nature causes a dilemma in classifying the lesion. Certain pathologists believe that these synovial lesions in and around joints and tendon sheaths of humans are reactions to repeated synovial trauma and bleeding.[6] This opinion is supported in part by the production of similar lesions in the stifle joints of dogs and rabbits following repeated injections of fresh blood or saline.[7,8] Unlike the natural disease, however, experimental lesions regress following cessation of injections. Some pathologists consider these lesions to be a variant of benign fibrous histiocytoma,[2,5] or *benign giant cell tumors of soft tissue.* They propose that the diffuse villonodular lesion of joints known as pigmented villonodular synovitis is a variant of benign fibrous histiocytoma involving a larger surface area of the synovium and having features of granulomatous inflammation. Further evidence that the disease is neoplastic rather than inflammatory is presented in a study of 81 human cases.[9]

Only occasional cases resembling human villonodular synovitis have been reported in animals. An 8-year-old Labrador retriever had presumptive lesions of villonodular synovitis in both coxofemoral joints,[10] and similar lesions were reported in the carpal joint of an 8-year-old dog.[11]

Pigmented Villonodular Synovitis of Joints

Classification

It is undetermined whether this lesion is a reaction to chronic injury and hemarthrosis or is a variant of benign fibrous histiocytoma. On the basis of the few cases examined by the authors, the lesion in animals appears to be a unique synovial response and possibly a variant of fibrous histiocytoma.

Incidence, Age, Breed, and Sex

Pigmented villonodular synovitis has been reported in the stifle joint of a 4-year-old Labrador retriever[12] and in both stifle joints of a 10-year-old crossbreed dog.[13] We have seen what we consider to be animal analogs of this disease in older dogs of both sexes from large and medium breeds. One putative lesion arose in the hock joint of an old male goat.

Clinical Characteristics

The lesion is first recognized because of joint distention or gradual onset of lameness. The affected joint is not initially warm or painful. Later, if there has been bony erosion along joint margins, pain due to joint instability may be recognized. The cases we have examined were initially thought to be examples of very low grade synovial sarcomas. In one older dog long-term "cure" followed limb amputation. Radical synovectomy was successful in another case. [13] The goat with this lesion was destroyed because of marked lameness brought about by chronic degenerative joint disease affecting several joints, including the joint with the synovial lesion.

Sites

Pigmented villonodular synovitis may potentially occur in any major weight-bearing joint. In dogs, three lesions were in hip joints, two in stifle joints, and one in the antebrachiocarpal joint. The published reports in two further dogs[12,13] also involved the stifle. The caprine lesion was located in a hock joint.

Gross Morphology

Most of the synovium of the joint was replaced by a thick, tan to dark brown, shaggy mat of villi. Amber-colored joint fluid was excessive in amount but retained its normal viscosity. In two dogs the abnormal synovial tissue produced superficial erosions in the femoral neck along the joint capsule insertion line. Bone erosion was not apparent in the other canine lesions. While all of the affected canine joints had mild gross changes of degenerative joint disease, similar degenerative changes were also present in the same joint of the opposite leg. In the goat, however, pigmented villonodular synovitis occurred in a hock joint affected with severe chronic degenerative joint disease. Marked fibrosis of the joint capsule and chronic adhesive tenosynovitis of the flexor tendons caudal to the hock joint suggested that joint infection probably preceded the development of the degenerative joint disease. The role, if any, that severe degenerative joint disease played in the development of pigmented villonodular synovitis in this joint was undetermined.

Radiographic Appearance

Several small and smoothly contoured erosions were present in the cortical surface of the femoral neck along the joint capsule insertion line of the hip joints in two canine cases. Massive intra-articular soft tissue proliferation, without bony involvement, was noted radiographically in the dog with bilateral villonodular synovitis.[13] Periarticular bone destruction was a more prominent feature in the tarsus of the goat. All affected joints that were radiographed showed distention of the joint capsule.

Histological Features

The affected synovium is several times greater than the normal thickness (fig. 4.3 A). Most synovial surfaces are altered by complex villous formation, while in other areas fused villi form a nodular surface. Deep areas have either a solid pattern or contain numerous irregular slits lined by synovial cells. The subsynovial cells are isochromic and without anaplastic features (fig. 4.3 B). Mitotic figures are occasionally found. Many synovial cells are ovoid, whether located on a surface or within the stroma, and some histiocyte-like synoviocytes contain fine granules of hemosiderin in their cytoplasm (fig. 4.3 C). Other synovial cells located within the stroma have a fusiform shape and can not always be distinguished from fibroblasts. Binucleate synoviocytes are not uncommon. A few multinucleated giant cells are present within the depths of the lesion. In a recent study of human villonodular synovitis, the multinucleated cells were shown to possess immunochemical characteristics of osteoclasts.[14] Macrophages, some of which are filled with hemosiderin, and small lymphocytes are scattered diffusely in small numbers throughout the lesion. Occasionally, both types of

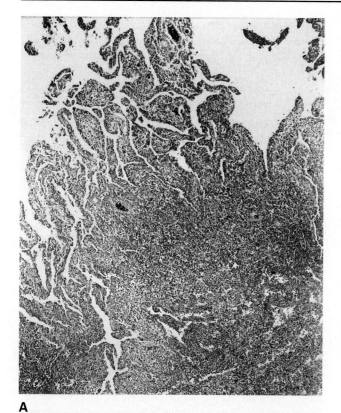

A

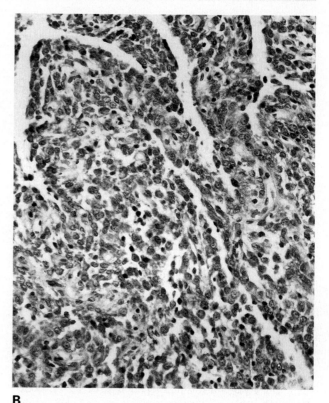

B

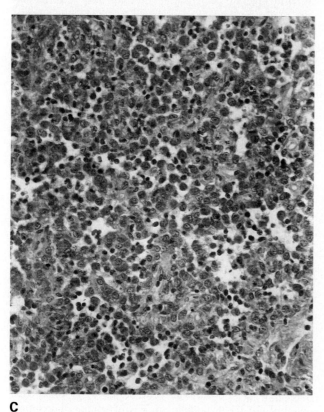

C

Fig. 4.3. Pigmented villonodular synovitis in the antebrachiocarpal joint of a dog. **A.** Hyperplastic synovium having a villous surface and both solid and slit-like patterns in deep tissues. **B.** Villi and clefts lined by synoviocytes. Subintimal synoviocytes and stromal cells are without anaplastic features. **C.** Solid area of subintima is populated by numerous large synoviocytes resembling histiocytes and by small lymphocytes.

inflammatory cells will form in dense clusters, especially at the border of the lesion. Proliferative synoviocytes spread into the fibrous layer of the joint capsule. They do not, however, extend beyond the joint capsule and do not invade the adjacent soft tissues in the specimens that we have examined. In some cases, the synovial response enters vascular channels in the periarticular bone along joint capsule insertion lines and mediates bone resorption by osteoclasts.

Differential diagnoses include chronic infectious synovitis, synovitis in response to hemarthrosis, reactive synovitis in response to osteoarthrosis, and low grade synovial sarcoma.

Growth and Metastasis

These are proliferative lesions that demonstrate slow but progressive enlargement. In humans, these lesions do not undergo malignant progression and do not metastasize.[5] In none of the animal lesions was there evidence of local vessel invasion or metastasis to local lymph nodes or to internal body organs. Long-term follow-up was available in only one case, a dog with pigmented villonodular synovitis of the hip joint. This dog was without local or systemic recurrence 6 years following amputation at the hip joint.

Localized Nodular Synovitis of Joints

Animal analogs of this human disorder have not been reported. The only purported example of this human disease is villonodular synovitis of the equine metacarpophalangeal joint (discussed in the following section). This unique equine lesion is most likely a synovial reaction to chronic trauma and is not a variant of fibrous histiocytoma, as has been proposed for humans.[2,5]

Villonodular Synovitis of the Equine Metacarpophalangeal Joint

Classification

This condition is characterized by hypertrophy of either the metacarpophalangeal or metatarsophalangeal joint capsule at its dorsoproximal attachment. It is considered to be a chronic inflammatory response involving the synovium, following repetitive trauma.[15,16] In the metacarpophalangeal joint of normal horses, a fold of tissue projects distally from the dorsal proximal attachment of the joint capsule.[16] In villonodular synovitis this fold of tissue becomes hypertrophic and develops into a nodular mass.[15,16]

Incidence, Age, Breed, and Sex

The condition was first reported in 1976,[15] and since then several cases per year are seen in any busy equine clinic treating race horses. Lesions are more commonly seen in racing thoroughbreds than in racing quarter horses. Both sexes are affected equally, and affected horses range in age from 2 to 13 years.[15]

Clinical Characteristics

Horses are presented because of an insidious onset of lameness and a soft tissue swelling over the dorsal surface of the distal end of the third metacarpal bone. The fetlock joint is distended and stiff. The degree of pain and lameness is accentuated when the joint is flexed and the horse is made to jog. In many cases, the joint has been treated unsuccessfully, prior to diagnosis, by firing, blistering, intra-articular injections of corticosteroids, and rest.

Gross Morphology

Lesions vary greatly in size and appearance, but all are centered on the synovial pad of fibrous and adipose tissue located between the dorsal articular margin of the distal end of the third metacarpal or metatarsal bone and the proximal insertion line of the joint capsule on the distal end of the bone. The lesion appears to be caused by trauma, when the pad is struck by the dorsal articular margin of the first phalanx during excessive dorsiflexion of the fetlock joint. Large lesions of a relatively short duration may have the gross appearance of an organizing hematoma of the synovial pad. Most lesions are pale, rubbery, lobulated, and pedunculated (fig. 4.4 A). They may involve the entire synovial pad or be located only on one side of the midline. In our experience many lesions are located on the medial side of the sagittal ridge of the cannon bone. The traumatized synovial pad with its pedunculated mass will often extend over the articular margin. When the lesion is removed, the underlying articular cartilage is pitted, and the surface of the dorsal cortex of the cannon bone is eroded.

Radiographic Appearance

The characteristic finding is a smoothly contoured erosion in the dorsal cortex of the distal end of the third metacarpal bone located just proximal to the articular margin. An intra-articular soft tissue mass centered in the proximal recess of the dorsal part of the fetlock joint can be demonstrated by positive contrast arthrography.

Histological Features

Microscopic appearance varies with the duration of the lesion. Acute lesions may have the features of an organizing hematoma. In these cases immature granulation tissue arising from the traumatized synovial pad invades the borders of the hematoma. Hemosiderin-laden macrophages are prominent. Subacute lesions (fig. 4.4 B) still have areas of necrosis and organizing hematoma, but the granulation tissue is orderly and mature. Chronic lesions are composed primarily of poorly vascularized, dense, irregular fibrous tissue covered on the joint surface by a thin layer of synoviocytes. Inflammatory cells, including plasma cells and macrophages are invariably present and are generally arranged in cuffs around blood vessels.

Growth and Metastasis

Most of these lesions enlarge over a period of a few weeks. Lesions with a history of rapid growth over a few days usually result from a hematoma. There is no morphological evidence of neoplasia. Excision of the mass appears to be curative, and prognosis for return to the previous level of performance is favorable.[15,16]

Localized Nodular Tenosynovitis

Classification

In humans, several terms have been used for this disorder, including giant cell tumor of tendon sheath, fibrous histiocytoma, xanthofibroma, benign synovioma,[1] benign giant cell tumor of soft tissue,[2] fibrous histiocytoma of tendon sheath, and nodular tenosynovitis.[5] Although there is no uniform agreement on the basic nature of the human lesion (reaction versus true neoplasm), the lesion undoubtedly arises in the synovium and has no metastatic potential.[1]

Although localized nodular tenosynovitis has been diagnosed only occasionally in dogs,[17] it is likely that many of the focal, nodular tumors of tendons previously diagnosed as benign synoviomas[18,19] were additional examples of this condition. The term *benign synovioma* is no longer in use.[2,20] It is possible that benign giant cell tumor of tendons and tendon sheaths, in addition to fibroma of tendons and tendon sheaths, are actually variants of localized nodular tenosynovitis, but until there is a greater

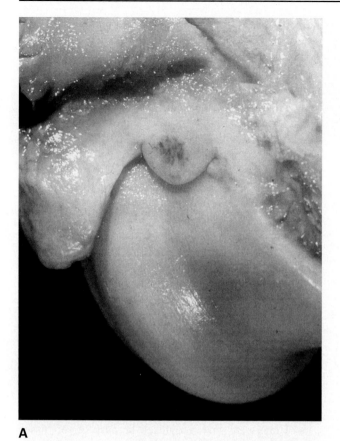

A

B

Fig. 4.4. Villonodular synovitis of the equine metacarpophalangeal joint. **A.** Pedunculated nodular lesion attached by a broad stalk to the dorsal proximal joint capsule (courtesy of S.E. Weisbrode). **B.** Area from margin of lesion showing necrosis, resolving inflammation, and fibroplasia.

understanding of the origin and nature of these tumor-like conditions, they are being considered separately.

Incidence

One report[17] describes nodular tenosynovitis in two dogs, a 9-year-old female Great Dane and an 8-year-old spayed female doberman pinscher. Additional likely examples or variants of the condition have been observed in six male and female dogs of medium and large breeds, ranging in age from 7 to 14 years.

Clinical Characteristics

The presenting sign is mild lameness that may be related to tendon dysfunction. This may result in partial loss of flexion or extension of the paw or splaying of digits. The tumor is palpated as a solitary movable mass associated with tendons of the legs. Dissection and complete surgical extirpation of the tumor can be curative, but local recurrence is common. In humans these tumors have no metastatic potential,[1] and this is probably also true for animal analogs.

Sites

Tendons and tendon sheaths of the extensors and flexors of the forefeet and hind feet , especially at the level of the metacarpus and metatarsus, are the most commonly affected sites. These solitary lesions, however, may also have a more proximal location in the limbs (e.g., the Achilles apparatus and the bursa surrounding the tendon of the long digital extensor muscle). By comparison, most of these tumors in humans are found between the wrist and the fingertips and between the ankle and the toetips.[5]

Gross Morphology

The masses in the Great Dane and the doberman pinscher measured $2.0 \times 2.0 \times 1.0$ cm and $0.5 \times 0.5 \times 1.0$ cm, respectively.[17] Both were firm, and in one case the lesion was firmly attached to a tendon. In one of our cases the tumor involved the bursa and the tendon of the long digital extensor muscle (fig. 4.5 A). This tumor was firm and had a pale nodular appearance on cut section. In two additional cases the tumors produced firm solitary nodules centered on tendons of the digits. On cut surface there were foci of mineralized cartilage within the villonodular centers of the tumor masses. Although tumors of this group appear to have discrete borders formed partly by compression of adjacent soft tissues, microscopic examination often shows infiltration of tumor tissue beyond the gross limits of the lesion.

Radiographic Appearance

Lesions were identified by soft tissue swelling and failed to induce bony responses in adjacent osseous tissue. Although these tumors are not malignant in humans, they may occasionally erode contiguous bone surface by pressure and/or cytokines produced by the inflammatory cells.[5]

Histological Features

The microscopic appearance of localized nodular tenosynovitis varies widely among different lesions and even within the same lesion. Although there is no typical pattern, most tumors will have at least a few cleft-like spaces lined by synoviocytes and moderately vascular areas of proliferating fibrous tissue (fig. 4.5 B). Cellular areas of the stroma often contain mainly synoviocytes, some multinucleated giant cells, a varying number of hemosiderin-laden macrophages, and clusters of mononuclear inflammatory cells (fig. 4.5 C). In some nodular areas, a spindle cell proliferation may resemble fibroma (fig. 4.5 D). In a few cases the spindle cell component may whirl around vessels and mimic the pattern of a hemangiopericytoma (fig. 4.6 A). While foam cells seen in human tumors[1] are not a common feature of animal tumors, some lesions will contain synoviocytes with highly vacuolated cytoplasm, apparently producing proteoglycan (fig. 4.6 B). An overlap in morphological features occurs between certain cases of localized villonodular tenosynovitis and benign giant cell tumor of tendons and tendon sheaths (fig. 4.6 C). The confusion lies in just how many giant cells must be present before a lesion can be called a benign giant cell tumor. Since there appears to be a continuum between the two, in the future we may recognize that the benign giant cell tumor of tendons and tendon sheaths is a variant of localized nodular tenosynovitis. Areas of hemorrhage and mineralization may be present. Two of the tumors we have examined had multiple areas of cartilage within the stroma of the lesion (fig. 4.6 D). The cartilage appeared to be formed by metaplasia from synoviocytes.

Growth and Metastasis

Enlargement occurs over a period of several weeks to a few months in most cases. Local recurrence is common following local resection. Infiltration of adjacent soft tissue occurs, but no malignant transformation or metastatic disease should be anticipated.

Benign Giant Cell Tumor of Tendons and Tendon Sheaths

Classification

These benign tumors arise from synovioblastic mesenchyme surrounding tendons and tendon sheaths and are characterized microscopically by the presence of numerous multinucleated giant cells. In humans, this entity is included under lesions of localized nodular tenosynovitis[1] and has been variously regarded as either a variant of fibrous histiocytoma[5] or classified as *benign giant cell tumor of soft tissues.*[2] Since this probably is the most common tumor of tendons and tendon sheaths of animals, and is a well-recognized entity in the veterinary literature, it is

included here as a separate entity even though it is recognized that it may eventually be classified as a variant of localized nodular synovitis.

Incidence, Age, Breed, and Sex

These tumors have been reported to occur infrequently in tendon sheaths of dogs and cats [18,19,21] and were formerly recognized as benign synovioma or benign giant cell synovioma. Since the term synovioma is no longer in use,[2,20] it is likely that these authors were describing benign giant cell tumors of tendons and tendon sheaths, although some of these lesions may have been examples of localized nodular tenosynovitis containing giant cells. The youngest affected animal was 6 years old, and tumors were found in both sexes. Too few cases have been studied to determine if breed and sex are factors.

Benign giant cell tumor is the most common tumor of tendons and tendon sheaths and ranks second only to synovial sarcoma of joints in the number of tumors affecting joints and tendons. Most tumors occurred in older dogs and cats; the youngest animal affected was a dog that was 2 years, 4 months of age. One example was found in a middle-aged horse.

Clinical Characteristics

Tumors are first recognized because of soft tissue swelling sometimes associated with a mechanical disturbance in tendon function. Most are firm to touch and are movable. Tumors centered on flexor tendons of the feet often produce skin erosions on the palmer and plantar surfaces of feet and become less movable. Prior to diagnosis by biopsy, many tumors of the feet were initially treated as inflammatory lesions. Much of the pain in these cases is probably due to secondary bacterial inflammation. Local recurrence following surgical excision is common.

Sites

The majority of benign giant cell tumors of tendons and tendon sheaths arise in association with the extensor and flexor tendons distal to the carpus and tarsus.

Gross Morphology

Tumors centered on a solitary tendon usually have a fusiform to ovoid shape and are loosely attached to the tendon (fig. 4.7 A). On cut surface they leave a fleshy appearance and borders are distinct. Tumors of the feet are more likely to form an irregular, pad-like tumor mass that entraps one or more of the digital branches of the extensor or flexor tendons (fig. 4.7 B). The tumor tissue feels firm or spongy. On cut surface the tumor mostly has a pale, nodular appearance, but usually there are also areas of soft mucoid tissue. The apparent distinctness of the border of the tumor is misleading since tumor tissue infiltrates the interstices of adjacent structures.

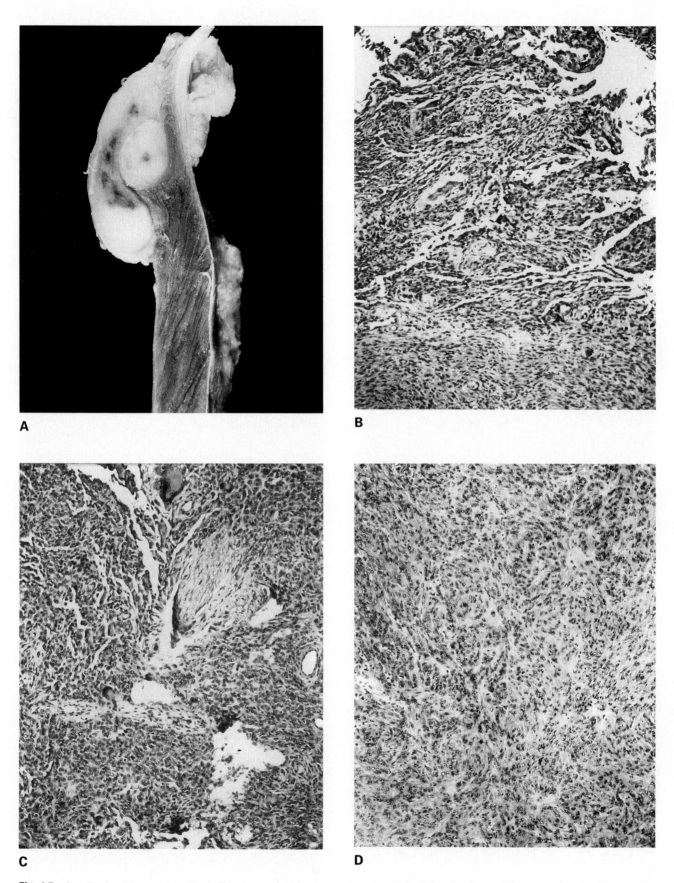

Fig. 4.5. Localized nodular tenosynovitis. **A.** Pale, firm, nodular tumor mass has arisen in the lining of the bursa of the tendon of origin of the long digital extensor muscle. **B.** Note cleft-like pattern in superficial tissues overlying solid areas at base. **C.** An area with numerous multinucleated giant cells scattered among synoviocytes and stromal cells. **D.** Nodular area formed by benign spindle shaped and polygonal cells resembling a fibroma.

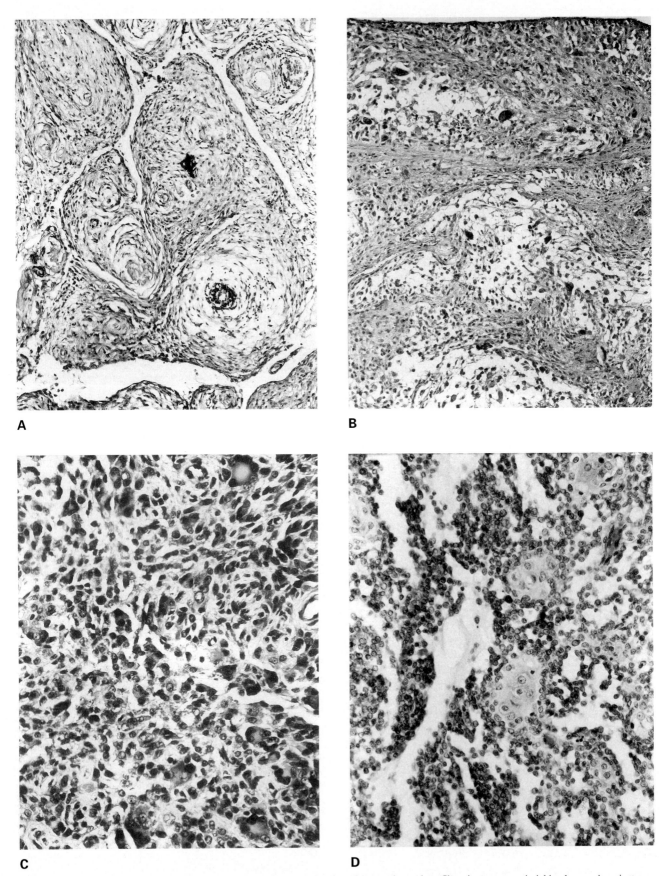

Fig. 4.6. Some patterns of localized nodular tenosynovitis. **A.** Stromal cells whirl around vessels or fibers in a pattern mimicking hemangiopericytoma. **B.** Benign tumor cells accompanied by giant cells produce proteoglycan rich islands separated by irregular septa of fibrous tissue. **C.** Area resembling benign giant cell tumor of tendons and tendon sheaths. **D.** Area in which benign tumor cells undergo metaplasia and form cartilage.

Radiographic Appearance

The tumor typically produces a soft tissue mass, often lying against a bone, but usually does not elicit a bony response.

Histological Features

A wide range of tissue patterns may be produced in these tumors, but all have in common the presence of large numbers of multinucleated tumor giant cells. The giant cells appear to result from fusion of proliferating synovioblastic mesenchymal cells. Small mononuclear inflammatory cells may be dispersed randomly in the tumor or concentrated at the border of the lesion. Some tumors have a solid pattern (fig. 4.7 C), whereas cleft-like spaces will be the predominant feature in other tumors (fig. 4.7 D). Most benign giant cell tumors of tendons and tendon sheaths have a mixture of both patterns. In these benign tumors the cells of the proliferating synoviocyte population do not have anaplastic features. While mononuclear synovoicytes have varying ovoid to fusiform shapes, their nuclei are open faced and isochromic. The appearance of the mononuclear synoviocytes is, in our experience, a better indication of biological behavior than is the confusing appearance presented by the giant cell population. Until further studies are done, however, the well-recognized caution in attempts to grade giant cell tumors of the bone[6] should also pertain to giant cell tumors of tendons and tendon sheaths.

Growth and Metastasis

Individual tumors will vary in their rate of growth after first recognition. These tumors are not believed to have metastatic potential, nor are they considered to undergo continuous malignant progression. Too few cases, however, have been followed closely to make that assumption with confidence. The major clinical problem is local recurrence following attempts at surgical removal.

Fibroma of Tendons and Tendon Sheaths

Classification

Solitary or multiple, discretely bordered nodular masses of dense fibrous tissue resembling fibromas of the dermis and subcutis of animals may arise from mesenchyme in the paratendon or tendon sheath. These tumors have been described in humans and in the horse.[22] Whether these are unique tumors or sclerotic variants of localized nodular tenosynovitis has not been determined.

Incidence, Age, Breed, and Sex

These uncommon lesions have been described in two immature quarter horse fillies.[22] Our series also includes three fibromas of tendons occurring in a 4-year-old male Welsh corgi dog.

Clinical Characteristics

Fibromas of tendons or tendon sheaths demonstrate slow but progressive enlargement over a period of several months. They may cease growth and remain asymptomatic. An animal may have more than one fibroma affecting the same tendon, or solitary fibromas may affect tendons of different legs in the same animal. These nodules are usually first discovered during grooming of the animal. Skin over the lesion is normal and freely movable. Fibromas are firm but are not warm or painful to palpation. They do not cause lameness, and their major importance is that of a blemish.

None of the three fibromas in the dog recurred following surgical removal. Incomplete removal of tendon fibromas on the dorsomedial surface of the hock of one horse was followed by regrowth of the lesion to its original size during the course of a year. However, neither further enlargement of the recurrent tumor mass nor lameness subsequently occurred. The second horse returned to racing 7 months after surgical removal of a solitary tendon fibroma on a foreleg. The tumor did not recur.

Sites

Extensor tendons at the level of the carpus and tarsus were affected in the two horses. The Welsh corgi had three separate fibromas, two involving the digital branches of the extensor tendon lying over the metacarpus of a forefoot and one involving the Achilles tendon of a hind leg.

Gross Morphology

Fibromas have distinct borders and may appear to have a fibrous capsule. They are not firmly attached to adjacent soft tissue structures and are ovoid to fusiform in shape. In one horse with multiple tendon fibromas the nodules varied from 2 to 4 cm in diameter. The solitary nodule in the second horse measured 3.5 × 5.5 cm. The largest of the three nodules in the dog was 1.5 cm in diameter. On cut surface the tumor tissue was white, firm, and solid.

In horses, the fibromas were so firmly attached to the tendon that the tumor could not be removed without causing tendon damage. All three tendon fibromas in the dog were freed from their tendon attachment by blunt dissection. While none of the fibromas had cavitations, canine tendon fibromas appeared to have remnants of the synovial lining between tendon attachment sites.

Radiographic Appearance

Tendon fibromas produce nodular soft tissue masses. In one affected horse[22] a tendon fibroma caused a depression in the cortex of the underlying radius.

Histological Features

These discretely bordered nodular tumors consist of solid masses of dense fibrous tissue having a low capillary density. In some lesions a histological pattern of coarse interwoven bundles of dense collagenous tissue

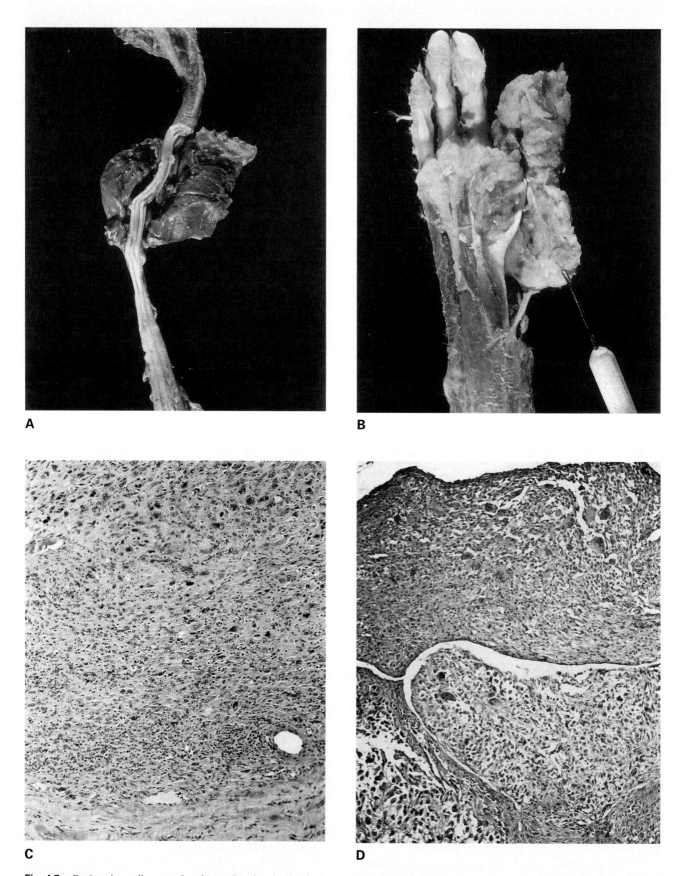

Fig. 4.7. Benign giant cell tumor of tendons and tendon sheaths. **A.** Tumor centered around the common digital extensor hind leg of a dog at the level of the talocrural joint. **B.** Tumor involving a digital branch of the flexor tendon of a cat's paw. **C.** Solid pattern with numerous benign multinucleated tumor cells and small lymphocytes. **D.** Clefts separate irregular nodules of tumor tissue. Numerous giant cells are found among pleomorphic tumor cells.

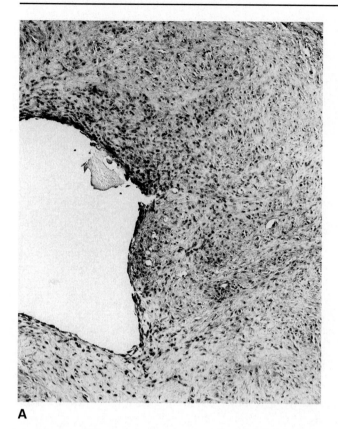

A

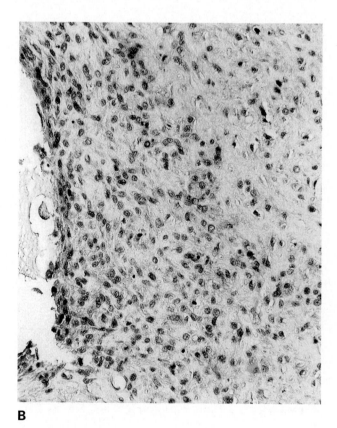

B

Fig. 4.8. Fibroma of a tendon sheath of a dog. **A.** Solid mass of unpatterned dense fibrous tissue lined by synovium. **B.** Polygonal and fusiform tumor cells are without anaplastic features and some resemble synovial lining cells.

predominates. Entrapped cells are mostly mature spindle-shaped fibroblasts. In other lesions (figs. 4.8 A,B), polygonal and fusiform cells are set in unpatterned fields of dense fibrous tissue. While cleft formation was not observed within the tendon fibromas of the horse and dog, remnants of a synovial surface, probably the lining of a synovial sheath, were present in cross sections through the canine fibromas. No synoviocytes, hemosiderin-laden macrophages, xanthoid cells, multinucleated giant cells, or adipose cells were recognized within the tumor masses. Inflammatory cells were also absent in these lesions. A differential diagnosis would include a fibrosed lipoma, a sclerotic variant of localized nodular tenosynovitis, a sclerotic Schwannoma, or a healed focal area of chronic tendon injury or infection.

Growth and Metastasis

Fibromas of tendons and tendon sheaths typically show slow, progressive growth over a period of months and then maintain their size and shape indefinitely. Since these nodular tumors do not produce lameness, they are not clinically important other than as a blemish. Total surgical excision of a fibroma may not be possible without producing a substantial disruption of the tendon, as was the case in one horse.[22] Incomplete removal of the tendon fibroma was followed by local regrowth of the nodule to its original size over a period of a few months. In the Welsh corgi described here and in the other horse,[22] surgical removal was curative. No malignant change was encountered in any of the fibromas.

REFERENCES

1. Fechner, R.F. (1976) Neoplasms and neoplasm-like lesions of the synovium. In Ackerman, L.V., Spjut, H.J., and Abell, M.R. (eds.), *Bones and Joints.* Williams and Wilkins Co., Baltimore, pp. 157–186.
2. Lattes, R. (1982) Tumors of the soft tissue. In *Atlas of Tumor Pathology.* 2nd series, fascicle 1, revised. Armed Forces Institute of Pathology, Washington, D.C.
3. Pool, R.R. (1990) Tumors and tumor-like lesions of joints and adjacent soft tissues. In Moulton, J.E. (ed.), *Tumors in Domestic Animals,* 3rd ed. University of California Press, Berkeley.
4. Johnston, A.D., and Parisien, M.V. (1979) Soft tissue tumors about the knee. *Orthop Clin N Amer* 10:253–279.
5. Ackerman, L.V., and Rosai, J. (1974) *Surgical Pathology,* 5th ed. Mosby Co., St. Louis.
6. Spjut, H.J., Dorfman, H.D. Fechner, R.E., and Ackerman, L.V. (1971) Tumors of bone and cartilage. In *Atlas of Tumor Pathology.* 2nd series, fascicle 5. Armed Forces Institute of Pathology, Washington, D.C.
7. Young, J.M., and Hudacek, A.G. (1954) Experimental production of pigmented villonodular synovitis in dogs. *Amer J Pathol* 30:799–812.
8. Roy, S., and Ghadially, F.N. (1969) Synovial membrane in experimentally produced chronic haemarthrosis. *Ann Rheum Dis* 28:402–411.
9. Rao, A.S., and Vigorita, V.J. (1984) Pigmented villonodular synovitis (giant cell tumor of the tendon sheath and synovial membrane). *J Bone Joint Surg* 66–A:76–94.

10. Kusba, J.K., Lipowitz, A.J., Wise, M., and Stevens, J.B. (1983) Suspected villonodular synovitis in a dog. *J Amer Vet Med Assoc* 182:390–392.

11. Hanson, J.A. (1998) Radiographic diagnosis—Canine carpal villonodular synovitis. *Vet Radiol Ultr* 39:15–17.

12. Somer, T., Sittnikow, K., Henriksson, K., and Saksela, E. (1990) Pigmented villonodular synovitis and plasmacytoid lymphoma in a dog. *J Amer Vet Med Assoc* 197:877–879.

13. Marti, J.M. (1997) Bilateral pigmented villonodular synovitis in a dog. *J Small Anim Pract* 38:256–260.

14. Darling, J.M., Goldring, S.R., Harada, Y., Handel, M.L., Glowacki, J., and Gravallese, E.M. (1997) Multinucleated cells in pigmented villonodular synovitis and giant cell tumor of tendon sheath express features of osteoclasts. *Amer J Pathol* 150:1383–1393.

15. Nickels, F.A., Grant, B.D., and Lincoln, S.D. (1976) Villonodular synovitis of the equine metacarpophalangeal joint. *J Amer Vet Med Assoc.* 168:1043–1046.

16. Rose, P. L. (1988) Villonodular synovitis of horses. *Comp Cont Educ* 10:649–654.

17. Carb, A., and Halliwell, W.H. (1982) Nodular tenosynovitis of the flexor tendon in two dogs. *J Amer Anim Hosp Assoc* 18:867–871.

18. Cotchin, E. (1954) Further observations on neoplasm in dogs with particular reference to site of origin and malignancy. *Brit Vet J* 110:274–286.

19. Davies, J.D., and Little, N.R.F. (1972) Synovioma in a cat. *J Small Anim Pract* 13:127–133.

20. Misdorp, W., and van der Heul, R.O. (1976) Tumors of bones and joints. *Bull WHO* 53:265–282.

21. Hulse, E.V. (1966) A benign giant cell synovioma in a cat. *J Pathol Bacteriol* 91:269–271.

22. Adams, S.B., Fessler, J.F., and Thacker, H.L. (1982) Tendon fibromas in two horses. *Equine Vet J* 14:95–97.

Metabolic Disorders of the Synovium

Biopsy tissues have been examined from several dogs with slowly progressive lameness centered in either a solitary point or a pair of major limb joints. The dogs were of different breeds, including a standard poodle, a doberman pinscher, an Irish setter, and a Labrador retriever. Both sexes were represented. The joints were not warm or very painful on palpation, but they were distended with joint fluid of normal color and consistency. During arthrotomy, to obtain an excisional biopsy, the clinicians observed marked villous hyperplasia of synovium in affected joints. Bilateral elbow joint disease in the poodle was progressive over a 2 year period, and the dog was euthanized without a necropsy or gross examination of the elbow joints. The doberman pinscher and the Irish setter were lost to follow-up. The Labrador retriever was the only immature dog in this group, and he was necropsied because marked epiphyseal dysplasia affected all major epiphyses of the long bones.

The histological appearance of the synovium varied among the cases, but all affected joints had a thickened synovium with villous hypertrophy. The synovium was distended by a localized proliferation of pale, foamy cells, presumably synoviocytes (figs. 4.9 A,B). Inflammatory cells and multinucleated giant cells were absent. The cases differed primarily in the morphological appearance of the foamy synoviocytes. These differences

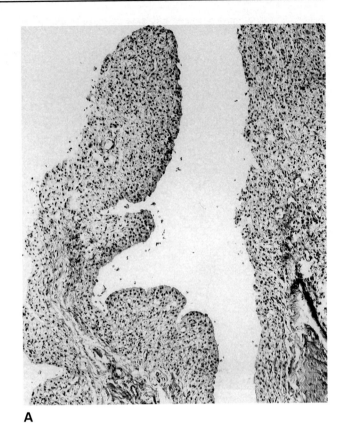

A

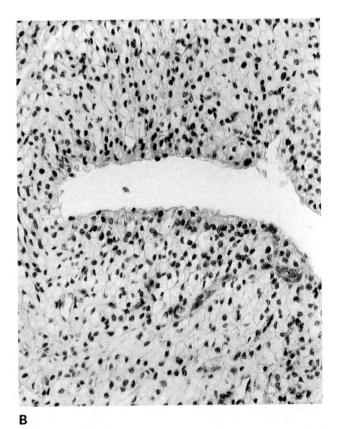

B

Fig. 4.9. Metabolic disorder of the synovium in the elbow joint of a dog. **A.** Hypertrophic villus of joint is heavily infiltrated with foamy cells. **B.** Foamy cells fill the subintima of the synovium.

included the location of the nucleus in the cell, the number and size of the cytoplasmic vacuoles, and whether there was granular material present within the cytoplasm. In the puppy with epiphyseal dysplasia the pale granular material occurring in the foamy cytoplasm of synoviocytes was also present in chrondrocytes of the deformed epiphyses. No similar foamy cells were present in lymph nodes draining the appendicular skeleton or in the bone marrow of this dog.

While we do not know the cause of these synovial lesions and can only assume that they have a metabolic basis, our intention in presenting them here is for a differential diagnosis for synovial tumors.

Myxoma of the Synovium

Classification

We have observed a morphologically unique lesion centered in the synovial linings of joints from three dogs. This lesion does not seem to belong to any of the existing categories of tumors or tumor-like conditions of animal joints. We have used the term *myxoma of the synovium* to identify this disorder until more is learned about the nature of this condition. The term *myxoma* reflects both the gross and microscopic appearance of the lesion and its biological behavior. A comparable entity does not appear to have been reported in humans, and there are no previous reports in animals.

Incidence, Age, Breed, and Sex

Myxoma of the synovium was found in synovial joints of three dogs. The affected dogs included a mature male doberman pinscher, a 16-year-old spayed female doberman pinscher, and a 9-year old spayed female English spaniel.

Clinical Characteristics

In the two doberman pinschers, the tumors produced cool, initially painless swellings that apparently caused mechanical lameness. In both cases, the synovial tumors involved a single stifle joint. In the mature male dog, synovectomy of the affected femoropatellar joint sac was apparently curative. Within a few months after surgery, the dog resumed its daily jogging routine with its owner, and no local or systemic disease has been observed in 2 years since surgery. The stifle lesion in the older female doberman was locally infiltrative and resulted in limb amputation. No local recurrence at the amputation stump or metastatic disease was found at necropsy a short time later.

The tumor in the English spaniel arose in ipsolateral apophyseal (synovial) joints of the second and third cervical vertebrae. Lesions in this case did not produce clinical signs and were discovered during a general necropsy for an unrelated condition. Tumor tissue had infiltrated beyond the joint capsule and had extended into adjacent muscle fascia, making surgical extirpation impossible.

Sites

The tumors affected one stifle joint from each of two dogs and two adjacent ipsolateral apophyseal joints (C-2 and C-3) in the cervical spine of a third dog.

Gross Morphology

Myxomas of the synovium were composed of multiple nodules of pale gelatinous tissue that replaced the synovial lining of the affected joints (fig. 4.10 A). There was no destruction of articular cartilage or of the joint margins. Joint fluid was excessive in amount but normal in color and consistency. In two cases the myxoid tumor tissue was observed to extend beyond the fibrous layer of the joint capsule and to infiltrate along facial planes of adjacent musculature.

Radiographic Appearance

There was no radiographic evidence of destruction of joint margins or periarticular new bone formation.

Histological Features

Most of the normal synovial architecture is replaced by pale, poorly vascularized myxoid nodules (fig. 4.10 B). These nodules are formed by stellate mesenchymal cells set in a loose matrix of delicate collagen fibrils and a large volume of proteoglycan. Large nodules arise by coalescence of smaller nodules. Cellularity and density of collagen fibrils increase at the borders of intrasynovial nodules. Once the tumor penetrates beyond the fibrous layer of the joint capsule, however, the border of the neoplasm is indistinct and tumor tissue extends along fascial planes. In parts of the synovium not replaced by myxoid nodules, the synovium is infiltrated with clusters of macrophages and other mononuclear inflammatory cells (fig. 4.10 C). This inflammatory response was a striking feature in the synovium of the male doberman pinscher whose joint was successfully treated by synovectomy.

True myxomas must be differentiated from areas of myxomatous change in Schwannomas, liposarcomas, rhabdomyosarcomas, mesenchymomas, and fibrous tumors.[1] The relative paucity of blood vessels and the retention by tumor cells of a stellate shape, even in areas of secondary fibrosis, support a diagnosis of myxoma.[1] Both features were present in these tumors of the synovium in dogs.

Growth and Metastasis

Growth in these few cases was slow but progressive. Once tumor tissue has extended beyond the fibrous layer of the joint capsule, it infiltrates along muscle fascial planes. In one case, synovectomy appeared to be curative, possibly because tumor tissue was still confined to the synovial lining and was removed along with the synovial membrane. Local recurrence should be anticipated in advanced cases. Metastases in true myxomas are exceedingly rare in humans.[1] It is likely that the metastatic potential for these canine lesions is also low.

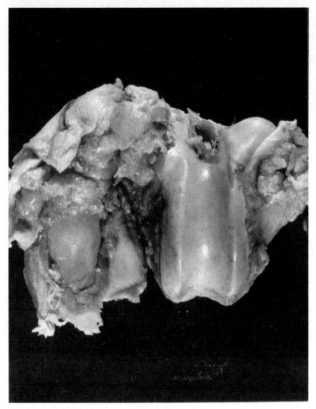

A

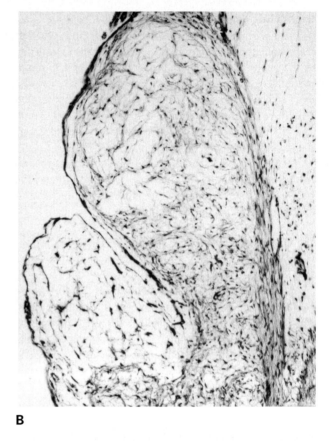

B

Fig. 4.10. *Myxoma* of the synovium of a canine stifle joint. **A.** Multi-nodular, pale gelatinous tissue replaces the normal synovial membrane. Note lack of articular cartilage destruction. **B.** Normal synovial subintima is replaced by nodular aggregations of poorly vasularized mucoid connective tissue. **C.** Area of chronic lymphocytic inflammation in a synovial myxoma.

C

Synovial Hemangioma or Vascular Hamartoma in the Tendon Sheath of the Horse

Benign vascular lesions involving the carpal and digital sheaths of the forelegs have been reported in young horses of several breeds.[2,3] There is some question whether these lesions are true hemangiomas or vascular hamartomas. The latter term was favored in a recent report of three cases involving the subcutis and deep tissues of the dorsal carpus in thoroughbred fillies ranging in age from 1 to 3 years.[3] In one case the mass over the lateral digital extensor tendon sheath had been apparent since the filly was several weeks of age and had slowly increased in size until it was 6 cm in diameter. There had been no lameness or radiographic evidence of bone involvement. In the 3-year-old filly, the lesion only became clinically apparent when a subcutaneous hematoma developed at the site.[3] In each case, the basic lesion consisted of abnormal vascular structures varying from large cavernous spaces containing thrombi to more disorderly vascular channels lined by plump endothelial cells. In one case, an initial diagnosis of possible malignancy was made on examination of a surgical biopsy.[3] This animal was euthanized on the basis of suspected malignancy and recurrence of the tumor after initial surgery. The diagnosis of vascular hamartoma was made after more detailed examination of the lesion.[3] Surgical removal was successful in the other two fillies but

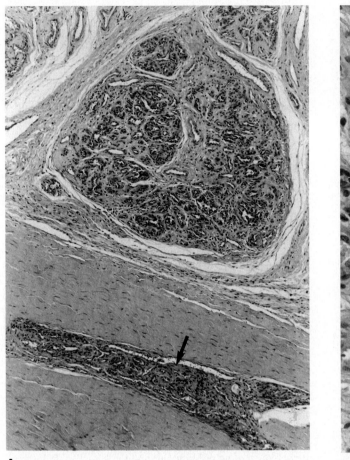

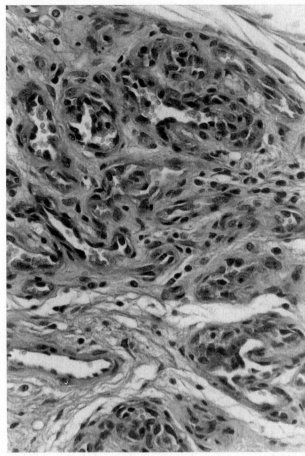

A   **B**

Fig. 4.11.   Vascular hamartoma of the tendon sheath in a 10-month-old standardbred colt (tissues courtesy of A.C. Johnstone). **A.** Clusters of capillary structures forming nodules adjacent to the superficial digital flexor tendon and, in one area (arrow), separating collagen bundles within the tendon. **B.** Same lesion at higher magnification. Proliferating endothelial cells are forming capillary structures but do not have features of malignancy.

required repeat surgery in one case due to incomplete removal at the first attempt.

It is possible that hemangiosarcomas reported in the tarsal synovial sheath of a 2-year-old standardbred colt[4] and a 10-month-old standardbred colt[5] were in fact benign vascular tumors that would be more appropriately classified as hemangiomas or vascular hamartomas. In one case,[4] the tendon sheath contained three circumscribed, sessile growths that were removed successfully at surgery. In the other case,[5] the diagnosis of malignancy was based on apparent invasion of the insertion of the superficial digital flexor tendon (fig. 4.11 A,B), but the author has subsequently reclassified the lesion as vascular hamartoma (personal communication).

In a case observed by one of the authors (R.R.P.), the condition was recognized because of filling of the affected sheaths with a blood stained fluid. No pain or lameness was evident. Surgical removal was attempted, but severe bleeding was a major problem. On surgical exploration of the tendon sheath, the tumor appeared as a solitary, deep red, multinodular structure that arose in the synovial lining of a recess in the tendon sheath. Clotted blood sometimes

adhered to the surface of the tumor. Bleeding into the sheath was apparently due to the trauma of locomotion. Microscopic examination showed that well-differentiated small caliber vessels tended to grow in nodular aggregations. Vascular nodules were randomly separated by septae of mature fibrous tissue. Endothelial cells lining the vessel walls did not have anaplastic features, and miotic figures were uncommon.

Similar clusters of well-differentiated capillaries separated collagen bundles near the insertion of the superficial digital flexor tendon in the 10-month-old standardbred colt (fig. 4.11 A,B).[5]

The occurrence of these lesions in young horses supports their classification as vascular hamartomas rather than hemangiomas, in spite of the fact that some cases were not recognized until the animals were 2 or 3 years of age. They are characterized by slow growth and, in some cases, by infiltration of adjacent structures, but they show no convincing microscopic features of malignancy and do not metastasize. Because of their location, surgical removal is often difficult and hemostasis presents a challenge, but recurrence is unlikely to follow complete excision.

Synovial Chondroma and Synovial Osteochondroma

Classification

Synovial chondromas are believed to represent metaplastic nodules of hyaline cartilage that develop in the synovial linings of bursae, tendon sheaths, and synovial joints. The stimulus for the metaplastic transformation of synovial cells into chondrocytes is unknown. Synovial osteochondromas are synovial chondromas that have undergone endochondral ossification.

Synovial chondromatosis is a condition in which the synovial lining of a bursa, tendon sheath, or joint has numerous synovial chondromas. If the majority of these metaplastic cartilage nodules have undergone bony replacement, the term *synovial osteochondromatosis* should be used to describe the lesion.

In humans it is unclear whether synovial chondromatosis is a neoplastic disease[6] or if synovial chondromas develop secondary to trauma, chronic irritation, inflammation, or other disturbances of the synovium. Although there is a widespread belief that synovial chondromas arise by metaplasia of synovial cells within the synovial membrane, an alternative hypothesis suggests that the cartilage nodules may in fact be derived from fragments of cartilage from the articular surface.[7] Such fragments released into the joint space may continue to enlarge as they derive their nutrients from the synovial fluid, and some may become incorporated into the synovial membrane. It is conceivable that the cartilage fragments could survive and continue to enlarge within the richly vascular synovial membrane and become ossified following vascular invasion. Primary (i.e., idiopathic) and secondary forms of the disorder occur in animals, with the secondary form being more common.

Incidence, Age, Breed, and Sex

Primary synovial chondromatosis and osteochondromatosis are rarely encountered in animals. One case involved the femorotibial bursa of a 16-year-old quarter horse mare.[8] We have seen a 5-month-old Arabian colt with synovial osteochondromatosis of both stifle joints. In humans the condition is twice as common in males as in females.

Lesions of secondary synovial chondromatosis and synovial osteochondromatosis are commonly encountered as incidental findings at necropsy in major limb joints of older horses and dogs affected with chronic secondary osteoarthritis. Sex and breed do not appear to be important factors in the secondary form of the disorder.

Clinical Characteristics

Neither horse with primary synovial osteochondromatosis exhibited lameness or pain on palpation of the affected structures. Lesions were recognized by local enlargement of the synovial structure, which resulted primarily from increased amounts of synovial fluid, and palpation of firm, nodular masses. Potential for creating

painful or mechanical lameness exists. Treatment in the horse with involvement of the femorotibial bursa[8] was complete surgical excision, and the lesion did not recur. No treatment was attempted in the young Arabian colt because there was extensive involvement of both stifle joints and because the femoropatellar pouches of the horse are not accessible to the surgeon for the extensive exposure that would have been required.

In contrast to animals, affected humans experience pain and limitation of motion. Synovial resection is the treatment of choice for humans[6] and is probably the appropriate therapy for symptomatic lesions in animals. Local recurrence is a problem in human cases and should be anticipated in animals since new nodules may continue to develop in the synovium.

Animals with the more common secondary form of the disorder often have pain, lameness, and limitation of motion, probably resulting from chronic degenerative joint disease. The nodular lesions (i.e., synovial chondromas or synovial osteochondromas) may be trapped between articular surfaces or break free to become joint bodies and produce painful or mechanical lameness. Surgical removal of the attached nodules or free joint bodies may give temporary relief but will not alter the predisposing condition.

Sites

Rare lesions of the primary form of synovial osteochondromatosis involved the femorotibial bursa of the left stifle region of an older horse[8] and the femoropatellar synovial sacs of both stifle joints of a colt.

In the secondary form of this disorder, solitary or multiple synovial chondromas and/or synovial osteochondromas may arise in any structure lined by a chronically irritated synovium. In dogs these synovial lesions are typically found in the linings of joints with advanced secondary osteoarthritis (fig. 4.12 A). These include shoulder joints having untreated lesions of osteochondrosis and elbow joints having a long-standing ununited anconeal or fragmented coronoid process. Synovial nodules and free bodies in horses are found in shoulder and stifle joints affected by chronic secondary osteoarthritis, often due to osteochondrosis. Solitary osteochondromas arising in traumatized synovium along the dorsal articular margin of the metacarpophalangeal joints of the forelegs of horses are often mistaken for displaced chip fractures of the proximal end of the first phalanx. Cartilage nodules are also found in the synovium of unstable stifle joints of dogs and horses with long-standing cruciate ligament disease. They may also be found in the synovial lining of chronically irritated bursae (e.g., cases of bicipital bursitis) or in the linings of adventitious bursae.

Gross Morphology and Radiographic Appearance

Synovial chondromas and osteochondromas are pale, hard nodules with smooth borders that are set in a thickened synovial membrane (fig. 4.12 A). They are small in dogs, ranging from microscopic dimensions to about 1 to 3 mm in diameter. In horses, they will sometimes reach 2 cm in diameter and may appear in grape-like clusters. Large solitary nodules may be pedunculated and are attached to the synovium by a thin fibrous thread. Sometimes numerous nodules with the appearance of rice grains will be set randomly within the synovium. Both large and small nodules can become free bodies within the affected joint, sheath, or bursa. Many cases of the secondary form of this disease are missed at necropsy unless the synovial membrane is removed and examined carefully.

On radiographic examination of the affected part, the primary form of the disorder is suspected when radiodense nodules are recognized in the lining of a synovial structure in which there is no evidence of a chronic, primary disease process. In the secondary form of the disorder, the radiodense nodules can not usually be distinguished radiographically from avulsion fractures of articular cartilage in a chronic osteoarthritic joint. Tumoral calcinosis involving the femorotibial joint capsule of horses probably can not be distinguished from synovial osteochondromatosis without a biopsy.

Histological Features

The diagnosis of this condition depends on the demonstration of cartilaginous nodules within the synovial membrane.[6] These nodules may range in size from a cluster of a few chondrocytes, set within a thickened synovial membrane, to large pedunculated nodules covered by flattened synovial lining cells. In any given case, none, some, or most of the synovial chondromas will have undergone endochondral ossification to form synovial osteochondromas (fig. 4.12 B). Actively growing chondromas are cellular. Chondrocytes grow in clusters or chondrones. Some chondrocytes will be enlarged, and binucleate cells may be present. These cytological features in synovial chondromas are considered to reflect active cartilage growth and are not indicative of malignancy, as would be the case if these features were found in a central cartilage tumor of bone (fig. 4.12 C).

In synovial osteochondromas, much of the original cartilage nodule may be replaced by cancellous bone, and the intervening marrow spaces may contain hematopoietic cells. Like the synovial chondroma, the attached synovial osteochondroma is covered by flattened synovial lining cells.

It is usually possible to distinguish detached synovial chondromas or osteochondromas from large fragments of

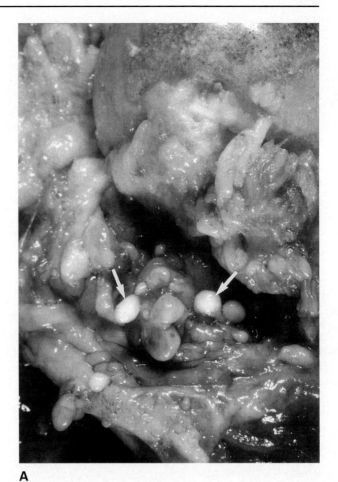

A

B

Fig. 4.12. Synovial chondromatosis. **A.** Hip joint of a 14-year-old dog with chronic degenerative joint disease. Several smooth oval to circular cartilaginous nodules (arrows) are present within or attached to the synovium (courtesy of R.A. Fairley). **B.** Synovial chondroma undergoing endochondral ossification to become an osteochondroma remains attached to the synovium. (continued)

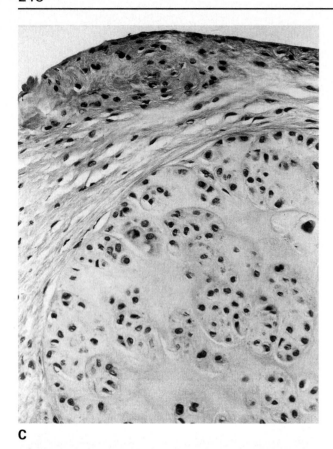

C

Fig. 4.12. (continued) **C.** Atypical chondrocytes in synovial chondromas are not indicative of malignancy.

articular cartilage that have recently become separated from deteriorated joint margins of osteoarthritic joints. The unique structure of articular cartilage usually remains recognizable in detached fragments of articular surfaces at least until they have been altered by continued growth within the synovial fluid or synovium. Bony spicules in synovial osteochondromas do not show the arrangement and maturity of bone tissue found in subchondral bone of marginal articular fractures. In both cases, the bone tissue and marrow spaces become ischemic after separation from their blood supply.

Growth and Metastasis

Synovial chondromas and synovial osteochondromas are slow growing benign lesions. The potential for malignant transformation to chondrosarcoma exists but is extremely unlikely.

REFERENCES

1. Lattes, R. (1982) Tumors of soft tissue. In *Atlas of Tumor Pathology.* 2nd series, fascicle 1, revised. Armed Forces Institute of Pathology, Washington, D.C.
2. Pool, R.R. (1990) Tumors and tumor-like conditions of joints and adjacent soft tissues. In Moulton J.E. (Ed.), *Tumors in Domestic Animals,* 3rd ed. University of California Press, Berkeley.
3. Colbourne, C.M., Yovich, J.V., Richards, R.B., Rose, K.J., and Huxtable, C.R. (1997) Vascular hamartomas of the dorsal carpal region in three young thoroughbred horses. *Aust Vet J* 75:20–23.
4. Van Pelt, R.W., Langham, R.F., and Gill, H.E., (1972) Multiple hemangiosarcomas in the tarsal synovial sheath of a horse. *J Amer Vet Med Assoc* 161:49–52.
5. Johnstone, A.C. (1987) Congenital vascular tumors in the skin of horses. *J Comp Pathol* 97:365–368.
6. Schajowicz, F. (1981) Tumors and tumor-like lesions of the synovial membrane. In *Tumors and Tumor-like Lesions of Bone and Joints.* Springer-Verlag, New York), pp. 519–567.
7. Kay, P.R., Freemont, A.J., and Davies, D.R.H. (1989) The etiology of multiple loose bodies, snow storm knee. *J Bone Joint Surg* 71:501–504.
8. Kirk, M.D. (1982) Radiographic and histological appearance of synovial osteochondromatosis of the femorotibial bursae in a horse: A case history report. *Vet Radiol* 23:168–170.

Tumoral Calcinosis

Classification

Tumoral calcinosis in humans is a disorder of undetermined etiology characterized by formation of nodular masses of calcareous material in soft tissues adjacent to a joint or joints.[1] The para-articular location is used to distinguish tumoral calcinosis from calcinosis circumscripta, calcinosis universalis, and hyperparathyroidism in which the subcutaneous calcareous deposits have a different pattern of distribution.

Tumoral calcinosis in animals has been recognized as *multicentric periarticular calcinosis* in vizsla puppies[2,3] and typically produces a focal lesion in the periarticular soft tissues over the tibiofibular joints of horses.[4,5]

The cause of the disorder in humans is unknown, although trauma and metabolic disorders have been proposed. In humans, the disease has a familial tendency.[1] Although the cause is also undetermined in animals, the lesions in vizsla dogs may be linked to a renal tubular defect in phosphorus transport.[3] In horses, repeated trauma has been suggested as a causative factor.[5]

Incidence, Age, Breed, and Sex

Both dogs affected with this disorder were immature and were of the vizsla breed.[2,3]

In a review of 18 cases in horses,[5] most affected animals were between 18 months and 4 years of age (range 1 to 13 years). Breeds most commonly affected were standardbreds (10 cases) and thoroughbreds (4 cases). Males (16 cases) were more commonly affected than females (2 cases).

Clinical Characteristics

The vizsla puppy[2] in one report was presented because of a progressive shoulder lameness. The pup was small for its age and had generalized muscle wasting. Limitation of joint motion in several joints was due to periarticular masses that were not painful or warm on palpation.

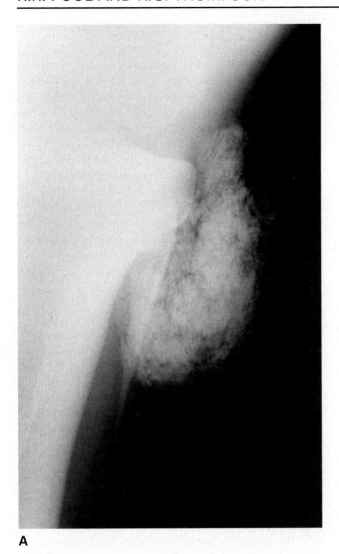

A

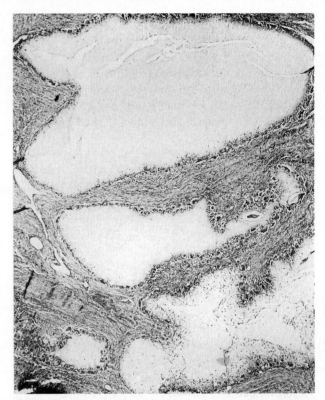

B

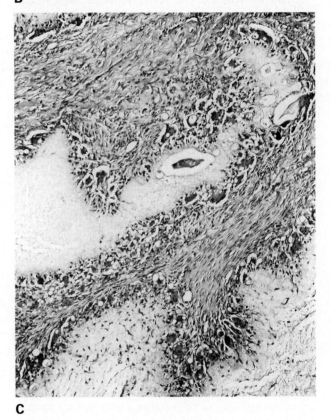

C

The cervical spine was rigid, and there was scoliosis of the thoracic spine. All other findings were normal.

The disease was recognized in horses because of the presence of one or more hard nodules in the subcutaneous tissue over the lateral surface of the femorotibial joint. The calcareous nodules were bound to the deeper structures, and the skin moved freely over their surface. In most cases lameness could not be associated with the presence of lesions. Surgical removal of the nodules was successful in several horses, and the lesions did not recur.[4,5]

Sites

In the vizsla puppy, para-articular soft tissues adjacent to the shoulder joints, synovial joints (C-1 and C-2) of the spine, both carpi, elbow joints, hip joints, and small joints of the feet had calcareous lesions.[2]

Of the 18 affected horses recorded in the literature,[5] 16 had lesions in the soft tissues over the lateral aspect of the femorotibial joint. In five horses the lesions were bilateral. One had bilateral lesions located in the shoulders, while another had multiple lesions involving the neck and pectoral regions and left hock joint.

Fig. 4.13. Tumoral calcinosis in the horse. **A.** Large, discrete, oval mass lateral to the femorotibial joint and containing multiple radiodense deposits. **B.** Decalcified section viewed at low magnification to demonstrate loculi, previously filled with calcareous material, that were separated by thin fibrous septa. **C.** Enlargement to show the multinucleated giant cells, macrophages, and fibroblasts that line the loculi.

Gross Morphology

The calcareous masses have a multilocular appearance. They are bordered by dense fibrous tissue from which thin fibrous septa divide the mass into irregular loculi. Chalky, paste-like material, white to yellow in color, fills the loculi. In both the dog[2] and the horse,[5] deep subcutaneous tissues, fasciae, and joint capsules are sites involved in this process.

Chemical analysis of this calcareous material in humans showed that it was mostly calcium carbonate, calcium phosphate, or a mixture of the two.[1] Analysis of the material from the vizsla puppy showed an ash content similar to that of bone mineral, but having a slightly higher calcium to phosphorus ratio.[2]

Radiographic Appearance

In the vizsla puppy there were stippled or punctate periarticular densities around most joints. In horses most lesions appeared as encapsulated soft tissue masses that were irregularly infiltrated with coalescing, highly radiodense granules. The equine lesions were located in soft tissues over the lateral aspect of the proximal fibula.

Histological Features

In decalcified tissue sections stained with hematoxlin and eosin, amorphous or feathery patterns remain in loculi formerly filled with calcareous material (figs. 4.13 A,B,C). Multinucleated giant cells, histiocytes, and fibroblasts form a cellular palisade along the margins of the loculi. Thin septa of immature fibrous tissue separate loculi of varying sizes and blend with a fibrous response bordering the lesion. Irregular foci of metaplastic bone and cartilage may be found within the fibrous tissue response. The histological lesion is similar to calcinosis circumscripta seen in subcutaneous tissues or the tongue.

Growth and Metastasis

These lesions are not neoplastic and do not undergo neoplastic transformation. Their importance is in differential diagnosis of synovial osteochondromatosis or a cartilage tumor.

Cystic Lesions of Joints, Tendon Sheaths, and Adjacent Soft Tissues

Ganglia

In humans, ganglia are described as tumor-like cystic masses usually attached to or adjacent to tendon sheaths of the hands, wrists, and feet, but sometimes within a tendon, muscle, or fibrocartilaginous meniscus of the knee joint.[6,7] The few ganglia we have seen in animals are encountered as incidental findings in the adipose tissue attached to the femorotibial synovial sacs of stifle joints of horses and dogs with severe secondary degenerative joint disease. In gross morphology the ganglia were small, yellow to tan, soft, ovoid, cystic structures embedded in the periarticular adipose tissue. Ganglia are formed by myxoid degeneration of fibrous tissue of the joint capsule or tendon sheath followed by softening and formation of unilocular or multilocular cysts.[6,7] The cysts are not lined by synovium and do not communicate with the joint cavity.[6] If the cyst has a synovial lining, then it must either be a synovial cyst or an adventitious bursa.[7] Figures 4.14 A and B show the formation of a ganglion from multilocular foci of connective tissue degeneration in the wall of the stifle joint of a dog with a ruptured cranial cruciate ligament.

The pathogenesis of ganglion formation is poorly understood.[7] The theory that they are formed following the development of a rent or herniation of the synovial lining of a joint or tendon sheath is not considered to be valid.[6,7]

Synovial Cysts

These cystic lesions are attached to the walls of synovial joints, tendon sheaths, and bursae (fig. 4.15 A,B). Synovial cysts are distinguished from ganglia by the presence of a synovial lining.[7] The most common example of a synovial cyst in humans is the Baker's cyst occurring in the popliteal space of the knee joint.[6] The cyst may form either by herniation of the synovial membrane of the knee joint through a rent in the posterior wall of the joint capsule or following the escape of joint fluid into the semimembranous bursa.[6] Any joint disease, such as chronic osteoarthritis, that stimulates excessive synovial fluid formation and causes elevated intra-articular pressure predisposes the joint to synovial cyst formation.

In animals, synovial cysts have been occasionally reported in dogs and cats.[8,9] The lesions in five affected dogs, ranging in age from 5 to 12 years, were described as cystic masses 2 cm or less in diameter adjacent to the carpus, tibiotarsus, or metatarsus.[8] None of the dogs had a history of joint disease or trauma to the area, and the lesions were incidental findings. The cysts contained clear viscous fluid and were lined by synovial cells. Recurrence following surgical excision had not occurred at 6 months to 5 years in three dogs where follow-up information was available.[8]

Synovial cysts have been reported in four cats,[8,9] all cases occurring in elderly animals (10 to 16.5 years of age) and involving the elbow joint. The lesions in all three cats of one report[9] were associated with radiographic evidence of elbow arthritis, and all recurred after surgical excision and drainage. The lesion in the other affected cat was not associated with an abnormality in the adjacent joint and had not recurred 9 months after excision.[8]

We have recognized synovial cysts in the walls of tendon sheaths of horses and in the walls of the apophyseal synovial joints of cervical vertebrae of horses with wobbler syndrome caused by chronic cervical instability. All affected joints had changes of chronic degenerative joint disease and distention of the joint capsule. We have never

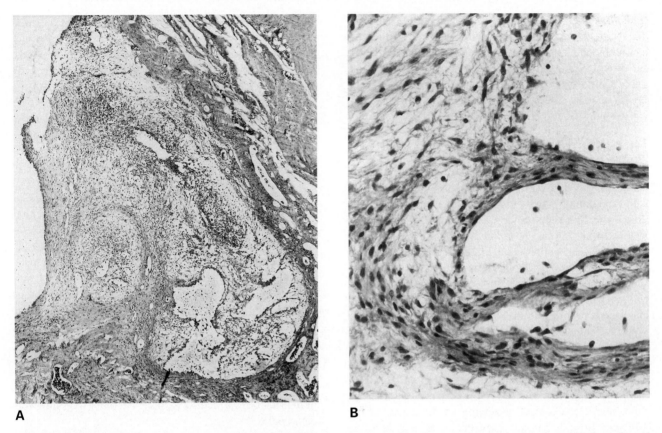

Fig. 4.14. Ganglion. **A.** Developing ganglion arises from multiloculated foci of connective tissue degeneration in the subsynovial tissues located between the femorotibial synovial sacs of the stifle joint of a dog with secondary osteoarthritis. **B.** Lining of ganglion is by adventitious fibroblasts and not synovial lining cells.

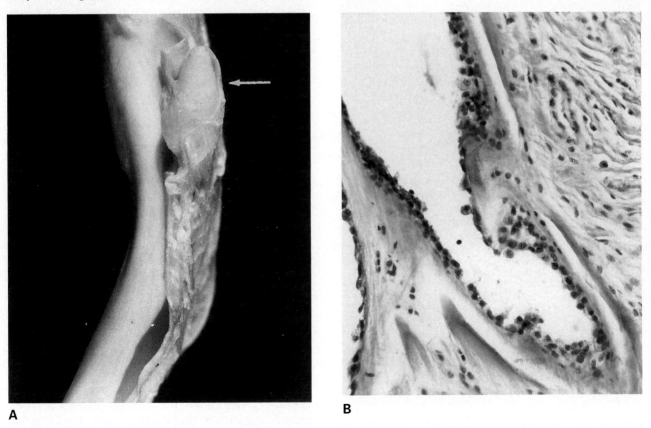

Fig. 4.15. Synovial cyst. **A.** Synovial cyst arising from the lateropalmar wall near the proximal end of the digital sheath in the foreleg of a horse. **B.** Ovoid cells identical to synoviocytes line the wall of the synovial cyst.

221

found Baker's cysts in the popliteal space of stifle joints of dogs with chronic degenerative disease of the stifle joints caused by cranial cruciate ligament disruption and meniscal disease. Synovial cysts, however, are present on the palmar surfaces of the antebrachiocarpal joints of small breeds of dogs suffering from chronic luxation of this joint caused by chronic rheumatoid arthritis.

Bursitis and Adventitious Bursitis

Bursae are normal anatomical structures having the appearance of thin walled, flattened sacs lined by attenuated synovium. Normal bursae are typically collapsed and difficult to find because they contain only a thin film of synovial fluid. Some are found at points of pressure and friction in deep periarticular locations and between tendons and bones, especially near tendon insertions. In superficial locations, the various subcutaneous bursae protect the skin from underlying bony protuberances. Natural bursae may become inflamed because of chronic trauma or septic inflammation. The synovial lining is usually lost, and the normally thin fibrous bursal wall becomes greatly thickened. Often the sac-like structure of the bursa is maintained, although the wall may be formed primarily of mature granulation tissue. The sac is distended with serous fluid, fibrin, or exudate, depending on the nature of the affliction. In some chronic cases, the bursae may be filled with fibrin concretions (fig. 4.16).

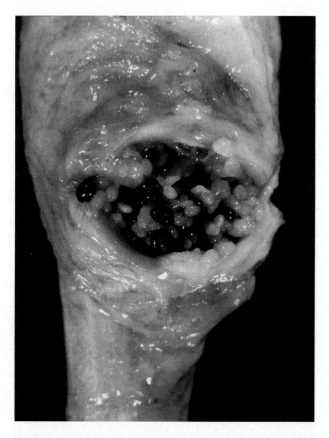

Fig. 4.16. Chronic carpal bursitis in a sheep. The bursa has a thickened fibrous wall and is filled with fibrin concretions. The darker concretions contain erythrocytes, reflecting the traumatic origin of the lesion.

Adventitious bursae, also called acquired subcutaneous bursae, develop in response to the constant pressure and movement at a specific site in the skin, in other words, a pressure point. Adventitious bursae appear to arise by cystic degeneration of chronically irritated connective tissue of the subcutis, and thus these bursae have a less well defined architecture than natural subcutaneous bursae. These reactive bursae present more of a diagnostic problem for the pathologist in their recognition. In gross morphology they may appear as irregular cavitary lesions in the subcutis that have shaggy linings with fibrous strands that cross the cavity. In chronic lesions, pale, hard nodular structures (synovial chondromas and synovial osteochondromas) may be attached to the lining or may be free bodies in the cavity of the bursa (fig. 4.16).On microscopic examination the lining cells may be seen to include cells considered to be adventitious fibroblasts. The bursal wall varies in thickness and maturity on the basis of the fibrous tissue response. Sometimes, the irregular slit-like structure of the wall, combined with the presence of a large number of tortuous capillary channels in the wall may give concern that a vascular neoplasm is present. Adventitious bursae may also become infected by pyogenic bacteria, and they have microscopic features resembling the cavitary lesions in the subcutis formed by foxtails and other migrating foreign bodies.

Adventitious bursitis of the hock is common in pigs, particularly those kept on slatted floors.[10] A study conducted on 21 properties in southwest England revealed an overall prevalence of 51 percent with a range of 10.1 to 84 percent.[10] The bursae are typically found immediately distal to the hock on the lateroplantar, plantar, and medial aspects of the joint. They are thought to arise through traumatic injury to lymphatic vessels and capillaries, followed by the accumulation of fibrinous exudate.

Heterotopic, Metaplastic, and Reactive Bone Formation in Soft Tissue

Heterotopic bone, which is bone tissue formed at an abnormal site, may occur in virtually any soft tissue location in the body. Heterotopic bone is produced by formerly uncommitted mesenchymal cells in interstitial tissues. Bone also arises by metaplasia, a process in which bone tissue is formed by transformation of cellular elements in mature fibrous tissue, such as in ligaments, tendons, joint capsules, organ capsules, fasciae, and cartilage tissue. Bony metaplasia also occurs in the stromal framework of muscle organs and glands. The precise conditions and biological signals for spontaneous heterotopic bone formation are poorly understood. This is also true for reactive bone production involving bone organs, where the initiating stimulus is often known. Recognition of heterotopic bone, osseous metaplasia, and reactive bone formation are important to diagnostic pathologists because they must often evaluate the nature of bone tissue present in a lesion.

Heterotopic bone can form at four kinds of sites. First, heterotopic bone may arise in nonskeletal soft tissues of animals. Examples include ossification of the spinal dura of dogs, bony pneumoliths in alveolar walls of the lungs, metaplastic bone in the mammary glands of cows and bitches, metaplastic bone in the walls of urinary bladders affected by chronic cystitis or carcinoma, and bone formed in the capsules of chronically inflamed salivary glands. Second, heterotopic bone may arise in nonosseous musculoskeletal tissues. Examples include ossifying myositis of quarter horses, localized myositis ossificans of dogs and cats, and generalized myositis ossificans of domestic cats and pigs. Third, heterotopic bone is commonly formed in entheses, which are bony sites of insertion of tendons, ligaments, and joint capsules. Examples include animals with chronic degeneration of synovial and amphiarthrodial joints and cats chronically exposed to toxic levels of vitamin A. Fourth, heterotopic bone is formed by paraskeletal tissues, which are tissues with osteogenic potential that lie adjacent to bone surfaces. Bony responses seen in hypertrophic osteodystrophy of dogs and in the organizing stages of subperiosteal hematomas are examples in this group.

Three disorders of animals in which heterotopic bone may be produced in muscle organs are discussed in greater detail in the following sections. They include fibrotic and ossifying myopathy of the horse, localized myositis ossificans of the dog and cat, and generalized myositis ossificans of the domestic cat and pig.

Fibrotic and Ossifying Myopathy of the Horse

Classification

Fibrotic myopathy is a condition caused by postinflammatory fibrosis of the caudal thigh muscles and the intervening intramuscular fascia.[11,12] The term *ossifying myopathy* is used to describe those cases in which metaplastic bone is formed in the fibrous tissue response.[11] Common initiating factors include work related trauma, especially in working quarter horses, external trauma,[11,12] and intramuscular injections.[12] A characteristic lameness develops following the organization of edema, both in muscle tissues and intramuscular fascia, into fibrous tissue, resulting in restrictive adhesions between affected muscle groups.

Incidence, Age, Breed, and Sex

Equine clinics will see one to several cases per year. The only large study of this condition[12] indicated that affected horses ranged from 3 to 15 years of age and involved primarily the quarter horse breed. There is no apparent sex predilection.

Clinical Characteristics

Restrictive adhesions produce a characteristic hindlimb gait abnormality sometimes referred to as *goose-stepping*. There is an abrupt shortening of the cranial phase of the stride, with the distal limb being jerked caudally just before the foot touches the ground. Often, the skin is adhered to the affected muscle group, resulting in a depression in the normal contour of the caudal thigh region. Affected muscle tissue and fascia are firm to hard on palpation. Surgical removal of the affected tissue usually produces some improvement in the gait.[12]

Sites

Caudal thigh muscles affected in this condition are primarily the semitendinosus muscle, less frequently the semimembranosus and biceps femoris muscles,[11,12] and rarely the gracilis muscle.[12,13]

Gross Morphology

The appearance of the affected tissue is related to the duration of the condition. In relatively early lesions there is edema separating fascicles in the muscle and in the adjacent fascia. Gradually, as the edema is organized by fibrous tissue, the connective tissue septa within the muscle organs become thicker, pale, and firm. Muscle fibers are replaced by fibrous tissue. The formerly loose tissue of the fasciae becomes filled with hard, white, dense connective tissue (fig. 4.17 A).

Histological Features

Within chronically affected muscle organs, muscle fibers atrophy and disappear, temporarily leaving behind adipose tissue and linearly oriented perimyseal tissue that formerly separated fascicles of muscle fibers (fig. 4.17 B). Gradually, the septa of perimyseal tissue thicken and obliterate the intervening adipose tissue (fig. 4.17 C). Epimyseum also undergoes a similar fibrotic change and merges with irregular dense fibrous tissue that has formed in the intermuscular fascia (fig. 4.17 D). There may be islands of metaplastic bone.

Growth and Metastasis

The lesion is a type of scar tissue that forms in and around muscle organs following aseptic inflammation resulting from mechanical trauma of work or repeated needle trauma from injections. The lesions may increase in size over a period of months. No progression to neoplasia is expected, although heterotopic bone may develop in the scar tissue as a result of metaplasia.

Localized Myositis Ossificans of the Dog and Cat

Classification

Localized myositis ossificans is a reactive lesion of dogs, cats, and humans occurring in soft tissues usually located adjacent to bones.[1,14-16] Some authors believe that the lesion in humans is initiated by trauma to paraskeletal

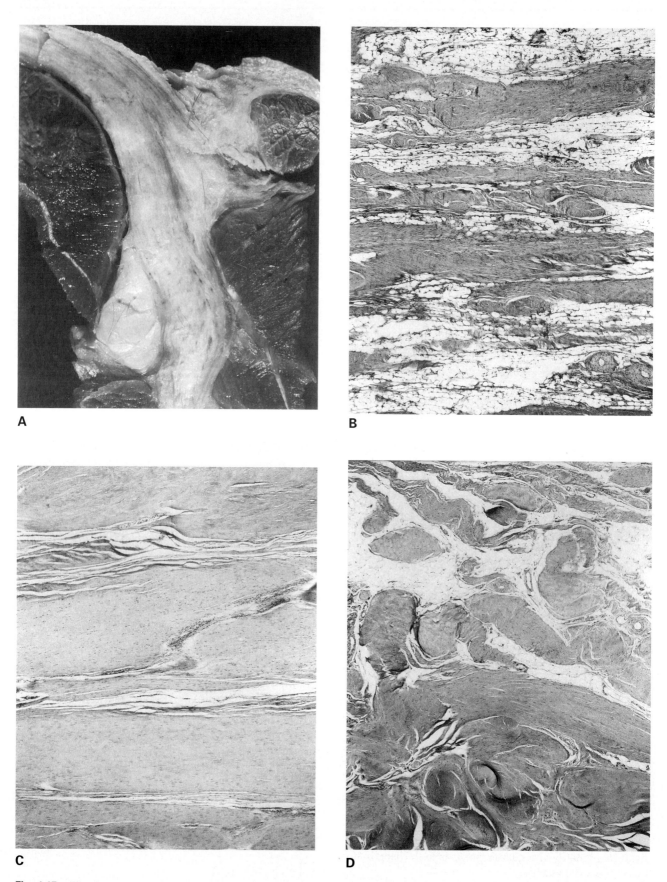

Fig. 4.17. Fibrotic myopathy of the horse. **A.** Septa of intermuscular fasciae are greatly thickened and hard. Abnormal fascia binds muscle groups together to prevent normal range of motion. **B.** Adipose tissue remains in muscle fascicles where muscle fibers have disappeared following chronic atrophy. Fibrous septa are remnants of perimysium. **C.** Area in which the greatly thickened perimysium obliterates intervening soft tissues. **D.** Merging of the irregularly thickened fibrous septa of muscle organs with abnormally thickened intermuscular fascia.

224

tissues, including muscle. The traumatized area contains a hematoma, disrupted fascia, and damaged muscle tissue. This area undergoes a unique pattern of organization and repair having a zonal arrangement in which metaplastic bone tissue forms at the periphery of the lesion. The name of this disorder was poorly chosen since muscle tissue is not always involved, no inflammation may be present, and bone formation is a late event in the development of the lesion.[1,6] The pathologist should be aware of this disorder since a biopsy specimen containing tissue from the center of a forming lesion may be confused with osteosarcoma.

Incidence, Age, Breed, and Sex

This condition is thought to be uncommon based on the paucity of reports in the veterinary medical literature; however, since it is not a life threatening disease and resolves eventually into a firm mass, few animals would be euthanized and submitted for postmortem examination because of the lesion. Localized myositis ossificans has been reported in a 2-year-old female Siamese cat,[14] two male German shepherd dogs 7 and 8 years of age,[15] and a 5-year-old male doberman.[16]

Clinical Characteristics

The affected animals had progressive weakness, muscle atrophy, pain, and loss of range of movement in the joints of the affected limbs. One of the dogs had a history of trauma to the affected leg about 2 months prior to presentation for this disorder.[15] Surgical removal was successful in one case where it was attempted.[16] The cat had firm bilateral nodular swellings in the common tendon of the triceps brachii muscle just proximal to its insertion onto the olecranon process of the ulna. Neither lesion recurred following surgical removal.[14]

Sites

The affected dogs had unilateral lesions involving the gluteal muscles, just caudal to the femoral neck of the right hind leg.[15,16] The cat developed bilateral nodular swellings involving the soft tissues surrounding the common tendon of the triceps brachii muscle proximal to its insertion onto the olecranon process of the ulna.[14]

Gross Morphology

The partially ossified masses removed from the gluteal muscles of the right hind legs of two dogs measured 4.5 × 3.2 × 2.9 cm and 24 × 6.9 × 10.8 cm, respectively.[15] The larger mass had a huge central hematoma. Adjacent muscle tissue was pale and fibrotic.

In the cat, the ossified masses in both forelegs measured about 1.4 × 2.5 cm and were centered on the soft tissues investing the common tendon of the triceps brachii muscle proximal to its insertion line on the olecranon of the ulna.[14]

Radiographic Features

A para-articular soft tissue radiodensity was located just caudal to the femoral neck of the right femur of each dog.[15,16] Radiographs of a necropsy specimen showed zonation in the mass with maximum radiodensity occurring at the periphery.

Radiographic studies of the cat showed radiodense masses located in the soft tissues proximal to the olecranon processes of both ulnas. Also present was a mild periosteal bony response on the left proximal ulna and a marked periosteal bony reaction on the distal humerus and proximal ulna of the right leg.[14] No cortical destruction of adjacent bones was observed in any of the affected animals.

Histological Features

A zonal pattern was evident histologically in the lesions of the dogs[15,16] and the cat.[14] An organizing hematoma is commonly found in the center of a lesion of localized myositis ossificans. The hematoma is bordered by a highly cellular and rapidly proliferating population of mesenchymal cells. Some cells have bizarre nuclei and may be found in areas where osteoid and cartilage matrix are being produced. Biopsy specimens taken from this area share many histological features with osteosarcoma. The proliferative zone is covered by a more mature fibrovascular response within which the osteoid is more abundant and orderly. In the maturing lesion the mass is covered by a thin bony shell formed by anastomotic trabeculae of woven bone. Peripheral to the shell of metaplastic bone, the soft tissues are fibrotic and may contain atrophic muscle fibers.

Growth and Metastasis

This is a rare and unique reactive lesion occurring in traumatized paraskeletal tissues. The lesion is self-limiting in humans[1] and probably also in animals. Pathologists should be aware of this lesion and distinguish it from parosteal osteosarcoma and extraosseous osteosarcoma.

Generalized Myositis Ossificans of the Pig and Cat

Classification

This is a nonneoplastic disease of the supporting connective tissues of muscle organs, attachments, fasciae, and aponeuroses. It is characterized by an abnormal proliferation of primitive connective tissue elements that undergo metaplastic bone formation and produce secondary degenerative changes in muscle tissue.[17] Examples of this rare disorder of children have been reported in a group of related pigs[18] and in two domestic cats.[19,20]

The etiology of this disorder is unknown. In children there is evidence that the disease may be hereditary,[17] as it appears to be in swine.[18] When the disease in children is recognized in the early fibroproliferative stage before ossification has begun, it is sometimes called progressive myositis fibrosa or hereditary polyfibromatosis.[7]

Incidence, Age, Breed, and Sex

The disease is rare in children and animals. Age of onset varies in children from infancy to adolescence. The affected boar was 9 months of age, and its 34 affected offspring ranged from 2 to 6 months of age at the time of initial onset of signs.[18] The breed of swine was not reported. The diseases occurred in both male and female pigs sired by this boar.

The affected cats were 10 months[19] and 2 years of age[20] at the time the disease was diagnosed.

Clinical Characteristics

The pigs developed rapidly progressive hind-leg paresis and loss of condition. Stiffness and reluctance to move accompanied the appearance and rapid growth of firm swellings in the soft tissues and musculature along the spine, hind legs, neck, shoulders, and tarsal regions.[18] One affected cat had a history of stiffness, pain, and progressive posterior paresis. A firm lump removed at 4 months of age from the musculature over the thoracic vertebrae recurred 3 months later. At this time numerous masses were also recognized in the musculature of all legs and later in the musculature of the ventral abdomen and back. Popliteal lymph nodes were greatly enlarged, and there was a neutrophilia with a left shift.[19] The other cat had a stiff forelimb gait and reduced movement of the shoulder joints due to a firm, bilateral subcutaneous mass extending from the dorsal cranial cervical area to the scapula.[20]

Sites

Location of bony masses varied in different pigs, but major sites affected in decreasing order of frequency were the musculature overlying the caudal, thoracic, and lumbar vertebrae and the neck, shoulder, and tarsal regions.[18] In both cats, the lesions were extensive, involving the musculature of the back, ventral abdomen, shoulders, forelegs, and caudal thighs.[19,20]

Gross Morphology

Lesions described in the pigs and cat are basically similar.[18-20] There is widespread replacement of muscle tissue by masses of cancellous bone and fibrous connective tissue. It is not always possible to distinguish between an extraosseous bony mass and the adjacent bone organ since they appear to fuse at some sites.

Histological Features

In sites of soft tissue involvement, muscle tissue is replaced by fibrous tissue and bone. Fatty tissue and some fibrous tissue fill the marrow spaces. In sites of bone organ involvement, the masses of heterotopic bone are continuous with the bony elements of the skeleton without obvious intervening remnants of the original cortex of periosteum. The boundary can usually be recognized by the abrupt transition from hematopoietic marrow filling marrow spaces of the bone organ to fatty marrow filling the cancellous bone spaces of the heterotopic bone.[18] Union of the heterotopic bone formed in the soft tissues to the adjacent bones apparently is the result of remodeling activities. Along the borders of the developing bony masses, there are cells in the fibrous tissue response that undergo metaplasia to osteoblasts. Soft tissues adjacent to the bony masses are fibrotic and often contain degenerating[19] and atrophic[18,20] muscle fibers.

Growth and Metastasis

This is a progressive, nonneoplastic, and fatal disorder of the interstitial tissue of muscle organs. Late in the course of the human disorder the person becomes virtually immobile due to the union of bony masses in different muscle groups and the formation of periarticular bony bridges that prevent joint motion.[17] Eventually death results from progressive involvement of the musculature of the thoracic cage, leading to respiratory failure or fatal pneumonia. None of the animals in the two reports were permitted to live to the end stage described for humans.

REFERENCES

1. Spjut, H.J., Dorfman, H.D., Fechner, R.E., and Ackerman, L.V. (1971) Tumors of bone and cartilage. In *Atlas of Tumor Pathology.* 2nd series, fascicle 5. Armed Forces Institute of Pathology, Washington, D.C.
2. Ellison, G.W., and Norrdin, R.R. (1980) Multicentric periarticular calcinosis in a pup. *J Amer Vet Med Assoc* 177:542–546.
3. Pedersen, N.C., Pool, R.R., and Morgan, J.P. (1983) Joint diseases of dogs and cats. In Ettinger, S.J. (ed.), *Textbook of Veterinary Internal Medicine, Diseases of the Dog and Cat,* 2nd ed. W.B. Saunders Co., Philadephia.
4. Dodd, D.C., and Raker, C.W. (1970) tumoral calcinosis (calcinosis circumscripta) in the horse. *J Amer Vet Med Assoc* 157:968–972.
5. Goulden, B.E., and O'Callaghan, M.W. (1980) Tumoral calcinosis in the horse. *N Z Vet J* 28:217–219.
6. Ackerman, L.V., and Rosai, J. (1974) *Surgical Pathology,* 5th ed. The C.V. Mosby Co., St. Louis.
7. Lattes, R. (1982) Tumors of soft tissue. In *Atlas of Tumor Pathology.* 2nd series, fascicle 1, revised. Armed Forces Institute of Pathology, Washington, D.C.
8. Prymak, C., and Goldschmidt, M.H. (1991) Synovial cysts in five dogs and one cat. *J Amer Anim Hosp Assoc* 27:151–154.
9. Stead, A.C., Else, R.W., and Stead, M.C.P. (1995) Synovial cysts in cats. *J Small Anim Pract* 36:450–454.
10. Mouttotou, N., Hatchell, F.M., and Green, L.E. (1998) Adventitious bursitis of the hock in finishing pigs: Prevalence, distribution and association with floor type and foot lesions. *Vet Rec* 142:109–114.
11. Adams, O.R. (1961) Fibrotic myopathy in the hindlegs of horses. *J Amer Vet Med Assoc* 139:1089–1092.
12. Turner, A.S., and Trotter, G.W. (1984) Fibrotic myopathy in the horse. *J Amer Vet Med Assoc* 184:335–338.
13. Bishop, R. (1972) Fibrotic myopathy in the gracilis muscle of a horse. *Vet Med Small Anim Clin* 67:270.
14. Liu, S.K., Dorfman. H.D., and Patnaik, A.K. (1974) Primary and secondary bone tumors in the cat. *J Small Anim Pract* 15:141–156.
15. Liu, S.K., and Dorfman, H.D. (1976) A condition resembling localized myositis ossificans in two dogs. *J Small Anim Pract* 17:371–377.
16. Bone, D.L., and McGavin, M.D. (1984) Myositis ossificans in the dog: A case report and review. *J Amer Anim Hosp Assoc* 21:135–138.

17. Goldman, A.B. (1994) Heritable diseases of connective tissue, epiphyseal dysplasias, and related conditions. In Resnick, D. (ed.), *Diagnosis of Bone and Joint Disorders*, 3rd ed. Vol. 6, ch. 87. W.B. Saunders, Philadelphia, pp.4095–4162.

18. Siebold, H.R., and Davis, C.L. (1967) Generalized myositis ossificans (familial) in pigs. *Pathol Vet* 4:79–88.

19. Norris, A.M., Pallet, L., and Wilcock, B. (1980) Generalized myositis ossificans in a cat. *J Amer Anim Hosp Assoc* 16:659–663.

20. Waldron, D., Pettigrew, V., Turk, M., Turk, J., and Gibson, R. (1985) Progressive ossifying myositis in a cat. *J Amer Vet Med Assoc* 187:64–65.

MALIGNANT TUMORS AND TUMOR-LIKE LESIONS IN AND AROUND JOINTS, TENDONS, AND DEEP FASCIAE

There are probably few other groups of tumors in animals subject to as much debate as those occurring in and around joints, tendons, and deep fascial tissues. Because of the infrequency with which these tumors occur in animals, their classification has understandably been based on extrapolation from the human literature. Unfortunately, the classification of certain malignant tumors involving periarticular tissues of humans is confusing and, in some cases, misleading. This is particularly true for synovial sarcomas, where there is convincing evidence that the tumor in affected humans is not of synovial origin.[1] This highlights the danger of attempting to force animal tumors into a classification system developed for humans. It is likely that the classification of these tumors in animals will evolve to a more accurate and widely accepted system following the use of immunohistochemistry to better characterize their histogenesis.

In this chapter, the malignant tumors and tumor-like conditions in and around the joints, tendons and deep fascia of animals will be discussed under the headings listed in table 4.2. This decision recognizes the fact that although there is not universal acceptance among veterinary pathologists of entities such as malignant fibrous histiocytoma and malignant giant cell tumor of soft parts, several reports of both tumors exist in the veterinary literature, and both are included in the most recent edition of the WHO bulletin on the histological classification of mesenchymal tumors of the skin and soft tissues of domestic animals.[2] Until an alternative classification system is developed,

TABLE 4.2. Malignant tumors and tumor-like lesions of joints, tendons, and deep fasciae

Synovial sarcoma
Malignant fibrous histiocytoma
Malignant giant cell tumor of soft parts or malignant giant cell tumor of the tendon sheaths
Histiocytic sarcoma
Musculoaponeurotic fibromatosis
Malignant mesenchymoma of the dog

preferably based on immunochemical staining or molecular biology techniques, the categories used here will no doubt continue to be employed by veterinary pathologists.

Most of the tumors and tumor-like lesions discussed in this section probably arise from undifferentiated mesenchyme found in the superficial and deep fasciae, synovium of joints, bursae and tendon sheaths, paratendon, and other deep connective tissues. These primitive cells are the surviving remnants of that portion of the fetal mesenchyme that underwent partial necrobiosis during the formation of cavities in joints and tendon sheaths and of fascial planes separating muscle groups. In a normal animal, these cells are recognized as a nondescript population of primitive cells varying in shape from ovoid to fusiform. They form the major cellular component of the subsynovial tissue, paratendon, and loose connective tissue of fascia. Normally, some of these cells produce proteoglycan to maintain suppleness and permit gliding movement within soft tissues. Some of them resemble fibroblasts and have a sustentacular role, but they assume the role of synoviocytes when located in the subsynovial tissues. If the environment of this cell population becomes edematous following trauma or inflammation, many cells transform into facultative fibroblasts and produce a fibrillar matrix.

Synovial Sarcoma

General Considerations and Classification

Synovial sarcoma in humans is described as a soft tissue tumor with a characteristic biphasic pattern comprising both mesenchymal and epithelial elements.[3-5] The epithelial cells typically form irregular cleft-like spaces (sometimes giving the tumor a *pseudoglandular* appearance) and are surrounded by neoplastic mesenchymal cells, forming areas indistinguishable from fibrosarcoma.[4,5] The mesenchymal component may predominate. The initial classification of these tumors as synovial sarcoma was based on their morphological resemblance with synovium, but there is convincing ultrastructural and immunochemical evidence that they are not derived from synovial lining cells.[1,6] Unlike synovial cells, the neoplastic epithelial cells of human synovial sarcoma are arranged on a basal lamina and possess tight junctions.[7] Furthermore, the cells stain positively with the epithelial markers cytokeratin and epithelial membrane antigen.[1,6] In contrast, normal synovial cells are vimentin positive (reflecting their mesenchymal origin) and stain negatively with epithelial markers. In addition, many human synovial sarcomas occur at sites remote from joints including the neck, head, retroperitoneum, and abdominal wall.[1,8] Even in cases that occur near joints, connection with the joint cavity is rare. There seems little justification therefore to classify synovial sarcomas in animals according to criteria used in human medicine.

Two types of synovial cells are recognized in the lining of joints and tendon sheaths. Type A cells originate in the bone marrow and migrate to the joint.[9] These cells resemble tissue macrophages and are phagocytic, being responsible for removing particulate matter from the joint. Type B cells, which comprise 70–80 percent of synovial cells, have ultrastructural characteristics of fibroblasts and are responsible for producing synovial fluid and the extracellular matrix of the synovium. Presumably, tumors may develop from either cell type, but in either case the tumor will be purely mesenchymal rather than containing a mixture of epithelial and mesenchymal components.

There appears to be some confusion as to whether true biphasic synovial sarcomas occur in animals. Although several reports describe intermingled synovioblastic (or *epithelioid*) and fibroblastic components,[10-13] there is little if any evidence to suggest that the epithelioid cells of animal synovial sarcomas correspond to the epithelial component of human synovial sarcomas. More likely, they represent either type A or type B synoviocytes. The cleft-like spaces that are a feature of many synovial sarcomas in animals are generally lined by an ill-defined layer of synovioblasts similar to that of the normal synovium, with no evidence of a basal lamina (see fig. 4.19 D). Most synovial sarcomas in animals are predominantly fibroblastic, and the presence of plump, oval, or polygonal cells in some areas may reflect regional pleomorphism of malignant mesenchymal cells, as occurs in many other tumor types, rather than a *biphasic* cell population. Perhaps this is an instance where veterinary pathologists have been too strongly influenced by the medical literature. To add to the confusion, pseudoglandular tumors resembling human synovial sarcomas are occasionally detected near the joints of dogs and cats. Whether these are analogous to the human synovial sarcoma or represent epithelial tumors of unknown origin is not clear, but they appear different from the majority of tumors diagnosed as synovial sarcoma in animals.

In this chapter, the term synovial sarcoma is restricted to mesenchymal tumors occurring in the region of joints or tendon sheaths and with microscopic features supporting a synovial origin. These tumors may be analogous to *monophasic synovial sarcomas* of human patients in which spindle cells predominate and the epithelial element is absent or poorly developed.[7,8] Synovial sarcoma in dogs should not be confused with histiocytic sarcomas (see later this chapter), which are probably derived from interstitial dendritic cells and may form extensive nodular lesions in and around joints.

Incidence, Age, Breed, and Sex

Synovial sarcoma is a rare tumor in animals, having been reported most frequently in dogs[10-15] and occasionally in the cat[16] and ox.[17,18] In dogs, the tumor occurs mainly in large but not giant breeds, and there is no specific breed predisposition.[11,13] It appears to be more common in males than in females (ratio approximately 3:2), the age range of

affected dogs is broad (12 months to 15 years), and it is most common in middle age.[10,11,13,15] This information is unavailable for the occurrence of synovial sarcoma in other species as there are too few reported cases, but the tumor is reported in a 9-year-old castrated male domestic shorthair cat,[16] a 3-year-old Jersey cow,[17] and a 10-year-old bullock.[18]

Clinical Characteristics

Most affected dogs are presented because of lameness associated with a nonpainful palpable mass located in the vicinity of a major weight-bearing joint or a tendon in one of the legs. The tumor mass is firm but may have soft fluctuant areas. A few synovial sarcomas will pursue an indolent course and slowly destroy the joint over a period of several months to more than 1 to 2 years. Conversely, a few tumors will suddenly appear and pursue a fulminating course, ending in euthanasia or death within a few weeks to a month. Most tumors, however, will be slow growing masses for several weeks to months and suddenly increase in size over a period of 2 to 3 weeks. The degree of lameness can usually be correlated with the degree of bone involvement seen radiographically. In one report[10] 7 of 18 dogs with synovial sarcomas affecting joints had extensive joint destruction. Dogs with synovial sarcomas originating from tendons or tendon sheaths may develop a slow growing, nodular mass that remains fixed to the deep structures of the leg.[15] Pitting edema of the leg may develop, and in some cases there is radiographic evidence of bone destruction or extension into a nearby joint. Local recurrence (following surgery) and metastatic disease are common developments, but some dogs will remain tumor free following amputation.

Sites

Synovial sarcomas involving the joints of dogs are most often located at or near one of the major weight-bearing joints. The stifle is the most frequent site, followed in decreasing order by the elbow, shoulder, tarsus, carpus, and hip.[13] There is one report of a synovial sarcoma involving the temporomandibular joint of a 12-year-old Irish setter[14] and another involving an apophyseal synovial joint of a cervical vertebra.[15] Synovial sarcomas of tendons or tendon sheaths generally involve flexor or extensor tendons of the limbs, usually proximal to the carpus and tarsus, but occasionally occurring in the metatarsal or digital regions.[15]

Gross Morphology

Synovial sarcomas of joints appear to be composed of confluent lobules of firm, tan-colored tissue. The borders are distinct and seem to be encapsulated (fig. 4.18 A). The cut surface exposes smooth textured tissue that often contains dark staining areas of hemorrhage and pale areas of necrosis. Cystic spaces filled with mucinous fluid are prominent features of some lesions. Tumor tissue infiltrates along fascial planes leading away from the affected

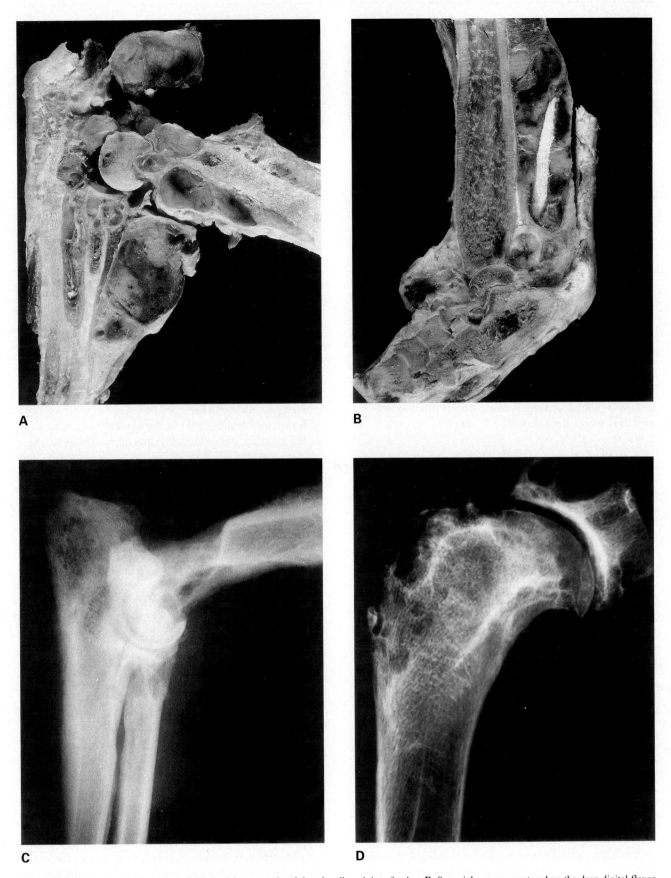

Fig. 4.18. Canine synovial sarcoma. **A.** Synovial sarcoma involving the elbow joint of a dog. **B.** Synovial sarcoma centered on the deep digital flexor tendon of a dog. **C.** Radiograph showing destructive lesions in the ends of all bones forming the elbow joint. **D.** Radiograph from the shoulder joint of a dog showing clinical signs for over 14 months and slow, clinical progression of the tumor. The sclerotic borders of the multiple areas of bone resorption reflect the indolent behavior of this synovial sarcoma.

joint. Most of the synovial membrane of the joint is infiltrated and effaced by tumor tissue. Unlike human tumors, the synovial sarcomas of dogs commonly encroach on the joint cavity, but the tumor does not appear to produce any direct damage to the articular cartilage. With aggressive tumors, however, the neoplastic tissue destroys the joint by eroding the articular margins and by invading the subchondral bone. Tumor tissue reaches the subchondral bone by infiltrating the joint capsule insertion line, and it frequently gains access to the epiphyseal cancellous bone by entering the bony vascular channels of the epiphyseal vessels. This process may lead to vessel occlusion and infarction of segments of subchondral bone and the epiphyseal spongiosa. Synovial sarcomas of tendons and tendon sheaths are fusiform masses, usually centered on a large caliber tendon and composed of confluent, soft tissue nodules.[15] The tumor tissue may extend along fascial planes and dissect between the underlying bone surface and the adjacent muscle. On cut surfaces (fig. 4.18 B), the tumor tissue is tan colored but may contain dark red areas of hemorrhage and necrosis. Cystic spaces containing viscous fluid may be present, and in some cases the tumor may contain extensive areas of soft, pale, gelatinous tissue. Nodules of mucoid tissue may infiltrate beyond the margins of the tumor, especially along the course of the tendon proximal to the main mass.

Radiographic Appearance

Most synovial sarcomas of canine joints appear as large nodular masses with discrete borders, often eccentrically oriented on a major joint of a limb. The tumor mass usually has a radiodensity similar to that of muscle tissue. In a few cases, and early in the course of many tumors, there are no radiographic signs of bone involvement. The earliest skeletal change may be an ill-defined periosteal reaction with cortical thinning.[6] With aggressive tumors this progresses to multiple foci of osteolysis involving the ends of all bones forming the joint (fig. 4.18 C). The two major radiographic patterns of permeative and punctate bone loss seen in affected joints of humans may occur as separate or combined patterns in canine joint tumors. It is our experience that when one examines the radiographs of a major limb joint of an older large breed dog and finds destructive lesions in the ends of the bones forming the joint, one should think first of synovial sarcoma. We have seen a few examples where metastatic tumors to the synovium of a joint have mimicked the pattern of a primary malignant joint tumor. Cases of osteomyelitis or inflammatory joint disease do not normally produce radiographic signs resembling malignant joint disease.

We occasionally encounter atypical cases of synovial sarcoma in which clinical progression is very slow, and the radiographic changes reflect this indolent behavior. Radiographs of these lesions show numerous discrete areas of bone resorption with sclerotic borders; these involve several bones of the affected joint (fig. 4.18 D). The ovoid radiolucencies appear to be the enlarged bony foramens of

vessels entering the bone organs along joint capsule insertion lines. Tumor tissue apparently mediates the bone resorption and in doing so creates a pathway for entering the ends of bones.

Histological Features

Most descriptions of histology of synovial sarcoma in animals refer to the presence of two cell populations, a synovioblastic or epitheloid cell type and a fibroblastic cell type, implying that there are two distinct cell types present. This concept seems to have been borrowed from descriptions of human synovial sarcoma, which typically possesses a biphasic histological character, but which is not considered to be of synovial origin.[1,7,9] It is debatable whether tumors analogous to human synovial sarcoma actually occur in animals, but if they do, they are probably extremely rare. Synovial sarcomas in animals consist of malignant mesenchymal cells, which may vary from fusiform spindle cells resembling fibroblasts to oval, polygonal, or even stellate cells with features more reminiscent of synovial cells. The variation in the shape of the cells does not imply a separate lineage; in fact, the variation is no greater than sometimes occurs in many other mesenchymal tumors, including osteosarcoma and hemangiosarcoma. Although there are two types of synovial cells with different histogenesis in the normal synovium, it is highly unlikely that both cell populations would undergo malignant transformation at the same time. One should therefore avoid comparisons with human synovial sarcoma and the use of the term *biphasic* in relation to synovial sarcoma of animals.

The relative proportion of the different shaped cells in canine synovial sarcoma varies between tumors, and even within the same tumor (fig. 4.19 A-D). In cases with a predominance of spindle cells, the tumor may be virtually indistinguishable from fibrosarcoma (fig. 4.19 A), but other tumors may consist predominantly of sheets of synovioblastic cells more closely resembling those of the normal synovial layer (fig. 4.19 B). Cavities or slit-like spaces lined by a poorly defined layer of malignant synovioblasts may form within sheets of tumor cells (fig. 4.19 C,D). The spaces may contain proteinaceous fluid or mucoid material.

The malignant synovioblastic cells of synovial sarcoma often have eccentric circular to oval nuclei, which vary in size and may contain one or more prominent nucleoli (fig. 4.20 A). The mitotic rate is highly variable, as is the frequency of binucleate and multinucleate giant cells. Individual cells may be surrounded by an eosinophilic matrix that resembles osteoid (fig. 4.20 A), leading to an incorrect diagnosis of osteosarcoma. In some canine synovial sarcomas, especially those involving tendons or tendon sheaths, nodules of myxomatous tumor tissue are scattered among areas that are more solid (fig. 4.20 B). The myxoid matrix may surround individual stellate tumor cells or clusters of tumor cells, or it may fill multiple spaces within the tumor. Synovial sarcomas with abundant

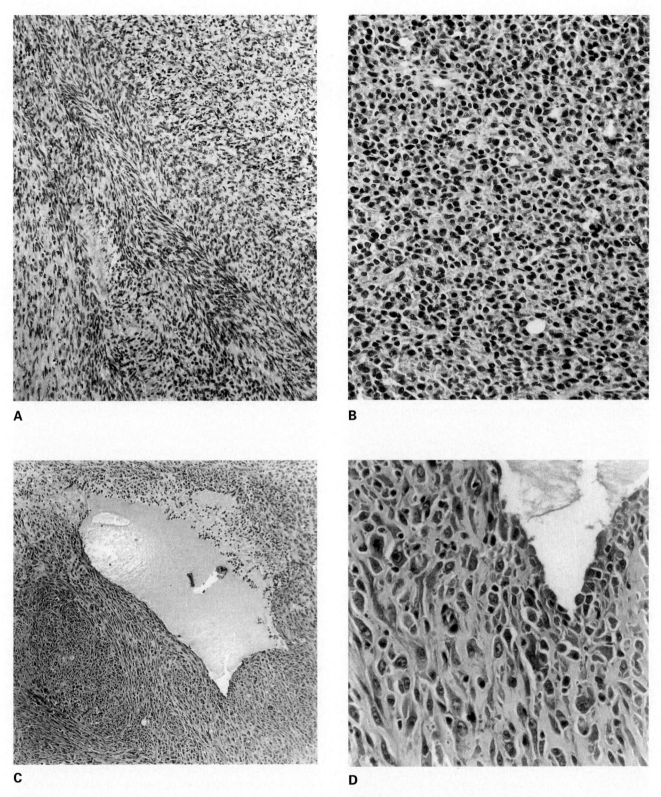

Fig. 4.19. Histological variations in synovial sarcoma of joints. **A.** Tumor in which the fibroblastic component predominates and mimics the interwoven pattern of fibrosarcoma. **B.** Sheets of malignant synovioblastic cells in another canine synovial sarcoma. **C.** Synovial sarcoma near the hock joint of a dog. Synovioblastic or epithelioid cells predominate and are forming occasional spaces lined by tumor cells and containing finely granular, eosinophilic fluid. **D.** Higher magnification of the same tumor showing plump synovioblastic cells lining the space. As with normal synovium, there is no suggestion that the lining cells are contained by a basal lamina.

231

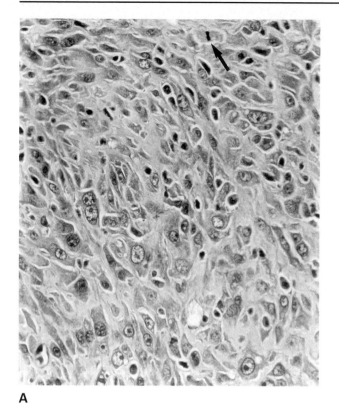

A

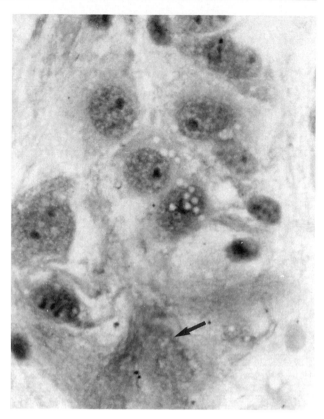

Fig. 4.21. Cytology of synovial sarcoma. Scraping prepared from tissue biopsy showing several plump, neoplastic mesenchymal cells closely associated with strands of brightly eosinophilic mucinous matrix (arrow). A diagnosis of synovial sarcoma cannot be made on the basis of cytology alone as similar cells can be harvested from other mesenchymal tumors, including chondrosarcomas and osteosarcomas.

myxoid change are difficult to differentiate from myxosarcoma or malignant peripheral nerve sheath tumors. The perivascular orientation of synovioblastic or fibroblastic tumor cells in some tumors might also cause confusion with hemangiopericytoma, especially in lesions where there is infiltration of the skin adjacent to the joint or tendon sheath.

As in human synovial sarcomas,[3] there appears to be no relationship in animals between the histological appearance of the tumor and its biological behavior.

Cytological examination of fine needle aspiration biopsies from a synovial sarcoma may reveal a population of plump, malignant mesenchymal cells with eccentric nuclei and basophilic cytoplasm[19] (fig. 4.21). Variable numbers of spindle cells and multinucleated giant cells may also be present. Malignant synoviocytes can not reliably be differentiated from malignant osteoblasts or certain other malignant mesenchymal cells on cytology alone, and histology is necessary for a definitive diagnosis.

Growth and Metastasis

In one review of canine synovial sarcomas,[13] 20 of 37 cases (54 percent) developed metastases at some stage, but there is considerable variation in the duration of clinical signs and the time to metastasis. The clinical course may vary from less than 1 month to greater than 1 year. Metas-

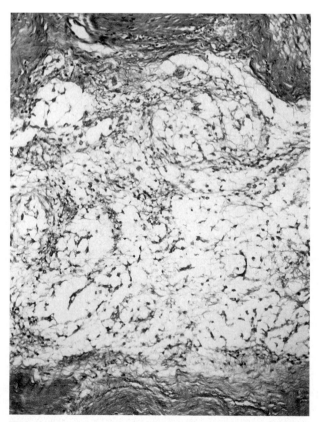

B

Fig. 4.20. Additional histological variations in canine synovial sarcoma. **A.** Sheets of malignant synovioblastic cells, many of which are angular and have eccentric nuclei. Nuclei vary in size and often contain prominent nucleoli. Occasional mitotic figures are present (arrow). Note the eosinophilic matrix around many of the cells. This might be mistaken for osteoid, leading to an incorrect diagnosis of osteosarcoma. **B.** Synovial sarcoma with abundant myxoid matrix resembling myxosarcoma.

tases were found most frequently in the lungs (10) and regional lymph nodes (10), and less often in the kidneys, spleen, thoracic pleura, liver, and heart.[13] Local recurrence following excision or amputation is common.[10,11]

REFERENCES

1. Miettinen, M. and Virtanen, I. (1984) Synovial sarcoma—A misnomer. *Amer J Pathol* 117:18–25.

2. Hendrick, M.J., Mahaffey, E.A., Moore, F.M., Vos, J.H., and Walder, E.J. (1998) *Histological Classification of Mesenchymal Tumors of the Skin and Soft Tissues of Domestic Animals.* World Health Organization. 2nd series, vol. 2. Armed Forces Institute of Pathology, American Registry of Pathology, Washington, D.C.

3. Cadman, N.L., Soule, E.H., and Kelly, P.J. (1965) Synovial sarcoma, an analysis of 134 tumors. *Cancer* 18:613–627.

4. Fechner, R.F. (1976) Neoplasms and Neoplasm-like lesions of the synovium. In Ackerman, L.V., Spjut, H.J., and Abell, M.R. (eds.), *Bones and Joints.* Williams and Wilkins Co., Baltimore, pp. 157–186.

5. Lattes, R. (1982) Tumors of soft tissue. In *Atlas of Tumor Pathology.* 2nd series, fascicle 1, revised. Armed Forces Institute of Pathology, Washington, D.C.

6. Salisbury, J.R., and Isaacson, P.G. (1985) Synovial sarcoma: An immunohistochemical study. *J Pathol* 147:49–57.

7. Dickersin, G.R. (1991) Synovial sarcoma: A review and update, with emphasis on the ultrastructural characterization of the nonglandular component. *Ultrastruct Pathol* 15:379–402.

8. Fox, R.I., and Kang, H. (1993) Structure and function of synoviocytes. In McCarty, D. (ed.), *Arthritis and Allied Conditions: A Textbook of Rheumatology,* 12th ed. Ch. 14. Lea and Febiger, p. 263.

9. Fisher, C. (1998) Synovial sarcoma. *Ann Diagn Pathol* 2:401–421.

10. Lipowitz, A.J., Fetter, Q.W., and Walker, M.A. (1979) Synovial sarcoma of the dog. *J Amer Vet Med Assoc* 174:76–81.

11. Madewell, B.R., and Pool, R.R. (1978) Neoplasms of joints and related structures. *Vet Clin N Amer* 8:511–521.

12. Bellah, J.R., and Patton, C.S. (1986) Non-weight bearing lameness secondary to synovial sarcoma in a young dog. *J Amer Vet Med Assoc* 188:730–732.

13. McGlennon, N.J., Houlton, J.E.F., and Gorman, N.T. (1988) Synovial sarcoma in the dog—A review. *J Small Anim Pract* 29:139–152.

14. Griffith, J.W., Frey, R.A., and Sharkey, F.E. (1987) Synovial sarcoma of the jaw in a dog. *J Comp Pathol* 97:361–364.

15. Pool, R.R. (1990) Tumors and tumor-like conditions of joints and adjacent soft tissues. In Moulton J.E. (ed.), *Tumors in Domestic Animals,* 3rd ed. Ch. 4. University of California Press, Berkeley.

16. Silva-Krott, I.U., Tucker, R.L., and Meeks, J.C. (1993) Synovial sarcoma in a cat. *J Amer Vet Med Assoc* 203:1430–1431.

17. Dungworth, D.L., Wilson, M.R., Gruchy, C.L., and McCallum, G. (1964) Malignant synovioma in a cow. *J Pathol Bacteriol* 88:83–87.

18. Gupta, P.P., and Singh, B. (1978) Synovial sarcoma in a bullock. *Indian Vet J* 55:831–832.

19. Baker, R., and Lumsden, J.H. (1999) *Color Atlas of Cytology of the Dog and Cat.* Mosby, St Louis.

Malignant Fibrous Histiocytoma

General Considerations and Classification

Although *tumors* in this section are categorized as separate entities, future studies may indicate a similar histogenesis for a visually diverse group and provide ancillary criterion that can be used to identify these interesting lesions. Malignant fibrous histiocytoma is a pleomorphic sarcoma centered more often in deep than in superficial connective tissues of adult humans. In its classic form the tumor is characterized by the presence of spindled (fibroblast-like) cells arranged in a storiform (*cartwheel* or *whirligig*) pattern and rounded (histiocyte-like) cells that are accompanied by pleomorphic multinucleated giant cells and, occasionally, by inflammatory cells.[1,2] Although subject to debate for many years, malignant fibrous histiocytoma is now widely regarded as a clinicopathological entity in humans and has been subclassified into five variants: storiform-pleomorphic, myxoid, giant cell, inflammatory, and angiomatoid.[2] More than one of these morphological types may exist within the same tumor, in which case classification is based on the predominant pattern. The tumor occurs in adults (peak incidence around 61 to 70 years) and may be located in the upper or lower extremities, abdominal cavity, or retroperitoneum.[1,2] Local recurrence is common, as is metastasis to the lungs and regional lymph nodes. Inflammatory cells, particularly lymphocytes, are present in greater than 50 percent of malignant fibrous histiocytomas in human patients.

The histogenesis of malignant fibrous histiocytoma remains controversial. Some authors suggest a histiocytic origin, while others suggest fibroblastic/myofibroblastic lineage. Studies using immunohistochemistry or electron microscopy have failed to provide a satisfactory resolution, but malignant fibrous histiocytoma is most likely a tumor of primitive mesenchymal cells capable of differentiating into either histiocytic or fibroblastic cell lines.

Malignant fibrous histiocytoma is uncommon in animals but has been reported with increasing frequency in dogs[3-10] and cats[3,6,11-15] and occasionally in the pig[16] and cow.[17] The tumors in animals have occurred at various locations, including the spleen, subcutis, bone, and periarticular tissues of the limbs. The storiform-pleomorphic variant is the most common form of malignant fibrous histiocytoma in dogs and in humans. The giant cell variant, which is believed to be analogous to the *giant cell tumor of soft parts,* predominates in cats[11-15] but has also been described in dogs[7,8] and horses.[18,19] It should be mentioned that although malignant fibrous histiocytoma is recognized as a distinct entity by many veterinary pathologists, this remains controversial, and the debate is likely to continue until it can be resolved by the use of immunochemical staining or other techniques in molecular biology. In the meantime, it will be included as an entity in this chapter.

Malignant Fibrous Histiocytoma in Dogs

Since the initial report of malignant fibrous histiocytoma in 2 dogs in 1979,[3] the tumor has been the subject of several reports.[4-10] Most dogs with malignant fibrous histiocytoma are middle-aged to old. In the only reports with sufficient numbers of cases to draw conclusions, the mean age of affected dogs varied from 8.4 to 9.4 years (range 1.5 to 17.5 years).[7,9] No sex predilection is apparent. In one study,[9] golden retrievers were overrepresented.

Malignant fibrous histiocytoma in dogs may occur as a single, expansile tumor, most often involving the skin or spleen, or may involve multiple organs, including the lungs, liver, lymph nodes, kidney, bones and periarticular tissues. Although metastases were not a feature of the initial report,[3] most subsequent reports describe malignant fibrous histiocytoma as an aggressive tumor that metastasizes via both lymphatic and vascular routes. Median survival time of 10 affected dogs in one study was 61 days.[7]

The tumors tend to be firm, unencapsulated, fleshy masses, sometimes containing areas of necrosis. Lytic bone lesions observed radiographically in the metaphyses of several long bones in one dog and in the axial skeleton of another[5] closely resembled the lesions of plasma cell myeloma. Periosteal proliferation may accompany tumors that occur in soft tissues adjacent to bone surfaces. Microscopically, malignant fibrous histiocytomas are pleomorphic neoplasms consisting of varying proportions of fibroblastic cells, mononuclear histiocytic cells, multinucleated giant cells, and nonsuppurative inflammatory cells. The histiocytic cells are rounded to polygonal and often possess very large nuclei with prominent nucleoli. Occasional very large mononuclear cells may be present in addition to variable numbers of binucleate and multinucleate cells. Mitotic figures are common and often bizarre. In some tumors, the fibroblastic component may dominate, suggesting the possibility of fibrosarcoma, but the presence of scattered histiocytic cells should cast doubt on this diagnosis. The fibroblasts may be arranged in the characteristic storiform (cartwheel) pattern, at least in some areas. Lymphocytes, plasma cells, and eosinophils are often present throughout the tumor and are a prominent feature in some cases. As in humans, malignant fibrous histiocytomas in dogs may be subclassified on the basis of the predominant pattern. The storiform-pleomorphic variant is the most common subtype in dogs, but inflammatory and giant cell subtypes are also recognized.

Differentiation of malignant fibrous histiocytoma from malignant histiocytosis, which occurs in dogs of similar age and breed,[9] is often difficult, especially in those cases where the histiocytic component is a dominant feature. In fact, tumors with features of both malignant fibrous histiocytoma and malignant histiocytosis are reported in a large survey in dogs.[9] It is suggested that these tumors may be derived from the same undifferentiated precursor that differentiates toward either malignant fibrous histiocytoma or malignant histiocytosis, sometimes resulting in a tumor with overlapping phenotypes. Malignant fibrous histiocytoma must also be differentiated from synovial sarcoma, which typically contains a mixture of fibroblastic and epithelioid elements. Because of the variation that may be present throughout malignant fibrous histiocytoma, the diagnosis is more reliable if the sections examined are representative of the entire mass.

Cytological examination of fine needle aspirates from a malignant fibrous histiocytoma may assist in the confirmation of malignancy, but it is unlikely to allow unequivocal diagnosis. It is important to be aware that the histiocytic cells and multinucleated giant cells are likely to exfoliate more readily than the neoplastic fibroblasts and that therefore cytological preparations may not be truly representative of the lesion. A definitive diagnosis requires histological assessment. In one report of malignant fibrous histiocytoma involving the deep musculature and fascia around the stifle joint of a dog,[10] cytological examination of joint fluid revealed neoplastic cells, including binucleate and occasional multinucleate forms. Many of the cells had multiple cytoplasmic vacuoles. The provisional diagnosis on the basis of cytology was chondrosarcoma or osteosarcoma.[10]

Malignant Fibrous Histiocytoma in Cats

The presence of abundant multinucleated giant cells is a feature of malignant fibrous histiocytoma in cats,[3,6,11-15] and the tumor in this species is considered analogous to the giant cell variant of malignant fibrous histiocytoma in humans. Postvaccinal sarcoma in the cat is also considered to represent a variant of malignant fibrous histiocytoma.[20] This giant cell type of malignant fibrous histiocytoma, which occurs in horses,[18,19] is commonly referred to as *malignant giant cell tumor of soft parts*. For convenience, the tumor will be discussed in detail in the following section.

Malignant Giant Cell Tumors of Soft Parts and Malignant Giant Cell Tumors of Tendon Sheaths

Classification

Malignant giant cell tumor of soft parts is a malignant tumor of superficial and deep connective tissue that has some of the microscopic features of malignant giant cell tumor of bone. The term was first used to describe 32 cases of this unique extraskeletal neoplasm in humans.[21] This tumor has also been reported in domestic animals.[3,11,18,19,22,23] The histogenesis of the tumor has not been determined. Earlier descriptions of this neoplasm in humans and in cats[22] indicated that some of the deeply seated tumors in the group may have originated in tendons or their sheaths, and the term *malignant giant cell tumor of the tendon sheath* was applied to those lesions.[21] Evidence to date does not, however, support the concept that malignant giant cell tumors of the tendon sheath constitute a specific entity, at least in humans.[21,24] In a survey of 32 cases in human patients,[21] although some deep-seated tumors involved the tendon apparatus, no tumor was completely localized to a tendon or tendon sheath. In fact the majority of the human tumors involved only deep fascia and skeletal muscles. These authors also observed that the malignant giant cell tumor of soft parts should not be regarded as the malignant counterpart of the benign giant cell tumor of tendons and tendon sheaths, and they pointed out that the two tumors occur in different anatomical sites. The similarity between the neoplastic mononuclear cells and normal histiocytes, together with the observation of phagocytic activity by both mononuclear and multinucleated tumor cells,[21] led the authors to suggest that the tumor originates from histiocytes or their precursors. It is now considered that the malignant giant cell tumor of soft parts in humans and domestic animals is a variant of malignant fibrous histiocytoma.[1,2,20]

Although malignant giant cell tumor of the tendon sheath is no longer considered a distinct entity in humans, giant cell sarcomas occasionally appear to arise within the mesenchyme of tendons and tendon sheaths of animals.[22,25] For this reason the term is preserved in this chapter, even though such tumors may eventually be shown to be analogous to malignant giant cell tumors of soft parts and, therefore, a variant of malignant fibrous histiocytoma.

Incidence, Age, Breed, and Sex

Malignant giant cell tumors of soft parts have been reported in several mature equidae, including quarter horses, standardbreds, an Arabian mare, and a mule.[18,19] In a study of six horses,[19] the average age was 6.8 years (range 3 to 12 years). The tumor appears to be more common in cats[3,6,11-15] than in horses. In one review of 16 previously published cases,[13] the average age of affected cats was 6.5 years (range 9 months to 12 years). Most were in domestic shorthair cats, but the tumor has also been recognized in domestic longhair, Persian, and tabby cats. No gender bias is apparent in either horses or cats with malignant giant cell tumors of soft parts. A series of 10 cases of the giant cell variant of malignant fibrous histiocytoma has been reviewed in dogs.[7] The breeds represented were golden retriever (four cases), rottweiler (two cases), Labrador retriever, pointer, miniature schnauzer, and a mixed breed (one case each). The median age was 8.4 years (range 3.0 to 10.3 years), and 7 of the 10 dogs were female. We have seen one further example of this tumor in an 8-year-old female doberman pinscher.

A case of malignant giant cell tumor, thought to be of tendon sheath origin,[22] was reported in an 8-year-old male domestic cat. It is possible that two of the cats in another report[3] were also afflicted with malignant giant cell tumors of the tendon sheath. We would also place the tumor involving the digit of a 2-year-old male cat in this category.[12] Two examples of this tumor in our collection occurred in mature male dogs.

Clinical Characteristics

Malignant giant cell tumors of soft parts appear in horses as firm, raised, solitary masses firmly attached to superficial subcutaneous tissue.[18-19] Although none of these tumors metastasized, excision was followed by local recurrence in three of seven cases. In two of three cats[18,23] and in the dog of our collection, the tumors were located in deep fascia. In one cat[11] the tumor formed a movable subcutaneous mass. The tumor recurred six times in this cat following surgery. Metastatic disease was not reported in the cats, but it was present at the time of diagnosis in 7 of 10 dogs with the giant cell variant of malignant fibrous histiocytoma.[7] Two further dogs in this report developed metastases during the course of treatment. In humans,[21] the superficial tumors are small, occur in the subcutis and superficial fascia, recur frequently after excision, and metastasize infrequently. The deep tumors are large and involve skeletal muscle, deep fascia, and tendons. About 70 percent of human patients with deeply seated tumors develop metastatic disease.

Malignant giant cell tumors of the tendon sheath form a painless cylindrical swelling of soft tissues following the course of a muscle-tendon apparatus. Usually, there is a history of rapid swelling and a rapidly progressive mechanical lameness. On initial examination the lesion is often thought to be an infection. Metastatic disease developed in one dog from our collection. Early diagnosis and amputation may control the tumor.

Sites and Gross Morphology

The superficial lesions of malignant giant cell tumors of soft parts reported in horses were located in the superficial fascia and subcutis of the jugular groove of the neck (two), thigh (two), stifle region (two), and shoulder (one).[18,19] The tumors were solitary, firm, raised, incompletely lobulated, ovoid masses, 1 to 4 cm in diameter, and they had a capsule. On cut surface they were pale and firm and had multiple small areas of hemorrhage and necrosis. The superficial lesion in one cat[11] was a mass 2 cm in diameter located in the subcutaneous tissue of the back between the shoulder blades.

The deep lesions of malignant giant cell tumors of soft parts formed a large ($3 \times 4 \times 12$ cm), glistening, lobulated mass obliterating the femoral canal on the medial side of the right hind limb of one cat[18] and a large mass involving the soft tissues of the right shoulder and axilla of a second cat.[23] The tumor has also been reported in the soft tissues of the distal forelimb in one cat[14] and the carpal region of another.[15] A firm, nodular, ovoid mass (2.5 cm in diameter) was located in the body of the triceps muscle of the left foreleg of a dog in our collection. Mineralized tissue was present within and at the borders of the canine tumor.

The malignant giant cell tumor of tendon sheaths in the cat[22] produced a cylindrical soft tissue swelling that extended from the elbow region to the carpus on the caudal side of the right foreleg. In our collection, the tumor produced a flattened, sac-like, doughy mass containing the digital flexor tendons on the plantar surface of the left metatarsal region of one dog; in the second dog it produced a fusiform swelling involving the tendon of the biceps brachii muscle and the biceps bursa (fig. 4.22 A). All three tumors were incompletely lobulated. Multiple hemorrhages were present in the sectioned tumors. The feline tumor was very firm. Both canine lesions were formed of soft, fleshy, tan to grayish white tissue. No mineralized tissue was apparent in any of the three tendon sheath tumors.

Histological Features

The characteristic cytological features occurring in both the malignant giant cell tumors of soft parts and malignant giant cell tumors of tendon sheaths include large multinucleated tumor giant cells, large pleomorphic mononuclear cells, histiocytes, neoplastic spindle cells, and fibroblasts (figs. 4.22 B,C,D). The multinucleated giant cells had as many as 60 nuclei per cell and appeared to arise from large mononuclear tumor cells or their precursors. Anaplastic features could be found in the multinucleated giant cells, the large mononuclear cells, and the spindle cell component. The latter cells often formed areas of fibrosarcomatous stroma at the periphery of the mass or in septa that partially divided the tumor into incomplete lobules.

The superficial malignant giant cell tumors of soft parts in humans are relatively small.[21] Mononuclear tumor cells have slight to minimal anaplastic features and a relatively low mitotic index. These features correlate with a low degree of malignancy of the superficial tumors in humans. Malignant bone tissue was formed in 4 of the 12 superficial human tumors. The pattern of the tumors described in horses[19] bore a striking similarity to the superficial human tumors, but no osteogenic tissue was found in the equine tumors.

In contrast, the deep types of malignant giant cell tumors of soft parts in humans are large.[21] The mononuclear tumor cells in these tumors exhibit moderate to marked anaplastic features and have a higher mitotic index than the superficial tumors. The fibrosarcomatous component is also increased. Areas of differentiation to malignant cartilage and bone were seen in 11 of the 20 deep tumors. It is likely that the deep types of tumors in the cat[11,18,23] and the dog of our collection are counterparts to the deeply seated tumors of humans. The dog had areas of metaplastic bone formed both within and at the borders of the tumor (fig. 4.22 C). We could find no evidence of malignant bone or cartilage tissue in the tumor.

The malignant giant cell tumors of two cats[12,22] and two dogs in our collection had histological features similar to those described for the deep types of malignant giant cell tumors of soft parts, with the exception that bone and cartilage tissues were absent. Although multinucleated giant cells and large mononuclear tumor cells were prominent features of these tumors, there were also large areas of spindle cell sarcoma that had the interwoven pattern of fibrosarcoma, especially along the borders and the poles of the fusiform tumor mass.

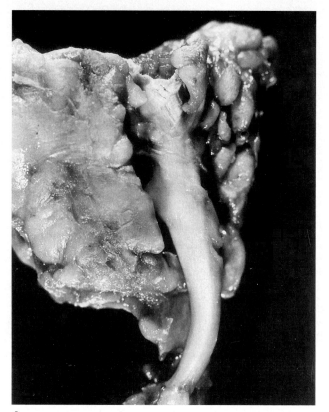

A

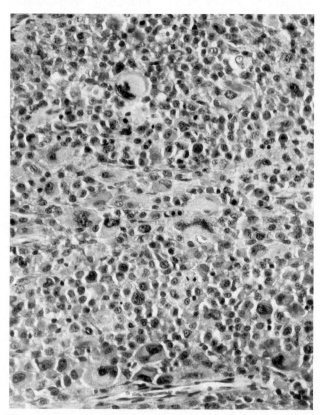

B

Fig. 4.22. Malignant giant cell tumors of soft parts and of tendon sheaths. **A.** Malignant giant cell tumor of the biceps bursa in a dog. Synovial lining of the bursa has nodular infiltrates of tumor cells. **B.** Numerous bizarre multinucleated tumor giant cells are among the infiltrate of large and small mononuclear cells. (continued)

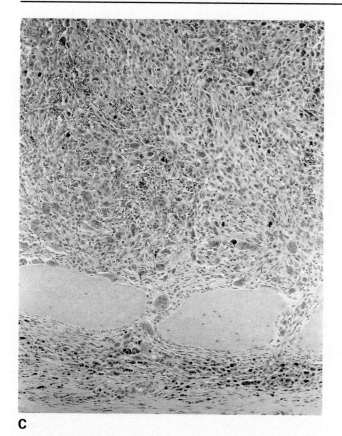

C

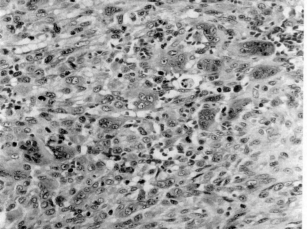

D

Fig. 4.22. (continued) **C.** Low magnification of a malignant giant cell tumor of soft parts located in the triceps muscle of a dog. Plates of metaplastic bone are located at the border of the tumor. **D.** Pleomorphic mononuclear cells, multinucleated giant cells, and spindled cells are major features of this sarcoma.

Growth and Metastasis

The superficial types of malignant giant cell tumors of soft parts as reported in horses[18,19] and humans[21] tend to be smaller, grow slower, and be less infiltrative than the more deeply seated types found in two cats,[18,23] the dog of our collection, and humans.[21] A superficial tumor in one cat,[11] however, recurred six times after local resection. Both the superficial and deep tumors tend to recur following surgery, but the deep form, at least in humans,[21] has a much higher metastatic potential.

The malignant giant cell tumors of tendon sheaths in two cats[12,22] and the two dogs of our collection grew rapidly in a few weeks' time. All four tumors appeared grossly to have a defined border, but infiltration of adjacent soft tissues was present microscopically in both canine cases. Metastasis to abdominal lymph nodes occurred in one of the dogs.

Canine Histiocytic Sarcoma

Histiocytic sarcoma in dogs is a rapidly growing, locally aggressive tumor that usually occurs on an extremity or in close proximity to a joint.[26] There is an apparent breed predilection, with flat-coated retrievers, golden retrievers, Labrador retrievers and rottweilers most commonly affected. An age range of 6–11 years is reported,[26] and the tumor occurs in both sexes. Although histiocytic sarcomas may arise from the skin or subcutaneous tissue and infiltrate underlying tissues, some cases appear to originate from deeper tissues, including the joint capsule. In such cases, the location of the tumor may lead to an incorrect diagnosis of synovial sarcoma. Histiocytic sarcoma and malignant histiocytosis in dogs are believed to represent malignancies of Langerhans cells,[26] probably derived from deep tissues rather than the epidermis.

Tumors with cytological and histological features of histiocytic sarcoma, apparently originating from joints, have also been recognized in three dogs, a 4-year-old Rottweiler, a 6-year-old black retriever, and a 13-year-old keeshond. All three were female, and all had been lame for 3–4 weeks before being presented for veterinary examination. The rottweiler had a soft tissue swelling around the right elbow joint and lytic lesions in the epiphysis of the distal humerus and metaphysis of the proximal radius. Surgical exposure of the elbow joint revealed marked nodular thickening and reddening of the synovial membrane. The retriever had a non–weight-bearing lameness centered on the right shoulder. This was associated with an 8 × 4 cm soft tissue mass medial to the joint and large lytic areas in the caudal aspect of the proximal humerus and the scapula. The joint capsule and synovial villi within the shoulder joint were markedly thickened (fig. 4.23 A). The mass extended dorsally along the medial side of the scapula and around the caudal aspect of the proximal humerus, where it was firmly adherent to the bone. The tumor tissue was firm, was gray/pink on cut surface, and contained focal areas of necrosis. In the keeshond, a soft tissue mass

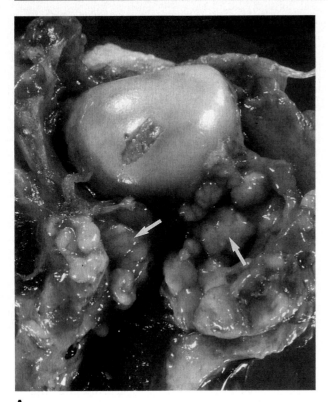

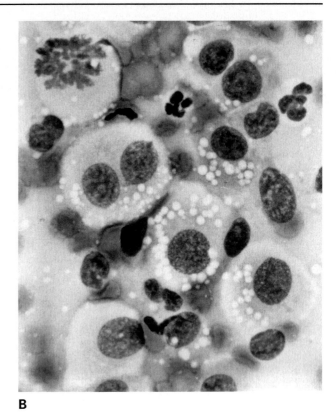

A

B

Fig. 4.23.   Histiocytic sarcoma involving the shoulder joint of a black retriever dog. **A.** There is nodular thickening of synovial villi (arrows) due to infiltration with tumor. The joint capsule is also thickened and fleshy, and the tumor extends into the skeletal muscle distal to the joint. The defect on the articular surface is artifactual. **B.** Scraping prepared from a cut surface of the tumor showing many large round cells with one or more nuclei and abundant, sometimes vacuolated, cytoplasm. One binucleate cell is present and another cell is undergoing mitosis. (continued)

surrounded the right stifle joint, infiltrating the synovium and joint capsule and extending into the adjacent muscles. Metastases were detected in the axillary lymph node of the retriever and in the popliteal and sublumbar lymph nodes of the keeshond. The keeshond also had metastases in the lungs, liver, and kidney.

Scrapings prepared for cytological examination from a cut surface of the tumor in the retriever revealed a monomorphic population of large round cells with circular to oval or indented nuclei and abundant cytoplasm, which often contained many discrete vacuoles (fig. 4.23 B). Multinucleated giant cells containing nuclei of various sizes were common, and there were many abnormal mitotic figures.

Histologically, the tumor in all three dogs had extensively infiltrated the joint capsule and synovial membrane, often causing nodular thickening of synovial villi (fig. 4.23 C). Sheets of tumor cells also separated muscle bundles adjacent to the affected joints and replaced the normal nodal architecture at sites of lymph node metastasis. The nuclei of the tumor cells varied considerably in size and shape and often contained large, irregularly shaped nucleoli (fig. 4.23 C,D). The cells had a moderate to large quantity of eosinophilic cytoplasm, which sometimes contained many small vacuoles (fig. 4.23 D). Multinucleated giant cells with variably sized nuclei were common, and the mitotic rate was high in many areas. Neutrophils,

eosinophils, lymphocytes, and plasma cells were present in varying numbers throughout the tumors in each dog. Sections of bone from the lytic area in the proximal radius of the rottweiler revealed sheets of tumor cells filling intertrabecular spaces, presumably due to direct invasion from the attachment of the joint capsule or the adjacent muscle.

Confirmation of the malignant cells in these tumors as histiocytic requires specific immunochemical staining. The tumor cells in the retriever and keeshond were both CD18 positive, but this antigen is present on all leukocytes and does not prove a histiocytic origin. These cases of suspected histiocytic sarcoma, and several others observed by Moore[27] in the vicinity of canine joints, await further immunochemical characterization before their histogenesis is proven beyond doubt.

The prognosis of histiocytic sarcoma is poor as the tumor is locally aggressive and may metastasize to regional lymph nodes or more distant sites. Early diagnosis followed by complete excision or amputation of the affected limb provides the best chance of a successful outcome.

REFERENCES

1. Lattes, R. (1982) Malignant fibrous histiocytoma: A review article. *Amer J Surg Pathol* 6:761–771.

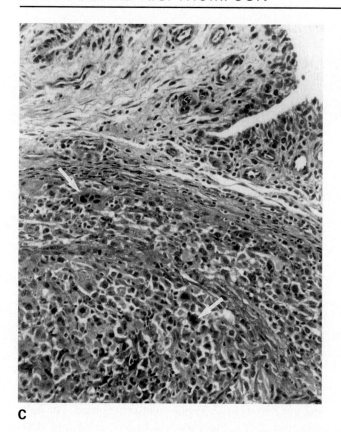

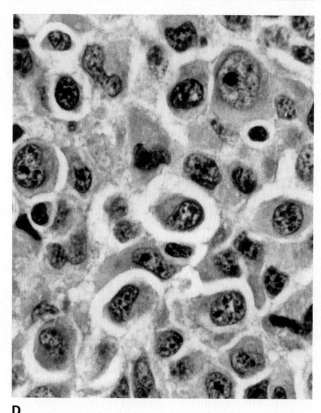

C   **D**

Fig. 4.23. (continued)   **C.** Sheets of tumor cells infiltrating the synovial membrane. Occasional binucleate cells and multinucleate giant cells (arrows) are present. **D.** Higher magnification of the same tumor showing a population of round cells with a moderate to large amount of cytoplasm, anisokaryosis, anisonucleoliosis, variable nuclear shape and variable N:C ratio.

2. Enzinger, F.M., and Weiss, S.W. (1988) Malignant fibrohistiocytic tumors. In *Soft Tissue Tumors,* 2nd ed. C.V. Mosby, St Louis), pp. 269–300,

3. Gleiser, C.A., C.A., Raulston, G.L., Jardine, J.H., and Gray, K.N. (1979) Malignant fibrous histiocytoma in dogs and cats. *Vet Pathol* 16:199–208.

4. Thomas, J.B. (1988) Malignant fibrous histiocytoma in a dog. *Aust Vet J* 65:252–254.

5. O'Brien, R.T., Hendrick, M.J., Evans, S.M., and Brooks, J.J. (1991) Pathological and radiological features of multicentric malignant fibrous histiocytoma in two dogs. *J Comp Pathol* 105:423–430.

6. Thoolen, R.J.M.M., Vos, J.H., van der Linde-Sipman, J.S., De Weger, R.A., van Unnik, J.A.M., Misdorp, W., and van Dijk, J.E. (1992) Malignant fibrous histiocytoma in dogs and cats: An immunohistochemical study. *Res Vet Sci* 53:198–204.

7. Waters, C.B., Morrison, W.B., DeNicola, D.B., Widmer, W.R., and White, M.R. (1994) Giant cell variant of malignant fibrous histiocytoma in dogs: 10 cases (1986–1993). *J Amer Vet Med Assoc* 205:1420–1424.

8. Hendrick, M.J., Brooks J.J., and Bruce, E.H. (1992) Six cases of malignant fibrous histiocytoma of the canine spleen. *Vet Pathol* 29:351–354.

9. Kerlin, R.L., and Hendrick, M.J. (1996) Malignant fibrous histiocytoma and malignant histiocytosis in the dog—Convergent or divergent phenotypic differentiation? *Vet Pathol* 33:713–716.

10. Booth, M.J., Bastianello, S.S., Jiminez, M., and van Heerden A. (1998) Malignant fibrous histiocytoma of the deep peri-articular tissue of the stifle in a dog. *J S Afr Vet Assoc* 69:163–168.

11. Confer, A.W., Enright, F.M., and Beard, G.B. (1981) Ultrastructure of feline extraskeletal giant cell tumor (malignant fibrous histiocytoma). *Vet Pathol* 18:738–744.

12. Renlund, R.C., and Pritzker, K.P.H. (1984) Malignant fibrous histiocytoma involving the digit in a cat. *Vet Pathol* 21:442–444.

13. Garma-Avina, A. (1987) Malignant fibrous histiocytoma of the giant cell type in a cat. *J Comp Pathol* 97:551–557.

14. Allen, S.W., and Duncan, J.R. (1988) Malignant fibrous histiocytoma in a cat. *J Amer Vet Med Assoc* 192:90–91.

15. Gibson, K.L., Blass, C.E., Simpson, M., and Gaunt, S.D. (1989) Malignant fibrous histiocytoma in a cat. *J Amer Vet Med Assoc* 194:1443–1445.

16. Tanimoto, T., Ohtsuki, Y., Sonobe, H., Takahashi, R., and Nomura, Y. (1988) Malignant fibrous histiocytoma in the spleen of a pig. *Vet Pathol* 25:330–332.

17. Sartin, E.A., Hudson, J.A., Herrera, G.A., Dickson, A.M., and Wolfe, D.F. (1996) Invasive malignant fibrous histiocytoma in a cow. *J Amer Vet Med Assoc* 208:1709–1710.

18. Ford, G.H., Empson, R.N., Plopper, C.G., and Brown, P.H. (1975) Giant cell tumor of soft parts: A report of an equine and a feline case. *Vet Pathol* 12:428–433.

19. Render, J.A., Harrington, D.D., Well, R.E., Dunstan, R.W., Turek, J.J., and Bosssinger, T.R. (1982) giant cell tumor of soft parts in six horses. *J Amer Vet Med Assoc* 183:790–793.

20. Hendrick, M.J., Mahaffey, E.A., Moore, F.M., Vos, J.H., and Walder, E.J. (1998) *Histological Classification of Mesenchymal Tumors of the Skin and Soft Tissues of Domestic Animals.* World Health Organization. 2nd series, vol, 2. Armed Forces Institute of Pathology, American Registry of Pathology, Washington D.C.

21. Guccion, J.G., and Enzinger, F.M. (1972) Malignant giant cell tumor of soft parts: An analysis of 32 cases. *Cancer* 29:1518–1529.

22. Neilsen, S.W. (1952) Extraskeletal giant cell tumor in a cat. *Cornell Vet* 42:304–311.

23. Alexander, J.W., Riis, R.C., and Dueland, R. (1975) Extraskeletal giant cell tumor in cat. *Vet Med Small Anim Clin* 70:1161–1166.

24. Fechner, R.F. (1976) Neoplasms and neoplasm-like lesions of the synovium. In Ackerman, L.V., Spjut, H.J., and Abell, M.R. (eds.), *Bones and Joints*. Williams and Wilkins Co., Baltimore, pp. 157–186.

25. Pool, R.R. (1990) Tumors and tumor-like conditions of joints and adjacent soft tissues. In Moulton J.E. (ed.), *Tumors in Domestic Animals*, 3rd ed. University of California Press, Berkeley.

26. Affolter, V.K. and Moore, P.F. (1997) Histiocytosis. *Proceedings of the European Society of Veterinary Dermatology 14th Annual Congress*, Pisa, Italy, 5-7 September, pp. 101–104.

27. Moore, P.F. personal communication.

Musculoaponeurotic Fibromatosis

Classification

Fibromatosis is a desmoid tumor that arises in the abdominal and extra-abdominal musculature of children and adult humans and infiltrates surrounding tissues.[1-3] In spite of their infiltrative and often aggressive clinical behavior, these lesions are benign.

Several human entities, which have a broad spectrum of clinical behavior ranging from harmless nodules to potentially life-threatening, highly infiltrative lesions, are included under the category of fibromatosis.[2] One of these conditions is musculoaponeurotic fibromatosis of shoulder girdle in humans.[1] A condition thought to be analogous to the human disorder was described in the horse.[4] Other reports of this lesion in animals include an aggressive fibromatosis in a cat[5] and an infantile desmoid type fibromatosis in an Akita puppy.[6] Although some cases of fibromatosis exhibit the highly infiltrative behavior of fibrosarcoma, they are regarded as tumor-like fibrous proliferations because of their benign histological appearance and failure to produce metastatic disease.[1-3] Trauma has been proposed as an initiating factor in the human disorder.[1]

Incidence, Age, Breed, and Sex

The disorder is rare in domestic animals, but since the original report of musculoaponeurotic fibromatosis of the pectoral muscle in a 15-year-old thoroughbred mare,[4] we have seen biopsy specimens from indurated pectoral masses of two mature horses with similar clinical and microscopic findings. An isolated case of aggressive extra-abdominal desmoid fibromatosis was reported in a 9-month-old male mixed breed cat,[5] and a case of infantile desmoid type fibromatosis was reported in a 10-week-old male Akita puppy.[6]

Clinical Characteristics and Sites

The pectoral swelling in affected horses has an insidious onset, and the period from first recognition by the owner to first physical examination may exceed 1 year. Firm, painless tumor masses are palpable in or near major skeletal muscles. As the mass enlarges, secondary complications may develop, including edema of the forelimbs and ulceration, accompanied by bacterial infection of the skin in the pectoral region. No attempt was made to surgically remove the fibrous tissue in the horse in the published case because of the size of the mass. A history of local trauma is common in human cases[1] and should be inquired about in the equine cases. The case of aggressive fibromatosis in the cat[5] presented with extensive swelling of the right forelimb from the toes to the shoulder joint. An ulcer, 2 cm in diameter, was present on the forearm. Radiographically, the radius and ulna were virtually absent. The cat had apparently been bitten on the limb, probably by another cat, two months previously. It had a positive blood test to FeLV antigen. The Akita puppy with infantile desmoid type fibromatosis[6] had a subcutaneous mass in the mid-ventral abdominal wall, extending from the xiphoid cartilage to midway between the umbilicus and the prepuce. An ulcer, 2.5 cm in diameter, was present in the skin overlying the mass adjacent to the umbilicus.

Gross Morphology

In the horse with musculoaponuerotic fibromatosis, parts of the pectoral and panniculus musculature of the ventral thoracic region were partially or totally replaced by fibrous tissue extending from a large, deeply seated, firm mass of fibrous tissue having no distinct borders. The overlying musculature, subcutaneous tissues, and dermis of the skin were partially indurated and hemorrhagic. The forearm of the cat with the aggressive form of fibromatosis was almost entirely replaced with firm, fibrous tissue, extending from the skin surface to the center of the limb.[5] Firm swellings were also present in the skin from the shoulders to the mandible.

Histological Features

The mass in affected horses is made up of highly indurated and poorly vascularized tissue in which a few uniform, spindle shaped cells separate randomly oriented collagen fibers (fig. 4.24 A). A more cellular zone of fibroblasts, producing relatively small amounts of collagen fibers, lies between the fibrous mass and the adjacent musculature. These cells are without anaplastic features, and mitotic figures are rare or absent. This cell population infiltrates between muscle fascicles and isolates individual muscle fibers (fig. 4.24 B). Entrapped muscle fibers may undergo atrophy or remain as elongated, multinucleated muscle giant cells. When the lesion extends to the skin, the dermis is infiltrated with thick, interlacing bands of collagen. Inflammatory cell exudate, necrosis, and hemorrhage are found at sites where ulcerated skin is infected. Similar microscopic changes are reported in the cat and the Akita puppy with other forms of fibromatosis. The tumor-like tissue consists of abundant collagen fibers and only sparse numbers of well-differentiated fibroblasts, surrounding muscle fibers, adipocytes, or other tissues located in the area. In the cat, some hypercellular areas contained multinucleated giant cells and immature fibroblasts.[5]

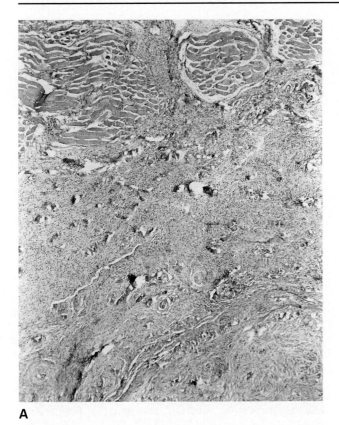

A

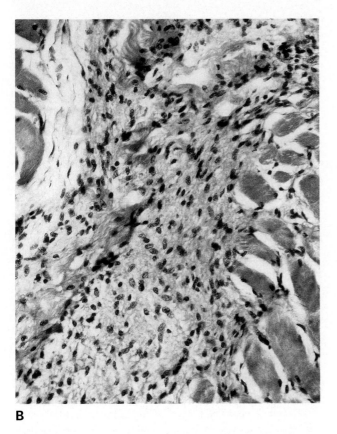

B

Fig. 4.24. Musculoaponeurotic fibromatosis in the pectoral region of a horse. **A.** Low magnification shows invasion between muscle bundles (top), an area of cellular proliferation (middle), and an area of dense collagen production (bottom). **B.** Spindle shaped cells without anaplastic features infiltrate a fascicle of muscle fibers.

Growth and Metastasis

Growth is slow and progressive but highly infiltrative. Although the lesion is regarded as a nonneoplastic fibrous proliferation, it should be diagnosed and treated by radical excision as soon as possible. In humans, multiple local recurrences following surgery are common, but neither metastatic disease nor transformation to fibrosarcoma has been documented.[1]

Malignant Mesenchymoma of the Dog

Classification

Malignant mesenchymoma is a tumor consisting of two or more different neoplastic cell lines of mesenchymal origin.[7] These tumors should be differentiated from certain sarcomas of soft tissues, such as synovial sarcoma, extraosseous chondrosarcoma, rhabdomyosarcoma, and liposarcoma, which contain an apparent malignant fibroblast-like component. They must also be differentiated from soft tissue sarcomas containing areas of metaplastic bone or cartilage formation.

Incidence, Age, Breed, and Sex

This rare tumor has been reported in an 8-year-old female German shepherd,[8] a 4-year-old male Irish setter,[9] and a 3-year-old female basset hound.[10] We have recognized this tumor in a 12-year-old spayed female Belgian sheepdog.

Clinical Characteristics

Clinical signs relate to the site and size of the lesion. In three cases, the lesions involved the limbs, and lameness and/or stiffness was associated with the presence of a large, firm, soft tissue mass. The tumor in the German shepherd occurred in the midshaft of the right femur, at the site of a previous fracture.[8] A large, radiodense lesion contained several cystic areas in the medullary region. In the Irish setter, a mass 6 cm in diameter had been removed from the thigh muscles and diagnosed as a malignant mesenchymoma approximately 6 months earlier.[9] The left hind limb was amputated by disarticulation at the hip joint, permitting the dog to survive for an additional 14 months. Metastatic lung disease became clinically apparent 13 months after amputation, when diffuse swelling of the forelimbs, indicative of hypertrophic osteopathy, was recognized. The dog was euthanized.

In the Belgian sheepdog, a firm, soft tissue mass 4 cm in diameter was first palpated in the fascia between the proximal thigh muscles and the left flank about 4 years earlier. In 3 years, the nodule grew to about 18 cm in diameter. In the 4 month period prior to clinical examination the mass showed rapid enlargement. The affected basset hound[10] was lethargic and inappetent and had a large, cyst-like intra-abdominal mass adhered to the dorsal aspect of the abdomen.

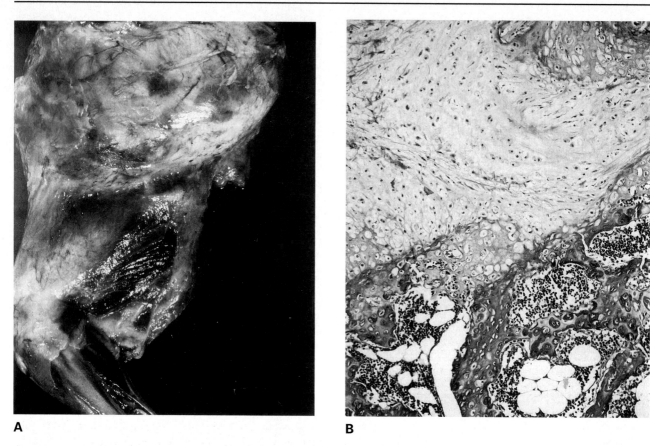

A   B

Fig. 4.25. Malignant mesenchymoma of the dog. **A.** Large, firm mass was adhered firmly to the dense fascia of the proximal thigh and outer abdominal wall. **B.** Central cartilage nodules of metaplastic and neoplastic cartilage that had undergone partial endochondral ossification. (continued)

Gross Morphology

The malignant mesenchymoma in the German shepherd[8] consisted of several irregularly sized, white/gray nodules that had invaded the cortex and medulla of the middle and proximal femur. Scattered, blood filled spaces were present in periosteal tissue.

The gross appearance of the recurrent tumor in the amputated leg of the Irish setter[9] was not described. However, an illustration of a cross section through the mass in the amputated limb shows a large, pale tumor mass that had apparently arisen in the superficial tissues of the thigh and had infiltrated and replaced most of the dorsal musculature of the proximal one-third of the thigh. The authors reported that the original mass occurred in the superficial soft tissues of the leg.

The tumor in the basset hound[10] was a smooth surfaced mass, 15 × 10 × 8 cm in size, extending from the right kidney to the left kidney and caudally to the bifurcation of the caudal vena cava. Approximately 10 cm of the caudal vena cava were incorporated into the tumor. On cut surface, the mass was granular, orange to brown, and had a multilayered structure. Following euthanasia, the body of the L₃ vertebra was found to be largely replaced with soft, brown tissue. Similar tissue was adherent to the spinal cord in the region of L₃ and appeared to be compressing the spinal cord.

Histological Features

All tumors consisted of anaplastic mesenchymal tissue differentiating along different cell lines. In the German shepherd, the tumor contained areas with microscopic features of liposarcoma and hemangiosarcoma, in addition to areas in which the tumor cells were forming either osteoid or chondroid matrix.[8] The neoplasm in the Irish setter included areas of chondrosarcoma and leiomyosarcoma with an abrupt interface between these tissue types.[9] Areas of osteoid and bone formation were scattered through the mass within bands of dense collagenous stroma. Interestingly, a pulmonary metastasis in this dog consisted of only chondrosarcoma. In the basset hound,[10] the tumor contained areas with features of both liposarcoma and osteosarcoma, in addition to areas of poorly differentiated mesenchymal cells with extensive necrosis and fibroplasia. Tumor cells were also found in the walls of several large blood vessels, including mesenteric veins and a thymic vein.

In the Belgian sheepdog, the central mineralized part of the tumor contained areas of metaplastic cartilage and low grade chondrosarcoma, both undergoing endochondral ossification (fig. 4.25 A,B). These areas were usually centered in dense fascia. There were several nodular areas of chondrosarcoma having more malignant features (fig. 4.25 C). No bone formation occurred in these areas. Small

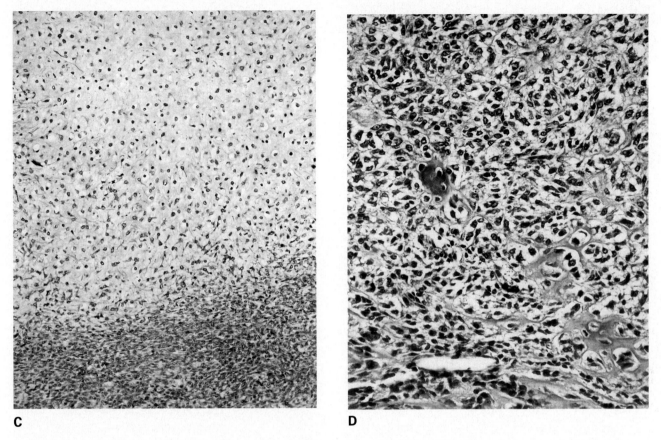

C   **D**

Fig. 4.25. (continued)   **C.** Nodular area of chondrosarcoma with a fibrosarcomatous component. **D.** Small area of osteosarcoma within the tumor.

areas of osteosarcoma were present (fig. 4.25 D), and vessel invasion was identified in one tissue section. The infiltrating tissue at the border of the mineralized tumor mass had features of a low grade fibrosarcoma containing foci of myxomatous change.

No metastatic disease was identified in the lung or regional lymph nodes of the Belgian sheepdog, although vessel invasion by osteosarcomatous tissue would have produced metastatic lung disease had the dog not been euthanized.

Growth and Metastasis

Malignant mesenchymomas are malignant tumors that have a much longer course than do most malignant tumors. They usually produce a large primary tumor mass before metastatic disease develops. Any one or all of the malignant components may metastasize. It appears that early recognition and complete surgical excision offers the best prognosis, but local recurrence should be anticipated because of the infiltrative nature of the malignant fibrous tissue component.

REFERENCES

1. Enzinger, F.M., and Shiraki, M. (1967) Musculo-aponeurotic fibromatosis of the shoulder girdle (extra-abdominal desmoid). *Cancer* 20:1131–1140.
2. Lattes, R. (1982) Tumors of soft tissue. In *Atlas of Tumor Pathology*. 2nd series, fascicle 1, revised. Armed Forces Institute of Pathology, Washington, D.C.
3. Resnick, D., and Niwayama, G. (1994) Soft tissues. In Resnick, D. (ed.), *Diagnosis of Bone and Joint Disorders*, 3rd ed. Vol. 6, ch. 95. W.B. Saunders, Philadelphia, pp.4491–4622.
4. Ihrke, P.J., Cain, G.R., and Stannard, A.A. (1983) Fibromatosis in a horse. *J Amer Vet Med Assoc* 10:1100–1102.
5. Motozwa, A., Yamazaki, H., and Kadota, K. (1992) Aggressive fibromatosis in a cat. *J Vet Med Sc* 54:329–333.
6. Cook, J.L., Turk, J.R., Pope, E.R., and Jordan, R.C. (1998) Infantile desmoid-type fibromatosis in an Akita puppy. *J Amer Anim Hosp Assoc* 34:291–294.
7. Stout, A.P., and Lattes, R. (1967) Malignant mesenchymoma. In *Tumors of Soft Tissues*. 2nd series, fascicle 1. Armed Forces Institute of Pathology, Washington, D.C., pp. 172–173.
8. Liu, S.K., Dorfman, H.D., Hurvitz, A.I., and Patnaik, A.K. (1977) Primary and secondary bone tumors in the dog. *J Small Anim Pract* 18:313–326.
9. Moore, R.W., Snyder S.P., Houchens, J.W., and Folk, J.J. (1983) Malignant mesenchymoma in a dog. *J Amer Anim Hosp Assoc.* 19:187–190.
10. Robinson, T.M., Dubielzig, R.R., and McAnulty, J.F. (1998) Malignant mesenchymoma associated with an unusual vasoinvasive metastasis in a dog. *J Amer Anim Hosp Assoc* 34:295–299.

5 Tumors of Bones

K. G. Thompson and R. R. Pool

Bones consist of a variety of mesenchymal tissues, any one of which has the potential to undergo neoplastic transformation. Primary tumors of bones may therefore be derived from precursors of bone tissue, cartilage, fibrous tissue, adipose tissue, or vascular tissue. Of these, tumors of bone and cartilage forming cell lines are the most common. Tumors arising from hematopoietic elements of the bone marrow are discussed in chapter 3. In humans, most primary tumors of bones are benign,[1] but this does not apply to all animal species. Several surveys and reviews of skeletal neoplasms in different species have been published.[2-11] In dogs, primary bone sarcomas, particularly osteosarcomas, greatly outnumber benign neoplasms of bones.[2,8,9] The proportions of benign and malignant neoplasms of bones are approximately equal in cats,[4] but in horses and cattle benign tumors of bones are much more common than sarcomas.[5] Secondary tumors of bones, especially metastatic carcinomas, are extremely common in human patients but are uncommon in animals. This may be partly due to less intense radiographic and pathological examination of the skeleton in animals, but the discrepancy does appear to be real.

The classification of primary tumors and tumor-like lesions of bones in domestic animals has recently been revised[12] and is presented in modified form in table 5.1. This system is based on the morphological characteristics of tumor cells, the matrix they produce, and their anatomic location. In reality, it can be difficult to confidently classify a skeletal tumor into one category or another. The predominant matrix component may vary throughout the tumor, and poorly differentiated mesenchymal cells in some tumors may show little evidence of their lineage. Generally, the tumor is classified based on identification of the most differentiated cells. However, since the prognosis of different bone tumors varies markedly, accurate classification by the pathologist will greatly assist the clinician or surgeon and is more than just an academic exercise.

GENERAL CONSIDERATIONS

The pathologist is ill-advised to rely purely on histological or cytological characteristics when diagnosing tumors of bones, particularly when dealing with small biopsy specimens. The clinical history of the animal and the radiographic appearance of the lesion are often crucial to an accurate diagnosis. Important clinical data include species, breed, age, the location of lesions, and the duration of the bone disorder. Certain bone tumors in man and animals have a tendency to occur in specific locations, hence the value of knowing the exact location of the tumor. It is also important to know if the animal has recently suffered from a systemic disease or soft tissue tumor, whether it is on immunosuppressive drug therapy, and whether there has been a previous fracture or infection at the site of the bone lesion.

Radiographic Examination

Radiographs provide valuable additional information on the extent, nature, and behavior of a bone tumor; they can be of considerable value to the surgeon or pathologist in establishing a list of likely differential diagnoses and in selecting sites for histological or cytological examination. Even at necropsy, a radiograph of a bone lesion will often provide more information of diagnostic relevance than gross examination of the affected bone. Morphologic features of value in the radiographic assessment of tumors and tumor-like lesions of bones include the pattern of bone destruction; the presence and nature of any visible tumor matrix or periosteal response; the pattern of cortical erosion, expansion, or penetration; and the presence of an adjacent soft tissue mass.[13-16] Radiographic examination of the lesion should note the following points:

- whether the lesion is monostotic or polyostotic,
- the exact location and extent of the lesion (e.g., epiphyseal, metaphyseal, or diaphyseal) and whether it is intramedullary, cortical, paracortical, periosteal, or juxtacortical in origin,
- the nature of the bony changes (e.g., focal or multifocal bone lysis and/or sclerosis),
- the density of the tumor tissue,
- the bone response to the tumor (e.g., whether the bony margins are well defined or indistinct and the nature of any periosteal reaction),
- the nature of any cortical changes, including cortical destruction and periosteal new bone formation,

- the involvement of adjacent soft tissues, and
- whether there is joint involvement.

Three main patterns of bone destruction are recognized: geographic, motheaten, and permeative. In the geographic pattern, which is the least aggressive, the lesion has well-defined margins and is clearly demarcated from the adjacent normal bone. A sclerotic margin may surround the lesion. Although most benign tumors demonstrate this pattern of bone destruction, it may also be present in some malignant tumors. The motheaten pattern has a more gradual transition from normal to abnormal bone and implies more aggressive bone destruction. Malignant bone tumors and osteomyelitis may demonstrate this pattern, but it is also found in some benign bone tumors. The permeative pattern reflects an aggressive bone lesion with rapid growth and invasion. The lesion is poorly demarcated, and it may be difficult to differentiate between affected and unaffected regions of bone. Highly malignant tumors such as osteosarcoma are most likely to display this pattern, as may some cases of osteomyelitis.

Knowledge of the growth rate of a bone tumor is of considerable importance in determining its aggressiveness. Serial radiographs are therefore of more value than a single radiograph. Radiodense areas within a tumor may reflect either calcification or ossification of the tumor matrix, but they may also be due to calcification of necrotic tumor tissue, callous formation in association with a pathologic fracture, or a sclerotic reaction in the adjacent normal bone.

Although the cortex provides an effective barrier to the lateral expansion of a benign tumor, fast growing malignant tumors and aggressive inflammatory lesions can readily penetrate it in one or several places. Cortical destruction will inevitably produce a periosteal response, the character of which can provide important information on the behavior of a bone tumor.[14,15] A slowly expanding tumor that is eroding the cortex from its endosteal surface is likely to stimulate the deposition of additional layers of bone beneath the periosteum, resulting in an expanded contour. More rapid tumor growth may stimulate the development of delicate spicules of woven bone on the periosteal surface. A triangular cuff, or *Codman's triangle,* may develop beneath an elevated periosteum at the edge of an invasive neoplasm (usually osteosarcoma) or infectious process. Osteosarcomas may also be accompanied by a *sunburst* appearance with spicules of periosteal bone, intermixed with tumor bone, radiating from a single focus. An *onion skin* appearance caused by several parallel layers of reactive periosteal bone generally indicates slower, or intermittent, expansion of the tumor.

It is seldom possible, on radiographic appearance alone, to reliably distinguish among primary tumors, secondary tumors, and inflammatory lesions of bones, especially in destructive monostotic lesions at locations not considered predilection sites for a primary bone tumor.

However, in cases of low grade fibrosarcoma and chondrosarcoma of bone, radiographs often provide a better indication of malignancy than microscopy. Radiographs may also indicate early malignant change in benign bone tumors such as osteochondroma.

Pathologic Examination

A primary requirement for making a correct microscopic diagnosis of a bone lesion is familiarity with the basic microscopic responses of bone and cartilage to various forms of injury. Equally important are properly fixed and decalcified tissue sections that can be oriented to the lesion in situ. Whenever possible, the pathologist should participate in selection of the biopsy site and take responsibility for processing the specimen so that optimal preservation of structure and orientation of the specimen are maintained. The reader is referred elsewhere[15,17] for a discussion of biopsy procedures, site selection, causes of unsatisfactory results, and problems of differential diagnosis. Surgical biopsy of a suspected bone tumor should never be attempted without reference to radiographs and should aim to include representative areas of the lesion, in particular, including areas of bone lysis.[17] Three samples are a minimum, and if the lesion is suspected to be an osteosarcoma, one or more of these samples must be from the endosteal area. The lytic areas will often contain the information of most value to the pathologist. Many biopsy samples submitted for microscopic examination contain only reactive bone and are nondiagnostic, even in cases where it is clear from radiographs that a more sinister lesion exists within the bone. In such cases, the pathologist must resist the temptation to make a diagnosis and must request a further biopsy. Based on the number of questionable reports in the veterinary literature, it is likely that the number of misdiagnoses is greater for tumors of bones than for tumors of any other organ system. This relates partly to the relative lack of experience of most veterinary pathologists with bone lesions, but also to the inadequacy of many routine diagnostic specimens. A good gross description of the lesion, including the appearance of the tumor tissue and the adjacent normal tissue observed at surgery or necropsy, contributes to making a definitive diagnosis.

Without an adequate clinical and radiographic evaluation of the lesion, and in the absence of tissue sections that can be structurally oriented to the bone abnormality, the pathologist may overinterpret or underdiagnose the bits and pieces of tissue presented for microscopic examination. Sections made tangential to an active front of granulation tissue or through the exuberant callus of an unstable fracture may be highly suggestive of primary bone sarcoma. Oblique tissue sections through an active, benign, periosteal response (e.g., a bony callus, a cuff of reactive bone, an actively forming osteophyte, an organizing subperiosteal hematoma, or the track of a biopsy punch) may mimic the cellular features and stromal patterns of osteosarcoma. This may also be true of fragmented tissue sections from a benign endosteal response obtained with a trephine (e.g., the active stage of canine panosteitis or the forming wall of a bone abscess in the spongiosa). Hemangiosarcoma of bone may go undetected in pieces of tissue from the site of a pathologic fracture, and conversely, small pieces of tissue taken from a large organizing hematoma in a spontaneous fracture may resemble hemangiosarcoma. The low cellularity, abundant fibrillar matrix component, and normochromic and isochromic properties of the spindle cells in a low grade fibrosarcoma of bone may belie its malignant behavior. Osteochondromas require proper orientation to determine their biphasic morphology and to distinguish them from exostoses. Although many anatomical pathologists are uncomfortable when interpreting cytological preparations, there is no doubt that some bone tumors can be accurately and rapidly diagnosed by this method. Fine needle aspirates can be collected with minimal discomfort to the patient, and preparations can be ready for examination within minutes. Cellular detail is generally far superior to that of histological sections, especially those subjected to decalcification. Cytology is most useful in tumors such as osteosarcoma and plasma cell myeloma, which exfoliate well and generally yield richly cellular preparations on fine needle aspiration or imprints. It is of limited value in the diagnosis of fibrosarcomas, chondrosarcomas, hemangiosarcomas, and benign tumors of bones, which exfoliate poorly, except in situations where scrapings can be prepared from an exposed lesion during surgery or at necropsy. It is important to remember that cytological preparations may not be fully representative of the lesion, and a diagnosis of malignancy can seldom be excluded on the basis of cytology alone. Both cytology and histology can be performed on the same lesion. This may increase the likelihood of making a definitive diagnosis by combining the attributes of both techniques.

Immunohistochemistry is not as widely used in the diagnosis of bone tumors as it is in tumors of soft tissues, but it may be useful in differentiating metastatic carcinomas and melanomas from primary bone tumors. Gentle decalcification can preserve antigenicity sufficiently for application of the commonly used markers. At present, little is known about the antigenic specificity of normal bone tissue and neoplastic bone cells, and reagents that detect bone specific antigens are not yet available.

It is important that the pathologist not feel pressured to make a definitive diagnosis in cases where either the history or the specimen is inadequate or where radiographic details are not available. The consequences of incorrectly diagnosing a tumor such as osteosarcoma, or excluding it inappropriately, can have particularly unfortunate conse-

quences for the patient. The morphological diagnosis must always be consistent with the clinical and radiographic findings in the case.

Throughout this chapter, the classification system presented in table 5.1 will be followed.

TABLE 5.1. Histological classification of tumors and tumor-like lesions of bones*

Benign tumors
 Osteoma
 Ossifying fibroma
 Myxoma of the jaw
 Osteochondroma
 Feline osteochondromatosis
 Chondroma
 Hemangioma

Malignant tumors
 Central
  Osteosarcoma
   poorly differentiated
   osteoblastic
    nonproductive
    productive
   chondroblastic
   fibroblastic
   telangiectatic
   giant cell type
  Chondrosarcoma
  Fibrosarcoma
  Hemangiosarcoma
  Giant cell tumor of bone
  Multilobular tumor of bone
  Liposarcoma
 Peripheral
  Periosteal chondrosarcoma
  Periosteal fibrosarcoma
  Maxillary fibrosarcoma (dogs)
  Periosteal osteosarcoma
  Parosteal osteosarcoma
 Tumors of bone marrow
  Plasma cell myeloma
  Malignant lymphoma

Tumor-like lesions
 Fibrous dysplasia
 Solitary (unicameral) bone cyst
 Aneurysmal bone cyst
 Subchondral (juxtacortical) bone cyst
 Epidermoid cyst of the phalanx
 Exuberant fracture callus

*Based on World Health Organization International *Histological Classification of Bone and Joint Tumors of Domestic Animals.*[12] (Tumors of joints are included in Chapter 4.)

REFERENCES

1. Schajowicz, F. (1981) *Tumors and Tumor-like Lesions of Bone and Joints.* Springer-Verlag, New York), pp. 1–23,
2. Brodey, R.S., Sauer, R.M., and Medway, W. (1963) Canine bone neoplasms. *J Amer Vet Med Assoc* 143:471–495.
3. Dorn, C.R., Taylor, D.O.N., Schneider, R., Hibbard, H.H., and Klauber, M.R. (1968) Survey of animal neoplasms in Alameda and

Contra Costa counties, California. II. Cancer morbidity in dogs and cats from Alameda County. *J Natl Cancer Inst* 40:307–318.

4. Engle, G.C., and Brodey, R.S. (1969) A retrospective study of 395 feline neoplasms. *J Amer Hosp Assoc* 5:21–31.

5. Jacobson, S.A. (1971) *The Comparative Pathology of the Tumors of Bone.* Charles C. Thomas, Springfield, Illinois.

6. Priester, W.A., and Mantel, N. (1971) Occurrence of tumors in domestic animals: Data for 12 United States and Canadian colleges of veterinary medicine. *J Natl Cancer Inst* 47:1333–1344.

7. Liu, S.K., Dorfman, H.D., and Patnaik, A.K. (1974) Primary and secondary bone tumors in the cat. *J Small Anim Pract* 15:141–156.

8. Misdorp, W., and van der Heul, R.O. (1976) Tumors of bones and joints. *Bull WHO* 53:265–282.

9. Liu, S.K., Dorfman, H.D., Hurvitz, A.L. and Patnaik, A.K. (1977) Primary and secondary bone tumors in the dog. *J Small Anim Pract* 18:313–326.

10. Priester, W.A., and McKay, F.W. (1980) *The Occurrence of Tumors in Domestic Animals.* Monograph No. 54, National Institutes of Health, Washington, D.C.

11. Alexander, J.W., and Patton, C.S. (1983) Primary tumors of the skeletal system. *Vet Clin N Amer Small Anim Pract* 13:181–195.

12. Slayter, M.V., Boosinger, T.R., Pool, R.R., Dämmrich, K., Misdorp, W., and Larsen, S. (1994) *Histological Classification of Bone and Joint Tumors of Domestic Animals.* World Health Organization. 2nd series, vol. 1. Armed Forces Institute of Pathology, American Registry of Pathology, Washington D.C.

13. Brodey, R.S., McGrath, J.T., and Reynolds, H.A. (1959) A clinical and radiological study of canine bone neoplasms. Part I. *J Amer Vet Med Assoc* 134:53–71.

14. Morgan, J.P. (1974) Systematic radiographic interpretation of skeletal diseases in small animals. *Vet Clin N Amer* 4:611–625.

15. Ling, G.V., Morgan, J.P., and Pool, R.R. (1974) Primary bone tumors in the dog: A combined clinical, radiographic, and histologic approach to early diagnosis. *J Amer Vet Med Assoc* 165:55–67.

16. Resnick, D. (1994) Tumors and tumor-like lesions of bone: Radiographic principles. In Resnick, D. (ed.), *Diagnosis of Bone and Joint Disorders,* 3rd ed. Vol. 6, ch. 82. W.B. Saunders, Philadelphia), pp. 3613–3627,

17. Wykes, P.M., Withrow, S.J., Powers, B.E., and Park, R.D. (1985) Closed biopsy for diagnosis of long bone tumors: Accuracy and results. *J Amer Anim Hosp Assoc* 21:489–494.

BENIGN TUMORS OF BONES

Benign bony, fibro-osseous, and cartilaginous lesions of animal bones are relatively uncommon and usually of no great clinical concern or economic significance. As a result, these lesions have been neglected by veterinary pathologists; consequently, they are inadequately documented, and their biological behavior is uncertain. Yet pathologists encounter tissue sections of these lesions with disconcerting regularity. Probably no single veterinary teaching institution has a sufficiently large collection of these conditions to allow authoritative characterization of these entities as they occur in the various domestic species. The descriptions and opinions offered here result from an examination of relatively few specimens from the following categories of lesions and may not accurately reflect the range of morphological variations or biological behavior that occur in any large population of animals. Furthermore, published reports of benign tumors of bones in animals often include only one or two animals, and the emphasis is more on the surgical approach to removal than on pathological characterization.

The lesions therefore are often poorly described and not sufficiently well illustrated to provide confidence for an accurate diagnosis. The morphological criteria used in this section are based on those described for similar tumors in humans.[1] Some benign bone tumors that are recognized as entities in humans (e.g., osteoid osteoma and osteoblastoma) are not well characterized in animals, although there are occasional references to them.[2,3] Analogous tumors probably exist in animals, but for convenience, most are probably "forced" into one of the more accepted categories.

Osteoma, Ossifying Fibroma, and Fibrous Dysplasia

General Considerations

Osteoma, ossifying fibroma, and fibrous dysplasia form a group of poorly understood benign lesions arising primarily from membranous bones. Although fibrous dysplasia is not truly a neoplasm of bones, it is included here among benign tumors of bones because of the need to differentiate it morphologically from osteoma and ossifying fibroma. All three diseases may occur in the jaw, but only ossifying fibroma seems to be restricted to that location. Osteomas are composed of dense accumulations of well-differentiated cancellous or compact bone with delicate intervening fibrous and vascular tissue (fig.5.1 A,B). In contrast, fibrous dysplasia has a major component of fibrovascular stroma separating equidistant, tenuous, curved trabeculae of poorly differentiated bone (fig.5.1 C). These trabeculae arise by metaplasia of fibrous connective tissue and are not typically lined by osteoblasts. The ossifying fibroma shows an intermediate architecture (fig.5.1 D). Some osteomas have features common to all three entities, which suggests the possibility that osteoma may be an end stage of more than one process. In fact, some physician pathologists consider that certain osteomas of the human skull are mature lesions of fibrous dysplasia and that ossifying fibroma is a form that fibrous dysplasia assumes in the mandible. This confounding problem in humans is not readily resolvable at present in animals. However, it is important that veterinary pathologists be aware of the morphology of these benign, proliferative, fibro-osseous processes if for no other reason than to separate them from sarcomas of bone.

Osteoma

Classification

An osteoma is a smoothly contoured, protruding mass of abnormally dense but otherwise normal bone originating from the periosteal surface of bones, usually those that form by intramembranous ossification. It has been suggested by some authors that they are hamartomas rather than true tumors, while others consider them to represent the sclerotic end stage of fibrous dysplasia.[4] They may resemble exostoses in structure, and at times the two entities can not be differentiated by microscopic examination.

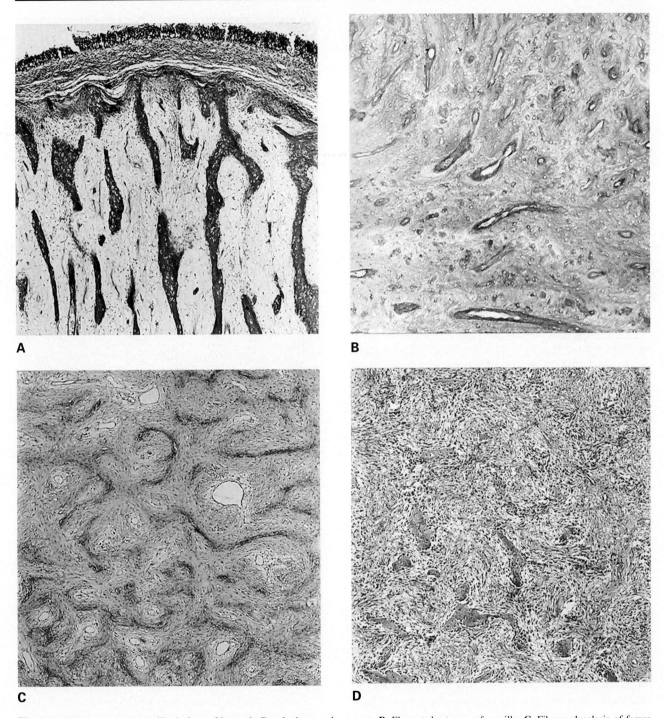

Fig. 5.1. Fibro-osseous tumor-like lesions of bone. **A.** Developing nasal osteoma. **B.** Eburnated osteoma of maxilla. **C.** Fibrous dysplasia of femur. **D.** Ossifying fibroma of mandible.

Incidence, Age, Breed, and Sex

These uncommon tumors appear in all domestic species but are more often recognized in horses and cattle. Most so-called osteomas of the canine head are really examples of multilobular tumors. Ossified canine epulides and tumors of tooth germ origin as well as craniomandibular osteopathy of intramembranous bones are excluded from this category. Too few cases of osteoma are docu-mented to permit proper evaluation of the influence of age, breed, or sex.

Clinical Characteristics

Osteomas demonstrate slow but progressive growth over a period of months, but they may then cease growth and remain quiescent for years. They cause disfigurement, obstruct natural passages in the head, place pressure on adjacent structures, disturb normal breathing, and interfere with prehension, mastication, and deglutition of food. They may recur locally following incomplete surgical removal.

Sites

Mandible, maxilla, nasal sinuses, and bones of the face and cranium are the most common sites of involvement in domestic animals. Massive benign bony growths resulting from unexplained chronic periosteal hyperplasia are occasionally found on the limbs, sternum, ribs, and skull of cats. These feline osteomas (see section on Parosteal Osteosarcoma, below) can be distinguished from osteochondromas and osteophytosis of vitamin A intoxication of cats on the basis of morphology, distribution, and history.

Gross Morphology and Radiographic Appearance

Osteomas typically have evenly contoured borders covered by a moderately vascularized layer of connective tissue, which tends to be mucoid or edematous in osteomas of the nasal cavity. In horse and cattle, osteomas (fig.5.2) may be more than 14 cm in diameter.[5] Many osteomas are so dense that they must be sectioned with a saw. On cut surface, mature osteomas are found to be composed of densely packed cancellous bone with fibrous and adipose connective tissue filling the marrow spaces.

Osteomas are typically monostotic, sclerotic lesions. They blend into contiguous normal bone structure and protrude from the bone surface while maintaining a distinct and regularly contoured border.

Histological Features

Osteomas are bony growths, initially formed of cancellous bone, that may become increasingly compact with time (figs. 5.1 A,B; 5.3 A,B). Soft tissue spaces between bony trabeculae contain one or more centrally located small caliber blood vessels, a sparse population of spindle cells, and a moderately fibrillar connective tissue matrix. Adipose tissue and hematopoietic elements may be present. The matrix of nasal osteomas frequently has a mucoid appearance. Actively growing osteomas are bordered by a layer of connective tissue resembling the periosteum, and newly formed bony trabeculae are slender and oriented perpendicular to the surface of the osteoma. Less superficial, older trabeculae are thicker and may show no surface orientation. Sclerotic or eburnated osteomas are produced by growth in diameter of individual bony trabeculae at the expense of tissue spaces (fig.5.1 B). In mature osteomas bony fusion of peripheral trabeculae produces a cortical margin of compact bone. Osteomas as a group show a variety of deviations from this pattern.

Many osteomas have an orderly zonal architecture. In actively growing osteomas the periosteum is well differentiated and is composed of both fibrous and osteogenic lay-

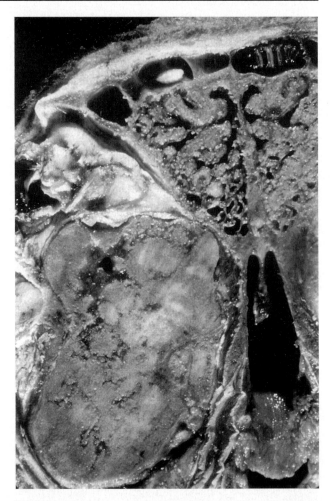

Fig. 5.2. Transverse section of the skull of a sheep showing a large, dense osteoma in the maxillary sinus. An *Oestrus ovis* larva is present in the frontal sinus.

ers. Peripheral trabeculae are formed of woven bone deposited by a border of typical osteoblasts. Deeper trabeculae are broader structures formed of finely fibered lamellar bone that partially or completely replaces woven bone following normal remodeling activity.

The pathologist will also encounter a number of less well structured osteomas (figs. 5.3 C,D). In some of these osteomas the periosteal covering is poorly differentiated and resembles only the fibrous layer of the periosteum. Recognizable osteoblasts are not present in the periosteum or on trabecular surfaces. The thin fibrous layer gives rise to peripheral trabeculae of immature woven bone by osseous metaplasia of fibrous connective tissue. Trabeculae are irregular in shape and size and show little or no orientation to the surface of the lesion. Even the older and deeper trabeculae are composed almost entirely of woven bone (fig. 5.3 B). Remodeling and replacement by lamellar bone is infrequent. Spindle cells in the mucoid matrix filling the tissue spaces account for appositional growth of the cancellous bone.

Osteomas occasionally arise from bones of the pelvis or tubular bones of the limbs and must be differentiated from osteochondromas. The presence of a cap of hyaline

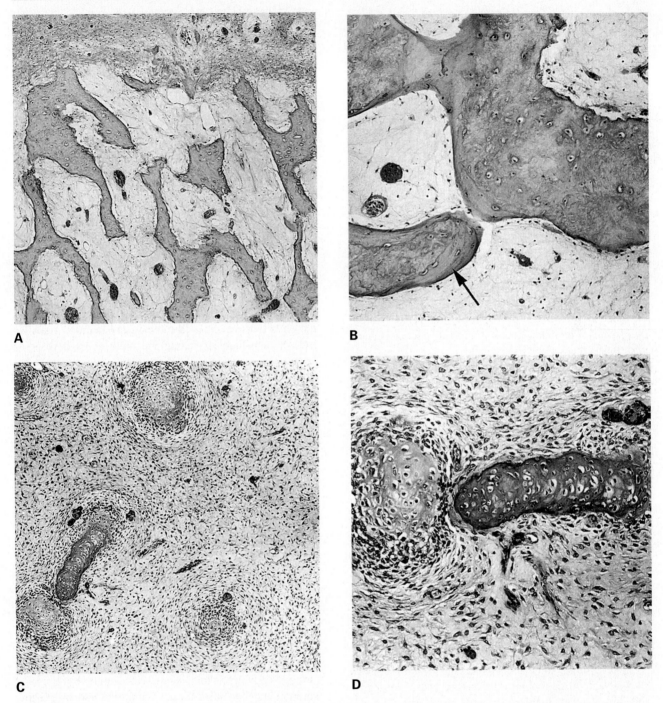

Fig. 5.3. Osteoma of the head. **A.** Nasal osteoma with poorly differentiated periosteal membrane. A few flattened cells line bone surfaces. **B.** Trabeculae consisting of central cores of woven bone with lamellar bone (arrow) deposited on the surface. **C.** Mandibular osteoma possibly arising from ossifying fibroma. **D.** Higher magnification of C showing condensation of cells along margins of crude bone spicules.

cartilage and/or continuity between the marrow cavity of the bone and the intertrabecular spaces of the tumor support a diagnosis of osteochondroma. The latter feature will usually be apparent radiographically. In some cases, the presence of plump mesenchymal cells in close association with irregular trabeculae of immature bone may suggest the possibility of osteosarcoma.[6]

Osteoid osteoma, a distinct form of osteoma in humans,[7] has also been reported in a cat.[3] The lesion is characterized by a discrete, intraosseous nidus of active bone formation in which disorganized trabeculae are surrounded by a rim of sclerotic bone. The trabeculae of immature bone are lined by plump osteoblasts but show no evidence of malignancy.

Growth and Metastasis

Osteomas exhibit slow, progressive growth over a period of months and then may maintain this size and shape indefinitely. Some nasal osteomas appear to arise by bony metaplasia of the fibrous stroma in nasal polyps. Such lesions, not arising from skeletal tissues, should probably not be designated as osteomas, but rather as metaplastic lesions. The site, size, and weight of osteomas cause clinical problems. Neoplastic transformation is unreported and not anticipated.

Ossifying Fibroma

Classification

This is a fibro-osseous lesion producing a tumor-like disease in the jaws of animals, particularly young horses. Because of an apparent predilection for the rostral mandible of young horses, it is suggested that the condition in this species be classified as equine juvenile mandibular ossifying fibroma.[8] A predilection for the mandible and maxillae also exists in humans, but a similar tumor occasionally occurs in tubular bones, particularly the tibia.[7] Differentiation of ossifying fibroma from fibrous dysplasia is important, at least in human patients, because of differing therapeutic indications.

Incidence, Age, Breed, and Sex

Ossifying fibroma is rare in all species but is reported most frequently in horses.[8] The tumor has also been reported in cats,[9] dogs,[10] greater kudus,[11] and sheep.[12] The age range in horses in one series was 2 months to 6 years, with most cases occurring in animals less than 1 year of age. In cats, the mean age of 13 reported cases was 6.5 years (range 2 to 12 years). The number of reported cases is too small for any breed or sex predilection to be apparent. Because of the morphological similarity between ossifying fibroma and some cases of osteoma and the possibility that ossifying fibroma may mature into osteoma, the true incidence of ossifying fibroma remains unclear. It is likely that some published cases, and no doubt some that do not make the literature, are misdiagnosed as osteosarcomas.

Clinical Characteristics and Sites

These large, solitary lesions in the jaw may replace alveolar and cortical bone. The disease causes loosening and loss of teeth, interference with mastication of food, and predisposition of the jaw to pathological fracture. Either the maxilla or mandible may be involved, and the lesions may be bilateral. There are occasional reports of ossifying fibroma involving bones of the limbs, pelvis, and chest wall in cats.[13]

Gross Morphology and Radiographic Appearance

Ossifying fibroma, unlike an osteoma that arises from a sessile base on the surface of a bone, produces an expansile lesion of the jaw bone and replaces normal bone tissue with fibro-osseous stroma. The abnormal tissue is dense and may be too well mineralized to be cut with a knife.

Ossifying fibroma presents as a sharply demarcated, solitary, mixed to moderately radiolucent lesion that expands the normal contours of the affected bone at the area of involvement (fig. 5.4 A). If the fibro-osseous process extends into adjacent soft tissue, the border of the lesion may be irregular, but without finger-like projections or a brush border. Possibly some of the more exuberant, large, productive bony lesions occasionally encountered at the mandibular symphysis of horses are examples of ossifying fibroma rather than osteoma or osteosarcoma.

Histological Features, Growth, and Metastasis

Irregularly shaped spicules of osteoid and bone rimmed with osteoblasts are randomly formed in a moderately vascularized, fibro-osseous stroma (fig. 5.4 B). The proliferative element is composed of isochromic spindle cells that resemble fibroblasts and undergo transformation to osteoblasts along the margins of developing bone spicules (fig. 5.4 C). Cartilage is not formed in the lesion. As the name of the disease implies, the morphology of the process is that of a fibroma in which bone forms by osseous metaplasia of the fibrous connective tissue component. Therefore, tissue spaces between bony trabeculae have a greater density of cells and fibers in ossifying fibroma than do the marrow spaces of an osteoma.

Zonation in the lesion, if present, is not obvious, and no recognizable periosteal membrane borders the lesion. Ossification occurs randomly through the lesion. Bone spicules are composed almost entirely of woven bone. In a few scattered areas, large, well developed, irregularly shaped bony trabeculae may be found. There may be osteoclastic resorption and some patchy deposits of lamellar bone. Soft tissue between bone spicules has a loss of cell and fiber density, so that in these small areas of the lesion there are foci resembling the major structure of an osteoma.

Proliferative tissue extends into adjacent soft tissue along a contoured front restrained, in part, by layers of compressed connective tissue. Within the jaw, preexisting bone is removed by osteoclastic activity.

Cellular and stromal microscopic features distinguish ossifying fibroma from osteosarcoma. In osteosarcoma the malignant cells have a high mitotic index and are more pleomorphic and hyperchromatic than cells in ossifying fibroma. Well-structured trabecular bone is seldom produced in osteosarcoma.

Ossifying fibromas destroy preexisting bone structure and produce expansile lesions of affected bones. They are not considered to be premalignant lesions. Recurrence is unlikely after complete excision of the lesion by rostral mandibulectomy but is reported after debulking.[14]

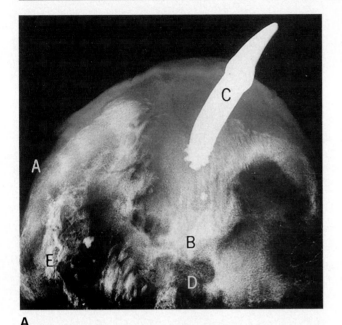

A

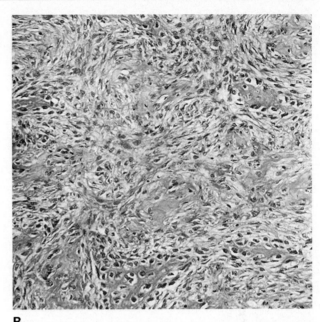

B

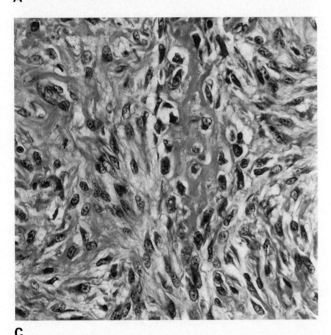

C

Fig. 5.4. Ossifying fibroma in a ruminant. **A.** Radiograph of section through bone lesion in the incisor region with an evenly contoured outer border *(A)*, residual bone *(B)*, and tooth *(C)*. Within the mandible there is irregular bone destruction *(D)* and random mineralization *(E)* of new bone matrix. **B.** Irregular trabeculae rimmed by osteoblasts arise in a benign fibro-osseous stroma. **C.** Proliferating cells are isomorphic and isochromic without the anaplastic features of osteosarcoma.

Fibrous Dysplasia

Classification

Although it is not a neoplasm, fibrous dysplasia is discussed here so that it will be included in the differential diagnosis of nonaggressive, radiolucent bone lesions con-

sisting of fibro-osseous connective tissue. It is considered to be a developmental abnormality of bone-forming mesenchyme[15,16] and is characterized by smoothly contoured, expanding fibro-osseous lesions involving one or several bones. Although well documented in humans, there are few reliable reports of fibrous dysplasia in animals. There seems little doubt, however, that the condition does occur in several animal species. In humans, extraskeletal abnormalities, including endocrine disturbances and patchy pigmentation of the skin are reported in association with fibrous dysplasia, but similar observations have not been made in animals.

Incidence, Age, Breed, and Sex

Fibrous dysplasia has been reported in horses,[13,17] dogs,[13,18] domestic cats,[3] and a Siberian tiger.[19] Some published reports of this lesion in animals are questionable, the lesions in some cases appearing more consistent with ossifying fibroma. Furthermore, a description of familial canine polyostotic fibrous dysplasia in three doberman pinscher pups[20] most likely represents a polyostotic form of unicameral bone cysts. It is also possible that some cases of fibrous dysplasia have been misdiagnosed as various tumors of bones. Although the true prevalence of the lesion in animals is unclear, there is no doubt that it is rare. As in humans, young animals are most commonly affected with fibrous dysplasia. Lesions resembling fibrous dysplasia have been found in the limbs of dogs in radionuclide toxicity studies.[21]

Clinical Characteristics

Clinical findings reflect the site of bone involvement and problems associated with an expansile bone lesion that causes loss of normal strength. Small lesions of fibrous dysplasia may remain asymptomatic for long periods. Clinical disease includes disfigurement, compression of adjacent structures, obstruction of natural cavities or passages, difficulty in eating, lameness, and pathological fracture.

Sites

The lesions may be monostotic or polyostotic. Solitary lesions reported in domestic animals include a mass in the sinuses of two horses[13,17;] tumor-like masses in the jaw, infraorbital bones, and nasal cavity of dogs[13,18;] and lesions in the ramus of the mandible and in the distal ulna of two cats.[3] In humans, monostotic fibrous dysplasia seldom causes severe bone deformity. In polyostotic forms an entire bone may be involved, resulting in pronounced deformity and reduced strength.[16]

Gross Morphology

Normal bone structure is replaced by a moderately dense, gritty, fibro-osseous stroma in which the bony component is usually not sufficiently dense to resist sectioning with a knife. A thin shell of dense bone laid down by the periosteum borders the lesion. Affected long bones may show fusiform expansion due to a central mass of firm, whitish tissue surrounded by a narrow rim of cortical bone, sometimes with an irregular periosteal reaction.[3]

Radiographic Appearance

The radiographic features of this disease in domestic animals have not been well characterized. In a cat with fibrous dysplasia of the ulna,[3] the expanded segment of bone showed marked homogeneous radiographic density and was accompanied by a periosteal reaction. In the solitary lesion of a Siberian tiger, there was sufficient fine bone trabeculation to give a faint, homogeneous radiodensity.[19] Periosteal bony response was minimal in the tiger as compared to the marked bony reaction in the ulnar lesion of a domestic cat.[3]

Histological Features

The unique microscopic feature of fibrous dysplasia is the presence of thin, arched trabeculae of poor quality woven bone that arise in a fibrous connective tissue stroma (fig. 5.5 A). These tenuous trabeculae tend to be equidistant and reflect the orientation of thin-walled blood vessels in the lesion. Spicules of woven bone arise within thin, linear condensations of fibrous tissue without transition of spindle cells of the stroma into recognizable osteoblasts (fig. 5.5 B). This is an important feature in differentiating fibrous dysplasia from ossifying fibroma. Rarely are trabeculae lined by osteoblasts, and only mature lesions contain deposits of lamellar bone.

No periosteal membrane or its equivalent, as seen in the osteoma, borders the diseased tissue. Trabecular bone formation occurs randomly within the lesion, and trabeculae show no orientation to the margin of the lesion. Within

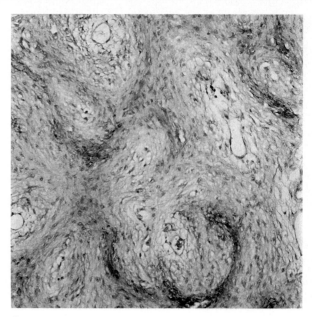

A

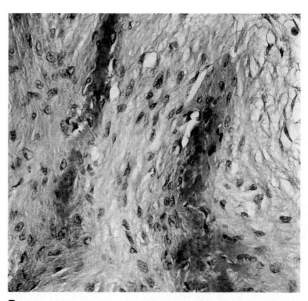

B

Fig. 5.5. Fibrous dysplasia of the distal femur. **A.** Thin, arched trabeculae of crude bone arise in a benign fibrous stroma. **B.** Unlike ossifying fibroma, no osteoblasts rim the spicules of bone in active areas of the disease process.

the affected bone, a zone of marked osteoclastic activity will often abruptly separate normal bone from the stroma of the lesion. Clusters of giant cells resembling osteoclasts are scattered throughout the lesion and probably represent vestiges of intense bone destruction.

It is important to remember that the typical lesion of fibrous dysplasia may become significantly altered should there be hemorrhage or pathological fracture at the site, both of which would be likely sequels to weakening of the bone by an expanding lesion.

Growth and Metastasis

Growth of the active lesion is by expansion. No normal bone structure remains in the affected area except a thin shell of bone produced by the intact periosteum. Malignant transformation occurs infrequently in humans and has not been reported to occur in animals.

REFERENCES

1. Spjut, H.J., Dorfman, H.D., Fechner, R.E., and Ackerman, L.V. (1971) Tumors of bone and cartilage. In *Atlas of Tumor Pathology.* 2nd series, fascicle 5. Armed Forces Institute of Pathology, Washington, D.C.

2. Misdorp, W., and van der Heul, R.O. (1976) Tumors of bones and joints. *Bull WHO* 53:265–282.

3. Liu, S.K., Dorfman, H.D., and Patnaik, A.K. (1974) Primary and secondary bone tumors in the cat. *J Small Anim Pract* 15:141–156.

4. Resnick, D., and Niwayama, G. (1994) Enostosis, hyperostosis and periostitis. In Resnick, D. (ed.), *Diagnosis of Bone and Joint Disorders,* 3rd ed. Vol. 6, ch. 93. W.B. Saunders, Philadelphia), pp. 4396–4466.

5. Rumbaugh, G.D., Pool, R.R., and Wheat, J.D. (1978) Atypical osteoma of the nasal passage and paranasal sinus in a bull. *Cornell Vet* 68:544–554.

6. Johnson, K.A., Cooley, A.J., and Darien, D.L. (1996) Zygomatic osteoma with atypical heterogeneity in a dog. *J Comp Pathol* 114:199–203.

7. Resnick, D., Kyriakos, M., and Greenway, G.D. (1994) Tumors and tumor-like lesions of bone: Radiographic principles. In Resnick, D. (ed.), *Diagnosis of Bone and Joint Disorders,* 3rd ed. Vol. 6, ch. 82. W.B. Saunders, Philadelphia), pp. 3613–3627.

8. Morse, C.C., Saik, J.E., Richardson, D.W., and Fetter, A.W. (1988) Equine juvenile mandibular ossifying fibroma. *Vet Pathol* 24:415–421.

9. Turrel, J.M., and Pool, R.R. (1982) Primary bone tumors in the cat: A retrospective study of 15 cats and a literature review. *Vet Radiol* 23:152–166.

10. Liu, S.K., Dorfman, H.D., Hurvitz, A.L., and Patnaik, A.K. (1977) Primary and secondary bone tumors in the dog. *J Small Anim Pract* 18:313–326.

11. Halliwell, W.H., and Hahn, F.F. (1980) Fibro-osseous lesions in the mandible and maxilla of greater kudus. In Montali, R.J., and Migaki, G. (eds.), *The Comparative Pathology of Zoo Animals.* Smithsonian Institute Press, Washington D.C., pp. 573–578.

12. Rogers, A.B., and Gould, D.H. (1998) Ossifying fibroma in a sheep. *Small Ruminant Res* 28:193–197.

13. Jacobson, S.A. (1971) *The Comparative Pathology of the Tumors of Bone.* Charles C. Thomas, Springfield, IL.

14. Richardson, D.W., Evans, L.H., and Tulleners, E.P. (1991) Rostral mandibulectomy in five horses. *J Amer Vet Med Assoc* 199:1179–1182.

15. Schajowicz, F. (1981) *Tumors and Tumor-like Lesions of Bone and Joints.* Springer-Verlag, New York, pp. 478–490.

16. Feldman, F. (1994) Tuberous sclerosis, neurofibromatosis, and fibrous dysplasia. In Resnick, D. (ed.), *Diagnosis of Bone and Joint Disorders,* 3rd ed. Vol. 6, ch. 92. W.B. Saunders, Philadelphia), pp. 4353–4395.

17. Livesey, M.A., Keane, D.P., and Sarmiento, J. (1984) Epistaxis in a standardbred weanling caused by fibrous dysplasia. *Equine Vet J* 16:144–146.

18. Wilson, R.B. (1989) Monostotic fibrous dysplasia in a dog. *Vet Pathol* 26:449–450.

19. Pool, R.R. (1990) Tumors of bone and cartilage. In Moulton J. E. (ed.), *Tumors in Domestic Animals,* 3rd ed. University of California Press, Berkeley.

20. Carrig, C.B., and Seawright, A.A. (1969) A familial canine polyostotic fibrous dysplasia with subperiosteal cortical defects. *J Small Anim Pract* 10:397–405.

21. Pool, R.R., Morgan, J.P., Parks, N.J., Farnham, J.E., and Littman, M.S. (1983) Comparative pathogenesis of radium-induced intracortical bone lesions in humans and beagles. *Health Phys* 44(Suppl. 1): 155–177.

Myxomatous Tumors of the Jaw

Classification

These are tumors of embryonal connective tissue producing destructive lesions in the jaws of large animals. In animals, these tumors are more common at soft tissue sites such as the skin, heart, and walls of viscera, but they also occur in the jaws of horses and cattle.[1] These tumors are characterized by a population of stellate tumor cells that produce an abundant gelatinous matrix composed mostly of proteoglycan and a loose network of reticulum and collagen fibers. It is reasonable that other bones of the skeleton could develop these tumors, but the authors are unaware of confirmed lesions.

Incidence and Sites

All reported cases have been centered on the dental arches of the molar region of the maxilla.[1] These are uncommon tumors and are seen far less frequently than tumors of tooth germ origin.

Clinical Characteristics

The tumors cause distortion of the affected maxilla. The jaw is swollen, and nasal passages may be compromised on the affected side. Loosening of cheek teeth and infection of the alveolar bone may occur. Myxomas usually produce slowly progressive clinical signs, but the course in one myxosarcoma was only 4 months.

Gross and Radiographic Appearance

Tumor tissue is characterized by a soft gelatinous or rubbery consistency. Small pockets in the pale tissue may be filled with slimy fluid. On cut section the tumor may be lobulated, with some lobules being separated by thin bony septa. In myxomas the external surface of the tumor mass is covered by a thin shell of periosteal new bone. The myxosarcoma was not lobulated, and gelatinous tumor tissue infiltrated the soft tissues on the side of the face. Radiographs of myxomas have a lobular pattern because bone tissue is remodeled along the borders of the slowly expanding tumor mass. The myxosarcoma had aggressive radiographic features marked by irregular bone lysis and a bizarre periosteal new bone response that also contained areas of bone destruction.[1]

Histological Features

Most tumor cells have a stellate shape and are set in an abundant intercellular matrix composed primarily of proteoglycan and lesser but variable amounts of collagen and reticular fibers. No fibrous capsule borders the lesion, but fine collagenous trabeculae may randomly divide the tumor mass into lobules. No cartilage should be formed by the tumor cells. Tumor cells retain their stellate shape in areas of secondary fibrosis, and this characteristic helps to differentiate pure myxomas from other tumors with areas of myxoid degeneration, such as fibrous tumors, rhabdomyosarcomas, liposarcomas, chondrosarcomas, and mesenchymomas.[2] Cells of myxomas were smaller, less pleomorphic, and less numerous than those in the myxosarcoma (figs. 5.6 A,B). Several veins were partially occluded with tumor cells in the myxosarcoma. In none of the cases examined was there any evidence of more differentiated patterns of matrix production.[1] There was a marked similarity of tumor tissue to mesenchyme of the dental papilla in the forming teeth of horses and cattle.

Growth and Metastasis

Because of the highly infiltrative nature of this tumor, local recurrence following resection is to be anticipated. While no metastatic lesions were found in one case of myxosarcoma, pulmonary metastases would have been expected had the animal lived longer. Since the distinction between myxoma and myxosarcoma of the jaw can not always be determined with confidence, and since local excision is not likely to be curative because of the infiltrative nature of the tumor, a guarded prognosis is warranted.

Osteochondroma of the Dog and Horse

Classification

An osteochondroma is a cartilage capped, exostotic, benign tumor arising from the surface of a bone formed by endochondral ossification. Osteochondromas present as either monostotic or polyostotic abnormalities and are called, respectively, solitary osteochondroma or osteochondromatosis (multiple cartilaginous exostosis). The polyostotic form is inherited as an autosomal dominant trait in humans, horses,[3] and dogs.[4] In spite of the benign nature of osteochondromas, malignant transformation to either chondrosarcoma or osteosarcoma occurs with some frequency in older dogs with osteochondromatosis.[5-7] This has not been reported in dogs with monostotic osteochondromas, but is reported in humans.[8]

There is debate as to whether osteochondromas are true neoplasms or manifestations of dysplastic physeal growth. The latter option is supported by the development of lesions from the margin of growth plates and the fact that they cease growing once the animal reaches skeletal maturity. Experimentally, osteochondromas can be reproduced by transplanting fragments of physeal growth plate

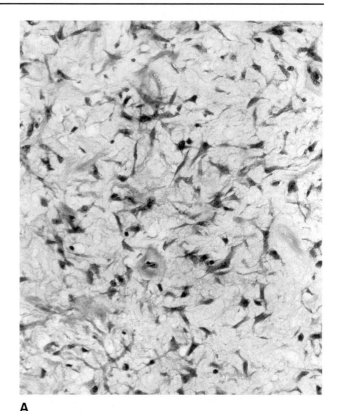

A

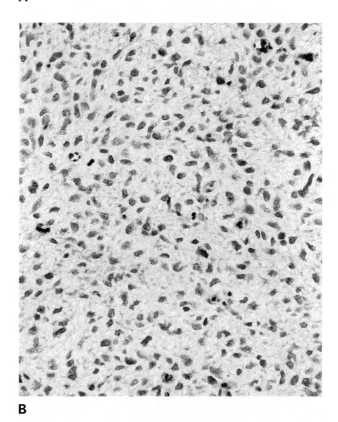

B

Fig. 5.6. Myxoma and myxosarcoma of the jaw. **A.** In the myxoma, small stellate cells are set in an abundant mucinous ground substance. **B.** In the myxosarcoma, the tumor cells are more numerous, pleomorphic, and mitotically active.

to the periosteal surface, adding further support to the hypothesis.

Self-limiting proliferations of cartilage occurring in soft tissues may undergo endochondral ossification and acquire the biphasic morphology of an osteochondroma. Such lesions are commonly found in the synovium of joints with chronic degenerative joint disease and in the trachea of dogs. Although the term *osteochondroma* is applied to these lesions, they should be distinguished from the developmental skeletal lesions and identified as osteochondromas of the synovium, trachea, and other areas.

Incidence, Age, Breed, and Sex

Osteochondromatosis is a relatively common disease in animals, although it is infrequently reported in the literature. Osteochondromas are often encountered as incidental findings in radiographic examinations of small animals. The disease appears to be more common in dogs than in cats or horses.

Typically, osteochondromatosis is first recognized in immature dogs and horses during the period of active bone growth, when exostoses are most likely to cause clinical abnormalities. Osteochondromas in most dogs and horses respond to the same trophic influences as do growth plates, and they gradually cease growth at skeletal maturity. No breed or sex predilection has been indicated for any domestic species.

Clinical Characteristics

Clinical signs depend on the size and location of the lesions and may include disfigurement, lameness, pain, paresis, and paralysis, due to compression or distortion of adjacent structures. Lesions on limbs may interfere with the function of tendons, muscles, vessels, and nerves in the area, resulting in lameness and pain. Vertebral involvement, especially in dogs, causes spinal cord compression and attendant neurologic deficits. Many animals have clinically silent osteochondromatosis, in which case the lesions may go undiscovered or be found during routine care of the animal. Malignant transformation of lesions, as occurs in some older dogs with osteochondromatosis, will obviously be accompanied by more severe clinical disease.

Sites

Osteochondromas may develop in any bone that forms by endochondral ossification, but they most commonly involve the scapula, ribs, vertebrae, and pelvis. Bilateral lesions occur often in dogs and horses. Osteochondromas should not arise from bones of the skull, which develop by intramembranous ossification.

Gross Morphology

Osteochondromas consist of a cap of cartilage, overlying cancellous bone, that is continuous with the marrow space of the parent bone (fig. 5.7 A). The narrow cortex at the base of an osteochondroma also blends imperceptibly with the cortex of the bone. Lesions on limbs tend to be pedunculated and point in the direction of muscle traction. They are located on the cortical surface in the metaphyseal region or toward the end of the diaphysis of a long bone, but they always spare the epiphysis. Osteochondromas on flat bones are often much larger than those involving tubular bones and have a broad, sessile base. They may form eccentric cuffs around the shafts of ribs and tend to be found adjacent to the costochondral junction. The outer surface of an osteochondroma is white to bluish white, reflecting the presence of the cartilaginous component.

Radiographic Appearance

Osteochondromas are exostoses with regular contours that merge into the substance of the bone from which they arise. Radiodensity of the tumor reflects the component of cancellous bone, while radiolucent areas represent areas of hyaline cartilage yet to undergo endochondral ossification. Loss of a smooth contour, with bone destruction or production along the margin or base of an osteochondroma may indicate malignant transformation. Large osteochondromas, during the active growth phase, may occasionally have an ominous mottled radiographic pattern and be initially suggestive of malignant bone tumor. Sequential radiographic studies or a bone biopsy will clarify the nature of the lesion.

Histological Features

Osteochondromas are orderly biphasic growths with an apical margin of hyaline cartilage and a base of cancellous bone with intervening marrow spaces (fig. 5.7 B). In young developing lesions the cartilage cap is a distinctive structure, but in maturing lesions the cap is discontinuous. In actively growing lesions the cartilage cap mimics a growth plate and produces bone by orderly endochondral ossification. Islands of cartilage, however, may be retained in cancellous bone within the base of the exostosis. Multiple islands of calcified cartilage scattered through large, rapidly growing osteochondromas produce a mottled radiographic pattern that may give concern for the presence of malignant bone tumor. A perichondrial membrane continuous with the periosteum of the host bone covers the surface of the osteochondroma. Chondrogenic activity of the membrane, followed by endochondral ossification, accounts for most of the growth of the osteochondroma. Some enlargement of the bony base is due to appositional growth by the periosteum.

Biopsies of osteochondromas must be properly oriented to reveal the architecture of the lesion. Sections taken tangentially through the cartilage cap of an actively growing lesion can be misleading and suggestive of chondrosarcoma. The pathologist should also realize that in mature osteochondromas, endochondral ossification may be completed, and little or no cartilage may remain at the apical surface. In some cases, the cartilage that remains is hyalinized, and the chondrocytes are poorly stained, necrotic, ghost-like remnants that can easily be overlooked.

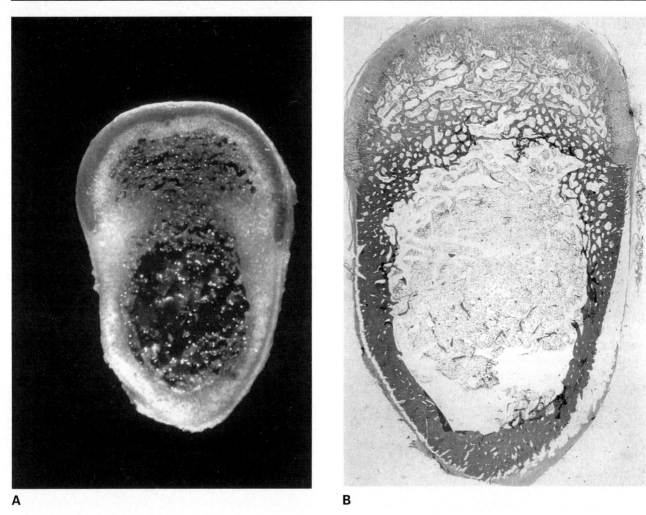

A   **B**

Fig. 5.7. Osteochondroma. **A.** Transverse section through the distal femur of a dog showing a cartilage capped mass firmly attached to the bone. The marrow cavity of the bone is continuous with that of the osteochondroma. **B.** Subgross of the same lesion showing the cap of cartilage giving rise to trabecular bone by endochondral ossification. The dense cortical bone of the femur merges with trabecular bone of the osteochondroma. (Photographs courtesy of S.E. Weisbrode.)

Growth and Metastasis

Osteochondromas typically continue to enlarge in synchrony with physeal growth and cease growing once the skeleton reaches maturity. Some lesions will cease growth at an earlier stage and may be either resorbed or incorporated into the enlarging metaphysis of the bone during modeling. In spite of this benign nature, the prognosis in dogs with the polyostotic form (multiple cartilaginous exostoses) is guarded to poor. In a survey of published cases in dogs,[7] 8 of 21 cases on which data was available were euthanized before 1 year of age due to progression of clinical signs related to the disease. Furthermore, malignant transformation occurred in a single lesion in five of the six dogs that survived to be more than 6 years of age. Pulmonary metastases were present in three of these dogs. Four of the malignancies were chondrosarcomas; the other was an osteosarcoma. Although malignant transformation of monostotic osteochondromas has not been reported in animals, it occurs in approximately 1 per-

cent of such lesions in humans.[8] The frequency of malignant transformation in human patients with multiple cartilaginous exostoses is approximately 25 percent. There are no reports of malignant transformation in horses with multiple cartilaginous exostoses.

Feline Osteochondromatosis

Classification

Osteochondromatosis of cats is presented separately from the disorder in dogs and horses bearing the same name because the disease in cats has a different clinical setting, a different skeletal distribution, and almost certainly a different cause. Unlike the cartilage capped exostoses of dogs and horses, which are developmental disturbances that cease growth at skeletal maturity, the osteochondromas of cats show progressive enlargement, a feature of true tumors.

Viral particles resembling the agent causing feline leukemia (FeLV) and transmissible feline sarcoma (FeSV) have been found consistently in the cartilage caps of cats with multiple cartilaginous exostoses.[9,10] Although the significance of the virus in the pathogenesis of the lesions is undetermined, a viral etiology with hematogenous localization in the periosteum at random sites could explain the different pattern of distribution and clinical setting of the disease in cats compared to dogs and horses. It is unfortunate that this disease of cats has been assigned the name osteochondromatosis, because the disease of dogs and horses clearly has many differences and can not be considered analogous.

Incidence, Age, Breed, and Sex

The incidence of osteochondromatosis in cats is unknown, but based on the frequency of published reports,[9-12] it appears to be less common than the disease of dogs. Affected cats ranged in age from 16 months to 8 years, but most were young adults, 2 to 4 years old at the time the exostoses were first discovered. There is no evidence of a breed or sex predilection and no hereditary pattern has been reported.

Clinical Characteristics

Initially, the lesions are asymptomatic, but continued growth of the nodules causes disfigurement, pain, encroachment on joints and tendons, and muscle atrophy. Additional lesions may be found during microscopic examination of the skeleton.[13] All cats tested for feline leukemia virus infection were positive, and all cases have occurred in animals with mature skeletons. Once the exostoses appear, they demonstrate progressive enlargement, a feature that is characteristic of a true tumor but does not appear in osteochondromatosis of dogs and horses.

Sites

Unlike osteochondromatosis in dogs, skeletal lesions in cats have a random distribution, including the development of exostoses in bones of the skull formed by intramembranous ossification. Sites of skeletal involvement in decreasing order of frequency are the rib cage, scapulae, vertebral column, skull, pelvis, and bones of the limbs. When exostoses occur on long bones, the lesions are random in distribution, with no affinity for the metaphysis.

Gross Morphology

Most feline osteochondromas are bulky masses, sometimes appearing to be formed by a coalescence of smaller nodules that are attached to the bone by a sessile base (fig. 5.8 A). Most of the mass is formed of cancellous bone, but a pale surface layer of cartilage can usually be recognized on cut surface.

Radiographic Appearance

Usually, osteochondromas of cats arise from bone surfaces as sessile excrescences with well defined, bosse-lated borders. Often, the outer third of a rapidly growing exostosis has an amorphous, mottled appearance. An aggressive radiographic pattern was present in an osteochondroma of a cervical vertebra that was shown histologically to have undergone malignant transformation.

Histological Features

Feline osteochondromas usually have a biphasic pattern, with a cap of cartilage giving rise to a bony base by endochondral ossification. However, the hyperplastic layer of periosteum may form bone instead of cartilage, a feature not seen in canine osteochondromas. Even when cartilage is formed by the periosteum, the cartilage tissue differs from that of the cartilage cap of the dog in being more cellular, forming fewer chondrones, and producing less ground substance. Endochondral ossification is less orderly than in the dog, and the cancellous bone is composed mostly of woven bone tissue (fig. 5.8 B). In time, the bony structures of many feline osteochondromas undergo remodeling, and the architecture becomes increasingly disorganized, with some stromal cells acquiring atypical features (fig. 5.8 C). The marrow spaces of the exostoses contain adipocytes, loose fibrous connective tissue, and islands of hematopoietic tissue, but unlike canine osteochondromas, the underling cortex remains intact, and there is no continuity between the marrow spaces of the tumor and the bone to which it is attached.[13]

Growth and Metastasis

Growth of feline osteochondromas is continuous. In a cat with numerous nodules of varying size and duration, lesions that undergo progressive transformation from periosteal hyperplasia to parosteal sarcoma can be identified. The proliferative response is thought to be caused by virus acting on cells of the periosteum (fig. 5.8 D). A grave prognosis should be given for any cat with this neoplasm since new lesions continue to appear in the skeleton throughout the course of the disease. Owners usually have the cat euthanized because of disfigurement and lameness caused by the enlarging lesions. Malignant transformation occurred in an osteochondroma of a cervical vertebra in one cat and the skull of another.[13]

Chondroma

Classification

A chondroma is a benign neoplasm of cartilage, but in veterinary medicine, the term has often been used loosely to include benign proliferations of cartilage in several extraskeletal tissues. In this chapter, its use is confined to lesions originating in bones. Primary chondromas of bone are separable into *enchondromas,* which originate within the medullary cavity of a bone, and *ecchondromas,* which arise from cartilage elsewhere in the skeleton. Both forms have been reported rarely in animals.[1,14] Enchondromas are sometimes polyostotic, in which case the syndrome is referred to as

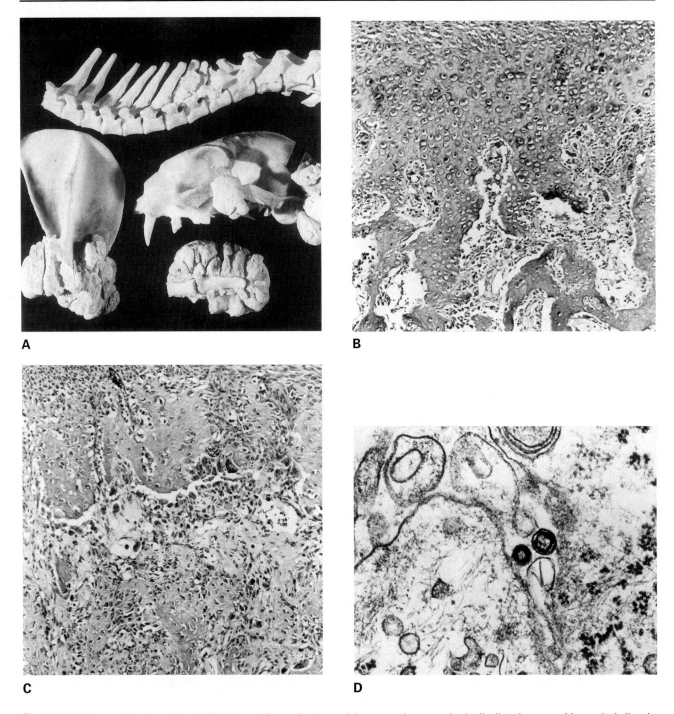

Fig. 5.8. Feline osteochondromatosis. **A.** Multiple, sessile, cartilage capped, bony growths are randomly distributed on several bones, including the skull, of a cat. **B.** Orderly endochondral ossification along base of cap. **C.** Disorganized architecture of osteochondroma with pleomorphism of stromal cells. **D.** Virus particles bud from plasmalemma of a chondrocyte in the cartilage cap.

enchondromatosis. Periosteal (or juxtacortical) chondromas, which develop beneath the periosteum adjacent to the cortical surface in humans,[8] have not been reported in animals. It is likely that many tumors diagnosed as chondromas in animals are in fact osteochondromas or low grade chondrosarcomas, especially in cases where the pathologist is not aided by an adequate history or access to radiographs of the lesion.

Incidence, Age, Breed, and Sex

Chondromas are rare in animals but have been reported in several domestic species, particularly aged dogs and sheep.[15] They occur much less frequently than their malignant counterparts. No breed or sex preference is reported, but the number of cases is too small for valid assessment.

Clinical Characteristics, Sites, and Gross Morphology

Chondromas demonstrate slow growth and deform affected bones. Clinical signs are related to size and location of the tumor. Although the lesions may become quite large, they are usually asymptomatic or accompanied by painless swellings.[8,14] Ecchondromas occur most commonly in flat bones, turbinates, and sternocostal cartilage complexes. In humans, enchondromas occur most commonly in the bones of the hands, especially the proximal phalanges. Few cases have been reported in animals, but sites include the proximal phalanx of a dog (fig. 5.9) and the distal tibia and distal fifth metatarsal of a rhesus monkey.[14]

Tumors vary in size. They are firm and generally have evenly contoured borders covered by a fibrous capsule. On cut surface chondromas are bluish white to milk white and have a multilobular structure.

Radiographic Appearance

Chondromas produce expansile bone lesions that attenuate the cortex while maintaining a smooth but discrete border (fig. 5.9). Evidence of osteolysis, production of reactive bone, soft tissue response, and change in radiographic appearance in a 2-week interval may indicate either malignant transformation or traumatic injury of the tumor.

Histological Features

These benign tumors consist of irregular lobules of hyaline cartilage. Neoplastic cartilage is composed of innocuous chondrocytes, tending to be rather uniform in size and shape, set in a matrix that on occasion has more fibrous stroma than is found in normal hyaline cartilage (fig. 5.10). Histological distinctions between chondroma and low grade chondrosarcoma are often equivocal, and it is important that the pathologist recognize the limitations of microscopy in making such decisions. The biological behavior of a cartilaginous bone tumor is often evaluated better by sequential radiographic studies than by biopsy.

Growth and Metastasis

Primary chondromas of bone grow by gradual expansion, often encroaching on adjacent or surrounding bone tissue. Although some chondromas may give rise to chondrosarcomas, it is currently believed that most chondrosarcomas of dogs arise de novo rather than from malignant change in a preexisting benign cartilage tumor.[16]

Hemangioma

Classification

Well-differentiated hemangiomas, similar to those occurring in soft tissues, occasionally arise in bones of animals and humans. There is debate as to whether these lesions are true tumors or hamartomas.

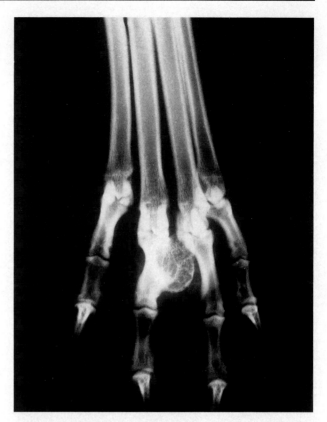

Fig. 5.9. Chondroma in a proximal phalanx of a dog. The tumor is an expansile, radiolucent growth with smooth outlines.

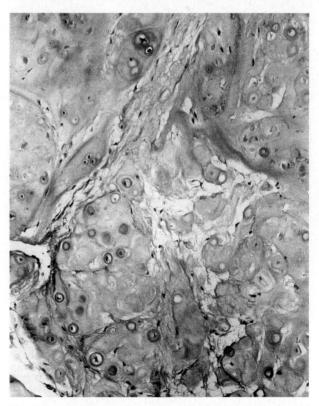

Fig. 5.10. Primary chondroma of bone. Encapsulated tumor of the mandible composed of irregular lobules of hyaline cartilage. Most tumor cells are small, isomorphic, and isochromic.

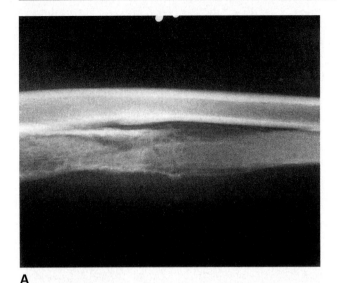

A

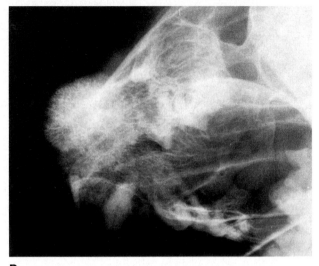

B

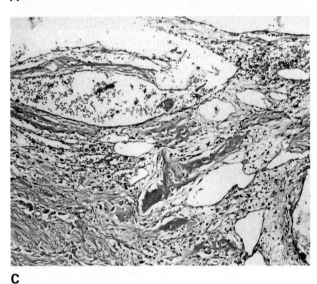

C

Fig. 5.11. Primary hemangioma of bone. **A.** Lytic lesion with persistent cortical shell of bone in an ulna of a dog. **B.** Productive lesion arising from the surface of the incisive bone of a cat. **C.** Vascular tumor composed of large caliber vessels with thin walls lined by a single flattened layer of endothelium.

Incidence, Age, Breed, and Sex

These rare tumors have been found in the skeletons of young to middle-aged dogs and cats and in a yearling horse.[17] Hemangiomas are much less common than primary hemangiosarcomas of bones. Too few cases have been described to know if age, breed, and sex are significant factors. The case reported in a yearling horse involved the distal phalanx and was considered to be congenital.[17]

Clinical Characteristics and Sites

Lesions are identified because of local swelling of the involved bone, lameness, and sometimes fracture. The course varies from a few weeks to more than 2 years.

Lesions occur in the skull, mandible, vertebral column, and long bones. The most common sites in human patients are vertebral bodies and the skull or facial bones. Hemangiomas can be detected in approximately 10 percent of human vertebral bodies at necropsy, but the lesions are generally small and asymptomatic.[8] Detailed examination of the skeleton of animals might also reveal a relatively high prevalence of clinically inapparent hemangiomas.

Gross Morphology

Skeletal hemangiomas are similar in appearance to those found in extraskeletal tissues. The tumor tissue is soft and dark red or purple. In the affected bone, the tumor replaces much of the cancellous bone except for small bony partitions. The cortex may bulge over the expanding tumor and be of reduced thickness, predisposing to pathologic fracture. A periosteal bony response is present in some cases.

Radiographic Examination

Lysis is the main pattern in most affected bones. Usually, the radiolucent lesions are well circumscribed and provoke no periosteal reaction. While the centers of some lesions are purely radiolucent (fig.5.11 A), others will have a honeycomb appearance. Hemangiomas of flat bones of the skull may produce an exuberant periosteal response mimicking the sunburst appearance characteristic of some osteosarcomas in animals (fig. 5.11 B).

Histological Features

Most tumors are composed of highly tortuous, cavernous vessels having thin walls (fig. 5. 11 C). Vascular spaces are typically filled with blood and lined by a single layer of endothelium. The vessels of some of these tumors have small diameters and thicker walls.

Growth and Metastasis

Lesions are slowly expansile. These tumors are benign and are not thought to undergo malignant progression.

REFERENCES

1. Pool, R.R. (1990) Tumors of bone and cartilage. In Moulton J. E. (ed.), *Tumors in Domestic Animals,* 3rd ed. University of California Press, Berkeley.

2. Stout, A.P., and Lattes, R. (1967) Tumors of the soft tissues. In *Atlas of Tumor Pathology.* 2nd series, fascicle 1. Armed Forces Institute of Pathology, Washington, D.C.

3. Shupe, J.L., Leone, N.C., Olson, A.E., and Gardner, E.J. (1979) Hereditary multiple exostoses: Clinicopathologic features of a comparative study in horses and man. *Amer J Vet Res* 40:751–757.

4. Chester, D.K. (1971) Multiple cartilaginous exostoses in two generations of dogs. *J Amer Vet Med Assoc* 159:895–897.

5. Owen, L.N., and Bostock, D.E. (1971) Multiple cartilaginous exostoses with development of a metastasizing osteosarcoma in a Shetland sheepdog. *J Small Anim Pract* 12:507–512.

6. Doige, C.E. (1987a) Multiple cartilaginous exostoses in dogs. *Vet Pathol* 24:276–278.

7. Jacobson, L.S., and Kirberger, R.M. (1996) Canine multiple cartilaginous exostoses: Unusual manifestations and a review of the literature. *J Amer Anim Hosp Assoc* 32:45–51.

8. Resnick, D., Kyriakos, M., and Greenway, G.G. (1994) Tumors and tumor-like lesions of bone: Imaging and pathology of specific lesions. In Resnick, D. (ed.), *Diagnosis of Bone and Joint Disorders,* 3rd ed. Vol. 6, ch. 83. W.B. Saunders, Philadelphia), pp. 3628–3938.

9. Pool, R.R., and Carrig, C.B. (1972) Multiple cartilaginous exostoses in a cat. *Vet Pathol* 9:350–359.

10. Pool, R.R., and Harris, J.M. (1975) Feline osteochondromatosis. *Feline Pract* 5:24–30.

11. Brown, R.J., Trevethan, W.P., and Henry, V.L. (1972) Multiple osteochondroma in a Siamese cat. *J Amer Vet Med Assoc* 160:433–435.

12. Riddle, W.E., and Leighton, R.L. (1970) Osteochondromatosis in a cat. *J Amer Vet Med Assoc* 156:1428–1430.

13. Doige, C.E. (1987b) Multiple osteochondromas with evidence of malignant transformation in a cat. *Vet Pathol* 24:457–459.

14. Silverman, J., Weisbrode, S.E., Myer, C.P., Biller, D.S., and Kerspack, S. (1994) Enchondroma in a rhesus monkey. *J Amer Vet Med Assoc* 204:786–788.

15. Sullivan, D.J. (1960) Cartilaginous tumors (chondroma and chondrosarcoma) in animals. *Amer J Vet Res* 21:531–535.

16. Brodey, R.S., Riser, W.H., and Van der Heul, R.O. (1974) Canine skeletal chondrosarcoma: A clinico-pathologic study of 35 cases. *J Amer Vet Med Assoc* 165:68–78.

17. Gelatt, K.J., Neuwirth, L., Hawkins, D.L., and Woodard, J.C. (1996) Hemangioma of the distal phalanx in a colt. *Vet Radiol Ultrasound* 37:275–280.

MALIGNANT TUMORS OF BONES

Veterinary pathologists are frequently required to examine cytological and histological preparations from bone lesions suspected of being malignant tumors. The diagnosis will often determine the clinical management of the case, frequently resulting in amputation of an affected limb, or even euthanasia of the animal. It is therefore important not only that a diagnosis of malignancy be based on appropriate microscopic changes, but also that the clinical, radiographic, and gross findings be consistent with this diagnosis.

General Considerations

Bones are organs composed of several different types of mesenchymal tissue, including bone, cartilage, fibrous tissue, adipose tissue, blood vessels, nerves, and hematopoietic tissue. Sarcomas may arise from mesenchymal precursors of any of these tissues in bones and are classified according to the tissue they most closely resemble. In reality, these malignant neoplasms present a spectrum of structural specialization ranging from sarcomas of undifferentiated mesenchyme to sarcomas closely mimicking one of the well differentiated types of connective tissue such as bone or cartilage. Confusion in morphological classification of certain bone sarcomas occurs because of a limited appreciation of the labile nature of neoplastic mesenchyme, a poor understanding of the interrelationships and transmutability among the several types of specialized connective tissues, and a desire to force even the most pleomorphic of these tumors into a rigid classification scheme. Malignant bone tumors mimicking each of the specialized connective tissues that occur in a bone organ have been reported in animals, but only the more common primary sarcomas of animal bones are discussed in this chapter and listed in table 5.1.

Recent advances in immunochemistry and molecular biology offer improved techniques for characterizing many soft tissue tumors, but these are not widely used in the diagnosis of bone tumors. No doubt specific antigenic markers will eventually become available, but in the meantime, classification of a tumor as osteoblastic, chondroblastic, or fibroblastic in origin is based on cellular morphology and on the nature of the matrix produced. Hyperplastic and neoplastic osteoblasts typically are pyriform cells with eccentric nuclei and basophilic cytoplasm, often with a clear Golgi zone adjacent to the nucleus (see figs. 5.23 A and 5.26 A,C). Their matrix (osteoid) consists predominantly of type I collagen fibers (approximately 90 percent), together with a mixture of proteoglycans and bone specific, noncollagenous proteins. Chondroblasts are ovoid to polyhedral and produce a matrix that also contains collagen (approximately 40 percent), but with a much larger quantity of proteoglycans. The collagen content of cartilage matrix is obscured in histological sections because it has a similar refractive index to the proteoglycan ground substance. Fibroblasts are ovoid to spindle shaped and produce a matrix composed almost entirely of collagen.

By definition, if malignant mesenchymal cells are seen to be producing osteoid, the tumor is an osteosarcoma, even if cartilage matrix is also present in some areas. However, it is often difficult in histological sections to distinguish between osteoid and the collagenous matrix of fibrous tissue, or chondroid, produced by neoplastic chondrocytes. This may be of considerable clinical importance because of the differences in prognosis among the various sarcomas of bone. Like fibrous connective tissue, osteoid is eosinophilic, but it is less fibrillar, more amorphous, and will often partly or completely surround plump tumor cells, entrapping them in lacunar spaces (see fig. 5.23 B,C). Osteoid will not necessarily be mineralized in neoplastic lesions, or even in the early stages of callous formation. The basophilic to amphophilic colors in the osteoid reflect its proteoglycan content and the immature nature of the osteoid, helping to differentiate it from mature trabeculae of osteoid that are usually devoid of these mosaic patterns. The osteoid in mature bone trabeculae is arranged in layers, and the osteocytes are in small, slit-like lacunae. In contrast, the osteoid produced by neoplastic osteoblasts is disorganized and may contain variable numbers of trapped tumor cells in large lacunae. Both osteoid and fibrous connective tissues are birefringent under polarized light, reflecting their collagen content. Fibrin in areas of hemorrhage may also be mistaken for osteoid, but it is not birefringent. The chondroid matrix produced by neoplastic chondrocytes is usually sufficiently basophilic to suggest its cartilaginous nature, but in some cases it may be tinctorially identical to osteoid. A matrix consisting of well-differentiated cartilage that transforms into an eosinophilic osteoid-like matrix without change in the cellular character is termed *chondro-osseous bone* (fig. 5.12). This is a consistent feature of fracture calluses and should not be confused with either a chondrosarcoma or an osteosarcoma, which may also contain both chondroid and osteoid.[1] Nonneoplastic bone may form in chondrosarcomas by the process of endochondral ossification, but in this case, the transition from one matrix to the other is abrupt, the cellular characteristics are different, and the bone formation is accompanied by vascular invasion of the tumor cartilage (see fig 5.30 B).

Reactive bone is commonly associated with primary and secondary bone tumors, either beneath an elevated periosteum or within the medullary cavity, and must be differentiated from the woven bone or lacy fragments of osteoid produced by malignant osteoblasts (see fig. 5.24 A,B). Unless there is convincing evidence that the tumor cells are manufacturing osteoid, a diagnosis of osteosarcoma should be resisted. Furthermore, it is important for the pathologist to recognize that an immature fracture callus, where primitive mesenchymal cells are proliferating rapidly and producing fragments of osteoid, may easily be confused with osteosarcoma. In fact, some published reports of unusual osteosarcomas almost certainly represent misdiagnosed fracture calluses. Such misdiagnoses are also likely to be common in submissions to veterinary diagnostic laboratories, especially in cases not supported by an adequate clinical history and radiographic description. This information, together with the histological organization of the lesion, is critical to an accurate diagnosis because cytological preparations from these proliferative lesions can contain undifferentiated and blastic appearing cells. Orderly maturation of undifferentiated cells into osteoblasts; their production of woven bone, gradually leading to trabeculae with embedded osteocytes; and continued maturation are events characteristic of periosteal

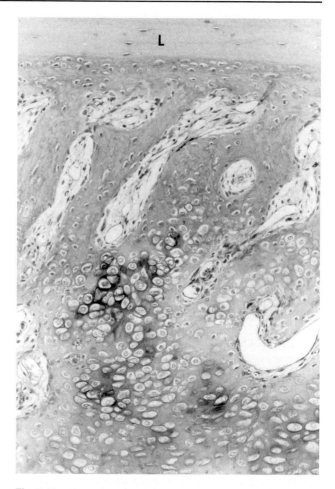

Fig. 5.12. Chondro-osseous bone in a fracture callus. Note the gradual transition of the hypercellular cartilaginous component, with its basophilic matrix, into tissue more closely resembling woven bone, but without alteration in the character of the cells. The mature lamellar bone *(L)* at the top of the field is part of the original cortex.

new bone formation and fracture repair. However, if such areas are sampled tangentially or at odd angles, this histological organization may be hidden. The sample then may need to be reoriented, or other areas of the lesions may need to be examined.

While the etiology of bone cancer is unknown, a number of contributory factors have been identified that are thought to play a role in the pathogenesis of bone sarcomas in humans and animals. These factors include ionizing radiation, bone tumor viruses, chemicals, chronic irritation in healing fractures repaired by metallic implants, bone infarcts, certain skeletal diseases or disorders, and host factors such as body size and sex. These risk factors and their putative role in bone tumor induction have been reviewed for humans[2] and for animals.[3-5]

It has been assumed by some veterinary cancer specialists that the same cytological criteria for malignancy and grading of human primary bone sarcomas, particularly chondrosarcomas, are directly applicable to animal bone cancer cases.[6,7] These criteria should be regarded only as useful guidelines to the veterinary pathologist until proper studies on large numbers of animals are concluded.

In current practice, complex hyphenated terms (e.g., osteo-chondro-fibrosarcoma) are no longer used to name a tumor. Because there are good data on survival rates of human patients with primary bone sarcoma, it has been determined that most primary bone sarcomas in humans can be categorized on the major type of tissue differentiation, resulting in distinct classes of tumors such as osteosarcoma, chondrosarcoma, and fibrosarcoma. As a class, each category of bone sarcoma exhibits a predictable clinical behavior. For example, osteosarcoma, as a class, pursues a more rapid clinical course with earlier lung metastasis than either chondrosarcoma or fibrosarcoma of bone. Although in most cases the major type of matrix differentiation reflects the clinical character of the tumor and also determines its histological classification, many bone tumor pathologists[8,9] consider it appropriate to name the tumor after a subdominant histological tissue pattern if the secondary tumor cell population is more malignant in character than the dominant histological component. For example, malignant mesenchyme of some canine bone sarcomas produces large volumes of neoplastic cartilage along with less prominent areas of osteosarcoma. These tumors should be designated as osteosarcoma or possibly chondroblastic osteosarcoma on the basis of anticipated clinical behavior. Subclassification of human osteosarcoma into osteoblastic, chondroblastic, and fibroblastic varieties based on the dominance of the major histological component has been related to differences in 5-year survival rates.[8] These varieties are seen in osteosarcomas and will be discussed and illustrated in this chapter. An attempt has been made to study their relationship to survival rate in dogs.[10]

Diagnosis of the tumor should be made on tumor tissue taken from the site of tumor origin within the bone organ. Malignant mesenchyme that penetrates the cortical surface of the bone may show a change in the histological quality of tumor matrix produced there, presumably in response to the different inductive environment (oxygen tension, physical tension) provided by the soft tissue surrounding the bone (fig. 5.13). Biopsies that obtain only tumor tissue lying outside the original cortical surface of a bone may show only neoplastic cartilage, while the more central tissue within the bone is osteosarcoma.

While histological diagnosis of primary bone sarcoma is based on the level of differentiation attained by the neoplastic matrix, prognosis is judged on the following criteria: the state of immaturity of the tumor cell population; the rate of tumor growth as indicated by the mitotic index or by the change measured in sequential radiographs; the ability of the host to contain the lesion as shown on radiographic studies; and the category of bone sarcoma, which, as previously mentioned, indicates the rapidity of the clinical course and the anticipated fate of the patient. There is disagreement regarding the validity of histological grading of osteosarcoma as a useful indicator of anticipated sur-

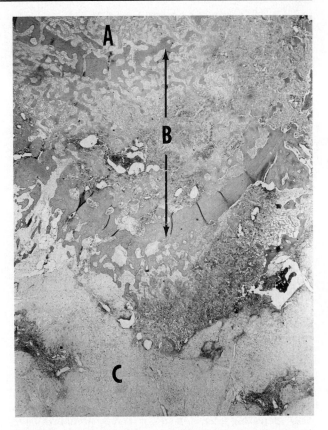

Fig. 5.13. Osteosarcoma of a dog's tibia. Transverse section through the cranial cortex at the tibial crest shows an osteosarcoma arising in the medullary cavity (A), invading the cortex (B), and producing cartilage on the surface (C) of the bone.

vival rate in humans,[9] although grading does appear correlated with survival rates in human fibrosarcoma and chondrosarcoma. Human patients with well-differentiated chondrosarcomas and fibrosarcomas of bone have a better prognosis than those with poorly differentiated tumors. By contrast, most reports indicate that the level of differentiation in human osteosarcoma has no prognostic value.[9]

Details of malignant bone disease in most domestic animals are cursory, but initial epidemiological studies have improved the estimates of the frequency with which the various types of bone sarcomas are distributed among the major animal species of veterinary concern.[10-12] Bone cancer is not a common disease in the animal population. One animal neoplasm survey found an incidence rate for bone cancer of 7.9 for dogs and 4.9 for cats per 100,000 individuals.[11] The disease is too rare in the other domestic species to determine an incidence rate. Of the major classes of animal bone sarcoma, osteosarcoma is by far the most common type occurring in dogs[13,14] and cats.[15-17]

In the dog, osteosarcoma (80 percent) and chondrosarcoma (10 percent) are the most common histological types. Fibrosarcoma and hemangiosarcoma together account for approximately 7 percent of the tumors. Lymphoid and myeloid tumors of the marrow are seen infrequently. Parosteal osteosarcoma and liposarcoma of bone marrow are very rare tumors of the dog and cat skeleton.

As the importance of breed variations in the development of primary bone neoplasia becomes better understood, clinicopathological studies will characterize the skeletal distribution of such lesions in different breeds. It has long been recognized that certain breeds of dogs are predisposed to bone neoplasia, and one study[14] has indicated that the pattern of skeletal involvement varies among several breeds of dogs. Certainly, the size of the dog is a major predisposing factor in the development of bone cancer.[18] Most skeletal maps depicting sites of predilection of canine bone sarcoma apply to large and giant breeds of dogs. Similar maps need to be made for the smaller canine breeds.

Influence of tumor site within the skeleton on biological behavior has not been fully evaluated. Osteosarcomas located below the knee and elbow joints in humans and occurring in the jaws are usually less aggressive and have less metastatic potential than osteosarcomas of other sites.[19] In a study on dogs from the Netherlands it was found that osteosarcomas of the hind legs have a poorer prognosis than those arising in other skeletal sites.[10] It is not known whether bone sarcomas of comparable histological appearance have the same growth rate and metastatic potential when located in the manus or pes as when situated in a more proximal site in the appendicular skeleton. With increasing interest in cancer therapy for animal bone tumors, new demands are being placed on the pathologist to characterize these tumors precisely and to provide morphological support in determining the efficacy of treatment of the several categories of mesenchymal neoplasms encountered in animal bone.

REFERENCES

1. Schwamm, H.A., and Millward, C.L. (1995) *Histologic Differential Diagnosis of Skeletal Lesions.* Igaku-Shoin, New York.
2. Pritchard, D.J., Finkel, M.P., and Reilly, C.A. (1975) The etiology of osteosarcoma. *Clin Orthop* 111:14–22.
3. Theilen, G.H., and Madewell, B.R. (1979) Tumors of the Skeleton. In Theilen, G. H., and Madewell, B. R. (eds.), *Veterinary Cancer Medicine.* Lea and Febiger, Philadelphia.
4. Stevenson, S., Hohn, R.B., Pohler, O.E.M., Fetter, A.W., Olmstead, M.L., and Wind, A.P. (1982) Fracture-associated sarcoma in the dog. *J Amer Vet Med Assoc* 180:1189–1196.
5. Pool, R.R., Morgan, J.P., Parks, N.J., Farnham, J.E., and Littman, M.S. (1983) Comparative pathogenesis of radium-induced intracortical bone lesions in humans and beagles. *Health Phys* 44(Suppl. 1): 155–177.
6. Brodey, R.S., Riser, W.H., and Van der Heul, R.O. (1974) Canine skeletal chondrosarcoma: A clinico-pathologic study of 35 cases. *J Amer Vet Med Assoc* 165:68–78.
7. Sullivan, D.J. (1960) Cartilaginous tumors (chondroma and chondrosarcoma) in animals. *Amer J Vet Res* 21:531–535.
8. Dahlin, D.C., and Coventry, M.B. (1967) Osteogenic sarcoma: A study of six hundred cases. *J Bone Joint Surg* 49A:101–110.
9. Spjut, H.J., Dorfman, H.D., Fechner, R.E., and Ackerman, L.V. (1971) Tumors of bone and cartilage. In *Atlas of Tumor Pathology.* 2nd series, fascicle 5. Armed Forces Institute of Pathology, Washington, D.C.
10. Misdorp, W., and Hart, A.A.M. (1979) Some prognostic and epidemiologic factors in canine osteosarcoma. *J Natl Cancer Inst* 62:537–545.
11. Dorn, C.R., Taylor, D.O.N., Schneider, R., Hibbard, H.H., and Klauber, M.R. (1968) Survey of animal neoplasms in Alameda and Contra Costa counties, California. II. Cancer morbidity in dogs and cats from Alameda County. *J Natl Cancer Inst* 40:307–318.
12. Priester, W.A., and Mantel, N. (1971) Occurrence of tumors in domestic animals: data for 12 United States and Canadian colleges of veterinary medicine. *J Natl Cancer Inst* 47:1333–1344.
13. Brodey, R.S., and Riser, W.H. (1969) Canine osteosarcoma: A clinico-pathologic study of 194 cases. *Clin Orthop* 62:54–64.
14. Brodey, R.S., Sauer, R.M., and Medway, W. (1963) Canine bone neoplasms. *J Amer Vet Med Assoc* 143:471–495.
15. Engle, G.C., and Brodey, R.S. (1969) A retrospective study of 395 feline neoplasms. *J Amer Hosp Assoc* 5:21–31.
16. Liu, S.K., and Dorfman H.D. (1974) The cartilage analogue of fibromatosis (juvenile aponeurotic fibroma) in dogs. *Vet Pathol* 11:60–67.
17. Turrel, J.M., and Pool, R.R. (1982) Primary bone tumors in the cat: A retrospective study of 15 cats and a literature review. *Vet Radiol* 23:152–166.
18. Tjalma, R.A. (1966) Canine bone sarcoma: Estimation of relative risk as a function of body size. *J Natl Cancer Inst* 36:1137–1150.
19. Dahlin, D.C., and Unni, K.K. (1977) Osteosarcoma of bone and its important recognizable varieties. *Amer J Surg Pathol* 1:61–72.

Sarcomas of Medullary Origin

Osteosarcoma

Sarcomas arising within bones are more common and consistently more malignant than sarcomas of periosteal origin. Osteosarcoma of central or medullary origin, as it occurs in the dog, is the most common primary bone tumor, and consequently, it is the only sarcoma of bone for which large numbers of cases have been available for gross and microscopic study. The description of osteosarcoma in this chapter pertains mainly to the disease as it appears in dogs.

Classification

Osteosarcomas are primary malignant bone tumors that arise in the medullary cavity and are characterized by the production of osteoid and/or immature bone by malignant osteoblasts. Various classification systems have been used for these tumors, both in man and in animals. The scheme used here is based on the nature of the matrix produced by the malignant cells and is consistent with that proposed in a bulletin of the World Health Organization[1] (see table 5.1). A similar classification system is used for osteosarcomas of humans.[2] Osteosarcomas are not a homogeneous group of tumors. They vary greatly in the amount and quality of matrix and in histological patterns, and they produce a wide range of radiographic changes. Often the radiographic and histological patterns will mimic those of the other major classes of primary bone tumor. Although there are no large studies in animals that conclusively prove differences in clinical behavior among the several subclasses of osteosarcoma, this classification scheme is useful for acquainting the veterinary pathology resident with the range of histological patterns produced in these tumors.

Incidence, Age, Breed, and Sex

Osteosarcoma accounts for over 80 percent of the malignant bone tumors in dogs and about 70 percent in cats.[3,4] Comparable data are not available for the other domestic animals since primary bone neoplasia is so uncommon in those species.

In dogs, the mean age at which osteosarcoma is first recognized is around 7.5 to 8 years, but the range is broad, and animals less than 2 years of age are sometimes affected.[3,5,6] Dogs of giant breeds generally develop osteosarcomas at a younger age than dogs of smaller breeds.[7] In some studies, differences are reported between the mean ages of dogs with osteosarcomas in different skeletal regions, but these reports are inconsistent, and the numbers of dogs with osteosarcomas involving the flat or irregular bones are often too few to allow reliable analysis. A mean age of 7 years was reported for dogs with osteosarcomas of the vertebral column in one study.[8] In another study of 116 tumors of the axial skeleton in dogs, osteosarcomas of the rib occurred at a significantly younger age (mean 5.4 years) than osteosarcomas of other axial skeletal sites, the overall mean being 8.7 years.[9]

Five breeds of dogs (boxers, Great Danes, Saint Bernards, German shepherds, and Irish setters) accounted for two-thirds of the cases in a study of dogs from Pennsylvania,[3] whereas Great Danes, rottweilers, German shepherds, and boxers were overrepresented in a study from the Netherlands.[7] The risks of primary bone sarcoma (primarily osteosarcoma) among giant (more than 80 pounds) and large (40 to 80 pounds) breeds of dogs are, respectively, 60.9 and 7.9 times the risk of small breeds (less than 20 pounds).[10] Osteosarcomas of the appendicular skeleton occur more often in male than in female dogs,[3,7,11,12] but this does not necessarily apply to osteosarcomas of the axial skeleton. In fact, females with axial osteosarcomas outnumbered males by 2.1:1 in one study,[9] although the incidence varied with tumor location.

Cats develop osteosarcoma at an older average age (10.5 years, range 3–18 years) than dogs.[4,13] The influence of breed predisposition is undetermined in cats. Male cats appear to be more commonly affected than female cats,[4,11,13] although in one study,[14] 12 of 15 affected cats were females.

Clinical Characteristics

In general, osteosarcoma is a rapidly progressive neoplasm leading to early mortality. Differential diagnoses include other primary bone tumors (malignant and benign), secondary bone tumors, mycotic and bacterial osteomyelitis, fracture, periostitis, arthritis, hypertrophic osteopathy, and metaphyseal osteopathy.[12,15] Clinical manifestations reflect the site of the lesion, but since the appendicular skeleton is most commonly affected, lameness is

the earliest sign in most cases.[12] Palpable swellings generally develop one or more weeks after pain has been present and are initially cool, but become increasingly warm and painful as the tumor enlarges and the periosteum is stretched.[12] Congestion, edema, fibroplasia, and periosteal bone formation accompany continued expansion of the tumor. In time, there is muscle atrophy in the affected limb, and the draining lymph nodes are often enlarged and firm. Older lesions tend to be less painful. Pathological fracture often complicates advanced cases, but fracture may also occur soon after the onset of clinical signs, especially in rapidly growing osteolytic osteosarcomas.

In the axial skeleton, tumors of the rib, cranial vault, zygomatic arch, and jaw usually are first recognized as firm bony enlargements. Osteosarcoma involving the nasal cavities or sinuses causes unilateral, bloody discharges that are sometimes purulent in character. Pain without neurological signs is the predominant initial finding with osteosarcoma of the vertebral column.[8]

In dogs[15] and cats[13] the duration of clinical signs prior to initial clinical examination is approximately 2 and 3 months, respectively. Some cases pursue a very rapid course, and the animal survives less than 1 month, but a few animals may survive without therapy for 6 months or longer following diagnosis. There is indication that the clinical course is slower in cats than in dogs.[4,13,16] One study of dogs treated surgically for osteosarcoma reported that 85 percent of 41 dogs were dead within 8 months following amputation of the limb.[3] Only one dog was alive and clinically free of tumor recurrence 6 years postsurgery. In another study, the median survival time of 162 dogs with appendicular osteosarcoma, treated by amputation, was 19.2 weeks.[17] The 1- and 2-year survival rates were estimated to be 11.5 percent and 2 percent, respectively. Most dogs either died or were euthanized because of problems related to metastatic spread of the tumor, usually to the lungs.[17] Despite this eventual high metastatic rate, only dogs with clinically and radiographically undetectable metastases received surgical amputation. Survival times for dogs with osteosarcomas of the axial skeleton are marginally better than those with appendicular tumors.[9] In particular, osteosarcomas of the maxilla and mandible do not metastasize as readily as those arising at other axial sites[9,18] and are more amenable to surgical removal. In comparison, four of five cats in one study were still alive 26 months after surgical excision or amputation of an osteosarcoma.[14] Results of another study reported a median survival time of 49.2 months in 12 cats with appendicular osteosarcoma treated by amputation.[16] Four of the 12 cats (33 percent) survived for 5 years or more after diagnosis. Cats with axial osteosarcoma had a much shorter median survival time (5.5 months), reflecting the difficulty of complete surgical removal of tumors in axial sites.[16]

Serum alkaline phosphatase activity is often increased in dogs and human patients with osteosarcoma. Increased activity of total alkaline phosphatase is more likely to reflect cholestatic liver disease or hyperadrenocorticism in a dog, but bone specific alkaline phosphatase may be a useful prognostic indicator. High activities of both total and bone specific alkaline phosphatase before surgery were significantly correlated with shorter survival time after surgery in a study of 75 dogs with appendicular osteosarcoma.[19] Surgical removal was accompanied by significant reductions in the activity of bone specific alkaline phosphatase. Failure of bone specific alkaline phosphatase to decrease following surgery was correlated with shortened survival time.[19] Similar results have been obtained in studies of human osteosarcoma.

Hypertrophic osteopathy (Marie's disease) is a relatively common sequel in dogs with pulmonary metastases of osteosarcoma or with large rib tumors that encroach on the thoracic cavity. In one report[15] the prevalence was 5 percent (7 of 130), but in another[3] 29 percent (12 of 41) of dogs were affected. The lesions of hypertrophic osteopathy developed 1–7 months after removal of the skeletal tumor, with average postsurgical times of 5.7 and 4.2 months in the two reports. The extent and severity of the bony lesions of hypertrophic osteopathy in dogs with pulmonary metastases of osteosarcoma depend on how long they survive. Common sites for the periosteal new bone formation characteristic of hypertrophic osteodystrophy are the abaxial surfaces of the second and fifth metacarpal and metatarsal bones. Later, the ends of the radius and ulna and of the tibia and fibula may be involved. In most dogs, the lesions are relatively mild, and no doubt, many cases are missed. Hypertrophic osteopathy is not reported in cats with metastatic osteosarcoma involving the lungs.[13,14]

Sites

Osteosarcomas in dogs have very strong site preferences. In fact, the location of a lesion, together with its radiographic appearance, may lead to a presumptive diagnosis of osteosarcoma. The appendicular skeleton is affected three to four times as often as the axial skeleton and the forelimbs approximately twice as often as the hind limbs (1.6 to 1.8 times).[3,5] This ratio closely corresponds to the ratio of weight distribution between the two pairs of limbs. In one study of the site incidence of canine osteosarcoma,[5] 68 percent of the tumors occurred in four long bones: radius (23 percent), humerus (19 percent), tibia (14 percent), and femur (14 percent). Certain sites in these bones were preferentially involved. In the radius, all of the tumors occurred in the distal metaphysis, and all but 1 of 60 tumors of the humerus occurred in the large proximal metaphysis. The distal ends of the tibia and femur had between two and three times the tumor frequency of the proximal ends of the bones. The region of the elbow joint is rarely involved in dogs, with only 7 of 98 osteosarcomas of the forelimb arising in this area.[3]

Although it is tempting to generalize when considering the site distribution of osteosarcomas in dogs, there are marked differences between breeds and between dogs of different size ranges.[3,10] For example, 67 percent of osteosarcomas in Great Danes occur in the distal radius,

while only 9 percent of tumors occur at that site in the boxer.[3] The ratio of appendicular to axial osteosarcomas decreases as the size of the dog decreases. It is probably no coincidence that the predilection sites for osteosarcomas, at least in the forelimb of large breeds, corresponds with the sites of most rapid early growth and latest physeal closure.[3,5] However, an analysis of tumor location and rate of bone growth in one study failed to demonstrate a significant relationship.[5] It was suggested that other factors, such as weight-bearing stress, might be important. While a single traumatic event does not appear to predispose to osteosarcoma, chronic irritation and repair associated with osteomyelitis, bone infarcts,[20,21] or the presence of an internal fixation device[22] is occasionally linked to tumor development (fig. 5.14). In such cases, the tumor may originate from the diaphyseal region of long bones or from other locations that are not considered predilection sites. Osteosarcomas are rarely reported in appendicular bones distal to the carpal or tarsal joints.[23]

Between 20 and 25 percent of canine osteosarcomas originate from bones of the axial skeleton.[3,5,9] Of these, approximately 50 percent occur in the head and 50 percent in the ribs, vertebrae, and pelvis. Breed differences again are important when one considers that osteosarcomas rarely occur in the skull or flat bones of Great Danes or Saint Bernards, while one-third of the osteosarcomas in boxers develop in flat bones. Also, the boxer is the breed most commonly affected by osteosarcoma of the skull. Most rib tumors arise near the costochondral junction.[9] Primary tumors of sternebrae are rare. While some reports indicate that osteosarcomas of the spinal column occur most often in lumbar vertebrae, thoracic vertebrae were more often involved in one study.[8] This difference may reflect the difficulty in radiographing the thoracic vertebrae to properly detect tumors there.

Predilection sites for osteosarcoma in cats are not as well defined as in dogs, partly because the tumor is less common in this species and there are fewer large scale studies. As in dogs, the appendicular skeleton is involved more often than the axial skeleton, but the ratio appears to be reduced, and there is no obvious predilection for the forelimbs.[4,13,16] In one study of 22 osteosarcomas in cats,[16] 67 percent of the tumors were in the appendicular skeleton. Of the 15 appendicular osteosarcomas, 5 were in either the distal femur or proximal tibia. A preference for the hind limbs was also identified in another study of 15 feline osteosarcomas,[14] where 9 were in the pelvic limb, and only 1 was in the forelimb. Of the remaining five, three were in the skull and one each involved the sacrum and coccyx. An association between osteosarcoma and fracture repair using an intramedullary pin is reported in the proximal femur of a cat.[24]

Osteosarcomas are rare in domestic animals other than dogs and cats but are reported occasionally in the head, particularly the mandible, of horses, cattle, and sheep.[11] Some osteosarcomas diagnosed in the mandible of large animals might in fact have been ossifying fibromas.

Gross Morphology

The gross and radiographic appearance of central (medullary) osteosarcomas is variable and is determined by the behavior of the tumor cells and the nature of the matrix they produce. Several subtypes are recognized on the basis of microscopic features and are discussed later in this chapter. In all cases, there is destruction of normal bone, formation of reactive bone by the endosteum and periosteum, and production of osteoid by the tumor. The variable extent to which these three processes occur is well illustrated in macerated and gross specimens (fig. 5.15 A,B,C). Some forms are predominantly *lytic* (figs. 5.15 A and 5.16 A), some are *productive* (fig. 5.16 B), and some are *mixed* forms containing both destructive and proliferative elements. These three patterns associated with bone tumors are very familiar to the radiologist, who also evaluates the radiographic patterns of altered bone mineral density.[25]

In lytic bone tumors the amount of cortical and cancellous bone destruction can be directly evaluated because the bone tumor matrix does not obscure resorbed bone surfaces. Periosteal new bone appears as a roughened bony

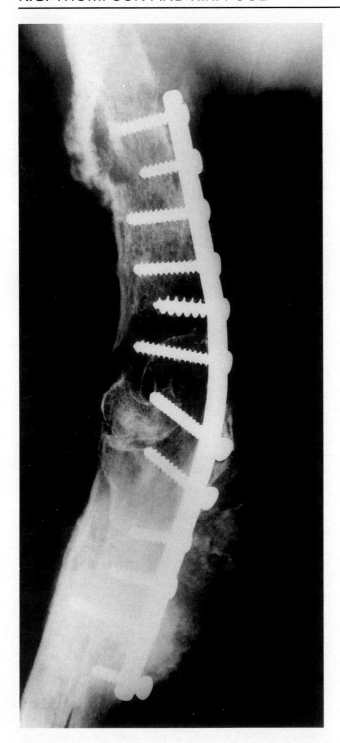

Fig. 5.14. Osteosarcoma involving the distal two-thirds of the humerus and the proximal half of the radius in a 6 1/2–year-old rottweiler. Arthrodesis of the elbow had been performed 4 years earlier using a metal plate that had not been removed. Note the extensive production of subperiosteal new bone on the shaft of the humerus and on the proximal radius and ulna. The tumor within the humerus is more lytic than that in the radius and ulna. The usual predilection sites for osteosarcoma in the forelimbs of dogs are the proximal humerus and the distal radius.

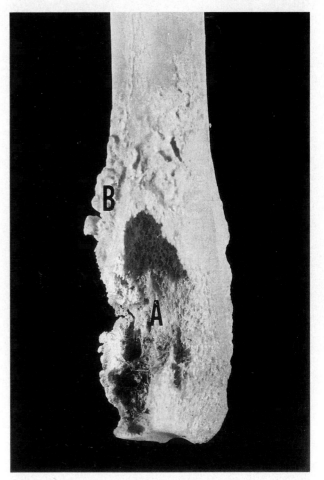

A

Fig. 5.15. Macerated specimens of canine osteosarcoma. **A.** Lytic tumor of distal radius showing lysis of most of the cancellous bone *(A)* and provoking a meager periosteal bony response *(B)*. (continued)

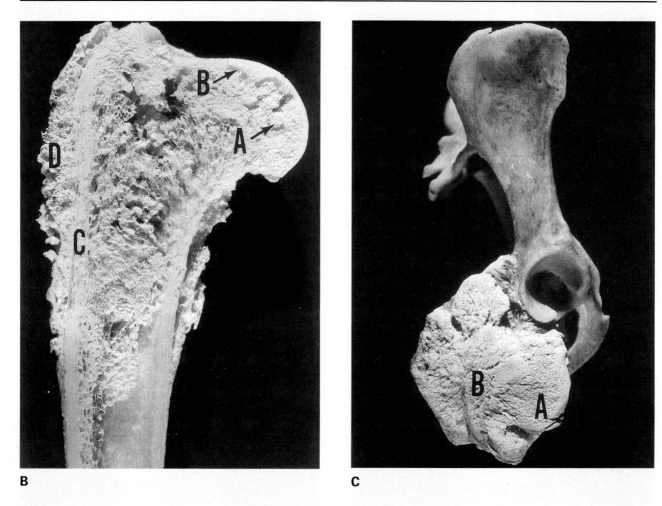

B   **C**

Fig. 5.15. (continued) **B.** Mixed tumor of proximal humerus. Note nodules of tumor bone *(A)*, lysis of subchondral bone *(B)*, areas of cortical bone destruction *(C)*, and a moderate periosteal bony response *(D)*. **C.** Productive tumor of the ischiatic table of the pelvis. Tumor bone *(A)* radiates away from a partially intact cortical surface of ischium *(B)*.

sheet or as a covering of irregular tufts or knobs of reactive bone matrix. The subtypes of osteosarcoma most often forming lytic lesions include poorly differentiated osteosarcoma, nonproductive osteoblastic osteosarcoma, some chondroblastic osteosarcomas, about 50 percent of the fibroblastic osteosarcomas, most telangiectatic and giant cell osteosarcomas, and some combined types. Some of the subtypes can be recognized by gross inspection. Poorly differentiated osteosarcoma, nonproductive osteoblastic osteosarcoma, and fibroblastic osteosarcoma (fig. 5.17 A,B) all have soft, pale matrix containing small, random areas of mucoid tissue, congestion, and necrosis. Differentiation of these three types therefore requires microscopic examination. Chondroblastic osteosarcoma and the combined type of osteosarcoma usually produce enough pale, glistening cartilage matrix to be detected grossly (fig. 5.18 A,B). Telangiectatic osteosarcomas (fig. 5.19 A,B) are readily recognized by their soft, bloody appearance, but they often can not be distinguished from either a primary or secondary hemangiosarcoma of bone.

Giant cell types of osteosarcoma (fig. 5.20 A,B) usually have a homogeneous, pale appearance, and the tumor matrix has the consistency of clay. Areas of hemorrhage and necrosis may predominate and confuse the pattern. These tumors grossly resemble primary giant cell tumors of bone.

In osteosarcoma characterized by a mixed pattern, there may be partial destruction of normal bone architecture in addition to considerable amounts of new bone matrix. The new bone tissue originates from three sources. First, tumor bone can be recognized as small nodular clusters of random, interlacing bony trabeculae that replace the lysed normal bone structures. Tumor bone can be found among the remaining trabeculae of cancellous bone, in resorbed segments of cortical bone, and within the periosteal new bone response. Second, the perturbed endosteum often attempts to form an abutment across the medullary cavity at the border of the expanding tumor mass. This same process can be found in bone infection, suggesting that it probably represents a form of response to

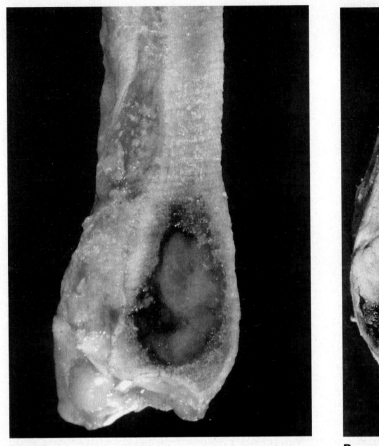

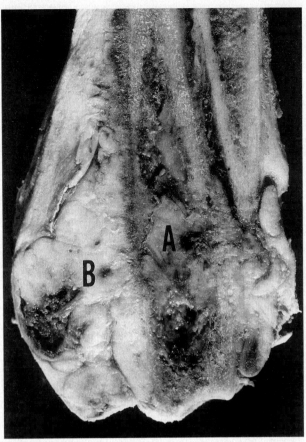

Fig. 5.16. **A.** Lytic osteosarcoma in the distal radius of a dog. The tumor has replaced most of the trabecular bone in the metaphyseal region but does not appear to have penetrated the cortex at this stage. (Photographs courtesy of R. A. Fairley.) **B.** Moderately productive osteosarcoma in the distal radius. In this case, the tumor has not only replaced the normal metaphyseal spongiosa *(A)*, but it has penetrated the cortex, forming a large soft tissue mass *(B)* on the bone surface.

a weakened bone, rather than an attempt to stop the extension of the disease process. Third, the periosteal new bone response is recognized as a roughened sheet or tufted covering of bone matrix, and this response is usually more marked (i.e., more productive) in tumors with a mixed pattern than in lytic tumors. The tumor subtypes of osteosarcoma most often associated with a mixed pattern include moderately productive osteoblastic osteosarcoma (fig. 5.16 B), most chondroblastic osteosarcomas (fig. 5.18 A), about 50 percent of the fibroblastic osteosarcomas, and most of the combined types of osteosarcoma. On gross inspection of sectioned fresh bone specimens, it is often not possible to distinguish between moderately productive osteoblastic osteosarcoma and fibroblastic osteosarcoma, or between chondroblastic osteosarcoma (fig. 5.18 A) and the combined type of osteosarcoma. However, one can often recognize a tumor from the latter pair if they contain enough glistening cartilage matrix.

Only a few osteosarcomas are primarily productive. Macerated specimens of these tumors (see fig. 5.15 C) show a dense, bony tumor, often centered on a flat surfaced bone such as the scapula, ilium, ischium, or mandible.

While the tumor destroys and penetrates the cortex, it spares enough compact bone that the cortex can still be recognized on cut surface. Amorphous bone tumor matrix fills the medullary cavity. Tumor bone on the periosteal surface, however, is arranged perpendicular to the cortical surface in an orderly pattern that mimics the massive overgrowth of periosteal new bone seen following trauma or infection. This pattern presents a major diagnostic problem for the radiologist when a productive osteoblastic osteosarcoma arises in the diaphysis of a long bone (see fig. 5.21 D). During the development of this tumor, the blood supply to the medullary cavity and cortex is lost, and tumor tissue within the diaphysis, as well as the diaphysis itself, is infarcted. Viable tumor and reactive periosteal new bone form a cuff of bone around the surface of the diaphysis. This confusing pattern may be misinterpreted as osteomyelitis, including fungal infection of the bone. The only subtype of osteosarcoma capable of forming this pattern is a productive osteoblastic osteosarcoma.

Representatives from any of the subtypes of osteosarcoma may occur at any skeletal site. In long bones of the

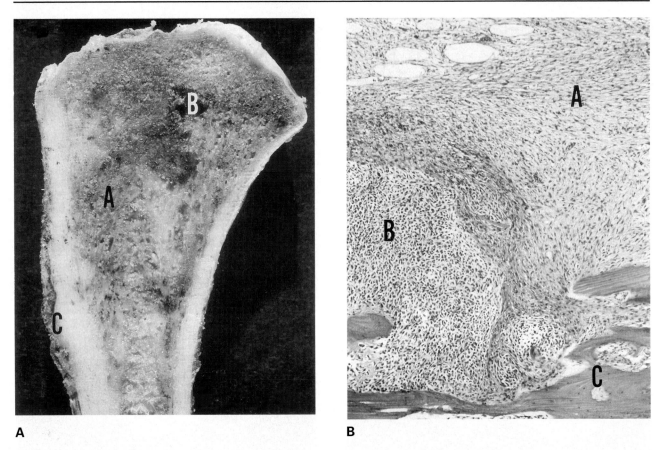

Fig. 5.17. Fibroblastic osteosarcoma of the proximal tibia. **A.** In this early lesion, tumor tissue primarily infiltrates marrow spaces of the metaphyseal spongiosa *(A)* without producing much bone lysis *(B)* and without provoking a prominent periosteal bony response *(C)*. **B.** In early cases the neoplasm is primarily a spindle cell sarcoma *(A)*, and areas of osteosarcomatous differentiation *(B)* with bone matrix formation may be uncommon. Note residual lamellar bone of cortex *(C)*.

limbs the tumors are typically centered in the metaphysis. Most osteosarcoma subtypes where osteolysis predominates destroy bone very rapidly and may be well advanced by the time they are diagnosed. Pathological fracture often occurs early in the disease and may be the reason for initial presentation to a veterinarian. The tumor subtypes most frequently associated with this aggressive course are poorly differentiated osteosarcoma, the nonproductive type of osteoblastic osteosarcoma, and telangiectatic osteosarcoma.[26] In these lesions, the tumor rapidly penetrates the cortex before significant periosteal and endosteal responses are made. The clinical course in untreated dogs with lytic osteosarcoma is usually shortened by the locally aggressive behavior of the tumor in the limb rather than by early development of metastatic disease. There is no evidence to indicate that dogs with lytic tumors develop metastatic disease earlier or more frequently than dogs with mixed or productive lesions caused by osteosarcoma. In contrast, the giant cell type of osteosarcoma that also produces a lytic pattern usually forms a much less aggressive, expansile bone lesion (fig. 5.20 A). Apparently, this tumor grows slowly, destroying the inner cortical surface at a rate that can be matched by periosteal new bone production. The periosteum lays down a thin shell of bone over the slowly expanding cortical surface of the affected bone. After a few weeks to months, the tumor penetrates the neocortex, and pathological fracture can result.

Most tumor subtypes forming the mixed patterns of production and destruction have a relatively slower initial growth rate than the more aggressive tumors forming the lytic bone lesions. The slow initial growth rate permits the bone organ to mount a periosteal containment response similar to a periosteal callus, to keep pace, at least temporarily, with cortical destruction. The bony endosteal abutment that develops across the medullary cavity, like the periosteal response, eventually becomes incapable of blocking the extension of tumor tissue. Often a continuous core or tongue of tumor tissue extends from the tumor mass along the medullary cavity of the bone for a few centimeters beyond the limits of the tumor as seen in radiographs. *Skip metastases,* which are tumors that spread within the medullary cavity of the bone organ, occur infrequently in human patients[27] and in dogs.

Radiographic Appearance

Moderately advanced cases of primary bone sarcoma of dogs can usually be recognized as malignant by clinical and radiological examination, but the final diagnosis rests

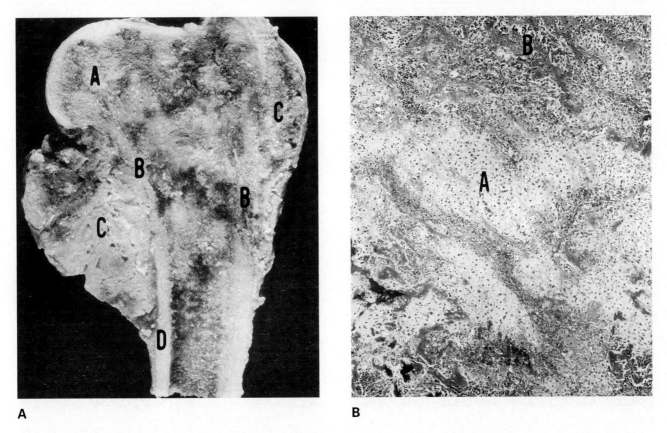

A

B

Fig. 5.18. Chondroblastic osteosarcoma of the proximal humerus. **A.** Sectioned proximal humerus showing nodular areas *(A)* of neoplastic bone and cartilage, cortical bone destruction *(B),* extraosseous tumor *(C),* and periosteal elevation (Codman's triangle) *(D).* **B.** Tumor cells produce an admixture of "malignant" cartilage *(A)* and bone *(B)* tissue.

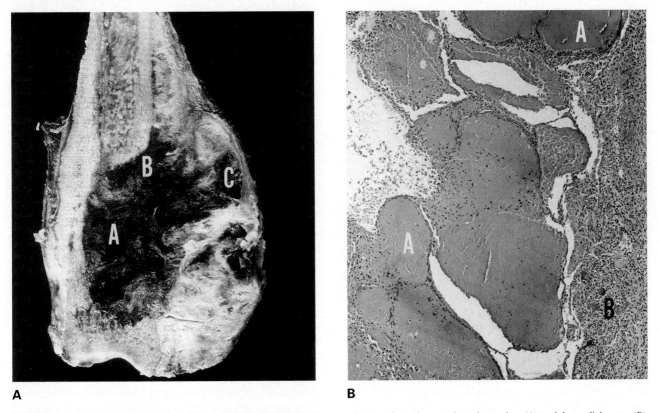

A

B

Fig. 5.19. Telangiectatic osteosarcoma of the distal radius. **A.** Soft bloody tumor tissue replaces the metaphyseal spongiosa *(A),* and the medial cortex *(B).* Tumor almost penetrates the periosteal cuff of reactive bone *(C)* covering the medial surface of the bone. **B.** Numerous large, blood filled spaces *(A)* lined by tumor cells, not endothelial cells, and small spicules of bone matrix *(B)* produced by tumor cells, are characteristic findings in this osteosarcoma subtype.

273

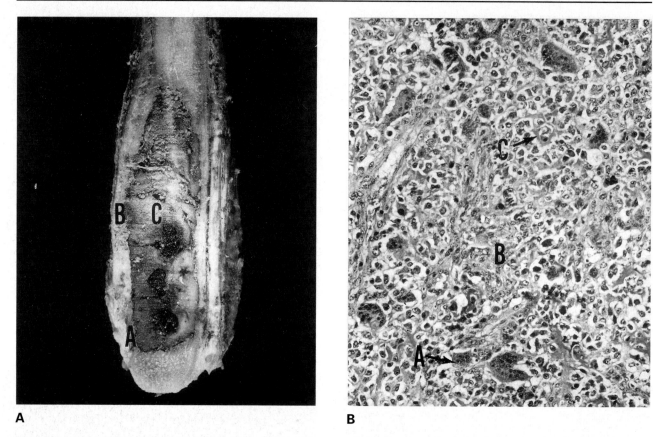

A

B

Fig. 5.20. Giant cell type of osteosarcoma of the distal radius. **A.** This expansile bone tumor has destroyed the cranial cortex *(A)*, but the tumor is covered by a smooth shell of periosteal new bone *(B)*. The soft pale tumor tissue *(C)* has necrotic areas containing blood. **B.** Tumor is characterized by numerous multinucleated tumor giant cells *(A)*, stroma of undifferentiated sarcoma *(B)*, and fields of malignant osteoblasts producing bone matrix *(C)*.

on cytological or histological findings since osteosarcoma, chondrosarcoma, and fibrosarcoma of bone do not produce pathognomonic radiographic patterns. In the initial stages of clinical bone disease, these three tumors produce similar radiographic changes: cortical destruction and periosteal response.[12]

As discussed in the previous section, the various subtypes of osteosarcoma can produce lytic, mixed (destructive and productive), or productive bone lesions, which are best distinguished by radiographic examination of the tumors. Unfortunately for the diagnostician, some of these patterns may also occur in other primary bone tumors, as well as in metastatic tumors of bone. For example, malignant primary bone tumors that may produce indistinguishable osteolytic radiographic patterns (fig. 5.21 A) include fibrosarcoma, hemangiosarcoma, giant cell sarcoma of bone, poorly differentiated osteosarcoma, a few of the chondroblastic osteosarcomas, about 50 percent of the fibroblastic osteosarcomas, most telangiectatic and giant cell type osteosarcomas, and some of the combined type osteosarcomas. Malignant bone tumors that may produce indistinguishable mixed radiographic patterns (fig. 5.21 B) include some higher grade chondrosarcomas, most moderately productive osteoblastic osteosarcomas, most chondroblastic osteosarcomas, about 50 percent of the fibrob-

lastic osteosarcomas, and most of the combined type osteosarcomas. A primarily productive radiographic pattern (fig. 5.21 C,D) is produced almost exclusively by the productive type of osteoblastic osteosarcoma, although this pattern can, rarely, be associated with a chondrosarcoma. In these tumors, the matrix is so dense that it causes ischemic necrosis both of the tumor and of the normal medullary and cortical structures. Viable tumor tissue, along with the periosteal new bone, forms a bony response of the cortical surface that has an almost orderly appearance mimicking that seen following trauma or infection. Persistence of the cortical shadow (fig. 5.21 C) may be secondary to bone ischemia and the inability of osteoclasts to reach the compact cortical bone in sufficient numbers to destroy it.

Most osteosarcomas occur as monostotic metaphyseal lesions in one of the predilection sites in the limbs of a large or giant breed dog. Narrowing of the cortical shadow is a common early sign and progresses rapidly to complete destruction as the tumor expands within the medullary cavity, replacing the normal metaphyseal architecture.[12,25] The lesion is poorly delimited due to a wide zone of transition between normal and abnormal bone, and is not accompanied by a sclerotic border. The periosteal response is not proportional to the degree of cortical destruction.[12] An early *brush* pattern may progress to a

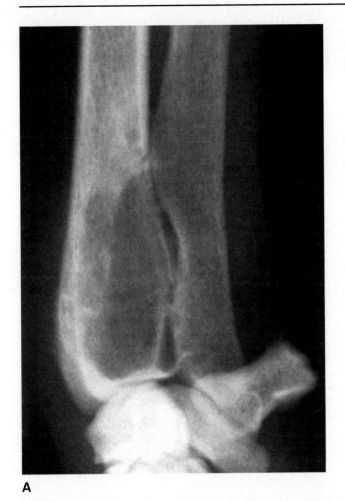

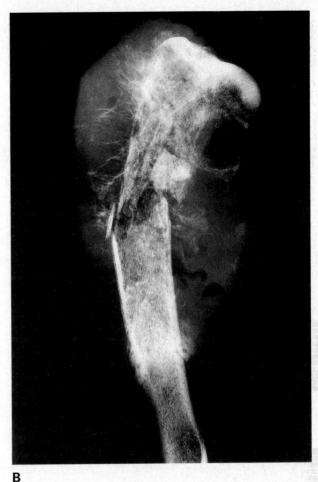

A   **B**

Fig. 5.21. Radiographic patterns of canine osteosarcoma. **A.** Osteolytic lesion in distal radius with minimal periosteal new bone or tumor bone production. **B.** Mixed lesion in proximal humerus with destruction of cranial and caudal cortices as well as the metasphyseal spongiosa. There is also pathological fracture and extension of bone matrix–producing tumor tissue into adjacent soft tissues. (continued)

coarser sunburst pattern characterized by radiating spicules of tumor bone perpendicular to the cortical surface. In dogs, the periosteal response to an osteosarcoma more often consists of amorphous bone matrix rather than a sunburst pattern.[12] Subperiosteal new bone, which develops beneath an elevated periosteum, forms a characteristic triangular mass of bone referred to as a Codman's triangle, which merges with the underlying cortex at the periphery of the tumor (see fig. 5.18 A). Osteosarcomas seldom spread through adjacent subchondral bone and articular cartilage to involve a joint space.

Osteosarcomas are dynamic lesions and may show dramatic change in radiographic appearance in as little as 7 to 10 days. Because these tumors present constantly evolving patterns, there appears to be little correlation between the type of radiographic pattern (i.e., osteolytic, mixed, or productive) and either the biological age or degree of malignancy of the tumor.[12]

Most osteosarcomas of the axial skeleton have radiographic features similar to those already described for the appendicular skeleton. Osteosarcomas of vertebrae are often osteolytic, but productive and mixed patterns are also seen.[8,12] These tumors may be overlooked because of problems associated with positioning, exposure and soft-tissue shadows. Osteosarcomas of ribs are generally located near costochondral junctions and tend to be osteoblastic.[12] In the head, osteosarcomas of the maxilla and zygomatic arch are usually osteolytic, while those involving the mandible are usually osteoblastic. Lytic osteosarcomas of the axial skeleton, particularly those in vertebral bodies may resemble plasma cell tumors.

Histological Features

Osteosarcomas may vary widely in their histological appearance, but in all cases a definitive diagnosis is based on the production of osteoid and/or bone by malignant mesenchymal cells. Because of the multipotential nature of primitive mesenchymal cells, the tumor matrix may contain variable quantities of cartilage, collagen, and osteoid, but even in tumors where the cartilage component predominates, the presence of osteoid denotes a diagnosis of osteosarcoma. This reflects the greater malignant potential

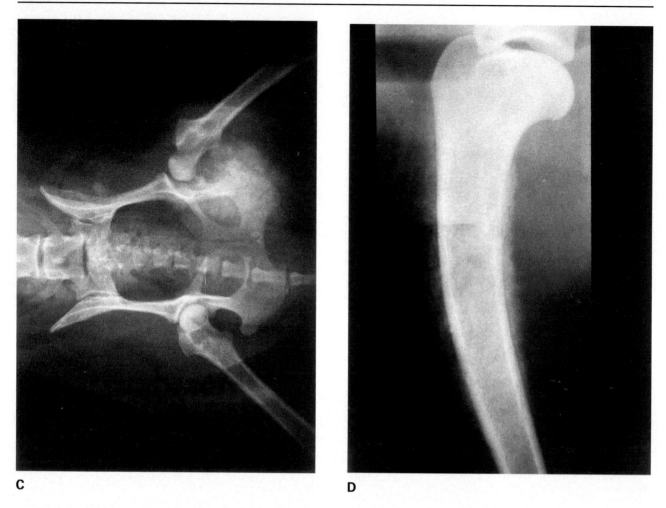

C

D

Fig. 5.21. (continued)   **C.** Productive lesion of ischium in which radiodense tumor tissue forms a contoured mass centered on the original bone but does not substantially destroy the cortical outline. **D.** Productive lesion of the proximal humerus characterized by no significant loss of bone and by production of a radiodense bony collar on the cortical surface that histologically is an admixture of tumor bone and periosteal reactive bone.

of mesenchymal tumors with osteogenic potential. Bone formation also occurs in some chondrosarcomas, but indirectly through endochondral ossification of tumor cartilage; bone formed in this way should not be mistaken for tumor bone. Similarly, osseous metaplasia of multipotential mesenchymal cells in tumors of nonosseous origin may create confusion. This is reported in association with intestinal adenocarcinoma of various species,[28] mammary carcinomas in dogs, and in an oral malignant melanoma in a dog,[29] probably due to the production by tumor cells of osteoinductive cytokines, such as those of the transforming growth factor–beta group.

It is important for the pathologist (and surgeon) to recognize that a biopsy sample submitted for histology from a suspected osteosarcoma may not be representative of the entire tumor. The presence of malignant mesenchymal cells producing a matrix of fibrous tissue or cartilage rather than osteoid does not exclude the possibility of osteosarcoma, especially if the lesion is at a known predilection site. Examination of several sections

from different areas of the tumor may be necessary before evidence of osteoid production is detected. Unfortunately, biopsies from bone lesions may be of inadequate size or quality to allow the pathologist to make a definitive diagnosis. In many cases, the specimen consists entirely of woven bone, indicating that the surgeon has sampled the periosteal or endosteal response rather than the tumor itself. Periosteal collars of new bone are often devoid of tumor tissue, which may still be confined to the medullary cavity and cortex.[12] Biopsy samples, collected following close examination of the radiograph, that include areas of medullary lysis and/or sclerosis are much more likely to be of value.

Low power microscopic examination of the lesion is important in determining the pattern and behavior of the tumor, in particular, whether there is evidence of destruction and/or permeation of preexisting bone tissue or bone marrow (fig. 5.22 A) and invasion of the cortex. At this magnification, it is also possible to gauge the variability within the tumor and identify areas for closer examination.

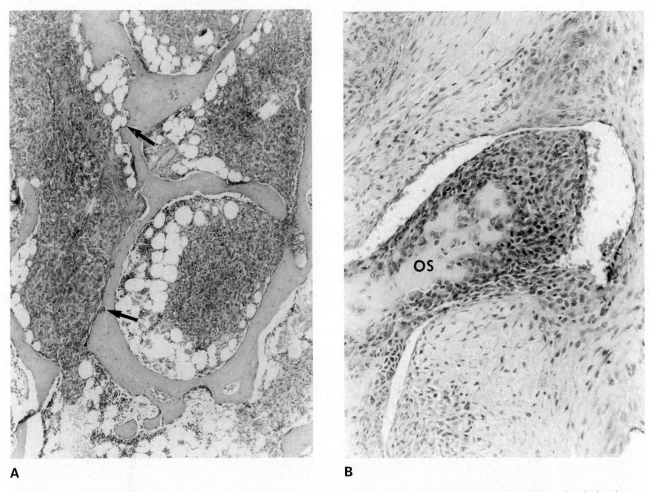

Fig. 5.22. **A.** Permeation of the marrow cavity by osteosarcoma. The tumor is infiltrating between preexisting bone trabeculae and replacing the normal architecture of the marrow cavity. The scalloped appearance of the bone trabeculae (lamellar bone) in some areas (arrows) reflects osteoclastic resorption, most likely triggered by the advancing tumor. **B.** Vascular invasion by osteosarcoma. A plug of tumor tissue, containing "tumor" osteoid (OS-woven bone), is present within a large vein at the margin of an osteosarcoma. Not surprisingly, metastases were detected in the lungs of this dog at necropsy.

Evidence of vascular invasion (fig. 5.22 B) or infiltration of adjacent tissues may also be apparent.

Malignant osteoblasts vary from pleomorphic, spindle shaped cells resembling fibroblasts to plump, oval, or rounded cells with basophilic cytoplasm and eccentric, hyperchromatic nuclei, more closely resembling nonneoplastic osteoblasts. Mitotic figures are often very common. The form and amount of osteoid is also highly variable. In some cases, it consists of hyaline, eosinophilic material arranged in thin strands or narrow ribbons among the malignant cells, producing a lace-like pattern (fig. 5.23 A). In others, the osteoid is present as irregular islands or spicules separated by malignant osteoblasts (fig. 5.23 B). In productive osteoblastic osteosarcomas the osteoid component of the tumor is abundant (fig. 5.23 C), while in nonproductive and moderately productive osteoblastic osteosarcomas (fig. 5.23 D) there is little osteoid production. Thin strands of osteoid may closely resemble collagenous fibrous tissue, and distinguishing the two forms of matrix may be impossible. Both are birefringent, reflecting their collagen content, and no histochemical stains allow reliable differentiation. In general, osteoid is less fibrillar than collagen, more amorphous, and often partly or completely surrounds the tumor cells, entrapping them in lacunar spaces (fig. 5.23 B,C). If the material is mineralized, it is probably osteoid rather than collagen, but this criterion can not be used with confidence when examining demineralized sections. Furthermore, the osteoid produced by rapidly proliferating malignant osteoblasts may not be mineralized. Fibrin in areas of hemorrhage may also be mistaken for osteoid, but is not birefringent.

Formation of endosteal and periosteal new bone is an expected response to a variety of inflammatory and neoplastic bone lesions, not just osteosarcoma. It is important, therefore, that spicules of nonneoplastic woven bone are not misinterpreted as tumor bone, leading to an incorrect diagnosis of osteosarcoma when the underlying process is much less sinister. There is no doubt that such errors occur, particularly when bone lesions are examined by inexperienced pathologists who may be unfamiliar with the manner in which bone responds to injury. In fact, occasional published reports describing unusual or atypical occur-

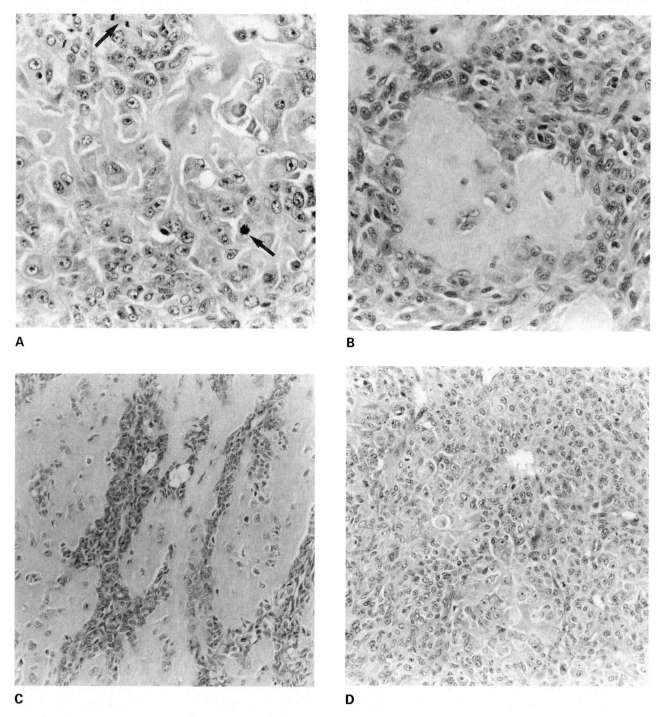

Fig. 5.23. Some histological patterns of osteosarcoma. **A.** Plump, malignant osteoblasts, many of which have eccentric nuclei and a prominent Golgi area, partly surrounded in some areas by lacy strands of osteoid. Mitotic figures (arrows) are common. **B.** Irregular islands of osteoid surrounded by malignant osteoblasts, some of which are incorporated in the osteoid. The tumor cells in this case are more fusiform than those in view A. **C.** Abundant osteoid in a productive osteoblastic osteosarcoma. Small clusters of malignant osteoblasts are often trapped within the tumor osteoid. **D.** Sheets of malignant osteoblasts with minimal osteoid formation in a moderately productive osteoblastic osteosarcoma.

rences of osteosarcoma are supported by photomicrographs that show reactive rather than neoplastic bone. Differentiation is often difficult, even for the experienced pathologist, and in some cases it is impossible. Irregular trabeculae of woven bone characterize both processes, but as a rule, the trabeculae of reactive bone are interconnected and lined by a single layer of plump osteoblasts, the spaces between them consisting of nonneoplastic connective tissue (fig. 5.24 A). In contrast, the spaces between spicules of tumor bone are filled with malignant osteoblasts, and the tumor cells are not organized in a layer along the surface of the tumor bone (fig. 5.24 B). Confusion may occur in areas where tumor cells are invading soft tissue spaces between trabeculae of reactive bone.

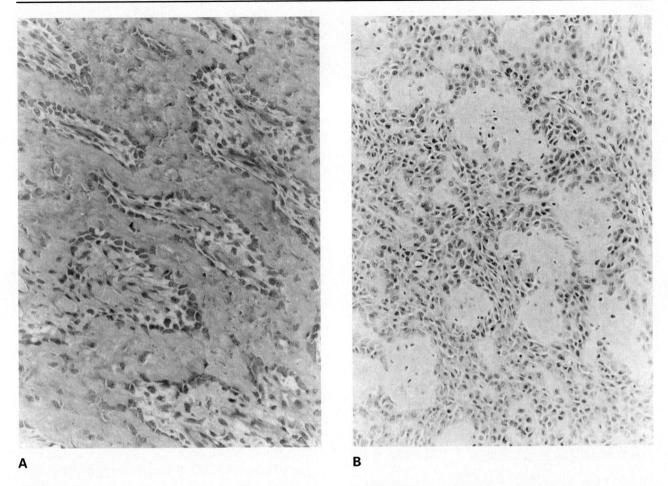

A   **B**

Fig. 5.24. Reactive and neoplastic bone tissue. **A.** Interconnected trabeculae of woven bone lined by a single layer of plump osteoblasts, typical of reactive bone. If cut in cross section this arborizing pattern of trabeculae would be lost, but the islands of osteoid would still be lined by osteoblasts. The spaces between trabeculae are filled with immature connective tissue showing no evidence of malignancy. **B.** In this section from an osteosarcoma, the malignant osteoblasts are producing irregularly shaped islands of "tumor" bone but do not line the bone forming surface the way they do in reactive bone, nor are the trabeculae connected in an orderly pattern.

The pathologist is presented with an even greater challenge in distinguishing between osteosarcoma and an early fracture callus. Rapidly proliferating, plump mesenchymal cells surrounding themselves with osteoid (fig. 5.25) are a feature of fracture repair, especially during the first few days, and may easily be confused with osteosarcoma. Evidence of maturation within the callus is a useful differentiating feature, and the cell population would be expected to have less atypia than most osteosarcomas. Another differentiating feature is the presence of chondro-osseous bone where highly cellular cartilage undergoes gradual transition to osteoid without abutment (see fig. 5.12). This is considered a feature of fracture calluses, not osteosarcomas.[30] In cases where pathological fracture has occurred in association with an osteosarcoma, interpretation of histological sections is even more difficult. Knowledge of the clinical history and radiographic findings are particularly important adjuncts to histology in such cases.

Multinucleate giant cells with features of osteoclasts are often scattered throughout osteosarcomas, sometimes in sufficient numbers to suggest a diagnosis of giant cell

tumor, but demonstration of osteoid production by the tumor cells allows exclusion of the latter option. In rapidly growing osteosarcomas, large areas of coagulation necrosis and hemorrhage are often present, probably due to localized ischemia.

Histologic grading of human osteosarcomas with respect to malignant potential has been attempted by some medical pathologists, but the marked variation that exists throughout many osteosarcomas and the rapid changes that can occur within the same tumor make this a questionable exercise. No system has been accepted as having prognostic significance,[31] and at present, no grading system is widely used for either human or animal osteosarcomas. Various classification systems for bone sarcomas, based on the predominant histological pattern, have been developed for humans and animals. The scheme used here (see table 5.1) is an adaptation of a system developed by Dahlin[2] and is well accepted by veterinary pathologists.[1,26] Such a classification system for this important group of tumors is justified in that it may lead to the identification of correlations between osteosarcoma subtype, prognosis, and sus-

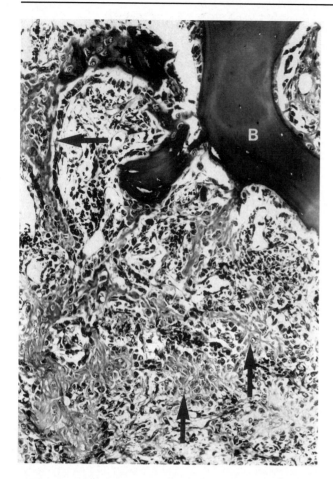

Fig. 5.25. Repairing fracture at 1 week. Disorganized condensations of plump mesenchymal cells are surrounding themselves with osteoid (vertical arrows) in a manner similar to some osteosarcomas. Some of the better developed bone spicules are lined by a single layer of osteoblasts (horizontal arrow), providing evidence that the bone is reactive rather than neoplastic. Others are attached to the mature (lamellar), preexisting bone *(B)*.

ceptibility to therapy. For example, in dogs, fibroblastic osteosarcomas have a relatively favorable prognosis,[7] while the prognosis for the telangiectatic form is very poor.[18] Similar observations have been made in human patients with these two tumor types. A significant difficulty in attempting to subclassify osteosarcomas is the inherent variability present within many tumors and the fact that a subdominant pattern may appear to be the most malignant. Classification into one of the six categories is determined by the predominant pattern in representative sections from the tumor,[26] but if no single pattern is dominant the tumor is best categorized as a *combined type osteosarcoma*. In cases where only small fragments of tissue are received for examination, the main aim should be to determine whether the tumor is an osteosarcoma, rather than what subtype it belongs to.

Poorly Differentiated Osteosarcoma

This primary bone tumor is produced by malignant cells that form at least small amounts of unequivocal osteoid and sometimes spicules of tumor bone. The malignant mesenchymal cells may vary in appearance from small cells resembling the reticular cells of bone marrow stroma to large, pleomorphic cells of undifferentiated sarcoma. Most are highly aggressive bone tumors that form lytic bone lesions. Pathological fracture may occur early in the clinical course.

Osteoblastic Osteosarcoma

Tumors of this subtype are formed by anaplastic osteoblasts and plump to spindle shaped osteogenic precursor cells (see fig. 5.23 A-D). Cells have hyperchromatic nuclei that are eccentrically positioned in dark-staining cytoplasm. Often the cells have angular borders. On the basis of the amount of tumor bone matrix that is produced by these tumors, they are further subcategorized as follows:

- Nonproductive osteoblastic osteosarcomas. These usually aggressive bone tumors form lytic bone lesions and tend to provoke little periosteal response. Pathological fracture may occur soon after onset of clinical signs.
- Moderately productive osteoblastic osteosarcoma. Mixed pattern of destruction and production characterizes the radiographic appearance of this subtype. Lytic areas may appear radiographically in areas that were radiodense a few days earlier because of replacement of a productive area by a less differentiated population of tumor cells that form little or no mineralized matrix (see fig. 5.23 D). In dogs, this is the most common subtype of osteosarcoma.
- Productive osteoblastic osteosarcoma. In this lesion, tumor cells produce abundant tumor matrix (see fig. 5.23 C) inside the bone organ as well as on its surface. Tumor bone formed on the cortical surface can be so regular in structure and arrangement, and the tumor cells so well differentiated, that the neoplastic tissue can microscopically mimic a reactive periosteal response.

Chondroblastic Osteosarcoma

Malignant mesenchymal cells in these tumors directly produces both osteoid and chondroid matrices. In most cases there is an intermingling of the bone and cartilage elements produced by the neoplastic cells (see fig. 5.18 B), but in a few lesions (see fig. 5.13) the two matrix patterns may be separate. In the latter case a biopsy taken from the cartilaginous part of the tumor would be given a diagnosis of chondrosarcoma. Examination of a radiograph of the tumor, however, would cast some doubt on the diagnosis since the tumor would most likely have a more aggressive, mixed pattern than would be usual for most chondrosarcomas.

Fibroblastic Osteosarcoma

These usually begin as lytic bone lesions, and about 50 percent will progress to the mixed pattern when the neoplastic spindle cells in this tumor increase their capacity to form mineralized bone matrix. In early lesions (see fig. 5.17 B) a spindle cell population resembling that of central fibrosarcoma will predominate, and areas of unequivocal bone formation by tumor cells may be difficult to find. Advanced lesions may have large areas of bone matrix formation by the spindle cell population. The amount and degree of mineralization of the spicules of neoplastic osteoid will determine the radiographic appearance of the tumor. In one study, the prognosis for dogs with this subtype of osteosarcoma was more favorable than for other forms.[7]

Telangiectatic Osteosarcoma

This tumor subtype characteristically produces an aggressive, osteolytic radiographic lesion, and the bloody, cystic lesions found on gross examination (see fig. 5.19 A) can not be distinguished from primary or metastatic hemangiosarcoma of bone. Microscopically, telangiectatic osteosarcoma can be differentiated from hemangiosarcoma by the presence of occasional spicules of osteoid among pleomorphic, malignant mesenchymal cells, although a careful search is often required to detect osteoid.[32] Also, the many small and large, blood filled spaces present throughout the tumor are lined by tumor cells, not endothelial cells, which are factor VIII positive (see fig. 5.19 B). Metastases of telangiectatic osteosarcomas generally resemble the primary tumor, containing many cystic spaces filled with blood. In human patients[2] and dogs,[18] this subtype is associated with a less favorable prognosis than all other forms of osteosarcoma.

Giant Cell Type Osteosarcoma

This variant usually produces an expansile, lytic bone lesion (see fig. 5.20 A). Microscopically, the tumor resembles nonproductive osteoblastic osteosarcoma except for large areas in which tumor giant cells predominate (see fig. 5.20B). The tumor must be differentiated from malignant giant cell tumor of bone. (p. 294).

Cytological Features

In general, cytology is less reliable than histology for assessment of mesenchymal tumors, but osteosarcomas can often be diagnosed with confidence on examination of fine needle aspiration or imprints prepared from tissue biopsy samples. Such preparations from osteosarcomas are usually more highly cellular than aspirates or imprints from soft tissue sarcomas, and the cells may have characteristic features of malignant osteoblasts. In many cases, the cytological features, together with clinical history and radiography, will be sufficient to allow a definitive diagnosis of osteosarcoma, but it is unwise to exclude a diagnosis of malignancy on the basis of cytology. Cytological preparations may not be representative of the lesion, and unless the sample is collected from lytic areas identified from radiographs, the tumor could easily be missed. Since most osteosarcomas originate from within the medullary cavity, shallow aspirates may be largely acellular or, at best, just contain reactive osteoblasts (fig. 5.26 A). It is worth

remembering that some productive subtypes of osteosarcoma with extensive tumor bone formation may not yield significant numbers of tumor cells to cytological preparations. Aspirates from telangiectatic osteosarcomas may be too heavily contaminated with blood to be of value. Furthermore, even in cases where a cytological diagnosis of osteosarcoma can be made, classification of the tumor into one of the subtypes listed above is not possible.

A highly cellular preparation (fig. 5.26 B) collected from a lesion with radiographic features of osteosarcoma should immediately raise concern unless the cells indicate inflammation. Malignant osteoblasts may be present individually or in clusters, sometimes closely associated with brightly eosinophilic strands or islands of osteoid.[33,34] They vary from round or oval to plump, fusiform cells and may vary markedly in size (fig. 5.26 C). The nucleus is often eccentric and the cytoplasm deeply basophilic, sometimes with a perinuclear Golgi such that the osteoblasts resemble plasma cells. The cytoplasm of some cells may contain variable numbers of small, clear, intracytoplasmic vacuoles and/or fine pink granules. Similar pink granules may also be present in tumor cells from chondrosarcomas or occasionally fibrosarcomas.[33,34] In anaplastic osteosarcomas there may be marked anisokaryosis, multiple large, irregularly shaped nucleoli, and a variable nuclear to cytoplasmic ratio. Mitotic figures are often common (fig. 5.26 B) and may be abnormal. On the other hand, well-differentiated osteosarcomas may consist largely of relatively uniform sized cells with many features of reactive osteoblasts. A similar population of reactive osteoblasts associated with strands of osteoid may be harvested from an early fracture callus, highlighting the importance of clinical history and knowledge of the radiographic appearance of the lesion. Unless the characteristics of malignancy are unequivocal, histological examination is recommended.

Growth and Metastasis

Central osteosarcoma is perhaps the most malignant group of tumors, at least in dogs, and the prognosis for all subtypes is very poor. Hematogenous metastasis to the lungs commonly occurs early in the disease, perhaps gaining access to the blood through the loose endothelial junctions of bone marrow sinusoids. Pulmonary metastases are detected radiographically in approximately 10 percent of canine appendicular and axial osteosarcomas at the time of initial diagnosis,[9,12] and it is likely that the actual percentage is much higher than this. In a long-term follow-up study of 162 dogs with appendicular osteosarcoma, treated by amputation alone,[6] 72.5 percent of the dogs died or were euthanatized because of problems related to metastases. It is likely that most dogs with osteosarcoma will develop metastases if their lives are prolonged by surgery or other forms of treatment.[15] In one study,[18] dogs with telangiectatic osteosarcoma had a 100 percent metastatic rate. The median survival time for dogs with appendicular skeletal osteosarcomas left untreated or treated with amputation

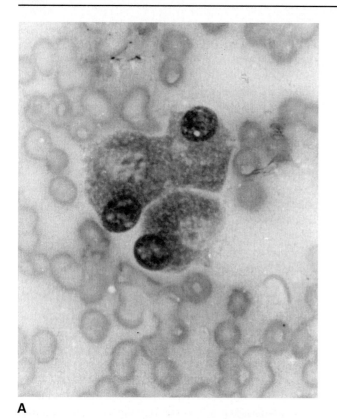

A

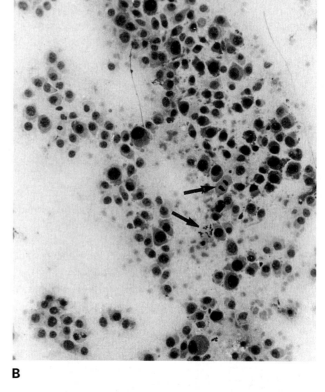

B

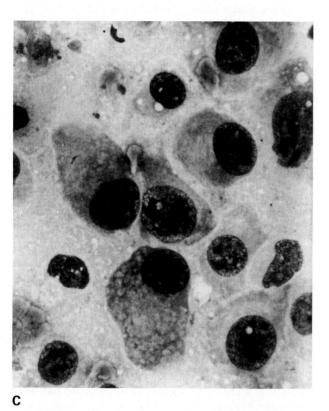

C

Fig. 5.26. Reactive and malignant osteoblasts in cytological preparations. **A.** Reactive osteoblasts with eccentric nuclei, abundant finely granular, basophilic cytoplasm, and a prominent Golgi zone reminescent of plasma cells. **B.** Scraping prepared from a core biopsy of an osteosarcoma. The sample is hypercellular, consisting of many round, oval, and occasionally spindle shaped cells showing moderate anisokaryosis. Many of the cells have an eccentric, hyperchromatic nucleus and a *plasmacytoid* appearance. Two mitotic figures (arrows) are present in this field. **C.** Higher power view of the same specimen showing malignant osteoblasts with hyperchromatic, eccentric nuclei and variable amounts of basophilic cytoplasm. Some cells have a well-defined Golgi area, and one cell has many intracytoplasmic vacuoles. These tumor cells are larger than the reactive osteoblasts shown in A, the two photographs being taken at the same magnification.

Although the lungs are easily the most common site for metastases of osteosarcoma, hematogenous spread to other organs, including the skeleton, also occurs.[6,15] Osseous metastases are reported in the vertebral column, ribs, long bones, pelvis, and sternum,[6] and their incidence may be underestimated because of the infrequency with which the skeleton is thoroughly examined radiographically or at necropsy. Osteosarcomas seldom spread to regional lymph nodes[15] but may be found in about 5 percent of dogs with large tumors extending into adjacent soft tissues.[26]

The incidence of metastasis in cats with osteosarcoma is considerably less than in dogs. In one study,[13] metastases were detected in 4 of 11 cats with osteosarcoma. The lungs were involved in three of the cats, the fourth having metastases only in the liver. In another study involving 22 cats,[16] no metastases were found at the time of initial diagnosis, and pulmonary metastases were detected in only one cat

alone is only 14 to 19 weeks.[3,6,15] Survival time is only marginally better (22 weeks) in dogs with osteosarcomas of the axial skeleton,[9] although those with osteosarcomas of the mandible[18,35] or osteoblastic tumors of paranasal sinuses and calvarium[12] generally have a better prognosis.

after amputation. Cats with osteosarcoma therefore have a more favorable prognosis than dogs. A median survival time of 49.2 months has been observed in cats with appendicular osteosarcoma following treatment by amputation, but the number of animals in the study was relatively small.[16]

REFERENCES

1. Slayter, M.V., Boosinger, T.R., Pool, R.R., DÑmmrich, K., Misdorp, W., and Larsen, S. (1994) *Histological Classification of Bone and Joint Tumors of Domestic Animals.* World Health Organization. 2nd series, vol. 1. Armed Forces Institute of Pathology, American Registry of Pathology, Washington D.C.

2. Unni, K.K. (1996) Osteosarcoma. In *Dahlin's Bone Tumors. General Aspects and Data on 11,087 Cases,* 5th ed. Ch. 11. Lippincott-Raven, Philadelphia, pp. 143–183.

3. Brodey, R.S., and Riser, W.H. (1969) Canine osteosarcoma: A clinico-pathologic study of 194 cases. *Clin Orthop* 62:54–64.

4. Turrel, J.M., and Pool, R.R. (1982) Primary bone tumors in the cat: a retrospective study of 15 cats and a literature review. *Vet Radiol* 23:152–166.

5. Wolke, R.E., and Nielsen, S.W. (1966) Site incidence of canine osteosarcoma. *J Small Anim Pract* 7:484–492.

6. Spodnick, G.J., Berg, J., Rand, W.M., et al. (1992) Prognosis for dogs with appendicular osteosarcoma treated by amputation alone: 162 cases (1978–1988). *J Amer Vet Med Assoc* 200:995–999.

7. Misdorp, W., and Hart, A.A.M. (1979) Some prognositic and epidemilogic factors in canine osteosarcoma. *J Natl Cancer Inst* 62:537–545.

8. Morgan, J.P., Ackerman, N., Bailey, C.S., and Pool, R.R. (1980) Vertebral tumors in the dog: A clinical, radiologic, and pathologic study of 61 primary and secondary lesions. *Vet Radiol* 21:197–212.

9. Heyman, S.J., Diefenderfer, D.L., Goldschmidt, M.H., and Newton, C.D. (1992) Canine axial skeletal osteosarcoma. A retrospective study of 116 cases (1986–1989). *Vet Surg* 21:304–310.

10. Tjalma, R.A. (1966) Canine bone sarcoma: Estimation of relative risk as a function of body size. *J Natl Cancer Inst* 36:1137–1150.

11. Jacobson, S.A. (1971) *The Comparative Pathology of the Tumors of Bone.* Charles C. Thomas, Springfield, IL.

12. Ling, G.V., Morgan, J.P., and Pool, R.R. (1974) Primary bone tumors in the dog: A combined clinical, radiographic, and histologic approach to early diagnosis. *J Amer Vet Med Assoc* 165:55–67.

13. Engle, G.C., and Brodey, R.S. (1969) A retrospective study of 395 feline neoplasms. *J Amer Hosp Assoc* 5:21–31.

14. Liu, S.K., and Dorfman, H.D. (1974) The cartilage analogue of fibromatosis (juvenile aponeurotic fibroma) in dogs. *Vet Pathol* 11:60–67.

15. Brodey, R.S., Sauer, R.M., and Medway, W. (1963) Canine bone neoplasms. *J Amer Vet Med Assoc* 143:471–495.

16. Bitetto, W.V., Patnaik, A.K., Schrader, S.C., and Mooney, S.C. (1987) Osteosarcoma in cats: 22 cases (1974–1984). *J Amer Vet Med Assoc* 190:91–93.

17. Spodnick, G.J., Berg, J., Rand, W.M., et al. (1992) Prognosis for dogs with appendicular osteosarcoma treated by amputation alone: 162 cases (1978–1988). *J Amer Vet Med Assoc* 200:995–999.

18. Hammer, A.S., Weeren, F.R., Weisbrode, S.E., and Padgett, S.L. (1995) Prognostic factors in dogs with osteosarcomas of the flat or irregular bones. *J Amer Anim Hosp Assoc* 31:321–326.

19. Ehrhart, N., Dernell, W.S., Hoffmann, W.E., Weigel, R.M., Powers, B.E., and Winthrow, S.J. (1998) Prognostic importance of alkaline phosphatase activity in serum from dogs with appendicular osteosarcoma: 75 cases (1990–1996). *J Amer Vet Med Assoc* 213:1002–1009.

20. Riser, W.H., Brodey, R.S., and Biery, D.N. (1972) Bone infarctions associated with malignant bone tumors in dogs. *J Amer Vet Med Assoc* 160:411–421.

21. Dubielzig, R.R., Biery, D.N., and Brodey, R.S. (1981) Bone sarcomas associated with multifocal medullary bone infarction in dogs. *J Amer Vet Med Assoc* 179:64–68.

22. Stevenson, S., Hohn, R.B., Pohler, O.E.M., Fetter, A.W., Olmstead, M.L., and Wind, A.P. (1982) Fracture-associated sarcoma in the dog. *J Amer Vet Med Assoc* 180:1189–1196.

23. Gamblin, R.M., Straw, R.C., Powers, B.E., Park, R.D., Bunge, M.M., and Withrow, S.J. (1993) Primary osteosarcoma distal to the antebrachiocarpal and tarsocrural joints in nine dogs (1980–1992). *J Amer Anim Hosp Assoc* 31:86–91.

24. Fry, P.D., and Jukes, H.F. (1995) Fracture association sarcoma in the cat. *J Small Anim Pract* 36:124–126.

25. Morgan, J.P. (1974) Systemic radiographic interpretation of skeletal diseases in small animals. *Vet Clin N Amer* 4:611–625.

26. Pool, R.R. (1990) Tumors of bone and cartilage. In Moulton, J.E. (ed.), *Tumors in Domestic Animals,* 3rd ed. University of California Press, Berkeley.

27. Enneking, W.F., and Kagan, A. (1975) "Skip" metastases in osteosarcoma. *Cancer* 36:2192–2205.

28. Head, K.W. (1990) Glandular tumors of the intestine. In Moulton, J.E. (ed.), *Tumors in Domestic Animals,* 3rd ed. University of California Press, Berkeley.

29. Chénier, S., and Doré, M. (1999) Oral malignant melanoma with osteoid formation in a dog. *Vet Pathol* 36:74–76.

30. Schwamm, H.A., and Millward, C.L. (1995) *Histologic Differential Diagnosis of Skeletal Lesions.* Igaku-Shoin, New York.

31. Resnick, D., Kyriakos, M., and Greenway, G.G. (1994) Tumors and tumor-like lesions of bone: Imaging and pathology of specific lesions. In Resnick, D. (ed.), *Diagnosis of Bone and Joint Disorders,* 3rd ed. Vol. 6, ch. 83. W.B. Saunders, Philadelphia, pp. 3628–3938.

32. Gleiser, C.A., Raulston, G.L., Jardine, J.H., Carpenter, R.H., and Gray, K.N. (1981) Telangiectatic osteosarcoma in the dog. *Vet Pathol* 18:396–398.

33. Mahaffey, E.A. (1999) Cytology of the musculoskeletal system. In Cowell, R.L., Tyler, R.D., and Meinkoth, J.H. (eds.), *Diagnostic Cytology of the Dog and Cat,* 2nd ed. Ch. 10. Mosby, St. Louis, MO, pp. 120–124.

34. Baker, R., and Lumsden, J.H. (1999) *Color Atlas of Cytology of the Dog and Cat,* Mosby, St. Louis.

35. Straw, R.C., Powers, B.E., Klausner, J., Henderson, R.A., Morrison, W.B., McCaw, D.L., Harvey, H.J., Jacobs, R.M., and Berg, R.J. (1996) Canine mandibular osteosarcoma: 51 cases (1980–1992). *J Amer Anim Hosp Assoc* 32:257–262.

Chondrosarcoma

Classification

A chondrosarcoma is a malignant neoplasm in which tumor cells produce varying amounts of neoplastic chondroid and fibrillar matrix but not osteoid. Although bone may be present in the tumor, the bone forms by endochondral ossification of tumor cartilage, rather than being produced by the malignant mesenchymal cells. A primary chondrosarcoma arises either de novo within a bone organ (central or medullary chondrosarcoma) or from the periosteum (peripheral chondrosarcoma). In animals most chondrosarcomas are considered primary bone tumors of medullary origin, and primary chondrosarcomas of periosteal origin are rare in animals (see Sarcomas of the Periosteum). Secondary chondrosarcomas of bone, by contrast, arise by malignant change in an antecedent lesion of bone (note that the term *secondary tumor* is sometimes used to indicate a metastatic tumor of bone). It has not yet been determined if malignant transformation of chondroma occurs in animals, and if so, what percentage of medullary chondrosarcomas have their origin in such lesions. However, secondary chondrosarcomas of the periosteum occasionally arise by malignant change in osteochondromas of animals (see Osteochondroma).

Incidence, Age, Breed, and Sex

Chondrosarcoma is reported most frequently in the dog,[1-3] where it accounts for approximately 10 percent of primary tumors of bones and is second only to osteosarcoma in incidence.[4] In most other domestic species, chondrosarcoma is a relatively rare tumor,[5] and too few cases are reported to provide reliable information on its clinicopathological features. In sheep, chondrosarcoma is considered to occur more frequently than osteosarcoma,[6] but it remains a rare tumor in this species.

In dogs, chondrosarcoma occurs most often in medium to large breeds weighing 20 to 40 kg,[3] particularly boxers, German shepherds, golden retrievers, and various mixed breeds, but is rare in small and giant breeds.[1-3] Although a broad age range is reported, the tumor is most common in middle-aged to older dogs, the mean age of affected animals varying from 5.9 to 8.7 years.[1-3] No sex predilection is recognized. There is less data on the age incidence of chondrosarcoma in cats, but in one review,[7] a mean age of 8.8 years (range 2 to 15 years) is reported. Most cases of chondrosarcoma in sheep are recognized in aged ewes, most likely reflecting the population distribution of farmed animals rather than a true sex prevalence.[6]

Sites

In all species, chondrosarcomas involve flat bones more often than long bones. In one canine study,[1] 69 percent of the 35 cases described involved the ribs, turbinates, or pelvis, although nasal chondrosarcomas were not detected in boxers. In another large retrospective study,[3] 61 percent of chondrosarcomas were in flat bones, particularly the nasal cavity and ribs. Chondrosarcomas may also occur in the appendicular skeleton of dogs,[3] including, but not restricted to, sites of predilection for osteosarcomas. Chondrosarcomas in cats are reported in both flat bones (especially the scapula) and long bones,[7-9] but in this species the published data is inadequate to draw reliable conclusions regarding site predilection. In sheep, the cartilages of the sternocostal complex were the most common site for chondrosarcoma, followed by the scapula and tuber coxae.[6] In cattle and horses, chondrosarcomas are found most often on flat bones, but long bones are occasionally affected.[5,6]

Gross Morphology

Chondrosarcomas typically form large masses when allowed to pursue a full clinical course without surgical intervention. Most chondrosarcomas have a convoluted surface with relatively distinct borders. On cut section tumor tissue of many chondrosarcomas will resemble hya-

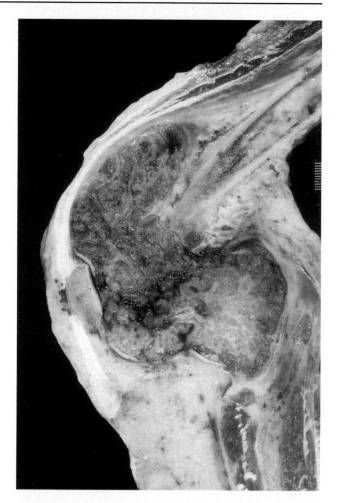

Fig. 5.27. Chondrosarcoma. Central chondrosarcoma of the distal femur in a dog. Extensive areas resembling hyaline cartilage are visible grossly. The tumor has virtually replaced the distal femur and is extending into adjacent tissues and encroaching on the joint space. (Photograph courtesy of K. Keel.)

line cartilage (fig. 5.27) . The tumor mass is composed of multiple small nodules of soft to moderately firm tissue that ranges from translucent to a white, grayish white, or bluish white. Often there are areas in the central region of the tumor that are gray to rust colored and have a slimy consistency. This mucoid character is a particular characteristic of some nasal chondrosarcomas. Irregular, chalky white foci of calcified tumor matrix are sometimes found. In some chondrosarcomas the tumor tissue is pale ivory, very firm, and tough, resembling fibrocartilage more than hyaline cartilage.

Nasal chondrosarcomas tend to destroy turbinates and fill the nasal cavity (see fig. 5.28 A,B,C) and may either spread into adjacent sinuses or penetrate overlying bone and infiltrate adjacent soft tissues.[1] Central chondrosarcomas of long bones usually demonstrate symmetric expansile growth until the tumor penetrates the cortex and supporting layers of reactive bone (fig. 5.27). The tumor may extend into the parosteal connective tissues through a rather small embrasure in the cortical surface. During cortical destruction, the periosteum may lay down a smoothly contoured periosteal collar of reactive bone several millimeters thick; this collar may eventually be penetrated at multiple sites by tumor tissue. Reactive bone can be very dense and is ivory colored. The tumor may extend for a variable distance through the medullary cavity of the diaphysis. In some cases, the limit of tumor invasion is marked by a transverse ridge of reactive bone that can be observed on clinical radiographs, but more often the tumor extends several centimeters beyond the limits observed in the radiograph. Chondrosarcomas of flat bones often demonstrate an eccentric manner of growth with costal and pelvic tumor masses, tending to protrude into body cavities, whereas scapular tumors are directed primarily in a dorsolateral direction. The central and basal areas of these tumors may contain bony tissue.

Clinical Characteristics

Clinical signs vary with the site of skeletal involvement. Tumors of the nasal cavity cause sneezing, unilateral and sometimes bilateral purulent to bloody discharges, and nasal obstruction, sometimes followed by bone destruction. Bone deformity may occur but is uncommon. Chondrosarcomas of the cranium may produce a palpable mass in the absence of neurologic signs, but as with tumors of the vertebrae, continuous growth of the tumor often leads to compression of nervous tissue and to development of attendant clinical signs. Rib tumors tend to cause the animal little pain unless there is a pathological fracture. These tumors show eccentric growth, especially in dogs, so that the major tumor mass projects into the thorax to produce some degree of pulmonary atelectasis. At times, pelvic tumors may be so large that they compress normal structures in the pelvic inlet. Most tumors in this location produce hind limb lameness. Chondrosarcomas of limbs are usually painful and cause lameness.

The duration of clinical signs may be relatively short in some cases of highly malignant chondrosarcoma, but many animals with chondrosarcoma survive for several months, with a few living for more than 2 years.[5] One cat with chondrosarcoma had signs for at least 6 years.[9] For dogs with primary chondrosarcoma of bone, the mean and median duration of clinical signs was 18 and 10 weeks, respectively.[1]

Surgical extirpation of chondrosarcomas located in accessible sites such as ribs or limbs can be curative,[1,3] but chondrosarcomas involving the nasal cavity tend to recur locally following surgery, and they usually demonstrate an increasingly malignant behavior with each clinical recurrence.

Radiographic Appearance

Chondrosarcomas present a variety of radiographic appearances (fig. 5.28A). Even in the dog, where more of these tumors have been examined than in any other domestic species, it is often impossible to differentiate between

chondrosarcoma and osteosarcoma on the basis of radiographic and clinical findings.[1] A biopsy is essential for establishing a definitive diagnosis. The earliest radiographic changes of cortical destruction and periosteal response are also initial features of primary osteosarcoma and fibrosarcoma of bone.[10] Tumors may be radiopaque or mostly radiolucent with flecks, irregular streaks, and floc-

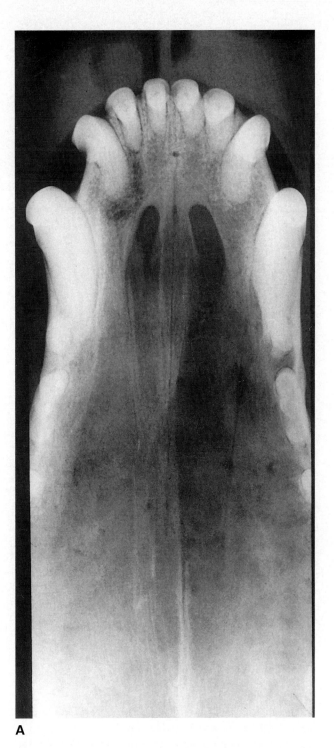

A

Fig. 5.28. **A.** Radiograph of the nasal cavity of the dog shown in B. The normal turbinate pattern is replaced by tumor tissue that has a radiodensity similar to soft tissue. (continued)

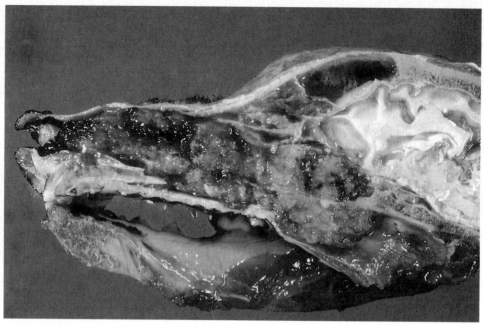

B

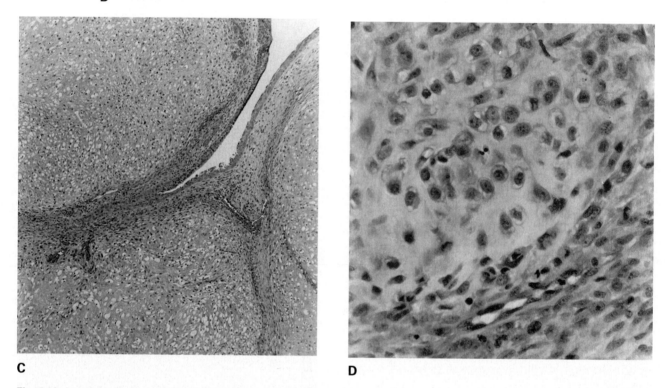

C   D

Fig. 5.28. (continued) **B.** Saggital section through the skull of the dog shown in A. Contiguous and coalescing nodules of tumor tissue resembling hyaline cartilage fill the nasal cavity and extend into the nasopharynx. The tumor is eroding into the presphenoid bone, cribriform plate and hard palate. **C.** Nasal chondrosarcoma from same dog has nodules of relatively well differentiated hyaline cartilage beneath the nasal mucosa and bulging into the attenuated lumen of the nasal cavity. **D.** Higher magnification of the same tumor showing an area of chondroid differentiation closely associated with densely packed spindle shaped stromal cells. This is a feature of mesenchymal chondrosarcomas, which appear to occur predominantly in the sinonasal region of dogs. (continued)

culent areas of increased radiodensity corresponding to sites of calcification and ossification.

In dogs, chondrosarcomas of ribs are located near the costochondral junction. They tend to be large, radiopaque masses with varying amounts of calcification and ossifica-

tion. Tumors of the nasal cavity displace the nasal septum and replace the normal turbinate pattern with an amorphous pattern having a radiodensity similar to that of soft tissue (fig. 5.28 B). Vertebral tumors tend to be small and produce osteolytic lesions. Scapular tumors are often large

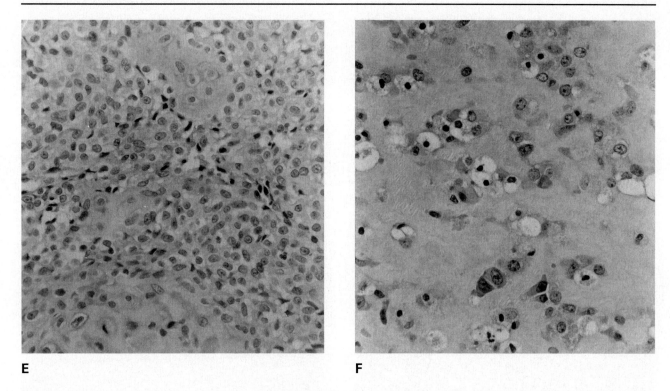

E

F

Fig. 5.28. (continued)   **E.** Nasal carcinoma from a cat with islands of hyaline cartilage forming within sheets of poorly differentiated mesenchymal cells. **F.** Chondrosarcoma from the metatarsus of a cow. Chondrocytes of various sizes and shapes are irregularly dispersed within an abundant chondroid matrix. Lacunae often contain two or more cells, some of which have large nuclei and prominent nucleoli.

bulky masses that are slightly more radiodense than adjacent soft tissue. Like rib tumors, they sometimes elicit bone proliferation along the cortical surface. Chondrosarcomas of long bones tend to be smaller and less productive than osteosarcomas. They may be very osteolytic and destroy the bony architecture of the metaphyseal spongiosa and cortex, while neither producing a radiodense matrix nor provoking a marked periosteal response.

Histological Features

Although a definitive diagnosis of chondrosarcoma requires histological examination of tumor tissue, the diagnosis is not always straightforward. Microscopically, well-differentiated chondrosarcomas closely resemble benign tumors of cartilage.[11,12] Fortunately for the veterinary pathologist, most chondrosarcomas in animals are well advanced before the owner seeks veterinary advice and biopsy samples are collected. Figures 5.28 C-F and 5.29 A,B illustrate many of the cellular features of chondrosarcoma discussed in this section. Usually, there is ample clinical and radiographic evidence of neoplasia, and the pathologist is only asked to indicate the type of neoplasm present. The tumor by this time usually has the microscopic features of a highly malignant tumor of cartilage. Since there are so few benign cartilage tumors in animals, and fewer yet that undergo malignant transformation to chondrosarcoma, the veterinary pathologist seldom has the task of distinguishing between a benign tumor and a well differentiated malignant tumor of cartilage. More

likely, the challenge is to decide whether a malignant mesenchymal tumor involving bone is a chondrosarcoma, osteosarcoma, or some other sarcoma. Such a decision is important, because of the differences in prognosis.

The microscopic features distinguishing benign from malignant cartilage tumors are fairly well established in human medicine. These features were arrived at, in part, by retrospective studies that followed the evolution of early cartilaginous lesions with subtle histological indications of malignant change into overt chondrosarcomas.[13] Such studies have not been conducted in animals. As a result, the histological diagnosis of chondrosarcoma in animals is generally based on criteria established for humans.[1,6]

The microscopic diagnosis of chondrosarcoma should be made only on viable tumor tissue in areas that are neither heavily calcified nor ossified. The tumor should be judged on the most malignant area present since the entire tumor will eventually resemble the tissue of this limited area. A cartilage tumor is considered to be malignant when the following features are found, even in small scattered areas: numerous cells with plump nuclei, more than an occasional cell with two plump nuclei, and the presence of large cartilage cells with single or multiple nuclei and clumps of heterochromatin. Other cellular features of malignancy, including prominent nucleoli and irregularly shaped nuclei also support a diagnosis of chondrosarcoma. Mitotic figures are seldom present in well-differentiated chondrosarcomas, and it has been suggested that even a single mitotic figure strongly supports a diagnosis of

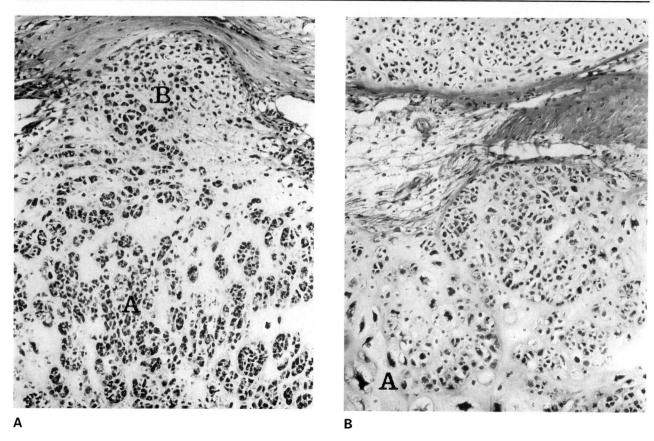

Fig. 5.29. Central chondrosarcoma of bone. **A.** Low grade chondrosarcoma has numerous disorganized, hypercellular chondrones containing hyperchromatic chondrocytes that vary little in size *(A)*; proliferative area compressing fibrous capsule *(B)*. **B.** More clearly malignant area from same tumor showing greater variation in cell size and hyperchromasia of nuclei; abnormal giant chondrocytes *(A)*.

malignancy in this tumor.[1] In poorly-differentiated, more malignant chondrosarcomas, mitotic figures may be relatively common.

These criteria for malignancy in cartilage tumors have been applied to primary cartilage neoplasms of bone in sheep and dogs. In a study of 20 chondrosarcomas of sheep, it was reported that in 10 cases there was good correlation between the gross indicators of malignancy (local invasion and metastatic disease) and microscopic features of malignancy.[6] In the remaining 10, the tumors were large, solitary, and well-circumscribed lesions, but met the microscopic criteria of chondrosarcoma.

In one study of chondrosarcomas in dogs, 35 tumors were examined microscopically and assigned a grade of histological malignancy.[1] There were nine Grade I chondrosarcomas composed of rather uniform tumor cells, often with double nuclei but lacking mitotic figures. No metastatic disease occurred in this grade. In only a few instances, the pathologist found some difficulty in determining if a tumor was chondrosarcoma or chondroma. Most neoplasms (22) were Grade II chondrosarcomas. These tumors were composed of pleomorphic cartilage cells, but no undifferentiated areas were present. Mitotic figures occurred in moderate numbers. Three of the neoplasms produced metastatic disease. Only four tumors were classified as Grade III chondrosarcomas. These contained areas of undifferentiated sarcoma. Nuclear pleomorphism was marked, and mitotic figures were numerous. One of the Grade III tumors produced pulmonary metastases. The degree of differentiation of chondrosarcoma is an important indicator of prognosis in humans[11] and may prove to be of similar value in animal chondrosarcomas as more cases are studied.

There is marked variation in cell density between different chondrosarcomas and, to a lesser extent, within an individual neoplasm. Tumor cells typically display a variation in size and shape in a malignant cartilage tumor. Cells may mimic the mesenchymal precursors of cartilage, embryonic cartilage of the developing bone model, or cells of mature hyaline cartilage. At times tumor cells acquire the spindle cell morphology of chondroblasts located in the chondrogenic layer of the fetal perichondrium, a feature also seen in some osteosarcomas and fibrosarcomas of bone. These tumors are referred to as *mesenchymal chondrosarcomas,* and are characterized by a transition between undifferentiated mesenchymal cells and a range of variously differentiated chondroid components.[14] Although rare in humans, mesenchymal chondrosarcomas were reported to comprise 24 of 34 chondrosarcomas of the sinonasal region of dogs in one study.[15] No distant

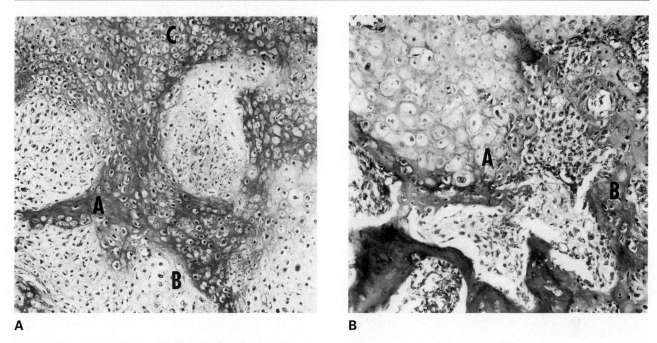

A   B

Fig. 5.30. Changes in the matrix of a chondrosarcoma. **A.** Hyalinized chondroid matrix *(A)* in a chondrosarcoma may be mistaken for osteoid. However, observe that the trabecular structures arise within a sheet of chondroid tissue and are not lined by osteoblasts *(B)*. Cells within these trabeculae resemble chondrocytes and not osteocytes *(C)*. **B.** Endochondral ossification occurs in many lower grade chondrosarcomas with replacement of "neoplastic cartilage" *(A)* by nonneoplastic bone tissue *(B)*.

metastases were found in any of the dogs with this form of chondrosarcoma, but there was extensive destruction and replacement of nasofrontal tissue.[15] The stromal cells in these tumors are generally small, densely packed and predominantly either spindle-shaped or round (fig. 5.28 C,D). The chondroid elements vary in amount and degree of differentiation and may be either eosinophilic or basophilic.[15]

The amount or nature of the matrix in chondrosarcomas appears to provide little indication of prognosis. However, when the malignant cartilage cells produce matrix that secondarily becomes fibrillar and hyalinized, resembling osteoid (fig. 5.30 A), or when chondroid matrix undergoes resorption and endochondral ossification (fig. 5.30 B), the pathologist may find it extremely difficult to decide between a diagnosis of chondrosarcoma and osteosarcoma. The decision is especially difficult, if not impossible, when only a small amount of tissue is available for examination. According to one report,[1] the distinction between chondrosarcoma and osteosarcoma may be assisted by the use of alcian blue stained sections. In chondrosarcoma, the osteoid, which forms indirectly in a mucochondroid matrix, stains pale blue and is surrounded by deeply blue–staining material. In osteosarcoma, this deep blue matrix does not surround the pale-staining osteoid.[1] Differentiation between chondrosarcoma and osteosarcoma is often a problem in large tumors of the ribs of dogs in which a considerable amount of cartilage and bone is produced. While these tumors have areas within them that microscopically resemble osteosarcoma, their biological behavior is more compatible with chondrosarcoma.

In making a microscopic diagnosis of chondrosarcoma, the pathologist should always determine if the morphological diagnosis is compatible with the clinical and radiographic findings. It is important to remember that some of the cytological features of malignancy in chondrosarcoma may be found in chondroblastic osteosarcomas, actively growing or traumatized osteochondromas, and a variety of nonmalignant responses of the periosteum and synovium to injury. Atypical chondrocytes can be found in a callus, some exostoses, traumatized ligament insertions, and in sites of chondro-osseous metaplasia in the linings of joints, tendon sheaths, and bursae. These present diagnostic problems primarily when the results of the clinical and radiographic studies are unavailable or inadequate, and when the pathologist is presented with a tissue specimen which can not be oriented to the lesion.

Cytological Findings

Fine needle aspiration biopsies from chondrosarcomas usually contain fewer cells than osteosarcomas, but on low power examination, lakes of bright pink chondroid matrix may be evident.[16] The tumor cells may be inconspicuous due to the abundant matrix. When visualized they are similar to those from osteosarcomas, varying from round to fusiform and possessing large, hyperchromatic nuclei and basophilic cytoplasm that sometimes contains fine pink granules (fig. 5.31). Anisokaryosis is generally a prominent feature, and there may be multinucleate tumor cells. Osteoclasts may also be present, reflecting tumor related osteolysis.

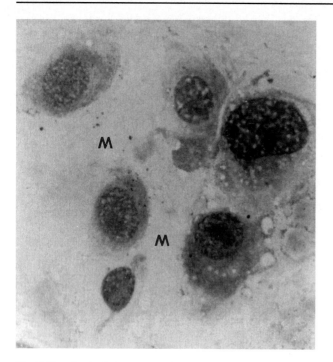

Fig. 5.31. Cytological preparation from a chondrosarcoma. The tumor cells vary from circular or oval to spindle shaped and possess large, hyperchromatic nuclei with prominent nucleoli. There is marked anisokaryosis and variation in the nucleus:cytoplasmic ratio. Some cells contain fine, metachromatic, intracytoplasmic granules, and there is abundant, faintly eosinophilic, extracellular matrix *(M)*. Typically there is more matrix than cells in cytological preparations of tumors of cartilage.

Although a presumptive diagnosis of chondrosarcoma may be possible in cytologic specimens, confirmation requires histopathology. Malignant chondroblasts and osteoblasts have too many features in common to allow reliable differentiation cytologically, and some osteosarcomas have extensive chondroid matrix. Furthermore, the possibility of malignancy can not be excluded following examination of cytologic specimens, as the samples may not adequately represent the lesion. The same also applies to tissue biopsies submitted for histopathology.

Growth and Metastasis

Chondrosarcoma in the dog,[1,2] cat,[7] and sheep[6] tends to grow more slowly, pursue a longer clinical course, and develop hematogenous metastasis later and with much less frequency than osteosarcoma. This is probably true for the other domestic species, but so few chondrosarcomas have been reported that little is known of their clinicopathological features.

Metastasis, when it does occur, is usually to the lungs, but distant organs such as the kidney, liver, heart, and skeleton may also be affected. The metastatic rate in dogs with chondrosarcoma is approximately 20 percent,[1-3] although chondrosarcomas of the sinonasal region in dogs appear to metastasize less frequently than those arising at other sites.[15] Local invasion is common, as is recurrence

following surgery, although removal of chondrosarcomas in accessible sites (such as the ribs) or amputation of an affected limb is curative more often than for osteosarcoma.

Fibrosarcoma

Classification

A central (medullary) fibrosarcoma of bone is a malignant neoplasm of fibrous connective tissue originating from stromal elements in the medullary cavity. Tumor cells produce varying amounts of collagenous matrix but no neoplastic bone or cartilage. This tumor must be differentiated from peripheral fibrosarcomas of bone and fibroblastic osteosarcomas of low osteogenic potential.

Incidence, Age, Breed, and Sex

The real incidence of central fibrosarcoma of bone in animals is undetermined, but it is seen less often than periosteal fibrosarcoma. Hemangiosarcoma and fibrosarcoma (peripheral and central) of bone together account for approximately 7 percent of the primary bone sarcomas of the dog. Central fibrosarcomas of bones are seen primarily in mature (1.5 to 12 years) male dogs of large and medium breeds.[4,5,10] They are rarely reported in other domestic animals.[5]

Clinical Characteristics

Central fibrosarcomas of bone fall into two general groups. The most common tumors produce bone destruction over a period of several months to a year and are generally slower to metastasize than primary osteosarcomas of bone. Amputation may be curative, but recurrence at the amputation stump can occur.[4] Less often, the pathologist will encounter aggressive, highly anaplastic fibrosarcomas that cause rapid and massive destruction of the affected bone. Evidence of metastatic disease is not invariably present at necropsy of these animals.

Sites

Too few cases are recorded in the veterinary literature to provide a skeletal pattern of site predilection for the tumor. In dogs, the metaphyses of long bones appear to be the most commonly affected skeletal sites for central fibrosarcomas,[4,5,10] but these tumors have also been reported in the mandible and the vertebral column.[5,17] This is in contrast to periosteal fibrosarcomas, which occur most commonly on bones of the skull (see below, this chapter).

Gross Morphology

In early or less aggressive lesions, the metaphyseal spongiosa may remain partially intact, and grayish white fibrous tissue fills the marrow spaces. In more aggressive tumors the bone is destroyed and replaced by soft to firm tumor tissue (fig. 5.32 A).[18] Destruction of the subchondral bone leads to extension of the neoplasm into the joint cav-

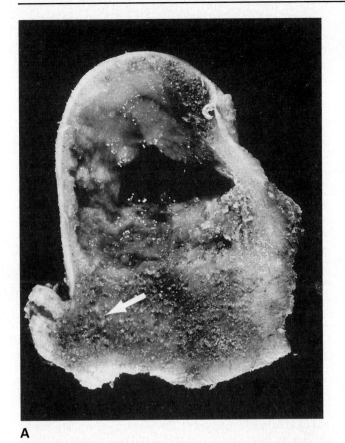

A

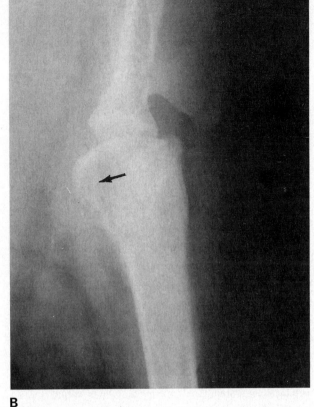

B

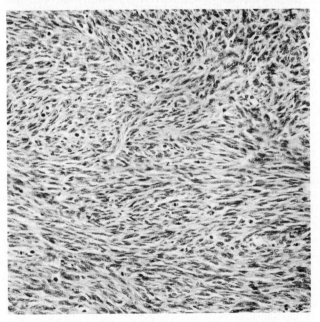

C

Fig. 5.32.   Central fibrosarcoma of bone. **A.** Pale, soft to firm tissue has replaced most of the spongiosa of the proximal humerus, undermined the subchondral bone, and infiltrated the marrow spaces of the remaining spongiosa (arrow). **B.** Radiograph of same humerus showing an osteolytic pattern (arrow). **C.** Anaplastic sarcoma of bone, probably a central fibrosarcoma of bone.

ity through fractures in the unsupported articular cartilage. Tumor tissue may also invade the fibrous layer of the joint capsule and involve the next bone without involving the joint cavity. The tumor is partially restrained from invasion of adjacent soft tissues by the fibrous periosteum. A bony periosteal response, if present, is usually mild and tends to be evenly contoured. Soft tissue swelling, however, may be marked.

Radiographic Appearance

Early lesions of fibrosarcoma produce the radiographic changes of bone lysis and cortical destruction found in primary osteosarcomas and chondrosarcomas of bone.[10,18] In many cases it may be impossible on the basis of radiographic appearance alone to differentiate between central fibrosarcoma of bone and one of several other bone tumors, including poorly differentiated osteosarcoma, nonproductive osteoblastic osteosarcoma, anaplastic chondrosarcoma, and hemangiosarcoma, since all of these tumors tend to produce a lytic radiographic lesion. Sequential radiographs of the lesion may be of diagnostic value because fibrosarcomas of bone, although they are primarily destructive (fig 5.32 B), usually progress more slowly than osteosarcomas or other highly malignant bone tumors.

Histological and Cytological Features

Most central fibrosarcomas of dogs have the moderately to well differentiated appearance of fibrosarcomas in soft tissue. In some fibrosarcomas the pathologist will encounter focal areas of dense collagen that closely resemble osteoid. In these instances, the distinction from fibroblastic osteosarcoma may be arbitrary if the decision is based solely on microscopic interpretation of a small biopsy specimen; the pathologist should therefore resist any temptation to diagnose primary fibrosarcoma of bone unless a significant quantity of tumor tissue is available for examination. In one study,[19] 6 of 11 tumors originally diagnosed as skeletal fibrosarcoma were reclassified as osteosarcoma following reexamination. Because of the poorer prognosis of the latter tumor, an accurate diagnosis carries considerable clinical relevance. Less commonly, fibrosarcomas are more anaplastic, highly cellular tumors composed of large, plump spindle cells with large hyperchromatic nuclei (fig. 5.32 C). Mitotic figures are numerous. At times, it may be impossible to distinguish these highly malignant tumors from other anaplastic sarcomas, including rhabdomyosarcomas and highly anaplastic osteosarcomas of low osteoblastic potential. In such instances, immunocytochemistry may be of value.

Histological grading of primary skeletal fibrosarcomas is considered a useful indicator of prognosis in human patients,[9] and there are indications that the same applies in dogs,[18] but the tumor is uncommon in this species, and the number of cases studied to date is small.

Cytological preparations are of limited value in diagnosing fibrosarcomas of bone. Fine needle aspiration biopsies may contain small to moderate numbers of plump spindle cells showing features suggestive of malignancy, but similar features may also be present during early fracture calluses and in granulation tissue. Scrapings will generally contain a greater number of cells, but differentiation from benign osseous lesions may still be difficult. Even in cases where there are convincing features of malignancy, the possibility of fibroblastic osteosarcoma can not be excluded on the basis of cytology.

Growth and Metastasis

Most central fibrosarcomas of animal bone tend to cause bone lysis, with local extension into soft tissue following destruction of the cortex. Well-differentiated fibrosarcomas usually do not produce metastatic disease, even when present for several months, and animals with these neoplasms are good candidates for ablative surgery. Less well-differentiated fibrosarcomas may, in time, produce hematogenous metastasis. Highly anaplastic fibrosarcomas tend to pursue a rapid clinical course with respect to the site of local bone involvement. Often, dogs with highly malignant fibrosarcomas are destroyed because of the poor prognosis that is given for all anaplastic sarcomas of bone, but at necropsy, metastatic disease is not invariably present. Amputation should be considered for highly malignant fibrosarcomas until statistical evidence is present that the survival rate following surgery is unacceptably low.

Hemangiosarcoma

Classification

Primary hemangiosarcoma (angiosarcoma) of bone is a malignant neoplasm arising from vascular endothelium within a bone organ.

Incidence, Age, Breed, and Sex

This is a relatively rare primary bone tumor in animals. It is seen mostly in dogs,[4,5,10,17,20] but it also has been found in horses and cattle.[5] Primary hemangiosarcoma of bone is slightly less common than primary fibrosarcoma of bone (peripheral and central), and together these two neoplasms constitute approximately 7 percent of the primary bone sarcomas of the dog. In one survey of 152 primary bone sarcomas in dogs, there were four hemangiosarcomas.[4]

A broad age range (2 to 16 years) is reported,[20,21] with a median age of 6 years in one study,[20] although not all hemangiosarcomas in this study were of primary skeletal origin. The tumor is found in large and medium-sized breeds, with boxers, German shepherds and Great Danes most commonly affected.[20] The sexes were equally represented in one study,[10] and a male to female ratio of 1.6:1 was reported in another.[20]

Clinical Characteristics

The tumor behaves like most aggressive primary sarcomas of bone, causing pain, lameness, soft tissue swelling, and bone destruction. However, the tumor tends to remain confined to the medullary cavity and may involve a relatively large area of bone before signs of pain become clinically apparent. Often, a pathological fracture through the tumor site is the first clinical sign of disease.

Sites and Gross Morphology

The proximal and distal one-third of long bones are the most common sites of involvement, followed by the pelvic bones, sternum, ribs, maxilla, and vertebral column.[4,5,10,17,20]

On cut section, the neoplasm is typically composed of dark, bloody, spongy tissue (fig. 5.33 A) but may also contain gray to tan areas with a rubbery consistency. Other primary lesions of bone that may be indistinguishable grossly from hemangiosarcoma are telangiectatic osteosarcoma and aneurysmal bone cysts. Furthermore, hemangiosarcomas of soft tissue origin may metastasize to bone and produce identical lesions. Postmortem examination of affected animals should therefore include a thorough inspection of the carcass for evidence of primary soft tissue hemangiosarcoma. In some cases with tumors at multiple sites, it is impossible to determine if the skeletal lesions are primary or secondary.

Primary hemangiosarcoma of bone destroys extensive areas of normal bone architecture including metaphyseal

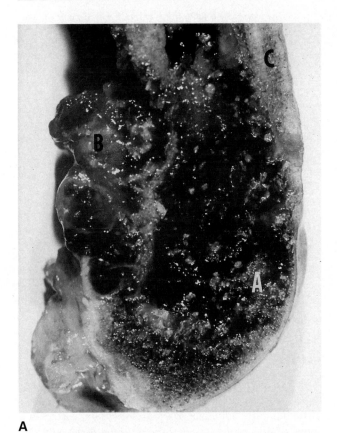

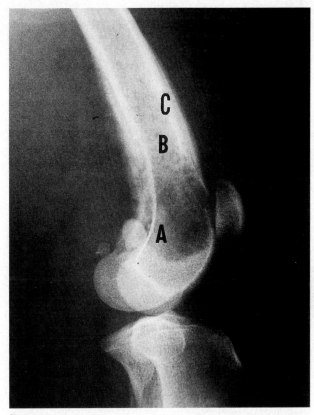

A

B

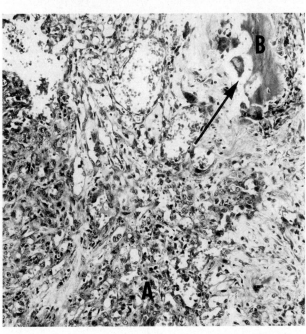

C

Fig. 5.33. Central hemangiosarcoma of bone. **A.** Spongy, dark, bloody tissue replaces the spongiosa of the distal femur *(A)* and extends through the cortex onto the caudal surface of the bone *(B)*. The periosteal response is smoothly contoured *(C, top)*. **B.** Radiograph of the tumor showing marked osteolysis in the distal femur *(A)* accompanied by a permeative pattern of bone destruction in the distal shaft *(B)*. Note the evenly contoured collar of periosteal new bone *(C)*. **C.** Tumor is composed of an irregular bed of proliferating neoplastic angioblasts *(A)* that are not producing osteoid. Bone *(B)* is being removed by osteoclastic resorption (arrow).

spongiosa and cortex, but most of these tumors provoke only a modest, smoothly contoured collar of periosteal new bone. Soft tissue swelling is often not as remarkable as that seen in most osteosarcomas.

Radiographic Appearance

The tumor produces a highly destructive lesion, often accompanied by pathological fracture. Hemangiosarcomas of long bones extend along the marrow cavity and destroy the cortical bone, but they tend not to extend into the soft tissue, as occurs in most primary sarcomas of bone (fig. 5.33 B). Usually the amount of extracortical reactive bone surrounding the lesion is minimal.[10]

Histological and Cytological Features

Tumor tissue resembles hemangiosarcoma of soft tissue. While much of the tumor may be composed of a poorly differentiated sarcoma, areas are found in which the neoplasm attempts to form vascular channels (fig. 5.33 C). Vascular spaces lined by atypical endothelial cells may form irregular clefts or more cavernous structures. The fibrous stroma supporting the vascular structures may, in some focal areas, become impregnated with blood proteins and cursorily resemble osteoid. The stroma of hemangiosarcoma does not form a calcifiable matrix. Telangiectatic osteosarcomas that have low osteoblastic potential are sometimes incorrectly diagnosed as hemangiosarcoma.[20] In telangiectatic osteosarcoma, malignant osteoblasts rather than endothelial cells line the blood filled spaces, but this distinction is not always straightforward, especially in biopsy samples collected from sites of pathological fracture. Depending on their degree of differentiation and antigenicity the malignant endothelial cells will be factor VIII positive.

Fine needle aspirates or scrapings from hemangiosarcomas are usually difficult to diagnose because they contain a large amount of blood and only a few nucleated cells, but they may also contain few to moderate numbers of spindle shaped cells with features of malignant mesenchymal cells.[16] Often, there are too few cells for a diagnosis of malignancy, and differentiation from telangiectatic osteosarcoma, other forms of osteosarcoma, and even certain nonneoplastic bone lesions, requires histopathology.

Growth and Metastasis

Hemangiosarcomas typically destroy an extensive area of bone before producing clinical signs. By this time most tumors have shed hematogenous metastases. While amputation may be curative in a few cases, there is no information currently available to suggest that an animal with an advanced primary tumor should be considered as a good candidate for ablative surgery.

REFERENCES

1. Brodey, R.S., Riser, W.H., and Van der Heul, R.O. (1974) Canine skeletal chondrosarcoma: A clinico-pathologic study of 35 cases. *J Amer Vet Med Assoc* 165:68–78.
2. Sylvestre, A.M., Brash, M.L., Atilola, M.A.O., and Cockshutt, J.R. (1992) A case series of 25 dogs with chondrosarcoma. *J Vet Comp Orthop Traum* 4:13–17.
3. Popovitch, C.A., Weinstein, M.J., Goldschmidt, M.H., and Shofer, F.S. (1994) Chondrosarcoma: A retrospective study of 97 dogs (1987–1990). *J Amer Anim Hosp Assoc* 30:81–85.
4. Brodey, R.S., Sauer, R.M., and Medway, W. (1963) Canine bone neoplasms. *J Amer Vet Med Assoc* 143:471–495.
5. Jacobson, S.A. (1971) *The Comparative Pathology of the Tumors of Bones.* Charles C. Thomas, Springfield, IL.
6. Sullivan, D.J. (1960) Cartilaginous tumors (chondroma and chondrosarcoma) in animals. *Amer J Vet Res* 21:531–535.
7. Turrel, J.M., and Pool, R.R. (1982) Primary bone tumors in the cat: A retrospective study of 15 cats and a literature review. *Vet Radiol* 23:152–166.
8. Engle, G.C., and Brodey, R.S. (1969) A retrospective study of 395 feline neoplasms. *J Amer Hosp Assoc* 5:21–31.
9. Liu, S.K., and Dorfman, H.D. (1974) The cartilage analogue of fibromatosis (juvenile aponeurotic fibroma) in dogs. *Vet Pathol* 11:60–67.
10. Ling, G.V., Morgan, J.P., and Pool, R.R. (1974) Primary bone tumors in the dog: A combined clinical, radiographic, and histologic approach to early diagnosis. *J Amer Vet Med Assoc* 165:55–67.
11. Spjut, H.J., Dorfman, H.D., Fechner, R.E., and Ackerman, L.V. (1971) Tumors of bone and cartilage. In *Atlas of Tumor Pathology.* 2nd series, fascicle 5. Armed Forces Institute of Pathology, Washington, D.C.
12. Schajowicz, F. (1981) *Tumors and Tumor-like Lesions of Bone and Joints.* Springer-Verlag, New York), pp. 109–204.
13. Lichtenstein, L., and Jaffe, H.L. (1943) Chondrosarcoma of bone. *Amer J Pathol* 19:553–589.
14. Resnick, D., Kyriakos, M., and Greenway, G.G. (1994) Tumors and tumor-like lesions of bone: Imaging and pathology of specific lesions. In Resnick, D. (ed.), *Diagnosis of Bone and Joint Disorders,* 3rd ed. Vol. 6, ch. 83. W.B. Saunders, Philadelphia), pp. 3628–3938.
15. Patnaik, A.K., Lieberman, P.H., Erlandson, R.A., and Liu, S. K. (1984) Canine sinonasal skeletal neoplasms: chondrosarcomas and osteosarcomas. *Vet Pathol* 21:475–482.
16. Baker, R., and Lumsden, J.H. (1999) *Color Atlas of Cytology of the Dog and Cat.* Mosby, St Louis.
17. Morgan, J.P., Ackerman, N., Bailey, C.S., and Pool, R.R. (1980) Vertebral tumors in the dog: A clinical, radiologic, and pathologic study of 61 primary and secondary lesions. *Vet Radiol* 21:197–212.
18. Peiffer, R.L., Rebar, A., and Burk, R. (1974) Fibrosarcoma involving the skeleton of the dog. *Vet Med Small Anim Clin* 69:1143–1148.
19. Wesselhoeft Ablin, L., Berg, J., and Schelling, S.H. (1991) Fibrosarcoma of the canine appendicular skeleton. *J Amer Anim Hosp Assoc* 27:303–309.
20. Bingel, S.A., Brodey, R.S., Allen, H.L., and Riser, W.H. (1974) Haemangiosarcoma of bone in the dog. *J Small Anim Pract* 15:303–322.
21. Pool, R.R. (1990) Tumors of bone and cartilage. In Moulton, J.E. (ed.), *Tumors in Domestic Animals,* 3rd ed. University of California Press, Berkeley.

Giant Cell Tumor of Bone

Although this is a well-established clinical and pathological entity in humans,[1] it is rare in animals, most reports involving only individual cases in dogs[2-6] and cats.[7-9] In a series of 403 primary bone tumors in the dog,[2] only one giant cell tumor was reported. No cases were reported in another series of 394 canine bone tumors.[10] In contrast, giant cell tumors comprised approximately 5 percent of cases in a large survey of human bone tumors.[1] Because there are so few documented cases of giant cell tumor in animals, there is inadequate information to provide an indication of the age, species, and site incidence or of biological behavior. Furthermore, some reported cases of giant cell tumor in animals are not convincing[2] and may, in fact, represent other bone lesions in which osteoclasts are a prominent feature.

Giant cell tumors in both man and animals typically cause expansile, osteolytic lesions near the ends of long bones,[1,4,7,8] often involving much of the subchondral epiphyseal bone (fig. 5.34 A). The tumor is usually surrounded by a thin shell of bone, even when the cortex is eroded, and may be subdivided by delicate bony trabeculae. Pathological fracture may occur at the site. Most reported giant cell tumors in animals have occurred near joints in long bones, but they are also reported occasionally in the cranium, ribs, and vertebrae.

The tumor is characterized by the presence of large numbers of multinucleated giant cells that resemble osteoclasts and are closely associated with neoplastic mononuclear cells (fig 5.34 B). The giant cells, which are often very large, are scattered uniformly throughout the tumor, and their nuclei resemble those of the mononuclear cells. The cytoplasmic borders of the giant cells are often indistinct. In some tumors there are areas of collagen and/or osteoid formation (fig.5.34 C), but this is not a prominent

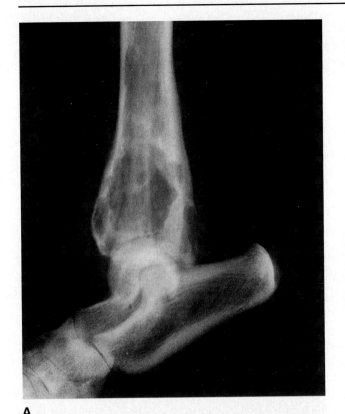

A

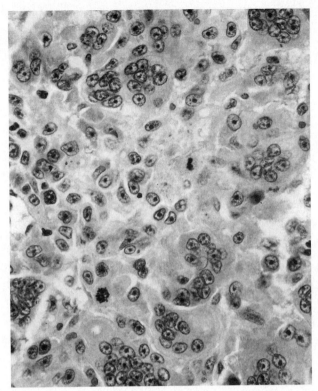

B

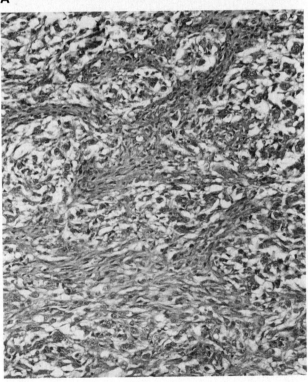

C

Fig. 5.34. Giant cell tumor of bone. **A.** Radiograph of an expansile, osteolytic lesion in the distal tibia of a dog. **B.** Tissues from a malignant giant cell tumor of the tibia. Tumor giant cells arise by fusion of rapidly proliferating neoplastic mononuclear cells. Note the similarity of nuclei in both cell populations and the indistinct borders of the giant cells. Lung metastases had a similar appearance. **C.** Less well differentiated area in same primary tumor but with smaller and less characteristic giant cells. Small spindle cells form anastomotic septa of collagenous tissue that sometimes contain spicules of bone matrix.

feature, and the matrix may be produced by reactive fibroblasts and/or osteoblasts, respectively, rather than by the tumor cells, particularly if the tumor is associated with a recent pathological fracture. The tumor is highly vascular and may contain cavernous spaces and areas of hemorrhage, leading to possible confusion with aneurysmal bone cyst, which also contains variable numbers of multinucleated giant cells. Osteosarcomas may also contain many osteoclasts in some areas and mistakenly be diagnosed as giant cell tumors.

Cytological examination of fine needle aspirates may be useful in the diagnosis of giant cell tumors. The presence of a relatively high percentage of multinucleated giant cells among many plump, spindle shaped or ovoid, mesenchymal cells suggests the possibility of giant cell tumor.[4] Giant cells may also be present in aspirates from other bone lesions, including osteosarcoma, chondrosarcoma, and even fibrosarcoma, but the percentage in giant cell tumors is likely to be much higher. In one report of this tumor in a dog,[4] 25 percent of all cells obtained by fine needle aspiration biopsy were multinucleated giant cells. However, definitive diagnosis still requires histological examination of sections from representative areas of the mass. A diagnosis of giant cell tumor should never be made on the basis of fragments of tissue collected for either histological or cytological examination.

The histogenesis of giant cell tumor is uncertain, but immunochemical staining suggests that the mononuclear tumor cells are of histiocytic origin and that the giant cells arise from their fusion.[1,11] C type viral particles were found to be budding from tumor cells in one feline giant cell tumor,[7] but their significance is unknown.

In humans, most giant cell tumors are benign, although an estimated 40–60 percent will recur locally following surgery.[12] Approximately 5–10 percent are malignant, metastasizing typically to the lungs.[12] Benign and malignant forms are also reported in animals, the former being most common.

Giant cell tumor is appropriate for a tumor in epiphysis, when giant cells are the number one feature and if osteoid production is absent or minimal. Osteosarcoma giant cell variant has obvious osteoid production, and although giant cells are prominent they are increased in regions rather than distributed uniformly through the tumor, as they are in giant cell tumors of bone.

Multilobular Tumor of Bone

Classification

Multilobular tumor of bone is a slow growing but potentially malignant tumor, occurring most often in the skull of dogs,[2,13-16] but occasionally in the cat[17] and horse.[18] Many alternative classifications have been proposed, including chondroma rodens,[2] cartilage analogue of fibromatosis,[13] calcifying aponeurotic fibroma, multilobular chondroma or osteoma, and multilobular osteochondrosarcoma.[16] The term *multilobular tumor of bone* is now preferred[19,20] as it avoids the confusion caused by the use of terms applied to similar, but not identical, tumors of man and recognizes the fact that these tumors may be either benign or malignant.

After initial thoughts that the lesion arose as a soft tissue tumor from dense fascia in the fronto-occipital or temporal regions of the skull[13] and resembled juvenile aponeurotic fibroma of children, a detailed study of 10 cases in dogs demonstrated that this is a unique, primary tumor of bone.[19] In histological sections, the tumor has a characteristic multilobular pattern; the lobules consist of islands of either crude bone or cartilage surrounded by a thin rim of poorly differentiated spindle cells. Disruption of the lobular pattern due to malignant transformation of bony, cartilaginous, or fibrous elements occurs in some cases and is associated with infiltrative growth into adjacent soft tissues, or metastatic spread to distant sites.[19]

The histogenesis of multilobular tumor of bone is unknown, but it is proposed that the tumors are derived from altered periosteal elements of the chondrocranium and viscerocranium, which share the same embryonic origin.[14] This would account for their occurrence primarily in the flat bones of the skull, although rare cases are reported at other sites.

Incidence, Age, Breed, and Sex

Multilobular tumor of bone is an uncommon neoplasm of the skull of dogs and is rare in other species. In dogs, it is primarily a disease of middle-aged to older animals, occurring most often in medium or large breeds, but rarely in giant breeds.[19] In one study of 39 cases in dogs,[16] the median age was 8 years (range 4 to 17 years) and the median weight was 29 kg, although four dogs weighed less than 25 kg.

Too few of these tumors have been found in noncranial sites of the canine skeleton or in the heads of cats and horses to know if age, breed, and sex are significant factors in these cases. Three cases have been recorded in cats varying in age from 9 months to 8 years.[2,17,19] The only reported case in a horse was in a 12-year-old thoroughbred mare.[18]

Clinical Characteristics

The dogs are usually presented because of a palpable, firm, unmovable mass arising from the surface of the bones of the skull. Less frequently, the owner's concern is directed toward a change in the dog's normal pattern of behavior. Signs are related to the degree that the tumor mass compresses and perturbs the function of adjacent structures. Some tumors may cause exophthalmia, sinus obstruction, interference with mastication, or loosening of teeth. A few tumors compress the brain and cranial nerves, causing neurological signs that mimic those of brain tumors. Local recurrence following surgical removal occurred in 47 percent of cases in one study,[16] but median time to recurrence was over 2 years, reflecting the slow rate of tumor growth. Not surprisingly, a significant reduction in time to local recurrence was reported in cases where surgical removal was incomplete. Furthermore, a better prognosis was recorded in cases where the tumor involved the mandible and other accessible sites that allowed complete removal.[16] In this same study, 56 percent of affected dogs developed metastases, mainly to the lungs. Because of the slow growth of the tumor, dogs can survive for several months with pulmonary metastases and may show no clinical signs of lung involvement. The metastatic lesions are usually small and in some cases are only detected histologically.[21] This is in contrast to metastatic osteosarcoma and chondrosarcoma, both of which grow rapidly, leading to death due to pulmonary metastasis. The lesion in the zygomatic process of the horse was successfully removed without local recurrence.[18]

Sites and Gross Morphology

In the report of 39 cases of multilobular tumor of bone in dogs,[16] 14 tumors occurred in the cranium, 11 in the maxilla and 10 in the mandible. Other sites include the orbit, tympanic bulla, and the base of the zygomatic process. The tumor has also been reported on the hard palate of dogs.[15,19]

The tumor is a hard, nodular mass with a discrete border (fig. 5.35 A). It is covered by a tough fibrous membrane when it projects into the soft tissues of the skull or by a thinner layer of intact epithelium or meninges when protruding into the nasal sinuses or cranial vault. Tumors ranging in size from 2 to more than 10 cm in diameter have produced clinical signs. On cut surface, the tumor is composed of numerous tiny, gray, gritty nodules and a few

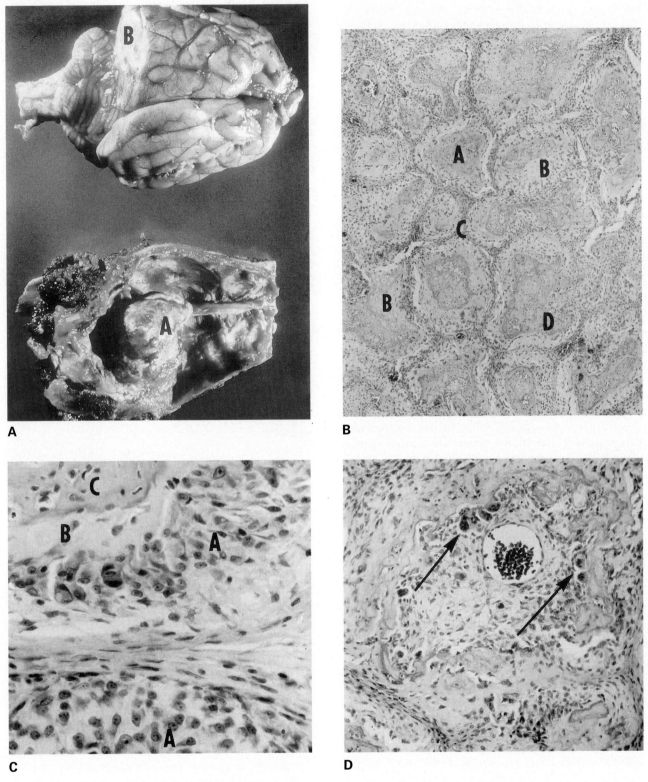

Fig. 5.35. Multilobular tumor of bone (chondroma rodens). **A.** Smoothly contoured intracranial mass *(A)* covered by an intact dura mater has compressed the caudal pole *(B)* of the left cerebral hemisphere. **B.** Multilobular pattern characteristic of this tumor. Crude bone *(A)* and/or cartilage *(B)* in the center of lobules, which are bounded by thin fibrous septa *(C)*. Blood vessels *(D)* in interstices between lobules. **C.** Plump cells resembling fetal osteoblasts *(A)* rim centrilobular islands of chondrois *(B)* and/or osseous matrix *(C)*. **D.** Remodeling of lobule with vascular invasion and osteoclastic resorption (arrows).

intersecting bands of fibrous tissue containing blood vessels. A lesion is typically centered in one of the flat bones of the skull and may exhibit symmetric or eccentric enlargement. Consequently, expansile growth directed primarily into a cavity (e.g., frontal sinus, orbit, or cranial vault) would not be palpable early in the course of the disease. Tumors protruding into cavities are covered by intact membranes, and they compress the brain without invading the meninges or nervous tissue (fig. 5.35 A).

Radiographic Appearance

Multilobular tumors of bone are solitary nodular lesions that have smoothly contoured, sharply demarcated borders (fig. 5.36 A). Normal bone structure in the affected area may be replaced by an amorphous pattern of increased radiodensity containing areas of granularity. A nodular to stippled pattern may be seen in tumors protruding into cavities or into the soft tissues of the head. The occurrence of large areas of lysis within the tumor or the development of a brush pattern along the borders of a tumor would suggest malignant change.

Histological Features

Multilobular tumors have a characteristic pattern of numerous contiguous lobules (fig. 5.35 B,C) bordered by thin septa of spindle cell mesenchyme. Vessels travel in interstices between adjacent lobules, but they may penetrate the centers of lobules undergoing endochondral ossification (fig. 5.35 D). The central two-thirds of a lobule may contain hyaline cartilage, tissue with matrix properties intermediate between bone and cartilage, or immature bone. The central island is typically surrounded by a zone of plump to ovoid cells that merge with fusiform septal cells. Hyperchromatic cells resembling primitive osteoblasts often form cellular palisades around the central islands of matrix. Mitotic figures are uncommon in most cases, and when present, they imply malignant transformation. While all of these tumors have the characteristic lobular pattern, the lobules may vary in their composition of cartilage and bone matrix. Some of the cartilaginous variants are so well differentiated that they may be mistaken for primary chondrosarcoma of the skull (fig. 5.36 B) unless adequate tumor tissue is available for inspection. Conversely, a few skull tumors will be so poorly differentiated that the lobular pattern and chondroid nature of the matrix may be overlooked(fig. 5.36 C).

In multilobular tumors of bone, the spindle cell component never predominates, nor are there mesenchymal cells forming the interwoven bundles or a *herringbone* pattern that would suggest a diagnosis of fibrosarcoma.[19] In some tumors, however, dedifferentiated spindle cells arising from the septal cells at the periphery of a tumor invade the soft tissue along muscle insertion lines.

Microscopic indicators of aggressive and malignant behavior include mitotic activity, loss of orderly lobular architecture, necrosis, hemorrhage, and overgrowth by one of the mesenchymal elements forming the lobular structure. A grading system based on these criteria and on the nature of the tumor margins has been proposed[21] and appears to provide useful prognostic information (see appendix) .[16,21] Grade III tumors were found to have shorter median times to local recurrence and metastasis and for survival than Grade I and Grade II tumors, but the range was broad and there was considerable overlap between grades.[16] In cases where metastatic lesions have been examined histologically, they possess the same lobular architecture as the primary tumor.[21,22]

Growth and Metastasis

These tumors exhibit slow, progressive growth, infiltrating locally and compressing adjacent structures such as the brain. Local recurrence following surgery is expected in approximately 50 percent of cases, depending on histological grade and on whether the tumor can be completely removed.[16,21] In a study of 39 dogs with multilobular tumor of bone, median time to local recurrence was 797 days (range 30 to 1332 days), and median time to metastasis was 542 days (range 0 to 1225 days).[16] Median time to death from the onset of recurrence or metastatic disease was 239 days (range 28 to 1280 days),[16] reflecting the relatively slow growth rate of these tumors compared to other malignant tumors of bone. In the single case reported in a horse,[18] surgical resection was apparently curative. A chondrosarcoma was reported to arise in a multilobular tumor in a cat.[17]

Liposarcoma

Liposarcoma of bone is a rare primary bone tumor in animals that arises from fat cell precursors in the marrow cavity. Few reports exist in the veterinary literature. A central (medullary) liposarcoma is described in an 18-month-old male Labrador retriever; it produced an osteolytic lesion in the distal two-thirds of the left humerus, with marked production of periosteal new bone and a firm, painless soft tissue swelling.[23] The tumor, consisting of gray fatty tissue, replaced bone marrow and eroded cortical and trabecular bone. The dog showed progressive lameness in the left forelimb for approximately 1 month before diagnosis. At necropsy 2 weeks later, there was no evidence of tumor beyond the primary site.

Liposarcoma of bone resembles its soft tissue counterpart. While much of the tumor tissue may be composed of well-differentiated signet ring cells and multivesicular cells (fig. 5.37), there may be foci of fibrosarcomatous differentiation or areas of undifferentiated spindle cell sarcoma. Central liposarcoma of bone should also be differentiated from central lipoma of bone, periosteal liposarcoma of bone,[2] and liposarcoma of soft tissues that secondarily involves bone.[24]

An infiltrating extradural angiolipoma surrounding the lumbar spinal cord and apparently invading L2 and L3 vertebrae was reported in a 12-year-old Labrador.[25] Histologically, the lesion was benign, consisting of mature adipocytes and scattered blood vessels, and should not be

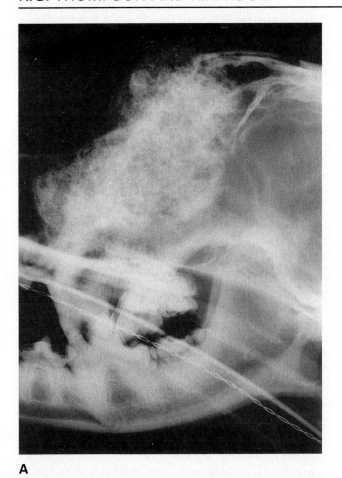

A

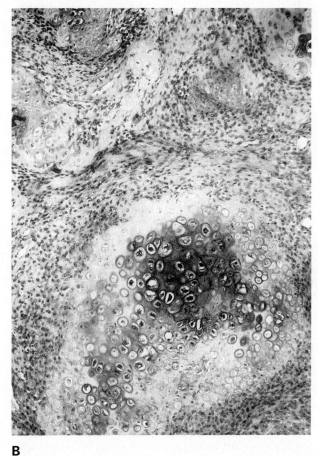

B

C

Fig. 5.36. Multilobular tumor of bone. **A.** Radiograph of large, productive, radiodense lesion having a smoothly contoured border and composed of multinodular densities. **B.** Disruption of nodular pattern (top) leads to confusion with chondrosarcoma. **C.** Multilobular pattern is difficult to recognize in some less well differentiated multilobular tumors. Note, however, the pattern formed by the septa and the presence of a chondrocyte (arrow).

confused with liposarcoma. The bone lysis was most likely due to local erosion and remodeling associated with the pressure of an expanding lesion within the confines of the spinal canal, rather than to active invasion by the tumor.[25]

Plasma Cell Myeloma of Bone

Plasma cell myeloma is a malignant tumor of plasma cells within the bone marrow, typically producing discrete, multicentric, lytic lesions in bones, especially those involved in active hematopoiesis.[26] The disease is uncommon in domestic animals but occurs more frequently in dogs[10,26,27] than in either cats[28,29] or horses.[30,31] The mean age of affected dogs is approximately 9.5 years (range 2.5 to 16 years), and males are affected more frequently than females.[26] In cats, the mean age of affected animals is 10.6 years, and as in dogs, there is a much higher incidence in males.[29] The median age of horses with plasma cell myeloma is 11 years, but the range is broad (3 months to

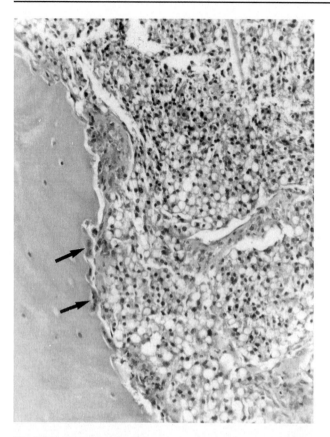

Fig. 5.37. Liposarcoma of bone in a dog. The marrow cavity is filled with relatively well differentiated neoplastic adipocytes containing either many small intracytoplasmic vacuoles or occasional large vacuoles. The bone surface is scalloped and lined by osteoclasts (arrows), indicating bone resorption in response to the advancing tumor.

22 years); no sex predilection is recognized in the small number of cases reported in horses.[31]

The clinical signs of plasma cell myeloma in dogs, cats, and horses depend on the site of the tumor but often include lameness, ill-defined pain, weight loss, and lethargy.[26,27,31] Involvement of vertebral bodies may result in paraplegia due to protrusion of tumor masses into the spinal canal, or secondary to pathological fractures of vertebral bodies.[27,31,32] Production of a homogeneous immunoglobulin or immunoglobulin fragment (paraprotein or M-component), which appears as a monoclonal spike on serum protein electrophoresis, is a consistent feature of plasma cell myeloma in all species.[10,26,31] Bence Jones proteinuria is present less often. Hyperviscosity syndrome is reported in some affected animals, as is hypercalcemia.[26-28] Hypercalcemia is only present in approximately 10 percent of affected dogs and is associated with a poorer response to chemotherapy.

Radiographic bone lesions are present in approximately two-thirds of dogs with plasma cell myeloma[27] but were detected in only 3 of 10 affected horses.[31] The lesions are typically discrete, *punched out* foci of osteolysis, varying in size and often involving multiple bones (figs. 5.38 A,B). No sclerotic, osteoblastic margins are

present. The principal sites of bone involvement in dogs are vertebrae, especially in the thoracolumbar region, femur, pelvis, humerus, and ribs.[10,26,27] Bones of the distal limbs are seldom involved in dogs, but in cats they appear to be involved as often as bones of the proximal extremities.[29] Bone lesions are reported in only three horses with plasma cell myeloma, two involving thoracic vertebrae and one with a lesion in the third metatarsal.[31]

On gross examination of sections through affected bones, the lytic foci consist of soft, fleshy or gelatinous, dark red nodules replacing trabecular bone. The lesions are often multiple and may be associated with a pathological fracture. Histological or cytological examination reveals a relatively pure, dense population of plasma cells (fig. 5.38 C), which may be either well-differentiated or large, anaplastic round cells with a high mitotic index. In less well differentiated tumors, there may be binucleated cells, and the characteristic features of plasma cells are difficult to find. Some tumor cells are so well differentiated they do not appear to be neoplastic, and it is their marked numbers, expansile growth, and clinical problems of osteolysis, serum protein abnormalities, and hypercalcemia that contribute to a definitive diagnosis.

Malignant Lymphoma of Bone

Malignant lymphoma may occur as a primary tumor of bone in humans[33] and dogs,[34] but such cases in animals are rare. More frequently, bone involvement occurs in association with multicentric lymphoma in dogs, cats, and cattle. It is likely that many animals with malignant lymphoma possess bone lesions that are not detected clinically or radiographically, but there are few published reports about dogs where lytic bone lesions are a prominent feature of the disease.[34-37] These cases are perhaps best referred to as *lymphoma primarily affecting bone,*[34,37] rather than as *primary lymphoma of bone.*

Although there are only nine reported cases where lymphoma primarily affects bone of dogs, six of the animals were less than 1 year of age.[37] This suggests that the age incidence may be much lower than in dogs with lymphoma primarily involving extraskeletal organs. Two of the nine dogs were boxers, and two were German shepherds, suggesting an increased prevalence in these breeds.

Most affected dogs have multiple, discrete, punched out lesions involving several bones of the appendicular and axial skeleton. In long bones, the lesions may involve either diaphyseal[35] or metaphyseal[36,37] regions and are radiographically and grossly indistinguishable from plasma cell myeloma. Pathological fractures are often associated with the lytic lesions,[37] and slipped epiphysis is reported in a pup with multiple metaphyseal involvement.[36] This pup was also hypercalcemic, but hypercalcemia was not reported in most other cases, even where bone lesions were extensive. Confirmation of a diagnosis of malignant lymphoma of bone requires either histopathology or cytological examination of fine needle aspiration biopsies from

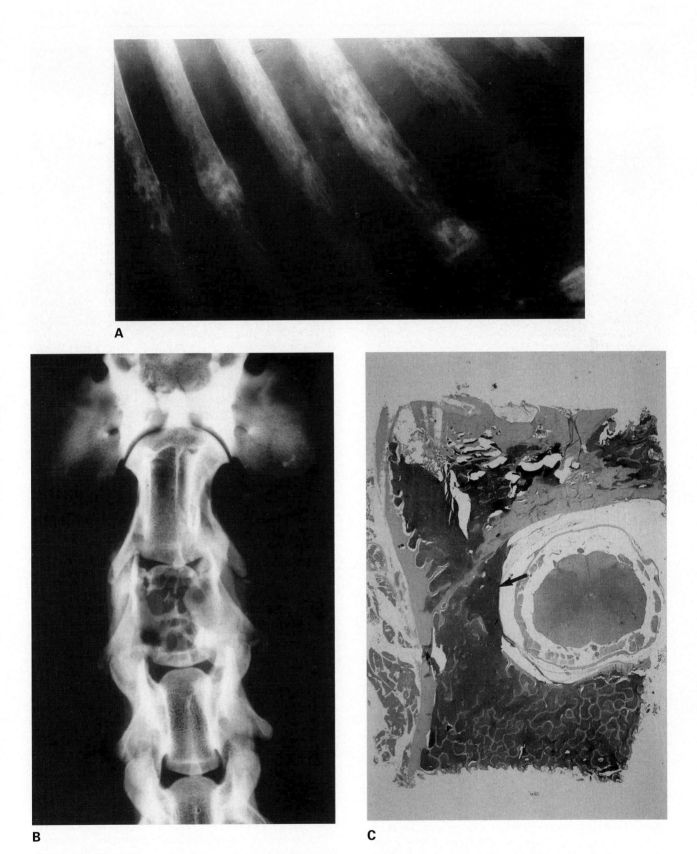

Fig. 5.38. Plasma cell myeloma. **A.** Multiple osteolytic foci in the ribs of a dog with multicentric plasma cell myeloma. Pathological fractures are present in some ribs. (Photograph courtesy of R.A. Fairley.) **B.** Discrete, punched out foci of osteolysis in the third cervical vertebra of another dog with plasma cell myeloma. **C.** Subgross photograph of vertebra showing extensive infiltration of marrow spaces with a dense population of neoplastic plasma cells. In some areas, trabecular bone has been replaced by tumor tissue and the tumor is starting to encroach on the spinal canal (arrow).

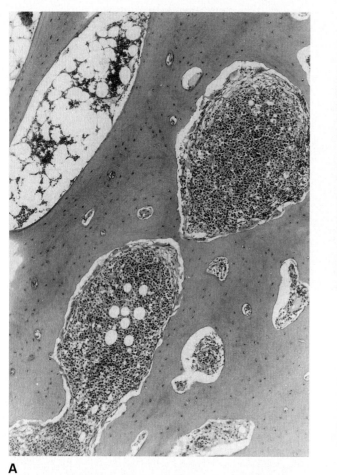

A

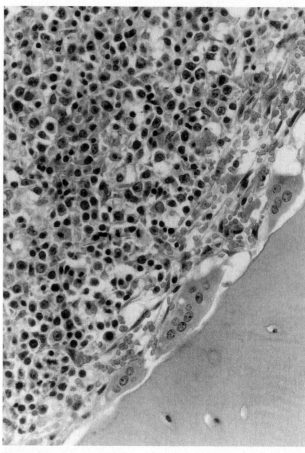

B

Fig. 5.39. Lymphoma in a 19-year-old quarter horse. (Sections courtesy of S.E. Weisbrode.) **A.** Large resorption cavities in the cortex of this bone are filled with tumor cells. **B.** A monomorphic population of round cells fill the marrow cavity. Activated osteoclasts are resorbing the adjacent bone.

lytic lesions. Histologically, sheets of monomorphic lymphoid cells fill marrow cavities, replacing hematopoietic tissue and bone trabeculae[34-37] in areas of radiographic bone lysis, and sometimes spread to involve adjacent tissues. Figure 5.39 A,B illustrates the infiltrative and lytic behavior of a malignant lymphoma in the bone of a horse.

Infiltration of bone marrow, together with multifocal to locally extensive bone infarction, is reported in calves with the sporadic form of malignant lymphoma.[38] Affected calves also have generalized lymph node enlargement and variable involvement of other organs, including liver, kidney, and spleen. The bone infarcts are readily visible grossly as discrete, pale areas (fig. 5.40), often surrounded by a red margin, but they are not detected unless the bones are sectioned during postmortem examination. The mechanism of the tumor associated bone marrow necrosis is not clear, but ischemia secondary to infiltration of the marrow with malignant cells is a likely explanation.[38]

REFERENCES

1. Unni, K.K. (1996) Giant cell tumor. In *Dahlin's Bone Tumors. General Aspects and Data on 11,087 Cases,* 5th ed. Ch. 19. Lippincott-Raven, Philadelphia, pp. 263–289.

2. Jacobson, S.A. (1971) *The Comparative Pathology of the Tumors of Bone.* Charles C. Thomas, Springfield, IL.

3. Garman, R.H., Powell, F.R., and Tompsett, J.W. (1977) Malignant giant cell tumor in a dog. *J Amer Vet Med Assoc* 171:546–548.

4. LeCouteur, R.A., Nimmo, J.S., Price, S.M., and Pennock, P.W. (1978) A case of giant cell tumor of bone (osteoclastoma) in a dog. *J Amer Anim Hosp Assoc* 14:356–362.

5. Crow, S.E., Hall, A.D., Walshaw, R., and Wortman, J.A. (1979) Giant cell tumor (osteoclastoma) in a dog. *J Amer Anim Hosp Assoc* 15:473–476.

6. Trigo, F.J., Leathers, C.W., and Brobst, D.F. (1983) A comparison of canine giant cell tumor and giant cell reparative granuloma of bone. *Vet Pathol* 20:215–222.

7. Popp, J.A., and Simpson, C.F. (1976) Feline malignant giant cell tumor of bone associated with C type virus particles. *Cornell Vet* 66:528–535.

8. Thornberg, L.P. (1979) Giant cell tumor of bone in a cat. *Vet Pathol* 16:255–257.

9. Turrel, J.M., and Pool, R.R. (1982) Primary bone tumors in the cat: A retrospective study of 15 cats and a literature review. *Vet Radiol* 23:152–166.

10. Liu, S.K., Dorfman, H.D., Hurvitz, A.L., and Patnaik, A.K. (1977) Primary and secondary bone tumors in the dog. *J Small Anim Pract* 18:313–326.

11. Yoshida, H., Akeho, M., and Yumoto, T. (1982) Giant cell tumor of bone. Enzyme histochemical, biochemical and tissue culture studies. *Virchows Arch* 395:319–330.

12. Resnick, D., Kyriakos, M., and Greenway, G.G. (1994) Tumors and tumor-like lesions of bone: Imaging and pathology of specific

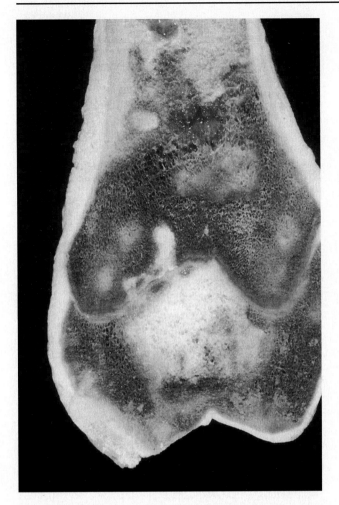

Fig. 5.40. Multiple, irregularly shaped, pale foci representing medullary infarcts in a young calf with the juvenile form of sporadic lymphoma. (Photograph courtesy of P.C. Stromberg.)

(1978–1988). *J Amer Vet Med Assoc* 195:1764–1769.

22. McLain, D.L., Hill, J.R., and Pulley, L.T. (1983) Multilobular osteoma and chondroma (chondroma rodens) with pulmonary metastasis in a dog. *J Amer Anim Hosp Assoc* 19:359–362.

23. Brodey, R.S., and Riser, W.H. (1966) Liposarcoma of bone: Case report. *J Amer Vet Radiol Soc* 7:27–33.

24. Brodey, R.S., Sauer, R.M., and Medway, W. (1963) Canine bone neoplasms. *J Amer Vet Med Assoc* 143:471–495.

25. Reif, U., Lowrie, C.T., and Fitzgerald, S.D. (1998) Extradural spinal angiolipoma associated with bone lysis in a dog. *J Amer Anim Hosp Assoc* 34:373–376.

26. Osborne, C.A., Perman, V., Sautter, J.H., Stevens, J.B., and Hanlon, G.F. (1968) Multiple myeloma in the dog. *J Amer Vet Med Assoc* 153:1300–1319.

27. van Bree, H., Pollet, L., Cousemont, W., Van Der Stock, J., and Mattheeuws, D. (1983) Cervical cord compression as a neurologic complication in an igg multiple myeloma in a dog. *J Amer Anim Hosp Assoc* 19:317–323.

28. Sheafor, S.E., Gamblin, R.M., and Couto, C.G. (1996) Hypercalcaemia in two cats with multiple myeloma. *J Amer Anim Hosp Assoc* 32:503–508.

29. Weber, N.A., and Tebeau, C.S. (1998) An unusual presentation of multiple myeloma in two cats. *J Amer Anim Hosp Assoc* 34:477–483.

30. Cornelius, C.E., Goodbarry, R.F., and Kennedy, P.C. (1959) Plasma cell myelomatosis in a horse. *Cornell Vet* 49:478–493.

31. Edwards, D.F., Parker, J.W., Wilkinson, J.E., and Helman, R.G. (1993) Plasma cell myeloma in the horse. A case review and literature review. *J Vet Int Med.* 7:167–176.

32. Braund, K.G., Everett, R.M., Bartels, J.E., and DeBuysscher, E. (1979) Neurologic complications of IgA multiple myeloma associated with cryoglobulinemia in a dog. *J Amer Vet Med Assoc* 174:1321–1325.

33. Schajowicz, F. (1981) *Tumors and Tumor-like Lesions of Bone and Joints.* Springer-Verlag, New York, pp. 267–280.

34. Giger, U., Evans, S.M., Hendrick, M.J., and Dudek, S.M. (1989) Orthovoltage radiotherapy of primary lymphoma of bone in a dog. *J Amer Vet Med Assoc* 195:627–630.

35. Rogers, K.S., Janovitz, E.B., Fooshee, S.K., Steyn, P.F., and Frankum, K.E. (1989) Lymphosarcoma with disseminated skeletal involvement in a pup. *J Amer Vet Med Assoc* 195:1242–1244.

36. Barthez, P.Y., Davis, C.R., Pool, R.R., Hornof, W.J., and Morgan, J.P. (1995) Multiple metaphyseal involvement of a thymic lymphoma associated with hypercalcemia in a puppy. *J Amer Anim Hosp Assoc* 31:82–85.

37. Langley-Hobbs, S.J., Carmichael, S., Lamb, C.R., Bjornson, A. P., Day, M.J. (1997) Polyostotic lymphoma in a young dog: A case report and literature review. *J Small Anim Pract* 38:412–416.

38. Doige, C.E. (1987) Bone and bone marrow necrosis associated with the calf form of sporadic bovine leukosis. *Vet Pathol* 24:186–188.

Sarcoma of the Periosteum

Sarcomas originating in the periosteum are much less common than primary bone sarcomas of central or medullary origin. Most are of low grade malignancy, exhibit slow growth, and may or may not invade underlying bone organs. They tend to recur locally following incomplete removal, but they pursue a long clinical course.

Periosteal Chondrosarcoma

Primary periosteal chondrosarcomas are cartilaginous neoplasms that arise de novo from a bone surface. They must be differentiated from secondary periosteal chon-

lesions. In Resnick, D. (ed.), *Diagnosis of Bone and Joint Disorders,* 3rd ed. Vol. 6, ch. 83. W.B. Saunders, Philadelphia, pp. 3628–3938.

13. Liu, S.K., and Dorfman, H.D. (1974) The cartilage analogue of fibroamtosis (juvenile aponeurotic fibroma) in dogs. *Vet Pathol* 11:60–67.

14. McCalla, T.L., Moore, C.P., Turk, J., Collier, L.L., and Pope, E.R. (1989) Multilobular osteosarcoma of the mandible and orbit in a dog. *Vet Pathol* 26:92–94.

15. Diamond, S.S., Raflo, C.P., and Anderson, M.P. (1980) Multilobular osteosarcoma in the dog. *Vet Pathol* 17:759–763.

16. Dernell, W.S., Straw, R.C., Cooper, M.F., Powers, B.E., LaRue, S.M., and Withrow, S.J. (1998) Multilobular osteochondrosarcoma in 39 dogs: 1979–1993. *J Amer Anim Hosp Assoc* 34:11–18.

17. Morton, D. (1985) Chondrosarcoma arising in a multilobular chondroma in a cat. *J Amer Vet Med Assoc* 186:804–806.

18. Richardson, D.W., and Acland, H.M. (1983) Multilobular osteoma (chondroma rodens) in a horse. *J Amer Vet Med Assoc* 182:289–291.

19. Pool, R.R. (1990) Tumors of bone and cartilage. In Moulton, J.E. (ed.), *Tumors in Domestic Animals,* 3rd ed. University of California Press, Berkeley.

20. Slayter, M.V., Boosinger, T.R., Pool, R.R., DÑmmrich, K., Misdorp, W., and Larsen, S. (1994) *Histological Classification of Bone and Joint Tumors of Domestic Animals.* World Health Organization. 2nd series, vol. 1. Armed Forces Institute of Pathology, American Registry of Pathology, Washington D.C.

21. Straw, R.C., LeCouter, R.A., Powers, B.E., and Withrow, S.J. (1989) Multilobular osteochondrosarcoma of the canine skull: 16 cases

drosarcomas, which develop as a result of malignant change in the cartilage cap of an osteochondroma. Primary periosteal chondrosarcomas are uncommon, and too few have been documented to determine if age, breed, and sex are significant factors. These tumors occur in older dogs and mature cats,[1] usually on bones with flat surfaces. Primary periosteal chondrosarcomas have been recognized at the following skeletal sites: proximal scapula, spinous processes of vertebrae, ribs, wings of pelvic bones, and the ends of long bones, especially the surfaces of the metaphyses, epiphyses, and the epicondyles.[1]

These tumors produce slow growing nodular masses on the surfaces of bones (fig. 5.41) and are slow to invade either the overlying soft tissues or the bone from which they arise. In one study,[1] several animals underwent multiple surgeries to debulk the tumor mass before eventual amputation or euthanasia. Metastatic disease was not observed, even in animals monitored for as long as 1 year, although the lesions often became locally aggressive.

Two dissimilar histological patterns may exist in these tumors. In the first pattern, the tumor tissue is identical with that of the central chondrosarcoma of bone (fig. 5.42 A), except that the tumor arises on the surface of the bone organ. Tumors with this pattern consist of multiple and often confluent lobules of neoplastic hyaline cartilage having cytological features of intermediate or low grade malignancy. Most of these tumors arise from the surface of a rib, the spinous process of a vertebra, the end of one of the pelvic bones, or the metaphyseal surface of a long bone.

In the second pattern, the tumor tissue usually lacks a lobular structure, and the chondrocytes have less anaplastic features throughout most of the tumor (fig. 5.42 B,C,D). Hyalinization of much of the cartilage matrix gives the appearance of bone tissue and may create the false impression that this is a mixed tumor of bone and cartilage (fig. 5.42 B). In some tumors this impression is enhanced by replacement of a part of the neoplastic cartilage with nonneoplastic bone through the process of endochondral ossification (fig. 5.42 C). In a few areas of such tumors, where most of the neoplastic cartilage tissue is replaced by apparently nonneoplastic bone (fig. 5.42 D), the lesion could be misinterpreted as a resolving periosteal reaction or a maturing callus. In more aggressive areas of some tumors there is dedifferentiation of the chondrogenic tumor cells, sometimes giving rise to an infiltrating spindle cell sarcoma. Tumors with this second pattern generally arise from the scapula and from the epicondyles and epiphyses of long bones.

Periosteal Fibrosarcoma

Periosteal fibrosarcomas are malignant fibroblastic tumors that arise from periosteal connective tissue and produce a slowly growing tumor mass intimately attached to the bone surface (fig. 5.43 A). In time, these tumors may

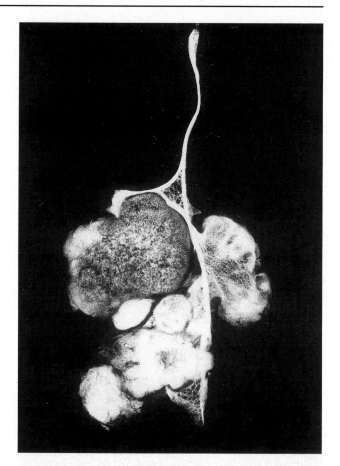

Fig. 5.41. Periosteal chondrosarcoma of a canine scapula. High detail radiograph of a transverse section through the middle of the scapula. Confluent nodules of partially ossified chondrosarcoma arise from the periosteal surface of the infraspinous fossa and the subscapular fossa.

locally erode and destroy adjacent bone organs. Affected bones, especially those covered by oral or nasal mucosa, are predisposed to pathological fracture and secondary inflammation. The tumor tends to recur locally following incomplete surgical removal. One survey of the veterinary literature[2] indicated that periosteal fibrosarcoma occurs in most domestic species and was most common in bones of the head. Periosteal fibrosarcomas of the mandible and maxilla of dogs appear to represent a distinct clinical entity and are discussed separately in the next section, but the tumor may also involve the scapula or long bones.[1] Fibrosarcomas of equine nasal sinuses and dental arcade may belong in this category, but the site of origin of most of these tumors is undetermined. Similarly, low grade fibrosarcomas involving the maxillary bones and paranasal sinuses are occasionally observed in cattle (fig. 5.44) and may represent periosteal fibrosarcomas. Periosteal fibrosarcomas arising from the surfaces of the maxilla, mandible, and other bones of the head in dogs and other species should be distinguished from the fairly common oral fibrosarcomas arising in the gingiva, labial and buccal mucosa, and mucosa of the palate. Although they seem to exhibit a similar biological behavior, with little tendency to metastasize, it is not always possible to differentiate

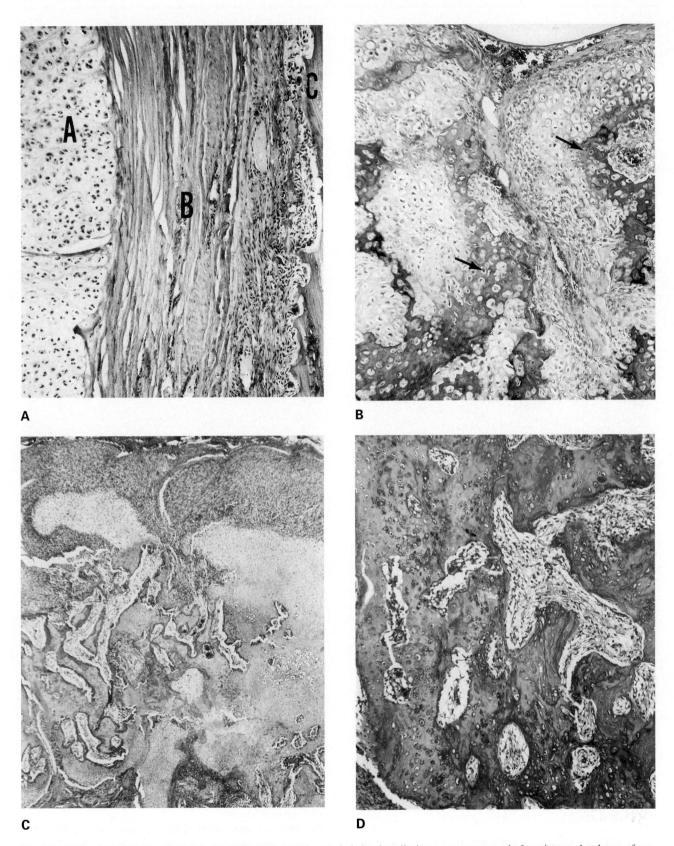

Fig. 5.42. Histological patterns found in periosteal chondrosarcoma. **A.** Lobulated cartilaginous tumor composed of contiguous chondrones of neoplastic chondrocytes *(A)* arises in the periosteum *(B)* on the cortical surface *(C)* of the bone. **B.** Areas of hyalinization (arrows) of chondroid tumor matrix may be mistaken for bone matrix. **C.** Complex matrix patterns result from endochondral ossification of tumor in which there is random replacement of low grade chondrosarcoma by nonneoplastic bone tissue. **D.** Area of tumor resembling an osteoma in which most of the tumor cartilage matrix has been replaced by nonneoplastic bone tissue.

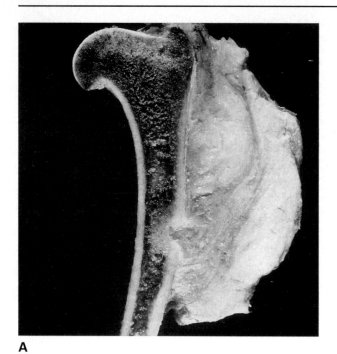

A

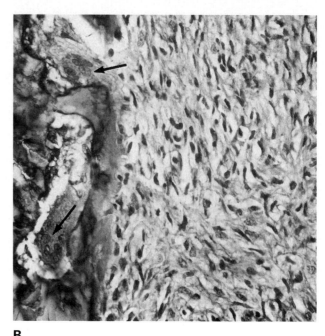

B

Fig. 5.43. Periosteal fibrosarcoma of bone. **A.** Slowly growing tumor firmly attached to the cranial surface of the humerus has invaded the cortex at mid-diaphysis. **B.** Undemineralized tissue section of moderately well differentiated fibrosarcoma beginning to invade the cortical surface as it follows resorption cavities cut by osteoclasts (arrows).

periosteal fibrosarcoma from a fibrosarcoma of soft tissue origin that secondarily involves bone. Blunt dissection of the tumor usually enables one to make this distinction in the earlier lesions, but not in more advanced cases. The radiographic appearance is primarily one of a soft tissue mass adjacent to the bone. There is a wide range in the amount of bone erosion present, from no apparent change to cortical destruction. There is little or no periosteal response.

The microscopic appearance of periosteal fibrosarcoma is typically one of a well differentiated and often highly collagenous stroma with only slight hyperchromasia and pleomorphism of the tumor cells (fig. 5.43 B). Mitotic figures are usually rare. It is often difficult to reconcile the relatively innocent histomorphology of some of these tumors with the radiographic evidence of massive bone destruction. Often, the affected animals are submitted to a series of biopsy procedures because the pathologist is unaware of the radiographic and clinical findings in the case and has underdiagnosed the lesion as fibroma or scar tissue.

Maxillary Fibrosarcoma of the Dog

These tumors are typically low grade fibrosarcomas that arise on the outer surface of the maxilla and slowly disfigure the dog's face. They are characterized in most instances by an innocuous histological appearance that belies their destructive nature. Although maxillary fibrosarcoma of the dog is technically a periosteal fibrosar-

coma, it is classified separately from other tumors of this type because of its more frequent occurrence and because there is evidence that it responds to combined radiation hyperthermia therapy.[3,4] Classification of these tumors as low-grade fibrosarcomas is based more on their invasive behavior than on their histological appearance. They are less cellular than conventional canine fibrosarcomas and lack the characteristic pattern of interwoven bundles, suggesting that they may eventually be reclassified as a variant of fibromatosis.[1]

Maxillary fibrosarcomas occur primarily in middle-aged dogs, usually around 7 years of age, and they appear to be most common in the golden retriever, Doberman pinscher and German shepherd breeds.[1] In one large survey of canine bone tumors,[5] 10 of 31 fibrosarcomas involved the maxilla.

Clinically, maxillary fibrosarcomas grow slowly and are initially recognized because of a firm swelling on the side of the face. In time, the tumors cause gross distortion of the face, loosening of teeth, and erosion of the maxilla. In advanced cases, tumor tissue may invade the nasal bone, nasal cavity, hard palate, and orbit (fig. 5.44). Disfigurement and local recurrence after surgery are the usual reasons for euthanasia.

At necropsy, after the skin and soft tissues are removed, the tumor mass remains tightly adhered to the surface of the maxilla (fig. 5.45 A). Transverse serial sections through the head also show that the bulk of the tumor mass lies on the external surface of the maxilla, although tumor tissue may invade the nasal passages at multiple sites and partially compress the turbinates.

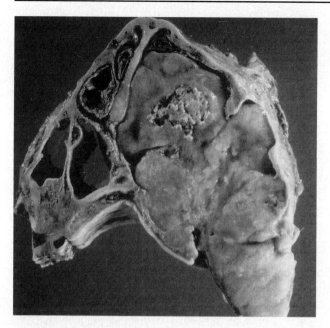

Fig. 5.44. Low grade fibrosarcoma involving the maxillary bone of an 8-year-old cow. The tumor has replaced much of the maxillary bone, filled the maxillary sinus, and encroached on the nasal cavity, replacing the turbinates on one side and causing deviation of the nasal septum. The surface of the maxillary bone has been expanded by the pressure of the tumor, reflecting its slow growth.

The histological appearance of these tumors is often deceiving, especially when one is examining small biopsy specimens. Most tumors are well-differentiated fibroblastic growths (fig. 5.45 B) that are not encapsulated. Tumor tissue slowly infiltrates the adjacent soft tissue and destroys the underlying maxillary bone (fig. 5.45 C). Biopsies of superficial tumor tissue are even more confusing because a mononuclear inflammatory cell infiltrate is often present, and there is fibrous tissue organization of edematous soft tissue in some tumors. In most tumors, areas of higher grade malignancy (fig. 5.45 D) can be found by sampling broadly. Metastasis occurs rarely.

Periosteal Osteosarcoma

These are osteosarcomas that arise on the surface of a bone, presumably from undifferentiated mesenchymal cells in the periosteum, and initially extend outward into the soft tissue. Later, the tumor may invade the underlying cortex and extend into the medullary cavity.

Periosteal osteosarcomas in human patients tend to arise more often on the surface of the diaphysis than on the metaphysis of long bones.[6] The histological pattern includes variable amounts of osteoid, cartilage, and fibrous tissue elements. In general, the neoplastic tissue in the periosteal osteosarcoma is intermediate in differentiation between the more malignant tissue of central osteosarcoma and the well-differentiated tissue of parosteal osteosarcoma. However, areas can be selected from periosteal osteosarcoma that can not be distinguished histologically from central osteosarcoma. Periosteal osteosarcomas are

not so well differentiated that tissue sections should be mistaken for reactive bone. In humans, periosteal osteosarcoma is accompanied by a better prognosis than central osteosarcoma, the incidence of metastasis being approximately 15 percent.[6] Two types of periosteal osteosarcoma have been recognized in dogs.[1] The first (fig. 5.46) is a highly aggressive tumor with the same histological features and biological behavior as central osteosarcoma. Such tumors may actually be central osteosarcomas that have arisen in the outer spongiosa of the metaphysis of a long bone and for some undetermined reason developed an eccentric growth pattern.

The second type of canine periosteal osteosarcoma more closely fits the description of this entity in humans. The number of cases reported in dogs is too small to determine age, sex, or site incidence. Two such tumors are reported on the metaphyseal surface of long bones,[1] rather than on the diaphyseal surface as in humans. Both tumors produced a dense bony matrix, and in neither dog were metastases detected after amputation.

Parosteal (Juxtacortical) Osteosarcoma

Classification

Parosteal osteosarcoma (juxtacortical osteosarcoma or parosteal sarcoma) is a sarcoma on the external surface of a bone and is composed typically of well differentiated but malignant fibrous, osseous, and in some cases cartilaginous, tissues. The neoplasm arises in bone-forming periosteal connective tissue and not in extraskeletal tissues beside the bone, as the name implies. In humans, these tumors are distinguished from the more common central or intramedullary osteosarcomas of bone by a longer clinical course and a higher survival rate. Four reports have indicated that a similar tumor exists in animals.[2,7-9] One of these authors[2] refers to this neoplasm as parosteal osteoma since the tumor is not as frankly malignant as typical cases of osteosarcoma. Currently, parosteal osteosarcoma is a poorly defined entity in domestic animals, and further study is necessary to determine whether this parosteal tumor of animals is analogous to human parosteal osteosarcoma in clinical behavior and in radiographic and histomorphological appearance.

Incidence, Age, Breed, and Sex

Parosteal osteosarcoma is a well recognized but rare tumor in humans, comprising only about 2 percent of primary malignant bone tumors.[10] Its true incidence in animals is unknown as too few cases have been reported. In fact, some large surveys of bone tumors in dogs and cats have not included mention of this tumor. It is unclear whether this reflects the rarity of parosteal osteosarcoma in animals, or it has gone unrecognized. It is also possible that at least some of the tumors diagnosed as parosteal osteosarcomas in animals are misdiagnoses of other primary bone tumors, such

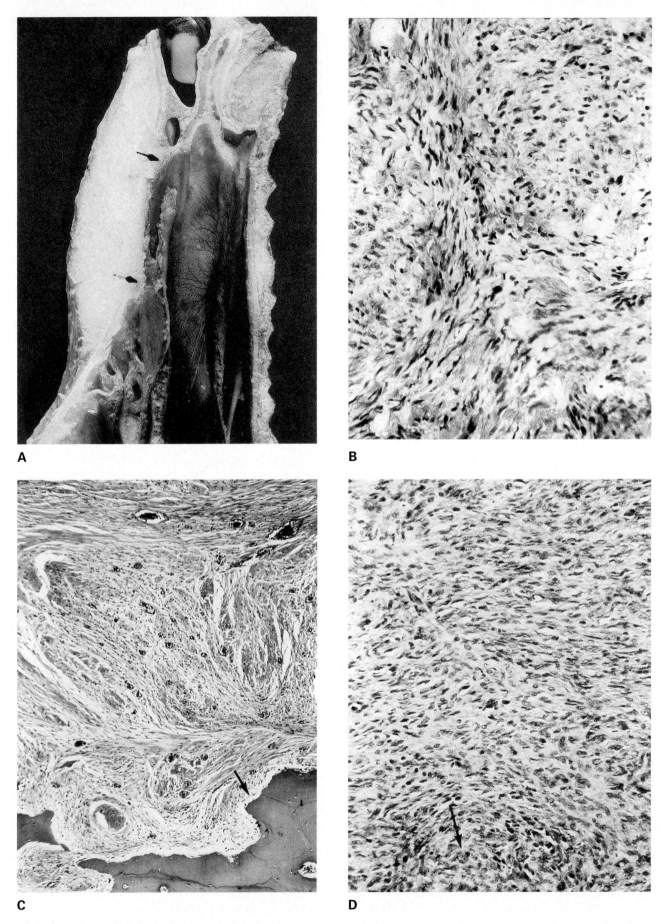

A

B

C

D

Fig. 5.45. Maxillary fibrosarcoma of the dog. **A.** Sagittal section showing intimate association of tumor mass with external surface of maxilla and nasal bones. Note areas of cortical destruction (arrows). **B.** Well-differentiated area of tumor is easily mistaken for reactive fibrosis. **C.** Note destruction of cortical bone (arrow) by well-differentiated fibrosarcoma. **D.** Anaplastic areas (arrow) may be found in some tumors producing very aggressive clinical lesions.

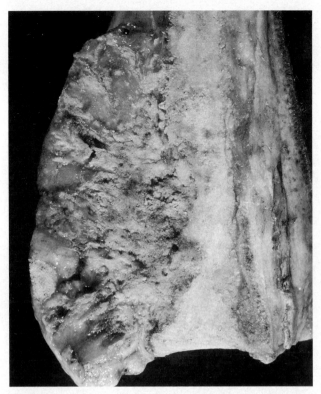

Fig. 5.46. Periosteal osteosarcoma of the distal radius. Rapidly growing, highly malignant osteosarcoma appears to originate in the periosteum, invade the radius, and extend into the soft tissue.

as osteochondroma. One report on the comparative pathology of bone tumors included 31 animal bone tumors fitting this category.[2] There were 14 cases in dogs ranging in age from 6 months to 13 years, with a mean age of 7 years. The dogs were mostly of the large and giant breeds, with about twice as many males as females represented. Eleven cases were found in cats ranging in age from 1 to 13 years, with a mean age of 7 years. Three parosteal osteosarcomas were diagnosed in horses and one each in a pig and a cow. It remains unclear how closely the animal tumors of this report resemble parosteal osteosarcoma of humans.

In a second report, parosteal osteosarcoma was diagnosed in a 10-year-old male German shepherd and a 14-year-old domestic shorthaired cat.[7] Further cases have been reported in six domestic cats ranging in age from 4 to 14 years.[8,9]

Clinical Characteristics

In humans parosteal osteosarcoma has a duration of months to years, producing a slowly expanding lesion that may or may not be painful and tender. Swelling and interference with locomotion can be the major complaints. The tumor tends to recur locally following surgical excision, but survival 5 years after the first surgery is 70–80 percent.[10]

In animals with tumors diagnosed as parosteal osteosarcoma the clinical course is of longer duration than that for central osteosarcoma of bone. The usual clinical finding in animals is the presence of a firm, slowly enlarging mass located on the surface of a bone. The lesion may

not be painful initially, but eventually it produces disfiguration, interferes with function, and may cause lameness. In the horse a tumor diagnosed as parosteal osteosarcoma of the cervical vertebrae caused staggering and partial paralysis.[2]

Sites

The vast majority of parosteal osteosarcomas in human patients occur on long bones, particularly the caudal aspect of the distal femur.[10] This site predilection is not a feature in animals, where parosteal osteosarcomas have been reported on various limb bones[7,8] and on bones of the skull.[9]

Gross Morphology

The surface of the tumor is generally smooth, but it may be multinodular with a dense fibrous capsule. Tumor tissue is firm to hard and gritty. The tumor arises on the cortical surface from either a sessile or pedunculated base. The cortex remains intact until late in the disease process, unlike periosteal osteosarcoma, where cortical invasion occurs relatively early.

Radiographic Appearance

The tumor is located on the surface of the bone (see fig. 5.36 A). It has an evenly contoured border and the underlying cortex and metaphyseal spongiosa remain intact for a long time. Tumor matrix typically makes an amorphous pattern with variations in radiodensity. The base of some tumors may be pedunculated or sessile after the manner of an osteochondroma, but in osteochondroma, the marrow cavity of the adjacent bone typically is continuous with that of the tumor.

Histological Features

In humans many parosteal osteosarcomas, especially early lesions, have an innocent histological character.[10,11] The fibro-osseous and occasionally the cartilaginous stromal elements more closely resemble reactive tissue than a neoplastic proliferation. Cellularity is generally low, but areas of moderate cell density are also present. There may be little or no pleomorphism of tumor cells, and typically no mitotic figures are found. Diagnosis is based in large part on the characteristic radiographic appearance of the lesion and appropriate clinical findings.

The microscopic appearance of parosteal osteosarcomas in animals needs further clarification. The diagnostic criterion in one study was the finding of a periosteal tumor with a neoplastic stroma in which the cells were too pleomorphic for a benign tumor, yet lacked the marked pleomorphism, cellular density, and mitotic activity of a frankly malignant tumor.[2] More advanced lesions approximated the gross and microscopic appearance of osteosarcoma. Chondrocytes with malignant features were present in the fibrocartilaginous and osseous tissues that made up the apical tissue, whereas the marrow spaces of the bony stalk contained fibrous tissue instead of fatty and hematopoietic marrow.

The histomorphology of the primary tumors of the feline and canine patients in another report resembled central osteosarcoma.[7] A biopsy of the lesion in the dog taken early in the course of the disease suggested osteosarcoma; however, at death the pulmonary metastases were those of chondrosarcoma. Parosteal osteosarcoma involving the humerus and distal scapula with pulmonary metastases is reported in one cat,[12] but no metastases were present in another cat with parosteal osteosarcoma involving the mandible.[9] The diversity in the histological descriptions and behavior of parosteal osteosarcoma in animals lends support to the possibility that not all such reports are of tumors that comfortably fit this classification.

In parosteal osteosarcomas examined by the authors (fig. 5.47 A,B,C), the tumor consists of haphazard fibro-osseous tissue centered on the cortical surface. Bony trabeculae formed by the fibrous tissue have no consistent pattern of orientation and tumor cells resembling fibroblasts have no anaplastic features (fig. 5.47 B,C).

Growth and Metastasis

Parosteal osteosarcomas demonstrate slow but continuous growth on the surface of a bone. In time, the tumor may acquire a more aggressive clinical behavior and will invade the cortex and extend into a medullary cavity. Pulmonary metastasis may occur, but only many months after the clinical disease first becomes apparent.

Extraskeletal Osteosarcoma

Osteosarcomas occasionally arise in soft tissue sites of dogs in the absence of a primary bone lesion.[13-15] In one report of 169 extraskeletal osteosarcomas over a 10-year period,[14] 64 percent were in the mammary gland, and the remainder originated in the gastrointestinal tract, subcutaneous tissues, spleen, urinary tract, liver, skin, muscle, eye, or thyroid gland. In another study, extraskeletal osteosarcomas comprised only about 1 percent of all osteosarcomas,[13] although osteosarcomas of mammary and thyroid origin were excluded from this survey. Osteosarcomas occurring in the esophagus in association with *Spirocerca lupi* infestation were also excluded. In general, extraskeletal osteosarcomas occur in older dogs than skeletal osteosarcomas (mean age 10.6–11.5 years) and show no apparent predilection for large breeds.[13-15] Although distant metastases are common, the lungs are involved less often than in skeletal osteosarcomas, and death is usually due to either local recurrence or euthanasia at the time of diagnosis. The mean survival time is reported to be lower than for skeletal osteosarcomas, in part due to the later detection of intra-abdominal tumors and limited surgical options for tumors at some sites.[14]

Extraskeletal osteosarcoma appears to be less common in cats than in dogs, but it has been reported in the eye of cats following ocular trauma[16,17] and in the mammary area of a 12-year-old cat.[18] In the latter case, the tumor recurred following surgical removal, and widespread lung metastases were detected at necropsy.

REFERENCES

1. Pool, R.R. (1990) Tumors of bone and cartilage. In Moulton J.E. (ed.), *Tumors in Domestic Animals,* 3rd ed., University of California Press, Berkeley.
2. Jacobson, S.A. (1971) *The Comparative Pathology of the Tumors of Bone.* Charles C. Thomas, Springfield, IL.
3. Slayter, M.V., Boosinger, T.R., Pool, R.R., DÑmmrich, K., Misdorp, W., and Larsen, S. (1994) *Histological Classification of Bone and Joint Tumors of Domestic Animals.* World Health Organization. 2nd series, vol. 1. Armed Forces Institute of Pathology, American Registry of Pathology, Washington D.C.
4. Brewer, W.G., and Turrel, J.M. (1982) Radiotherapy and hyperthermia in the treatment of fibrosarcomas in the dog. *J Amer Vet Med Assoc* 181:146–150.
5. Liu, S.K., Dorfman, H.D., Hurvitz, A.L., and Patnaik, A.K. (1977) Primary and secondary bone tumors in the dog. *J Small Anim Pract* 18:313–326.
6. Bertoni, F., Boriani, S., Laus, M., and Campanacci, M. (1982) Periosteal chondrosarcoma and periosteal osteosarcoma. Two distinct entities. *J Bone Joint Surg* 64B:370–376.
7. Banks, W.C. (1971) parosteal osteosarcoma in a dog and a cat. *J Amer Vet Med Assoc* 158:1412–1415.
8. Turrel, J.M., and Pool, R.R. (1982) Primary bone tumors in the cat: A retrospective study of 15 cats and a literature review. *Vet Radiol* 23:152–166.
9. Liu, S.K., and Dorfman, H.D. (1974) The cartilage analogue of fibromatosis (juvenile aponeurtoic fibroma) in dogs. *Vet Pathol* 11:60–67.
10. Schajowicz, F. (1981) *Tumors and Tumor-like Lesions of Bone and Joints.* Springer-Verlag, New York, pp. 95–103.
11. Resnick, D., Kyriakos, M., and Greenway, G.G. (1994) Tumors and tumor-like lesions of bone: Imaging and pathology of specific lesions. In Resnick, D. (ed.), *Diagnosis of Bone and Joint Disorders,* 3rd ed. Vol. 6, ch. 83. W.B. Saunders, Philadelphia, pp. 3688–3697.
12. Griffith, J.W., Dubielzig, R.R., Riser, W.H., and Jezyk, P. (1984) Parosteal osteosarcoma with pulmonary metastases in a cat. *Vet Pathol* 21:123–125.
13. Patnaik, A.K. (1990) Canine extraskeletal osteosarcoma and chondrosarcoma: A clinicopathologic study of 14 cases. *Vet Pathol* 27:46–55.
14. Lagenbach. A., Anderson, M.A., Dambach, D.M., Sorenmo, K.U., and Shofer, F.D. (1998) Extraskeletal osteosarcoma in dogs: A retrospective study of 169 cases (1986–1996). *J Amer Anim Hosp Assoc* 34: 113–120.
15. Kuntz, C.A., Dernell, W.S., Powers, B.E., and Withrow, S. (1998) Extraskeletal osteosarcomas in dogs: 14 cases. *J Amer Anim Hosp Assoc* 34:26–30.
16. Woog, J., Albert, D.M., Gonder, J.R., and Carpenter, J.L. (1983) Osteosarcoma in a phthisical feline eye. *Vet Pathol* 20:209–214.
17. Miller, W.W., and Boosinger, T.R (1987) Intraocular osteosarcoma in a cat. *J Amer Anim Hosp Assoc* 23:317–320.
18. Easton, C.B. (1994) Extraskeletal osteosarcoma in a cat. *J Amer Anim Hosp Assoc* 30:59–61.

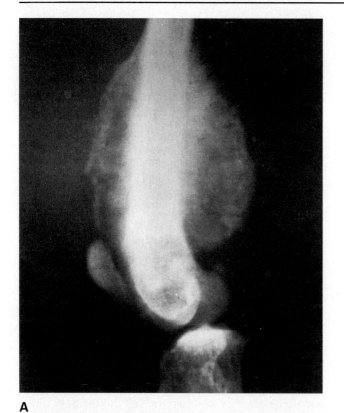

A

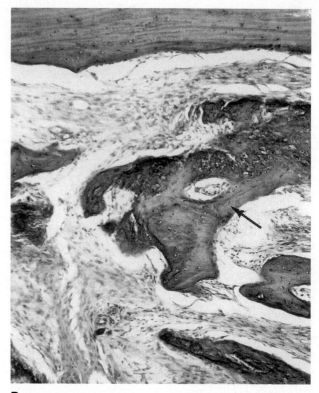

B

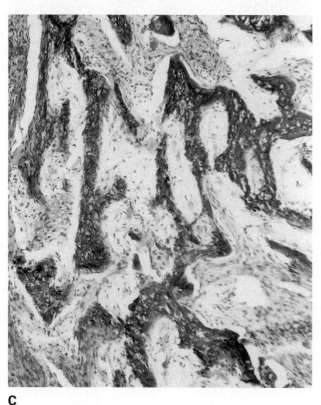

C

Fig. 5.47. Parosteal osteosarcoma. **A.** Radiograph of tumor arising from the cortical surface of the distal femur. Note the evenly contoured surface of the tumor. **B.** Tumor lying adjacent to the cortical surface (top) is a low grade spindle cell tumor that produces crude spicules of woven bone, some of which have been remodeled and partially replaced by lamellar bone tissue (arrow). **C.** Tissue from periphery of tumor is composed of a haphazard pattern of woven bone spicules formed by fusiform tumor cells without anaplastic features.

SECONDARY TUMORS OF BONE

Malignant neoplasms originating in soft tissues or in the skeleton itself may secondarily involve bones either by direct extension or by hematogenous metastasis. Secondary bone tumor may also refer to a bone tumor that has arisen in a preexisting lesion, for example, malignant transformation of an osteochondroma to a chondrosarcoma or an osteosarcoma as discussed previously in this chapter. In this section, discussion will be restricted to metastatic and invasive tumors involving bones, although invasion of a soft tissue tumor into an adjacent bone is not always considered to represent a secondary bone tumor.

Local bone destruction is a feature of many infiltrating neoplasms, especially tumors arising in mucous membranes of the heads of animals. Familiar examples are malignant melanoma, carcinoma, and fibrosarcoma of the oral cavity and carcinoma of the nasal cavity and conjunctiva. Soft tissue tumors that are less common causes of local bone destruction include carcinoma of the nail bed of dogs and cats, fibrosarcoma, hemangiosarcoma, rhabdomyosarcoma, and synovial sarcoma. These tumors are centered on soft tissue and tend to produce bone destruction late in the course of the disease. With the possible exception of certain nasal tumors, the clinician can usually distinguish between invasive tumors of soft tissue and primary bone tumor.

Metastatic Bone Disease

The skeleton is one of the most frequent sites of tumor metastasis in humans.[1] In fact, skeletal metastases of mammary, prostatic, and pulmonary carcinomas are more common than primary bone tumors.[1] In contrast, metastatic tumors of the skeleton of animals are generally considered much less common than primary bone tumors.[2,3] Although there does appear to be a genuine difference between the frequency of skeletal metastases in humans and domestic animals, metastatic bone disease in animals is likely to be much more common than realized. The skeleton of animals with malignancies at other sites is seldom examined in detail, either radiographically or during necropsy, and skeletal metastases could easily be missed.[2,3] Skeletal metastases were identified in 5.8 percent of dogs with metastatic carcinoma in one survey,[4] but since less than 20 percent of the dogs underwent bone scan, skeletal radiography, or necropsy, the true prevalence was considered to be much greater. In another study,[5] 98 dogs with a variety of carcinomas were subjected to thorough examination of the skeleton at necropsy. The spine, pelvis, and long bones were sectioned longitudinally, and the ribs were inspected visually. Macroscopic metastases were detected in 21 (21.4 percent) of the 98 dogs, and presumably, the prevalence would have been even higher had the bones been scanned or radiographed. Furthermore, only macroscopically visible lesions were examined histologically, and the presence of micrometastases was not evaluated.[5] The most common primary tumor sites in dogs with skeletal metastases are the mammary gland, thyroid, prostate, ovary, and lung, but metastatic carcinomas and sarcomas from a variety of other organs have been detected in the skeleton.[2-6] In dogs, metastatic sarcomas of bone are less common than carcinomas.[5] Information on the prevalence of skeletal metastases in cats is scarce, but there are occasional reports of pulmonary and mammary carcinomas metastasizing to the bones of cats.[3,7,8]

In dogs, the most frequent sites for bone metastases are the ribs, vertebrae, and proximal long bones.[2-6] As in humans,[1] metastases are uncommon in bones distal to the elbow or stifle of dogs. This may, at least partly, reflect the greater vascular supply of bones involved in active hematopoiesis, but anatomical characteristics are also likely to be involved. For example, anastomoses between the venous drainage of the prostate gland and paravertebral veins may account for the high prevalence of vertebral metastases in men with prostatic carcinoma.[9] A predilection for the vertebral column is also seen for osseous metastases of prostatic carcinoma in dogs.[5] The skeletal distribution of metastatic carcinoma in cats more frequently involves the distal limbs (acrometastases).[7,8] In one study,[7] multiple digital metastases were found in four of nine cats with metastatic bronchial carcinoma. Metastasis of a mammary carcinoma to the talus of a cat is also reported.[8] The reason for this apparent species difference is not clear, but it may relate either to an increased blood flow to the limbs of cats, in order to dissipate body heat from the footpads, or possibly to hemodynamic changes associated with traumatic injury to the feet.[8]

Secondary bone tumors generally produce osteolytic lesions that are difficult, if not impossible, to distinguish radiographically from the lesions of primary bone tumors.[2,3] This may contribute to the underdiagnosis of secondary bone tumors in cases where the radiographic diagnosis is not confirmed by histological or cytological examination of biopsy specimens. In a report of 20 metastatic bone tumors in dogs,[3] the radiographic diagnosis was primary bone tumor in all but one case. Most lesions were osteolytic and were accompanied by extensive periosteal new bone formation.[3] In some cases, a proliferative osteoblastic reaction within the tumor is associated with areas of increased radiographic density.

Dogs with skeletal metastases tend to be older than dogs with primary tumors of bones (median age 8.5 to 10 years), and there is no obvious breed or size predilection.[2,4-6] Unlike primary bone sarcomas, metastatic skeletal carcinomas were found most commonly in dogs weighing less than 25 kg.[4] Approximately 30 percent of such tumors can be found in small dogs weighing less than 15 kg.[2,4,5] Clinical signs vary with the bone involved and the stage of the disease, but in many cases signs relating to the bone lesions, including lameness, progressive paresis, and pathological fracture, will be the initial clinical manifestation.[4]

Definitive diagnosis of metastatic bone tumor requires cytological or histological examination of fine needle aspirates or tissue biopsies, respectively, but in most cases these techniques will not provide a reliable indication of the tissue of origin. Even after thorough postmortem examination, the primary site of metastatic skeletal carcinomas is often not apparent.[4] However, malignant epithelial cells within a skeletal lesion (fig. 5.48 A,B) can only be derived from an extraskeletal carcinoma. In one report, all carcinomas that metastasized to bone also metastasized to soft tissues[5]. Poorly organized reactive bone is commonly present in association with both primary and metastatic bone tumors (fig. 5.48 A) and should not be misinterpreted as tumor bone, leading to an incorrect diagnosis of osteosarcoma. The histological appearance may be further complicated in cases where a metastatic tumor has predisposed to pathological fracture, as the early fracture callus has many features in common with osteosarcoma.

Osteosarcomas may metastasize from the bone of origin to other skeletal sites, in which case the secondary lesions may be in atypical locations and may appear to have been present for different lengths of time.[6] For some sarcomas, such as hemangiosarcoma, which may originate in bone or other tissues, it may be impossible to determine whether skeletal involvement is primary or secondary. If the tumor is present in several skeletal sites, metastasis is more likely; but in reality, the distinction is purely academic.

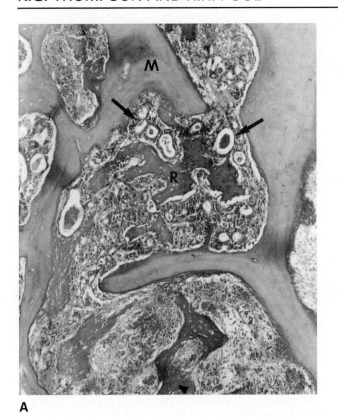
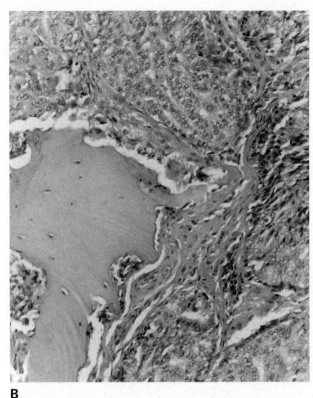

A   **B**

Fig. 5.48.   Gastric carcinoma metastatic to the vertebral body of a dog. **A.** Tumor cells are forming glandular structures (arrows) in the marrow cavity between trabeculae of mature bone *(M)* and more basophilic spicules of reactive woven bone *(R)*. Poorly organized reactive bone forms in response to many types of bone injury, including neoplastic and inflammatory conditions, and should not be misinterpreted as "tumor" bone. **B.** Higher magnification showing closely packed cords of neoplastic epithelial cells replacing the normal marrow tissue. The fragment of lamellar, trabecular bone is undergoing resorption as indicated by its scalloped border and the presence of osteoclasts.

Invasive Tumors of Bones

Malignant tumors in soft tissues adjacent to a bone may penetrate the bone by direct extension. Although not generally regarded as secondary tumors of bone, some types of tumor appear to have an affinity for bone invasion and warrant mention in this section. Squamous cell carcinoma of the digits and oral cavity in dogs and cats are aggressive tumors, which frequently invade the periosteum of the underlying bone, erode the cortex, and penetrate the medullary cavity.[6,10,11] In dogs, bone invasion is reported to occur in 77 percent of oral squamous cell carcinomas.[12] Radiographic changes include cortical erosion, periosteal new bone formation, and variable lysis of medullary bone. Histologically, columns of anaplastic epithelial cells, showing evidence of squamous differentiation, permeate the osseous and extraosseous tissues; they are accompanied either by an osteoblastic reaction or a prominent fibroblastic response with osteoclastic resorption of adjacent bone (figs. 5.49).[10,11] Squamous cell carcinomas of the canine digit not only invade bone but also metastasize to local lymph nodes, and eventually to the lungs.

Malignant melanomas of the oral cavity of dogs invade bone in approximately 50 percent of cases,[12] in addi-tion to metastasizing by both the lymphatic and hematogenous routes. Similarly, fibrosarcomas of the canine skull and long bones frequently invade the adjacent bone.[6,11,12] Bone invasion is reported in 68 percent of oral fibrosarcomas in dogs.[12] However, some of these cases probably represent periosteal or maxillary fibrosarcomas and could therefore be considered primary rather than secondary tumors of bone. Tumors of dental origin, including acanthomatous epulis, ameloblastoma, and fibroameloblastoma, may also extend to involve the maxilla or mandible of dogs and cats.

Benign soft tissue tumors in close contact with bone surfaces may induce a reactive periosteal response and cortical erosion without invading the bone. This occurs in parosteal lipoma of humans, a rare form of lipoma that originates close to the periosteal surface of bones. This tumor has also been reported in a dog.[13] These lipomas are similar to those occurring in the subcutis, and their effect on the adjacent bone presumably relates to local pressure rather than to any invasive tendency. In humans, noninfiltrating and infiltrating forms of angiolipoma are reported in the spinal canal,[14] the latter being characterized by pressure erosion and infiltration of adjacent vertebrae. Extradural angiolipoma associated with lysis of the second

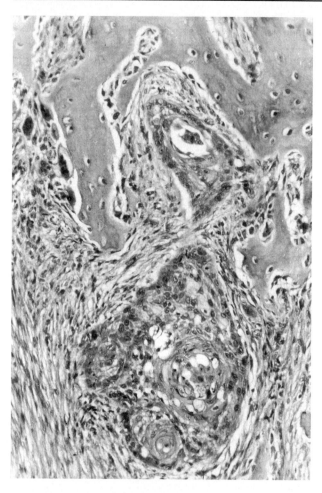

Fig. 5.49. Squamous cell carcinoma invading the maxilla of a cat. Clusters of neoplastic epithelial cells undergoing squamous differentiation are present within the bone. The prominent fibroblastic response generally accompanies osseous invasion by this tumor.

lumbar vertebra has been reported in a dog with paraparesis.[15] Radiographic and macroscopic changes suggested malignancy, but histologically the tumor appeared benign. The bone lysis associated with such tumors is probably due to chronic pressure atrophy and remodeling rather than to aggressive invasion.

REFERENCES

1. Resnick, D., and Niwayama, G (1994) Skeletal metastases. In Resnick, D. (ed.), *Diagnosis of Bone and Joint Disorders,* 3rd ed. Vol. 6, ch. 85, W.B. Saunders, Philadelphia, pp. 3991–4064.
2. Brodey, R.S., Reid, C.F., and Sauer, R.M. (1966) Metastatic bone neoplasms in the dog. *J Amer Vet Med Assoc* 148:29–48.
3. Kas, N.P., van der Heul, R.O., and Misdorp, W. (1970) Metastatic bone neoplasms in dogs, cats and a lion. *Zbl Vet Med* A17:909–919.
4. Cooley, D.M., and Waters, D.J. (1998) Skeletal metastasis as the initial clinical manifestation of metastatic carcinoma in 19 dogs. *J Vet Int Med* 12:288–293.
5. Goedegebuure, S.A. (1979) Secondary bone tumors in the dog. *Vet Pathol* 16:520–529.
6. Russell, R.G., and Walker, M. (1983) metastatic and invasive tumors of bone in dogs and cats. *Vet Clin N Amer Small Anim Pract* 13:163–180.
7. May, C., and Newsholme, S.J. (1989) Metastasis of feline pulmonary carcinoma presenting as multiple digital swelling. *J Small Anim Pract* 30:302–310.
8. Waters, D.J., Honeckman, A., Cooley, D.M., and DeNicola, D. (1998) Skeletal metastases in feline mammary carcinoma: case report and literature review. *J Amer Anim Hosp Assoc* 34:103–108.
9. Orr, F.W., Sanchez-Sweatman, O.H., Kostenuik, P., and Singh, G. (1995) Tumor-bones interactions in skeletal metastasis. *Clin Orthop Rel Res* 312:19–33.
10. Liu. S.K., and Dorfman, H.D. (1974) The cartilage analogue of fibromatosis (juvenile aponeurotic fibroma) in dogs. *Vet Pathol* 11:60–67.
11. Liu, S.K., Dorfman, H.D., Hurvitz, A.L., and Patnaik, A.K. (1977) Primary and secondary bone tumors in the dog. *J Small Anim Pract* 18:313–326.
12. Todoroff, R.J., and Brodey, R.S. (1979) Oral and pharangeal neoplasia in the dog: A retrospective survey of 361 cases. *J Amer Vet Med Assoc* 175:567–571.
13. Doige, C.C. (1980) Parosteal lipoma in a dog. *J Amer Anim Hosp Assoc* 16:87–92.
14. Pagni, C.A., and Canavero, S. (1992) Spinal epidural angiolipoma: Rare or unreported? *Neurosurgery* 31:758–763.
15. Reif, U., Lowrie, C.T., and Fitzgerald, S.D. (1998) Extradural spinal angiolipoma associated with bone lysis in a dog. *J Amer Anim Hosp Assoc* 34:373–376.

TUMOR-LIKE LESIONS OF BONE

There are several nonneoplastic conditions in man and animals that simulate primary or secondary bone tumors. The most common of these are included here as differential diagnoses for bone tumors.

Fibrous Dysplasia

One such lesion is fibrous dysplasia, which is probably a developmental abnormality of bone-forming mesenchyme rather than a neoplasm. Fibrous dysplasia is discussed earlier in this chapter in association with osteoma and ossifying fibroma because of its morphological similarity to those two tumors.

Exuberant Fracture Callus

An exuberant fracture callus may also resemble certain bone tumors on radiographic and gross appearance. Furthermore, histological and cytological examination of biopsy specimens from an early fracture callus may be mistakenly interpreted as osteosarcoma by an inexperienced pathologist, especially if the sample is not accompanied by an adequate history.

Cysts

Solitary (Unicameral) Bone Cysts

Cysts of various types occur in bones and may be difficult, or impossible, to distinguish from certain bone tumors radiographically. Solitary or unicameral bone cysts are reported in the metaphyses of long bones in young dogs[1,2] and in children.[3] A breed predisposition has been suggested in doberman pinschers.[1] The lesions, which may be monostotic or polyostotic, are generally lytic and expansile, with narrowing of the cortex and little or no periosteal new bone formation. In radiographs, shelves of bone often project from the cyst wall, but in most cases these are incomplete and the cysts are unicameral.[1] Pathological fracture is often associated with the lesion due to the localized bone destruction. The cyst cavity is filled with clear or sanguineous fluid and lined by a connective tissue membrane of variable thickness, with scattered multinucleate giant cells and hemosiderin-containing macrophages. Unicameral cysts seldom recur after surgical drainage and curettage.[1] Their pathogenesis is uncertain, but current opinion favors impaired venous drainage from sites of active endochondral ossification.[3]

Aneurysmal Bone Cysts

Aneurysmal bone cysts occur much less often in animals than in people, but they have been reported rarely in dogs,[4-6] cats,[7-9] and horses[10-12] and in a bull.[13] Radiographically, they appear as expansile, osteolytic lesions contained by a thin, *ballooned* periosteum; they have an internal *soap-bubble* appearance (fig. 5.50 A). Pathological fracture may be present. Such lesions must be differentiated from osteosarcoma, hemangiosarcoma, fibrosarcoma, and plasma cell myeloma. In humans, aneurysmal bone cysts occur most often in the tubular bones and spine, within the first three decades of life.[3] Too few cases are reported in animals to establish an age or site prevalence, although lesions are described in bones of both the axial and appendicular skeleton. The gross appearance of aneurysmal bone cysts closely resembles telangiectatic osteosarcoma and hemangiosarcoma, typically exuding blood from the cut surface, and may contain solid areas in addition to multiple, blood filled cysts. Fine needle aspiration biopsies are unlikely to yield diagnostically useful samples from either aneurysmal or unicameral bone cysts. Confirmation of the diagnosis requires histopathological examination of biopsy specimens. The cavernous spaces of aneurysmal bone cysts are separated by septa of loosely arranged spindle cells with scattered multinucleate giant cells and hemosiderin-containing macrophages (fig. 5.50 B,C), similar to the lining of unicameral bone cysts. Osteoid may be present in some areas, but it is typical of that produced in reactive bone lesions. The pathogenesis of these lesions is not known, but altered blood flow, perhaps secondary to trauma or some other bone disease such as malignancy, is believed to play a role.[3] The majority of human cases however, arise de novo, without any evidence of a predisposing lesion. In one equine case,[12] the demonstration (by immunohistochemical staining) of alpha–smooth muscle actin in the wall of an aneurysmal bone cyst supported a vascular origin, possibly through passive dilation of an arteriovenous shunt or interference with venous drainage.

Subchondral (Juxtacortical) Bone Cysts

Subchondral (juxtacortical) bone cysts occur in young horses,[14] pigs, and less commonly, in other species as a manifestation of osteochondrosis. The lesions are typically 5 to 10 mm in diameter and may be multilocular. In horses, subchondral cysts are found most frequently beneath the articular surfaces of phalanges, but they also occur in femoral condyles and a range of other bones. The cysts may develop either from residual nodules of epiphyseal cartilage or within foci of subarticular hemorrhage. Histologically, the lesions are not always cystic, instead consisting of fibrous tissue with extensive myxoid matrix or, in some cases, degenerate cartilage. Cystic spaces lined by fibrous tissue and containing fluid, possibly of synovial origin, are present within some lesions. In humans, subchondral cysts occur in association with degenerative joint disease and are thought to be secondary to either synovial fluid intrusion or bony contusion.[15]

Intraosseous Epidermoid Cysts

Intraosseous epidermoid cysts are reported rarely as a cause of lytic lesions in the distal phalanx of dogs[16,17] and must be differentiated from nail bed carcinomas, malignant melanomas, and osteomyelitis. One case is also reported in the tenth thoracic vertebral body of a dog.[16] Similar lesions occur in the distal phalanx and skull of humans.[3] Radiographically, there may be a sclerotic reaction around one or more lytic foci and extensive proliferation of periosteal bone (fig. 5.51 A). The cut surface of an affected bone reveals multilocular cysts containing pale cream, crumbly material. Histologically, the cysts are lined by well-differentiated, stratified squamous, keratinizing epithelium and filled with layers of keratinized squames (fig. 5.51 B). The squamous epithelium may show marked pseudoepithelomatous hyperplasia and could be mistaken for squamous cell carcinoma if an inadequate biopsy sample is received for microscopic examination. The cysts are generally supported by a dense fibrous stroma and surrounded by thickened bone trabec-

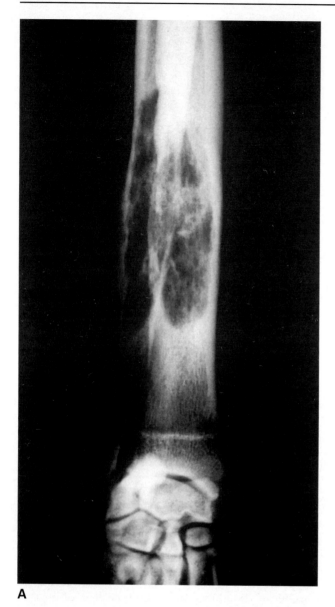

A

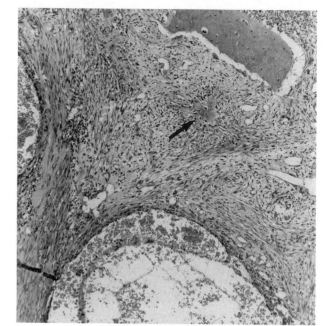

B

C

Fig. 5.50. Aneurysmal bone cyst in a 1-year-old Labrador retriever. **A.** Expansile, osteolytic lesions involving the distal diaphyseal regions of the radius and ulna. **B.** Cavernous spaces containing blood are surrounded by sheets of loose connective tissue within which there are occasional foci of reactive bone (arrow). The larger island of bone is a remnant of either cortical or trabecular bone. **C.** Lining of one of the cysts with a fibroblastic stroma and scattered multinucleate giant cells (arrows).

ulae. The pathogenesis of intraosseous epidermoid cysts is uncertain, but the digital lesions are believed to be secondary to a penetrating wound, with traumatic implantation of epidermal fragments into the underlying bone.[3] Cysts involving the skull of humans and vertebral body of a dog may represent nests of heterotopic ectoderm that have become sequestered along lines of closure during embryonic development.

REFERENCES

1. Carrig, C.B., and Seawright, A.A. (1969) A familial canine polyostotic fibrous dysplasia with subperiosteal cortical defects. *J Small Anim Pract* 10:397–405.
2. Schrader, S.C, Burk, R.L., and Liu, S.K. (1983) Bone cysts in two dogs and a review of similar cystic lesions in the dog. *J Amer Vet Med Assoc* 182:490–495.

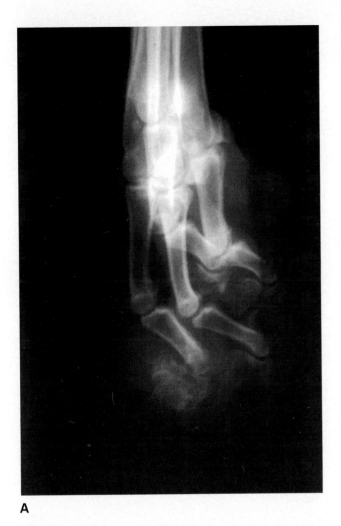

A

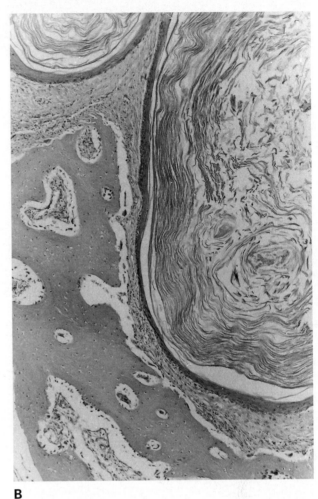

B

Fig. 5.51. Intraosseous epidermoid cysts in a dog. **A.** The third phalanx in one of the digits is replaced by a proliferative bony reaction, which contains several lytic foci. **B.** Large cystic space filled with keratinized squames and lined by a stratified squamous epithelium.

3. Resnick, D., Kyriakos, M., and Greenway, G.G. (1994) Tumors and tumor-like lesions of bone: Imaging and pathology of specific lesions. In Resnick, D. (ed.), *Diagnosis of Bone and Joint Disorders,* 3rd ed. Vol. 6, ch. 83. W.B. Saunders, Philadelphia, pp. 3628–3938.

4. Bowles, M.H.Y., and Freeman, K. (1986) Aneurysmal bone cyst in the ischia and pubes of a dog: A case report and literature review. *J Amer Anim Hosp Assoc* 23:423–427.

5. Pernell, R., Dunstan, R., and DeCamp, C. (1992) Aneurysmal bone cyst in a 6-month-old dog. *J Amer Vet Med Assoc* 201:1897–1899.

6. Shiroma, J.T., Weisbrode, S.E., Biller, D.S., and Olmstead, M.L. (1993) Pathological fracture of an aneurysmal bone cyst in a lumbar vertebra of a dog. *J Amer Anim Hosp Assoc* 29:434–437.

7. Liu, S.K., Dorfman, H.D. (1974) The cartilage analogue of fibromatosis (juvenile aponeurotic fibroma) in dogs. *Vet Pathol* 11:60–67.

8. Walker, M.A., Duncan, J.R., Shaw, J.W., and Chapman, W.W. (1975) Aneurysmal bone cyst in a cat. *J Amer Vet Med Assoc* 167:933–934.

9. Biller, D.S., Johnson, G.C., Birchard, S.J., and Fingland, R.B. (1987) Aneurysmal bone cyst in the rib of a cat. *J Amer Vet Med Assoc* 190:1193–1195.

10. Steiner, J.V., and Rendano, V.T. (1982) Aneurysmal bone cyst in the horse. *Cornell Vet* 72:57–63.

11. Lamb, C., and Schelling, S. (1989) Congenital aneurysmal bone cyst in the horse. *Equine Vet J* 21:130–132.

12. Momiyama, N., Tagami, M., et al. (1999) Aneurysmal bone cyst in a colt. *Equine Vet Educ* 11:243–246.

13. Belknap, E.B., Brodie, S., Lowry, J., and Getzelman, R. (1992) Aeurysmal bone cyst in a Holstein bull. *J Amer Vet Med Assoc* 201:1413–1415.

14. McIlwraith, C.W. (1982) Subchondral cystic lesions (osteochondrosis) in the horse. *Comp Cont Educ* 4:S282–S291.

15. Resnick, D., and Niwayama, G. (1994) Degenerative disease of extraspinal locations. In Resnick, D. (ed.), *Diagnosis of Bone and Joint Disorders,* 3rd ed. Vol. 3, ch. 39. W.B. Saunders, Philadelphia, pp. 1271–1278,

16. Liu, S.K., and Dorfman, H.D. (1974) Intraosseous epidermoid cysts in two dogs. *Vet Pathol* 11:230–234.

17. Homer, B.H., Ackerman, N., Woody, B.J., and Green R.W. (1992) Intraosseous epidermoid cysts in the distal phalanx of two dogs. *Vet Radiol Ultrasound* 33:133–137.

6 Tumors of Muscle

B. J. Cooper and B. A. Valentine

Muscle tissue occurs within many systems of the body and includes both striated (skeletal and cardiac) and smooth muscle. Skeletal muscle forms the postural, loco-motory, abdominal, and respiratory muscles (diaphragm, intercostal, and laryngeal) as well as part of the digestive system (tongue, pharynx, and part of the esophagus in the dog and cat). Cardiac muscle occurs only within the heart. Smooth muscle is widely dispersed throughout the body and is found in the tunics of the gastrointestinal and geni-tourinary tracts, in the tracheobronchial tree, in the vascular system, in the skin associated with hair follicles (arrector pilae muscles), and even within the uveal tract of the eye. As a result, there is a wide range of possible expression of myogenic tumors within the body.

The use of cell culture techniques and specific cell markers has indicated that pluripotential cells of such diverse lineage as germ cell, neural crest, and mesenchyme can undergo myogenic differentiation. Although light microscopic features are still useful for identification of myogenic tumors, in many instances a definitive diagnosis may rely on application of electron microscopic and/or immunohistochemical techniques. Separate sections describe both the electron microscopic features and the most useful immunohistochemical procedures for diagnosis and differentiation of tumors of smooth muscle and of striated muscle.

The information provided in this chapter is based on a review of the literature, the authors' own experience, and a search conducted of the pathology files of the College of Veterinary Medicine at Cornell University for a period of 20 years, during which time approximately 83,000 tumor diagnoses were made. All tumors with a diagnosis of rhabdomyoma or rhabdomyosarcoma were reviewed and subjected to immunohistochemical studies, but only a representative sample of the smooth muscle tumors were reviewed and immunostained.

TUMORS OF SMOOTH MUSCLE
General Considerations
Classification and General Histological Features

Tumors composed primarily of smooth muscle have been traditionally divided into benign tumors (leiomyomas) or malignant tumors (leiomyosarcomas). The recent recognition of fibroblastic and/or neural differentiation in gastrointestinal tumors designated as tumors of smooth muscle origin by routine light microscopy has resulted in the entirely new classification of nonlymphoid mesenchymal tumors of the gastrointestinal tract as gastrointestinal stromal tumors.[1] Smooth muscle tumors (leiomyoma and leiomyosarcoma) are, however, still the most common type of gastrointestinal stromal tumor. The differentiation of leiomyoma from leiomyosarcoma can generally be made with reasonable certainty based on gross and light microscopic features. Mitotic index and determination of nucleolar organizer regions have both been shown to be useful in distinguishing benign from malignant smooth muscle tumors.[2] Mitotic index is clearly more easily determined as a routine procedure.

Leiomyomas are discrete, nonencapsulated, noninvasive tumors. Characteristic features are a relatively homogeneous population of densely packed spindle cells with indistinguishable cytoplasmic borders and elongate, blunt-ended (cigar shaped) nuclei, arranged in broad interlacing fascicles that mimic normal smooth muscle tissue (figs. 6.1 A-C). Fascicles are often described as intersecting at 90 degree angles, forming a *herringbone* pattern, but in our experience this feature is neither consistent nor pathognomonic. There may be alternating "bands" created by cutting cells longitudinally or transversely. The cytoplasm may be strongly eosinophilic. Vacuolization, similar to that seen in

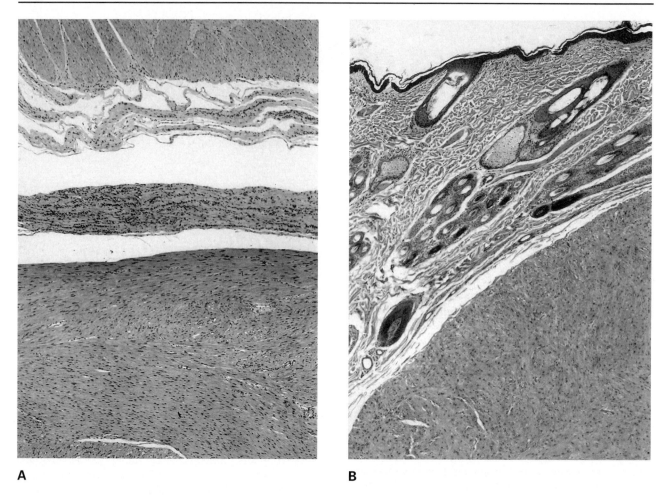

A   B

Fig. 6.1.   Leiomyoma. **A.** Gastric leiomyoma from a dog showing clear demarcation between the tumor at the bottom of the figure and the normal gastric smooth muscle at the top. **B.** Cutaneous leiomyoma from a ferret forming a compressive encapsulated dermal nodule. (continued)

hypertrophic smooth muscle, may also be seen. Variation from this "typical" histological pattern occurs, however, particularly in cutaneous leiomyomas, in which cells may be more heterogeneous, with scattered binucleate or multinucleate cells and moderate anisokaryosis (fig. 6.1 D). Mitoses are uncommon; in one study the average mitotic index of canine leiomyomas was only 0.05 [5 mitoses/ 100 high power (HP)(400x) fields].[2] Although large tumors may have surface ulceration, these tumors do not typically undergo necrosis. Well-differentiated leiomyomas may be difficult to distinguish from normal smooth muscle, but the presence of a nodular mass, often with some degree of disorientation of cells, characterizes the mass as a tumor.

Leiomyosarcomas, in contrast, are nonencapsulated and frequently invasive tumors. Histological features are quite variable. These tumors may be formed by densely packed, relatively homogenous spindle cells that retain many features of normal smooth muscle cells and tissue, or by more pleomorphic spindle to ovoid or round cells with variable histological patterns. Mitoses are present and may be numerous. An average mitotic index of 1.65 (1–2 mitoses/400x field) has been reported in canine leiomyosar-

comas.[2] Well-differentiated leiomyosarcomas may be composed of spindle cells with elongate nuclei with granular chromatin and abundant eosinophilic cytoplasm, forming broad interlacing fascicles (fig. 6.2 A); only evidence of invasion, mitotic index, and/or areas of tumor necrosis distinguish them from leiomyoma. Less well differentiated leiomyosarcomas appear much more cellular due to diminished cytoplasm and closely packed nuclei that may be round to elongate, with chromatin that may be granular or markedly dispersed (figs. 6.2 B, 6.3). The cells may retain the typical broad interlacing fascicular pattern; however fascicles may be short and narrow, forming more of a *basketweave* pattern, or interlacing fascicles may be inapparent in many areas of the tumor. Binucleate, multinucleate, and bizarre cells are common in more poorly differentiated leiomyosarcomas (fig. 6.4). Areas of tumor necrosis are common, and areas of necrosis and inflammation can result in marked edema and distortion of histological features. A dispersed or plexiform pattern of growth or a microcystic change within the tumor can also obscure the typical leiomyosarcoma pattern of broad interlacing fascicles, leaving pleomorphic and often attenuated cells interspersed in a collagenous or edematous stroma (fig. 6.5 A,B). Areas of

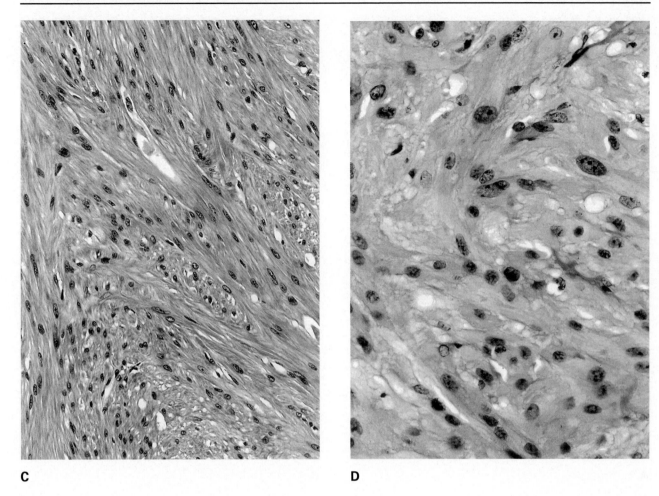

C   D

Fig. 6.1. (continued)   **C.** Gastric leiomyoma from a dog. The tumor cells form broad interlacing fascicles that mimic normal smooth muscle. **D.** Nuclear and cellular pleomorphism in a cutaneous leiomyoma from a ferret.

hemorrhage may also occur. In some instances it may be difficult to distinguish between a leiomyoma and a well-differentiated leiomyosarcoma. The most useful features suggesting malignancy are (1) a mitotic index of 1/10 400x HP fields or more, (2) evidence of invasion, and (3) areas of tumor necrosis.

Metastatic spread of leiomyosarcoma is probably more common than previously recognized; up to 50 percent of leiomyosarcomas may undergo metastasis. A 50 percent incidence of metastasis (6 of 12) of canine leiomyosarcoma was reported in one study.[2] As described in the following text, certain sites of origin appear to have a higher incidence of metastasis (e.g., duodenum, spleen, and liver in the dog), but we know of no studies of leiomyosarcoma that have attempted to identify histopathologic factors predictive of metastatic behavior, nor have preferential sites of metastasis been identified. If these tumors arise within abdominal organs or viscera, they may achieve a large size before becoming clinically apparent. Metastasis may be obvious at the time of diagnosis or may become evident months to years later. Metastatic leiomyosarcoma may occur as an expansile tumor nodule within the affected organ. Metastatic foci

within the lung and liver, however, often have a locally infiltrative growth pattern, dissecting between hepatic cords and growing along alveolar walls, similar to what may be seen in metastatic hemangiosarcoma in these sites (fig. 6.3 B). It must be pointed out, however, that although these tumors demonstrate the interlacing bundles of spindle cells considered characteristic of leiomyosarcoma, in our experience immunohistochemical procedures often fail to demonstrate convincing smooth muscle differentiation, and it is quite possible that some of these tumors are actually undifferentiated sarcomas or malignant gastrointestinal stromal tumors.

When these tumors occur within well-recognized anatomic sites of smooth muscle, such as the intestinal and genitourinary system, a diagnosis of a putative smooth muscle tumor is readily made. In some cases it may be difficult to distinguish these tumors from other mesenchymal spindle cell tumors, especially when collagenous tissue is a large component of the tumor or when tumors arise from sites such as the arrector pilae muscles of the skin, smooth muscle within the hepatobiliary system, or smooth muscle within organ capsules and trabeculae. Special stains, such as Masson's trichrome, Gomori's trichrome, and Van

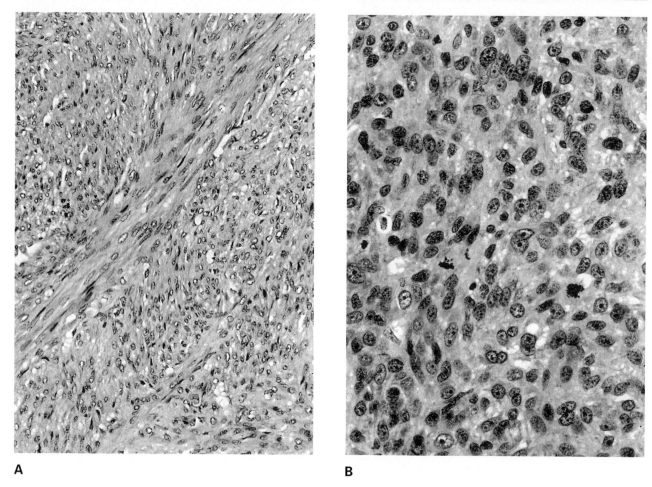

Fig. 6.2.   Leiomyosarcoma. **A.** Well-differentiated intra-abdominal leiomyosarcoma from a ferret. **B.** Vaginal leiomyosarcoma from a dog with haphazardly arranged spindle cells and scattered mitoses.

Gieson stains, which differentially stain muscle and collagenous elements, may be of some value in the diagnosis of relatively well differentiated leiomyomas, but they should not be considered reliable indicators of muscle origin and are not useful in the diagnosis of leiomyosarcoma. Stains such as phosphotungstic acid hematoxylin (PTAH), used to distinguish myofibrils, have not proven to be useful for identification of smooth muscle tumors in our hands. Suspect cases may require electron microscopy and/or immunohistochemical procedures for a definitive diagnosis. Immunohistochemical procedures are rapidly replacing electron microscopy in the determination of tumor cell origin or differentiation, due to their ease of implementation and their sensitivity and specificity. Many spindle cell tumors and tumor-like lesions may have histological features reminiscent of smooth muscle differentiation; fibroma, fibrosarcoma, collagenous nevus (dermatofibroma), Schwannoma, malignant nerve sheath tumor, vaccine-associated sarcoma in the cat, hemangiosarcoma, hemangiopericytoma, sarcoid, rhabdomyosarcoma, and undifferentiated sarcoma can be misdiagnosed as leiomyoma or leiomyosarcoma. Although the prognosis may not be different in some cases in which a spindle cell

tumor of non–smooth muscle origin is misdiagnosed as a leiomyoma or leiomyosarcoma (or vice versa), there are cases in which this distinction is important. For example, recurrence of equine sarcoid is common, but regression may be achieved following various local therapies. Again, the tumor site is an important consideration. Leiomyosarcoma of the oral cavity and subcutis is likely to be over-diagnosed in veterinary pathology; although it is possible that a smooth muscle tumor could arise within the oral cavity, we have been unable to confirm this diagnosis with immunohistochemical staining; smooth muscle tumors of the skin and subcutis are extremely uncommon, and most of those identified appear to be benign.

As discussed above, gastrointestinal tumors containing proliferating smooth muscle admixed with other elements such as proliferating fibroblastic and/or neural crest cells are most appropriately designated as stromal tumors[1] (fig. 6.5 C). The simple presence of fibrous connective tissue, however, does not, in the authors' opinion, warrant designation as a separate entity; hence those female genital tract tumors previously designated as fibroleiomyomas are discussed under the heading of leiomyoma and multicentric leiomyomas/leiomyosarcomas. In many of these

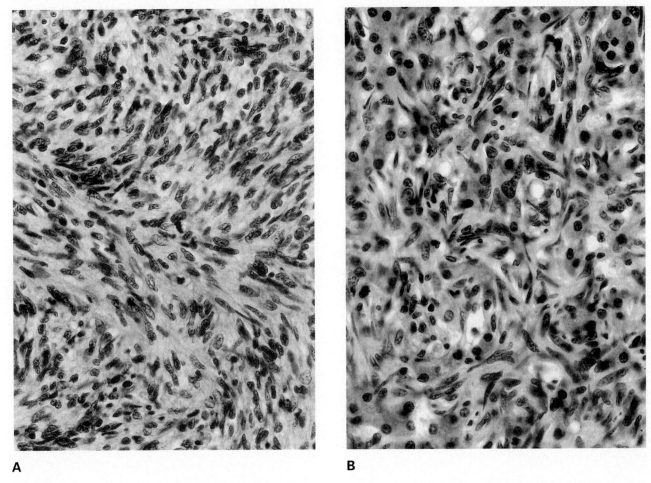

A   **B**

Fig. 6.3. Canine splenic leiomyosarcoma with metastasis to the liver. **A.** Interlacing fascicles of densely packed spindle cells in the splenic tumor. **B.** Infiltrative growth of tumor cells metastatic to the liver.

female genital tract tumors, differentiation of a neoplastic from a reactive process has not been firmly established. Similarly, dispersed cutaneous leiomyoma may in fact be hamartomatous rather than neoplastic in nature (fig. 6.6). Lastly, there are entities in which a mixture of cell and tissue types, including smooth muscle and vascular elements, has given rise to terms such as angioleiomyoma.[3]

The relatively recent recognition of the capacity of fibroblastic cells to differentiate to form myofibroblasts, expressing actin, within tumors as well as within granulation tissue where myofibroblasts were first identified, adds another layer of complexity to the classification of connective tissue tumors. Such tumors are, however, considered by the authors to be primarily of fibroblastic origin and will not be discussed in this chapter.

Clinicopathologic Features

Cytologic evaluation of tumors of smooth muscle origin typically reveals a spindle cell population rendering a diagnosis of mesenchymal tumor, but cytologic features do not allow for a more definitive diagnosis.

A smooth muscle tumor–associated paraneoplastic syndrome has been recently recognized; 12 dogs with intra-abdominal smooth muscle tumors have presented with profound hypoglycemia with resultant clinical signs of weakness and/or seizures.[4-7] Blood insulin levels have been either low[4-6] or normal.[4,5] Both leiomyoma and leiomyosarcoma have been associated with hypoglycemia, and resection of the tumor resulted in normalization of blood glucose levels. Tumors reported have been in the stomach (six cases), jejunum (three cases), duodenum (one case), spleen (one case), and liver (one case). It is interesting to note that this syndrome has not been reported associated with smooth muscle tumors of the genitourinary system. Immunohistochemical staining of four tumors for insulin and glucagon indicated that all tumors were negative for insulin production, but three out of four stained positively for glucagon.[5] The mechanism by which these tumors produce hypoglycemia is not clear, as glucagon production would not be expected to do so. Possible mechanisms include increased utilization of carbohydrates by tumor cells and, for tumors within the liver, hepatic dysfunction. Neither of these explanations is considered

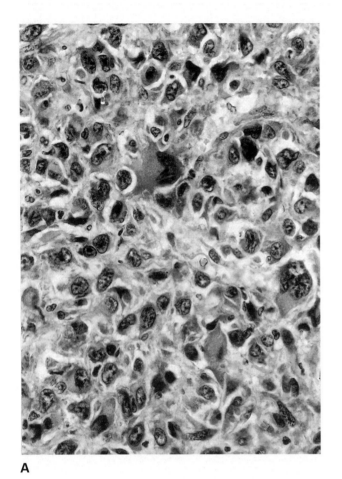

A

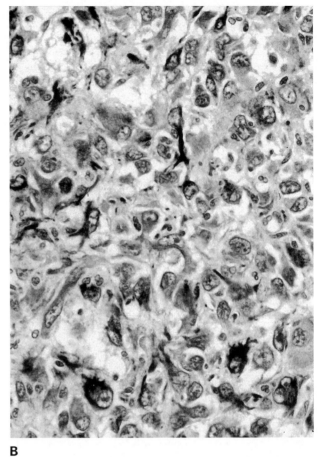

B

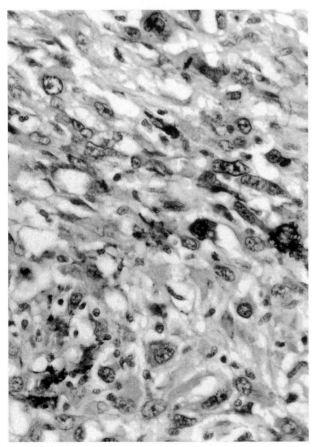

C

Fig. 6.4. Pleomorphic leiomyosarcoma from the spleen of a dog. **A.** Round to spindle cells exhibiting marked cellular and nuclear pleomorphism. **B.** Same tumor with scattered cells demonstrating dense intracytoplasmic desmin expression. **C.** Same tumor with scattered cells demonstrating dense intracytoplasmic expression of smooth muscle actin.

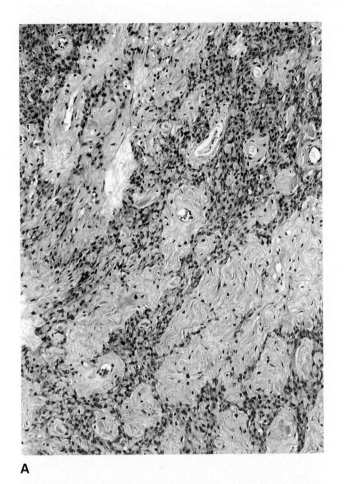

A

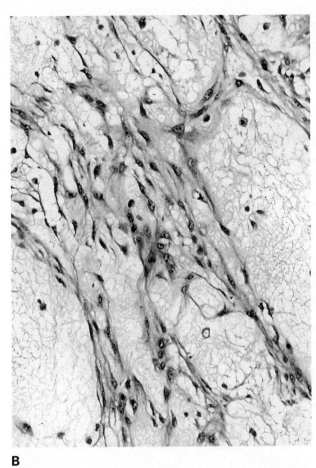

B

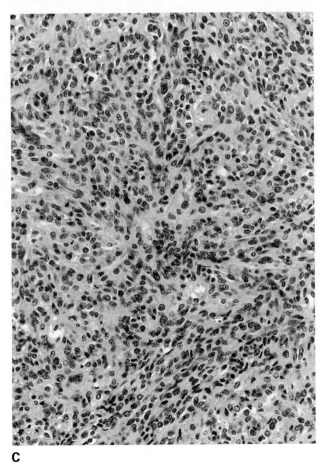

C

Fig. 6.5. Patterns of leiomyosarcoma and gastrointestinal stromal tumors. **A.** Plexiform pattern of leiomyosarcoma with admixed dense collagen in a canine vaginal leiomyosarcoma. **B.** Microcystic change within a colonic leiomyosarcoma from a dog. **C.** Densely cellular arrangement of plump spindle cells in an equine gastrointestinal stromal tumor.

325

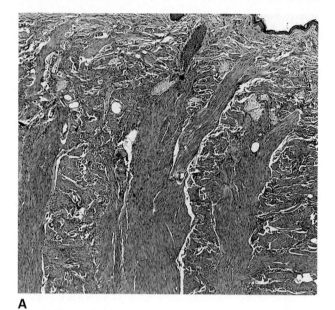

A

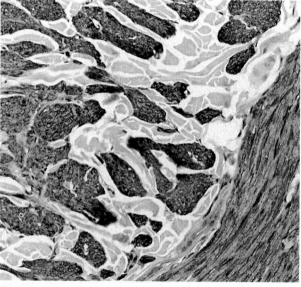

B

Fig. 6.6. Canine cutaneous leiomyoma. **A.** Dispersed pattern of tumor cells mimicking arrector pilae muscles in the dermis. **B.** Diffuse expression of desmin within tumor cells.

likely, and the most likely explanation is believed to be production of an insulin-like molecule, such as insulin-like growth factor 2 (IGF-2), resulting in altered glucose homeostasis.[4,5] Increased IGF-2 levels in serum and tumor tissue of a dog with gastric leiomyoma have been reported.[7]

REFERENCES

1. LaRock, R.G., and Ginn, P.E. (1997) Immunohistochemical staining characteristics of canine gastrointestinal stromal tumors. *Vet Pathol* 34:303–311.

2. Johnson, G.C., Miller, M.A., and Ramos-Vara, J.A. (1995) Comparison of argyrophilic nucleolar organizer regions (AgNORs) and mitotic index in distinguishing benign from malignant canine smooth muscle tumors and in separating inflammatory hyperplasia from neoplastic lesions of the urinary bladder mucosa. *J Vet Diag Invest* 7:127–136.

3. Carpenter, J.L., and Hamilton, T.A. (1995) Angioleiomyoma of the nasopharynx in a dog. *Vet Pathol* 32:721–723.

4. Bagley, R.S., Levy, J.K., and Malarkey, D.E. (1996) Hypoglycemia associated with intra-abdominal leiomyoma and leiomyosarcoma in six dogs. *J Amer Vet Med Assoc* 208:69–71.

5. Beaudry, D., Knapp, D.Q., Montgomery, T., Sandusky, G.S., Morrsion, W.B., and Nelson R.W. (1995) Hypoglycemia in four dogs with smooth muscle tumors. *J Vet Int Med* 9:415–418.

6. Bellah, J.R., and Ginn, P.E. (1996) Gastric leiomyosarcoma associated with hypoglycemia in a dog. *J Amer Anim Hosp Assoc* 32:283–286.

7. Boari, A., Venturoli, M., and Minuto, F. (1992) Non-islet-cell tumor hypoglycemia in a dog associated with high levels of insulin-like growth factor II. XVII World Small Animal Veterinary Association Congress Proceedings, pp. 678–679.

Electron Microscopic Features

Cytoplasmic filaments with plasma membrane associated dense bodies are the most characteristic ultrastructural feature of smooth muscle tumors (fig. 6.7).[1] Other features that may be seen are intercellular attachment plaques and pinocytotic vesicles.[1-4] A basal lamina may be present and may be either complete[1] or incomplete.[2,4] The cells of gastrointestinal stromal tumors may or may not have evidence of smooth muscle differentiation, and they may contain only cells with features of fibroblasts, primitive mesenchymal cells, and/or Schwann cells.[5] The one equine intestinal stromal tumor that we have studied ultrastructurally included cells with smooth muscle (cytoplasmic filaments with associated dense bodies; fig. (6.7) and features suggestive of Schwann cell differentiation (formation of basal laminae in the absence of cytoplasmic filaments and associated dense bodies), as well as undifferentiated cells.[6]

Immunohistochemical Features

The information in this section pertains to immunohistochemical studies utilizing formalin fixed, paraffin embedded tissues and is derived from results of immunohistochemical characterization of selected smooth muscle tumors in the Cornell files and from a review of the literature. As a general rule, all immunohistochemical procedures should include positive control tissue as well as negative control sections in which the primary antibody has been either deleted or replaced by an irrelevant antibody. Internal control tissue is ideal, and the ubiquitous presence of vascular smooth muscle accomplishes this and allows for ease of interpretation of results of smooth muscle–reactive antibody preparations. If no vascular smooth muscle staining is visible, either there was a procedural error, or the tissue tested is unsuitable for immunohistochemical staining for the antibody and technique employed. Special techniques such as trypsinization or microwave exposure of the section may "unmask" hidden antigens. On the other hand, nonspecific background staining that may occur with

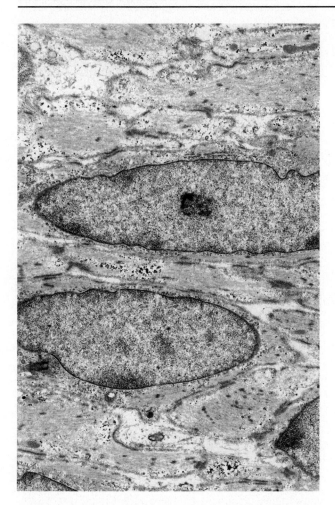

Fig. 6.7. Ultrastructural features of smooth muscle differentiation in an equine gastrointestinal stromal tumor. Cells exhibit bundles of cytoplasmic filaments with associated dense bodies, partial basal lamina, and surface attachment plaques. (Photograph courtesy of Dr. John Cummings and Dr. Fabio Del Piero.)

these procedures can also render accurate interpretation impossible. Although reports of immunohistochemical studies of tumors often imply that interpretation of such preparations is clear-cut, our experience suggests that in some cases, a definitive interpretation of results may not be possible. Obviously, more differentiated tumors express many markers more effectively, and the results of immunohistochemistry can be straightforward. Less differentiated tumors, however, may have a relatively small percentage of cells that react positively. In these cases, using multiple antibodies, changing antibody concentrations, changing incubation times, or employing additional techniques such as transmission electron microscopy may all be necessary to definitively rule in or rule out muscle origin. Care must also be taken not to interpret staining of vascular smooth muscle in highly vascular tumors or, especially, entrapped smooth or skeletal myofibers as evidence for smooth muscle origin of the tumor in question. Tumors of myofibroblasts or tumors with myofibroblasts present as a reactive process will also express muscle specific actin and alpha–smooth muscle actin; interpretation must therefore

always take into account the context in which cells expressing muscle actin are encountered. The use of immunohistochemical preparations can not ever replace the instincts of an experienced pathologist.

Antibodies to desmin and muscle specific actin, which recognize both skeletal and smooth muscle actins, detect cytoskeletal proteins specific for muscle differentiation, but they do not distinguish among tumors of smooth muscle, cardiac muscle, and skeletal muscle. In one study of canine smooth muscle tumors, 14 of 22 tumors identified histologically as leiomyoma or leiomyosarcoma stained positively for desmin. Only 2 of 11 tumors diagnosed as leiomyomas failed to stain positively, whereas 4 of 11 leiomyosarcomas were negative for desmin, and two gave equivocal results.[7] However, no mention was made of internal control (vascular smooth muscle) staining in this report to validate the negative findings. The two leiomyomas that did not stain with desmin were vaginal and perineal, and it is possible that these tumors were fibromas rather than leiomyomas. The leiomyosarcomas that did not stain with desmin were reported to have occurred within the abdomen or intestine and may, in fact, have been gastrointestinal stromal tumors lacking smooth muscle differentiation. In a study of 19 bovine myogenic tumors, 14 of 15 tumors identified as either leiomyoma or leiomyosarcoma stained positively with muscle specific actin.[8] It has been our experience that desmin may be a less reliable antibody than muscle specific actin for diagnosis of tumors of smooth muscle in routinely processed tissue. Therefore, for differentiation of myogenic and nonmyogenic tumors, we prefer to rely on antibodies to muscle specific actin. Poorly differentiated smooth muscle tumors may, however, react with antibodies to either desmin or muscle specific actin, but not both; therefore, use of both antibodies may be prudent. Antibodies to both desmin and muscle specific actin bind *diffusely* and *uniformly* to cells of leiomyomas (fig. 6.6 B), and either diffuse or patchy staining of varied intensity is often seen in leiomyosarcoma (fig. 6.4 A).

Alpha–smooth muscle actin is a specific marker for smooth muscle differentiation and can distinguish smooth muscle tumors from tumors of skeletal or cardiac muscle. It has been used successfully to study routinely processed animal tumors.[6,8-10] In our experience, antibodies to alpha–smooth muscle actin react in a similar pattern to, but more intensely than, antibodies to muscle specific actin (fig. 6.4 C). For routine diagnostic purposes, however, histopathologic features of most cases accurately distinguish smooth muscle tumors from tumors of striated muscle. Therefore, use of this antibody can be reserved for those tumors in which rhabdomyoma or rhabdomyosarcoma are on the list of differential diagnoses, as tumors of striated muscle origin almost always express desmin and/or muscle specific actin but rarely express alpha–smooth muscle actin. Furthermore, identification, by electron microscopic examination, of primitive myofibrils resembling sarcomeric structures will differentiate these tumors (see

Special Diagnostic Procedures in chapter section on Tumors of Striated Muscle).

Vimentin is an intermediate filament expressed by many tumor cells of mesenchymal origin and may even be expressed by cells of poorly differentiated epithelial tumors. When applied to tumors of suspected smooth muscle origin, vimentin is considered a nonspecific marker more commonly expressed in less well differentiated tumors,[1,8] but this expression may be quite variable. For example, we have found strong vimentin expression in cutaneous leiomyomas but not in leiomyomas in other sites. The major utility of vimentin may be in differentiating fibroblastic and undifferentiated mesenchymal tumors from smooth muscle tumors (i.e., tumors that are positive for vimentin but that do not express desmin or muscle specific actin are most likely to be fibrosarcomas, undifferentiated sarcomas, or gastrointestinal stromal tumors), but even here the value of vimentin expression is questionable due to its nonspecificity. Vimentin may also be useful as a control for the "stainability" of the tissue, although the vascular elements provide an internal positive control for muscle actin and smooth muscle actin.

Gastrointestinal stromal tumors that appear to have smooth muscle differentiation at the light microscopic level may or may not contain cells expressing muscle or smooth muscle markers, but they often express vimentin[5] and may express S-100, neuron specific enolase, and c-kit protein.[5,6,11]

REFERENCES

1. Rosai, J. Soft tissues. (1996) In *Ackerman's Surgical Pathology,* 8th ed. Mosby, New York, pp. 2083–2087.
2. Anjiki, T., Takeya, G., Hashimoto, N., and Kadota, K. (1991) An ultrastructural study of vulval myofibroblastoma in a cow. *J Vet Med A* 38:770–775.
3. Seely, J.C., Cosenza, S.F., and Montgomery, C.A. (1978) Leiomyosarcoma of the canine urinary bladder, with metastases. *J Amer Vet Med Assoc* 172:1427–1429.
4. Hanzaike, T., Ito, I., Ishikawa, T., Ishikawa, Y., and Kadota, K. (1995) Leiomyosarcoma of soft tissue in a cow. *J Comp Pathol* 112:237–242.
5. Banerjee, M., Lowenstine, L.J., and Munn, R.J. (1991) Gastric stromal tumors in two Rhesus macaques. *Vet Pathol* 28:30–36.
6. Del Piero, F., Summers, B.A., Credille, K.M., Cummings, J.F., and Mandelli, G. (1996) Gastrointestinal stromal tumors in *Equidae. Vet Pathol* 33:611.
7. Andreason, C.B., and Mahaffey, E.A. (1987) Immunohistochemical demonstration of desmin in canine smooth muscle tumors. *Vet Pathol* 24:211–215.
8. Une, Y., Shirota, K., and Nomura, Y. (1993) Immunostaining of bovine myogenic tumors. *Vet Pathol* 30:455.
9. Johnson, P. J., Wilson, D.A., Turk, J.R., Pace, L.W., Campbell-Beggs, C., and Johnson, G.C. Disseminated peritoneal leiomyomatosis in a horse. *J Amer Vet Med Assoc* 205:725–728.
10. Brunnert, S.R., Herron, A.J., and Altman, N.H. (1990) Subcutaneous leiomyosarcoma in a Peruvian squirrel monkey *(Saimiri sciureus). Vet Pathol* 27:126–128.
11. Hafner, S. , Harmon, B.G., and King, T. (2001) Gastrointestinal stromal tumors of the equine cecum. *Vet Pathol* 38:242–246.

Gastrointestinal Stromal Tumors (GIST)

Similar to recent findings in humans,[1-3] immunohistochemical studies of nonlymphoid mesenchymal tumors within the gastrointestinal tract of animals are proving that tumors previously designated as of smooth muscle origin are actually a heterogeneous group of tumors. Smooth muscle differentiation can be demonstrated in most, but not all, tumors, despite a similar appearance on routine light microscopic examination. One study found evidence of smooth muscle differentiation in 14 of 15 gastrointestinal tumors designated as leiomyoma, in 17 of 18 tumors diagnosed as leiomyosarcoma, and in one of two tumors diagnosed as sarcoma.[4] Forty-nine percent of these tumors expressed S-100, with or without concurrent evidence of smooth muscle differentiation, and the authors concluded that, although the majority of canine gastrointestinal stromal tumors have evidence of smooth muscle differentiation, subgroups of these tumors may have a more complex histogenesis or differentiation.[4,25] Similar conclusions have been made following studies of similar tumors of the equine intestinal tract.[5,25] Two gastric tumors in nonhuman primates with light microscopic features suggestive of smooth muscle origin were found not to express smooth muscle markers (following immunohistochemical staining) or ultrastructural features of smooth muscle.[6] Our studies of a small number of canine gastrointestinal tumors with light microscopic features suggestive of origin from smooth muscle have confirmed that these tumors in the dog are heterogeneous, and that not all express smooth muscle markers. Therefore the term *gastrointestinal stromal tumors,* of which leiomyoma and leiomyosarcoma are the most common subset, is the most appropriate designation.

Gastrointestinal stromal tumors can not be distinguished from smooth muscle tumors in H&E stained sections. Although similar light microscopically, they are a heterogeneous group of lesions via immunohistochemistry. Some, but not all, will stain with S100 or neuron specific enolase or synaptophsin or c-kit protein and other immunohistochemical markers.[4-6,25] GISTs are proposed to originate from the interstitial cells (myofibroblasts) of Cajal, which are precursors to the pacemaker cells of the intestinal wall.[25] Some of these tumors express neural markers (in humans), and it has been proposed that this subset of human GISTs be called gastrointestinal autonomic nerve tumors (GANT). Additional studies may clarify whether these subsets are clearly distinct entities and if these divisions are predictive of biological behavior. We know from studies of mesenchymal tumors in the subcutis that the morphological diagnosis is not as predictive of biological behavior as are mitoses and other generic microscopic assessments. Similar studies should be performed on the various subsets of intestinal mesenchymal tumors. Although the following sections describe gastrointestinal leiomyoma and leiomyosarcoma, bear in mind that this classification is based on the diagnosis made on routine light microscopic features alone and that immunohisto-chemistry would be necessary to confirm smooth muscle differentiation.

Leiomyoma

Incidence, Age, Breed, and Sex

Although uncommonly reported, benign nonlymphoid mesenchymal gastrointestinal tumors with features of leiomyoma are commonly encountered at necropsy, especially in the dog. These tumors occur in mature to aged dogs. In one report, 2 of 20 canine gastric neoplasms were diagnosed as leiomyomas.[7] In a study of laboratory beagles, esophageal/gastric leiomyoma occurred with equal incidence in males and females and was age-related, with tumors found in 82 percent of dogs 17–18 years of age.[8] Increased incidence of gastric leiomyomas in aged animals was also reported in one study in which 15 of 17 gastric leiomyomas were diagnosed in dogs 11 years of age or older, with an average age of 16 years.[9] A strong male predominance was found in this study,[9] but not in a later study.[8] A search of the Cornell pathology files (Table 6.1) found 309 canine leiomyomas in which the system of origin was recorded, and almost half (162 cases) occurred within the gastrointestinal tract. Although leiomyoma occurred in many breeds, the poodle and chihuahua appeared to be overrepresented. More evidence for an apparent breed predilection is found in one study[9] in which poodles were the breed most commonly affected by gastric leiomyoma (5 of 17), followed by chihuahuas (3 of 17). In the Cornell files, leiomyomas were also common in German shepherds, Labrador retrievers, golden retrievers, and beagles, although this may reflect the popularity of these breeds. Interestingly, leiomyoma at these sites was uncommon in the boxer dog.

Leiomyoma of the gastrointestinal tract is much less common in other species. In the Cornell files, gastrointestinal leiomyomas occurred in 11 cats, with no apparent breed or sex predisposition. Intestinal leiomyomas have been reported in the horse,[10-14] in which ages ranged from 2 years to 15 years. Sixteen leiomyomas of the equine gastrointestinal tract were found in the Cornell files. These occurred in several breeds including mixed breeds; although many were quarter horse related breeds and thoroughbreds, this may represent the popularity of these breeds. These tumors are uncommonly reported in the cow, perhaps due to the relatively young age at which most cattle are necropsied. A leiomyoma of the spiral colon has been reported in a 10-year-old cow.[15] We have also seen a leiomyoma of the omasum in a goat.

Clinical Characteristics and Sites

These tumors are most often encountered in the dog as incidental findings at necropsy. Large masses may cause clinical signs of obstruction, particularly if they occur at outflow sites such as the esophageal/gastric area or pylorus or at sites such as the colorectal or anorectal region, where

TABLE 6.1. 366 leiomyomas of the dog, cat, cow, and horse in which the specific site of origin was identified in the Cornell files from 1977 to 1997

Site	Dog	Dog,% by Site	Cat[a]	Cow	Horse
Esophagus	18	6	0	0	0
Stomach	77	25	6	0	2
Small intestine	21	7	4	0	12
Ileocecal	0	0	1	0	0
Large intestine (including rectum and anus)	43	14	0	0	1
Cecum	3	1	0	0	1
Gall bladder	10	3	1	0	NA
Urinary bladder	29	9	5	0	1
Vulva	16	5	0	0	1
Vagina/cervix	58	19	1	3	3
Uterus	25	8	5	2	2
Ovary	2	0.5	1	0	0
Testis	0	0	0	0	4
Skin	5	2	0	0	0
Spleen	2	0.5	0	0	0
Iris	0	0	1	0	0
Total	**309**	**100.0**	**25**	**5**	**27**

NA = Not applicable.
[a]Includes two exotic cats.

signs of obstruction and/or obvious tumor occur. They may be multiple, especially in the stomach wall. In one report, canine leiomyomas were most common at the esophageal/gastric junction.[8] In another report, 5 of 14 canine gastrointestinal leiomyomas occurred in the stomach.[9] The stomach was the most common site of gastrointestinal canine leiomyoma in the Cornell pathology files (77 cases). The large intestine was the second most frequent site of canine leiomyomas (46 cases), and large intestinal leiomyomas were most common in the colorectal or anorectal region, although 3 were found in the cecum. Leiomyoma of the esophagus and of the small intestine occurred at about equal frequency in the dog (18 and 21 cases, respectively). Interestingly, no intestinal leiomyomas were diagnosed in one study of 64 dogs with intestinal tumors.[9] We have also recognized leiomyoma of the gall bladder as an incidental finding at necropsy in three dogs, and seven canine gall bladder leiomyomas were diagnosed following biopsy.

In the Cornell files, feline gastric and small intestinal leiomyomas occurred with about equal frequency (six and four cases, respectively). One feline leiomyoma occurred at the ileocecal junction, but none was diagnosed in more distal large intestine. In the horse, intestinal leiomyomas may occur in either the small or large intestine and may cause obstruction and colic[12] or intussusception,[11,14] or they can be an incidental finding.[13] A small intestinal obstruction caused by an equine jejunal leiomyoma resulted in gastric rupture.[10] Leiomyoma of the stomach was found as an incidental finding at necropsy in two horses at Cornell, and equine leiomyomas were more common in the small intestine (12 cases) than in the large intestine (two cases). The spiral colon leiomyoma in the cow resulted in ruminal stasis and melena,[15] and the omasal tumor in the goat was an incidental finding at necropsy.

Gross Morphology

These tumors within the gastrointestinal tract can be seen to arise from within the smooth muscle tunics and are generally broad based, sessile tumors that frequently bulge into the lumen or from the external wall of the affected organ. These tumors are not encapsulated but are discrete. Neither mucosal ulceration nor tumor necrosis are characteristic, although the large size of many leiomyomas may result in mechanical ulceration. On section, these masses are semifirm to firm, solid, and pale pink to tan. The edges of the tumor may be distinct or may blend with the adjacent smooth muscle.

Histological Features, Growth, and Metastasis

Histological features of gastrointestinal leiomyomas are as described above under Classification and General Histological Features. The degree of fibrous connective tissue admixed with smooth muscle varies considerably, and defining a leiomyoma as a well-differentiated spindle cell tumor with minimal fibrous stroma is inappropriate, as leiomyomas may have a substantial collagen component. A proliferating population of fibroblasts, however, is not typical of leiomyoma, and if present, the tumor is more appropriately classified as a gastrointestinal stromal tumor. Gastrointestinal stromal tumors may contain a mix of smooth muscle, neural tissue, and fibroblasts. Gastrointestinal leiomyomas are noninvasive and do not metastasize; therefore surgical excision of the tumor and any associated devitalized bowel is generally curative.

Leiomyosarcoma

Incidence, Age, Breed, and Sex

Leiomyosarcoma is most common in the dog, and is second only to epithelial malignancy within the canine gastrointestinal tract.[9,16] A review of records for a 5-year period at The Animal Medical Center found that 23 of 44 leiomyosarcomas in dogs occurred within the gastrointestinal tract (16 of 44 were in the spleen).[16] Results of review of the Cornell cases of leiomyosarcoma are presented in table 6.2. Of the 158 total canine leiomyosarcomas in the Cornell files, 100 (61 percent) were reported as occurring in the gastrointestinal tract, and approximately 50 percent of these were in the small intestine. An earlier study reported that leiomyosarcoma of the intestine occurred in female dogs approximately twice as frequently as in males,[9] but a similar female predisposition was not found in a subsequent study,[16] and no sex predisposition was apparent following review of the Cornell files. Although an intestinal leiomyosarcoma was diagnosed in a 17-month-old dog,[17] the majority of cases occurred in dogs 10 years of age or older. The average age of dogs with gas-

TABLE 6.2. 182 leiomyosarcomas of the dog, cat, and horse in which the specific site of origin was identified in the Cornell files from 1977 to 1997

Site	Dog	Dog,% by Site	Cat	Horse
Esophagus	1	0.5	0	0
Stomach	11	7	2	0
Small intestine	46	29	6	1
Ileocecal	3	2	3	1
Large intestine (including rectum and anus)	15	10	3	0
Cecum	24	15	0	0
Spleen	21	13	2	0
Liver	1	0.5	0	0
Urinary bladder	15	10	4	0
Ureter	1	0.5	0	0
Vulva/vagina	13	8	0	0
Uterus	1	0.5	1	0
Perineal/pelvic canal	6	4	1	0
Total	**158**	**100.0**	**22**	**2**

tric leiomyosarcoma was reported to be 7 years, and it was 11 years for dogs with intestinal leiomyosarcoma.[9] Intestinal leiomyosarcoma occurs in all breeds and may be more common in mixed breeds,[9] but no breed predisposition for leiomyosarcoma was reported in a study of 44 cases.[16] One study suggested that German shepherds may be predisposed to leiomyosarcoma,[9] and German shepherds and poodles were the most common breeds diagnosed with this tumor in the Cornell files. This may simply reflect the popularity of these breeds. The cases in German shepherds, however, included a 3- and a 4-year-old dog, suggesting that these tumors may occur at a younger age in this breed.

Gastrointestinal leiomyosarcoma is much less common in other species. Of the 22 feline leiomyosarcomas in the Cornell files, 14 occurred within the gastrointestinal tract; this is slightly higher than the number of feline gastrointestinal leiomyomas (11). Feline cases occurred in domestic cats as young as 2 years of age, but they were most common in middle-aged to aged cats. No apparent sex or breed predisposition was found. Gastrointestinal leiomyosarcomas in two horses were found in the Cornell files, and there are four reported cases in the literature.[18-20] One case occurred in a 4-year-old horse,[20] but all others occurred in horses 10 years of age or older. No sex predisposition is apparent, and breeds include thoroughbred (three), cob (two), and quarter horse (one). Gastrointestinal leiomyosarcoma is apparently very rare in ruminants and pigs, as no cases were found in the literature or in the Cornell files.

Clinical Characteristics and Sites

Gastrointestinal leiomyosarcomas most often cause clinical signs of gastrointestinal dysfunction (i.e. vomiting and/or diarrhea, which may contain blood), and intestinal tumors have been associated with intussusception of the involved segment. Tumors may result in intestinal perforation and fever, lethargy, and anorexia due to septic peritonitis.[21] In contrast to leiomyoma, canine leiomyosarcoma more commonly occurs in the intestine than in the stomach. In the Cornell files, 88 percent of canine gastrointestinal leiomyosarcomas occurred within the intestine (46 percent in the small intestine, 39 percent within the large intestine, and 3 percent at the ileocecal junction), and only 11 percent occurred in the stomach. In a study of 20 gastric tumors in the dog, only one leiomysarcoma was reported.[7] Of tumors in which the involved segment of intestine was identified, the jejunum accounted for just over half of the canine small intestinal leiomysarcomas at Cornell (17 cases), followed by the duodenum (11 cases), with only rare involvement of the ileum (3 cases). The cecum was the second most frequent site (24 cases), followed by, in decreasing order, colon or rectum (15 cases), and ileocecal junction (3 cases), which is similar to an earlier report.[9] Leiomyosarcoma of the esophagus is rare, and only one was found in the Cornell files.

In the cat, the small intestine was the most common site of gastrointestinal leiomyosarcoma (6 of 14) in our files; four of six cases occurred in the jejunum, one was in the duodenum, and the specific site of origin was not specified in one case. Feline leiomyosarcoma occurred with equal frequency (three cases each) in the large intestine/rectum and the ileocecal junction. Only two gastric leiomyosarcomas were recorded in cats. No reported cases of feline gastrointestinal leiomyosarcoma were found in a literature search. Equine gastrointestinal leiomyosarcoma has been reported to involve the duodenum (two cases),[18] stomach (one case),[19] and rectum (one case).[20] The two equine cases in the Cornell files were in the jejunum and at the ileocecal junction. Colic was the presenting sign for equine intestinal leiomyosarcomas,[18] and the gastric leiomyosarcoma caused anorexia and weight loss.[19] The rectal tumor intermittently protruded through the anus.[20]

Gross Morphology

Tumors can be seen to arise within the muscular tunic of the involved organ and can become quite large, resulting in considerable narrowing of the lumen of the affected segment (fig. 6.8). Smaller tumors can be seen growing from the muscular tunic and are still covered by an intact mucosa. Mural thickening may be annular or nodular. Tumors may be relatively well circumscribed or may extend into the adjacent omentum. Necrosis and hemorrhage of either the mucosal or serosal surface, with associated inflammation, is common. Leiomyosarcomas of the rectum are locally invasive and may fill the pelvic canal. The rectal leiomyosarcoma in the horse was polypoid and pedunculated,[20] suggesting that this case may in fact represent a rectal leiomyoma, as no light microscopic features were reported. On section, leiomyosarcomas are firm, generally solid, cream colored, and may have obvious interstitial fibrosis and/or hemorrhage. Multiple areas of necrosis may give leiomyosarcomas a cystic or multicystic appearance.

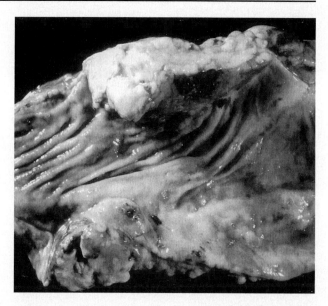

Fig. 6.8. Irregular thicking of the small intestinal wall by leiomyosarcoma in a dog.

Histological Features, Growth, and Metastasis

Histological features are as described above in the classification and general histological features section. These tumors are frequently described as locally invasive but slow to metastasize; however, metastasis may be more common than previously recognized, and its occurrence is probably underestimated due to lack of follow-up information. In the Cornell files, 16 percent of all canine leiomyosarcomas (27 cases) had evidence of metastasis, and of those for which a primary site was recorded, metastasis was recorded for 14 percent of all canine gastrointestinal leiomyosarcomas. In some cases metastasis was evident at the time of surgery, and in others metastasis was detected at varying times, from 1 to 2 months to 2 years following initial diagnosis. Metastasis of small intestinal leiomyosarcoma was most common (eight cases). Although small intestinal leiomyosarcoma occurred most commonly in the jejunum (17 cases), duodenal leiomyosarcoma was more likely to metastasize; 4 of 11 (36 percent) canine duodenal leiomyosarcomas metastasized. In the literature, metastasis of duodenal leiomyosarcoma was present at the time of diagnosis in one dog[22] and occurred within 1 month after surgery in another dog,[23] providing further evidence that a cautious prognosis must be given for duodenal leiomyosarcoma in the dog. Two of 17 canine jejunal tumors metastasized (12 percent), and only 1 of 11 canine gastric leiomyosarcomas underwent metastasis (9 percent). Of tumors of the lower intestinal tract in the dog, metastasis of cecal leiomyosarcoma was most common and was recorded in 4 of 24 tumors (17 percent). One of three ileocecal leiomyosarcomas underwent metastasis (33 percent), and metastasis of 1 of 15 colonic/rectal leiomyosarcomas

(7 percent) was recorded. In a study of 44 canine leiomyosarcomas, 31 percent of gastric and small intestinal tumors metastasized, and 20 percent of cecal leiomyosarcomas metastasized, although one dog was alive and well 3 years following surgery, despite evidence of peritoneal metastasis at the time of surgery.[16] Evidence of metastasis of feline gastrointestinal leiomyosarcoma was not found in the Cornell files, although no follow-up studies of biopsy diagnoses were attempted. One feline colonic leiomyosarcoma was apparently multicentric. Evidence of metastasis was not found in the reported equine gastrointestinal leiomyosarcomas, but metastasis of an ileocecal leiomyosarcoma was found at necropsy in one horse in the Cornell files. Metastasis to liver and to mesenteric lymph nodes was most common in all cases of metastatic gastrointestinal leiomyosarcoma, although pulmonary, splenic, omental/mesenteric, and renal metastases were also seen.

Multiple Gastrointestinal Stromal Tumors

A unique presentation of gastrointestinal stromal tumors is the recognition of a subset of tumors that occurs as multicentric tumors within the intestinal tract (fig. 6.9). A report of multiple tumors described as peripheral nerve sheath tumors in the small intestinal wall of a young adult horse, in which tumor cells expressed S-100, GFAP (glial fibrillary acidic protein), and desmin,[24] appears similar to a case of multicentric stromal tumors in the small intestine of an adult horse,[5] and we consider that multiple intestinal stromal tumors is a more appropriate classification for these tumors. A case of multiple stromal tumors in the colon of an adult cat was found in the Cornell files. The nerve sheath tumor[24] is similar to a subset of GIST, gastrointestinal autonomic nerve tumors (GANTs), characterized in humans. These tumors are composed of a mixture of cell types, which may (but do not necessarily) include myogenic (smooth muscle actin positive) as well as neurogenic

(S-100 positive) and/or undifferentiated mesenchymal elements. Some tumors appear to arise within myenteric plexi, whereas others form within the smooth muscle wall. These tumors can cause clinical signs of colic, and excision of the affected intestine in one horse was apparently curative.[24] None of these tumors showed evidence of metastasis.

GISTs of the equine cecum have recently been described and characterized.[25] The tumors were multinodular and consisted of mesenchymal spindle cells arranged in interconnected trabeculae that were separated by mucinous fluid. Tumor cells were immunopositive for vimentin, neuron specific enolase, and c-kit protein, with focal staining for smooth muscle actin, but were negative for S-100 or desmin. The tumors were in the wall of the cecum, and there was no mucosal ulceration grossly or microscopically.[25] Tumors appeared to grow by expansion rather than invasion, a fibrous capsule was present, mitotic rate was markedly low, and no metastases were reported. Too few mesenchymal tumors have been classified as GIST and followed clinically to determine their biological behavior in domestic animals.

REFERENCES

1. Franquemont D.W., and Frierson, H.F. (1992) Muscle differentiation and clinicopathologic features of gastrointestinal stromal tumors. *Amer J Surg Pathol* 16:947–954.
2. Franquemont, D.W. (1995) Differentiation and risk assessment of gastrointestinal stromal tumors. *Amer J Clin Pathol* 103:41–47.
3. Ma, C.K., De Peralta, N., Amin, M.B., Linden, M.D., Dekovich, A.A., Kubus, J.J., and Zarbo, R.J. (1997) Small intestinal stromal tumors. A clinicopathologic study of 20 cases with immunohistochemical assessment of cell differentiation and the prognostic role of proliferation antigens. *Amer J Clin Pathol* 108:641–651.
4. La Rock, R.G., and Ginn, P.E. (1997) Immunohistochemical staining characteristics of canine gastrointestinal stromal tumors. *Vet Pathol* 34:303–311.
5. Del Piero, F., Summers, B.A., Credille, K.M., Cummings, J.F., and Mandelli, G. (1996) Gastrointestinal stromal tumors in *Equidae*. *Vet Pathol* 33:611.
6. Banerjee, M., Lowenstine, L.J., and Munn, R.J. (1991) Gastric stromal tumors in two Rhesus macaques (*Macaca mulatta*). *Vet Pathol* 28:30–36.
7. Sautter, J.H., and Hanlon, G.F. (1975) Gastric neoplasms in the dog: A report of 20 cases. *J Amer Vet Med Assoc* 166:691–696.
8. Culbertson, R., Branam, J.E., and Rosenblatt, L.S. (1983) Esophageal/gastric leiomyoma in the laboratory Beagle. *J Amer Vet Med Assoc* 183:1168–1171.
9. Patnaik, A.K., Hurvitz, A.I., and Johnson, G.F. (1977) Canine gastrointestinal neoplasms. *Vet Pathol* 14:547–555.
10. Hanes, G.E., and Robertson, J.T. (1983) Leiomyoma of the small intestine in a horse. *J Amer Vet Med Assoc* 182:1398.
11. Collier, M.A., and Trent, A.M. (1983) Jejunal intussusception associated with leiomyoma in an aged horse. *J Amer Vet Med Assoc* 182:819–821.
12. Kasper, C., and Doran, R. (1993) Duodenal leiomyoma associated with colic in a two-year-old horse. *J Amer Vet Med Assoc* 202:769–770.
13. Haven, M.L., Rottman, J.B., and Bowman, K.F. (1991)Leiomyoma of the small colon in a horse. Vet Surg 20:320–322.
14. Wilson, T., Modransky, P., and Savage, C.J. (1994) Small intestinal intussusception in a mule. *Equine Prac* 16:36–38.

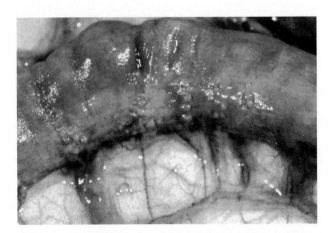

Fig. 6.9. Multiple nodular serosal tumors in the small intestine of a horse with multiple gastrointestinal stromal tumors. (Photograph courtesy of Dr. Kelly Credille.)

15. Saidu, S.N.A., and Chineme, C.N. (1979) Intestinal leiomyoma in a cow. *Vet Rec* 104:388–389.

16. Kapatkin, A.S., Mullen, H.S., Matthiesen, D.T., and Patnaik, A.K. (1992) Leiomyosarcoma in dogs: 44 cases (1983–1988). *J Amer Vet Med Assoc* 201:1077–1079.

17. Laratta, L.J., Center, S.A., Flanders, J.A., Dietze, A.E., and Castleman, W.L. (1983) Leiomyosarcoma in the duodenum of a dog. *J Amer Vet Med Assoc* 183:1096–1097.

18. Mair, T.S., Taylor, F.G.R., and Brown, P.J. (1990) Leiomyosarcoma of the duodenum in two horses. *J Comp Pathol* 102:119–123.

19. Gardiner Boy, M., Palmer, J.E., Heyer, G., and Hamir, A.N. (1992) Gastric leiomyosarcoma in a horse. *J Amer Vet Med Assoc* 200:1363–1364.

20. Clem, M.F., DeBowes, R.M., and Leiopold, H.W. (1987) Rectal leiomyosarcoma in a horse. *J Amer Vet Med Assoc* 191:229–230.

21. Eckerlin, R.H. (1974) Perforated duodenum associated with nonobstructive leiomyosarcoma in a dog. *J Amer Vet Med Assoc* 165:449–450.

22. Weller, R.E., and O'Brien, E. (1979) Intestinal leiomyosarcoma in a dog. *Mod Vet Prac* 60:621–623.

23. Kolaja, G.J., and Fairchild, D.G. (1973) Leiomyosarcoma of the duodenum in a dog. *J Amer Vet Med Assoc* 163:275–276.

24. Kirchhof, N., Scheidemann, W., and Baumgärtner. (1996) Multiple peripheral nerve sheath tumors in the small intestine of a horse. *Vet Pathol* 33:727–730.

25. Hafner, S., Harmon, B.G., and King, T. (2001) Gastrointestinal stromal tumors of the equine cecum. *Vet Pathol* 38:242–246.

Smooth Muscle Tumors (Leiomyoma) of the Gall Bladder

Incidence, Age, Breed, and Sex

Although uncommonly reported, benign smooth muscle tumors of the gall bladder are encountered at necropsy, especially in the dog. Ten leiomyomas of the gall bladder were found in the Cornell files, occurring in mature to older dogs. These tumors are much less common in other species; only one leiomyoma of the gall bladder was found in an adult cat. Not surprisingly, no leiomyomas of the gall bladder have been seen in horses.

Clinical Characteristics

These tumors may be encountered as an incidental finding at necropsy, however large masses may cause clinical signs of obstruction. The Cornell files contained three dogs in which a leiomyoma of the gall bladder was an incidental finding at necropsy and seven dogs in which the tumor was diagnosed following exploratory surgery and biopsy. The feline case was associated with cholecystitis, biliary obstruction, and jaundice.

Gross and Histological Features, Growth, and Metastasis

Tumors within the biliary tree arise from within the smooth muscle wall, and the gross morphology is similar to leiomyomas within the gastrointestinal tract. Histological features of leiomyomas of the gall bladder are as described in Classification and General Histological Features, above. We are not aware of any diagnoses of leiomyosarcoma within the biliary tree of domestic animals. These tumors are noninvasive; therefore, surgical excision of the tumor is generally curative, provided a patent biliary tree can be maintained.

Smooth Muscle Tumors of the Urinary System

Leiomyoma

Incidence, Age, Breed, and Sex

Leiomyoma of the urinary system most commonly occurs in the adult dog and has no apparent sex predisposition. Twenty-nine leiomyomas of the canine urinary system were recorded in the Cornell files. Mesenchymal tumors are much less common in this system than are epithelial neoplasms; in one study only 2 of 115 canine urinary tract tumors were reported as leiomyomas,[1] and in another study of tumors of the canine urinary bladder, only 1 of 21 tumors was reported as leiomyoma.[2] Another report found five leiomyomas and three fibroleiomyomas in 130 canine urinary bladder tumors; the mean age of the dogs was 12.5 years for leiomyoma, but no information was available regarding the age of dogs with fibroleiomyoma.[3] Of the 1547 urinary bladder tumors recorded in dogs in table 10.4, there were 57 (4 percent) leiomyomas and 18 (1 percent) leiomyosarcomas.

This tumor is much less common in other species. In the Cornell files only five leiomyomas of the urinary system were identified in adult cats; one feline urinary bladder leiomyoma in a 12-year-old cat was reported in a series of nine feline urinary bladder tumors;[3] and one is reported in a 5-year-old cat.[4] We have seen only one leiomyoma of the urinary bladder in *Equidae,* and that was an aged pony.

Clinical Characteristics and Sites

The wall of the urinary bladder is by far the most common site of leiomyoma of the urinary system, and all canine and feline urinary tract leiomyomas in the Cornell files were in the urinary bladder, as were two reported canine leiomyomas[1] and one feline leiomyoma.[3] Leiomyomas within the urinary bladder and urethra may cause hematuria and, if large enough, dysuria. Leiomyoma of the urethra is uncommon, but urethral leiomyoma was reported to cause postrenal failure in a 12-year-old dog[5] and urinary obstruction in a 13-year-old cat.[6] Leiomyoma of the kidney was reported as an incidental finding in an adult male dog.[7]

Gross and Histological Features, Growth, and Metastasis

Leiomyomas within the urinary system generally have a similar gross and histological appearance to leiomyomas within the gastrointestinal tract. One reported feline urinary bladder leiomyoma was unique in that the tumor demonstrated intraluminal growth in markedly dilated veins and lymphatics and was thought to have arisen within venous smooth muscle. This tumor was highly cellular, composed of spindle and round cell bundles with infrequent mitoses, and leiomyoblastoma was also considered as a diagnosis in this unusual case.[4] Leiomyomas are discrete tumors that, if adequately excised, do not recur.

Leiomyosarcoma

Incidence, Age, Breed, and Sex

Leiomyosarcoma represents only a very small proportion of tumors arising in this system. A study of 115 canine bladder and urethral tumors found only one leiomyosarcoma,[1] and none were reported in a study of 21 canine urinary bladder neoplasms.[2] Another study found four leiomyosarcomas in 130 urinary bladder neoplasms, occurring in dogs from 2 to 11 years of age, with a mean age of 7 years.[3] No leiomyosarcomas were observed in a report of nine feline urinary bladder tumors.[3] The Cornell files contained 16 leiomyosarcomas of the urinary system in dogs, four in cats, one in a cow, one in a skunk, and one in a woodchuck. Leiomyosarcoma of the urinary system is most common in the dog, followed by the cat. This tumor is rare in other species. This tumor occurs in middle-aged to older animals, with no apparent breed or sex predisposition.

Clinical Characteristics and Sites

The urinary bladder is by far the most common site of leiomyosarcoma in the urinary system. In the Cornell files, 15 of the canine urinary tract leiomyosarcomas were in the urinary bladder, and only one was in the ureter. The tumor reported in the study of 115 canine urinary tract tumors was a leiomyosarcoma of the urinary bladder.[1] A urinary bladder leiomyosarcoma was reported in a cat,[8] and all four feline urinary tract leiomyosarcomas in the Cornell files occurred in the bladder. The bovine leiomyosarcoma also occurred in the urinary bladder. The most common clinical signs are hematuria and/or dysuria, although a ureteral leiomyosarcoma in a dog resulted in anorexia, lethargy, and an acutely painful abdomen.[9] If large enough to be obstructive, azotemia, uremia,[8] or pelvic limb edema[9] may be evident.

Gross Morphology

Leiomyosarcoma of the urinary bladder often results in irregular and nodular thickening of the affected wall and can compromise the patency of the ureters and/or urethra. The ureteral leiomyosarcoma was a large lobulated mass in the retroperitoneal space intimately associated with a ureter.[9]

Histological Features, Growth, and Metastasis

Histological features of urinary tract leiomyosarcomas are similar to those at other sites, although in our experience urinary bladder leiomyosarcomas may have a prominent multinucleate giant cell component and can be mistaken for botryoid rhabdomyosarcoma of the bladder. Metastasis is uncommon; none were recorded in the Cornell files, and only one report was found of a canine urinary bladder leiomyosarcoma that underwent widespread metastasis to abdominal and thoracic organs.[10] The extensive local infiltration, rendering complete surgical excision difficult, results in frequent recurrence following excision, necessitating euthanasia.

REFERENCES

1. Norris, A.M., Laing, E.J., Valli, V.E.O., Withrow, S.J., Macy, D.W., Ogilvie, G.K., Tomlinson, J., McCaw, D., Pidgeon, G., and Jacobs, R.M. (1992) Canine bladder and urethral tumors: A retrospective study of 115 cases (1980–1985). *J Vet Int Med* 6:145–153.
2. Strafuss, A.C., and Dean, M.J. (1975) Neoplasms of the canine urinary bladder. *J Amer Vet Med Assoc* 166:1161–1163.
3. Osborne, C.A., Low, D.G., Perman, V., and Barnes, D.M. (1968) Neoplasms of the canine and feline urinary bladder: Incidence, etiologic factors, occurrence and pathologic features. *Amer J Vet Res* 29:2041–2055.
4. Patnaik, A.K., and Greene, R.W. (1979) Intravenous leiomyoma of the bladder in a cat. *J Amer Vet Med Assoc* 175:381–383.
5. Blackwood, L., Sullivan, M., and Thompson, H. (1992) Urethral leiomyoma causing post renal failure in a bitch. *Vet Rec* 131:416–617.
6. Swalec, K.M., Smeak, D.D., and Baker, A.L. (1989) Urethral leiomyoma in a cat. *J Amer Vet Med Assoc* 195:961–962.
7. Mills, J.H.L., Moore, J.T., and Orr, J.P. (1977) Canine renal leiomyoma—An unusual tumor. *Can Vet J* 18:76–78.
8. Burk, R.L., Meierhenry, E.F., and Schaubhut, C.W., Jr. (1975) Leiomyosarcoma of the urinary bladder in a cat. *J Amer Vet Med Assoc* 167:749–751.
9. Berzon, J.L. (1979) Primary leiomyosarcoma of the ureter in a dog. *J Amer Vet Med Assoc* 175:374–376.
10. Seely, J.C., Cosenza, S.F., and Montgomery, C.A. (1978) Leiomyosarcoma of the canine urinary bladder, with metastases. *J Amer Vet Med Assoc* 172:1427–1429.

Smooth Muscle Tumors of the Genitalia

Leiomyoma

Incidence, Age, Breed, and Sex

Leiomyomas of the genitalia occur far more frequently in females than males, and they are among the most commonly encountered tumors of the female reproductive system in almost all domestic species. They are most common in older intact females. There were 326 canine leiomyomas in the Cornell files in which the specific site of origin was recorded, and almost one-third of these (101 cases) occurred in the female reproductive tract. In a survey of vulvar and vaginal tumors in 99 dogs, almost one-third were classified as leiomyoma (26 cases), and tumors occurred most frequently in intact female dogs.[1] A survey of tumors of the reproductive tract in 90 intact female dogs found 66 vulvar/vaginal and 10 uterine leiomyomas in dogs averaging 10.8 years of age.[2] Boxers were overrepresented. There is some confusion in the literature regarding differentiation of leiomyoma, fibroleiomyoma, myofibroblastoma, and fibroma. Fibroma is easily distinguished by a lack of myogenic differentiation following appropriate immunohistochemical staining; in our opinion the presence of myogenic differentiation qualifies the tumor as leiomyoma, although there is some justification for considering that some fibroblastic tumors may have a myofibroblastic component.

Five bovine genital leiomyomas were recorded in the Cornell files. In cattle, large uterine wall leiomyomas are frequently encountered in abbatoir samples, possibly due to interference with reproductive ability in affected cows. A report of 71 connective tissue tumors from a survey of 9.5 million cattle, sheep, and pigs examined at slaughter indicated that all of the smooth muscle tumors (eight) occurred within the female reproductive system. Five of eight were considered to be leiomyomas, which represented approximately 6 percent of all connective tissue tumors identified in cattle, 8 percent of connective tissue tumors in sheep, and 16 percent of connective tissue tumors identified in pigs.[3] In a survey of tumors of the genitalia of sows,[4] leiomyoma was reported in 6 of 1445 sows and accounted for 50 percent of the total tumors in this system. We have seen similar tumors in the uterus and vagina of the cat and horse, as well as in nonhuman primates, ferrets, rabbits, and elephants. Seven leiomyomas of the feline female reproductive tract and six in the equine female reproductive tract were found in the Cornell files. No breed predisposition was apparent. Leiomyomas of the male reproductive system occur, but they are far less frequent in all species than those in the female genitalia; only four leiomyomas of the male genitalia have been recorded at Cornell, all in horses. One leiomyoma of the male reproductive tract has been reported in a dog,[5] and a search of the Veterinary Medical Data Base for 20 years found three leiomyomas of the prostate in 1397 canine prostatic tumors.[6]

Clinical Characteristics and Sites

Leiomyomas in all species occur most frequently in the uterus, cervix, or vagina and may interfere with reproductive function. If large enough, they may also result in urinary or colonic obstruction. It may be difficult to distinguish the exact site of origin of very large tumors within the pelvic canal. In the Cornell files, leiomyoma of the canine vagina and cervix was approximately twice as common (58 cases) as leiomyoma of the uterus (25 cases) or vulva (16 cases). The most common clinical presentation of vaginal, vulvar, and cervical leiomyomas is vulvar discharge and/or a protruding vulvar mass.[1,2] In the Cornell files, five feline leiomyomas occurred in the uterus, and one was present in the cervix of a lion. The five bovine leiomyomas occurred in the uterus (two cases) and in the vagina (three cases). In the horse, vaginal, uterine, and vulvar leiomyomas were found with almost equal frequency (two uterine, three vaginal, and one vulvar). A

leiomyoma within the testis has been reported in an aged ram,[7] and leiomyoma of the testicular tunica albuginea has been reported in a 7-year-old horse[8] and in a dog.[5] Prostatic leiomyoma has been reported in three dogs.[6] Leiomyoma of the ovary is uncommon; one ovarian leiomyoma has been reported in a sow.[3] Two canine ovarian leiomyomas and one in the ovary of a leopard were found in the Cornell files.

Gross Morphology

Leiomyomas of the genitalia often have a similar appearance to those in the gastrointestinal tract. Leiomyomas arising from the vagina, cervix, or vulva may, however, be polypoid and/or pedunculated.[1,2] Caudal vaginal tumors often protrude through the vulva and may become ulcerated and secondarily inflamed. The testicular leiomyoma in the ram was a circumscribed, red-brown, multilobular, soft tumor arising within the testis,[7] and the canine testicular tunic leiomyoma resulted in hydrocele and atrophy of the affected testis.[5]

Histological Features

Histological features of leiomyomas within the genitalia are similar to those of the gastrointestinal tract, although there may be a more prominent fibrous component. In the past, the term *fibroid* has been applied to leiomyomas of the uterus and vagina in humans and animals, but this is no longer considered an appropriate designation for these smooth muscle tumors. If smooth muscle is present, even with a large fibrous component, the diagnosis is leiomyoma or leiomysarcoma.

Growth and Metastasis

There is evidence to suggest that leiomyomas within the female reproductive tract have a hormonal basis. In women it is suggested that some uterine leiomyomas may regress after menopause.[9] A similar hormonal basis for tumor growth is evident in studies of multicentric smooth muscle tumors within the female reproductive tract in animals. Leiomyomas are noninvasive and do not metastasize.

Leiomyosarcoma

Incidence, Age, Breed, and Sex

Almost all cases of leiomyosarcoma of the genitalia that we are aware of have occurred in females and are most common in intact females. One case of testicular leiomyosarcoma occurred bilaterally in retained testes in an 11-month-old thoroughbred,[10] and prostatic leiomyosarcoma has been reported in a 10-year-old intact male boxer dog.[6] Genital leiomyosarcoma is most common in dogs. In a study of vulvar and vaginal tumors in the dog, leiomyosarcoma accounted for 10 of 99 tumors, and only one occurred in a spayed female.[1] A study of genital tumors in 90 intact female dogs aged 9–15 years reports 11 uterine and three vaginal leiomyosarcomas.[2] In the

Cornell files, 14 of 163 canine leiomyosarcomas occurred in the genital tract. There is no apparent breed predisposition.

Only one feline genital leiomyosarcoma was found in the Cornell files, and one was recorded in a rabbit. Genital leiomyosarcoma has been reported in three cows[3,11] and a pig.[3] Multicentric tumors in dogs, cats, goats, and cows are discussed in the section on Multicentric Leiomyomas/Leiomyosarcomas.

Clinical Characteristics and Sites

Vulvar and vaginal leiomyosarcomas accounted for 13 of 14 canine genital leiomyosarcomas in the Cornell files, whereas the feline genital leiomyosarcoma occurred in the uterus. The uterus appears to be the most common reported site of bovine leiomyosarcoma,[3,11] but none were found in the search of our files. Similarly to leiomyomas, leiomyosarcomas may cause reproductive failure or urinary or colonic obstruction. Vulvar and vaginal leiomyosarcomas may be extensively ulcerated.

Gross and Histological Features, Growth, and Metastasis

These tumors may show marked infiltrative growth within the vaginal or uterine wall and can occlude the pelvic canal. Areas of necrosis are common. Histological features are similar to those of leiomyosarcomas at other sites. Metastases were not recorded in any canine or feline genital leiomyosarcomas in the Cornell files. A vulvar leiomyosarcoma in an aged poodle recurred at the site and metastasized to abdominal lymph nodes, lungs, and cervical spinal cord.[12] The vulvar tumor in this case contained multiple foci of osseous metaplasia. Metastasis of bovine uterine leiomyosarcoma has been reported in three cases.[3,11] Metastases most frequently involved iliac and abdominal lymph nodes,[3,11] but widespread metastasis to abdominal organs, lung, and heart has also been described.[11] A vaginal leiomyosarcoma in a 15-year-old dog was reported to have splenic metastases.[2] There was widespread metastasis of the equine testicular leiomyosarcoma[10] and of the canine prostatic leiomyosarcoma,[6] involving multiple lymph nodes and internal organs.

Multicentric Leiomyomas/Leiomyosarcomas of the Female Genital Tract (Leiomyofibromatosis/Fibroleiomyomas/Myofibroblastomas)

A variety of terms has been applied to multicentric smooth muscle–containing tumors within the female genital tract. These tumors may have a prominent fibrous and/or myofibroblastic component and have also been called *fibroleiomyomas* or *myofibroblastomas*. We propose that if smooth muscle differentiation is apparent, the terms *leiomyoma* or *leiomyosarcoma* be applied. The differentiation of genital leiomyosarcoma from leiomyoma relies on the same histological features that distinguish these tumors in other locations, that is, mitotic index, cellular pleomorphism, tumor necrosis, and evidence of invasion. We recognize that, given the suspect hormonal basis for many of these tumors and the lack of evidence of metastasis, the designation of leiomyosarcoma in some cases may be controversial.

Incidence, Age, Breed, and Sex

A syndrome of multiple smooth muscle tumors has been recognized in the genital tract of mature intact females of many species. In dogs and cats, these tumors have features consistent with leiomyoma. Although described as common in the dog,[13] only a few cases of canine multicentric leiomyomas were found in the Cornell files, and all occurred within the vagina. In a survey of genital tumors in 90 intact female dogs, there were three dogs with both vaginal and uterine leiomyomas, and three dogs with multiple vaginal leiomyomas.[2] Multiple leiomyomas of the ovary and uterine horn were reported in a lion,[14] and we have also seen multicentric leiomyomas in the vagina, uterus, cervix, broad ligament, and ovaries of a snow leopard (fig. 6.10 A). A review of the literature and of the Cornell files indicates that this syndrome of multiple genital tract smooth muscle tumors may be most common in the goat, and multicentric vaginal and cervical tumors variously known as *leiomyomas, leiomyofibromatosis,* or *leiomyosarcomas* have been recognized (fig. 6.10 B).[15,16] Nine goats with genital smooth muscle tumors were found in the Cornell files. This syndrome occurs primarily in older female goats, appears to be more common in Saanen goats and, based on its occurrence in two related does, may have a hereditary component. A similar condition involving the vulva, vagina, and anus, in which tumors were reported as myofibroblastomas, has been described in a pregnant cow.[17]

Clinical Characteristics and Gross Morphology

These tumors within the uterus are generally not associated with clinical signs, although they may interfere with reproductive capacity. Systemic illness may be seen if uterine inflammation (endometritis/pyometra) is present. Those arising from the vagina are often pedunculated and may protrude through the vulva and be associated with bleeding and inflammation as described for solitary vaginal leiomyomas. Bleeding in the goat may be severe and life threatening. A hormonal basis for these tumors is supported by the reported history of polycystic ovaries, cystic endometrial hyperplasia, and inappropriate lactation in one

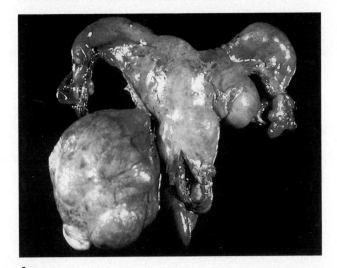

A

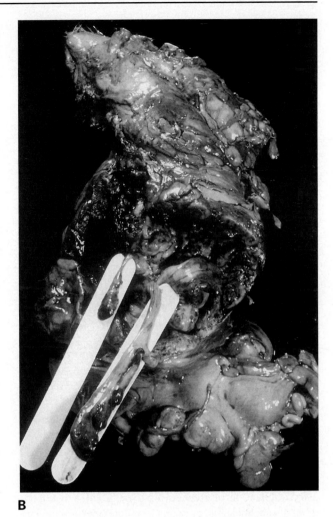

B

Fig. 6.10. Multicentric smooth muscle tumors of the female genital tract. **A.** Multiple large uterine leiomyomas from a snow leopard. (Photograph courtesy of Dr. Matthew Jacobson.) **B.** Multiple vaginal and cervical leiomyosarcomas, often forming smaller and long pedunculated masses, in an aged goat. (Photograph courtesy of Dr. Katharine Whitney.)

goat[15] and cystic endometrial hyperplasia, endometritis, and pseudopregnancy in another.[16] The snow leopard exhibited signs of lethargy and anorexia and was also found to have cystic endometrial hyperplasia, endometrial polyps, and chronic endometritis.

Histological Features, Growth, and Metastasis

Histological features may be similar to those of solitary leiomyomas, although there is often a more pronounced fibrous and/or myofibroblastic component. These tumors are generally slow growing and, due to their location, may become quite large before becoming clinically apparent. As this syndrome is believed to have a hormonal basis, ovariectomy (or ovariohysterectomy) should be considered, as this procedure may cause regression of growths[15] and should markedly reduce the likelihood of similar growths arising. The tumors in the cow appeared to regress following parturition,[17] and leiomyomas of the uterus in women may regress following menopause.[9] The resolution of growths following ovariectomy, parturition, or menopause is evidence that at least some of these growths are not truly neoplastic. In the older goat, multicentric tumors arising from the cervix and/or vaginal wall can be invasive and may result in considerable bleeding, sometimes leading to death by exsanguination. In these cases, the invasive nature of the tumors, as well as the presence of multifocal tumor necrosis and cellular atypia, probably justifies their classification as low grade leiomyosarcomas.[16] Metastasis of these caprine tumors, however, has not been seen.

REFERENCES

1. Thacher, C., and Bradley, R.L. (1983) Vulvar and vaginal tumors in the dog: A retrospective study. *J Amer Vet Med Assoc* 183:690–692.
2. Brodey, R.S., and Roszel, J.F. (1967) Neoplasms of the canine uterus, vagina, and vulva: A clinicopathologic survey of 90 cases. *J Amer Vet Med Assoc* 151:1294–1307.
3. Anderson, L.F., and Sandison, A.T. (1969) Tumours of connective tissues in cattle, sheep and pigs. *J Pathol* 98:253–263.
4. Akkermans, J.P.W.M., and van Beusekom, W.J. (1984) Tumors and tumor-like lesions in the genitalia of sows. *Vet Quarterly* 6:90–96.
5. Patnaik, A.K., and Liu, S.K. (1974) Leiomyoma of the tunica vaginalis in a dog. *Cornell Vet* 65:228–231.
6. Hayden, D.W., Klausner, J.S., and Waters, D.J. (1999) Prostatic leiomyosarcoma in a dog. *J Vet Diag Invest* 11:283–286.
7. Foster, R.A., Ladds, P.W., and Hoffman, D. (1989) Testicular leiomyoma in a ram. *Vet Pathol* 26:184–185.
8. Johnson, R.C., and Steinberg, H. (1989) Leiomyoma of the tunica albuginea in a horse. *J Comp Pathol* 100:465–468.
9. Zaloudek, C., and Norris, H.J. (1994) Mesenchymal tumors of the uterus. In Kurman, R.J.(ed.), *Blaustein's Pathology of the Female Genital Tract*, 4th ed. Springer-Verlag, New York, pp.488–490.
10. Allison, N., and Moeller, R.B., Jr. (1999) Bilateral testicular leiomyosarcoma in a stallion. *J Vet Diag Invest* 11:179–182.
11. Noordsy, J.L., Cook, J.E., and Downing, C.W. (1973) Leiomyosarcoma of the uterus in a Holstein cow. *Vet Med Small Anim Clin* 68:176–179.
12. Helphrey, M.L., and Meierhenry, E.F. (1978) Vulvar leiomyosarcoma metastatic to the spinal cord in a dog. *J Amer Vet Med Assoc* 172:583–584.

13. Hulland, T.J. (1990) Tumors of the muscle. In Moulton, J.E. (ed.), *Tumors in Domestic Animals,* 3rd ed. University of California Press, Berkeley, pp. 88–101.

14. Norris, H.J., Garner, F.M., and Taylor, H.B. (1969) Pathology of feline ovarian neoplasms. *J Pathol* 97:138–143.

15. Haibel, G.K., Constable, P.D., and Rojko, J.L. (1990) Vaginal leiomyofibromatosis and goiter in a goat. *J Amer Vet Med Assoc* 196:627–629.

16. Whitney, K.M., Valentine, B.A., and Schlafer, D.H. (2000) Caprine genital leiomyosarcoma. *Vet Pathol* 37:89–94.

17. Anjiki, T., Takeya, G., Hashimoto, N., and Kadota, K. (1991) An ultrastructural study of vulval myofibroblastoma in a cow. *J Vet Med A* 38:770–775.

Leiomyoma/Leiomyosarcoma of the Skin and Subcutis

Cutaneous leiomyoma occurs most frequently in dogs and ferrets. Leiomyosarcomas of the skin and subcutis are extremely rare, however, although this diagnosis may be made based on light microscopic features reminiscent of smooth muscle differentiation. Light microscopic differentiation of cutaneous and subcutaneous leiomyoma and leiomyosarcoma from other connective tissue tumors is difficult. Electron microscopic and/or immunocytochemical techniques are often necessary to confirm that a tumor is of smooth muscle origin. In the dog, a misdiagnosis of leiomyoma or leiomyosarcoma is most often made on tumors such as hemangiopericytoma, fibroma, fibrosarcoma, collagenous nevus (dermatofibroma), Schwannoma, malignant nerve sheath tumor, undifferentiated sarcoma, and malignant fibrous histiocytoma. In the cat, a distinctive dermal, subcutaneous, or gingival spindle cell tumor occurs that has been diagnosed as leiomyoma or leiomyosarcoma. We have undertaken immunohistochemical studies of approximately 30 of these tumors, and in only one case were we able to confirm a smooth muscle origin. Although the precise cell of origin of these distinctive feline subcutaneous tumors remains undetermined, many had patchy to diffuse staining with S-100, suggesting that they may be of Schwann cell or perineurial cell origin; however, this stain is not specific for just these cells.

Incidence, Age, Breed, and Sex

Leiomyoma of the skin is an uncommon tumor, and there is not sufficient data to allow for determination of age, breed, or sex predilections. The majority of these tumors are thought to arise from the smooth muscle of arrector pilae. We have recognized this tumor in the skin of five dogs aged 8 to 14 years (two mixed breeds, one each poodle, German shepherd, and golden retriever) and three ferrets aged 4.5 to 8 years, and immunohistochemical studies confirmed origin from smooth muscle. A cutaneous smooth muscle tumor has been reported in a 12-year-old cat.[1] A tumor with both fibrous and immature smooth muscle elements (fibroleiomyoma) has been reported in the skin of an 11-month-old pig.[2] A subcutaneous leiomyosar-

coma has been reported in a cow[3] and in a Peruvian squirrel monkey.[4] Leiomyomas and leiomyosarcomas also occur in the perineal region of dogs and cats. The exact site of origin of these perineal tumors is often not clear; vaginal, rectal, or even anal sac origin is possible. A dermal intravascular leiomyosarcoma has been reported in an adult cat.[5]

Clinical Characteristics, Sites, and Gross Morphology

Cutaneous tumors occur as solitary, raised, minimally to nonulcerated, nodular to multinodular, solid, firm tumors within the dermis. Canine tumors may be discrete expansile masses; nonexpansile infiltrative but still localized masses; or more dispersed within the skin, involving multiple tumor nodules within a localized area. The piloleiomyoma in the cat was more dispersed and was thought to arise within arrector pilae muscle. Although described as a single multinodular mass, the tumor was diagnosed as multiple piloleiomyomas.[1] Those in the ferret have been discrete expansile lesions. The young sow was reported to have a nodular scab-like lesion in the skin of the ear. On section the tumor was gray-white with numerous small blood vessels in the center.[2] The bovine leiomyosarcoma, confirmed by electron microscopy and immunohistochemistry, was reported to be a rapidly growing mass in the soft tissue of the neck.[3] The leiomyosarcoma in the monkey was a rapidly growing mass in the subcutis of the thorax near the sternum.[4] Large perineal tumors may ulcerate and/or cause urinary or fecal obstruction. The subcutaneous intravascular leiomyosarcoma in the cat occurred in the tissues of the distal digit, and it was an expansile, locally invasive tumor.[5]

Histological Features, Growth, and Metastasis

Discrete cutaneous leiomyomas occur within the dermis as slow growing, expansile nodules with three distinct histological patterns. One is of homogeneous spindle cells with features similar to leiomyomas in other sites (fig. 6.1 B). This pattern is most common in tumors of the perineal region. The second pattern is of loosely to densely arranged, mildly pleomorphic, plump ovoid to elongate cells with intensely eosinophilic cytoplasm and frequent cytoplasmic vacuolization forming broad interlacing bundles. Nuclei are central to occasionally eccentric, plump, oval to elongate, with granular to dispersed chromatin. Binucleate and multinucleate cells may be seen, but are not prominent. Anisokaryosis is common (fig. 6.1 D), and scattered nuclei may contain prominent vacuoles, presumed to be due to cytoplasmic invaginations. Small to large foci of perivascular lymphocytic infiltration are common. These tumors strongly resemble normal to hypertrophied arrector pilae muscles. This histological pattern is also seen in the more dispersed cutaneous leiomyomas (fig. 6.6). The third pattern is of loosely arranged, markedly attenuated spindle cells forming small irregularly arranged bundles. Cells have pale eosinophilic cytoplasm, and nuclei are remarkably elongate with granular chromatin and blunt to elongate ends. This tumor pattern is very similar to that seen in tumors of neural origin. The more dispersed form of cutaneous leiomyoma, formed by multiple nests of disarrayed smooth muscle cells within the dermis (fig. 6.6), begs the question of whether this is a true neoplasm or a hamartoma that becomes apparent only in adulthood. The piloleiomyomas in the cat demonstrated prominent osteoid metaplasia within tumor fascicles.[1] The tumor in the young sow consisted of disarrayed collagen bundles admixed with immature smooth muscle cells that often formed the walls and filled the adventitial zones of small atypical muscular arteries.[2] This tumor was thought to have arisen within vascular smooth muscle and may be similar to the angioleiomyoma of the nasopharynx reported in a young dog.[6] The histological features of leiomyosarcoma of the skin and subcutis are similar to those seen in leiomyosarcoma at other sites. The leiomyosarcoma in the neck of the cow contained metaplastic trabeculae of bone and osteoid.[3] Leiomyoma and leiomyosarcoma of the perineum are histologically similar to those tumors within the gastrointestinal and genitourinary tract. Invasion of leiomyoma or metastasis of leiomyosarcomas of the skin and subcutis is uncommon, and wide excision is apparently curative. The feline digital leiomyosarcoma was unique, composed of closely packed bland and relatively homogeneous, oval to spindle cells with small amounts of eosinophilic cytoplasm. The mass was multilobular, with large nests of cells clearly contained within large dilated vascular channels resembling lymphatics (fig. 6.11),[5] very similar to the intravenous leiomyoma reported in the bladder of a cat.[7] This unusual dermal tumor was initially thought to be an undifferentiated carcinoma or carcinoid with lymphatic invasion, but special stains, including immunohistochemistry, indicated clear-cut smooth muscle differentiation (muscle actin and smooth muscle actin positivity) of the tumor cells. The diagnosis of leiomyosarcoma in this case was based on the presence of more than 1 mitosis per 10 HP fields and on local invasion. Endothelial cells lining the vascular channels were strongly positive for factor VIII–related antigen, more consistent with a venous than with a lymphatic origin. This tumor recurred at the site, with invasion proximally around, but not into, the bone of the third phalanx. Metastasis was not apparent.[5]

Leiomyoma/Leiomyosarcoma of the Spleen and Liver

To our knowledge, immunohistochemical or ultrastructural studies have not been performed in any reported

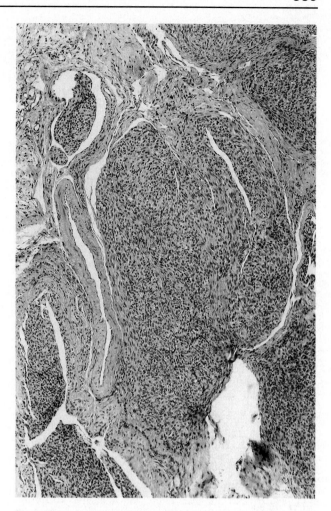

Fig. 6.11. Cutaneous intravascular leiomyosarcoma from a cat. Densely cellular tumor nodules occur within dilated vascular spaces. (Photograph courtesy of Dr. Matthew Jacobson.)

splenic or hepatic leiomyosarcoma in animals. The immunohistochemical studies performed on cases diagnosed at Cornell confirmed all cases diagnosed as leiomyoma, but they failed to provide convincing evidence of smooth muscle differentiation in many of the splenic and hepatic leiomyosarcomas. Therefore a diagnosis of undifferentiated sarcoma may be more appropriate. The light microscopic features of these tumors are, however, so characteristic of leiomyosarcoma that, in the absence of immunohistochemical studies, there is no doubt that a diagnosis of leiomyosarcoma will be made. Given the light microscopic findings and the documented aggressive behavior of these tumors, we are still reporting these tumors as *leiomyosarcomas.*

Incidence, Age, Breed, and Sex

Leiomyomas and leiomyosarcomas may arise within the vascular or interstitial smooth muscle of the spleen, causing splenic enlargement. Two canine splenic leiomyomas were found in the Cornell files. The spleen was the second most common site of leiomyosarcoma in a study of 44 dogs, accounting for 16 of 44 cases.[8] Splenic leiomyosarcoma accounted for 21 of 163 canine leiomyosarcomas in the Cornell files. Reviews of all canine splenic lesions indicate that leiomyosarcoma accounts for 1 percent[9] to 4 percent[10] of all lesions, whereas a study of nonangiogenic and nonlymphomatous canine splenic sarcomas found a 5.5 percent incidence of leiomyosarcoma.[11] We found no hepatic leiomyomas occurring outside of the biliary tree, and primary hepatic leiomyosarcoma is uncommon. In one report, 5 of 44 canine leiomyosarcomas occurred within the liver,[8] and only one primary canine hepatic leiomyosarcoma was found in the Cornell files. Mean age of diagnosis of primary canine splenic leiomyosarcoma has been reported as 7.3 years[10] and 10.3 years.[8] Mean age of primary canine hepatic leiomyosarcoma was reported to be 9 years.[8] There is no apparent breed or sex predisposition.

Primary splenic and hepatic leiomyosarcomas are uncommon in other species. In the Cornell files, 2 of 22 feline leiomyosarcomas occurred in the spleen. Primary splenic or hepatic leiomyosarcoma was not found in any other domestic species.

Clinical Characteristics and Gross Morphology

Clinical signs of primary splenic leiomyosarcoma are nonspecific and include anorexia, lethargy, vomiting, weight loss, distended abdomen, and diarrhea.[8] Clinical signs of primary hepatic leiomyosarcoma include lethargy, anorexia, and vomiting.[8] Gross morphology is similar to leiomyosarcoma at other sites (fig. 6.12).

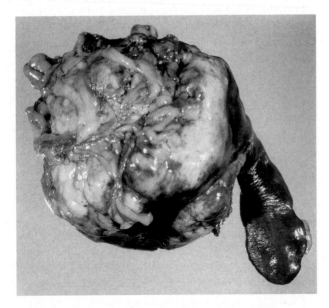

Fig. 6.12.   Splenic leiomyosarcoma from a dog.

Histological Features, Growth, and Metastasis

Despite our inability to demonstrate convincing smooth muscle differentiation with immunohistochemistry, the histological features of tumors diagnosed as leiomyosarcoma of the spleen and liver are similar to those at other sites (fig. 6.3 A). The aggressive behavior of these tumors, however, warrants discussion under a separate heading. In the Cornell files, 38 percent of canine splenic leiomyosarcomas had metastasis to intra-abdominal lymph nodes and serosal surfaces, and there were occasional pulmonary metastasis, usually noted at the time of diagnosis. Hepatic metastasis was recorded for one of two feline splenic leiomyosarcomas. Although one report concluded that the prognosis in dogs with leiomyosarcoma of the spleen is good to excellent if surgery is performed, these authors also report that 82 percent of the affected dogs eventually died due to metastatic disease.[8] Another report describes evidence of metastasis at the time of surgery for three of four splenic leiomyosarcomas in dogs.[10] In one report, all five dogs with primary hepatic leiomyosarcoma had evidence of diffuse intra-abdominal metastasis at surgery,[8] and the dog with primary hepatic leiomyosarcoma in the Cornell files had intrahepatic and mesenteric metastases at the time of surgery. These data suggest that a guarded to poor prognosis following diagnosis of splenic or hepatic leiomyosarcoma is warranted.

Smooth Muscle Tumors (Leiomyoma) of the Respiratory Tract

Incidence, Age, Breed, and Sex

Smooth muscle tumors arising within the respiratory tract are extremely rare. Only one case in a 7-year-old ferret was found in the Cornell files. Two tracheal leiomyomas have been reported in aged dogs,[12,13] one male and one female. Interestingly, one dog was a poodle and one was a poodle mix, but clearly there is insufficient data to provide age, breed, or sex predilections. An angioleiomyoma has been reported in the nasopharynx of a 1-year-old male golden retriever.[6] No cases of leiomyosarcoma of the respiratory tract were found in the Cornell files or in the literature.

Clinical Characteristics and Gross Morphology

The dogs with tracheal leiomyomas presented with severe respiratory distress due to airway compromise. The gross morphology was of smooth, firm masses arising from the tracheal smooth muscle and growing into the tracheal lumen.[12,13] The angioleiomyoma was a polypoid mass with a narrow base that resulted in clinical signs of sneezing and nasal discharge.[6] The ferret tumor was intimately associated with the outer surface of the trachea and was an incidental finding at necropsy.

Histological Features, Growth, and Metastasis

The histological features of tracheal leiomyomas were typical of leiomyomas occurring in the gastrointestinal tract and genitourinary system. In one case of tracheal leiomyoma, surgical excision required tracheal resection,[13] whereas the other case could be excised with only an incision into the trachea.[12] Recurrence was not observed. Leiomyosarcoma of the respiratory tract has not been reported, and none were found in the Cornell files. The canine angioleiomyoma was composed of papillary growths with scattered islands of woven bone, with a stroma consisting of numerous vascular structures, both arteriolar and venous, with many elongate, eosinophilic, occasionally binucleate, cells and cellular areas of small pleomorphic cells that blended with adjacent vascular smooth muscle. This tumor was thought to have arisen within vascular smooth muscle. It recurred following initial excision, but wide excision was apparently curative.[6] Given the features of this case, and the young age of the dog, we would also consider the possibility that this may have been a reactive or hamartomatous lesion.

Leiomyomas and Leiomyosarcomas at Other Sites

A large intra-abdominal smooth muscle tumor diagnosed as leiomyoma (leiomyomatosis) in a 6-year-old mare resulted in anorexia, weight loss, intermittent fever, and abdominal enlargement and was compared to disseminated peritoneal leiomyomatosis that occurs in women of childbearing age.[14] The origin of this tumor appeared to be the omentum. We have seen a similar tumor within the omentum of a dog. Surgical excision of the mass in the mare was apparently curative. We have also seen a leiomyoma within the iris of a cat. Leiomyosarcomas are occasionally found either as large masses within the abdomen or as disseminated intra-abdominal tumors (in which a primary site cannot be determined) in the mesentery and along serosal surfaces. In the Cornell files, a large intra-abdominal leiomyosarcoma associated with the omentum was found in a 4-year-old spayed female ferret, and a large intra-abdominal leiomyosarcoma was found in an 8-year-old female lemur (nonhuman primate). These cases are interesting and are somewhat similar to the case reported in the young adult mare.[14] A retroperitoneal leiomyosarcoma was found as a large sublumbar mass in an 8-year-old spayed female cat in which metastases were found in the heart, lungs, and urinary bladder; however, it is possible that this malignant tumor arose within the urinary bladder.[15]

REFERENCES

1. Finnie, J.W., Leong, S.-Y., and Milios, J. (1995) Multiple piloleiomyomas in a cat. *J Comp Pathol* 113:201–204.
2. Nakamura, T., Fukagawa, S., and Kiryu, K. (1987) Fibroleiomyoma on a sow ear. *Jpn J Vet Sci* 49:1177–1179.
3. Hanzaike, T., Ito, I., Ishikawa, T., Ishikawa, Y., and Kadota, K. (1995) Leiomyosarcoma of soft tissue in a cow. *J Comp Pathol* 112:237–242.
4. Brunnert, S.R., Herron, A.J., and Altman, N.H. (1990) Subcutaneous leiomyosarcoma in a Peruvian squirrel monkey *(Saimiri sciureus)*. *Vet Pathol* 27:126–128.
5. Jacobsen, M.C., and Valentine, B.A. (2000) Dermal intravascular leiomyosarcoma in a cat. *Vet Pathol* 37:100–103.
6. Carpenter, J.L., and Hamilton, T.A. (1995) Angioleiomyoma of the nasopharynx in a dog. *Vet Pathol* 32:721–723.
7. Patnaik, A.K., and Greene, R.W. (1979) Intravenous leiomyoma of the bladder in a cat. *J Amer Vet Med Assoc* 175:381–383.
8. Kapatkin, A.S., Mullen, H.S., Mattiesen, D.T., and Patnaik, A.K. (1992) Leiomyosarcoma in dogs: 44 cases (1983–1988). *J Amer Vet Med Assoc* 201:1077–1079.
9. Day, M.J., Lucke, V.M., and Pearson, H. (1995) A review of pathological diagnoses made from 87 canine splenic biopsies. *J Small Anim Prac* 36:426–433.
10. Johnson, K.A., Powers, B.E., Withrow, S.J., Sheetz, M.J., Curtis, C.R., and Wrigley, R.H. (1989) Splenomegaly in dogs. Predictors of neoplasia and survival after splenectomy. *J Vet Int Med* 3:160–166.
11. Weinstein, M.J., Carpenter, J.L., and Mehlhaff Schunk, C.J. (1989) Nonangiogenic and nonlymphomatous sarcomas of the canine spleen: 57 cases (1975–1987). *J Amer Vet Med Assoc* 195:784–788.
12. Black, A.P., Liu, S., and Randolph, J.F. (1981) Primary tracheal leiomyoma in a dog. *J Amer Vet Med Assoc* 179:905–907.
13. Bryan, R.D., Frame, R.W., and Kier, A.B. (1981) Tracheal leiomyoma in a dog. *J Amer Vet Med Assoc* 178:1069–1070.
14. Johnson, P.J., Wilson, D.A., Turk, J.R., Pace, L.W., Campbell-Beggs, C., and Johnson, G.C. (1994) Disseminated peritoneal leiomyomatosis in a horse. *J Amer Vet Med Assoc* 205:725–728.
15. Speakman, C.F., Pechman, R.D. Jr., and D'Andrea, G.H. (1983) Aortic thrombosis and unilateral hydronephrosis associated with leiomyosarcoma in a cat. *J Amer Vet Med Assoc* 182:62–63.

TUMORS OF STRIATED MUSCLE

General Considerations

Neoplasms that differentiate to form striated muscle are called *rhabdomyomas,* in the case of benign lesions, and *rhabdomyosarcomas,* when malignant. Although these tumors may arise in skeletal muscle, where they are presumably derived from the nesting myoblasts, or satellite cells, they can arise in any part of the body, including sites that normally lack striated muscle. In such locations it has been suggested that they arise from nests of primitive mesenchymal cells capable of differentiation into striated muscle cells.[1]

Neoplasms of striated muscle are rare. In our 20-year retrospective search of records at Cornell University, 58 of approximately 83,000 cases of neoplasia were diagnosed as rhabdomyoma or rhabdomyosarcoma. However, misdiagnosis was common. Of the 58 cases, only 16 could be confirmed using contemporary methods (table 6.3). Misdiagnosis appeared most commonly to be based on the presence of multinucleate giant cells in what was otherwise obviously a sarcoma. For confirmation of the diagnosis of striated muscle tumors, the use of immunohistochemistry, and possibly electron microscopy, is important. Furthermore, the true incidence of these neoplasms is difficult to determine, due to the difficulty of finding cases that were, in fact, rhabdomyomas or rhabdomyosarcomas but were misdiagnosed as something else.

Classification and General Histological Features

A well-established scheme exists for the classification of tumors of striated muscle in humans.[2-4] The same classification can generally be applied to animal tumors and is summarized as follows.

Rhabdomyoma

Benign tumors of striated muscle, rhabdomyomas, are much rarer in humans than their malignant counterpart. Based on the literature and the records at Cornell University, this is true also in animals. Three different forms of rhabdomyoma are recognized in humans: *adult type, fetal type,* and *genital type.*[2,5] Only the adult type was recognized in the Cornell material.

Adult rhabdomyoma in humans occurs in older patients, predominantly in males, and usually in the head and neck region. They sometimes protrude into the larynx

or pharynx and may be comparable to some of the laryngeal tumors that occur in dogs, described later in this section. These neoplasms are composed of closely packed, round to polygonal cells, with deeply eosinophilic and finely granular cytoplasm. Cells are separated by a fine vascular stroma, and the mass is generally well circumscribed or encapsulated. Many of the tumor cells are vacuolated as a result of the presence of glycogen that is removed during processing. Heavily vacuolated cells with thin radiating cords of cytoplasm are referred to as *spiderweb cells.* Mitotic figures are rare or absent. Cross striations may be present, but are usually difficult to identify. Poorly developed myofibrils may be recognized ultrastructurally, and immunostaining for markers of skeletal muscle differentiation, such as desmin and myoglobin, is positive.

Fetal rhabdomyoma is a very rare tumor occurring mainly in young, male children, but it can occur at any age. These neoplasms occur mainly in the subcutaneous tissue in the head and neck region. Histologically they are composed of primitive muscle fibers, or myotubes. These cells, which may be multinucleate, are admixed with spindle shaped cells and a variably myxoid matrix. Well-differentiated muscle fibers are often more numerous at the periphery of the tumor, these cells often showing cross striations. These tumors are usually well demarcated from surrounding tissue, and mitotic figures are rarely seen. Because of variation in cellularity, it may be difficult to differentiate this tumor from rhabdomyosarcoma. We have found no examples corresponding to this tumor in the veterinary literature or in our files.

TABLE 6.3. Sixteen cases of rhabdomyoma or rhabdomyosarcoma

Case	Diagnosis	Sex	Age	Site	Vim	CK	msA	smA	srcA	Des	Mb
1	Emb RMS	M	1.5y	Hard palate	+	–	+	–	+	+	–
2	RMA	Fs	10y	Larynx	+/–	–	+	–	+	+	+
3	Pleo RMS	M	3y	Neck	+	–	+	–	+	+	+
4	Bot RMS	F	1y	Bladder	+	–	+	–	+	+	+
5	Bot RMS	F	6mo	Bladder	+	–	ND	–	+	+	+
6	RMA (adult)	M	11y	Skin of abdomen	+	–	ND	–	+	+	+
7	Emb RMS	F	Adult	Mammary gland	+	–	+	–	+	+	+
8	Emb RMS	F	9y	Leg muscle	+	–	+	–	+	+	–
9	Emb RMS	F	11y	Tongue	–	+/–	+–	–	+	+	+
10	Emb RMS	M	4y	Muscle of flank	+	–	+	–	+	+	+
11	RMA (adult)	M	14y	Skin of foot	+	–	+/–	+	+	+	+
12	Alv RMS	M	7y	Hip	+/–	–	+	+/–	–	+	+
13	Emb RMS	F	12y	Tongue	+	–	+	–	+	+	+
14	RMA	M	8y	Larynx	ND	ND	+	ND	+	+	ND
15	Emb RMS	M	6y	Perirenal	+	ND	ND	–	+	+	+/–
16	Emb RMS	F	14y	Axilla	+	–	+	–	+	+	+

These cases were retrieved from 20 years of archived material. Case 8 was a cat, all others were dogs; no obvious breed predisposition was identified.
Tests: Vim = vimentin; CK = cytokeratins, msA = muscle specific actin; smA = smooth muscle actin; srcA = sarcomeric actin; Des = desmin; Mb = myoglobin. **Test Results:** + = positive; – = negative; +/– = weak or doubtful staining; ND = not done. **Diagnosis:** RMA = rhabdomyoma; RMS = rhabdomyosarcoma; Emb = embryonal; Bot = botryoid; Pleo = pleomorphic; Alv = alveolar.

Genital rhabdomyoma is a rare tumor occurring in the vagina or vulva of young to middle-aged women. They generally form polypoid masses that, histologically, contain haphazardly organized, well-differentiated muscle fibers. We have found no examples in animals corresponding to this neoplasm.

Rhabdomyosarcoma

Rhabdomyosarcomas, malignant tumors of striated muscle, are classified as *embryonal, botryoid, alveolar,* and *pleomorphic*.[2,4] In humans, pleomorphic rhabdomyosarcoma, overall the least common variant, is almost exclusively a neoplasm of adults.[6] Although any rhabdomyosarcoma may be pleomorphic, the diagnosis of the pleomorphic variant should be reserved for those tumors that are pleomorphic *and* lack areas of embryonal or alveolar pattern.[6] The presence of such areas, even if limited in extent, justifies the corresponding diagnosis. The accurate classification of these tumors in humans is prognostically important, with the best outcomes associated with botryoid rhabdomyosarcoma and the worst with alveolar rhabdomyosarcoma. Embryonal forms have an intermediate prognosis. There is presently insufficient information on clinical outcome to make such prognostic predictions in animals, but development of such information will depend on accurate and consistent classification.

Embryonal rhabdomyosarcoma is the most common variant in humans. It is typically a tumor of children, but it may occur also in adults. It may occur in the head and neck region, the urogenital tract, the retroperitoneum, and the limbs. This tumor is characterized by relatively primitive myogenic cells, with two main forms being recognized. In the first variant, the neoplastic cells are small and round, with variable numbers of large, well-differentiated rhabdomyoblasts. In the second, the neoplastic cells are elongate and resemble myotubes in developing muscle. Cross striations may be present. Some of these tumors may be pleomorphic and may be difficult to differentiate from pleomorphic rhabdomyosarcoma.

Botryoid rhabdomyosarcoma is regarded as a variant of embryonal rhabdomyosarcoma.[2] It grows in a polypoid, grape-like pattern, typically projecting into a mucosa lined organ. In humans these tumors typically contain a sparse population of cells suspended in a myxoid matrix. Variable numbers of rhabdomyoblasts and/or elongate muscle cells may be present. The presence of a densely cellular *cambrium layer* beneath the mucosa is an important diagnostic feature.

Alveolar rhabdomyosarcoma is a less common form in humans. It is a tumor of adolescents and young adults. Histologically this type is composed of aggregates of poorly differentiated cells separated by fibrovascular stroma. The cells in the center of the aggregates are poorly cohesive and become degenerate, separating from one another, thus producing the alveolar pattern. Viable cells often line the fibrous stroma. Differentiated rhabdomyoblasts are relatively uncommon in alveolar rhabdomyosarcoma, and cross striations are rarely recognized. However, multinucleate giant cells are commonly found. An additional variant, solid alveolar rhabdomyosarcoma, has now been recognized in humans. This variant has dense sheets of neoplastic cells, cytologically similar to other alveolar rhabdomyosarcomas, but with only focal areas of fibrosis. The neoplasm in humans referred to as alveolar soft-part sarcoma may also represent alveolar rhabdomyosarcoma, as many cases stain with markers for muscle differentiation.

Pleomorphic rhabdomyosarcoma, although often perceived as being the classic type of rhabdomyosarcoma, is the least common variant in humans.[2,4,6] Although it has been reported in patients of varying ages, it typically occurs in adults and is now regarded as extremely rare or nonexistent in children. Typically, this variant occurs in large muscles of the limbs and histologically contains a very pleomorphic cell population. Some of the neoplastic cells have abundant eosinophilic cytoplasm, but in humans, this type of rhabdomyosarcoma generally lacks cells with cross striations. The cells of pleomorphic rhabdomyosarcoma often contain glycogen.

REFERENCES

1. Parham, D.M., Kelly, D.R., Donnelly, W.H., and Douglass, E.C. (1991) Immunohistochemical and ultrastructural spectrum of hepatic sarcomas of childhood: Evidence for a common histogenesis. *Mod Pathol* 4:648–53.
2. Enzinger, F.M., and Weiss, S.W. (1988) *Soft Tissue Tumors,* 2nd ed. CV Mosby Co., Washington, D.C.
3. Tsokos, M. (1994) The diagnosis and classification of childhood rhabdomyosarcoma. *Sem Diag Pathol* 11:26–38.
4. Newton, W.A., Jr. (1995) Classification of rhabdomyosarcoma. In Harms, D., and Schmidt, D., (eds.) *Current Topics in Pathology.* Springer-Verlag, Berlin.
5. Willis, J., Abdul-Karim, F.W., and di Sant'Agnese, P.A. (1994) Extracardiac rhabdomyomas. *Sem Diag Pathol* 11:15–25.
6. Hollowood, K., and Fletcher, C.D.M. (1994) Rhabdomyosarcoma in adults. *Sem Diag Pathol* 11:47–57.

Clinicopathologic Features

Reports of striated muscle tumors in animals rarely include information on cytology. However, given the variable histological features of these neoplasms, cytologic findings would also be expected to be variable. The presence of multinucleate, elongate cells, possibly with cross striations, could suggest the diagnosis,[1,2] but in many cases cytologic features will be nonspecific. In one pleomorphic rhabdomyosarcoma reported in a horse, cytology revealed individual and clustered pleomorphic cells with variable nuclear to cytoplasmic ratio, variably shaped nuclei, and variable numbers of nucleoli.[3] In a laryngeal rhabdomyosarcoma in a dog, cytology was nonspecific and revealed atypical cells with abundant irregular cytoplasm, some with purple intracytoplasmic granules, and variably sized nuclei.[4] No confirmed cases in the Cornell files were examined cytologically.

REFERENCES

1. Bundza, A., and Greig, A.S. (1981) Cytological, cytochemical, light and ultrastructural studies of a bovine rhabdomyosarcoma. *Bov Prac* 2:24–27.
2. Alleman, A.R., Raskin, R.E., Uhl, E.W., and Senior, D.R. (1991) What is your diagnosis? (Botryoid rhabdomyosarcoma of the urinary bladder). *Vet Clin Pathol* 20:44.
3. Hanson, P.D., Frisbie, D.D., Dubielzig, R.R., and Markel, M.D. (1993) Rhabdomyosarcoma of the tongue in a horse. *J Amer Vet Med Assoc* 202:1281–1284.
4. Henderson, R.A., Powers, R.D., and Perry, L. (1991) Development of hypoparathyroidism after excision of laryngeal rhabdomyosarcoma in a dog. *J Amer Vet Med Assoc* 198:639–643.

Special Diagnostic Procedures

The age-old criterion for confirmation of a diagnosis of rhabdomyosarcoma is the identification of cross striations in tumor cells. This is still a useful criterion, but it can involve use of special stains and long hours of searching, often without success. As has been indicated, many confirmed rhabdomyosarcomas lack demonstrable cross striations. This difficulty has in the past led to the use of electron microscopy for confirmation of diagnosis. This is still a useful tool, and ultrastructural features of rhabdomyomas and rhabdomyosarcomas will be discussed. However, electron microscopy has largely been supplanted by the use of immunohistochemistry, which is less expensive, quicker, and provides more effective sampling.

Ultrastructural Features of Tumors of Striated Muscle

Electron microscopic examination has been carried out in several published cases.[1-5] Ultrastructurally the most useful diagnostic feature is the presence of myofilaments, that is, the presence of actin and myosin filaments. These are most meaningful when they are organized into parallel bundles, or myofibrils, with recognizable electron dense Z bands (see fig. 6.16). These are the ultrastructural equivalent of light microscopic cross striations. However, bundles of myofilaments that may be too small and disorganized to be recognized at the light microscopic level may be apparent ultrastructurally. Other common ultrastructural features of rhabdomyosarcomas are the presence of numerous mitochondria, which may be aligned in rows between myofibrils, large euchromatic nuclei, ribosomes occurring singly or as polysomes, and glycogen. The sarcoplasmic reticulum is usually poorly developed and difficult to identify. Poorly differentiated mesenchymal cells in these tumors contain similar euchromatic nuclei, mitochondria, and ribosomes but lack convincing evidence of myofibril formation.

Immunohistochemistry of Tumors of Striated Muscle

Immunohistochemistry is now the preferred diagnostic technique for confirmation of the diagnosis of rhabdomyoma or rhabdomyosarcoma. It has been utilized in a number of recent case studies.[6-13] Antibodies that have proven useful in these studies include those against vimentin, desmin, actin, myoglobin, myosin, and titin. The same control procedures described for smooth muscle tumors are appropriate for suspect rhabdomyomatous tumors. It is important to use a panel of antibodies for immunohistochemical characterization of these tumors because the various antigens are expressed differentially, depending on the degree of differentiation of the neoplastic cells. This reflects the expression of proteins in developing muscle. For example, vimentin, desmin, fast myosin, and myoglobin are expressed in that order.[14] Vimentin is expressed early but is later lost as muscle fibers develop, while desmin and the sarcomeric isoform of actin are also expressed early but persist.[15] Myoglobin, on the other hand, is expressed later than desmin, and poorly differentiated rhabdomyosarcomas may express desmin but lack myoglobin.[16] A corollary of this is that immunohistochemical staining of rhabdomyosarcomas is usually heterogeneous, and in some cases only occasional cells, usually the well-differentiated large rhabdomyoblasts or strap cells, are positive, particularly for myoglobin.

Most of these markers are not specific for striated muscle differentiation.[17] Besides skeletal muscle, desmin is expressed in cardiac and smooth muscle cells; actin is expressed in cardiac muscle, smooth muscle, and many other cells, including myofibroblasts; and myosin is expressed in both cardiac and smooth muscle. Many of these proteins exist in relatively tissue specific isoforms, and antibodies have been developed to those forms. Thus, antibodies to actin that are available include muscle specific actin, smooth muscle actin, and sarcomeric actin. To complicate matters, neoplasms may express unexpected proteins. For example, rhabdomyosarcomas occasionally express smooth muscle actin,[17] although we have observed this in only one of the tumors in the Cornell series.

A panel of antibodies was used on the Cornell cases, including vimentin, cytokeratins, desmin, muscle specific actin (which stains smooth muscle, cardiac, and skeletal muscle cells, as well as some other cells, most importantly myofibroblasts), alpha–smooth muscle actin (which stains smooth muscle and certain other cells, including myofibroblasts), alpha–sarcomeric actin, and myoglobin. Of these, myoglobin and alpha–sarcomeric actin are the only markers that can be regarded as specific for striated muscle differentiation. The results for the 16 cases of rhabdomyoma and rhabdomyosarcoma are shown in table 6.3. Summarizing these results, the "typical" staining pattern for rhabdomyoma or rhabdomyosarcoma is vimentin, negative or weakly reactive; cytokeratin, negative; desmin, positive; muscle specific actin, positive; smooth muscle actin, negative; sarcomeric actin, positive; and myoglobin, positive (fig.6.13 A-F). Some variation in these results will be found depending on the techniques and antibodies used. For example, cytokeratins are said to be fairly commonly expressed in human rhabdomyosarcomas,[17] but they were invariably absent in our cases. This is likely to be due to differences in the antibodies used and to the cytokeratin isoforms they recognize.

Care is required too in interpreting these immunostains. For example, staining, even though specific, may be focal. In some cases only a few cells stain (fig. 6.13 B,E), but if the stain lacks background and the appropriate cells stain (often the large well-differentiated rhabdomyoblasts), the rhabdomyogenic nature of the neoplasm can be confidently identified. Not all markers may be positive. This is particularly a problem with myoglobin, but the inclusion of desmin and alpha–sarcomeric actin in the panel should minimize this difficulty. Smooth muscle actin is expressed in perivascular and interstitial cells, and care must be taken not to confuse this with a positive result. However, expression of alpha–smooth muscle actin in rhabdomyosarcomas is documented in human cases[17] and occurred in one of our cases. This does not rule out the diagnosis. Similarly, vimentin is often expressed in interstitial cells but is usually absent from well-differentiated rhabdomyoblasts. It may be expressed in small, poorly differentiated neoplastic rhabdomyoblastic cells. Vimentin is not a particularly useful marker for determination of histogenetic origin of tumors, but it is always included in our panel, if for no other reason than to establish that the tissue is amenable to the immunostaining techniques in use. Failure of the vimentin stain to work on interstitial cells indicates a problem with the technique or with blocks or tissues that have been stored for prolonged periods in formalin.

Two markers that have recently become useful for the diagnosis of rhabdomyosarcoma in humans are *myo*D1 and myogenin.[17] *Myo*D1 is a regulatory gene product expressed in the nucleus, preceding the expression of other markers such as desmin. Myogenin is a similar regulatory gene product. Both appear to be specific for the striated muscle phenotype. *Myo*D1, in particular, has proven useful for the identification of poorly differentiated rhabdomyosarcomas where other markers are negative. They have not yet been applied in veterinary medicine but should prove useful for the recognition of poorly differentiated rhabdomyosarcoma.

REFERENCES

1. Peter, C.P., Kluge, J.P. (1970) An ultrastructural study of a canine rhabdomyosarcoma. *Cancer* 26:1280–1288.
2. Meyvisch, C., Thoonen, H., and Hoorens, J. (1977) The ultrastructure of rhabdomyosarcoma in a dog. *Zbl Vet Med A* 24:542–551.
3. Pospischel, A., Weiland, F., von Sandersleben, J., Hänichen, T., and Schäffler, H. (1982) Endemic ethmoidal tumours in cattle: Sarcomas

and carcinosarcomas. A light and electron microscopic study. *Zbl Vet Med A* 29:628–636.
4. Bundza, A., and Greig, A.S. (1981) Cytological, cytochemical, light and ultrastructural studies of a bovine rhabdomyosarcoma. *Bov Prac* 2:24–27.
5. Meuten, D.J., Calderwood Mays, M.B., Dillman, R.C., Cooper, B.J., Valentine, B.A., Kuhajda, F.P., and Pass, D.A. (1985) Canine Laryngeal rhabdomyoma. *Vet Pathol* 22:533–539.
6. Brown, P.J. (1987) Immunohistochemical localization of myoglobin in connective tissue tumors in dogs. *Vet Pathol* 24:573–574.
7. Andreasen, C.B., White, M.R., Swayne, D.E., and Graves, G.N. (1988) Desmin as a marker for canine botryoid rhabdomyosarcomas. *J Comp Pathol* 98:23–29.
8. Moore, A.S., Madewell, B.R., and Lund, J.K. (1989) Immunohistochemical evaluation of intermediate filament expression in canine and feline neoplasms. *Amer J Vet Res* 50:88–92.
9. Matsui, T., Imai, T., Han, J.S., Awakura, T., Taniyama, H., Osame, S., Nakagawa, M., and Ono, T. (1991) Bovine undifferentiated alveolar rhabdomyosarcoma and its differentiation in xenotransplanted tumors. *Vet Pathol* 28:438–445.
10. Martín de las Mulas, J., Vos, J.H., and Van Mil, F.N. (1992) Desmin and vimentin immunocharacterization of feline muscle tumors. *Vet Pathol* 29:260–262.
11. Clegg, P.D., and Coumbe, A. (1993) Alveolar rhabdomyosarcoma: An unusual cause of lameness in a pony. *Equine Vet J* 25:547–549.
12. Hanson, P.D., Frisbie, D.D., Dubielzig, R.R., and Markel, M.D. (1993) Rhabdomyosarcoma of the tongue in a horse. *J Amer Vet Med Assoc* 202:1281–1284.
13. Sarnelli, R., Grassi, F., Romagnoli, S. (1994) Alveolar rhabdomyosarcoma of the greater omentum in a dog. *Vet Pathol* 31:473–475.
14. Carter R.L., Jameson C.F., Philp E.R., and Pinkerton C.R. (1990) Comparative phenotypes in rhabdomyosarcomas and developing skeletal muscle. *Histopathology* 17:301–309.
15. Wijnaendts, L.C.D., van der Linden, J.C., van Unnik, A.J., Delemarre, J.F., Voute, P.A., and Meijer, C.J. (1994) The expression pattern of contractile and intermediate filament proteins in developing skeletal muscle and rhabdomyosarcoma of childhood: Diagnostic and prognostic utility. *J Pathol* 174:283–292.
16. Carter R.L., McCarthy K.P., Machin L.G., Jameson C.F., Philp E.R., and Pinkerton C.R. (1989) Expression of desmin and myoglobin in rhabdomyosarcomas and in developing skeletal muscle. *Histopathology* 15:585–595.
17. Brooks, J.S.J. (1996) Immunohistochemistry in the differential diagnosis of soft tissue tumors. In Weiss, S.W., and Brooks, J.S.J. (eds.), *Soft Tissue Tumors.* Williams and Wilkins, Baltimore, pp. 65–128.

Rhabdomyoma

Incidence, Age, Breed and Sex

Apart from the laryngeal tumors described below, rhabdomyomas are very rare in the veterinary literature, and it is difficult to retrospectively classify those that have been reported. Because of this it is impossible to make generalized statements about incidence and clinical characteristics. One report exists of rhabdomyomas occurring in four female cats, aged 6–7 years.[1] A cystic tumor diagnosed as a rhabdomyoma was found at necropsy in a 2-year-old female horse.[2] Of the 16 striated muscle tumors in the Cornell material, four were classified as rhabdomyomas, two of which were laryngeal and two subcutaneous (table 6.3). All were of the adult type, and all occurred in aged male dogs.

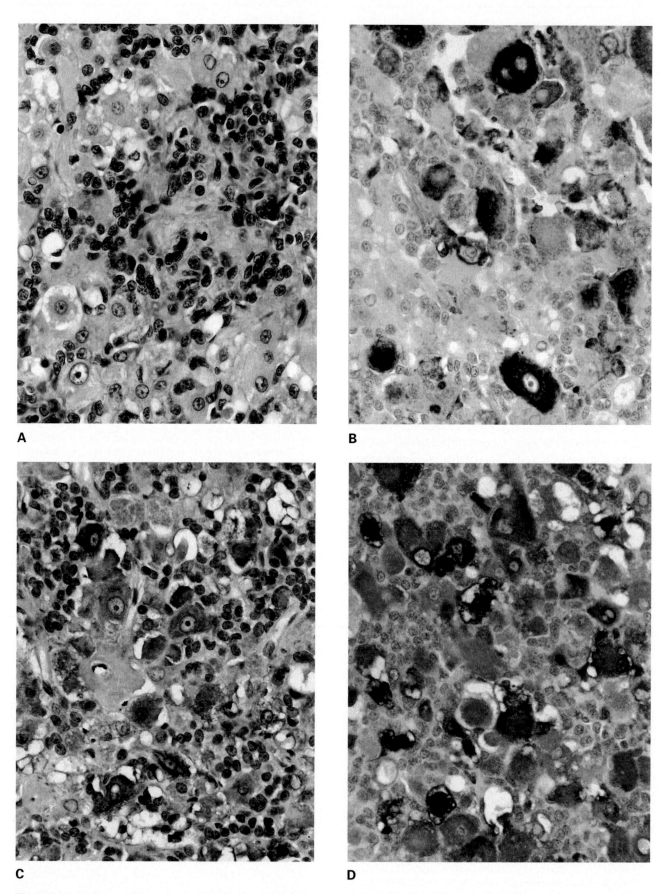

Fig. 6.13. Histochemical panel, embryonal rhabdomyosarcoma from a dog. **A.** Tumor composed of a mixture of large rhabdomyoblasts and small round cells. Some of the rhabdomyoblasts are vacuolated, producing a spiderweb pattern. The tumor is positive for **B.** Muscle specific actin, **C.** Sarcomeric actin, **D.** Myoglobin, and (continued)

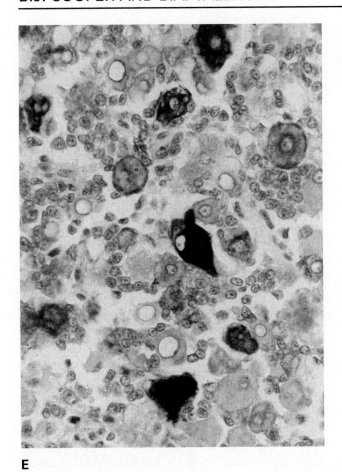

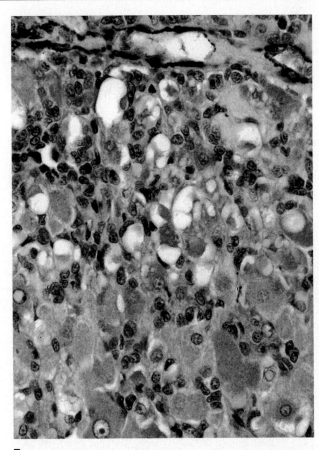

E

F

Fig. 6.13. (continued) **E.** Desmin. **F.** It is negative or weakly reactive for smooth muscle actin. Note the contrasting strong staining of the vessel wall for smooth muscle actin.

Clinical Characteristics and Sites

These lesions present either as noticeable masses or with signs referable to their location. The feline lesions presented as nonulcerated discoid masses protruding from the convex surface of the pinna, which in all of the cases was white.[1] The equine case presented with dyspnea and dependent edema.[2] Both of the adult rhabdomyomas in the Cornell series presented as subcutaneous masses, one on the abdomen and one on a foot. The most common site for rhabdomyoma in animals, based on published reports, is in the larynx. The tumors are discussed separately below.

Gross Morphology

Most rhabdomyomas would be expected to form pale, fleshy masses of variable size. The feline cases[1] and the rhabdomyomas in the Cornell series were 1–2 cm in diameter. The equine tumor was large (30 x 20 x 20 cm), was located in the posterior ventral mediastinum, and was attached by a stalk to the diaphragm.[2]

Histological Features, Growth, and Metastasis

Histologically, the nonlaryngeal rhabdomyomas in the Cornell series were consistent with adult rhabdomy-

oma of humans. They were discrete, with well-demarcated borders, but not encapsulated. In one case the tumor was divided into lobules by a fine fibrovascular stroma. They were dominated by large round to polygonal cells, so-called rhabdomyoblasts, with abundant, strongly eosinophilic cytoplasm (fig. 6.14 A,B). Some cells were vacuolated, forming the spiderweb appearance. Cell size varied, and one tumor had moderate cellular and nuclear pleomorphism. Binucleate and multinucleate cells were present. Nuclei were generally euchromatic with one or more prominent nucleoli. Smaller cells with minimal to moderate cytoplasm and dense, heterochromatic nuclei were interspersed between the large rhabdomyoblasts. Mitoses were rare. The neoplastic cells were positive by immunohistochemistry for striated muscle markers (table 6.3).

Histologically the reported feline tumors were well circumscribed and nonencapsulated and consisted of whorls and bundles of spindle shaped cells.[1] Mitotic figures were rare. PTAH staining revealed evidence of cross striations in a few neoplastic cells, although the tumors were not studied by immunohistochemistry or electron microscopy. The equine tumor was made up of elongate fibers in which cross striations were demonstrated by PTAH staining.[2] Moderate numbers of mitotic figures were present. In view of the reported mitoses, the basis for clas-

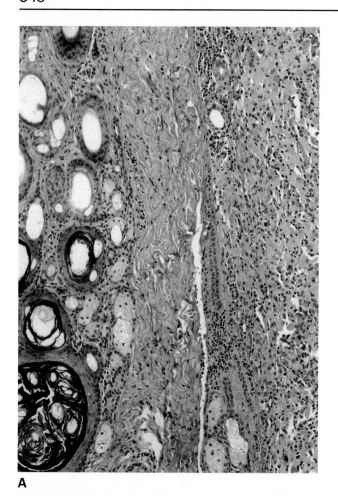

A

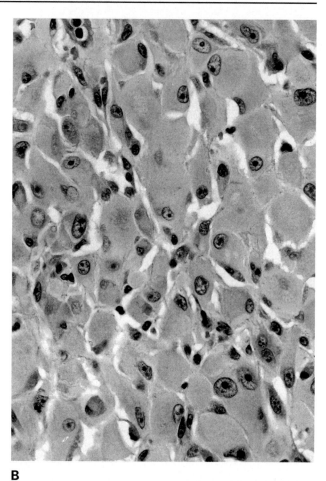

B

Fig. 6.14.   Cutaneous rhabdomyoma from a dog. **A.** Note that the mass is demarcated from the adjacent dermis. **B.** The tumor is made up of uniformly large, round, mononuclear cells; these cells have abundant eosinophilic cytoplasm and vesicular nuclei with prominent nucleoli (so-called owl's eye nuclei). There are no mitoses.

sification of this lesion as benign is not clear, but classification may have been based on the pedunculated nature of the mass. Without the opportunity to review these cases, it is difficult to classify them into one of the three recognized types of rhabdomyoma.

Although little data is available, one would expect these neoplasms to be slow growing and noninvasive and to not metastasize. In all four of the feline cases surgical excision resulted in apparent cure, with no recurrence after 2–3 years.[1]

Laryngeal Rhabdomyoma and Rhabdomyosarcoma

Incidence, Age, Breed, and Sex

This tumor forms a recognizable clinicopathologic entity in the dog. Four cases have been reported in the literature.[3,4] In addition, 2 of the 16 Cornell cases were classified as laryngeal rhabdomyoma. Young animals may be affected by this tumor, and ages in reported cases range from 2 to 10 years. There is no apparent breed predisposition. There is a suggestion of a sex predilection: four of the

six cases were females, one a male, and one of unstated sex. Similar tumors in the larynx and pharynx have been diagnosed as rhabdomyosarcomas, although the basis for the designation of malignancy is not always clear.

Clinical Characteristics, Gross Morphology, and Sites

Typically these neoplasms occur as masses protruding into the lumen of the larynx, and one case was described as a mass in the laryngeal pharynx.[5] Presenting signs are typically dyspnea, stridor, and/or dysphonia. The masses may show local infiltration but are usually covered by an intact mucosal epithelium.

Histological Features, Growth, and Metastasis

These tumors also have features consistent with adult rhabdomyoma and are made up of moderately pleomorphic, large, round or polygonal rhabdomyoblasts, which have abundant eosinophilic, sometimes granular or vacuolated, cytoplasm (fig. 6.15 A,B,C,D). Some tumors have

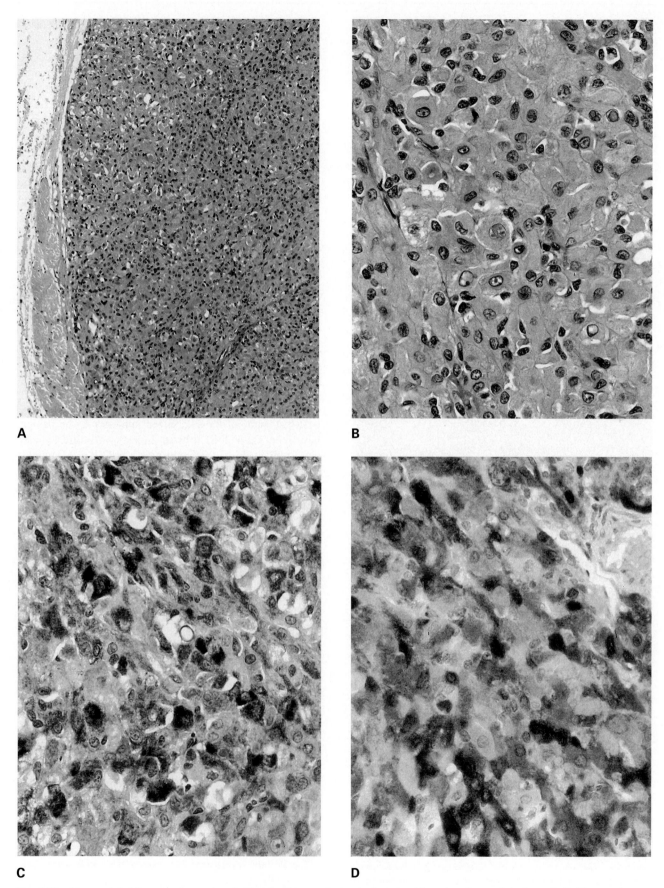

Fig. 6.15. Laryngeal rhabdomyoma from a dog. **A.** Note that the mass is sharply demarcated from the adjacent skeletal muscle. **B.** The mass is composed of uniformly large cells with abundant eosinophilic cytoplasm and generally vesicular nuclei with prominent nucleoli. The tumor is immunohistochemically positive for: **C.** Muscle specific actin, **D.** Myoglobin.

349

been misdiagnosed initially as oncocytomas based on their granular, eosinophilic cytoplasm and numerous mitochondria.[3] The tumors may contain a fine fibrovascular stroma dividing them into lobules. Interspersed between the large rhabdomyoblasts are variable numbers of small cells. Nuclei of the large rhabdomyoblasts are typically vesicular and contain one or more prominent nucleoli as well as occasional inclusions resulting from invagination of cytoplasm. The small cells contain denser, heterochromatic nuclei. Multinucleate and elongate strap-like cells may be present, as may cross striations, particularly in these cells. Mitotic figures are rare. Some cells are positive for glycogen using the PAS stain.[3] In some cases tumor cells locally infiltrate adjacent skeletal muscle fibers. Necrosis, hemorrhage, and hemosiderosis may be present.

Ultrastructurally the large rhabdomyoblasts contain myofilaments, poorly developed myofibrils, and Z bands, features that may be used to confirm the diagnosis (fig. 6.16). Numerous mitochondria, rough endoplasmic reticulum, and glycogen granules may also be present. A basal lamina is often associated with these cells. The smaller, less differentiated cells lack myofilaments and myofibrils. Laryngeal rhabdomyomas are positive for immunohisto-

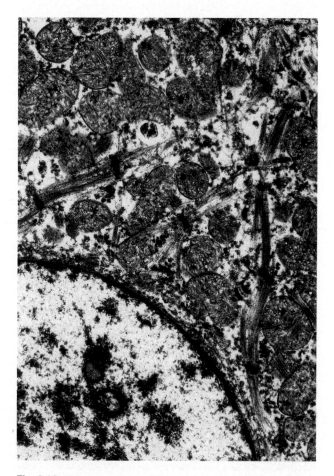

Fig. 6.16. Electron micrograph from a canine laryngeal rhabdomyoma showing part of the euchromatic nucleus and numerous mitochondria. Note the presence of disorganized myofibrils with obvious Z line structures. The myofibrils provide definitive evidence of striated muscle differentiation. [Reproduced, with permission, from reference 3.]

chemical markers for skeletal muscle (table 6.3), with staining being strongest in the large rhabdomyoblasts.

These tumors apparently have a benign course. The tumor free postsurgical period in the reported cases ranges from 15 to 42 months. One case recurred five months after initial surgery and was removed a second time.[3] The tumor had not recurred 24 months after the second surgery.

Five cases diagnosed as laryngeal rhabdomyosarcoma have been reported in the literature, all in the dog.[5-9] In general, presenting signs and histological features are similar to those of laryngeal rhabdomyoma. The designation of malignancy has usually been based on infiltration of adjacent tissues and may be debatable in some cases. Histological features, as described in these reports, are similar to those of laryngeal rhabdomyoma. Some of the reported tumors were circumscribed, were said to have low mitotic indices, and did not recur after surgery. However, in one case an apparent single hepatic metastatic lesion was found at necropsy 22 months after laryngectomy, despite the absence of local recurrence at the site of the original tumor.[6]

It is difficult, given the small number of cases in the literature, to provide firm guidelines for making the distinction between laryngeal rhabdomyoma and rhabdomyosarcoma. Given current experience, we would suggest that many of these laryngeal tumors may be benign, based on their low mitotic index, well-differentiated appearance, limited invasiveness, and clinical course. Malignancy may be suspected if the tumors are very pleomorphic with many small, undifferentiated cells, have a high mitotic index, or are locally very aggressive.

REFERENCES

1. Roth, L. (1990) Rhabdomyoma of the ear pinna in four cats. *J Comp Pathol* 103:237–240.
2. Hamir, A.N. (1982) Striated muscle tumours in horses. *Vet Rec* 111:367–368.
3. Meuten, D.J., Calderwood Mays, M.B., Dillman, R.C., Cooper, B.J., Valentine, B.A., Kuhajda, F.P., and Pass, D.A. (1985) Canine laryngeal rhabdomyoma. *Vet Pathol* 22:533–539.
4. Liggett, A.D., Weiss, R., and Thomas, K.L. (1985) Canine laryngopharyngeal rhabdomyoma resembling an oncocytoma. Light microscopic, ultrastructural and comparative studies. *Vet Pathol* 22:359–365.
5. Ladds, P.W., and Webster, D.R. (1971) Pharyngeal rhabdomyosarcoma in a dog. *Vet Pathol* 8:256–259.
6. Henderson, R.A., Powers, R.D., and Perry, L. (1991) Development of hypoparathyroidism after excision of laryngeal rhabdomyosarcoma in a dog. *J Amer Vet Med Assoc* 198:639–643.
7. Madewell, B., Lund, J., Munn, R., and Pino, M. (1988) Canine laryngeal rhabdomyosarcoma: An immunohistochemical and electron microscopic study. *Jap J Vet Sci* 50:1079–1084.
8. Block, G., Clarke, K., Salisbury, S.K., DeNicola, D.B. (1995) Total laryngectomy and permanent tracheostomy for treatment of laryngeal rhabdomyosarcoma in a dog. *J Amer Anim Hosp Assoc* 31:510–513.
9. Saik, J.E., Toll, S.L., Diters R.W., et al. (1986) Canine and feline laryngeal neoplasia: A 10-year survey. *J Amer Anim Hosp Assoc* 22:359–365.

Rhabdomyosarcoma

Rhabdomyosarcomas constitute the most commonly encountered neoplasms of striated muscle in animals, although they are still rare. They have been most commonly diagnosed in the dog, but a variety of species is involved, as discussed here. The different variants of rhabdomyosarcoma, as defined earlier, will be discussed, but it should be understood that this classification was not followed in many of the reported cases, and it is difficult to reclassify some cases based on the descriptions given.

Embryonal Rhabdomyosarcoma

Incidence, Age, Breed, and Sex

Embryonal rhabdomyosarcoma was the most common variant encountered in the Cornell material, with 8 of the 14 rhabdomyosarcomas being classified in this group. Seven of these cases were in dogs, and one in a cat. There is no obvious breed or sex predilection. Although these tumors can occur in young animals, as young as 1.5 years in the Cornell material, the majority of our cases were in older animals (see table 6.3).

Relatively few of the published cases have been classified as embryonal rhabdomyosarcoma, but this may be due to changes over the years in classification schemes and the failure to subclassify the reported tumors at all. A 1.5-year-old male bassett hound was reported with embryonal rhabdomyosarcoma involving the temporal muscle.[1] A case was reported in the paraspinal muscles of a 1-year-old female Hampshire sheep.[2] Two sheep, one a 3-month-old lamb and one of unknown age, were reported to have pulmonary rhabdomyosarcoma.[3,4] Both had features suggestive of embryonal rhabdomyosarcoma of the myotubular type, although the presence of tubular epithelial structures, if they were not entrapped bronchioles, raises the possibility of a mixed embryonal tumor. In one, metastasis to a mediastinal lymph node occurred.[4] An embryonal rhabdomyosarcoma of the trachea was reported in a 4-month-old male dog.[5] However, based on the data in the report, there is cause to speculate that this tumor was benign, as it was reported to contain few mitotic figures and had not recurred 34 months after resection. It may be that this tumor is related to the laryngeal rhabdomyomas already discussed.

A series of seven rhabdomyosarcomas in cats was reported in a paper whose principal objective was immunohistochemical characterization.[6] It is difficult to classify those tumors, but based on the histological description and the illustration of one of the tumors, at least some of them were embryonal rhabdomyosarcomas. No other information regarding age, sex, and so forth was given. An unusual tumor, diagnosed as embryonal rhabdomyosarcoma, was reported in the liver of a 2-year-old male cat.[7] Although that tumor undoubtedly showed evidence of rhabdomyoblastic differentiation, based on histological features and immunostaining, it was also multifo-

cally positive for S-100 protein and for neuron specific enolase. This raises the possibility that it represented a primitive mesenchymal tumor with both neuronal and muscle differentiation, although rhabdomyosarcoma in humans can express S-100.[8]

A remarkable cluster of rhabdomyosarcoma cases was reported in 25 piglets.[9] These tumors occurred in skeletal muscle at various sites in piglets less than 1 month old, and they probably represented embryonal rhabdomyosarcomas. Subsequently, additional cases were found on other farms, and a genetic cause was proven.[10] This is an interesting corollary to rhabdomyosarcoma in humans, where associated cytogenetic abnormalities are common.

A rhabdomyosarcoma was reported in the maxillary sinus, extending to the orbit, of a 9-year-old Swiss brown cow.[30] Based on the morphologic description and the photomicrograph, this case also would be classified as embryonal rhabdomyosarcoma.

Clinical Characteristics and Sites

Most cases are presented because of the observation of a mass lesion. Embryonal rhabdomyosarcoma can arise in a variety of sites, including areas in which striated muscle normally is not found. As in humans, a common site of occurrence is the head region, with three of the eight Cornell cases being in this area (one on the hard palate, two on the tongue). Both of the reported canine cases were in the head region.[1] Three of the Cornell cases were associated with large muscle masses, one (the feline case) being on a limb, one in the flank, and one in the axilla. One lesion occurred as a perirenal mass. In the cases in lambs, one was associated with the paraspinal muscles,[2] and two were pulmonary lesions.[3-4]

Gross Morphology

These tumors generally present as pale white to tan, fleshy, firm masses. Necrosis and hemorrhage may be present in the mass. In many cases no description of the gross appearance is available, presumably because many are received by the pathologist already excised and fixed.

Histological Features, Growth, and Metastasis

Histological features of embryonal rhabdomyosarcoma in animals closely resemble those summarized above. As in human cases, two types can be identified, those composed predominantly of round cells, and those composed predominantly of primitive myotubes. The majority of the Cornell cases were of the round cell type, with only two being classified as the myotubular type.

Typically, embryonal rhabdomyosarcomas of the round cell type contain large, round to polygonal, deeply eosinophilic round cells (rhabdomyoblasts) (fig. 6.17 A, fig. 6.13 A) intermixed with smaller cells with much less cytoplasm. The proportions of the two cell types vary, and

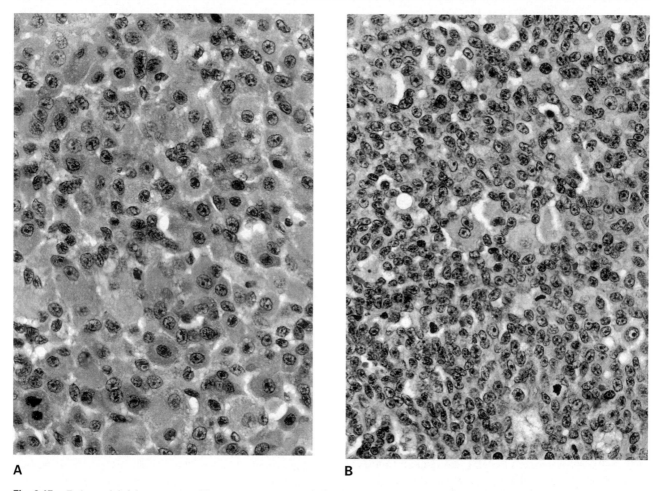

A   B

Fig. 6.17. Embryonal rhabdomyosarcoma. These tumors are composed of a mixture of large, round rhabdomyoblasts, which predominate in some areas, and small cells, which predominate in other areas. **A.** Tumor from cat. Note predominance of large rhabdomyoblasts. **B.** Tumor from a dog. Small cells are predominant. Some rhabdomyoblasts are vacuolated. Note the presence of mitotic figures.

there may be only occasional large rhabdomyoblasts (fig. 6.17 B). However, recognition of the large rhabdomyoblasts can be of great diagnostic assistance, and these are the cells that are most likely to be positive for immunohistochemical markers (fig. 6.13). Cells of intermediate size may be present. The larger cells are referred to as rhabdomyoblasts, but based on the results of immunohistochemistry, these are the more fully differentiated cells. In the opinion of the authors, the smaller cells represent the less differentiated, proliferative population. There may be considerable pleomorphism, and binucleate or multinucleate cells, some containing dozens of nuclei, may be present. Some of these cells may adopt the strap cell morphology. Cross striations are uncommon and difficult to find, but when present, are most easily seen in strap cells. Special stains such as PTAH may be helpful to demonstrate cross striations, but immunohistochemistry is more dependable. Some cells may be vacuolated and may resemble spiderweb cells, and some cells stain for glycogen using the PAS stain. The larger rhabdomyoblasts usually contain large, vesicular nuclei with one or more

prominent nucleoli, while the nuclei of the small cells are more basophilic. Mitotic index varies from low (about 1/HP field) to very high (> 10/HP field). Areas of necrosis and hemorrhage or hemosiderosis may be present. Many embryonal rhabdomyosarcomas show infiltration of adjacent muscle and connective tissue, although in our experience vascular or lymphatic invasion is uncommon. One particularly aggressive case reported in the literature[1] showed widespread vascular invasion.

One immunohistochemically confirmed embryonal rhabdomyosarcoma from the Cornell cases was in the hind limb muscles of a cat (fig. 6.17 A). It had multifocal osseous and chondroid metaplasia as well as multifocal lymphoid aggregates in and around the tumor. No vaccine adjuvant was found associated with the lesion.

The myotubular type of embryonal rhabdomyosarcoma is made up of cells resembling primitive muscle cells or myotubes, similar to those seen in developing muscle. This form is uncommon, except for the botryoid rhabdomyosarcomas of the urinary bladder, described below. Three cases consistent with this type have been reported in sheep, one of which had two embryonal rhabdomyosarcomas, one being of the round cell type.[2-4] The lesions in one of these cases were made up of either stellate or spindle shaped cells with abundant myxoid matrix, or long, myotubular fibers, some of which showed cross striations.[2] The lesions in the other two ovine cases were made up of well-differentiated, long, thin muscle fibers.[3,4] One unusual case in the Cornell material was from a 14-year-old, female springer spaniel dog with an extremely mucoid mass in the axilla. The tumor was composed of small bipolar to stellate cells embedded in copious myxoid matrix (fig. 6.18 A,B). Occasionally cells were arranged in denser clumps, often near blood vessels, and many of the spindle cells overlapped to form short chains. Occasional cells with two or a few nuclei were present, with rare cells forming short, blunt-ended straps. Nuclei were moderately pleomorphic, and there was a moderately high mitotic index. These cells were very reminiscent of muscle cells in culture. This tumor was immunohistochemically confirmed and was classified as an embryonal rhabdomyosarcoma of the myotubular type. The differential diagnosis for this type of lesion is myxosarcoma, and it is possible, or even likely,

that similar cases have been misdiagnosed as such.

Because of the relatively few cases reported in the literature, and the lack of follow-up on the Cornell cases, it is difficult to provide objective criteria for establishing a prognosis for these tumors. However, embryonal rhabdomyosarcomas should be regarded as being invasive, with some potential to metastasize. One of the cases reported in dogs showed widespread metastasis, and one of the cases in a lamb had metastasized to a lymph node.[1,4] One of the Cornell cases occurring in muscles of the flank histologically had peripheral infiltration and recurred some months later. One of the myotubular lesions in the Cornell cases proved to be very aggressive and had infiltrated much of the thoracic wall within 3 weeks of initial biopsy, following which the dog was euthanized. In the absence of objective data, we suggest that the most useful criteria for determination of malignancy and for establishing the prognosis are the mitotic index and the presence of aggressive infiltration of surrounding tissue. The presence of more than an occasional mitosis should be taken as an unfavorable prognostic indicator, and a high mitotic index warrants a poor prognosis.

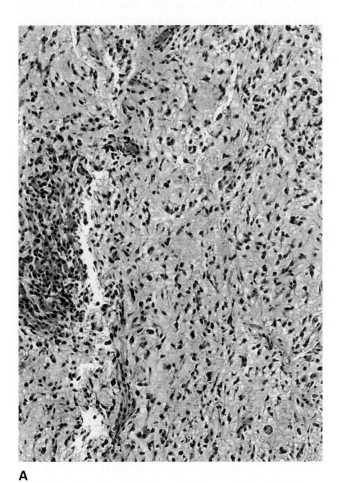

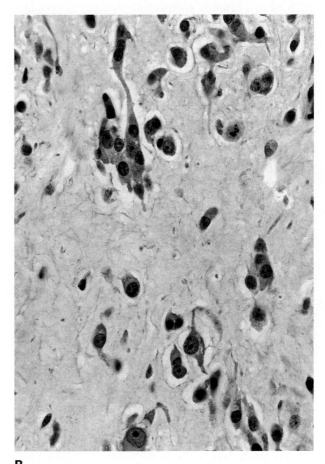

A

B

Fig. 6.18. Embryonal rhabdomyosarcoma, myotubular type, from a dog. **A.** This tumor is composed of small cells embedded in copious myxoid matrix, with clusters of more densely packed cells. **B.** The neoplastic cells are round to spindle shaped and rarely form short, multinucleate straps. This tumor was immunohistochemically positive for muscle markers.

Botryoid Rhabdomyosarcoma

Incidence, Age, Breed, and Sex

Botryoid rhabdomyosarcoma has been most commonly reported in the urinary bladder of the dog, in which species it constitutes a distinct entity. Nevertheless, this is an uncommon neoplasm. In one series of 130 cases of neoplasia of the urinary bladder in the dog, only one was a rhabdomyosarcoma.[11] Of the 83,000 tumor cases in our 20-year survey of the Cornell files, 63,000 were in dogs. Of those, 520 were urinary bladder tumors of which only two (2 of the 16 striated muscle tumors) were botryoid rhabdomyosarcoma. The lesion is fairly commonly reported in the literature, giving a false impression of its frequency, both absolutely and with reference to other forms of rhabdomyosarcoma.[11-21] This is probably because of the characteristic nature of this tumor, which makes it readily recognizable.

Typically these neoplasms occur in young large breed dogs (with the St. Bernard being overrepresented), almost invariably under 2 years of age. The average age of published cases, including those in the Cornell series, is 1.7 years, with only one animal over 2 years (a 5-year-old St. Bernard). Females predominate, outnumbering males 2:1. Botryoid rhabdomyosarcoma also has been reported in the urinary bladder of a 2-year-old filly and in the uterus of a yearling filly.[12,13]

Clinical Characteristics and Sites

Animals with botryoid rhabdomyosarcoma of the urinary bladder typically present with signs relating to obstruction of urinary outflow, including dysuria, stranguria, and hematuria. These signs may be present for some weeks before the presence of a tumor is recognized, and it is common for them to be treated initially as cystitis. In the case of uterine rhabdomyosarcoma in a filly, the animal presented because of a bloody vaginal discharge.[13]

Botryoid rhabdomyosarcoma of the bladder in most cases is located at or near the trigone, although in a few cases the mass was in the bladder wall not associated with the trigone.[14] The uterine mass reported in a filly was large (18 kg), projected into the lumen of the uterus, and was occasionally visible at the vagina.[13] In the dog, hypertrophic osteopathy appears to be a relatively common complication of botryoid rhabdomyosarcoma of the bladder, with three such cases having been reported.[17,20,21]

Gross Morphology

The tumor typically projects into the lumen of the bladder as a polypoid mass, often referred to as grape-like, thus leading to the term botryoid. In some cases the lesion extends into the body of the bladder, and it may fill the urethra. Obstruction of the ureters may result in hydroureter and hydronephrosis. In some cases the mucosal surface is ulcerated. The masses are usually described as white to tan on cut surface, may have areas of hemorrhage and necrosis, and may be firm or friable.

Histological Features, Growth, and Metastasis

Botryoid rhabdomyosarcoma is regarded as a variant of embryonal rhabdomyosarcoma, and its histological appearance is consistent with this view. However, botryoid rhabdomyosarcoma typically has a morphologic appearance consistent with the myotubular form of embryonal rhabdomyosarcoma. Typically these tumors are made up of spindle shaped or stellate cells of variable density, forming a loose myxoid arrangement in some areas, often described as being central in the tumor, and more compact arrangements in other areas, often at the periphery (fig. 6.19 A). This is reminiscent of the cambrium layer in human cases. The presence of multinucleate cells is common. Strap-like cells are present in many cases, and there are often myotubes, which may form long, relatively well differentiated muscle fibers of small diameter. Cells with cross striations are present in about half the cases and are most obvious in the long, multinucleate muscle fibers (fig. 6.19 B). Nuclei are usually round to oval, or even elongate, and may be located centrally or, in the well-differentiated myofibers, peripherally. In larger or in multinucleate cells the nuclei are vesicular and usually have a prominent nucleolus; in smaller, less differentiated cells they are denser, and nucleoli may not be apparent. Mitoses are commonly observed and are typically present in the small cell population. Necrosis may be present in confluent areas or in single cells. Infiltration of adjacent tissue may be present if the sample is suitable.

It is stated in some papers describing botryoid rhabdomyosarcoma that metastasis does not commonly occur. However, in veterinary cases this is difficult to judge, as affected animals are often euthanized shortly after the discovery of the tumor. Of 14 canine cases (including published cases and the two Cornell cases) five were euthanized at initial diagnosis; three were euthanized later due to tumor complications; one was reported to have recurred; and one was reported to have recurred and metastasized widely within 3 months. Outcome was not known for four of the cases. The longest recorded survival time after tumor diagnosis is 5 months, but it should be noted that some animals had signs for weeks or even months before definitive diagnosis.[15] The poor survival rate is presumably related to the difficulty of complete resection of tumors occurring in the neck of the bladder. Regardless, this tumor carries a poor prognosis.

In the two reported equine cases, the outcome was equally poor. The filly with botryoid rhabdomyosarcoma of the bladder died 3 months after surgery to debulk the tumor and was found at necropsy to have metastatic disease.[12] The filly with the uterine tumor died of postsurgical complications.[13]

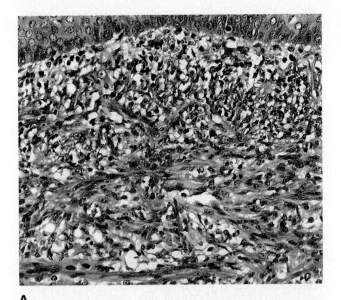

A

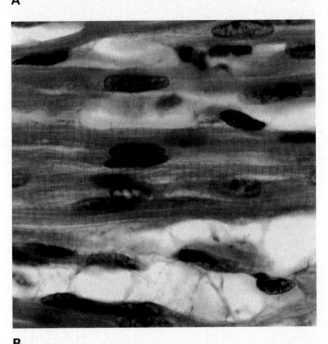

B

Fig. 6.19. Botryoid rhabdomyosarcoma of the bladder from a dog. **A.** The transitional epithelium is shown at the top. The tumor is composed of small round to spindle shaped cells most densely packed beneath the epithelium. **B.** Well-differentiated, long myotubes are apparent deeper in the mass. These cells have obvious cross striations and closely resemble immature skeletal muscle fibers.

Alveolar Rhabdomyosarcoma

Incidence, Age, Breed, and Sex

Several cases of alveolar rhabdomyosarcoma in animals have been reported in the literature. Two cases have been reported in dogs, one a 2-year-old mixed breed and the other a 9-year-old female of unstated breed.[22,23] One of

the 16 Cornell cases, a dog, was classified as this type. Two cases have also been reported in horses, one in a 19-year-old New Forest gelding and the other in a 2-year-old Appaloosa filly.[24,25] One case has been reported in a 7-year-old holstein cow.[26]

Clinical Characteristics and Sites

Of the canine cases, one presented with a firm subcutaneous mass in the maxillary area, which caused the eyeball and periocular tissue to protrude from the orbit.[22] The other presented with a palpable abdominal mass, which was found to be in the omentum.[23] The Cornell case presented as a mass on the hip. Of the equine cases, one was presented with lameness due to a mass on the hock, which involved the deep digital flexor muscle, while the other presented because of progressive enlargement of a hind limb, with involvement of muscle proximal to the hock.[24,25] The bovine case presented because of emaciation and was found to have multiple abdominal masses.[26]

Gross Morphology

Again, it is difficult to generalize about the appearance of these neoplasms. Cases have been reported as white, yellow-gray, red-brown, or "fish-flesh" in color, with areas of necrosis and hemorrhage.

Histological Features, Growth, and Metastasis

The classic histological appearance of alveolar rhabdomyosarcoma is one in which the tumor cells form alveoli supported on a framework of fairly dense fibrous septa.[27] The central cells in these alveolar structures frequently lose cohesiveness and become separated from one another (fig. 6.20 A). Many of these "floating" cells are degenerate. More viable cells remain attached to the septa, forming an adenocarcinoma-like pattern. The cells making up the neoplasm are generally uniform, small, poorly differentiated cells with round to oval hyperchromatic nuclei. Large eosinophilic rhabdomyoblasts are less commonly found in alveolar rhabdomyosarcoma than in embryonal types. Neoplastic cells associated with the fibrous septa are often spindle shaped and may occasionally demonstrate cross striations. In human material, the presence of large, round to oval, multinucleate cells with peripherally placed nuclei and pale eosinophilic cytoplasm are a diagnostically useful feature of alveolar rhabdomyosarcoma.[27] These cells rarely if ever show cross striations. Only one reported case of alveolar rhabdomyosarcoma in animals demonstrates the classic features of this variant (fig. 6.20 A).[23] The tumor was described as consisting of poorly differentiated small cells lacking cross striations. However, the case was immunohistochemically confirmed using antibodies to desmin and myoglobin.

The remaining published cases, and the one case from the Cornell material classified as the alveolar variant, are

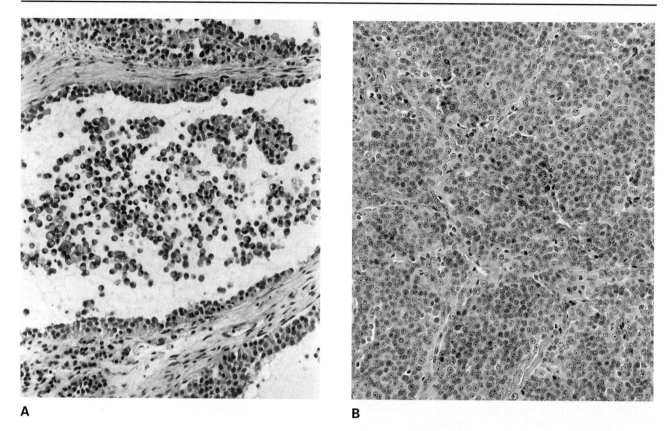

A   B

Fig. 6.20. Alveolar rhabdomyosarcoma variants, from two dogs. **A.** The classical alveolar pattern with relatively uniform round cells supported on collagenous septae. In the central cavity of the alveoli there are loose, often degenerate, desquamated cells. [Reproduced, with permission, from reference 23.] **B.** An immunohistochemically positive rhabdomyosarcoma, classified as solid alveolar pattern. It is composed of clusters or packets of relatively uniform, intermediate sized cells separated by fine collagenous septa.

of a solid alveolar pattern (fig. 6.20 B). In humans, even classic alveolar rhabdomyosarcoma may have areas in which the tumor cells form solid cellular lobules separated by fibrous septa, and some cases are entirely composed of this pattern.[27]

Identification of this variant can be difficult, as other forms of rhabdomyoma, rhabdomyosarcoma, and other neoplasms (neuroendocrine) may be divided into lobules by a fine fibrovascular stroma. The most useful criterion for identification of solid alveolar rhabdomyosarcoma is the lack of features of embryonal rhabdomyosarcoma and the uniformity of the constituent cells, with large eosinophilic rhabdomyoblasts being rare or absent. In humans, the distinction is important, because alveolar rhabdomyosarcomas carry a particularly poor prognosis. Clearly, more experience with this variant in animals is required to improve the criteria for diagnosis and for establishment of the prognosis.

Pleomorphic Rhabdomyosarcoma

Incidence, Age, Breed, and Sex

As in humans, pleomorphic rhabdomyosarcoma appears to be the least common form of this tumor in animals. Of the 16 Cornell cases, only one was classified as

the pleomorphic variant, which is at odds with the impression many pathologists may have. The reason, in part, is that virtually all rhabdomyosarcomas show some cellular pleomorphism, or at least marked variation in cell size, but any case having *any* areas characteristic of embryonal or alveolar rhabdomyosarcoma should be classified as such, not as the pleomorphic type.[28] Indeed, there are a number of reports in the literature that describe "pleomorphic" tumors that, from photomicrographs, should be classified as embryonal. One case classified as pleomorphic rhabdomyosarcoma has been reported in a 5-year-old quarter horse mare.[29] In the Cornell material there was one case in a 3-year-old, male, mixed breed dog.

Clinical Characteristics and Sites

It is difficult to develop a comprehensive summary of the clinical presentation of this tumor, given its rarity. If comparison to human cases is of any value, this tumor would be expected to occur in adult animals, most often in the larger muscle masses of the limbs.[27] The reported equine case occurred in the tongue, and the animal presented with nasal discharge and dysphagia,[29] while the case in the Cornell files occurred in the muscles of the neck and was presumably presented because of an obvious mass lesion.

Gross Morphology

No information is available regarding the gross appearance of these neoplasms, but they would be expected to present as pale, white to tan, fleshy masses.

Histological Features, Growth, and Metastasis

In practice it can be difficult to differentiate pleomorphic rhabdomyosarcoma from embryonal and alveolar rhabdomyosarcoma, especially in those cases in which areas of considerable pleomorphism occur. We have followed contemporary criteria applied to human cases, in which any areas of clear-cut embryonal or alveolar type lead to that diagnosis, even in tumors with areas of pleomorphism.

Pleomorphic rhabdomyosarcoma is characterized by the presence, throughout the tumor, of haphazardly arranged, interlacing, plump, spindle cells (fig. 6.21). Multinucleate cells and strap or racket cells may be present. Large, round rhabdomyoblasts are also present. Larger cells have abundant eosinophilic cytoplasm. In human

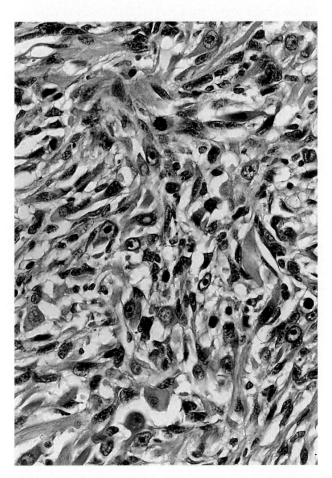

Fig. 6.21. Pleomorphic rhabdomyosarcoma in a dog. This tumor is composed of highly pleomorphic cells, including spindle or stellate cells and strap-like cells. They have large vesicular nuclei with prominent nucleoli. A mitotic figure is present in the field. This tumor was uniformly of this pattern.

cases cross striations are said to be rare. However, in the Cornell case we were able to find cells with cross striations. There is minimal collagenous connective tissue. Nuclei are large, round to oval, and vesicular and have one or more prominent nucleoli. The Cornell case had a high mitotic index and showed clear invasion of adjacent muscle and thus was considered malignant. However, no follow-up information in this case was available.

REFERENCES

1. Kim, D.-Y., Hodgin, E.C., Cho, D.-Y., and Varnado, J.E. (1996) Juvenile rhabdomyosarcomas in two dogs. *Vet Pathol* 33:447–450.
2. Tanaka, K., and Stromberg, P.C. (1993) Embryonal rhabdomyosarcoma in a sheep. *Vet Pathol* 30:396–399.
3. Donnelly, W.J.C., and Hamilton, A.F. (1972) Fatal pulmonary rhabdomyosarcoma in a lamb. *Vet Rec* 91:280–282.
4. O'Donahoo, R., and Seawright, A.A. (1971) Rhabdomyosarcoma of the lungs of a sheep. *Aust Vet J* 47:572.
5. Yanoff, S.R., Fuentealba, C., Boothe, H.W., and Rogers, K.S. (1996) Tracheal defect and embryonal rhabdomyosarcoma in a young dog. *Can Vet J* 37:172–173.
6. Martín de las Mulas, J., Vos, J.H., and Van Mil, F.N. (1992) Desmin and vimentin immunocharacterization of feline muscle tumors. *Vet Pathol* 29:260–262.
7. Minkus, G., and Hillemans, M. (1997) Botryoid-type embryonal rhabdomyosarcoma of liver in a young cat. *Vet Pathol* 34:618–621.
8. Brooks, J.S.J. (1996) Immunohistochemistry in the differential diagnosis of soft tissue tumors. In Weiss, S.W., and Brooks, J.S.J. (eds.), *Soft Tissue Tumors.* Williams and Wilkins, Baltimore, pp. 65–128.
9. Vos, J.H., Borst, G.H.A., Martín de las Mulas, J., Ramaekers, F.C.S., van Mil, F.N., Molenbeek, R.F., Ivanyi, D., and van den Ingh, T.S.G.A.M. (1993) Rhabdomyosarcomas in young pigs in a swine breeding farm: A morphologic and immunohistochemical study. *Vet Pathol* 30:271–279.
10. Van de Loop, F.T.L., Bosma, A.A., Vos, J.H., Mirck, M.H., Schaart, G., van den Ingh, T.S.G.A.M., and Ramaekers, F.C.S. (1995) Cultured pig rhabdomyosarcoma cells with a deletion of the Xq24-qter chromosome region: An immunochemical and cytogenetic characterization. *Amer J Vet Res* 56:1062–1069.
11. Osborne, C.A., Low, D.G., Perman, V., and Barnes, D.M. (1968) Neoplasms of the canine and feline urinary bladder: Incidence, etiologic factors, occurrence and pathologic features. *Amer J Vet Res* 29:2041–2055.
12. Turnquist, S.E., Pace, L.W., Keegan, K., Andrew-Jones, L., Kreeger, J.M., Bailey, K.L., Stogsdill, P.L., and Wilson, H.A. (1993) Botryoid rhabdomyosarcoma of the urinary bladder in a filly. *J Vet Diag Invest* 5:451–453.
13. Torbeck, R.L., Kittleson, S.L., and Leathers, C.W. (1980) Botryoid rhabdomyosarcoma of the uterus of a filly. *J Amer Vet Med Assoc* 176:914–916.
14. Kelly, D.F. (1973) Rhabdomyosarcoma of the urinary bladder in dogs. *Vet Pathol* 10:375–384.
15. Stamps, P., and Harris, D.L. (1968) Botryoid rhabdomyosarcoma of the urinary bladder of a dog. *J Amer Vet Med Assoc* 153:1064–1068.
16. Andreasen, C.B., White, M.R., Swayne, D.E., Graves, G.N. (1988) Desmin as a marker for canine botryoid rhabdomyosarcomas. *J Comp Pathol* 98:23–29.
17. Halliwell, W.H., and Ackerman, N. (1974) Botryoid rhabdomyosarcoma of the urinary bladder and hypertrophic osteoarthropathy in a young dog. *J Amer Vet Med Assoc* 165:911–913.
18. Pletcher, J.M., and Dalton, L. (1981) Botryoid rhabdomyosarcoma in the urinary bladder of a dog. *Vet Pathol* 18:695–697.

19. Stone, E.A., George, T.F., Gilson, S.D., and Page, R.L. (1996) Partial cystectomy for urinary bladder neoplasia: Surgical technique and outcome in 11 dogs. *J Small Anim Prac* 37:480–485.

20. Teunissen, G.H.B., and Misdorp, W. (1968) Rhabdomyosarcoma of the urinary bladder and fibromatosis of the extremities in a young dog. *Zbl Vet Med A* 15:81–88.

21. Brody, R.S. (1971) Hypertrophic osteoarthropathy in the dog: A clinicopathologic survey of 60 cases. *J Amer Vet Med Assoc* 159:1242–1256.

22. Seibold, H.R. (1974) Juvenile alveolar rhabdomyosarcoma in a dog. *Vet Pathol* 11:558–560.

23. Sarnelli, R., Grassi, F., and Romagnoli, S. (1994) Alveolar rhabdomyosarcoma of the greater omentum in a dog. *Vet Pathol* 31:473–475.

24. Clegg, P.D., and Coumbe, A. (1993) Alveolar rhabdomyosarcoma: An unusual cause of lameness in a pony. *Equine Vet J* 25:547–549.

25. Finocchio, E.J., Coffman, J.R., and Strafuss, A.C. (1969) Rhabdomyosarcoma in a horse. *Vet Med Small Anim Clin* 64:494–496.

26. Matsui, T., Imai, T., Han, J.S., Awakura, T., Taniyama, H., Osame, S., Nakagawa, M., and Ono, T. (1991) Bovine undifferentiated alveolar rhabdomyosarcoma and its differentiation in xenotransplanted tumors. *Vet Pathol* 28:438–445.

27. Enzinger, F.M., and Weiss, S.W. (1994) *Soft Tissue Tumors,* 2nd ed. CV Mosby Co., Washington, D.C.

28. Hollowood, K., and Fletcher, C.D.M. (1994) Rhabdomyosarcoma in adults. *Sem Diag Pathol* 11:47–57.

29. Hanson, P.D., Frisbie, D.D., Dubielzig, R.R., and Markel, M.D. (1993) Rhabdomyosarcoma of the tongue in a horse. *J Amer Vet Med Assoc* 202:1281–1284.

30. Pospischil, A., Weiland, F., von Sandersleben, J., Hänichen, T., and Schäffler, H. (1982) Endemic ethmoidal tumours in cattle: sarcomas and carcinosarcomas. A light microscopic study. *Zbl Vet Med A* 29:628–636.

Cytogenetic and Genetic Abnormalities in Rhabdomyosarcoma

In humans, certain consistent cytogenetic and molecular abnormalities have been identified in patients with rhabdomyosarcoma, even to the extent that specific abnormalities can be associated with particular histological tumor types.[1-3] In animals, little work has been done to search for similar abnormalities. However, a very interesting cluster of cases of rhabdomyosarcomas in piglets, apparently progeny of a single boar, has been observed.[4] Cultures of rhabdomyosarcoma cells were established from one of those animals, and a deletion of Xq24-qter, the long arm of the X chromosome, was found. No further information is yet available about what genes might contribute to the genesis of rhabdomyosarcoma in these cases. Increased expression of c-*myc,* without evidence of structural abnormalities in the gene, has been reported in a canine rhabdomyosarcoma.[5] However, the tumor in that case was not proven to be a rhabdomyosarcoma.

REFERENCES

1. Fletcher, J.A. (1996) Cytogenetics and molecular biology of soft tissue tumors. In Weiss, S.W., Brooks, J.S.J. (eds.), *Soft Tissue Tumors.* Williams and Wilkins, Baltimore, pp. 37–64.

2. Parham, D.M. (1994) The molecular biology of childhood rhabdomyosarcoma. *Sem Diag Pathol* 11:39–46.

3. Rydholm, A. (1996) Chromosomal aberrations in musculoskeletal tumours: Clinical importance. *J Bone Joint Surg* 78B:501–506.

4. Van de Loop, F.T.L., Bosma, A.A., Vos, J.H., Mirck, M.H., Schaart, G., van den Ingh, T.S.G.A.M., and Ramaekers, F.C.S. (1995) Cultured pig rhabdomyosarcoma cells with a deletion of the Xq24-qter chromosome region: an immunochemical and cytogenetic characterization. *Amer J Vet Res* 56:1062–1069.

5. Engström, W., Barrios, C., Willems, J.S., Möllermark, G., Kängström, L.E., Eliasson, I., and Larsson, O. (1987) Expression of the *myc* protooncogene in canine rhabdomyosarcoma. *Anticancer Res* 7:1109–1110.

Myogenic Tumors of the Heart

Cardiac Rhabdomyoma

Incidence, Age, Breed, and Sex

Cardiac rhabdomyoma has been reported most frequently in swine.[1-4] Typically, it is found as an incidental lesion at necropsy or during meat inspection, most commonly in young animals. Several breeds have been affected, but a higher frequency of the lesion was reported in red wattle pigs than in other breeds.[3] The sex of the affected animals is not always identified, but there appears to be a preponderance of females. This lesion has also been reported in sheep,[1,5] cattle, and dogs.[6] No cases of cardiac rhabdomyoma were encountered in the Cornell material.

Clinical Characteristics and Sites

This lesion is generally clinically silent, most cases occurring as incidental findings. The lesion occurs in the ventricular wall, with the left ventricle being the most common site.

Gross Morphology

The lesions occur as well-demarcated, nonencapsulated, white to yellowish-gray or tan, single or multiple nodules embedded in the ventricular wall. They are more common in the left ventricular wall than the septum and least common in the right ventricular wall.[4] They can vary from barely visible to about 3 cm in diameter. Most reports describe nodules 1–1.5 cm in diameter.

Histological Features, Growth, and Metastasis

Histologically, cardiac rhabdomyomas are well circumscribed, but generally not encapsulated. They are composed of large, vacuolated, cardiac myocytes with cytoplasm that is eosinophilic but may be less intensely stained than the surrounding normal myocardium. They contain large nuclei with one or two nucleoli. Binucleate cells may be observed, but mitoses are not present. The cytoplasmic vacuoles can form spider cells, or spiderweb cells. Most authors report some diastase sensitive staining of the cells by PAS, indicating that they contain glycogen, but often the vacuoles appear empty. The cells making up the tumor typically contain cross striations, indicating that they are derived from cardiac myocytes. There is minimal stroma in the nodules. In the cases described in red wattle pigs, histological examination revealed additional lesions that were not grossly apparent.[3]

The true nature of cardiac rhabdomyomas is in question. There is general agreement that they are not true neoplasms, and several authors offer the opinion that they represent hamartomas. Studies using ultrastructure and immunohistochemical techniques demonstrated that these lesions are derived from cardiac muscle and/or Purkinje cells, suggesting that they are dysplastic.[4] Despite the fact that these authors demonstrated expression of PCNA in cardiac rhabdomyomas, all reports agree that mitotic figures are absent. It is likely that these lesions enlarge, if at all, because of enlargement of the constituent cells.

Cardiac Rhabdomyosarcoma

Incidence, Age, Breed, and Sex

Cardiac rhabdomyosarcoma is extremely rare, with a total of three cases having been reported in dogs. One case was in a 14-month-old female golden retriever,[7] one in a 7-year-old male Labrador retriever,[8] and the third in a 7-year-old doberman.[9] Rhabdomyosarcomas metastatic to the heart have also been described.[10] No cardiac rhabdomyosarcomas were confirmed in the Cornell material, although three cases had initially been diagnosed as such. These could not be confirmed on review with immunohistochemical staining.

Clinical Characteristics and Sites

Two of the reported cases showed clinical signs related to cardiac dysfunction, one presenting with syncope,[7] and the second with lethargy and dyspnea.[8] The lesions in the third animal were an incidental finding.[9]

Gross Morphology

Lesions were reported in one case as a white to tan mass at the apex of the heart, with cystic masses in the right ventricle and extending from the left ventricle into the aorta.[7] In another case the lesion was described as a white pedunculated mass on the epicardial surface of the right ventricle.[8] The third case, had multiple masses in the atrial septum and both ventricles.[9]

Histological Features, Growth, and Metastasis

Histological descriptions are available for two of these cases. In one, the neoplastic tissue was described as being composed of pleomorphic cells, with elongate and strap-like cells interspersed among embryonic cells.[7] Neoplastic tissue had invaded vessels in some areas. There

were few mitoses. A few myoglobin positive cells were detected among the tumor cells by immunohistochemistry, and ultrastructural features were consistent with muscle cells. No metastases were reported. In the second case, the neoplasm was described as being highly invasive and was composed of anaplastic cells arranged in either dense sheets or loosely in a myxomatous matrix.[8] The cells varied from round with an eccentric nucleus, to spindle, stellate, or elongate strap-like cells with centrally placed, multiple nuclei. Nuclei were large, round to oval, with prominent nucleoli, and mitoses were common. These cells were reported to be immunohistochemically positive for vimentin and sarcomeric actin. Although no necropsy was performed, no other abnormalities were observed at surgery.

The histogenesis of these lesions is debatable. As mature cardiac myocytes do not have the capacity for mitosis, it is likely that these tumors, like many other rhabdomyosarcomas, arise from mesenchymal cells that retain the capacity for rhabdoid differentiation.

REFERENCES

1. Bradley, R., and Wells, G.A.H. (1980) Ovine and porcine so-called cardiac rhabdomyoma (hamartoma). *J Comp Pathol* 90:551–558.
2. Omar, A.R. (1969) Congenital cardiac rhabdomyoma in a pig. *Vet Pathol* 6:469–474.
3. McEwen, B.J.E. (1994) Congenital cardiac rhabdomyomas in red wattle pigs. *Can Vet J* 35:48–49.
4. Tanimoto, T., and Ohtsuki, Y. (1995) The pathogenesis of so-called cardiac rhabdomyoma in swine: A histological, immunohistochemical and ultrastructural study. *Virchows Arch* 427:213–221.
5. Cordes, D.O., and Shortridge, E.H. (1971) Neoplasms of sheep: A survey of 256 cases recorded at Ruakura Animal Health Laboratory. *N Z Vet J* 19:55–64.
6. Hadlow, W.J. (1962) Diseases of skeletal muscle. In Innes, J.R.M., and Saunders, L.Z. (eds.), *Comparative Neuropathology*. Academic Press, London, pp. 224–225. Cited in Ref. 1.
7. Krotje, L.J., Ware, W.A., and Niyo, Y. (1990) Intracardiac rhabdomyosarcoma in a dog. *J Amer Vet Med Assoc* 197:368–371.
8. Gonin-Jmaa, D., Paulsen, D.B., and Taboada, J. (1996) Pericardial effusion in a dog with rhabdomyosarcoma in the right ventricular wall. *J Small Anim Pract* 37:193–196.
9. Camy, G. (1986) Tumeur intracardiaque (rhabdomyosarcoma). *Pratique Medicale et Chirirgicale de l'Anirnale de Compagne* 21:229–230. Cited in ref. 2.
10. Girard, C., and Odin, P.H. (1999) Intrapericardial neoplasia in dogs. *J Vet Diag Invest* 11:73–78.

MUSCLE PSEUDOTUMORS

As the name suggests, muscle pseudotumors are nonneoplastic masses that form within skeletal muscle.[5] In the broadest sense, any reactive or degenerative process that results in a tumor-like enlargement of skeletal muscle may be classified as a muscle pseudotumor. Sclerosis associated with an underlying tumor involving muscle may also result in a histopathologic diagnosis of muscle pseudotumor if the underlying neoplasm is not present on the samples examined. In humans, some muscle pseudotumors are thought to be due to localized muscle injury.[1] We have recognized a condition in dogs that qualifies as muscle pseudotumor. Disorders that may also result in tumor-like lesions involving muscle include myositis ossificans, musculoaponeurotic fibromatosis (desmoid tumor), and equine fibrotic myopathy. As these somewhat diverse entities may, in the broadest sense, be considered muscle pseudotumors, they will be discussed briefly in this section.

Incidence, Age, Breed, and Sex

Muscle pseudotumors are uncommon and are most often seen in adult horses. Musculoaponeurotic fibromatosis appears to be most common in young adult horses, whereas fibrotic myopathy may affect horses of any age, with older horses predominating in the cases we have examined. We have also recognized muscle pseudotumors in two adult Great Dane dogs, and myositis ossificans was seen in an adult doberman pinscher. There is no apparent sex predisposition.

Clinical Characteristics and Sites

In the horse, a localized muscle pseudotumor has been recognized in the triceps muscle (Huxtable, personal communication). Musculoaponeurotic fibromatosis (desmoid tumor) involving the pectoral musculature has been reported in three horses.[2] We have seen four horses with disorders consistent with musculoaponeurotic fibromatosis. In one horse the pectoral muscle was affected, and in a second the lateral cervical musculature was affected. In the third horse, the lesion began in the area of the withers and extended ventrally through the shoulder musculature to the triceps, and in the fourth the lesion occurred within the triceps muscle. We have also examined one case of a recurrent mass in the triceps muscle of a dog that was diagnosed as musculoaponeurotic fibromatosis. Musculoaponeurotic fibromatosis may present either with an enlarging but localized swelling (*tumor*) within the affected muscle or with progressive induration of the affected area.[5] Equine fibrotic myopathy most commonly affects the semimembranosus/semitendinosus muscles and may result in a localized mass within the distal muscle in the popliteal area. Affected horses have a characteristic gait in which the swing phase of the affected limb is remarkably shortened, and the limb is placed on the ground in a stabbing motion.[3] In the dog, myositis ossificans most commonly presents as a firm nodule within the muscle over bony prominences, and the two muscle pseudotumors in the Great Dane dogs both presented as swellings in the dorsal scapular area.

Gross Morphology

Muscle pseudotumors may appear similar to the surrounding muscle, but paler and firmer. Musculoaponeurotic fibromatosis results in a poorly localized region of muscle mixed with dissecting fibrous tissue. In two equine cases in which an attempt was made to remove the mass, one or more internal pockets of apparently sterile serous fluid were found. In one advanced case of musculoaponeurotic fibromatosis of the pectoral region, the lesion extended to and involved the sternal periosteum. Myositis ossificans is a discrete lesion within muscle that has a cartilagenous and/or bony consistency. In the muscle pseudotumors in the Great Dane dogs, one mass was described as encapsulated but attached to underlying muscle, and the other was described as a lighter colored mass within the muscle that was attached to the scapular spine.

Histological Features, Growth, and Metastasis

Musculoaponeurotic fibromatosis of the horse is characterized by infiltrating loose to dense fibrovascular tissue dissecting among myofibers. The myofibers may be markedly atrophied but are otherwise normal. In the two cases in which a thorough examination of the extent of the lesion was made, one or more deep internal cavities containing proteinaceous fluid with scattered foamy macrophages and intact neutrophils were seen. Loose granulation tissue containing myofibroblasts surrounded these cavities, with formation of more mature dissecting connective tissue at the periphery. In the canine case the lesion consisted of spindle cells resembling smooth muscle cells dissecting along intramuscular fascial planes. There was little atypia, and mitoses were rare. The cells at the periphery of the dissecting bands (the least mature cells) were positive for smooth muscle actin, supporting the contention that they were myofibroblastic in nature.

The masses within muscle in equine fibrotic myopathy are distinctly different: there is marked angular atrophy of myofibers; angular atrophied fibers often occurring in small to large groups, admixed with hypertrophied fibers; and there is extensive fibrous replacement. Fibrotic myopathy has been classically described as being secondary to muscle injury,[3] but in the three horses with fibrotic myopathy that we have examined carefully, intramuscular nerves were markedly depleted of myelinated fibers, and the myofiber atrophy and fibrosis were determined to be secondary to denervation.[4] Denervation atrophy and subsequent muscle contracture in these cases are thought to have resulted in the palpable mass and abnormal stride. Myositis ossificans consists of discrete areas of chondroid and/or osteoid metaplasia within fibrous connective tissue. The muscle pseudotumors in the dogs were relatively discrete; they consisted of markedly disarrayed muscle fibers of varying diameter and shape with both myopathic changes (vacuolization, internal nuclei, fiber splitting) and scattered fiber necrosis (fig. 6.22). There were small scattered foci of lymphocytes and neutrophils. It is thought that an abnormal response to muscle trauma may be the underlying cause of musculoaponeurotic fibromatosis, myositis ossificans, and muscle pseudotumor. In humans, musculoaponeurotic fibromatosis lesions may recur repeatedly but never metastasize. The canine case

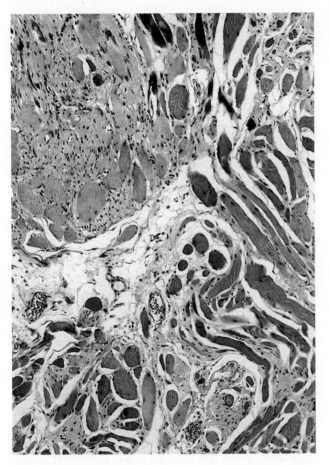

Fig. 6.22. Muscle pseudotumor from a dog. This mass is composed of haphazardly arranged mature skeletal muscle fibers admixed with smaller spindle cells, loose connective tissue, and some adipose tissue.

described above also recurred. If possible, wide excision of these lesions will likely be curative. Resection of the affected muscle in equine fibrotic myopathy is not always possible and obviously will not correct any underlying neuropathy. However, either resection of the muscle or severing the tendon of insertion of the affected muscle may result in a more normal stride.

REFERENCES

1. Kakulas, B.A. (1982) Muscle trauma. In Mastaglia, F.L., and Walton, J. (eds.), *Skeletal Muscle Pathology.* Churchill Livingstone, New York, pp. 599–602.
2. Pool, R.R. (1990) Tumors and tumor-like lesions in joints and adjacent soft tissues. In Moulton, J.E. (ed.), *Tumors in Domestic Animals,* 3rd ed. University of California Press, Berkely, pp. 129–130.
3. Adams, O.R. (1961) Fibrotic myopathy and ossifying myopathy in the hindlegs of horses. *J Amer Vet Med Assoc* 139:1089–1092.
4. Valentine, B.A., Rouselle, S.D., Sams, A.E., Edwards, R.B., III. (1994) Denervation atrophy in three horses with fibrotic myopathy. *J Amer Vet Med Assoc* 205:332–336.
5. Rosai, J. (1996) *Ackerman's Surgical Pathology,* 8th ed. Mosby, St. Louis, p.2031–2033.

GRANULAR CELL TUMOR (GRANULAR CELL MYOBLASTOMA)

Granular cell tumor (GCT), once called *granular cell myoblastoma,* is a neoplasm of uncertain origin. As the old name implies, it was once thought to be of myoblast origin, but it is now considered to be nonmyogenic. For completeness, this entity will be discussed briefly here.

Incidence, Age, Breed, and Sex

Granular cell tumor is an uncommon tumor but has been reported most frequently in the dog and in the horse. It also occurs in cats, birds, and laboratory rodents. It is found typically in mature to aged animals. There is no obvious sex or breed predisposition.

Clinical Characteristics and Sites

In the dog, GCT occurs mostly in the tongue, but cases have been reported on the ear, the lip, the palate, the cerebral cortex and/or meninges, the heart, lymph node, orbit, and skin.[1-6] In the feline cases tumors have been reported in the tongue, the palate, the vulva, and the digits.[5-6] These cases typically present clinically as mass lesions.

In the horse, GCT appears to be exclusively a tumor of the lung in mature to aged animals. It can occur as single or multiple nodules. Those occurring as multiple nodules may be localized to a limited area or may be disseminated throughout the lung. The masses are typically associated with bronchi and may bulge into the lumen. The common presenting complaint is dyspnea, which sometimes leads to a clinical diagnosis of chronic obstructive pulmonary disease, or heaves.

Histological Features, Growth, and Metastasis

The cells of GCT have been described as round to spindle shaped. The tumors are generally well circumscribed, with nests of tumor cells separated by fine collagenous stroma. The common histological feature is the presence of prominent cytoplasmic granules that are PAS positive and diastase resistant. Ultrastructurally these granules have been interpreted as secondary lysosomes. Some granular cell tumors have features of epithelial cells, in particular of basal cell tumors. Immunohistochemically, one study of granular cell tumors showed that most cases stained with antibodies to neuron specific enolase (NSE), and some stained with antibodies to S-100.[5] In humans, similar results contribute to the current opinion that many GCTs are of Schwann cell origin. Those tumors showing features of basal cell tumors were positive for cytokeratins. Two of six canine tumors stained with vimentin, but all eight cases were negative for desmin, making a myogenic origin very unlikely.[5] One feline GCT failed to stain with any of these antibodies. In another study the results of immunohistochemical staining were very variable, emphasizing the heterogeneous nature of tumors diagnosed as GCT.[6] The biologic behavior of GCT is difficult to assess because of a lack of follow-up in reported cases. The circumscribed nature of many of the tumors and a lack of mitotic activity might suggest a benign course. However, some reported GCTs have had features of invasion and or mitotic activity. It would seem prudent, with our current understanding, to assess biologic behavior from first principles, namely the presence or absence of invasion, mitoses, and features of pleomorphism.

In the horse, cells of GCT are round or polyhedral, with poorly defined cell borders.[7-10] Nuclei are round to oval with stippled to vesicular chromatin and centrally placed nucleoli. The cytoplasm contains numerous coarse eosinophilic granules. The cells often form clusters or rows separated by sparse stroma. The cytoplasmic granules in equine GCT are variably PAS positive and were reported in one series to stain strongly with luxol fast blue (LFB).[10] However, in another study, the granules were LFB negative.[9] Where immunohistochemistry has been done, these tumors have been found consistently to be positive for S-100.[9-10] In one series all six cases were NSE positive,[10] while in a second study all three cases were negative.[9] The reasons for these discrepancies are unclear, but they may involve the antibodies and techniques used.

The histogenesis of GCT is unclear and may be variable. In humans it is currently felt that most GCTs originate from Schwann cells or Schwann cell precursors. Unfortunately, this diagnosis can be a "fall back" for tumors of uncertain nature having granular cytoplasm. Indeed, a review of some cases from the Cornell files that were diagnosed as GCT revealed a heterogeneous group of neoplasms. The diagnosis of GCT should probably be reserved for tumors whose cells contain abundant eosinophilic, PAS positive, diastase resistant granules and are immunohistochemically negative for muscle markers and positive for either NSE or S-100 or both. Even so, it is likely that this represents a heterogeneous group.

REFERENCES

1. Wyand, D.S., and Wolke, R.E. (1968) Granular cell myoblastoma of the canine tongue: Case reports. *Amer J Vet Res* 29:1309–1313.
2. Parker, G.A., Botha, W., Van Dellen, A., and Casey, H.W. (1978) Cerebral granular cell tumor (myoblastoma) in a dog: Case report and literature review. *Cornell Vet* 68:506–520.
3. van de Gaag, I., and Walvoort, H.C. (1983) Granular cell myoblastoma in the tongue of a dog: A case report. *Vet Quarterly* 5:89–93.
4. Sandord, S.E., Hoover, D.M., and Miller, R.B. (1984) Primary cardiac granular cell tumor in a dog. *Vet Pathol* 21:489–494.
5. Geyer, C., Hafner, A., Pfleghaar, S., and Hermanns, W. (1992) Immunohistochemistry and ultrastructural investigation of granular cell tumours in dog, cat, and horse. *J Vet Med B* 39:485–494.
6. Patnaik, A.K. (1993) Histologic and immunohistochemical studies of granular cell tumors in seven dogs, three cats, one horse, and one bird. *Vet Pathol* 30:176–185.
7. Misdorp, W., and Nauta-van Gelder, H.L. (1968) 'Granular cell myoblastoma' in the horse. A report of 4 cases. *Vet Pathol* 5:385–394.
8. Scarratt, W.K., Crisman, M.V., Sponenberg, D.P., Dubbin, E.S., and Talley, M.R. (1993) Pulmonary granular cell tumour in 2 horses. *Equine Vet J* 25:244–247.
9. Bouchard, P.R., Fortna, C.H., Rowland, P.H., and Lewis, R.M. (1995) An immunohistochemical study of three equine pulmonary granular cell tumors. *Vet Pathol* 32:730–734.
10. Kelley, L.C., Hill, J.E., Hafner, S., and Wortham, K.J. (1995) Spontaneous equine pulmonary granular cell tumors: Morphologic, histochemical, and immunohistochemical characterization. *Vet Pathol* 32:101–106.

DIFFERENTIAL DIAGNOSIS AND APPROACH TO DIAGNOSIS OF TUMORS OF MUSCLE

The diagnosis of a smooth muscle tumor may appear to be quite straightforward in the case of a spindle cell tumor showing what appear to be clear-cut features of smooth muscle differentiation arising in the smooth muscular wall of the intestine or urinary bladder. However, results of immunohistochemical staining of such gastrointestinal tumors, which reveal a range of cellular differentiation, clearly indicates that such tumors may or may not be true smooth muscle tumors. A similar situation appears to be true for most, if not all, of the splenic and hepatic spindle cell tumors that mimic leiomyosarcoma. Conversely, what may appear to be round cell or undifferentiated tumors in sites such as the dermis and subcutis may, with immunohistochemical staining, prove to be of smooth muscle origin. It would seem prudent to advise including a muscle marker such as muscle specific actin or desmin in every immunohistochemical panel of antibodies applied to a poorly differentiated tumor. Fortunately, most, if not all, of the mesenchymal tumors arising in the urogenital system appear to be truly of smooth muscle origin.

The differential diagnosis for rhabdomyoma and rhabdomyosarcoma depends on the pattern of the tumor in question. For those having a predominant cell population of large eosinophilic round cells, the differential diagnosis includes oncocytoma, liposarcoma, and carcinoma. For those with predominantly small round cells the differential diagnosis includes neuroendocrine and round cell tumors, such as lymphoma. For pleomorphic varieties the differential diagnosis includes any poorly differentiated pleomorphic sarcoma, including fibrosarcoma, pleomorphic leiomyosarcoma, hemangiosarcoma, malignant fibrous histiocytoma, and malignant histiocytic lesions. Those embryonal rhabdomyosarcomas having predominantly a myxoid pattern could be confused with myxosarcoma. Finally, alveolar rhabdomyosarcoma could be confused with carcinoma or adenocarcinoma.

There are certain presentations that should arouse suspicion of rhabdomyosarcoma. These include the following: any round cell sarcoma arising in young animals, particularly in the head and neck region, suggests rhabdomyosarcoma; neoplasms at the trigone of the bladder in very young dogs are, clinically, botryoid rhabdomyosarcoma until proven otherwise; and tumors of the larynx, particularly in the dog, should be considered as potential rhabdomyomas or rhabdomyosarcomas. There are certain misconceptions that need to be overcome to arrive at the potential diagnosis as well. The most common of these are that rhabdomyosarcomas arise in skeletal muscle and that they are typically spindle cell tumors with marked pleomorphism, giant cells, and strap cells. The latter is true only for pleomorphic rhabdomyosarcoma, the least common variant. Indeed, the most likely reasons for misdiagnosis of other sarcomas as rhabdomyosarcoma in the Cornell series (based on their failure to stain with immunohistochemical markers) was location of the mass in striated muscle and/or the presence of multinucleate giant cells.

Any potential tumor of muscle, smooth or striated, should be subjected to immunohistochemical study. It can be expensive to subject every case to a full panel such as the one suggested above. A useful approach is to utilize a screening panel first, followed by a more complete panel, as suggested by the initial results. In the screening panel, antibodies to vimentin, cytokeratins, desmin, and muscle specific actin should be included. For those tumors reacting with either desmin or muscle specific actin, additional stains should include alpha–smooth muscle actin, alpha–sarcomeric actin, myoglobin, and when they become more generally available, myoD1 and myogenin. Pleomorphic leiomyosarcoma should be distinguished from rhabdomyosarcoma by the staining of the latter for alpha–sarcomeric actin and, if well enough differentiated, myoglobin. A tumor positive for desmin and muscle specific actin and strongly positive for alpha–smooth muscle actin, yet negative for alpha–sarcomeric actin and myoglobin can be assumed to be of smooth muscle origin.

Finally, we urge that every effort be made to classify the neoplasm according to the currently accepted schemes for muscle tumors and to obtain clinical follow-up information. At present, knowledge of clinical behavior of some of these tumors is woefully inadequate.

7 Tumors of the Respiratory Tract

D. W. Wilson and D. L. Dungworth

TUMORS OF THE UPPER RESPIRATORY TRACT

Nasal Cavity and Paranasal Sinus Tumors of the Dog

General Considerations

Classification

The many different types of tissue in the walls of the nasal cavity and paranasal sinuses give rise to a wide variety of tumors (table 7.1). Most of the mesenchymal tumors in this region do not differ histologically from their counterparts in other locations but are significant because of their frequency in this site and the need for consideration in differential diagnosis. Epithelial tumors of the nasal cavity are generally thought to arise from the nasal epithelium. Normal nasal epithelium exhibits divergent differentiation based on anatomic location within the nasal cavity. The most rostral nasal epithelium is stratified, squamous, and nonkeratinized. The respiratory epithelium lining the majority of the central nasal cavity is separated from the squamous portion by a region containing highly pseudostratified, tall columnar, secretory epithelium that lacks ciliated cells. This latter region is described as transitional epithelium. While the patterns that characterize nasal epithelial neoplasms reflect similarities to the morphology of the normal epithelium, their occurrence does not necessarily imply origin from these sites. As in much of the respiratory lining, there is considerable plasticity in the differentiation of nonneoplastic epithelium in reaction to stimuli. Other than tumors evidently arising from olfactory epithelium, it is likely that patterns of nasal tumors represent the diversity of cell types making up normal respiratory epithelium.

Prevalence

Only approximations can be provided for prevalence data because of variations in populations sampled, sample bias, inconsistencies in diagnosis, or a combination of these factors. Figures for overall prevalence of sinonasal tumors

TABLE 7.1. Classification of sinonasal tumors

Epithelial Tumors
  Benign
    Papilloma
  Malignant
    Squamous cell carcinoma
      Spindle cell variant
    Transitional carcinoma
    Adenocarcinoma
    Acinic cell carcinoma
    Adenoid cystic carcinoma
    Adenosquamous (mucoepidermoid) carcinoma
    Undifferentiated (anaplastic) carcinoma

Mesenchymal Tumors
  Fibroma/fibrosarcoma
  Chondroma/chondrosarcoma
  Osteosarcoma
  Hemangioma/hemangiosarcoma
  Angioleiomyoma
  Leiomyosarcoma
  Rhabdomyoma/rhabdomyosarcoma
  Malignant mesenchymoma
  Myxosarcoma
  Myoepithelioma
  Undifferentiated sarcoma

Other Tumors and Tumor-like Lesions
  Olfactory neuroblastoma (esthesioneuroblastoma)
  Neuroendocrine carcinoma
  Ethmoid hematoma
  Polyps
  Paranasal meningioma
  Malignant peripheral nerve sheath tumor (malignant Schwannoma)
  Lymphoid and mast cell tumors
  Malignant fibrous histiocytoma
  Canine transmissible venereal tumor
  Malignant melanoma

vary according to whether frequency is based on total population of dogs, on medical admissions in a large hospital, or on total canine tumors. The only estimate for a population based incidence reports a rate of 2.5 sinonasal tumors per 100,000 dogs.[1] Data from surveys of hospital admissions have been used to calculate rates of 81 per 100,000 dogs at risk[2] or 38 per 100,000 medical admissions.[3] Based on data from pathology laboratories, the prevalence of primary sinonasal tumors has been reported as from 0.8 percent of all necropsies[4] to between 0.8 and 1 percent of all tumors.[5,6] Dorn et al.[7] reported that 0.3 percent of all canine tumors

365

from a mostly urban clinic population was from the nasal region. This lower figure probably reflects, at least in part, the higher proportion of sinonasal tumors in cases referred to major hospitals.

Occupational associations of wood dust, glues, and adhesives with nasal carcinomas in humans suggests the potential for chemical carcinogenesis in animal tumors.[8] Detailed studies on the pathogenesis of formaldehyde induced nasal squamous cell carcinoma in rats[39-41] have not been extended to other species. It has been suggested that environmental factors increase the risk of nasal tumors in dogs,[3,9] but a separate study[10] reported no significant difference in frequency between urban and rural dogs. The possible influence of environmental factors therefore remains debatable.

Tumor Location

Data in published reports varies according to the thoroughness of evaluation and how early in the disease process the lesions were evaluated. The largest pooled data set contained 504 canine carcinomas, of which 88 percent originated in the nasal cavity, 6 percent originated in the sinuses, and 6 percent were multicentric.[3] An earlier report using similar pooled data for all types of sinonasal tumors listed 81 percent of 239 tumors arising from the nasal region and 19 percent from the paranasal sinuses.[2] These data were pooled from diagnoses made from clinical, radiological, and pathological observations and therefore provide only an approximate guide.

In a series of 110 cases of malignant sinonasal tumors where accurate postmortem information on tumor location was available, approximately half (50.9 percent) of the dogs had bilateral involvement.[4] The proportional distribution of lesions in the main anatomic locations were nasal cavity, 24 percent; frontal sinuses, 18 percent; nasofrontal regions, 30 percent; and nasal and/or frontal regions with invasion of the cranial cavity, 28 percent. These distributions do not reflect initial site of development because necropsies were done at advanced stages of the disease.

The conclusion is that the large majority of tumors (approximately 80 percent) arise in the nasal cavity, but by the time accurate mapping is possible the actual site of origin is obscured by the amount of growth and local invasion by the neoplasm. The impression is that the tumors arise predominantly from caudal regions of the nasal cavity.

Tumor Type

Pooled data from major veterinary hospitals revealed that of 239 recorded tumors, 82 percent were malignant and 18 percent were benign.[2] The percentage of benign tumors in this series was higher than is normally experienced and probably reflected the fact that a miscellaneous group of nonepithelial tumors constituted the majority (74 percent) of the benign lesions listed, some of which

might not have been strictly of sinonasal origin. Reports that have focused exclusively on malignant tumors indicate that 60 percent of the tumors were carcinomas and 40 percent were of mesenchymal or other origin [4,11-14]. The frequency of carcinomas in moderately large series reported in connection with treatment trials has generally been in the region of 75 percent, but here selection bias plays a role.[15,-17]

Adenocarcinomas predominate among the carcinomas, followed by transitional carcinomas (nonkeratinizing squamous cell carcinomas) and squamous cell carcinomas. The relative frequencies of the various types of carcinoma recorded in one series were adenocarcinoma, 53 percent; nonkeratinizing squamous cell carcinoma (transitional carcinoma), 32 percent; and keratinizing squamous cell carcinoma, 15 percent.[4] For comparison, the relative frequency in another series was adenocarcinoma, 33 percent; transitional carcinoma, 26 percent; squamous cell carcinoma, 26 percent; and undifferentiated carcinoma, 15 percent.[17] Chondrosarcoma is clearly the most frequent sarcoma. Fibrosarcoma, osteosarcoma, and lymphoma are the next most frequent types; their order of frequency depends on the population sampled and the type of sampling.

Age, Breed, and Sex

The greatest risk for canine sinonasal tumors occurs approximately between 10 and 15 years of age.[2,3] The mean age of affected dogs has ranged from 8.7 to 10.7 years,[2,17] but nasal tumors have been observed in dogs less than 6 months to greater than 16 years of age.[3,18] Chondrosarcomas occur at a slightly younger age, with a mean of 7 to 8.7 years, depending on the series reported.[12,19] There is some evidence that neuroendocrine carcinomas and olfactory neuroblastomas occur at a later age than other types of tumor, but this needs to be confirmed because of the small numbers reported.[4]

Certain breeds of dog are unquestionably at greater risk for sinonasal tumors. Whether the observed difference among various breeds can lead to the conclusion that longskulled (dolichocephalic) breeds are more at risk than those breeds with medium (mesaticephalic) or short skulls (brachycephalic) is controversial. The largest available set of pooled data reveals that breeds with significantly increased risk of nasal carcinoma are, in decreasing order, Airedale terrier, basset hound, Old English sheepdog, Scottish terrier, collie, Shetland sheepdog, and German shorthair pointer.[3] All of these breeds but the collie and Shetland sheepdog are mesaticephalic. Although pooled risk estimates of all dolichocephalic breeds indicated a significantly increased risk over other breeds, this was essentially due to the preponderance of collies and Shetland sheepdogs in the case series.[3] It is therefore not possible to conclude that dolichocephalic breeds as a whole are at increased risk. Brachycephalic breeds, however, are at decreased risk with the exception of the Boston terrier.

Whether male dogs are at higher risk for sinonasal tumors than females is debatable. Pooled hospital data comprising the largest reported series of carcinomas gave a male to female ratio of 1.3:1.[3] The male to female ratio varied considerably among breeds and was reversed in a number of them. The implication of the varied male to female ratios among pure breeds is uncertain because of the small numbers involved. The next largest series reported were all from one center and included epithelial and other types of tumors.[4] An overall male predominance was found, but there were exceptions for different types of tumor. The male to female ratio was greatest for olfactory neuroblastoma (4.0:1) and least for adenocarcinoma (1.2:1). The significance of this is unknown. Pooled data from large series of sinonasal tumors therefore show a slightly greater risk in males. The numbers of cases in small series are insufficient to reveal this consistently. There also appear to be exceptions according to the breed of dog and tumor type.

Clinical Characteristics

Clinical signs are referable to a slowly and insidiously expanding, space occupying mass in the sinonasal region, with attendant invasion and destruction of adjacent structures and associated loss of function. The most common sign is unilateral or bilateral nasal discharge, which is commonly mucopurulent and may be bloodstained. Other signs include sneezing, dyspnea, and ocular discharge. Advanced cases tend to cause facial deformity and exophthalmos.[20,21] Occasionally, presenting signs are predominantly neurologic, with little or no clinical evidence of nasal disease.[22,23] One or more of seizures, behavioral changes, circling, visual deficits and ataxia are the most common neurologic signs in such cases and are associated with preferential invasion of the tumor through the cribriform plate into the cranial vault and brain.

The presenting signs, whether relating to upper respiratory tract, neurologic abnormalities, or both, are not specific for sinonasal neoplasia. Differential diagnoses of upper respiratory signs should include rhinitis, especially chronic bacterial and fungal infections, foreign body impaction, osteomyelitis, and periodontal abscess. The approach to differential diagnosis has been reviewed.[21] The development of a paraneoplastic syndrome is not expected with sinonasal tumors, but there has been one report of an associated erythrocytosis[24] and one of hypercalcemia.[25]

Radiography and computed tomography can often provide a high probability of diagnosis of sinonasal tumors. Computed tomography provides more detailed information and is especially useful in early stages.[26-29] Definitive diagnosis depends on histopathologic examination of an adequate sample of the primary nasal lesion. Examination of cells obtained by nasal swabs or flushes is not a reliable diagnostic method. Although surgical biopsy specimens provide the most representative samples of the lesion, most initial clinical approaches use core needle biopsies. To ensure that the core biopsy accurately samples the primary lesion, the biopsy instrument should be directed to the appropriate site by radiography or computed tomography, and at least three to four samples should be taken. Because of the common association with rhinitis and the frequency of tumors in the caudal portions of the nasal cavity, false negative biopsies lacking tumor may occur. Frozen sections can aid in ensuring adequate sampling.

Growth and Metastasis

Malignant sinonasal tumors typically grow slowly. They cause their effects mainly by space occupation and local destruction and invasion. More extensive destruction and invasion is usual with carcinomas, neuroendocrine carcinomas, and olfactory neuroblastomas (esthesioneuroblastomas) than with sarcomas.[4] Neuroendocrine carcinomas and olfactory neuroblastomas are particularly prone to invade the cribriform plate, cranial cavity, and brain.

Metastasis of malignant sinonasal tumors is uncommon and usually late. An overall metastasis rate of 41 percent in 120 necropsies of advanced cases has been reported; however, the majority of the cases in which metastasis was considered to have occurred were actually local extensions into the cranial cavity and brain.[4] If metastasis to regional lymph nodes or lung is taken as the index of metastasis, then only 16 percent of 68 carcinomas had metastases in regional nodes, and 12 percent has metastases in the lung.[4] Sarcomas are much less likely to metastasize to discontinuous sites. Only 3 of 37 (8 percent) sarcomas had pulmonary metastases, and one had nodal metastasis. A higher overall percentage of metastases might occur in dogs with recurrence following radiotherapy,[15,17] but this needs to be substantiated.

Treatment and Prognosis

Essentials of treatment are reviewed elsewhere.[20,21] For epithelial and usual mesenchymal tumors, the only treatment regimen that has proved to be of benefit is radiotherapy, with or without surgical debulking. Lymphomas are a special case and are dealt with elsewhere. With specific reference to the influence of pathologic diagnosis, it is important to note that there are conflicting reports about the prognostic value of tumor staging and histological typing. A modified staging scheme has been reported to be useful,[17] but the staging recommended by the World Health Organization has not been of value.[17,30] The only treatment regimen that has proved to be of benefit is radiotherapy, with or without surgical debulking. A comparison of survival times in dogs with nasal adenocarcinoma found that neither chemotherapy protocol nor surgical procedure influenced survival time, while dogs given radiotherapy had significantly increased survival time.[31] Tumor stage and invasiveness was not predictive of survival time in this study, but the presence of distant metastasis at the time of diagnosis was significantly predictive of shortened survival times. Current evidence indicates that staging is of limited value and will remain so unless protocols with proven effectiveness can be developed. As far as tumor type is concerned, some evidence exists that dogs with sarcomas respond better to treatment than those with carcinomas,[15,17] but other studies have failed to confirm this as a significant factor.[16,30,32]

Gross Morphology

Papillomas of the nasal or sinus cavities can be solitary or multiple. They are small verrucous or papillary projections from the mucous membrane. Adenomas are usually well-circumscribed lesions and are often small. Carcinomas and sarcomas are generally irregular, bulky masses by the time they are diagnosed. Initially they tend to be unilateral and conform to the cavities in which they grow, but at necropsy considerable invasion and destruction of adjacent structures is usually observed (fig. 7.1). Secondary infection, necrosis, and hemorrhage is common. Carcinomatous tissue is usually soft, friable or fleshy, and pink to off-white with dark red mottling. Occasionally, carcinomas will be firm when extensive scirrhous response has developed. Sarcomas have a gross appearance similar to counterparts in other regions of the body. Because the tumors grow into a cavity, they develop edema and other vascular complications due to obstructed venous and lymphatic outflow. They therefore tend to be soft and juicy regardless of whether they are carcinomas or sarcomas. Gross appearance is therefore not a reliable discriminator between carcinomas and sarcomas in most instances.

Histological Features

Nonepithelial tumors are similar to their counterparts at other sites and are described in relevant chapters. Typical patterns of malignant epithelial tumors are shown in figure 7.2.

Papilloma

The surface epithelium of the papilloma is predominantly of the well-differentiated squamous type with an intact basement membrane unless secondary ulceration has occurred. Sometimes, other cell types such as mucous cells can be interspersed among the squamous epithelium, or less commonly, the epithelium may resemble normal pseudostratified respiratory epithelium. Nasal papillomas are uncommon. Differential diagnosis from nasal polyps is important and will be addressed under that heading later in this chapter. While adenomas within the nasal mucosa occur in rats exposed to carcinogens,[41] they are rare in domestic species, and no good background information on them exists.

Adenocarcinoma

Adenocarcinomas (fig. 7.2 A) are characterized by the presence of glandular structures which usually contain secretory products. The most common glandular patterns

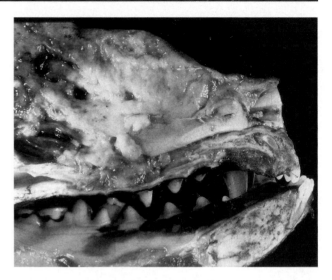

Fig. 7.1. Carcinoma of the nasal cavity in the dog. Invasion of hard palate, extension into ethmoturbinates, and invasion and distortion of the nasal and maxillary bones.

are papillary, tubulopapillary, and acinar. Mixed patterns are fairly frequent. Low grade adenocarcinomas have glandular spaces or papillary fronds lined by cuboidal to columnar cells in a single layer or perhaps with pseudostratified appearance. The cells have uniform round or oval nuclei and inconspicuous nucleoli. Cytological atypia is minimal, and mitoses are uncommon. High grade adenocarcinomas have irregular glandular spaces and more solid sheets of cells. Cellular pleomorphism, nuclear atypia, and a high mitotic index are present. Mucus is the most common type of secretion in adenocarcinomas, but serous material predominates in some tumors. Retention of secretion can lead to a cystic appearance.

Adenocarcinomas can be further subdivided according to some dominant feature other than the papillary, tubulopapillary, or acinar pattern. Published examples include the mucinous adenocarcinoma and adenocarcinoma with marked desmoplasia,[11] but no one, to our knowledge, has followed up or extended this subdivision. Five cases of adenocarcinoma originating in the olfactory glands have been reported.[36] It is unclear within which histological subtype of adenocarcinoma these fit.

Transitional Carcinoma

The name *transitional carcinoma* (fig. 7.2 B) was originally applied because the stratified arrangement of nonkeratinizing cuboidal cells resembles the transitional epithelium in the urinary tract. The recognition of a distinctive zone of transitional epithelium lying between the rostral squamous epithelium of the nose and the more caudal respiratory epithelium[34] confirms the appropriateness of the term for the corresponding type of nasal tumor. Other terms in the literature which have been used to diagnose transitional carcinomas are *respiratory epithelial carcinoma,*[35] *nonkeratinizing squamous cell carcinoma,*[11] and *undifferentiated carcinoma.*[1]

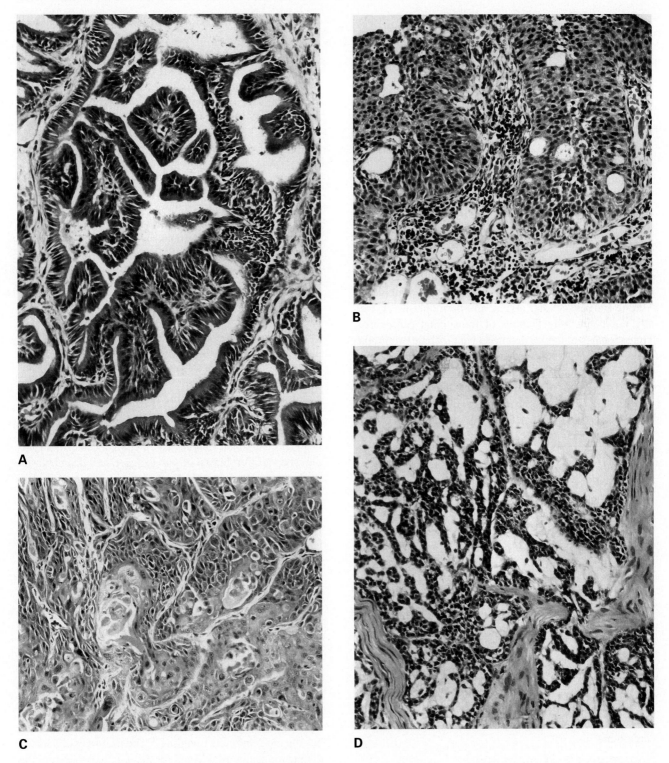

Fig. 7.2. Patterns of nasal carcinomas. **A.** Adenocarcinoma. Simple columnar to pseudostratified epithelial cells overlie fibrovascular stalks that form branching fronds within cystic spaces of nasal submucosa. **B.** Transitional. Palisaded tall columnar epithelium with marked pseudostratified appearance due to vertically staggered placement of nuclei. **C.** Squamous. Lobular aggregates of polygonal cells enlarge and become more differentiated toward individual keatinocytes, occasionally forming cysts of keatinaceous debris. **D.** Adenoid cystic. Simple to attenuated columnar epithelium forms irregular glandular cysts containing residual strands of seromucinous secretory material.

Transitional carcinomas typically consist of thick stratified layers of cells. Large tumors have complex infolding or pleating of epithelial layers that are separated by delicate fibrovascular septa. The cells in large tumors are mostly cuboidal to polyhedral in shape. These tumors may have a characteristic palisading arrangement of columnar cells that is most apparent perpendicular to the basement membrane. The cells have a small to moderate amount of pale cytoplasm, medium size nuclei with stippled chromatin and one or two prominent nucleoli, and indistinct cell boundaries. A well-defined basement membrane is present beneath the stratified layers of neoplastic cells. Microcysts are sometimes present within the epithelial layers of transitional carcinomas. They are often associated with necrosis and "drop out" of cells. When these microcysts are prominent and contain precipitated protein or cell debris, they superficially resemble glandular acini and can lead to the mistaken diagnosis of adenocarcinoma. Mitotic figures, cellular atypia, and desmoplasia are usually not noteworthy features of transitional carcinomas. Transitional carcinomas described here include two human tumor types described separately: the cylindrical cell type of sinonasal carcinoma and the nonkeratinizing, differentiated, nasopharyngeal carcinoma.[33] Whether there is advantage to separating the transitional carcinomas in dogs into two types remains to be determined.

Mixed phenotypic expression is fairly common in nasal carcinomas, especially if multiple sections are examined. Transitional carcinomas, therefore, sometimes have scattered foci of squamous differentiation and/or focal adenocarcinomatous pattern, but the great preponderance of transitional components warrants a diagnosis of transitional carcinoma rather than squamous cell or adenosquamous carcinoma.

For accuracy of classification, though not for prognostic purposes as far as we know, differentiation needs to be made between transitional carcinomas in which the basal layer of cells is columnar and tumors that are more appropriately designated nonkeratinizing squamous cell carcinomas. Although the separation is not absolute, in the nonkeratinizing squamous cell carcinomas there is progression within the epithelial layers from the basal columnar cells to more central keratinocytes with ample acidophilic cytoplasm and sometimes detectable intercellular bridges. Such progression is not a feature of transitional carcinomas.

Squamous Cell Carcinoma

Squamous cell carcinomas (fig. 7.2 C) of the sinonasal region have the same range of histological features as those arising elsewhere in the body, although they tend to be poorly keratinized. The characteristic tumor cells have abundant eosinophilic cytoplasm and large pale nuclei with one or more distinct nucleoli. Some degree of differentiation is usually detectable from basal to central regions, and in well-differentiated carcinomas, there can be close resemblance to the normal sequence of squamous

differentiation. Intercellular bridges and keratinization are easy to discern in well-differentiated squamous cell carcinomas but might be difficult to resolve in poorly differentiated ones. Immunostaining with antibodies to high molecular weight cytokeratins characteristic of squamous epithelium are a diagnostic aid in poorly differentiated cases. The degree of cellular and nuclear atypia and the frequency of mitotic figures increase with the degree of malignancy. Invading tumor cells are usually associated with a florid desmoplastic response.

Spindle Cell Carcinoma

The spindle cell carcinoma is an unusual variant of squamous cell carcinoma described in humans; it is nonkeratinizing, and the majority of the tumor is composed of spindle shaped cells similar to those of a spindle cell sarcoma. Careful search of several sections is often needed to reveal transition from recognizable squamous cell carcinoma. Spindle cell carcinomas can also resemble transitional carcinomas in which some columnar cells appear slightly spindle shaped, but in the spindle cell carcinoma there is a monomorphic accumulation of spindle shaped (sarcoma-like) cells. Positive immunohistochemical staining for cytokeratins and a negative reaction for vimentin in tumor cells is the most certain way of differentiating between spindle cell squamous carcinoma and a sarcoma of fibroblastic or other origin. Care also has to be taken to distinguish spindle cell carcinoma cells from spindle shaped fibroblasts of an exaggerated desmoplastic response. In the desmoplastic response, a separate population of inciting neoplastic cells and desmoplastic cells should be evident, and in difficult cases, immunohistochemical distinction between carcinomatous and desmoplastic cells should be possible. No mixed tumor (carcinosarcoma) of spindle cell type such as occurs in humans[33] has been recorded in domestic animals.

Adenosquamous Carcinoma

These are malignant tumors with intermixing of both adenocarcinomatous and malignant squamous cell components. Adenosquamous carcinomas with abundant mucin secreting tumor cells are also referred to as mucoepidermoid carcinomas. In humans, a distinction is made between mucoepidermoid and adenosquamous carcinomas according to the degree of intermingling of glandular and squamous components. The mucoepidermoid carcinoma has the more intimate mingling.[33] The usefulness of such a distinction is not established for the dog, and therefore the term *adenosquamous* is preferred.

Both glandular and squamous components in an adenosquamous carcinoma have the expected cytological features of malignancy, regardless of their respective proportions. The term adenocarcinoma with squamous metaplasia should only be used for an adenocarcinoma in which there are minor portions with regular squamous differentiation. Adenosquamous carcinoma tends to be among the more highly invasive nasal carcinomas.

Acinic Cell Carcinoma

These are very rare sinonasal tumors and have only been reported once.[11] The tumors are composed mainly of cells resembling serous cells of salivary glands and are presumed to be derived from minor salivary glands in the region. The cells are typically polyhedral or wedge shaped and are arranged in discrete lobules separated by delicate stroma. The lobules have solid, acinar, or trabecular patterns. The cells have small basally located hyperchromatic nuclei and abundant amphophilic cytoplasm with diastase resistant, PAS positive granules. The tumors occasionally have features of salivary serous glands such as basophilic cells, oncocytoid changes and duct-like structures. These tumors are reported to be of low grade malignancy associated with slow infiltrative growth and a tendency to recur after excision. Further documentation of this type of canine sinonasal tumor is required.

Adenoid Cystic Carcinoma

Adenoid cystic carcinoma (fig.7.2 D) is also a rare nasal tumor. The tumor typically consists of small, uniform cords and/or solid nests. The tumor cells tend to be surrounded by basophilic mucoid or hyaline material, and cystic spaces filled with the same material occur within cellular aggregates. The effect is to produce a characteristic cribriform pattern. The basaloid cells have hyperchromatic nuclei and a small amount of indistinct basophilic cytoplasm. Mitoses are rare. Myoepithelial-like cells are also present in stromal regions. The amount of mucoid material, and therefore the prominence of the cribriform pattern, varies from tumor to tumor and from one lobule to another within a single tumor.

Adenoid cystic carcinomas are believed to originate from submucosal glands or minor salivary glands.

Undifferentiated (Anaplastic) Carcinoma

These tumors are characterized by sheets or highly packed clusters of round to polyhedral cells with no discernible features of the more differentiated adenocarcinomas. Some degree of cellular atypia and pleomorphism are usually present, as are fairly frequent mitoses. These features help to distinguish undifferentiated carcinomas from poorly differentiated transitional carcinomas, although the boundary between the two tumors is not well defined. The absence of easily definable carcinomatous characteristics in undifferentiated carcinomas also makes for difficult separation from tumors such as olfactory neuroblastomas, neuroendocrine carcinomas, amelanotic malignant melanomas, lymphoid tumors, poorly differentiated mast cell tumors, and undifferentiated sarcomas. This situation requires the use of immunohistochemical markers for phenotypic characteristics, as described under the specific tumors. The distinction between undifferentiated carcinomas, olfactory neuroblastomas, and neuroendocrine carcinomas is not sharp, however, because of the overlap of ultrastructural and immunohistochemical features.

Olfactory Neuroblastoma (Esthesioneuroblastoma)

These tumors typically have nests or sheets of spherical to columnar cells separated by delicate fibrovascular stroma. The cells usually have a small amount of poorly defined cytoplasm and round nuclei with evenly distributed chromatin. An important feature in the better differentiated neuroblastomas is the presence of eosinophilic fibrillar material (neuropil) between cells. Boundaries between cells and fibrillar material are indistinct. The fibrillar material contains nerve processes that can be revealed by silver stains (e.g., Bodian) or demonstrated ultrastructurally. An important ultrastructural feature is the presence of microtubules within the cell processes. Additional ultrastructural features are the occasional presence of intracytoplasmic neurofilaments and membrane bound, dense-core vesicles. The latter are argyrophilic (Grimelius positive) by light microscopy. Some degree of palisading of tumor cells around blood vessels can occur, but a more useful diagnostic feature, when present, is the formation of rosettes where the tumor cells are arranged around a central accumulation of fibrillary material (Homer-Wright rosettes) or a well-defined clear lumen (Flexner-Wintersteiner type rosettes). Rosettes are only occasionally found in canine tumors but are a frequent finding in cats. Rosettes are not pathognomonic for neuroblastomas, however, because they can be present in some other tumors, including neuroendocrine carcinomas, which also occur in the olfactory region.

Immunohistochemically, cells of olfactory neuroblastomas can be positive for a variety of neural and glial markers including neuron specific enolase (NSE) and S-100 protein, the latter especially at the periphery of cell accumulations. Other markers that have been used, at least in humans, are those for glial fibrillary acidic protein (GFAP), neurofilament protein, synaptophysin, microtubule associated protein, and class III beta tubulin.[37] The full range of immunohistochemical markers has not been studied in animals. In a total of 10 canine and feline cases, immunohistochemical staining for NSE, GFAP, and S-100 protein did not reveal a consistent pattern useful for diagnostic purposes.[38] Only a few tumor cells stained for NSE, S-100 positivity was indistinct, and GFAP was negative. Further immunohistochemical investigation of olfactory neuroblastomas in cats and dogs is therefore required in order to determine the most useful markers.

Because of their origin from the olfactory region, olfactory neuroblastomas almost always invade the cranial cavity and brain. Olfactory neuroblastomas need to be differentiated from other highly cellular tumors of the region; for example, neuroendocrine carcinomas, undifferentiated carcinomas, lymphoid tumors, and amelanotic melanomas. The presence of rosettes is a useful, but not absolute, diagnostic aid for olfactory neuroblastomas and is mostly applicable to the cat. Most specific is the ultrastructural demonstration of neural processes containing microtubules.

Immunohistochemical identification of NSE, S-100 protein, and possibly GFAP and other neural and glial markers referred to earlier, should differentiate neuroblastomas from undifferentiated carcinomas, lymphomas, and melanomas. Differentiation of olfactory neuroblastomas from neuroendocrine carcinomas will also be considered further in the next section.

Neuroendocrine Carcinoma (Carcinoid)

The term *neuroendocrine carcinoma* is preferred to *carcinoid*. Neuroendocrine carcinomas of the nasal cavity are extremely rare in domesticated animals and have only been reported to occur in the dog.[11] They are characterized by sheets, nests, or cords of small to medium size cells separated by delicate fibrovascular stroma to give an *endocrine type packeting*. The stroma is more dense in some regions. The tumor cells are round to polyhedral with rounded, centrally placed nuclei and distinct granular, eosinophilic cytoplasm. Nuclei can be small and dense, have coarsely clumped chromatin, or be slightly vesiculate with a prominent nucleolus. Peripheral palisading of tumor cells and formation of rosettes similar to neuroblastomas has been described, as has variable distribution of mitotic figures, and necrosis and mineralization in the centers of large tumor masses.[11]

Differential diagnosis from other highly cellular tumors of the region can be difficult. It is particularly difficult to distinguish poorly developed neuroendocrine carcinomas from olfactory neuroblastomas. The extent to which poorly differentiated forms of these two tumors are separable is questionable because of overlap of phenotypic characteristics and possibility of close histogenetic relationships. By conventional light microscopy, the endocrine type packeting and distinct granular cytoplasm of the neuroendocrine carcinoma differ from the indistinct cytoplasm merging with neurofibrillary material in the olfactory neuroblastoma. The usefulness of rosette formation is unclear because they have been described in neuroendocrine carcinomas.[11] Prominent rosettes such as occur in the cat, however, are a useful indicator of olfactory neuroblastoma. Definitive separation of olfactory neuroblastomas and neuroendocrine carcinomas requires ultrastructural evaluation. This has not been done for the dog, so we can only speculate from the reported data from human tumors that neuroendocrine carcinomas should lack cell processes containing microtubules, which are a feature of olfactory neuroblastomas.[33,37] Immunohistochemically, there is considerable overlap, but neuroendocrine carcinomas would be expected to stain more regularly for cytokeratins, chromogranin, and various peptides (e.g., calcitonin, calcitonin–gene-related peptide, and vasoactive intestinal peptide). Positive staining for epithelial membrane antigen and negative staining for microtubule related components (e.g., tubulin) are features of some human neuroendocrine carcinomas.[33,37] The situation in animals awaits investigation.

REFERENCES

1. Schneider, R. (1990) General considerations. In Moulton, J.E. (ed.), *Tumors in Domestic Animals,* 3rd ed. University of California Press, Berkeley, pp. 308–346.
2. Madewell, B.R., Priester, W.A., Gillette, E.L., and Snyder, S.P. (1976) Neoplasms of the nasal passages and paranasal sinuses in domesticated animals as reported by 13 veterinary colleges. *Amer J Vet Res* 37:851–856.
3. Hayes, H.M., Wilson, G.P., and Fraumeni, J.F. (1982) Carcinoma of the nasal cavity and paranasal sinuses in dogs: Descriptive epidemiology. *Cornell Vet* 72:168–179.
4. Patnaik, A.K. (1989) Canine sinonasal neoplasms: Clinico-pathological study of 285 cases. *J Amer Anim Hosp Assoc* 25:103–114.
5. Brodey, R.S. (1970) Canine and feline neoplasia. *Adv Vet Sci Comp Med* 14:311–354.
6. Cotchin, E. (1959) Some tumours of dogs and cats of comparative veterinary and human interest. *Vet Rec* 71:1040–1050.
7. Dorn, C.R., Taylor, D.O.N., Schneider, R., Hibbard, H.H., and Klauber, M.R. (1968) Survey of animal neoplasms in Alameda and Contra Costa counties. II. Cancer morbidity in dogs and cats from Alameda County. *J Natl Cancer Inst* 40:307–318.
8. Luce, D., Gaerin, M., Leclerc, A., Morcet, J.F., Brugaere, J., and Goldberg, M. (1993) Sinonasal cancer and occupational exposure to formaldehyde and other substances. *Intl J Cancer* 53:224–231.
9. Hayes, H.M., Hoover R., and Tarone, R.E. (1981) Bladder cancer in pet dogs: A sentinel for environmental cancer? *Amer J Epidemiol* 114:229–233.
10. Reif, J.S., and Cohen, D. (1971) The environmental distribution of canine respiratory tract neoplasms. *Arch Environ Health* 22:136–140.
11. Patnaik, A.K. (1983) Canine and feline nasal and paranasal neoplasm: Morphology and origin. In Reznik, G., and Stinson, S.F. (eds.), *Nasal Tumors in Animals and Man,* Vol. 2, *Tumor Pathology.* CRC Press, Boca Raton, FL, pp. 199–228.
12. Patnaik, A.K., Lieberman, P.H., Erlandson, R.A., and Liu, S.K. (1984) Canine sinonasal skeletal neoplasms: Chondrosarcomas and osteosarcomas. *Vet Pathol* 21:475–482.
13. Patnaik, A.K., Lieberman, P.H., Erlandson, R.A., et al. (1986) Paranasal meningioma in the dog: A clinicopathologic study of ten cases. *Vet Pathol* 23:362–368.
14. Patnaik, A.K. (1989) Canine sinonasal neoplasms: Soft tissue tumors. *J Amer Anim Hosp Assoc* 25:491–497.
15. Adams, W.M., Withrow, S.J., Walshaw, R., Turrell, J.M., Evans S.M., Walker, M.A., and Kurzman, I.D. (1987) Radiotherapy of malignant nasal tumors in 67 dogs. *J Amer Vet Med Assoc* 191:311–315.
16. Evans, S.E., Goldschmidt, M., McKee, L.J., and Harvey, C.E. (1989) Prognostic factors and survival after radiotherapy for intranasal neoplasms in dogs: 70 cases (1974–1985). *J Amer Vet Med Assoc* 194:1460–1463.
17. Theon, A.P., Madewell, B.R., Harb, M.F., and Dungworth, D.L. (1993) Megavoltage irradiation of neoplasms of the nasal and paranasal cavities in 77 dogs. *J Amer Vet Med Assoc* 202:1469–1475.
18. Keller, E.T., and Madewell, B.R. (1992) Locations and types of neoplasms in immature dogs: 69 cases (1964–1989). *J Amer Vet Med Assoc* 200:1530–1532.
19. Popovitch, C.A., Weinstein, M.J., Goldschmidt, M.H., and Shofer, F.S. (1994) Chondrosarcoma: A retrospective study of 97 dogs (1987–1990). *J Amer Anim Hosp Assoc* 30:81–85.
20. Madewell, B.R., and Theilen, G.H. (1987) Tumors of the respiratory tract and thorax. In Theilen, G.H., and Madewell, B.R. (eds.), *Veterinary Cancer Medicine,* 2nd ed. Lea and Febiger, Philadelphia, pp. 535–566.

21. Theisen, S.K., Hosgood, G., and Lewis, D.D. (1996) Intranasal tumors in dogs: Diagnosis and treatment. *Comp Cont Educ Pract Vet* 18:131–138.

22. Smith, M.O., Turrel, J.M., Bailey, C.S., and Cain, G.R. (1989) Neurologic abnormalities as the predominant signs of neoplasia of the nasal cavity in dogs and cats: Seven cases (1973–1986). *J Amer Vet Med Assoc* 195:242–245.

23. Moore, M.P., Gavin, P.R., Kraft, S.L., DeHaan, C.E., Leathers, C.W., and Dorn, R.V. (1991) MR, CT and clinical features from four dogs with nasal tumors involving the rostral cerebrum. *Vet Radiol* 32:19–25.

24. Couto, C.G., Boudrieau, R.J., and Zanjani, E.D, (1989) Tumor-associated erythrocytosis in a dog with nasal fibrosarcoma. *J Vet Int Med* 3:183–185.

25. Wilson, R.B., and Bronstad, D.C. (1983) Hypercalcemia associated with nasal adenocarcinoma in a dog. *J Amer Vet Med Assoc* 182:1246–1247.

26. Thrall, D.E., Robertson, I.D., McLeod, D.A., Heidner, G.L., Hoopes, P.J., and Page, R.L. (1989) A comparison of radiographic and computed tomographic findings in 31 dogs with malignant nasal cavity tumors. *Vet Radiol* 30:59–66.

27. Burk, R.L. (1992) Computed tomographic imaging of nasal disease in 100 dogs. *Vet Radiol Ultrasound* 33:177–180.

28. Park, R.D., Beck, E.R., and LeCouteur, R.A. (1992) Comparison of computed tomography and radiography for detecting changes induced by malignant nasal neoplasia in dogs. *J Amer Vet Med Assoc* 201:1720–1724.

29. Codner, E.C., Lurus, A.G., Miller, J.B., Gavin, P.R., Gallina, A., and Barbee, D.D. (1993) Comparison of computed tomography with radiography as a noninvasive diagnostic technique for chronic nasal disease in dogs. *J Amer Vet Med Assoc* 202:1106–1110.

30. McEntee, M.C., Page, R.L., Heidner, G.L., Cline, J.M., and Thrall, D.E. (1991) A retrospective study of 27 dogs with intranasal neoplasms treated with cobalt radiation. *Vet Radiol* 32:135–139.

31. Henry, C.J., Brewer, W.G., Tyler, J.W., Brawner, E.R., Henderson, R.A., Hankes, G.H., Royer, N. (1998) Survival in dogs with nasal adenocarcinoma: 64 cases (1981–1995). *J Vet Int Med* 12:436–439.

32. Morris, J.S., Dunn,K.J., Dobson, J.M., White, R.A.S. (1994) Effects of radiotherapy alone and surgery and radiotherapy on survival of dogs with nasal tumours. *J Small Anim Pract* 35:567–573.

33. Shanmugaratnam, K., Sobin, L.H., Barnes, L., et al. (1991) *Histological Typing of Tumours of the Upper Respiratory Tract and Ear*, 2nd ed. (World Health Organization International Histological Classification of Tumours). Springer-Verlag, Berlin, Heidelberg, New York, pp. 35–69.

34. Adams, D.R., and Hotchkiss, D.K. (1983) The canine nasal mucosa. *Zbl Vet Med C Anat Histol Embryol* 12:109–125.

35. Confer, A.W., and DePaoli, A. (1978) Primary neoplasms of the nasal cavity, paranasal sinuses and nasopharynx in the dog. A report of 16 cases from the files of the AFIP. *Vet Pathol* 15:18–30.

36. Zaki, F.A., and Liu, S.-K. (1974) Adenocarcinoma of the olfactory gland in the dog. *Vet Pathol* 11:138–143.

37. Burger, P.C., and Scheithauer, B.W. (1994) Tumors of the central nervous system. *Atlas of Tumor Pathology*. 3rd series, fascicle 10. Armed Forces Institute of Pathology, Washington, D.C., pp. 200–202.

38. Hafner, A. (1997) Electronemikroskopische und immunhistochemische Untersuchung der neuralen Elemente der Riechschleimhaut des Hundes und lichtmikroskopische und immunhistochemische Charakterisierung spontaner Reichschleimhauttumoren bei Hund und Katze. Thesis, University of Munich, p. 119.

39. Recio, L., (1997) Oncogene and tumor suppressor gene alterations in nasal tumors. *Mutat Res* 380:27–31.

40. Bermudez, E., Chen, Z., Gross, E.A., Walker, C.L., Recio, L., Pluta, L., and Morgan, K.T., (1994) Characterization of cell lines derived from formaldehyde-induced nasal tumors in rats. *Molec Carcinogen* 9:193–199.

41. Haseman, J.K., and Hailey, J.R., (1997) An update of the National Toxicology Program database on nasal carcinogens. *Mutat Res* 380:3–11.

Nasal Cavity and Paranasal Sinus Tumors in Other Species

Cat

The incidence of nasal tumors in cats relative to dogs differs significantly from survey to survey. While one comparative survey found a lower incidence in cats,[1] comparison of frequencies from hospital and necropsy records suggests that cats have a slightly higher incidence than dogs. The prevalence of feline sinonasal tumors in a clinic population has been reported to be 23 tumors per 10,000 cats.[2] Sinonasal tumors are reported to be 8.4 percent of all feline tumors.[2] These figures are probably higher due to the inclusion of squamous cell carcinomas, many of which presumably originated from the nasal planum rather than within the sinonasal region proper.[2,4] Even when squamous cell carcinomas of the nasal planum are eliminated, the hospital based incidence of intranasal tumors in cats can be calculated to be 11 per 10,000 admissions compared with 4 per 10,000 canine admissions in other surveys.[3] As in dogs, the risk for sinonasal tumors increases with age. The mean age of affected cats is around 10 years. Squamous cell carcinomas of the nasal planum tend to occur at a later age (mean 12.1 years) than tumors within the sinonasal region (mean 8.7 years). Neutered cats of both sexes, especially males, have increased risk.[2] Clinical signs, diagnostic workup, and treatment are similar to those described for dogs.[5-7]

The relative frequency of tumor types differ between the cat and dog. In cats, as many as half the recorded tumors are squamous cell tumors of the nasal planum.[2,4] Within the nasal cavity, adenocarcinomas are the most frequent carcinoma.[2,7,8] In contrast to the dog, transitional carcinomas have not been recorded for the cat. Lymphoma usually predominates among the nonepithelial tumors in the cat, and chondrosarcomas are uncommon. Olfactory neuroblastomas are observed occasionally, and they tend to have prominent rosette formation (see description under canine tumors). The finding of type C viral particles in olfactory neuroblastoma that resemble those of the feline leukemia virus raises unanswered questions about a causal association.[9]

It has been our observation that, compared to the dog, the cat has a larger proportion of tumors of nondescript round cell type, for which differential diagnosis is difficult, particularly among undifferentiated carcinomas, sarcomas, lymphomas, mast cell tumors, and olfactory neuroblastomas. This fact could lead to an overreporting of lymphoma in some series.

Horse

Sinonasal tumors are rare in horses.[1,10] Most occur in horses over 15 years of age.[1] The paranasal sinuses are an important site for development of sinonasal tumors in the horse, particularly the superior maxilary sinus. In one series, 9 of 22 tumors (41 percent) originated in paranasal sinuses.[1] Squamous cell carcinomas are the most frequent tumor, but adenocarcinomas, undifferentiated carcinomas, and a variety of mesenchymal tumors have been reported.[1,10-12] A few tumors have been reported in foals: congenital ethmoid carcinoma,[13] osteoma of the paranasal sinus,[14] and fibrosarcoma of the maxillary sinus.[15]

Cow, Sheep, and Pig

Apart from endemic ethmoid tumors, there is limited information on nasal tumors. Since an early review complete through 1967,[10] there has been one report of a mixed mesenchymal tumor and an undifferentiated carcinoma in nasal cavities of cows.[16] Another survey only had one bovine tumor, a fibrosarcoma of paranasal sinuses, among the 300 pooled cases from a variety of species.[1] A description of a squamous cell carcinoma in the nasal cavity of a cow mentioned the importance of differentiation of bovine nasal tumors from nasal granulomas, especially in young animals.[17]

REFERENCES

1. Madewell, B.R., Priester, W.A., Gillette, E.L., and Snyder, S.P. (1976) Neoplasms of the nasal passages and paranasal sinuses in domesticated animals as reported by 13 veterinary colleges. *Amer J Vet Res* 37:851–856.
2. Cox, N.R., Brawner, W.R., Powers, R.D., Wright, J.C. (1991) Tumors of the nose and paranasal sinuses in cats: 32 cases with comparison to a national database (1977 through 1987). *J Amer Anim Hosp Assoc* 27:339–347.
3. Hayes, H.M., Wilson, G.P., and Fraumeni, J.F. (1982) Carcinoma of the nasal cavity and paranasal sinuses in dogs: Descriptive epidemiology. *Cornell Vet* 72:168–179.
4. Moulton, J.E. (1990) Tumors of the respiratory system. In Moulton, J.E. (ed.), *Tumors in Domestic Animals,* 3rd ed. University of California Press, Berkeley, pp. 308–346.
5. Ogilvie, G.K., and LaRue, S.M. (1992) Canine and feline nasal and paranasal sinus tumors. *Vet Clin N Amer Small Anim Pract* 22:1133–1144.
6. O'Brien, R.T., Evans, S.M., Wortman, J.A., and Hendrick, M.J. (1996) Radiographic findings in cats with intranasal neoplasia or chronic rhinitis: 29 cases (1982–1988). *J Amer Vet Med Assoc* 208:385–389.
7. Theon, A.P., Peaston, A.E., Madewell, B.R., and Dungworth, D.L. (1994) Irradiation of nonlymphoproliferative neoplasms of the nasal cavity and paranasal sinuses in 16 cats. *J Amer Vet Med Assoc* 204:78–83.
8. Patnaik, A.K. (1983) Canine and feline nasal and paranasal neoplasm: Morphology and origin. In Rezik, G., and Stinson, S.F. (eds.), *Nasal Tumors in Animals and Man,* vol. 2, *Tumor Pathology.* CRC Press, Boca Raton, FL, pp. 199–228.
9. Schrenzel, M.D., Higgins, R.J., Hinrichs, S.H., Smith, M.O., and Torten, M. (1990) Type C retroviral expression in spontaneous feline olfactory neuroblastomas. *Acta Neuropathol* 80:547–553.
10. Cotchin, E. (1967) Spontaneous neoplasms of the upper respiratory tract in animals. In Muir, C.S., and Shanmugaratnam, K. (eds.), *Cancer of the Nasopharynx.* International Union Against Cancer, Monograph Series No.1. Medical Examination Publishing Co., Flushing, NY, pp. 203–259.
11. Noack, P. (1956) Die Geschwulste der oberen Atmungswege bei den Haussaugetieren (Teile I, Teile II). *Wiss Z Humboldt-Univ* pp. 293–314, 373–391.
12. Leyland, A., and Baker, J.R. (1975) Lesions of the nasal and paranasal sinuses of the horse causing dyspnoea. *Brit Vet J* 131:339–346.
13. Acland, H.M., Orsini, J.A., Elkins, S., Lee, J.W., Lein, D.H., and Morris, D.D. (1984) Congenital ethmoid carcinoma in a foal. *J Amer Vet Med Assoc* 184:979–981.
14. Peterson, F.B., Martens, R.J., and Montali, R.J. (1978) Surgical treatment of an osteoma in the paranasal sinuses of a horse. *J Equine Med Surg* 2:279–283.
15. Hultgren, B.D., Schmotzer, W.B., Watrous, B.J., Hedstrom, O.R., Schmitz, J.A., Wagner, P.C., Kaneps, A.J., and Gallagher, J.A. (1987) Nasal-maxillary fibrosarcoma in young horses: A light and electron microscopic study. *Vet Pathol* 24:194–196
16. Becker, M., Pohlenz, J., and Ammann-Mann, M. (1972) Zum Vorkommen von Nasentumoren beim Rind. *Schweizer Arch Tierheilk* 114:404–412.
17. Pycock, J.F., Pead, M.J., and Longstaffe, J.A. (1984) Squamous cell carcinoma in the nasal cavity of a cow. *Vet Rec* 114:542–543.

Endemic Ethmoid Tumors (Enzootic Intranasal Tumors)

Endemic tumors of the ethmoid region have been recognized in animals in many countries for most of this century. Cases have been reported in sheep, goats, cattle, pigs, horses, and buffaloes.[1,2] Multiple cases occur in a few flocks or herds and can continue to occur over several years. More than one species are occasionally affected on individual farms. *Enzootic intranasal tumor* is the term usually applied in recent literature, although it offers no advantage over its predecessor, *endemic ethmoid tumor.*

Sheep and Goats

Enzootic intranasal tumors of sheep occur widely throughout the world, but in goats they have only been reported from France, Spain, Italy, and India. The tumors are believed to originate from Bowman's glands in the ethmoid mucosa.[3] In goats, they might also originate in serous glands.[4] There is ample evidence that type D–like retroviruses are implicated in causing the tumors in both sheep and goats. The ovine tumor was first transmitted experimentally from sheep to sheep by using tumor homogenates filtered free of cells and bacteria.[5] Retrovirus-like particles were later demonstrated ultrastructurally in ovine tumor cells[3] and in caprine cells.[6] Viral particles were subsequently detected in nasal fluid and tumor tissue of goats. These viral particles possessed reverse transcriptase activity and contained a protein which cross-reacted with a protein from Mason-Pfizer monkey virus, an established type D retrovirus.[7] Particles containing a protein cross-reacting with Mason-Pfizer monkey virus have also been found in nasal fluid of affected sheep.[8] Experimental transmission has now been achieved in goats using retrovirus concentrated from nasal fluids of diseased goats.[9]

Clinically, affected sheep and goats have profuse seromucinous nasal exudate, dyspnea, stertorous breathing, and coughing. Openmouthed breathing, exophthalmos, and facial deformity are possible complications. Grossly, the tumors are unilateral or bilateral, polypoid to confluent masses centered on the ethmoid region. Their origin from ethmoid mucosa is sometimes still evident. Tumor tissue ranges from whitish to pink to dark red and from firm to friable. A granular or papillary surface covered by mucus often covers polypoid masses. Advanced tumors cause local bone destruction, invade frontal or maxillary sinuses, and can invade gingiva and orbit. Occasionally, tumor tissue can protrude through the anterior nares or into the nasopharynx. Nonneoplastic nasal polyps adjacent to neoplastic tissue are reported for goats.[4]

Histologically, the tumors have variously been called adenomas[5,10,11] or adenocarcinomas[12,13] (fig. 7.3). The papillary subtype is common, although mucinous, tubular, and acinar patterns are also seen. The tumors in goats are interpreted to be well-differentiated (low grade) carcinomas, also with papillary, tubular, or acinar patterns.[4] The tumors in sheep and goats do not appear to differ significantly in histological type. Whether they are called adenomas or well-differentiated carcinomas is a matter of interpretation. The regularity of the neoplastic epithelium, lack of obvious cellular atypia, usually very low mitotic index, and lack of stromal or vascular invasion and metastasis leads some authors to prefer the diagnosis of adenoma. Others view the progressive infiltrative and destructive growth as indicative of a well-differentiated adenocarcinoma. The occasional occurrence of metastases in goats[14] and the transplantability of cultured caprine tumor cells into nude mice[15] support the interpretation of low grade malignancy, at least in the goat.

Cattle

Endemic ethmoid tumors in cattle were mainly observed in Sweden in the early part of this century and apparently no longer occur in that region.[16] The tumors were more diverse than those of sheep and goats. Undifferentiated carcinomas, adenocarcinomas, sarcomas, and mixed tumors (carcinosarcomas) were described. More recently, these tumors were reported to be endemic in the Dominican Republic.[16,17] Adenocarcinomas and squamous cell carcinomas are most common, but various sarcomas and occasional carcinosarcomas occur. Viral etiology was hypothesized, but no evidence was found to support the hypothesis.[17] Contamination of feeds with mycotoxins was also speculated to play a role in causing these tumors.[17]

Horse and Pig

Endemic ethmoid tumors of horses were reported from Scandinavia earlier this century, often in association with bovine cases.[1] As in cattle, a diverse range of tumor

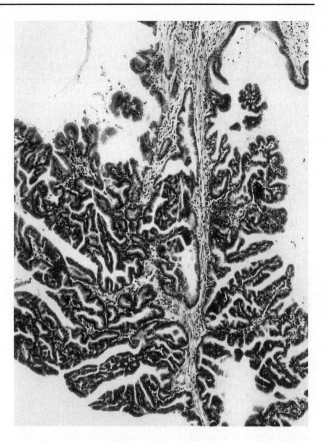

Fig. 7.3. Ovine caprine epizootic nasal tumors. Exophitic papillary growths of nasal mucosa arising in epithelium overlying nasal turbinates.

types was observed. There have not been recent reports of the condition in horses.

Endemic nasal adenocarcinomas have been reported to occur in pigs from Brazil, China, Ghana, and India.[2,18,19] No current information is available.

REFERENCES

1. Cotchin, E. (1967) Spontaneous neoplasms of the upper respiratory tract in animals. In Muir, C.S., and Shanmugaratnan, K. (eds.). *Cancer of the Nasopharynx.* International Union Against Cancer, Monograph Series No.1. Medical Examination Publishing Co., Flushing, NY, pp. 203–259.

2. Rajan, A. (1987) Carcinoma of the mucosa of the domestic animals. *Ann Rech Vet* 18:13–17.

3. Yonemichi, H., Ohgi, T., Fujimoto, Y., Okada, K., Onuma, M., and Mikami, T. (1978) Intranasal tumor of the ethmoid olfactory mucosa in sheep. *Amer J Vet Res* 39:1599–1606.

4. De las Heras, M., Garci de Jalon, J.A., and Sharp, J.M. (1991) Pathology of enzootic intranasal tumor in thirty-eight goats. *Vet Pathol* 28:474–481.

5. Cohrs, P. (1953) Infectiose Adenopapillome der Reichschleimhaut beim Schaf. *Berl Muench Tierarztl Wochenschr* 66:225–228.

6. De las Heras, M., Garcia de Jalon, J.A., Balaguer, L., and Badiola, J.J. (1988) Retrovirus-like particles in enzootic intranasal tumors in Spanish goats. *Vet Rec* 123:135.

7. De las Heras, M., Sharp, J.M., Garcia de Jalon, J.A., Dewar, P. (1991) Enzootic nasal tumur of goats: Demonstration of a type D–related retrovirus in nasal fluids and tumours. *J Gen Virol* 72:2533–2535.

8. De las Heras, M., Sharp, J.M., Ferrer, L.M., Garcia de Jalon, J.A., and Cebrian, L.M. (1993) Evidence for a type D–like retrovirus in enzootic nasal tumor of sheep. *Vet Rec* 132:441.

9. De las Heras, M., Garcia de Jalon, J.A., Minguijon, E., Gray, E.W., Dewar, P., and Sharp, J.M. (1995) Experimental transmission of enzootic intranasal tumors of goats. *Vet Pathol* 32:19–23.

10. Njoku, C.O., Shannon, D., Chineme, C.N., and Bida, S.A. (1978) Ovine nasal adenopapilloma: Incidence and clinicopathologic studies. *Amer J Vet Res* 39:1850–1852.

11. Perl, S., Yakobson, B., Orgad-Klopfer, U., Abramson, M., and Nobel, T. (1987) Enzootic nasal tumor of sheep. *Vet Quarterly* 9:118–122.

12. Young, S., Lovelace, S.A., Hawkins, W.W., and Catlin, J.E. (1961) Neoplasms of the olfactory mucous membrane of sheep. *Cornell Vet* 51:97–112

13. Duncan, J.R., Tyler, D.E., Van Der Maaten, M.J., and Andersen, J.R. (1967) Enzootic nasal adenocarcinoma in sheep. *J Amer Vet Med Assoc* 151:732–734.

14. Rajan, A., Sulochana, S., Sreekumaran, T., Reddi, M.V., and Nair, M.K. (1980) Tumours of the ethmoid mucosa in goats (*Capra hircus*). *Indian J Cancer* 17:196–199.

15. Torres, R. (1984) Activitie tumorigene chez la souris d'une lignee cellulaire issue d'une tumeur des sinus de chevre. *Ann Rech Vet* 15:129.

16. Pospischil, A., Haenichen, T., and Schaeffler, H. (1979) Histological and electron-microscopic studies of endemic ethmoidal carcinomas in cattle. *Vet Pathol* 16:180–190.

17. Pospischil, A., Weiland, F., van Sandersleben, J., Haenichen, T., and Schaffler, H. (1982) Endemic ethmoidal tumor in cattle: sarcoma and carcinosarcomas: A light- and electron-microscopic study. *Zentralblt Veterinaermed(A)* 29:628–636.

18. Amaral, L.B.S., and Nesti, A, (1963) Incidencia de cancer em bovinos e suinos. *Biologico* 29:30–31.

19. Vohradsky, F. (1974) Adenocarcinoma of the olfactory mucosa of sheep and pigs in Ghana. *Acta Vet (Brno)* 43: 243–249.

Nasal and Nasopharyngeal Polyps

These polyps are nonneoplastic, usually pedunculated, growths arising from the mucosal surface of the nasal cavity or nasopharynx. In the cat, they can also arise from the lining of the auditory canal or middle ear. The cause and pathogenesis of polyps is unknown. They are associated with hyperplasia of the mucous membrane and some degree of chronic inflammation of the underlying connective tissues, but the causal relationship between these two features is uncertain. After attaining a certain size, they can become self-perpetuating because of impairment of venous and lymphatic drainage in the stalk and development of edematous stroma.

Differentiation of polyps from polypoid tumors, particularly fibromas, papillomas, and hemangiomas, is usually fairly clear because a polyp lacks any regions with consistent and characteristic features of neoplasia (see earlier descriptions), and most of the lesion is formed by chronically inflamed, edematous stroma. One differential diagnosis to be considered in the dog is angioleiomyoma.[1] Differentiation between polyps and tumors can sometimes be very difficult and requires either careful search of numerous sections or, in the case of biopsy material, examination of recurrent lesions.

Polyps occur infrequently. They are seen most often in the cat and horse, usually in the form of one of the entities described below. Grossly, polyps are moist, glistening, and spherical, ovoid, or elongated. They are often pedunculated. The growths are firm or rubbery and commonly have a slimy, smooth or roughened surface, which might be ulcerated. The color is off-white, pink, or red. Polyps are sometimes multiple (polyposis). Polyps can attain a size sufficient to produce respiratory difficulty. They can also cause complications by becoming secondarily infected. Removal of a polyp can be followed by recurrence, especially if excision was incomplete.

Histologically, polyps consist of edematous fibrous tissue covered by regular respiratory epithelium or stratified squamous epithelium (fig. 7.4 A). Some degree of subepithelial accumulation of chronic inflammatory cells is present (fig. 7.4 B). Venous and lymphatic dilation is usual except when there are regions of granulation or scarring. These latter regions are usually found underlying mucosal ulceration.

Nasopharyngeal and Middle Ear Polyps in Cats

These polyps typically occur in cats less than a year old and lead to progressive increase in clinical signs associated with nasopharyngeal obstruction. The polyps can originate from mucous membrane of the nasopharynx, auditory canal, or tympanic bulla. Polyps arising in the auditory canal frequently extend back up into the middle ear or down into the nasopharynx. Gross and microscopic features are as described previously in this section. Cause of the feline polyps is unknown. A congenital factor has been proposed, but without solid evidence. The role of infection and inflammation is more plausibly suspected. More detailed clinicopathologic features of the condition have been published.[2-5] A nasopharyngeal polyp in a young dog, possibly analogous to the polyps in cats, has been described[6].

Progressive Ethmoid Hematoma of the Horse

This condition was first described in 1974,[7] and the lesions were later described as hemorrhagic nasal polyps.[8] The polyps typically arise unilaterally from the ethmoid region and can be large enough to reach the nostril or choanae. Except for surface hemorrhage or ulceration and secondary infection, the polyps have a smooth surface. The cut section appears hemorrhagic or mottled pale, brown, and hemorrhagic. Histologically, the polyps are highly vascular and have a distinctive appearance resulting from repeated hemorrhage, hemoglobin breakdown, and organization by fibrous tissue (fig. 7.5). There is extensive hemosiderin deposition, lipofuscin accumulation, and prominent ferruginous and calcareous encrustations of collagen fibers and vessel walls. Giant cells and hemosiderin laden

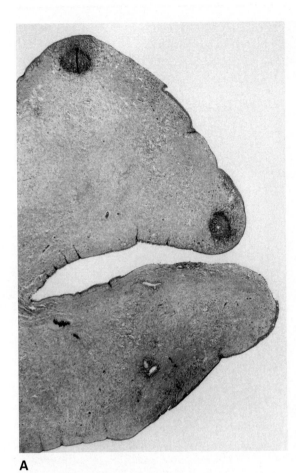

A

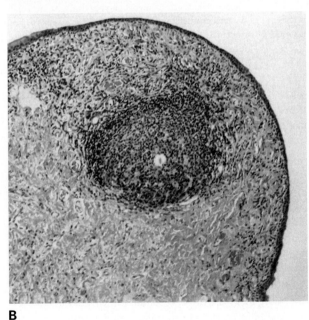

B

Fig. 7.4. Feline nasopharyngeal polyp. **A.** Low magnification illustrating solid irregular exophytic growth of connective tissue lined by stratified squamous nonkeratinizing epithelium. **B.** Higher magnification illustrating the dense collagenous matrix forming the bulk of the lesion and the presence of lymphohistiocytic nodules.

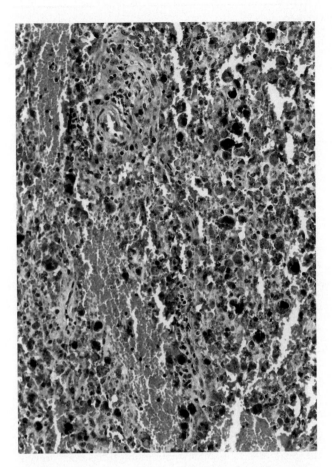

Fig. 7.5. Equine progressive hematoma. Cellular components include a predominace of macrophages, many of which are distended by abundant hemosiderin, that are loosely aggregated by poorly formed, highly vascularized connective tissue and occasional dilated, blood filled spaces.

macrophages are common. In one reported case[8] the lesion involved the mucous membrane of a paranasal sinus and more resembled a hemangioma composed of an extensive capillary network. Ethmoid hematomas are differentiated from vascular tumors on the basis of the former having the expected features of response to repeated hemorrhages, whereas the latter have substantial portions composed of neoplastic vascular components (see descriptions of hemangioma and hemangiosarcoma elsewhere in this book). The differential diagnosis of hemangiosarcoma and progressive hematoma has been addressed.[9]

Tumors of the Larynx and Trachea

Neoplasms of the larynx and trachea are very rare, and most published reports are of single cases. Information is therefore fragmentary. Any tissue in or adjacent to the walls of these structures can give rise to tumors, so a variety of epithelial and mesenchymal tumors has been found.

377

Larynx

Cases in the earlier literature have been reviewed.[10] The most comprehensive report is more recent and refers to canine and feline laryngeal tumors.[11] The authors reviewed the literature and described an additional 24 cases (13 in dogs and 11 in cats) compiled over a 10-year period. Laryngeal tumors were 0.02 percent of all biopsy and necropsy specimens in dogs and 0.14 percent in the cat. The higher frequency in the cat was mainly due to the preponderance of lymphoma. Ages of affected animals ranged from 2 to 12 years for dogs and 2 to 17 years for cats. Males outnumbered females by more than 2 to 1 in both dogs and cats. No one tumor type predominated in the dog, since 11 different types of tumor were recorded. In contrast, the majority of tumors in the cat (8 of 11) were lymphomas. There were no squamous cell carcinomas among the 13 canine laryngeal tumors.[11] This contrasts with an earlier report in which four primary laryngeal tumors in dogs were all squamous cell carcinomas.[12] Reasons for the apparent difference are not known.

Chondromas (fig. 7.6) or osteochondromas occasionally originate from laryngeal or tracheal cartilages.[13,14] The osteochondromas are usually cartilaginous nodules with central endochondral ossification. They are derived from perichondrial proliferation of developmental, inflammatory, or neoplastic nature. It is often difficult to decide what the basic process is in any one tumor. It has been argued that the lesions should be classified as osteochondral dysplasia, but the term osteochondroma is well established and can be used without implying specific pathogenesis.

The histological appearance of laryngeal tumors resembles that of the same tumor types found elsewhere. The tumor deserving of discussion here is the canine oncocytoma because it has been reported to occur predominantly in the laryngeal region and because of the confusion which has occurred with respect to differentiating it from tumors of striated muscle origin.

Laryngeal Rhabdomyoma/ Oncocytoma of the Dog

Oncocytomas are generally considered benign neoplasms, although they can cause death by laryngeal obstruction. The diagnosis of these tumors is based on characteristic ultrastructural findings of cells with abundant cytoplasm filled with enlarged, closely packed, mitochondria. In humans, oncocytomas occur most often in the kidney, where antigenic markers suggest they arise from tubular epithelium.[15] Tumors with similar ultrastructure occur in various other sites including lacrimal sacs,[16] adrenal glands,[17] salivary glands[18] and nasal cavity.[19] Whether oncocytes represent a specific cell type or a manifestation of mitochondrial alterations in a variety of cell types remains uncertain.

Tumors originally diagnosed as laryngeal oncocy-

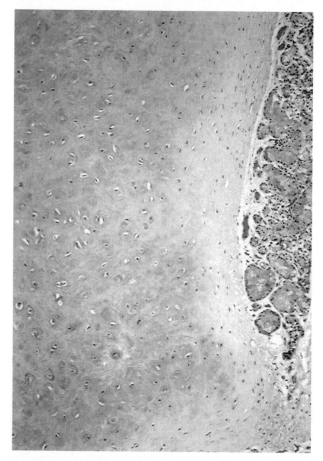

Fig. 7.6. Laryngeal chondroma (equine): Laryngeal glands are compressed by multilobular proliferations of well differentiated chondrocytes in a cartilaginous matrix.

tomas in dogs[20,21] were later determined to be of muscle origin[22] These tumors presented as solitary nodules that originated in the submucosal tissues of the larynx and protruded into the laryngeal lumens, thus causing dyspnea and stertorous respiration. Ages of three affected dogs ranged from 2 to 8 years. Grossly, the tumors were pink, fleshy masses with occasional areas of hemorrhage. Histologically, the tumors consisted mostly of lobular accumulations of variously sized and shaped cells with abundant finely granular or foamy cytoplasm. Some cells contained large, clear, cytoplasmic vacuoles. Nuclei were round to oval and had one distinct nucleolus or several small ones. Cytoplasmic invaginations into nuclei were common; mitotic figures were rare. Important ultrastructural features were packing of cytoplasm with mitochondria and intermitochondrial accumulations of rough endoplasmic reticulum and glycogen granules.

Since two of the tumors originally reported as oncocytomas[21] were subsequently found to be rhabdomyomas,[22] it remains uncertain whether oncocytoma is a tumor that exists in the dog. Histologically, there is no easy way to distinguish clearly between oncocytoma and poorly differentiated striated muscle tumors since both have cells with ample granular or foamy eosinophilic cytoplasm (fig. 7.7 A). While the *strap cells* of rhabdomyosarcomas are unusual, multinucleate cells are often present as a small proportion of the population (fig. 7.7 B). Careful search might reveal cross striations in cells with elongated eosinophilic cytoplasm, preferably in sections stained with phosphotungstic acid hematoxylin (PTAH), and this would indicate muscle origin. Definitive separation requires ultrastructural and immunohistochemical examinations.[22,23] Ultrastructurally, the presence of intracytoplasmic myofibrils containing occasional electron-dense lines (Z lines) is diagnostic for rhabdomyoma. Immunohistochemically, positive staining for myoglobin and desmin are diagnostic for rhabdomyomas. They should also be positive for myosin and actin, but there is no information on this for laryngeal tumors in dogs. The conclusion is that, when rigorous diagnostic criteria are applied, there is some uncertainty as to whether true oncocytomas have been characterized, at least in the canine larynx.

An "oncocytoma" that metastasized to the tracheobronchial lymph node has been diagnosed in a canine lung (Dr. F.Y. Schulmann, Armed Forces of Pathology, personal communication), and there is a report of one from the subcutis on the face of a cat.[24] These have not been thoroughly examined to distinguish them from the rhabdomyomas described earlier.

Trachea

There are even fewer reports of tracheal tumors than of laryngeal tumors. A variety of epithelial and nonepithelial tumors is possible, but examples occur very rarely.[10] Recent reports of canine cases include leiomyomas,[25,26] osteosarcoma,[27] chondrosarcoma,[28] and a mast cell tumor.[29] Two adenocarcinomas and a lymphoma were found in cats.[30,31] Tracheal osteochondromas in young dogs represent a slightly more definitive syndrome.[13,32] These cartilagenous tumors likely represent dysplasia of cartilage ring formation. A definitive connection to tracheal rings may or may not be evident. Some of these apparently benign growths may have central endochondral ossification with marrow space formation. Surgical removal is generally curative. An association with multiple cartilagenous lesions has been suggested.[13]

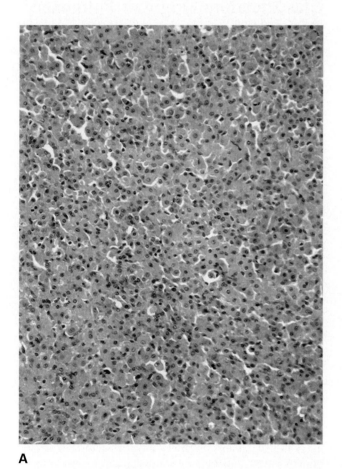

A

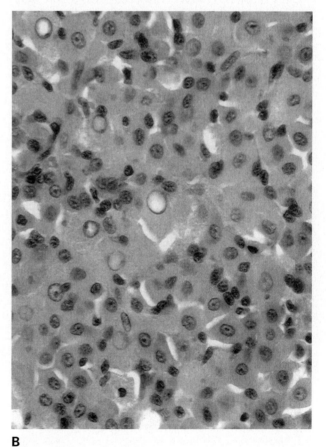

B

Fig. 7.7. Laryngeal oncocytoma/rhabdomyosarcoma. **A.** Rhabdomyosarcoma. Diffuse sheet of infiltrative polygonal cells with abundant homogenous cytoplasm. **B.** Rhabdomyosarcoma. Round to polygonal cells with abundant cytoplasm and spherical vesicular central nuclei have occasional mutinucleate cells, some of which have nuclei in rows. Intranuclear cytoplasmic inclusions (invaginations) are often seen in the neoplasm.

REFERENCES

1. Carpenter, J.L., and Hamilton, T.A. (1995) Angioleiomyoma of the nasopharynx in a dog. *Vet Pathol* 32:721–723.

2. Lane, J.G., Orr, C.M., Lucke, V.M., and Gruffydd-Jones, T.J. (1981) Nasopharyngeal polyps arising in the middle ear of the cat. *J Small Anim Pract* 22:511–522.

3. Bradley, R.L., Noone, K.E., Saunders, G.K., and Patnaik, A.K. (1985) Nasopharyngeal and middle ear polypoid masses in five cats. *Vet Surg* 114:141–144.

4. Kapatkin, A.S., Matthiesen, D.T., Noone, K.E., Church, E.M., Scavelli, T.E., and Patnaik, A.K. (1990) Results of surgery and long-term follow-up in 31 cats with nasopharyngeal polyps. *J Amer Anim Hosp Assoc* 26:387–392.

5. Bradley, R.L. (1990) Removal of nasopharyngeal and middle ear polyps in the cat. In Bojrab, M.J. (ed.) *Current Techniques in Small Animal Surgery,* 3rd ed. Lea and Febiger, Philadelphia, pp. 187–189.

6. Fingland, R.B., Gratzek, A., Vorhies, M.W., and Kirpensteijn, J. (1993) Nasopharyngeal polyp in a dog. *J Amer Anim Hosp Assoc* 29:211–314.

7. Cook, W.R., and Littlewort, M.C.G. (1974) Progressive haematoma of the ethmoid region in the horse. *Equine Vet J* 6:101–108.

8. Platt, H. (1975) Haemorrhagic nasal polyps of the horse. *J Pathol* 115:51–55.

9. Chan, C.W., and Collins, E.A. (1985) Case of angiosarcoma of the nasal passage of the horse—Ultrastructure and differential diagnosis from progressive haematoma. *Equine Vet J* 17:214–218.

10. Cotchin, E. (1967) Spontaneous neoplasms of the upper respiratory tract in animals. In Muir, C.S., and Shanmugaratnam, K. (eds.), *Cancer of the Nasopharynx.* International Union Against Cancer, Monograph Series No. 1. Medical Examination Publishing Co.,Flushing, NY, pp. 203–259.

11. Saik, J.E., Toll, S.L., Diters, R.W., and Goldschmidt, M.H. (1986) Canine and feline laryngeal neoplasia: A 10-year survey. *J Amer Anim Hosp Assoc* 22:359–365.

12. Wheeldon, E.B., Suter, P.F., and Jenkins, T. (1982) Neoplasia of the larynx in the dog. *J Amer Vet Med Assoc* 180:642–647.

13. Carb, A., and Halliwell, W.H. (1981) Osteochondral dysplasias of the canine trachea. *J Amer Anim Hosp Assoc* 17:193–199.

14. Trotter, G.W., Aanes, W.A., and Snyder, S.P. (1981) Laryngeal chondroma in a horse. *J Amer Vet Med Assoc* 178:829–830.

15. Kovacs, G., Welter, C., Wilkens, L., Blin, N., and Deriese, W. (1989) Renal oncocytoma. A phenotypic and genotypic entity of renal parenchymal tumors. *Amer J Pathol* 134:967–971.

16. Tomic, S., Warner, T.F., and Brandenburg, J.H. (1995) Malignant oncocytoma of the lacrimal sac: Ultrastructure and immunocytochemistry. *Ear Nose Throat J* 74:717–720.

17. Waters, P.R., Haselhuhn, G.D., Gunning, W.T., Phillips, E.R., and Selman, S.H. (1997) Adrenocortical oncocytoma: Two case reports and review of the literature. *Urology* 49:624–628.

18. Corbridge, R.J., Gallimore, A.P., Dalton, C.G., and O'Flynn, P.E. (1996) Oncocytomas of the upper jaw. *Head Neck* 18:374–380.

19. Comin, C.E., Dini, M., and Lo, R.G. (1997) Oncocytoma of the nasal cavity: Report of a case and review of the literature. *J Laryngol Otol* 111:671–673.

20. Pass, D.A., Huxtable, C.R., Cooper, B.J., Watson, A.D.J., and Thompson, R. (1980) Canine laryngeal oncocytomas. *Vet Pathol* 17:672–677.

21. Calderwood Mays, M.B. (1984) Laryngeal oncocytoma in two dogs. *J Amer Vet Med Assoc* 185:677–679.

22. Meuten, D.J., Calderwood Mays, M.B., Dillman, R.C., Cooper, B.J., Valentine, B.A., Kuhajda, F.P., and Pass, D.A. (1985) Canine laryngeal rhabdomyoma. *Vet Pathol* 22:533–539.

23. Liggett, A.D., Weiss, R., and Thomas, K.L. (1985) Canine laryngopharyngeal rhabdomyoma resembling an oncocytoma: Light microscopic, ultrastructural and comparative studies. *Vet Pathol* 22:526–532.

24. Berry, K.K., Wilson, R.W., Holscher, M.A., and Crisp, J. (1988) Oncocytoma in a cat. *Comp Anim Pract* 2:16–18.

25. Black, A.P., Liu, S., and Randolph, J.F. (1981) Primary tracheal leiomyoma in a dog. *J Amer Vet Med Assoc* 179:905–907.

26. Bryan, R.D., Frame, R.W., and Kier, A.B. (1981) Tracheal leiomyoma in a dog. *J Amer Vet Med Assoc* 178:1069–1070.

27. Brodey, R.S., O'Brien, J.A., Berg, P., and Rozel, J.F. (1969) Osteosarcoma of the upper airway in the dog. *J Amer Vet Med Assoc* 155:1460–1464.

28. Aron, D.N., DeVries, R., and Short, C.E. (1980) Primary tracheal chondrosarcoma in a dog: A case report with description of surgical and anesthetic techniques. *J Amer Anim Hosp Assoc* 16:31–37

29. Harvey, H.J., and Sykes, G. (1982) Tracheal mast cell tumor in a dog. *J Amer Vet Med Assoc* 180:1097–1100.

30. Beaumont, P.R. (1982) Intratracheal neoplasia in two cats. *J Small Anim Pract* 23:29–35.

31. Cain, G.R., and Manley, P. (1983) Tracheal adenocarcinoma in a cat. *J Amer Vet Med Assoc* 182:614–616.

32. Dubielzig, R.R., and Dickey, D.L. (1978) Tracheal osteochondroma in a young dog. *Vet Med Small Anim Clin* 73:1288–1290.

TUMORS OF THE LUNG

General Considerations

Classification: Origin of Pulmonary Tumors

Neoplasia can arise from every component of the lung. Tumors of clinically significant incidence, however, mostly arise from epithelium of the conducting airways or alveolar parenchyma. Various approaches to classification of lung tumors in both humans and animals have used site of origin (bronchogenic, bronchial gland, or bronchioloalveolar), histological pattern (adenoid, squamous, large cell, small cell), or combinations thereof. Unfortunately, there is significant overlap in the histological pattern of tumors from various sites of origin within the lung. Further complications arise because the site of origin is often obscured by aggressive tumor growth by the time tumors are examined and by transdifferentiation from one phenotype to another at various stages in the neoplastic process. Phenotype is, therefore, not a completely reliable indication of histogenesis.

Tumors derived from the large airway epithelium are more often located near the hilus of the lung, while tumors of parenchymal origin tend to be peripheral. Tumors of large airway origin predominate in humans and are associated with inhalation of carcinogens, particularly cigarette smoke, while tumors of the bronchioloalveolar region are more common in the dog, where they can be multicentric. Based on a higher frequency of hilar masses with predominately adenocarcinomatous histological pattern, cats are more likely to have tumors of airway origin than tumors arising from the distal lung. Reports of spontaneous tumors in other species are too limited to predict likely sites of origin. Histological patterns of tumor growth from both regions can overlap with a combination of glandular, solid, and squamous phenotypes, sometimes within the same neoplasm.

Previous classifications of pulmonary tumors in domestic animals have attempted to distinguish bronchogenic neoplasms from bronchioloalveolar tumors.[1, 2] The overlap in histological pattern and the difficulties in determining site of origin in the airways has made this approach unworkable. The recently revised WHO guidelines[3] classify primary lung tumors of animals largely by histological pattern without reference to site of origin and are the basis for the classification used here (table 7.2). The exception is the recognizable pattern of well-differentiated bronchioloalveolar tumors. These tumors form a characteristic papillary growth of simple cuboidal epithelium on a network of fibrovascular stroma that recapitulates the appearance of fetal or reparative alveolar epithelium. Epithelial cells in these tumors can have ultrastructural characteristics of either alveolar type II cells (lamellar granules) or Clara cells (dense protein secretory granules). Given the apparent bipotential differentiation of type II and Clara cells, these differences do not necessarily imply origin from parenchyma versus small airways.

Despite the difficulty in definitively identifying tumors as of large airway origin, specific features can be highly suggestive. Tumors of large airway origin tend to grow near the hilus and are often aggressive, solitary, large masses that may have smaller metastatic foci, while bronchioloalveolar tumors are peripheral and can appear multicentric. Increasing evidence in human airway neoplasia suggests that the multistep process of transformation is manifest in airway epithelium as recognizable preneoplastic foci. Similar hyperplastic/dysplastic changes can be seen in some animal tumors of airway origin.

Prevalence

Pulmonary neoplasia is an infrequent finding in domestic animals, with the exception of dogs and cats. Pulmonary neoplasia in colony raised dogs has an increasing age specific incidence,[4] with up to 25 percent of aged colony housed dogs having some form of lung carcinoma.[5] This latter study demonstrated a crude incidence of 8.8 percent of all animals in a life span study. Frequencies reported from pathology accessions in the overall canine population are significantly lower, with estimates that range from 0.1 to 0.9 percent of dogs that were necropsied at veterinary schools.[6-8] The estimate of populational incidence of pulmonary carcinoma based on a two-county survey of animals admitted to veterinary clinics in California was 4.2 per 10,000 dogs per year.[9]

The prevalence of lung tumors in the cat appears similar to or slightly higher than that in the dog. A survey of records of cases submitted for pathological evaluation at the University of California found pulmonary neoplasia represented 0.75 percent of all feline accessions and 0.58 percent of all canine cases.[10]

Tumor Type

The frequency of histological tumor types differs among dogs, cats, and humans. In humans, 75 percent of lung cancers are non–small cell types, which represent approximately equal numbers of adenocarcinoma and adenosquamous or squamous cell tumors. Tumors of squamous differentiation are presumably of bronchial origin and related to cigarette smoking.[11] Bronchioloalveolar tumors are more prevalent in the dog, with a presumption that they arise from the lung periphery in both species. Adenocarcinomas, adenosquamous, and squamous cell tumors are less common in the dog, representing 13–15 percent of primary lung tumors in two different surveys, with the remainder being bronchioloalveolar tumors.[5,12] In the cat, the predominant pattern is adenocarcinoma, with lesser numbers of adenosquamous or squamous and bronchioloalveolar tumors. Frequency of adenocarcinomas ranged from 60 to 70 percent of all feline lung tumors in three surveys, while bronchioloalveolar tumors represented 10–27 percent and squamous/adenosquamous tumors 8–14 percent of all primary lung tumors.[10,13,14] Small cell carcinomas, which represent 25 percent of human pulmonary neoplasms, are rare in domestic animals, and reports in dogs have been limited to individual cases.

Primary lung tumors appear to be quite rare in cattle, with slaughter surveys finding from 2 to 20 cases per million cattle.[15,16] The majority of bovine tumors appear to be adenocarcinomas with the typical pattern of well-differentiated papillary growths of mucous filled goblet cells. Other tumors reported in the cow include pulmonary blastomas[17] and an anaplastic small cell carcinoma.[18]

The only pulmonary tumor of note in the horse is the granular cell tumor. While this rare tumor has been the subject of case reports,[19] no information on its incidence is available.

TABLE 7.2.   Classification of pulmonary tumors

Epithelial Tumors
Papillary adenoma
Bronchioloalveolar adenoma
Adenocarcinoma
　　Acinar adenocarcinoma
　　Papillary adenocarcinoma
Bronchioloalveolar carcinoma
Squamous cell carcinoma
Adenosquamous carcinoma
Combined carcinoma
Large cell carcinoma
Small cell carcinoma
Neuroendocrine or carcinoid tumor
Pulmonary blastoma
Ovine retroviral pulmonary carcinoma

Mesenchymal Tumors
Osteosarcoma
Chondrosarcoma
Undifferentiated sarcoma
Granular cell tumor
Malignant histiocytosis
Lymphomatoid granulomatosis
Mesothelioma

Age, Breed, and Sex

The reported average age of dogs with primary lung tumors from several studies over the last three decades is fairly consistent at approximately 10.8 years.[1,6,8,12] These tumors are relatively rare in dogs less than 6 years of age. Anaplastic carcinomas tend to occur at a younger age than other tumor types.[1] The aforementioned age specific increase in incidence in colony housed dogs has apparently not yet been studied in the pet population.

There is no apparent predisposition based on sex. Breeds reported to have higher than expected incidences of primary pulmonary epithelial neoplasia include the boxer,[6] doberman pinscher, Australian shepherd, Irish setter, and Bernese mountain dog.[12]

The average age of incidence in the cat is consistently reported as 12–13 years in several surveys. This is slightly older than the mean for dogs. No breed or sex predilections have been found in cats with pulmonary tumors.

Tumor Location

Where single primary growths are present in the dog, they are more frequent in the right lobes, with an additional predilection for the caudal lung. Multifocal growths in one or more lung lobes are fairly common occurrences, particularly in bronchioloalveolar tumors. A compilation of all cases cited in three surveys shows 39 percent of reported tumors to be multifocal in the lung at time of necropsy.[7,12,20] Given the aggressive growth of many pulmonary malignancies, location within a lung lobe is often difficult to ascertain as the entire lobe may be involved. Bronchioloalveolar tumors tend to arise in the periphery of the lung. Hilar tumors are more likely to be derived from airway epithelium or possibly bronchial glands; histologically, they are adenocarcinomas, squamous cell carcinomas or adenosquamous carcinomas. Bronchioloalveolar tumors are also more likely to be multifocal, while hilar tumors are more often recognized as solitary masses.

There appears to be no preference in cats for left or right lung, but a predilection for caudal lung lobes was evident in one survey.[13] The hilar location and histological pattern of the adenocarcinomatous lesions in cats has led to the suggestion that most of these tumors are of bronchial or bronchial gland origin.[2,13,14] The adenocarcinomatous pattern in cats is often of the combined type, wherein mixtures of glandular elements and oval to spindle cells contribute to the neoplastic mass. Immunohistochemical evaluation demonstrates the oval cell component to be of epithelial origin, most likely derived from basal cells. These tumors often form cystic spaces lined by stratified layers of large epithelial cells with abundant cytoplasm.[10] This pattern may contribute to the higher incidence of radiographically evident cavitary lesions in cats.[14]

Clinical Characteristics

The most frequent clinical sign associated with pulmonary carcinoma in one large survey done by the Veteri-

nary Cooperative Oncology Group was cough (52 percent), followed by dyspnea (24 percent), lethargy (18 percent), and weight loss (12 percent).[8] Interestingly, 25 percent of these cases were incidental findings in dogs that had no evident clinical signs of respiratory disease before diagnosis. These relatively nonspecific respiratory signs require additional diagnostic tests for specific diagnosis. Thoracic radiographs demonstrate a majority of tumors (77 percent of the Oncology Group survey); other diagnostic techniques used less frequently include surgical biopsy, bronchoscopic biopsy, closed core biopsy, transtracheal washes, and fine needle aspiration.

Paraneoplastic syndromes associated with primary lung tumors in domestic animals include hypertrophic osteopathy and hypercalcemia.[30] Fever unassociated with infections and ACTH secretion occurs in humans but is not described in animal lung tumors. All of these syndromes are relatively infrequent complications. While hypertrophic osteopathy is fairly often associated with primary lung tumors, (30 percent of affected dogs had lung carcinoma in one survey[21]), it is reported to occur in fewer than 3 percent of lung tumors.[8]

While many cases in the cat may present as nonproductive cough and dyspnea, clinical manifestations of pulmonary neoplasia in cats are more likely to include nonspecific problems of ill thrift, weight loss, lethargy, and inappetence.[13] A frequent presentation is lameness due to skeletal metastases.[14,22-24] Cases of primary pulmonary neoplasia have been discovered by recognition of metastatic lesions of the adenocarcinoma to the digits.[22,24] Occasionally, regurgitation is seen secondary to esophageal involvement.[25] Hypertrophic osteopathy is generally not seen,[13] and only one case was reported in the literature.[26]

Clinical abnormalities include pleural effusion (30–60 percent of reported series[13,14,25]), normochromic normocytic nonregenerative anemia, and neutrophilic leukocytosis.[13] Clinical diagnosis is accomplished largely by radiography demonstrating solitary or multiple pulmonary masses, with confirmation by biopsy or fine needle aspirates. Cats more frequently have cavitating pulmonary masses than do dogs and may exhibit radiographic evidence of calcification.[14] Fine needle aspirates appear to give fairly accurate diagnostic information (20 of 25 cases in one study were identified[13]). Cytology reveals oval carcinoma cells in rafts or acinar arrays. These cells have deeply basophilic cytoplasm and variable nuclear to cytoplasmic ratio and may have cytoplasmic vacuoles suggestive of secretion.[27]

Growth and Metastasis

Pulmonary carcinomas spread by local invasion and metastasize through lymphatic routes to other sites in the lung and hilar lymph nodes.[8,30] Transcoelomic metastasis to multiple sites in the thoracic cavity is also occasionally evident (fig. 7.9 C). Intrapulmonary metastasis to form multifocal tumor masses is postulated to occur, either through vascular/lymphatic spread or intra-airway seeding. Alternatively, the frequency of multiple tumors in multiple lung lobes raises the possibility of a process of multicentric transformation. This is made further plausible by the development of multiple chemically induced tumors in carcinogen treated rodents.[28] Resolution of this question awaits definitive demonstration of clonality in multifocal tumors.

In one survey, 71 percent of anatomically malignant pulmonary tumors had evidence of local vascular or lymphatic invasion, and 23 percent had distant metastasis beyond hilar lymph nodes.[12] Higher rates of metastasis are reported for squamous cell and anaplastic carcinomas, while adenocarcinomas and bronchioloalveolar carcinomas metastasize less frequently. Metastasis of neuroendocrine tumors has not been reported, and the morphology of these rare tumors suggests that they are benign.[31]

Pulmonary tumors in cats appear to have a high rate of metastasis. Whether this represents biologic differences due to the high incidence of adenocarcinomas or the occult nature of the clinical manifestations of these tumors is uncertain. In one survey, 76 percent of feline pulmonary tumors had evidence of metastatic disease.[13] These included lesions in bronchial lymph nodes (30 percent), intrathoracic metastases (30 percent), and a variety of extrathoracic sites (16 percent).[13] While several authors report a predilection for bony metastases, the evidence for this varies among surveys. Metastasis of primary pulmonary tumors to bone, particularly the digits, is a recognized syndrome in cats.[22,24] These cases often are discovered from biopsies of pedal lesions that contain adenocarcinomas. Evidence of pulmonary origin includes the occasional presence of ciliated cells and mucous secretion in these metastatic foci.

Treatment and Prognosis

Treatment of pulmonary carcinomas is largely by surgical excision. In general, surgical removal by lobectomy of relatively small solitary lesions has a good prognosis.[29] In one survey, 72 percent of surgically treated dogs underwent remission. Dogs with recurrence had significantly shortened survival times, averaging 28 days postsurgery. Lack of detectable lymph node metastasis at surgery was significantly correlated with remission.[30] In dogs with inoperable tumors or in which surgery is otherwise contraindicated, chemotherapy with cisplatin and vindesine[29] or doxorubicin or mitoxantrone[31] has been used. Prognosis for long-term survival is best predicted by evaluating the lymph node metastasis and differentiation state of the tumor rather than its histological type. Useful histological features in predicting clinical behavior based on tumor differentiation include cellular organization and polarity, incidence of mitotic figures, nuclear pleomorphism, size of nucleolus, extent of desmoplasia, and evidence of invasion at the tumor periphery. Surgical and pathological evaluation of lymph nodes is of great importance in forming a prognosis based on significant risk for shortened survival in dogs with nodal metastasis in two large surveys.[30,31]

Lobectomy for extirpation of pulmonary tumors is also the treatment of choice in cats, but the prognosis is generally worse than for the dog. A greater number of feline tumors are classified as inoperable at diagnosis, either as a result of extensive disease or metastasis or due to intercurrent decompensated cardiomyopathy.[23]

Gross Morphology

Primary pulmonary tumors vary from solid discrete masses that displace large portions of single lung lobes (fig. 7.8) to multiple masses that can be difficult to distinguish from metastatic neoplasia (fig. 7.9). They may grow in an expansile or infiltrative manner. Adjacent regions of lung are often atelectatic. While generally composed of solid tissue that may be dissected by connective tissue septa, many times they become necrotic and resemble granulomas or diffuse pulmonary consolidation from other inflammatory processes. Central necrosis may also give these tumors an umbilicated appearance. Diffuse involvement may occur from coalescence of multiple areas of growth, particularly in bronchioloalveolar tumors. Obstruction of large airways or mucous secretion by the tumor itself may lead to accumulations of mucus in cystic spaces within the mass. Bronchioloalveolar tumors tend to be peripheral in the lung and more often are located near

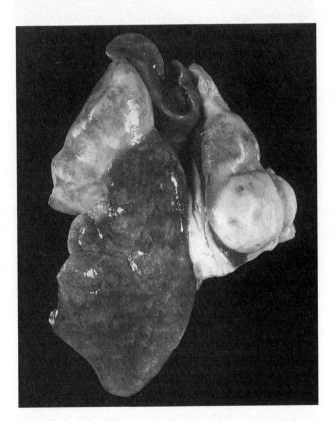

Fig. 7.8. Adenosquamous carcinoma in the cat. The left lung lobes are reduced in size and the pleura thickened by fibrous connective tissue. The parenchyma is replaced by creamy white to yellow friable tissue.

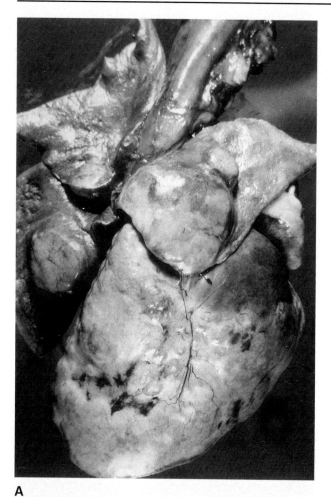

A

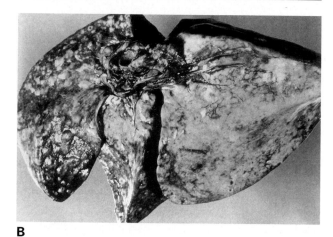

B

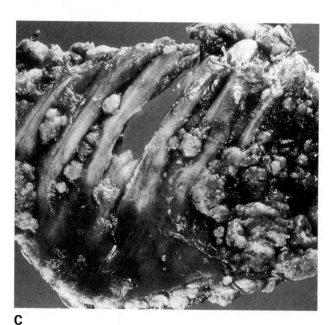

C

Fig. 7.9. Bronchioloalveolar carcinoma of lung (gross) with transceolomic metastasis. **A.** Diffuse mass involving most of the right caudal and middle lung lobes as well as the left caudal lobe. **B.** Multiple coalescing nodules of neoplasm evident on diaphagmatic surface of caudal lobe. **C.** Transceolomic metastasis to parietal pleura.

the pleura. Tumors presumably of large airway origin appear to arise near the hilus but may extend to involve most of a lobe or multiple lobes. Since the lung is a frequent location for metastasis of tumors from other sites, a principal caveat in the examination of suspected primary lung tumors is that complete evaluation of other potential sources of metastatic lesions should be done.

Gross appearance of feline pulmonary tumors is not different from those in dogs, with the exception of the increased frequency of cavitary lesions in cats.[14]

Histological Features

The histological features presented below are used to classify spontaneous tumors in all domestic species. Primary lung tumors must be distinguished from the frequent metastatic lesions of epithelial malignancies arising from other tissues. Solitary lesions of the lung in the absence of other systemic neoplastic lesions are fairly obvious, but this information may not always be available to the surgical

pathologist. Primary lung malignancies which metastasize widely through the lung can be particularly challenging to distinguish from systemic spread of other carcinomas. Features supporting a diagnosis of primary lung tumor include (1) presence of a principal large mass involving a selected region of lung or a single lobe, (2) evidence of bronchioloalveolar growth pattern or Clara cell differentiation of neoplastic epithelial cells, (3) involvement of airways in the neoplastic process either by location or evidence of preneoplastic "field change" in adjacent airway epithelium, and (4) often, in primary lung tumors, a spectrum of progression of neoplastic transformation within the tumor. Metastases tend to be more uniformly differentiated, and metastatic lesions are more uniform in their size and distribution in the lung. Metastatic lesions also may show evidence of intravascular embolization and spherical growth, although this must be interpreted with caution since primary lung tumors with intrapulmonary dissemination can have similar behavior.

Benign Tumors of Epithelial Origin

Papillary Adenoma

Adenomas of the lung other than the bronchioloalveolar adenoma described below are rare. The best documented type is the papillary adenoma of cattle[16] (fig. 7.10). These tumors are composed of tubulopapillary formations of columnar epithelial cells arranged on a moderate arborizing connective tissue stroma. They are distinguished from bronchioloalveolar growths by location adjacent to airways and the predominant mucous goblet cell differentiation of the neoplastic epithelium. Given the low incidence of these lesions, there is no information as to whether they might progress. Their origin is speculated to be associated with airways, but whether they represent tumors of airway epithelium or glands is also undetermined.

Bronchioloalveolar Adenoma

These tumors have a simple alveolar pattern that is lined by cuboidal to columnar epithelial cells. They do not differ histologically from bronchioloalveolar carcinomas described below except for the lack of invasive behavior

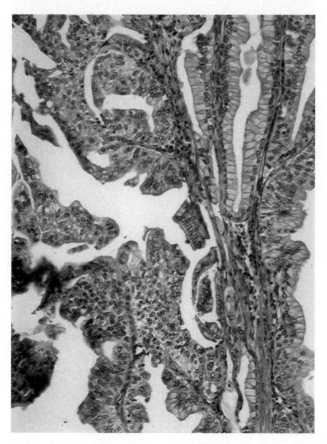

Fig. 7.10. Papillary adenoma of lung (bovine). Well-differentiated simple columnar goblet cells with basally polar nuclei line a thin connective tissue stroma in an arborizing pattern.

and the discrete nature of their growth. Characteristics differentiating hyperplasia from benign and malignant forms of this tumor and its likely progression toward papillary adenocarcinoma are given in the section on carcinomas. Bronchioloalveolar adenomas are fairly common in dogs, but malignant forms are more frequently diagnosed. Often the adenomas are clinically silent incidental findings in radiographic and necropsy surveys, so their true frequency may be underestimated.

Malignant Tumors of Epithelial Origin

Adenocarcinoma

This pattern encompasses a variety of phenotypic manifestations of tumors of divergent histogenesis. Tumors composed entirely or largely of coarse distorting and irregular papillary, acinar, solid, or mixed glandular structures are classified as adenocarcinomas. They may or may not contain PAS positive secretory material and can potentially be derived from airways, bronchial glands, or the bronchioloalveolar region of the lung. These tumors are often highly destructive and invasive. Multiple foci of tumor growth often develop within the lung, and widespread dissemination through pulmonary lymphatics is common. Distant metastases beyond mediastinal lymph nodes is, however, infrequent. Two common growth patterns, papillary and acinar, can be distinguished.

Papillary Adenocarcinoma

The characteristic of this pattern is a distorting and irregular arborizing growth of epithelial cells overlying a connective tissue core (fig. 7.11 A). Papillary adenocarcinomas may be divided into lobules by thicker connective tissue septa. Epithelial cells in papillary adenocarcinomas are columnar and may secrete mucus. While the better differentiated tumors maintain a simple epithelium lined by epithelial cells with basal polarity, they may become stratified and demonstrate increasingly disorderly growth and variant cytological differentiation in less well differentiated growths. This progression is suggestive of more aggressive behavior. The principal distinction to be made is between papillary adenocarcinoma and bronchioloalveolar carcinomas, which may also have regions of papillary growth. Key features of adenocarcinomas are the disorderly arrangement of fronds of tumor growth that exhibit a destructive and infiltrative growth and the diverse differentiation of the neoplastic epithelial cells in columnar to stratified layers. Regions of papillary growth in bronchioloalveolar carcinomas are more regular and are lined by simple cuboidal epithelium.

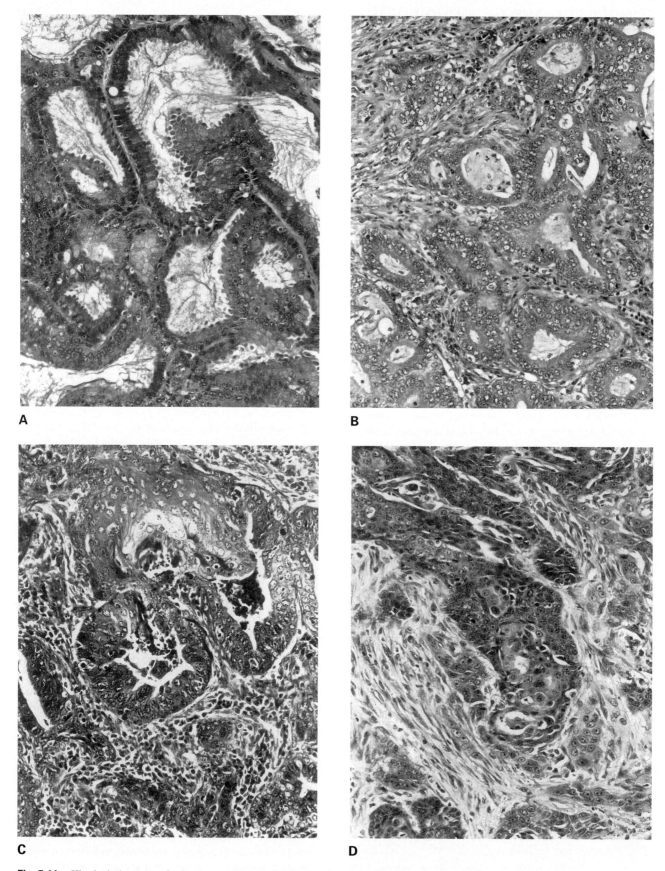

Fig. 7.11. Histological patterns of pulmonary carcinomas. **A.** Adenocarcinoma, papillary. Simple tall columnar epithelium with numerous goblet cells in a papillary growth containing abundant mucus. **B.** Adenocarcinoma, acinar. Simple to focally stratified growth of cuboidal epithelial cells forms acini separated by a thick connective tissue stroma. **C.** Adenosquamous carcinoma. Mixtures of glandular epithelium forming acini blend with more solid cords with evident stratified squamous differentiation. **D.** Squamous cell carcinoma. Majority of neoplastic epithelium forms solid cords of spherical to polygonal cells with abundant cytoplasm and indistinct cell borders.

Acinar Adenocarcinoma

These tumors are primarily tubuloacinar growths with a predominance of glandular formation (fig. 7.11 B). Tubular cords of epithelial cells are surrounded by connective tissue stroma that can be extensive and desmoplastic. Evidence of synthesis of mucus by neoplastic cells may or may not be present. Ciliated cells are unusual but are occasionally seen. More anaplastic variants exhibit increasing stratification of neoplastic epithelium. Ultrastructurally, adenocarcinomas are composed of pseudostratified secretory cells whose granules have the homogenous, moderately electron dense character of mucous glycoprotein, short surface microvilli, and apical zonula adherens/occludens junctional complexes (see fig.7.13 A).

Squamous Cell Carcinoma

These tumors have a significant component or predominance of solid carcinoma containing moderate to large amounts of homogenous amphophilic to eosinophilic cytoplasm and round to oval, centrally placed nuclei (fig. 7.11 D). While evidences of keratinization and intercellular bridges may be present, not all tumors classified as squamous contain these histological features. Confirmation of the differentiation toward keratinocytic cells is based on the ultrastructural presence of tonofilament bundles and a large component of uniformly distributed desmosomal junctions between neoplastic cells (see fig.7.13 D). Expression of cytokeratin profiles similar to those in epidermal keratinocytes also distinguishes these tumors.

Adenosquamous Carcinoma

In practice, many pulmonary carcinomas demonstrate a spectrum of adenomatous to squamous patterns. Tumors with significant components of both acinar and squamous cell differentiation are classified as adenosquamous. Often these tumors have interspersed regions of each phenotype (fig. 7.11 C). Selective cytokeratin staining demonstrates expression profiles characteristic of epidermal keratinocytes or glandular epithelium in regions of squamous or acinar differentiation, respectively.

Bronchioloalveolar Carcinoma

Based on their location in the lung periphery and histological appearance resembling alveoli and small airway epithelium, the majority of canine lung tumors are of bronchioloalveolar origin. While most respiratory tumors are currently classified based solely on their histological pattern, the architecture, cytology, and location of some tumors arising from the bronchioloalveolar region are characteristic enough for these neoplasms to be diagnosed as bronchioloalveolar tumors. The principal characteristic of this pattern is recapitulation of alveolar growth and extension to the surface of preexisting alveolar structures (fig. 7.12). The neoplastic epithelial cells are cuboidal to low columnar and fairly universally of single cell thick-

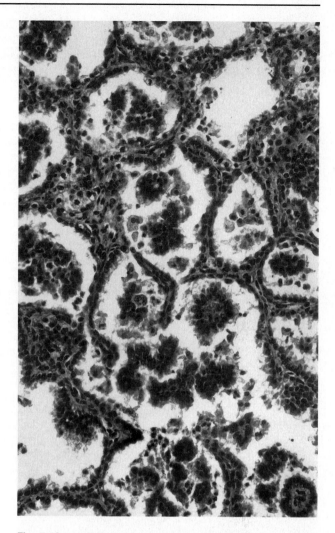

Fig. 7.12. Bronchioloalveolar carcinoma. Cuboidal epithelium lines regular polygonal spaces formed by thin connective tissue in a pattern reminiscent of fetal alveoli.

ness. In many of these tumors, regions can be found which mimic the appearance of immature fetal alveoli or the hyperplastic responses of epithelium in repair of alveolar injury. In the most common form, the epithelial cells are simple, low, cuboidal cells with slightly projecting apical cytoplasm and a lower profile at intercellular junctions. Tumors which demonstrate differentiation toward Clara cells (nonciliated bronchiolar epithelium) are more columnar, have a greater surface area of cell to cell contact, and have evident apical projections of amphophilic cytoplasm similar to those seen in normal airways. Ultrastructurally, Clara cell differentiation, manifest as SER accumulations in the apical cytoplasmic blebs, can be mixed with surfactant granule formation (fig. 7.13 B) or the more dense secretory granules characteristic of Clara cell secretory glycoprotein.

Regions of delicate arborizing papillary growth are common in bronchioloalveolar carcinomas. Tumors with a predominance of papillary growth but containing significant regions with characteristic alveolar formation can best be described as papillary adenocarcinomas of bronchi-

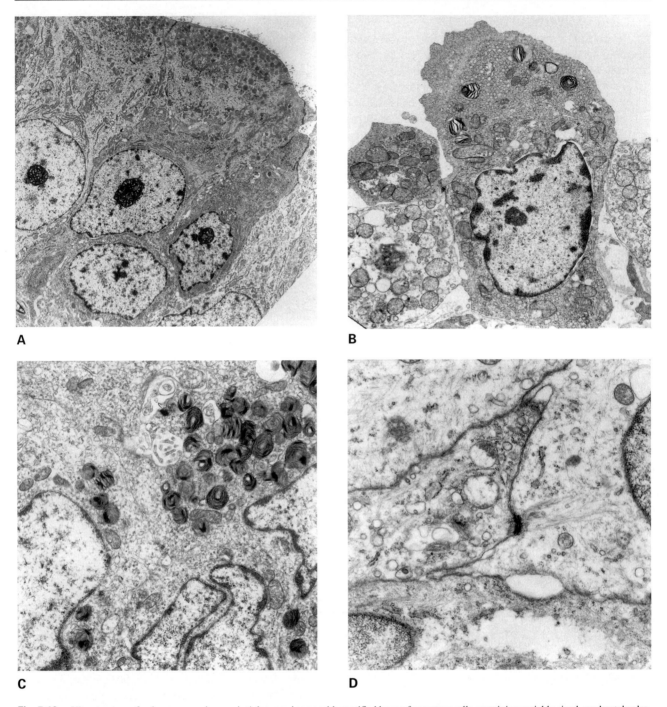

Fig. 7.13.   Ultrastructure of pulmonary carcinoma. **A.** Adenocarcinoma with stratified layer of secretory cells containing variably sized, moderately electron dense, secretory granules and apical microvilli. Apical junctional complexes between cells are composed of layered adherens and occludens junctions typical of secretory epithelium. **B.** Bronchioloalveolar carcinoma composed of a simple cuboidal epithelium containing electron-lucent lamellar secretory granules. There is a significant amount of apical SER, suggestive of differentiation toward Clara cells. **C.** High magnification of bronchioloalveolar tumor demonstrating typical lamellar granules of surfactant. **D.** Desmosome and tonofilaments in an adenosquamous tumor.

oloalveolar origin. Confimation of alveolar type II cell differentiation can be made by ultrastructural demonstration of surfactant granule formation (fig.7.13 C). The potential exists for confirmation of alveolar or Clara cell–like differentiation using immunohistochemical stains for Clara cell secretory protein and surfactant apoprotein A, but this is currently not done in veterinary diagnostic practice.

Regions of differentiation toward mucous goblet cells may be present, and some tumors may have intralumenal accumulations of mucoid secretion. Necrotic regions frequently contain foci of cholesterol cleft formation. Some tumors may have small intralumenal calcific nodules resembling psammoma bodies or corpora amylacea.

Solitary, discrete, and well-encapsulated tumors with a

predominance of simple epithelium in tubuloalveolar growths are benign. The tendency of these tumors to grow along the preexisting alveolar structures at their periphery should not be confused with invasive properties as many discrete and well-differentiated adenomas will exhibit this pattern rather than encapsulation. Adenomas must be distinguished from foci of type II cell hyperplasia (see Bronchioloalveolar Hyperplasia, below). The latter may be present overlying interstitial granulation and scarring. Groups of alveoli lined by hyperplastic type II cells are also present in lungs of some older dogs. Whether or not these represent preneoplastic lesions remains to be determined.

Progression toward more stratified or solid growth and capsular invasion are often seen regionally within these tumors and are evidences of malignant transformation. Increased proportion of papillary growth, epithelial stratification, or mucous secretion also occur as bronchioloalveolar tumors progress toward malignancy. Progression from a bronchioloalveolar pattern to the more distorted and dysplastic growth characteristic of papillary adenocarcinoma is evident in some tumors. Other evidences of malignancy include increased desmoplastic stroma and lymphatic invasion. Metastases of bronchioloalveolar tumors must be differentiated from multiple primary growths that can occur. It is unknown whether these represent multicentric transformation in a sensitive cell population or intrapulmonary implants via airway, lymphatic, or transcoelomic metastasis.

Bronchioloalveolar Hyperplasia

Bronchioloalveolar hyperplasia is a very common response to many forms of pulmonary injury, particularly in subacute to chronic phases. The epithelium can be predominantly of either bronchiolar or alveolar type, or a combination might be present. There is frequently an associated remodeling of bronchioloalveolar structures and interstitial fibrosis. Prominent, postinflammatory epithelial lining of alveolar sized spaces has misleadingly been referred to as adenomatosis. The term *adenomatosis* was appropriately used for viral induced pulmonary adenomatosis in sheep, although now the condition is being referred to as carcinomatosis because it behaves like a low grade carcinoma.

Confusion between bronchioloalveolar hyperplasia and neoplasia mostly arises when there is exaggerated hyperplasia in the absence of inflammatory components, such as occurs in foci of scarring. Histological features indicative of hyperplasia are (1) multifocal, often subpleural and segmental distribution of lesions, (2) epithelial-lined airspaces that are remodeled and distorted by scarring, (3) epithelial proliferation present only in locations where there is underlying interstitial fibrosis and/or interstitial inflammation, (4) lack of a strongly convex border to the lesion, and (5) regular characteristics of epithelial population. With regard to the last feature, when the cells are stratified they represent metaplasia toward nonkeratinizing squamous epithelium.

Combined Tumors

The apparent dual components of these tumors include a population of small oval to spindle shaped cells that are relatively unorganized or tend to be arranged in a slightly storiform pattern about more obvious glandular elements (fig. 7.14 A,B). These tumors seem to arise in the region of large airways, but it is not always apparent that they are associated with changes in the airway lumenal epithelium. Immunohistochemically, the two populations are distinguishable based on differential cytokeratin expression; the glandular population expresses markers for pulmonary epithelium, and the smaller cells express cytokeratins expressed exclusively in basal cells of the pulmonary airways and differentiating epidermal keratinocytes.[10] Many of these tumors become cystic but not necessarily through necrosis. Occasional well differentiated and encapsulated tumors can be considered benign, but the majority of these tumors exhibit invasive and metastatic properties of malignancy. These tumors are distinguishable from adenosquamous tumors based on the presence of a dual population rather than on a transition from glandular to solid nests of cells with evident squamous differentiation.

Large Cell Carcinoma

This is an extremely rare and poorly documented tumor in domestic animals. The tumors consist of large, rounded to polyhedral cells occupying and effacing alveolar parenchyma. The cells have ample eosinophilic, sometimes foamy, cytoplasm and large, round, oval, or distorted nuclei. Infiltrative growth along adjacent airways is often a striking feature. Transition from bronchioloalveolar carcinoma is seen in a few cases. A few cases of the giant cell variant of large cell carcinoma have been diagnosed in the dog, but at least some of these were actually cases of malignant histiocytosis. Accurately identified cases of large cell carcinoma, of giant cell or any other type, are therefore extremely rare. There is no current justification for separate listing of giant cell or clear cell types, but pathologists should be aware that these terms may be used.

Any suspect case of large cell carcinoma of the lung must be established to be primary and of epithelial origin, (e.g., cytokeratin positive). In cases where giant cells are prominent, the possibility of malignant histiocytosis should be excluded by demonstrating that the cells are immunohistochemically negative for lysozyme, alpha-1-antitrypsin, and other monocyte macrophage markers.

Small Cell Carcinoma

These unusual tumors are classified based on their histological similarity to human small cell carcinomas. They are solid masses composed of small round to oval neoplastic cells, with modest to slight cytoplasm, that generally do

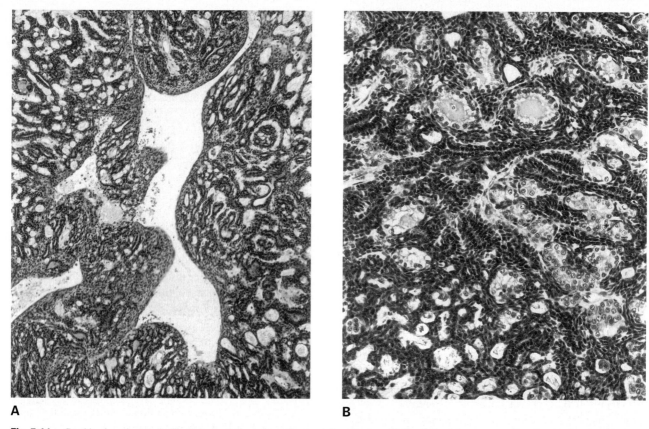

Fig. 7.14. Combined carcinoma. **A.** Glandular formation surrounding central cystic space. **B.** Small glandular structures lined by simple cuboidal epithelium are separated by an oval to spindle shaped population of cells with scant, indistinct, cytoplasm.

not form apparent acinar or papillary structure (fig. 7.15). While the tumors often appear as diffuse sheets of fairly uniform cells, close inspection often reveals organization in aggregates by fine fibrovascular stroma. This packeting is sometimes interpreted as filling of preexisting alveolar structures by the neoplastic population. This pattern helps in distinguishing these tumors from lymphoma. Small cell carcinomas in humans are thought to arise from airway neuroendocrine cells, and a variety of neuropeptide components can be recognized immunohistochemically. While examples of this pattern are presented in compilations of animal tumors,[3] there are presently no publications characterizing ultrastructure or expression of cytokeratin or neuroendocrine markers for these tumors in domestic animals.

Neuroendocrine/Carcinoid Tumors

These rare tumors are characterized by their histological similarity to neuroendocrine growths, with round to polygonal cells grouped in small solid aggregates by a thin fibrovascular stroma. Neoplastic cells have regularly sized, spherical, centrally placed nuclei and modest, lightly amphophilic cytoplasm. These tumors are proposed to arise from neuroendocrine cells in the airway epithelium, although immunohistochemical stains for markers such as bombesin and calcitonin gene regulatory peptide are negative, and electron microscopy to demonstrate intracytoplasmic granules has not been done.[32]

Pulmonary Blastomas

These tumors are rare aggressive growths of mixed cell type recapitulating embryonic pulmonary development. They have been described in humans,[33,34] cattle,[17] and as single case reports, in the dog[35] and laboratory rat.[36] Gross descriptions in the cow emphasize smooth white firm masses disseminated through the lungs and involving the mediastinal and prescapular lymph nodes as well as the parietal pleura. These tumors are characterized by a diffuse mesenchymal growth embedded with tubular structures lined by simple cuboidal to columnar epithelium (fig. 7.16). Foci of irregularly clumped blast-like epithelial cells without evident tubular formation are found randomly distributed in the mesenchymal mass. These features resemble the primitive state of the fetal lung. Early descriptions of the human lesion recognized the similarity to nephroblastoma. Immunocytochemical markers used in bovine tumors demonstrated expression of cytokeratins in the epithelial cells lining tubules, whereas the mesenchymal-like cells were cytokeratin negative but positive for vimentin, muscle specific actin, and smooth muscle specific actin. The nests of blast-like cells appear to be a less differentiated form of epithelial cell that does not express cytokeratin but does express vimentin, neuron specific enolase, and muscle specific actin.[17]

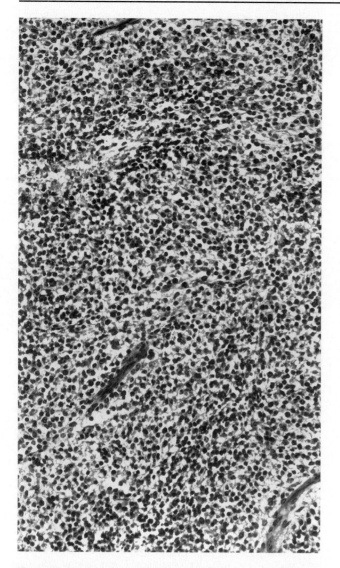

Fig. 7.15. Small cell carcinoma. Solid masses of small round to polygonal epithelial cells with scant cytoplasm are partially compartmentalized by thin connective tissue septa.

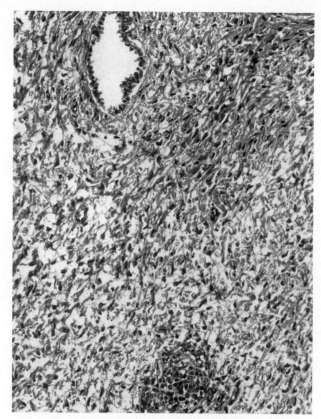

Fig. 7.16. Pulmonary blastoma. The principal component of the neoplasm is a background growth of oval to spindle shaped cells. Embedded are occasional small glandular structures lined by immature cuboidal epithelium and focal aggregates of undifferentiated epithelial cells without architectural organization.

Molecular Lesions Associated with Pulmonary Neoplasia in Domestic Animals

A variety of alterations in biologically active molecules have been documented in human lung cancer. These include alterations in growth factor expression, mutations in oncogenes, chromosomal deletions, and mutations and altered expression of tumor suppressor genes. Many of these changes are associated with prognosis and survival time in humans. The most significant alterations include increased expression of epidermal growth factor (EGF), transforming growth factor beta, the EGF receptor encoded by c-*erbB*-1, the *ras* gene family, loss of the short arm of chromosome 3, loss or altered retinoblastoma tumor suppresser gene (*Rb*) product, or missense mutations in the tumor suppresser gene

p53.[11] Some of the genetic lesions underlying altered oncogene or tumor suppresser gene activity are either specific to histological types or are different in tumors from smokers than in those from nonsmokers. For example, different alterations in codon 12 of the K-*ras* oncogene are detected in smokers and can be detected in sputum before clinically evident neoplasia is present.[37] Amplification of the *myc* gene family is generally limited to small cell tumors.[38] Missense mutations in *p53* occur in both small cell and non–small cell tumors but are more common in small cell tumors in humans and represent a different genetic alteration than is present in adenocarcinomas.[11]

Surveys of genetic alterations in lung tumors of domestic animals are still relatively limited. Lung tumors from colony raised beagles, some of which had been exposed to $^{239}PuO_2$ by inhalation, have been shown to express altered p53 protein in a relatively small proportion of cases (14 percent), almost exclusively in adenosquamous or squamous tumors. Mutations in K-*ras* were also evident in codons 12, 13, or 61 in 19 percent of all lung tumors in this survey. No mutational differences between tumors from $^{239}PuO_2$ exposed dogs and those from controls were evident.[39]

K-*ras* mutations have been documented to occur in spontaneous tumors from the general canine population. Nineteen percent of malignant tumors of a variety of anatomic types had K-*ras* mutations; the most common alteration was a G to A transition in the second position of codon 12. The frequency and type of mutation more closely matched those for tumors from human nonsmokers with K-*ras* mutations than those from smokers.[12]

REFERENCES

1. Stunzi, H., Head, K.W., and Nielsen, S.W., (1974) Tumours of the lung. *Bull WHO* 50:9–19.
2. Moulton, J.E., von Tscharner, T.C., and Schneider, R. (1981) Classification of lung carcinomas in the dog and cat. *Vet Pathol* 18: 513–528.
3. Dungworth, D.L., Haenichen, T., Hahn, F.F., Hauser, B., Harkema, J.R., and Wilson, D.W. (1999) Histological classification of respiratory tract tumors of domestic animals. In Schulman, F.Y. (ed.), *WHO International Histological Classification of Tumors of Domestic Animals.* 2nd series, vol. IV. Armed Forces Institute of Pathology, Washington D.C.
4. Taylor, G.N., Shabestari, L., Angus, W., Lloyd, R.D., and Mays, C.W. (1979) Primary pulmonic tumors in beagles. *Amer J Vet Res* 40:1316–1318.
5. Hahn, F.F., Muggenburg, B.A., and Griffith, W.C. (1996) Primary lung neoplasia in a beagle colony. *Vet Pathol* 33: 633–638.
6. Brodey, R.S. and Craig, P.H. (1965) Primary pulmonary neoplasms in the dog: A review of 29 cases. *J Amer Vet Med Assoc* 147:1628–1643.
7. Nielsen, S.W., and Horava, A. (1960) Primary pulmonary tumors of the dog. *Amer J Vet Res* 21:813–830.
8. Ogilvie, G.K., Haschek, W.M., Withrow, S.J., Richardson, R.C., Harvey, H.J., Henderson, R.A., Fowler, J.D., Norris A.M., Tomlinson, J., McCaw, D., Klausner, J.S., Reschke, B.S., and McKiernan, B.C. (1989) Classification of primary lung tumors in dogs: 210 cases (1975–1985). *J Amer Vet Med Assoc* 195:106–108.
9. Dorn, C.R., Taylor, D.O., Frye, F.L., and Hibbard, H.H. (1968) Survey of animal neoplasms in Alameda and Contra Costa counties, California. I. Methodology and description of cases. *J Natl Cancer Inst* 40:295–305.
10. Wilson, D.W. (1997) Pulmonary neoplasia in cats. *Vet Pathol* 34:485A.
11. Johnson, B.E., (1995) Molecular biology of lung cancer. In Mendelsohn, J., et al. (eds.), *The Molecular Basis of Cancer.* W.B.Saunders Co., Philadelphia, pp. 317–339.
12. Griffey, S.M., Kraegel, S.M., Madewell, B.R. (1998) Rapid detection of K-ras gene mutation in canine lung cancer using single-strand conformational polymorphism analysis. *Carcinogenesis* 19:959–963.
13. Hahn, K.A., and McEntee, M.F. (1997) Primary lung tumors in cats: 86 cases (1979–1994). *J Amer Vet Med Assoc* 211:1257–1260.
14. Koblik, P.D. (1986) Radiographic appearance of primary lung tumors in cats. *Vet Radiol* 27:66–73.
15. Monlux, A.W., Anderson, W.A., and Davis, C.L. (1956) A survey of tumors occurring in cattle, sheep and swine. *Amer J Vet Res* 17:646–677.
16. Migaki, G., Helmboldt, C.F., and Robinson, F.R. (1974) Primary pulmonary tumors of epithelial origin in cattle. *Amer J Vet Res* 35:1397–1400.
17. Kelley, L.C., Puette, M., Langheinrich, K.A., and King, B. (1994) Bovine pulmonary blastomas: Histomorphologic description and immunohistochemistry. *Vet Pathol* 31:658–662.
18. Piercy, D.W.T., Cranwell, M.P., and Wannacott, B.J. (1993) Anaplastic small cell carcinoma of the lung in a six month old Friesian calf. *Vet Rec* 132:386–387.
19. Kelley, L.C., Hill, J.E., Hafner, S., and Wortham, K.J. (1995) Spon-
taneous equine pulmonary granular cell tumors: Morphologic, histochemical, and immunohistochemical characterization. *Vet Pathol* 32:101–106.
20. Monlux, W.S. (1952) Primary pulmonary neoplasms in domestic animals. *Southwestern Vet J* 6:131–133.
21. Brodey, R.S. (1971) Hypertrophic osteoarthropathy in the dog: A clinicopathologic survey of 60 cases. *J Amer Vet Med Assoc* 159:1242–1256.
22. Pool, R.R., Bodle, J.E., Mantos, J.J., and Ticer, J.W. (1974) Primary lung carcinoma with skeletal metastasies in the cat. *Feline Pract* 4:36–41.
23. Melhaff, C.J., and Mooney. S. (1985) Primary pulmonary neoplasia in the dog and cat. *Vet Clin N Amer Small Anim Pract* 15:1061–1068.
24. May, C., and Newsholme, S.J. (1989) Metastasis of feline pulmonary carcinoma presenting as multiple digital swelling. *J Small Anim Pract* 30:302–310.
25. Barr, F., Gruffydd-Jones, T.J., Brown, P.J., and Gibbs, C. (1987) Primary lung tumors in the cat. *J Small Anim Pract* 28:1115–1125.
26. Gram, W.D., Wheaton, L.G., Snyder, P.W., Losonsky, J.M., and Whiteley, H.E. (1990) Feline hypertrophic osteopathy associated with pulmonary carcinoma. *J Amer Anim Hosp Assoc* 26:425–428.
27. Rebar, A.H., DeNicola, D.B. (1988) The cytologic examination of the respiratory tract. *Sem Vet Med Surg (Small Anim)* 3:109–121.
28. Witschi, H., Wilson, D.W., Plopper, C.G. (1993) Modulation of N-nitrosodiethylamine-induced hamster lung tumors by ozone. *Toxicology* 77:193–202.
29. Mehlhaff, C.J., and Mooney, S. (1985) Primary pulmonary neoplasia in the dog and cat. *Vet Clin N Amer Small Anim Pract* 15:1061–1067.
30. Ogilvie, G.K., Weigel, R.M., Haschek, W.M., Withrow,S.J., Richardson, R.C., Harvey, H.J., Henderson, R.A., Fowler, J.D., Norris, A.M., Tomlinson, J., McCaw, D., Klausner. J.S., Reschke, B.S., and McKiernan, B.C. (1989) Prognostic factors for tumor remission and survival in dogs after surgery for primary lung tumor: 76 cases (1975–1985). *J Amer Vet Med Assoc* 195:109–112.
31. McNiel, E.A., Oglivie, G.K., Powers, B.E., Hutchison, J.M., Salman, M.D., and Withrow, S.J. (1997) Evaluation of prognostic factors for dogs with primary lung tumors: 67 cases (1985–1992). *J Amer Vet Med Assoc* 211:1422–1427.
32. Harkema, J.R., Jones, S.E., Naydan, D.K., Wilson, D.W. (1992) An atypical neuroendocrine tumor in the lung of a beagle dog. *Vet Pathol* 29:175–179.
33. Bodner, S.M., and Koss, M.N. (1996) Mutations in the *p53* gene in pulmonary blastomas: Immunohistochemical and molecular studies. *Human Pathol* 27:1117–1123.
34. Larsen, H. Sorensen,J.B., (1996) Pulmonary blastoma: A review with special emphasis on prognosis and treatment. *Cancer Treat Rev* 22:145–160.
35. Watson, A.D., Young, K.M., Dubielzig, R.R., and Biller, D.S. (1993) Primary mesenchymal or mixed-cell-origin lung tumors in four dogs. *J Amer Vet Med Assoc* 202:968–970.
36. Chen, H.C., and Frame, S.R. (1991) Pulmonary blastoma in a rat. *Vet Pathol* 28:255–257.
37. Slebos, R.J., Hruban, R.H., Dalesio, O., Mooi, W.J., Offerhaus, G.J., and Rodenhuis, S. (1991) Relationship between K-*ras* oncogene activation and smoking in adenocarcinoma of the human lung. *J Natl Cancer Inst* 83:1024–1027.
38. Brennan, J., et al. (1991) *myc* family DNA amplification in 107 tumors and tumor cell lines from patients with small cell lung cancer treated with different combination chemotherapy regimens. *Cancer Res* 51:1708–1712.
39. Tierney, L.A., Hahn, F.F., and Lechner, J.F. (1996) *p53, erbB-2* and K-*ras* gene alterations are rare in spontaneous and plutonium-239–induced canine lung neoplasia. *Radiat Res* 145:181–187.

Retroviral Pulmonary Tumors of Sheep: Ovine Pulmonary Carcinoma

History and Clinical Characteristics

Infectious multicentric tumors of alveolar epithelium in sheep first gained prominent recognition when large scale outbreaks in Iceland developed in the 1930's. The initial outbreak on a farm containing karakul rams imported from Germany led to involvement of one-third of the sheep in the country.[1] Ovine pulmonary carcinoma (OPC) has since been eradicated from Iceland (through extreme depopulation measures requiring slaughter of 600,000 to 700,000 sheep) but continues to exist in most sheep raising areas of the world, with the notable exception of Australia. Its long incubation period and consequent potential for flock carriers to induce high infectivity leads to a high prevalence, approaching 20 percent of some infected flocks. While OPC is a sporadic disease of low incidence in the United States, it remains a significant economic problem in Scotland, South Africa, and Peru, where annual mortalities reach 2 percent of adult sheep.[2,3]

Several regionally recognized syndromes of chronic respiratory disease in sheep that lead to progressive dyspnea have now been distilled into two retrovirally induced diseases, ovine progressive pneumonia caused by ovine lentivirus, and OPC caused by Jaagsiekte retrovirus (JSRV). Clinical distinction between the nonneoplastic ovine progressive pneumonia (also called maedi, zwoegerzidkte, bouhite, Montana progressive pneumonia, and Marsh's progressive pneumonia) and OPC (synonyms: pulmonary adenomatosis, Jaagsiekte) remains difficult due to the insidious onset of similar respiratory signs and the lack of a specific diagnostic test applicable in the field. Specific diagnosis is dependent on histopathologic features characteristic for each disease. Recent research suggests that confirmation by antibody tests that recognize specific epitopes or molecular biologic techniques such as polymerase chain reaction will soon be possible.[4]

Sheep with OPC generally have poor body condition and dyspnea that is accentuated by exercise. Animals without intercurrent infections have normal temperatures and continue to eat. Sheep with progressive pneumonia present with similar signs, and the only distinguishing clinical characteristic of OPC is the production of excessive lung fluid that is evident as a copious, watery, nasal discharge. Elevating the hindquarters of affected sheep to lower the head can induce a marked nasal outpouring of this fluid. Recent understanding of the molecular biology of the JSRV agent is promising for more accurate diagnostic test development in the near future. Details of the biology and etiopathogenesis of retrovirally induced small ruminant respiratory neoplasms have been reviewed.[4]

Age, Breed, and Sex

The long incubation period before clinical signs are evident makes OPC a disease of adult sheep, with 2- to 4-year-olds most commonly affected. Experimental inoculations in lambs can lead to dyspnea in as little as 3 weeks, and the disease has been diagnosed in lambs as young as 3 months. While there is no apparent sex related susceptibility, ewes are generally kept to an older age than rams, resulting in a higher incidence in females from affected flocks.

Epidemiological evidence from South Africa and the Icelandic outbreak suggested that there are genetic and breed differences in susceptibility. Gottorp and merino sheep have an apparently higher incidence than the Adalbol and ramboulliet breeds.[5] Incidence data from Scotland, however, does not support breed susceptibility differences.[6]

Gross Morphology

Gross lesions of OPC predominate in the anterioventral regions of the lung but may be present throughout the lobes. The right lung is more commonly affected than the left. The tumors are evident as large to coalescing gray masses that are associated with regions of atalectasis (fig. 7.17 A). Some cases may have smaller nodules in less affected regions of lung (fig. 7.17 B). This reflects the appearance of early or experimental cases where multiple small foci of white to gray-red nodules may be present.

Affected regions of lung have a solid appearance and tough consistency due to fibroplasia, which may be extensive. Lungs with significant involvement weigh three or more times normal (up to 2 kg) and often exude clear fluid from affected sections. This fluid may also be found as frothy material in bronchi or the trachea. In advanced cases, the lungs fail to collapse when the thorax is entered, and chronic pleuritis may be present. Evidence of tumor necrosis or secondary bacterial infection may also occur. Regional lymph nodes may be enlarged, edematous, or firm if metastasis has occurred.

Histological Features

OPC lesions are those of a well-differentiated, multicentric, bronchioloalveolar carcinoma. Ultrastructural characterization of the component epithelial cells shows a predominance of alveolar type II cell morphology with microvilli, desmosomes, and intracellular lamellar bodies.[7-10] Cytoplasmic dense bodies suggestive of Clara cell differentiation can also be present in some cases, and these cells may coexist with cells of type II cell morphology. The tumor grows as a simple cuboidal to columnar epithelium on a thin connective tissue stroma forming acinar or papillary architecture (fig. 7.18 A). These masses tend to com-

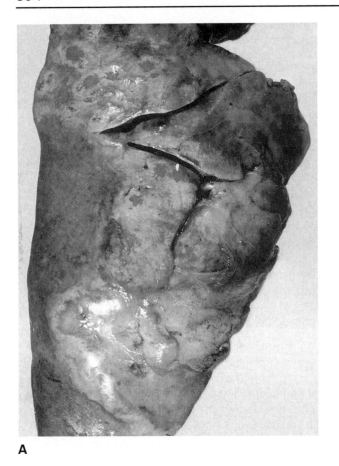

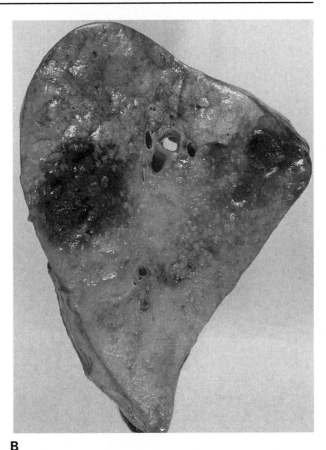

A

B

Fig. 7.17. Ovine pulmonary carcinoma. **A.** Coalescing areas of pulmonary consolidation in sheep with ovine pulmonary carcinoma. **B.** Section of lung with multiple poorly delimited regions of neoplastic involvement of parenchyma.

press adjacent alveoli and may be associated with a moderate lymphohistiocytic alveolar infiltrate. Adjacent alveolar septa may also have significant collagen deposition, with regions of overt fibrosis. Some cases may have prominent peribronchiolar lymphoid hyperplasia, but this is likely to represent coinfection with ovine lentivirus. A distinguishing feature of the OPC lesion is the cuboidal lining of alveoli at the periphery of the neoplastic nodules. This recapitulates the early stages of tumor development where alveolar type II cell proliferation is the initial change (fig. 7.18 B). Approximately 10 percent of OPC affected animals have metastasis to regional pulmonary lymph nodes.[3] Metastasis to heart and skeletal muscle has also been reported.[6]

Lesions of OPC (JSRV) must be differentiated from progressive pneumonia (lentivirus). While both can have type II cell hyperplasia and interstitial fibrosis, the ovine lentivirus induced lesion has a prominent peribronchiolar and perivascular lymphoid inflammation and lacks the papillary alveolar ingrowths of epithelium present in early OPC lesions. These distinctions are important because dual infections with JSRV and ovine lentivirus are present in many flocks.[2]

Etiology

Although as yet uncultivated and without confirming evidence of infectivity, there is strong evidence that the etiology of OPC is a retrovirus.[11] A retroviral genome for a new retrovirus, Jaagsiekte sheep retrovirus (JSRV) has been cloned and sequenced from lung washings of affected sheep. Sequence analysis suggests relationships to both the type B and type D retroviral groups. The retroviral genome does not appear to code for an oncogene, and the mechanism of neoplastic transformation remains undetermined.[12] Complicating the etiopathogenesis of this infectious pulmonary neoplasm is the existence of multiple copies of related endogenous sheep retroviral loci that hybridize to JSRV DNA probes.[13] Endogenous JSRV sequences are expressed in a number of tissues from a wide species range of domestic sheep, wild sheep, and goats. Sequences within the JSRV *gag* gene have been identified as specific to the exogenous virus and have been shown to be present exclusively in tumor tissues or lung secretions from affected animals but not nontumor tissues or in unaffected animals.[14] Further analysis of this specific segment has identified two genotypes of JSRV in a survey of neoplasms from three continents.[15]

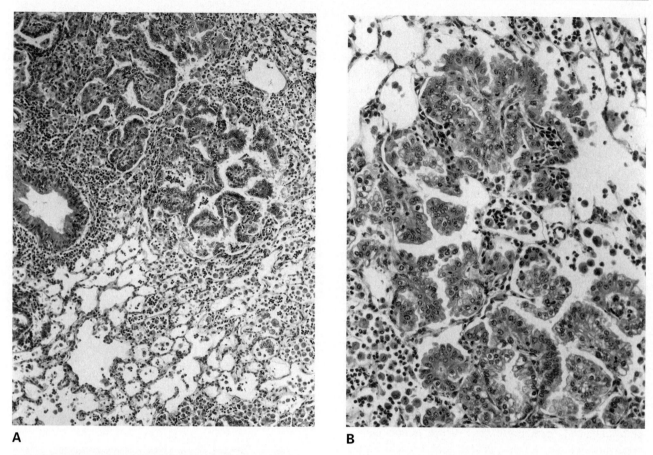

Fig. 7.18. Ovine pulmonary carcinoma. **A.** Papillary growth infiltrates adjacent alveolar parenchyma containing mixed mononuclear interstitial and alveolar inflammatory cells. **B.** Papillary growths composed of simple cuboidal to low columnar, polarized, epithelial cells similar to those in bronchioloalveolar tumors.

REFERENCES

1. Dungal, N., Gislason, G., and Taylor, E.L. (1938) Epizootic adenomatosis in the lungs of sheep: Comparisons with Jaagsiekte, verminous pneumonia, and progressive pneumonia. *J Comp Pathol* 51:46–68.

2. Snyder, S.P., DeMartini, J.C., Ameghino, E., and Caletti, E. (1983) Coexistence of pulmonary adenomatosis and progressive pneumonia in sheep in the central sierra of Peru. *Amer J Vet Res* 44:1334–1338.

3. Demartini, J.C., Rosadio, R.H., and Lairmore, M.D. (1988) The etiology and pathogenesis of ovine pulmonary carcinoma (sheep pulmonary adenomatosis). *Vet Microbiol* 17:219–236.

4. DeMartini, J.C., and York, D.F. (1997) Retrovirus-associated neoplasms of the respiratory system of sheep and goats. Ovine pulmonary carcinoma and enzootic nasal tumor. *Vet Clin N Amer Food Anim Pract* 13:55–70.

5. Dungal, N. (1946) Experiments with Jaagsiekte. *Amer J Pathol* 22:737–759.

6. Hunter, A.R., and Munro, R. (1983) The diagnosis, occurrence and distribution of sheep pulmonary adenomatosis in Scotland 1975 to 1981. *Brit Vet J* 139:153–164.

7. Cutlip, R.C., and Young. S. (1982) Sheep pulmonary adenomatosis (jaagsiekte) in the United States. *Amer J Vet Res* 43:2108–2113.

8. Nisbet, D.I., Mackay. J.M., Smith, W., and Gray, E.W. (1971) Ultra-

9. Perk, K., Hod, I., and Nobel, T.A. (1971) Pulmonary adenomatosis of sheep (Jaagsiekte). I. Ultrastructure of the tumor. *J Natl Cancer Inst* 46:525–537.

10. Rosadio, R.H., Sharp, J.M., Lairmore, M.D., Dahlberg, J.E., and De, M.J. (1988) Lesions and retroviruses associated with naturally occurring ovine pulmonary carcinoma (sheep pulmonary adenomatosis). *Vet Pathol* 25:58–66.

11. He, Y., Hecht, S.J., and DeMartini, J.C. (1992) Evidence for retroviral capsid and nucleocapsid antigens in ovine pulmonary carcinoma. *Virus Res* 25:159–167.

12. Hecht, S.J., Sharp, J.M., and Demartini, J.C. (1996) Retroviral aetiopathogenesis of ovine pulmonary carcinoma: A critical appraisal [see comments]. *Brit Vet J* 152:395–409.

13. Bai, J., Zhu, R.Y., Stedman, K., Cousens, C., Carlson, J., Sharp, J.M., and DeMartini, J.C. (1996) Unique long terminal repeat U3 sequences distinguish exogenous Jaagsiekte sheep retroviruses associated with ovine pulmonary carcinoma from endogenous loci in the sheep genome. *J Virol* 70:3159–3168.

14. Palmarini, M., Cousens, C., Dalziel, R.G., Bai, J., Stedman, K., DeMartini, J.C., and Sharp, J.M. (1996) The exogenous form of Jaagsiekte retrovirus is specifically associated with a contagious lung cancer of sheep. *J Virol* 70:1618–1623.

15. Hecht, S.J., Stedman, K.E., Carlson, J.O., DeMartini, J.C. (1996) Distribution of endogenous type B and type D sheep retrovirus sequences in ungulates and other mammals. *Proc Natl Acad Sci USA* 93:3297–3302.

structure of sheep pulmonary adenomatosis (Jaagsiekte). *J Pathol* 103:157–162.

Mesenchymal Tumors Primary to Lung

While connective tissue tumors such as osteosarcoma, chondrosarcoma, fibrosarcoma, and undifferentiated sarcoma do, on rare occasions, occur in the lung without evident other primary sources, these lesions have little difference from their morphology in other sites and will not be described here. Description of other mesenchymal tumors that are uniquely associated with pulmonary lesions follows.

Granular Cell Tumors

Granular cell tumors are a group of rare neoplasms characterized by a distinctive, variably PAS positive, cytoplasmic granularity that is not argyrophilic. While granular cell tumors are associated with specific sites that vary between species, primary granular cell tumors of the lung occur in humans (in addition to other sites) and as the only reported site in the horse. While granular cell tumors are reported in the tongue and other sites in dogs, granular cell tumors of the respiratory system in the dog are limited to one case report of a multifocal pleural tumor.[1] In the horse, granular cell tumors are airway associated peri- and endobronchial tumors that frequently are multiple but generally are histologically benign growths.[2,3] These tumors have a propensity for the lower tracheae and bronchi, often resulting in airway obstruction and disruption of airway cartilage.

Granular cell tumors are circumscribed, expansile masses that are usually centered around bronchi and bronchial structures and displace bronchial epithelium luminally to occlude the airways. The tumor has limited organization, with sheets of cells that are sometimes loosely arranged in nests or rows by sparse collagen bundles. Neoplastic cells are large, round to polyhedral cells with abundant cytoplasm and poorly defined cell borders. They have regular, oval nuclei that are central to eccentrically placed and have stippled chromatin and a single central nucleolus. The cytoplasm is filled with characteristic eosinophilic granules (fig. 7.19 A). These granules are variably PAS positive, fairly consistently luxol fast blue (LSB) positive, and uniformly negative with silver stains. The LSB staining is reportedly consistent with the presence of choline based phospholipds and suggests the presence of a myelin-like product.[2] Results of immunohistochemical stains also support a neural origin for these tumors. They stain positively for S-100 protein but negatively for cytokeratins, muscle specific actin, and lysozyme.[2,3] Ultrastructural evaluation of human and one equine granular cell tumors characterizes the cytoplasmic granules as small granules associated with an active Golgi apparatus and larger granules characteristic of multivesicular autophagocytic vacuoles (fig. 7.19 B).[4,5] Results of ultrastructural and immunohistochemical studies have lead to the general acceptance of these tumors as arising from either Schwann cell or possibly neuroendocrine origins.

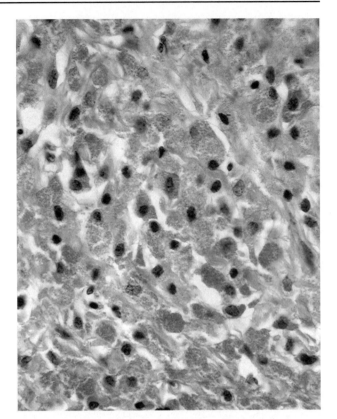

A

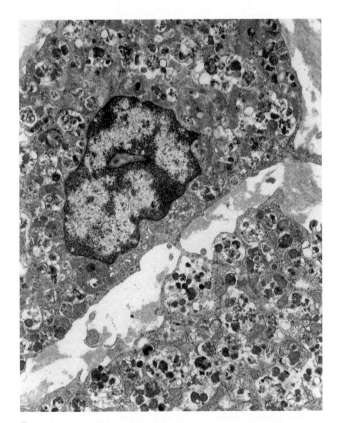

B

Fig. 7.19. Granular cell tumor (equine). **A.** Irregular oval to angular polygonal cells have abundant, prominent, fine cytoplasmic granules. **B.** Ultrastructure of equine granular cell tumor demonstrates multiple, membrane bound, autophagocytic bodies containing irregular dense deposits and membranous debris.

Lymphomatoid Granulomatosis

Lymphomatoid granulomatosis is an angiocentric and destructive pulmonary lymphoid neoplastic disorder that can affect dogs of all ages without an apparent sex or breed predisposition.[6] Clinical signs referable to chronic respiratory disease are accompanied by radiographic evidence of multiple pulmonary mass lesions and hilar lymphadenopathy. Grossly, solitary to multiple, firm, homogenous, light tan masses are present. These masses have a tendency to coalesce. Infiltrates of similar consistency are often present in hilar lymph nodes. Involvement of peripheral lymph nodes is only occasionally seen, and involvement of other systemic lymphoid organs is rare.

Histologically, nodules of lymphomatoid granulomatosis are composed of angiocentric infiltrates of pleomorphic mononuclear cells that spread into adjacent alveolar parenchyma (fig. 7.20). These cells are cytologically heterogeneous with respect to size and chromatin content but tend to be large, hyperchromatic cells with scant to moderate eosinophilic to amphophilic cytoplasm. Angioinvasion and vascular obliteration with subsequent thrombosis is commonly observed and can lead to large regions of necrosis in infiltrated parenchyma.[6] Infiltrates may be accompanied by neutrophils and eosinophils. Cells in the lymphomatoid infiltrates do not react immunohistochemically for lysozyme, suggesting that they most likely are of lymphocytic rather than histiocytic origin.[7] No cases demonstrating definitive lymphocyte markers have been published. The angiocentric orientation of infiltrates and lack of lysozyme immunostaining as well as cytological features distinguish lymphomatoid granulomatosis from malignant histiocytosis.

Malignant Histiocytosis

Originally described as a histiocytic neoplasm, often primary to the lung, of Bernese mountain dogs,[8] malignant histiocytosis is recognized in other breeds as well,[9] with some increased incidence in flat-coated retrievers and rottweilers. Incidence is highest in older male animals and appears to be genetically related to the systemic histiocytic disorder in the Bernese breed. Gross lesions of large, solitary, firm white masses can replace entire lung lobes, or lesions can be multiple with random distribution. Tracheobronchial lymph nodes are often involved, and pleural effusions can occur. Involvement of other organs, including the liver, spleen, central nervous system, and other lymph nodes, by multiple masses occurs in many cases.[8] It has been associated with hypercalcemia.

Histologically, these masses are poorly organized infiltrates that obliterate normal architecture. Neoplastic infiltrates are composed of large pleomorphic mononuclear cells and frequent multinucleated giant cells dispersed in a fine fibrovascular stroma (fig. 7.21). This histological pattern has led to incorrect diagnoses of anaplastic carcinoma or giant cell carcinoma. Nuclei are extremely variably sized and are often quite large with

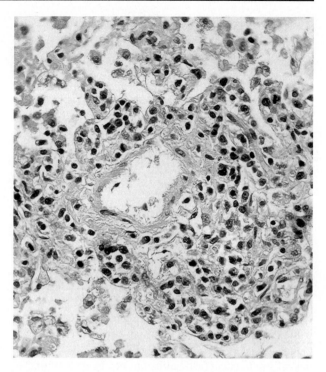

Fig. 7.20. Lymphomatoid granulomatosis. Angiocentric infiltrates of large lymphocytes extend into adjacent alveolar parenchyma.

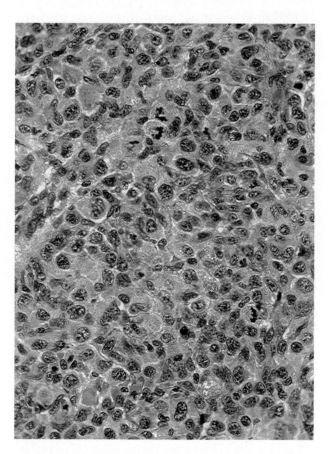

Fig. 7.21. Malignant histiocytosis. Pleomorphic population of irregularly arranged, large, histiocytic cells has frequent multinucleate cells and a high incidence of mitotic figures.

multiple nucleoli. Mitotic figures, often abnormal, are frequent. Cytoplasmic volume also varies and can be abundant, with frequent vacuolation. Phagocytosis of erythrocytes, neutrophils, and other tumor cells by both mononuclear and multinucleate forms are characteristic features of this neoplasm. Further evidence for the histiocytic origin of this tumor is positive immunostaining of neoplastic cells for lysozyme.[7,9] These latter features distinguish malignant histiocytosis from lymphomatoid granulomatosis.

Mesothelioma

Pleural mesothelioma may occur as an isolated neoplasm or in combination/extension of mesothelioma of the pericardium or peritoneum. These appear to be relatively unusual lesions in the dog, with most published descriptions including modest numbers of cases. Most cases are recognized when effusion of the affected serous cavity is evaluated. Pericardial mesothelioma presents with signs referable to pericardial effusion. Cytological diagnosis can be very difficult because reactive mesothelial cells in nonneoplastic effusions can be very similar to neoplastic cells. Incidence in larger groups of neoplasms ranges from 0.5 to 0.8 percent of canine tumors.[10,11] Review of case records of the Teaching Hospital of the University of California–Davis finds mesothelioma in 0.2 percent of all canine cases submitted for pathological evaluation; 35 percent are limited to pericardium, 26 percent are limited to pleura, and 18 percent involved both pericardium and pleura. Nine percent of mesotheliomas were present in the peritoneum, and 3 percent were present in all three serous cavities. An additional 9 percent involved the spermatic cord.

Fairly strong evidence links pleural mesotheliomas in humans with exposure to asbestos. More limited studies suggest a similar association for dogs where increased amounts of asbestos fibers (ferruginous bodies) have been isolated from lungs of affected dogs compared with control dogs.[12] Asbestos related occupations or hobbies of owners of dogs with mesothelioma were significantly associated with mesothelioma incidence in another study.[13]

Grossly, mesothelioma appears as diffuse granular or velvety plaques covering mesothelial surfaces (fig. 7.22). Firm, discrete nodules may also be present, and some cases may have a significant scirrhous component (scirrhous mesothelioma). Histologically, these growths recapitulate their gross appearance as plaque-like proliferations of arborizing to papillary structures lined by cuboidal basophilic mesothelial cells over a fibrovascular supporting framework (fig. 7.23 A). Invaginations of mesothelial growths can give an acinar appearance resembling adenocarcinoma (fig. 7.23 B). Mesothelial cells are cuboidal to polygonal with large oval nuclei, abundant granular eosinophilic cytoplasm, and distinct cell borders. More aggressive tumors elicit a marked scirrhous response that may isolate islands of neoplastic

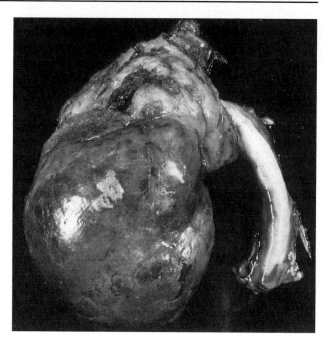

Fig. 7.22. Pericardial mesothelioma. The heart base is expanded by diffuse proliferation of white, firm, dense and fibrous tissue with an irregular nodular surface. Plaques of similar tissue are present on the epicardium overlying the right ventricle.

mesothelial cell aggregates. Ultrastructural features are fairly characteristic for mesothelial cells, which have abundant, long, surface microvilli that may be present around the circumference of the cell and are joined to other cells by numerous desmosomes. The cytoplasm contains numerous bundles of tonofilaments arranged circumferentially around the nucleus. Immunohistochemical stains are also useful in differentiating these tumors since mesothelial cells uniquely express both epithelial cytokeratins and mesenchymal markers such as vimentin.[14]

REFERENCES

1. Foley, G.L. (1988) Intrathoracic granular cell tumour in a dog. *J Comp Pathol* 98:481–487.
2. Kelley, L.C., Hill, J.E., Hafner, S., and Wortham, K.J. (1995) Spontaneous equine pulmonary granular cell tumors: Morphologic, histochemical, and immunohistochemical characterization. *Vet Pathol* 32:101–106.
3. Bouchard, P.R., Fortna, C.H., Rowland, P.H., and Lewis, R.M. (1995) An immunohistochemical study of three equine pulmonary granular cell tumors. *Vet Pathol* 32:730–734.
4. Sobel, H.J., Schwarz, R., Marquet, E. (1973) Light and electron-microscopic study of the origin of granular cell myoblastoma. *J Pathol* 109:101–111.
5. Turk, M.A.M., and Breeze, R.G. (1981) Histochemical and ultrastructural features of an equine pulmonary granular cell tumor (myoblastoma) in the lung of a horse. *J Comp Pathol* 91:471–481.
6. Berry, C.R., Moore, P.F., Thomas, W.P., Sisson, D., and Koblik, P.D. (1990) Pulmonary lymphomatoid granulomatosis in seven dogs (1976–1987). *J Vet Int Med* 4:157–166.
7. Moore, P.F. (1986) Utilization of cytoplasmic lysozyme immunore-

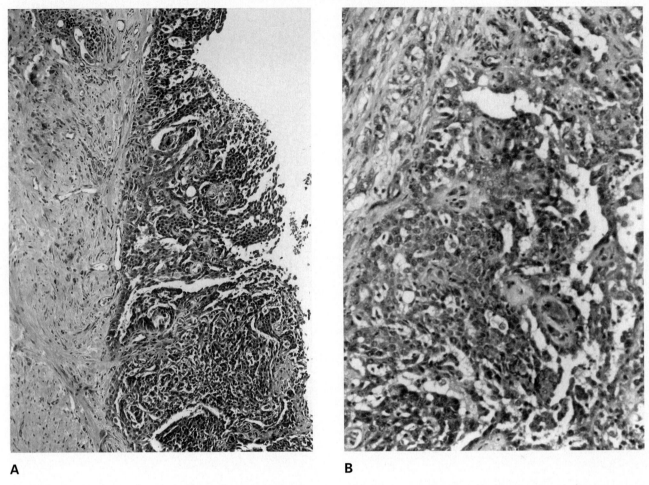

A   **B**

Fig. 7.23. Mesothelioma. **A.** Plaques of disorganized mesothelial and stromal growth overlie granulation tissue containing nests of malignant cells in the thickened pleura. **B.** Pleomorphic plump and occcasionally irregularly stratified mesothelial cells form clefts and villous-like structures on a poorly organized connective tissue stroma.

activity as a histiocytic marker in canine histiocytic disorders. *Vet Pathol* 23:757–762.

8. Moore, P.F., and Rosen, A. (1986) Malignant histiocytosis of Bernese mountain dogs. *Vet Pathol* 23:1–10.

9. Moore, P.F. (1986) Utilization of cytoplasmic lysozyme immunoreactivity as a histiocytic marker in canine histiocytic disorders. *Vet Pathol* 23:757–762.

10. Ogilvie, G.K., Obradovich, J.E., Elmslie, R.E., Vail, D.M., Moore, A.S., Straw, R.C., Dickinson, K., Cooper, M.F., and Withrow, S.J. (1991) Efficacy of mitoxantrone against various neoplasms in dogs. *J Amer Vet Med Assoc* 198:1618–1621.

11. Ogilvie, G.K., Haschek, W.M., Withrow, S.J., Richardson, R.C., Harvey, H.J., Henderson, R.A., Fowler, J.D., Norris, A.M., Tomlinson, J., McCaw, D., Klausner, J.S., Reschke, B.S., and McKiernan, B.C. (1989) Classification of primary lung tumors in dogs: 210 cases (1975–1985). *J Amer Vet Med Assoc* 195:106–108.

12. Harbison, M.L., and Godleski, J.J. (1983) Malignant mesothelioma in urban dogs. *Vet Pathol* 20:531–540.

13. Glickman, L.T., Domanski, L.M., Maguire, T.G., Dubielzig, R.R., and Churg A. (1983) Mesothelioma in pet dogs associated with exposure of their owners to asbestos. *Environ Res* 32:305–313.

14. McDonough, S.P., MacLachlan, N.J., and Tobias, A.H. (1992) Canine pericardial mesothelioma. *Vet Pathol* 29:256–260.

8 Tumors of the Alimentary Tract

K. W. Head, R. W. Else, and R. R. Dubielzig

INTRODUCTION

K.W. Head and R.W. Else

The alimentary tract is a tube extending from the lips to the anus. It is composed of many types of lining and supporting cells, each of which can give rise to a specific tumor type with its own behavior pattern. It is useful for diagnosis and clinical management of these tumors to divide the tract into sections: mouth and pharynx; esophagus and stratified squamous lined stomach; glandular stomach; intestine; rectum and anus.

Since the last edition of this text over 1000 articles have been published on these subjects. An exhaustive reference list has not been attempted. Those publications that are listed will give the reader access to the wider literature that covers the recent progress that has been made in the fields of gastrointestinal tumor histogenesis, carcinogenesis, and patient management.

It is usually easy to recognize the cell lineage of benign tumors but this becomes increasingly difficult with the progressive anaplasia shown by malignant tumors. The development of molecular biology has in part unraveled the multifactorial nature of carcinogenesis: extrinsic or intrinsic carcinogens initiate cellular changes in an animal that is susceptible because of the composition of its genome, then these cells are promoted to their full neoplastic growth potential when internal or external environmental factors operate. One of the mechanisms that has been discovered is that of the protein produced by the *p53* gene that normally stops DNA replication in the G_1 phase of the cell cycle to allow DNA repair, or if the damage to the DNA is excessive, it initiates apoptosis. Cells with mutant *p53* or those that lack *p53* continue to divide, perpetuating the mutation and allowing other mutations to accumulate in the neoplastic clone. Squamous cell carcinoma of the equine palate and stomach, of the bovine phar-

ynx, and of the feline tongue and palate have given positive results for mutant p53 protein.[1,2] This mechanism cannot be demonstrated in all tumors.[1]

Animal management changes may lead to the prevention of tumor initiation and promotion by avoiding exposure to causative factors. In addition to the established methods of surgery, cryosurgery, radiotherapy, and hyperthermia, chemotherapy[3] and immunotherapy[4] have been used in the treatment of alimentary tumors. To assess these treatment regimes, attention has been focused on the clinical staging of tumors, and this in turn necessitated consideration of the relative values of histological examination of wedge or large needle core biopsies as compared to cytology of fine needle aspiration smears. In veterinary pathology changes in the cytoplasm and nucleus that reflect the degree of malignancy are usually assessed visually by the microscopist, but semi-automated image analyzing systems are increasingly being used for morphometric measurements of cells and their components (e.g., nuclear:cytoplasmic ratio, nuclear size, AgNOR numbers, etc.).[5]

REFERENCES

1. Johnston, H.M., Thompson, H., and Pirie, H.M. (1996) p53 immunohistochemisty in domestic animal tumors. *Eur J Vet Pathol* 2:135–140.
2. Teifke, J.P., and Lohr, C.V. (1996) Immunohistochemical Detection of p53 overexpression in paraffin wax-embedded squamous cell carcinomas of cattle, horses, cats and dogs. *J Comp Pathol* 114:205–210.
3. Helfand, S.C. (1990) Principles and applications of chemotherapy. *Vet Clin N Amer Small Anim Pract* 20:987–1013.
4. Arlinghaus, R.B. (1989) Vaccines against tumor antigens. *Adv Vet Sci Comp Med* 33:377–395.
5. Roels, S., van Diest, P.J., Beliën, J.A.M., and Ducatelle, R. (1998) Computerized image analysis in diagnostic veterinary pathology. *Eur J Vet Pathol* 4:21–27.

ODONTOGENIC TUMORS AND CYSTS

R.R. Dubielzig

Tumors of odontogenic origin in domestic animals are rare but interesting tumors that present several challenges to accurate diagnosis. Classification systems have been put forward that emphasize the tissue differentiation exhibited in the neoplasm, and the classification scheme put forward here is based on that same principle.[1-5] Odontogenesis begins with the ingrowth of oral ectoderm into the mesenchyme of the jaw. Subsequent events affect the morphology of both the epithelium and the surrounding mesenchyme. The classification system used in this chapter (table 8.1) largely follows that suggested by Gardner for naming odontogenic tumors in animals.[5] *Fibromatous epulis of periodontal ligament origin* was given a separate category because periodontal ligament stroma is not part of the inductive process.

There is considerable confusion over the use of the term epulis in the veterinary literature. The term epulis simply refers to a tumor or tumor-like lesion of the gingiva. The term *fibromatous epulis of periodontal ligament origin* was first used in 1958.[6] Gorlin used the term not only for fibromatous epulis of periodontal ligament origin but for tumors with the features of what we are now calling *acanthomatous ameloblastoma (acanthomatous epulis)*.[7] Subsequent nomenclature proposed three types of epulis, *fibromatous epulis of periodontal ligament origin, acanthomatous epulis* (now called *acanthomatous ameloblastoma*), and *ossifying epulis*. The unifying feature was evidence of periodontal ligament stroma within the mass. Subsequently, others have proposed classifications that include proliferative lesions without periodontal ligament stroma. The system proposed here includes only one tumor, the *fibromatous epulis of periodontal ligament origin,* to be designated by the term *epulis.*

The odontogenic epithelium gives rise to ameloblastomas and odontomas (table 8.1). Tumors can arise centrally, within the jaw bone, or peripherally, within the gingiva. Tumors can be derived from the original enamel organ, the cell rests of Malassez, or from odontogenic epithelium incorporated into the gingival epithelium. The unifying feature is the presence of odontogenic type epithelium. The histological features (fig. 8.1) that suggest a neoplastic epithelium is of odontogenic origin are (1) peripheral palisading of epithelial cells, (2) location of the nucleus at the apical pole of the palisaded cell, (3) basilar epithelial cytoplasmic clearing, and (4) the connection of nonbasilar epithelial cells by long intercellular bridges reminiscent of the stellate reticulum. The decisive features in naming odontogenic neoplasia are the presence or absence of a dental pulp-like mesenchyme, dentin, cementum, or enamel matrix.

REFERENCES

1. Thoma, K.H., and Goldman, H.M. (1946) Odontogenic tumors: A classification based on observations of the epithelial, mesenchyma, and mixed varieties. *Amer J Pathol* 22:433–471.
2. Pinborg, J.J., and Clausen, F. (1958) Classification of odontogenic tumours. *Acta Odontolog Scandv* 16:293–331.
3. Hoffman, J., Jacoway, J.R., and Krolls, S.O. (1987) Intraosseous and periosteal tumors of the jaws. Armed Forces Institute of Pathology, Washington, D.C., pp. 92–93.
4. Kramer, I.R.H., Pinborg, J.J., and Shear, M. (1992) *Histologic Typing of Odontogenic Tumors,* 2nd ed. Springer-Verlag, Berlin, pp. 7–9.
5. Gardner, D.G. (1992) An orderly approach to the study of odontogenic tumors in animals. *J Comp Pathol* 107:427–438.
6. Gorlin, R.J., Clark, J.J., and Chaudhry, A.P. (1958) The oral pathology of domesticated animals. *Oral Surg Oral Med Oral Pathol* 11:500–535.
7. Gorlin, J.J., Barron, C.N., Chaudhry, A.P., and Clark, J.J. (1959) The oral and pharyngeal pathology of domestic animals: A study of 487 cases. *Amer J Vet Res* 20:1032–1061.

TUMORS OF ODONTOGENIC EPITHELIUM WITHOUT ODONTOGENIC MESENCHYME

Ameloblastoma and Keratinizing Ameloblastoma

Ameloblastoma and keratinizing ameloblastoma are rare tumors in domestic animals, with variants occurring in dogs,[1-4] cats, and horses.[5-8] Ameloblastoma (fig. 8.1) is derived from odontogenic epithelial cells found near the tooth (central) or in the gingival epithelium (peripheral). Previous reports combined tumors that might be considered amyloid-producing odontogenic tumors or calcifying epithelial odontogenic tumors today.[1] *Adamantinoma* is a term used in much of the original veterinary literature, and it is considered synonymous with *ameloblastoma.*

TABLE 8.1. Tumors derived from odontogenic epithelium

Ameloblastoma/keratinizing ameloblastoma
Amyloid-producing odontogenic tumor
Canine acanthomatous ameloblastoma
Ameloblastic fibroma-ameloblastic fibro-odontoma
Feline inductive odontogenic tumor–inductive fibroameloblastoma
Complex odontoma

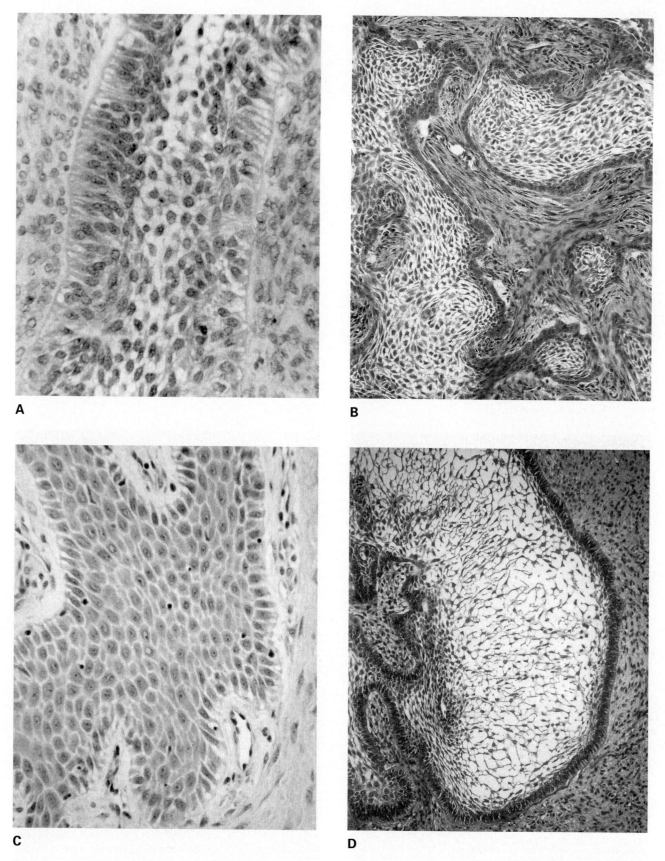

Fig. 8.1. **A.** The characteristic morphological features of odontogenic epithelium in a neoplasm are (1) peripheral palisading, (2) location of the nucleus at the apical pole, (3) basilar epithelial clearing, and (4) central cells connected by long intercellular bridges. **B.** Canine ameloblastoma with odontogenic epithelium. **C.** Photomicrograph of the characteristic epithelium from acanthomatous ameloblastoma (acanthomatous epulis). There are peripheral palisading and central acanthocytes connected by prominent intercellular bridges. **D.** Bovine ameloblastic fibroma with well-differentiated odontogenic epithelium resembling enamel and a cellular mesenchymal stroma resembling dental pulp.

Gross Morphology and Histological Features

Ameloblastoma and keratinizing ameloblastoma are the same tumor, but with varying degrees of keratinization. They are typically slowly progressive tumors within the dental arcade and are no metastatic risk. These tumors are seen in dogs, cats, and horses. Most tumors are characterized by a swelling of the affected jaw with an osteolytic mass within the jaw bone delineating the tumor (figs. 8.2, 8.3). Tumors within the jaw are designated as *central,* and tumors of the gingiva, which are rare, are designated as *peripheral.* The tumors can be solid or cystic, and they are usually discrete (fig. 8.2). The characteristic feature is the presence of odontogenic epithelium as the major component of the neoplasm (see fig. 8.1). Odontogenic epithelium has the following characteristics: (1) peripheral palisading of epithelial cells, (2) location of the nucleus at the apical pole of the palisaded cell, (3) basilar epithelial cytoplasmic clearing, (4) nonbasilar epithelial cytoplasmic clearing, (5) nonbasilar epithelial cells connected by intercellular bridges reminiscent of the stellate reticulum. If there is a prominent tendency toward keratin expression, the term *keratinizing ameloblastoma* should be used. Keratinized epithelial cells are often round and hypereosinophilic. Keratin pearls are seldom seen, but when seen are of no diagnostic significance. Rarely, ameloblastoma and keratinizing ameloblastoma may be pigmented.

Amyloid-Producing Odontogenic Tumor

Amyloid-producing odontogenic tumor,[9] also designated calcifying epithelial odontogenic tumor,[2,3,10,11] is a tumor of both dogs and cats, also derived from odontogenic epithelium. It shares biological features with ameloblastoma and keratinizing ameloblastoma, but histologically there are variable amounts of amyloid matrix between neoplastic epithelial cells (fig. 8.4). The name calcifying epithelial odontogenic tumor suggests a similarity to the human odontogenic tumor with the same name; however, histologically the tumors are quite distinct, and for that reason, the name amyloid-producing odontogenic tumor is preferred.[9]

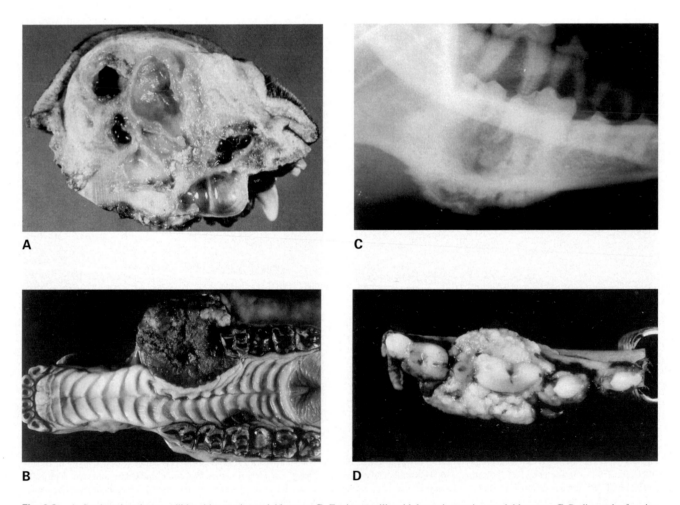

A   **C**

B   **D**

Fig. 8.2. **A.** Sectioned canine mandible with a cystic ameloblastoma. **B.** Equine maxilla with large destructive ameloblastoma. **C.** Radiograph of canine mandible that has a destructive osteolytic ameloblastoma. **D.** Acanthomatous ameloblastoma (acanthomatous epulis) forming an exophytic verrucous mass on both sides of the dental arcade.

Canine Acanthomatous Ameloblastoma

Acanthomatous ameloblastoma[12] is a common tumor of the canine dental arcade. Other names used for this tumor include *acanthomatous epulis*,[13] *peripheral ameloblastoma*,[14] *basal cell carcinoma*,[15] and *adamantinoma*.[16] The name put forward here correctly classifies this lesion as a tumor of odontogenic epithelial origin, based on morphology, and borrows the descriptive term acanthomatous to emphasize the prominent feature of acanthocytes in this tumor.

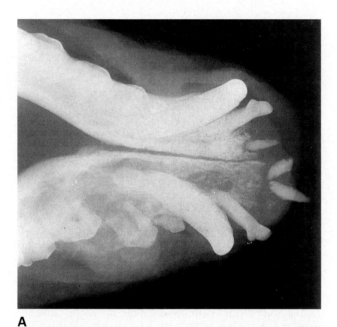

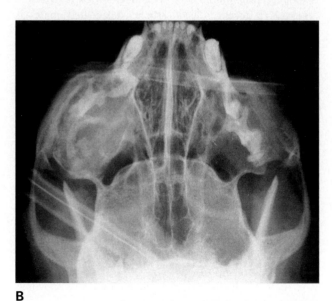

Fig. 8.3. **A.** Radiograph of acanthomatous ameloblastoma (acanthomatous epulis) demonstrating marked osteolysis in a 10-year-old dog. The tumor was infiltrative and recurred twice after surgical excision. **B.** Feline inductive odontogenic tumor (feline inductive fibroameloblastoma) has induced marked osteolysis in left maxillae.

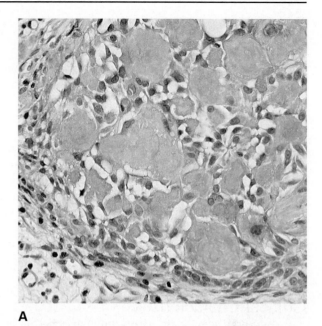

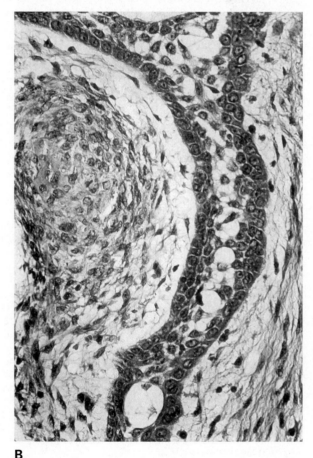

Fig. 8.4. **A.** Photomicrograph of amyloid-producing odontogenic tumor showing extracellular amyloid deposits that characterize the tumor. **B.** Feline inductive odontogenic tumor (feline inductive fibroameloblastoma) in which the odontogenic epithelium cradles highly cellular round mesenchymal aggregates.

Gross Morphology and Histological Features

Acanthomatous ameloblastoma presents an exophytic verrucous mass often occurring on both sides of the dental arcade of the mandible or maxilla in dogs (fig. 8.2 D). In advanced cases, radiographs reveal osteolysis in adjacent bone (fig. 8.3 A).

Tumors are characterized by the presence of broad interconnecting sheets of nonkeratinizing odontogenic epithelium with peripheral palasading and prominent central acanthocytic formation with intercellular bridges typical of stellate reticulum (see fig. 8.1 C). In early cases, a mesenchyme typical of periodontal ligament is seen. The mesenchyme is highly cellular, with stellate fibroblasts in a dense fibrillar collagen background with regularly positioned, empty blood vessels.

Clinical Characteristics

Advanced tumors are locally infiltrative but never metastasize. Surgical excision with histological confirmation of free borders is the treatment of choice. These tumors respond favorably to radiation therapy; however, an unacceptably high percentage of animals develop new tumors at the irradiated site. The recurrent tumor is most frequently squamous cell carcinoma, but fibrosarcoma and osteosarcoma have been reported.[17]

REFERENCES

1. Dubielzig, R.R., and Thrall, D.E. (1982) Ameloblastoma and keratinizing ameloblastoma in dogs. *Vet Pathol* 19:596–607.
2. Walsh, K.M., Denholm, L.J., and Cooper, B.J. (1987) Epithelial odontogenic tumors in domestic animals. *J Comp Pathol* 97:503–521.
3. Poulet, F.M., Valentine, B.A., and Summers, B.A. (1992) A survey of epithelial odontogenic tumors and cysts in dogs and cats. *Vet Pathol* 29:369–380.
4. Gardner, D.G., and Dubielzig, R.R. (1993) The histologic features of canine keratinizing ameloblastoma. *J Comp Pathol* 109:423–428.
5. Vaughan, J.T., and Bartels, J.E. (1968) Equine mandibular adamantinoma. *J Amer Vet Med Assoc* 153:454–457.
6. Hanselka, D.V., Roberts, R.E., and Thompson, R.B. (1974) Adamantinoma of the equine mandible. *Vet Med Small Anim Clin* 69:157–160.
7. Weber, A., Ligthem, A.J., and Verstraete, F.J.M. (1981) Primary intraosseous carcinoma of the maxilla in a horse. *J Comp Pathol* 104:443–448.
8. Gardner, D.G. (1994) Ameloblastomas in the horse: A critical review and report of an additional example. *J Oral Pathol* 23:41–44.
9. Gardner, D.G., and Dubielzig, R.R. (1994) The so-called calcifying epithelial odontogenic tumour in dogs and cats (amyloid-producing odontogenic tumor) *J Comp Pathol* 111:221–230.
10. Langham, R.F., Bennett. R., and Koestner, A. (1984) Amyloidosis associated with a calcifying ameloblastoma (calcifying epithelial odontoma) in a cat. *Vet Pathol* 21:549–550.
11. Abbott, D.P., Walsh, K., and Diters, R.W. (1986) Calcifying epithelial odontogenic tumors in three cats and a dog. *J Comp Pathol* 96:131–136.
12. Gardner, D.G., and Baker, D.C. (1993) The relationship of the canine acanthomatous epulis to ameloblastoma. *J Comp Pathol* 108:47–55.
13. Dubielzig, R.R., Goldschmidt, M.H., and Brodey, R.S. (1979) The nomenclature of periodontal epulides in dogs. *Vet Pathol* 16:209–214.
14. Verstraete, F.J.M., Ligthelm, A.J., and Weber, A. (1992) The histological nature of epulides in dogs. *J Comp Pathol* 106:169–182.
15. Bostock, D.E., and White, R.A.S. (1987) Classification and behavior after surgery of canine epulides. *J Comp Pathol* 97:197–206.
16. Langham, R.F., Koahey, K.K., Mostosky, U.V., et al. (1965) Oral adamantinoma in the dog. *J Amer Vet Med Assoc* 146:474–480.
17. Thrall, D.E., Goldschmidt, M.H., and Biery, D.N. (1981) Malignant tumor formation at the site of previously irradiated acanthomatous epulides in four dogs. *J Amer Vet Med Assoc* 178:127–132.

TUMORS OF ODONTOGENIC EPITHELIUM WITH ODONTOGENIC MESENCHYME

Ameloblastic Fibroma and Ameloblastic Fibro-Odontoma

Ameloblastic fibroma and ameloblastic fibro-odontoma are variations of the same tumor derived from odontogenic epithelium and pulpal mesenchyme. They are rare in all species, but they are the most common odontogenic neoplasm in cattle. Tumors are seen as mass-like lesions interfering with mastication in young cattle.[1-4] Although these tumors have been given different names in the past, a recent review article[4] designated these as *ameloblastic fibroma* or *ameloblastic fibro-odontoma*. Radiographs reveal osteolysis and variable complex intralesional mineralization. Histologically, there are long cords of well-differentiated odontogenic epithelium in a background of loose mesenchymal tissue reminiscent of dental pulp (see fig. 8.1D). Areas of ameloblastic differentiation can be associated with deposition of dentin or enamel matrix. The presence of dentin and enamel differentiates ameloblastic fibro-odontoma from ameloblastic fibroma (no dentin or enamel).

Feline Inductive Odontogenic Tumor

Feline inductive odontogenic tumor is also known as inductive fibroameloblastoma. The name *feline inductive odontogenic tumor* is meant to designate this as a specific entity in *cats* and avoids the inaccurate use of the term *fibroameloblastoma*. This rare tumor of the dental arcade is the most common dental tumor of young cats.[5-9] Tumors occur most often on the rostral maxilla and present as osteolytic masses that interfere with mastication or distort the facial features (see fig. 8.3 B).

Histological Features

Histologically, these tumors are characterized by the presence of both odontogenic epithelium and localized aggregates of mesenchymal differentiation. Neoplastic epithelial cells tend to form circular aggregates around clusters of highly cellular mesenchyme in a pattern reminiscent of the cap stage of odontogenesis (see fig. 8.4 B). Local reoccurrence has been reported in incompletely excised tumors, but metastasis does not appear to occur.[9]

Complex Odontoma

Complex odontoma is a mass-like lesion associated with fully differentiated dental components but not forming tooth-like structures. These tumors are rare in all species, but they are most commonly seen in young horses[10-12] and young dogs.[6,7,13-15] Tumors present as radiodense mass lesions in the jaw of young animals. The gross specimen is often very hard, and the sectioned specimen reveals jumbled dental matrix (fig. 8.5). The lack of organized tooth formation is the feature that distinguishes between complex odontoma and compound odontoma. Histologically, there is well-differentiated dentin and enamel matrix formation, often with fully mineralized enamel present. These tumors can have variable amounts of odontogenic epithelium. The presence of an odontogenic epithelium should not distract the pathologist into a diagnosis of ameloblastoma. Tumors in horses also show abundant cemental deposition, which is not seen in dogs or humans. These tumors are treated successfully by surgical extraction, and they do metastasize.

Compound Odontoma

Compound odontoma presents as a mass lesion of the jaw of young canines and is associated radiographically and grossly with the presence of large numbers of abnormally shaped tooth-like structures (denticles) originating from within the mass (fig. 8.5). Histologically, all components of normal odontogenesis occur in a configuration suggestive of normal tooth development, and the result is large numbers of denticles forming within the mass. Histologically, there may be remnants of odontogenic epithelium, but in older more mature lesions, the epithelial tissue may be absent. Extraction with debridement is usually curative even of large apparently destructive masses. Some would argue that complex and compound odontoma would be correctly classified as hamartomas rather than neoplasia. I have seen one case of compound odontoma in a dog reoccur after removal as an aggressive carcinoma; therefore I prefer to think of these as neoplasms.

REFERENCES

1. Cheema, A.H., and Shanin, H. (1974) Congenital ameloblastoma in a calf. *Vet Pathol* 11:235–349.
2. Chalmers, G.A., and Shaklady, E.M. (1991) Ameloblastic odontoma in a calf. *Can Vet J* 32:366–367.
3. Masegi, T., Kudo, T., Kawada, M., et al. (1994) Ameloblastic fibroodontoma in the mandibular incisor of a cow. *J Vet Med Sci* 56:157–159.
4. Gardner, D.G. (1996) Ameloblastic fibromas and related tumors in cattle. *J Oral Pathol* 25:119–124.
5. Dubielzig, R.R., Adams, W.M., and Brodey, R.S. (1979) Inductive fibroameloblastoma, an unusual dental tumor of young cats. *J Amer Vet Med Assoc* 174, 720–722.
6. Walsh, K.M., Denholm, L.J., and Cooper, B.J. (1987) Epithelial odontogenic tumors in domestic animals. *J Comp Pathol* 97:503–521.
7. Poulet, F.M., Valentine, B.A., and Summers, B.A. (1992) A survey of epithelial odontogenic tumors and cysts in dogs and cats. *Vet Pathol* 29:369–380.
8. Nyska, A., and Dayan, D. (1995) Ameloblastic fibroma in a young cat. *J Oral Pathol* 24:233–236.
9. Gardner, D.G., and Dubielzig, R.R. (1995) Feline inductive odontogenic tumor (feline inductor fibroameloblastoma) a tumor unique to cats. *J Oral Pathol* 24:185–190.
10. Peter, C.P., Myers, V.S., and Ramsey, F.K. (1968) Ameloblastic odontoma in a pony. *Amer J Vet Res* 29:1495–1498.
11. Lingard, D.R., and Crawford, T.B. (1970) Congenital ameloblastic odontoma in a foal. *Amer J Vet Res* 31:801–804.
12. Dubielzig, R.R., Beck, K.A., Levine, S., et al. (1986) Complex odontoma in a stallion. *Vet Pathol* 23:633–635.
13. Langham, R.F., Mostosky, U.V., and Schirmer, R.G. (1969) Ameloblastic odontoma in the dog. *Amer J Vet Res* 30:1873–1876.
14. Nold, J.B., Powers, B.E., Eden, E.L., and McChesney, A.E. (1984) Ameloblastic odontoma in a dog. *J Amer Vet Med Assoc* 185:996–998.
15. Valentine, B.A., Lynch, M.J., and May, J.C. (1985) Compound odontoma in a dog. *J Amer Vet Med Assoc* 186:177–179.

TUMORS COMPOSED PRIMARILY OF ODONTOGENIC ECTOMESENCHYME

Cementoma

Cementomas are benign mass-like lesions associated with excess cementum deposition. Although these tumors are rarely seen in dogs and cats, I have seen several cases as reactive lesions associated with inflammatory disease in domestic herbivores. When seen in association with inflammation, cementoma should not be considered a true neoplasm. Proliferating cemental tissue is seen as a mass in the jaw or a mass extending into the nasal cavity or maxillary sinus. Traumatic tooth fracture, impacted infundibulum, or periodontitis can predispose to cementoma formation. Cementum is characterized histologically by the many basophilic lines that give it a mosaic appearance and by the anchoring of Sharpey's fibers into the margins of the cemental matrix. In reactive cementoma the

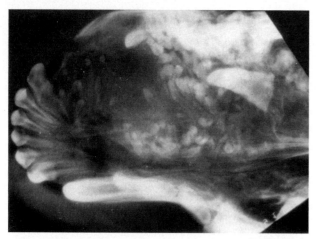

A

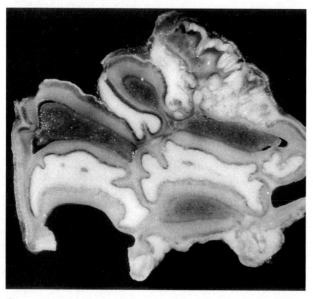

C

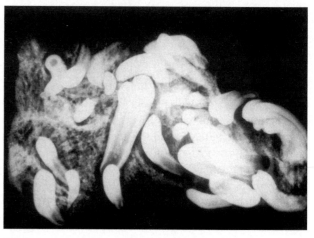

B

Fig. 8.5. **A.** Radiograph of canine maxilla with large compound odontoma has countless toothlike structures (denticles). **B.** High detail radiograph of a surgical fragment from the same tumor as view A demonstrates denticles embedded in the bone. **C.** Sectioned complex odontoma from a young horse with jumbled but well-differentiated odontogenic matrices. The white is cementum, the gray is dentin, and the almost transparent matrix is fully mineralized enamel.

cemental matrix is seen with inflammation and fibrosis. Cementoblastoma, which is occasionally seen in animals, is an expansile, truly neoplastic, lesion showing cemental differentiation.

Cementifying Fibroma

Cementifying fibroma is a rare tumor of the jaw seen in horses and dogs. The tumor is analogous to ossifying fibroma, but the matrical component of the tumor shows complex basophilic lines typical of cementum.

Fibromatous Epulis of Periodontal Ligament Origin

Fibromatous epulis of periodontal ligament origin is common adjacent to the dental arcade in dogs. Dogs of all ages can be affected; however, it is rare in dogs less than 3 years of age. The tumor has also been called peripheral odontogenic fibroma because the tumor in

dogs shares some features of the human tumor.[1-3] The term *fibromatous epulis of periodontal ligament origin* is preferred because it correctly identifies the stroma as having features of the periodontal ligament, whereas *peripheral odontogenic fibroma* has a cellular fibrous stroma with no features of periodontal ligament.[4] Other authors offer the opinion that these lesions are reactive hyperplastic lesions classified as plexiform epithelial hyperplasia.[5] A similar multifocal lesion is seen rarely in young cats.[6]

Gross Morphology and Histological Features

These tumors are epithelial covered, rounded, tan to pink masses that arise immediately adjacent to the tooth from the gingiva. They vary in size from incidental masses to large masses several centimeters in size and interfering with normal mastication (fig. 8.6).

The characteristic histological feature of the fibromatous epulis of periodontal ligament origin is the presence of a mesenchyme suggesting the periodontal ligament (fig. 8.6). Periodontal ligament mesenchyme is characterized by a dense cellularity composed of small stellate to spindle fibroblast cells regularly positioned in a dense fibrillar collagen background. Localized deposition of collagen matrix is often seen, and the matrix can have characteristics of bone, cementum, or dentin. Large empty blood vessels are evenly spaced in the stroma. Odontogenic epithelium is frequently seen in fibromatous epulis of periodontal ligament origin and is considered a secondary feature. The epithelium forms long fronds that can occasionally be seen attaching to the surface epithelium; however,

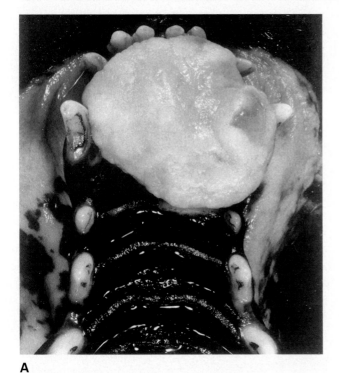

A

these tumors do not always extend to the surface gingiva, and the epithelial cords may also be derived from the cell rests of Malassez within the periodontal ligament. When the entire jaw is available for histopathologic evaluation, decalcified sections that include the periodontal ligament confirm the continuity of the mass with the periodontal ligament. Downward growth with destruction of alveolar bone is not a feature, and local excision is usually curative.

REFERENCES

1. Bostock, D.E., and White, R.A.S. (1987) Classification and behavior after surgery of canine epulides. *J Comp Pathol* 97:197–206.
2. Gardner, D.G., and Baker, D.C. (1991) Fibromatous epulis in dogs and peripheral odontogenic fibroma in humans: Two equivalent lesions. *Oral Surg Oral Med Oral Pathol* 71:317–321.
3. Verstraete, F.J.M., Ligthelm, A.J., and Weber, A. (1992) The histological nature of epulides in dogs. *J Comp Pathol* 106:169–182.
4. Dubielzig, R.R., Goldschmidt, M.H., and Brodey, R.S. (1979) The nomenclature of periodontal epulides in dogs. *Vet Pathol* 16:209–214.
5. Reichart, P.A., Philpsen, H.P., and Durr, U-M. (1989) *J Oral Pathol Med* 18:92–96.
6. Colgin, L.M.A., Schulman, F.Y., and Dubielzig, R.R. (2001) Multiple epulides in 13 cats. *Vet Pathol* 38:227–229.

CYSTS OF THE JAW

Clinically significant cysts of the jaw are rare in domestic animals, but pathologists may be called upon to distinguish between cystic and neoplastic lesions. Cysts usually present as a swelling of the jaw or because of interference with mastication. Radiographically, cysts are rounded masses with a smooth bony outer lining and a radiolucent center. Occasionally, jaw cysts in domestic species fail to meet the morphological criteria for the designated conditions listed below. In these cases, unless there is a compelling reason to use another name, the designation odontogenic cyst as a generic term for epithelium lined, noninflammatory cysts is appropriate. Odontogenic cysts probably arise from the cell rests of Malassez.[1] Tumors are often mistaken for cysts, and care should be taken to rule out neoplasia.

Dentigerous Cyst

Dentigerous cyst is an epithelium lined cyst forming around tooth remnants. The characteristic feature of the epithelial cyst is attachment of the epithelium to the tooth remnants at the neck portion of the tooth, with the crown extending into the cyst (fig. 8.7A). The cyst develops when the reduced-enamel epithelium is retained. Fluid develops between the epithelium and the crown of the tooth. Cysts are usually lined by stratified squamous epithelium; however, localized segments of ciliated epithelium or mucus-producing epithelium can also be seen.[2] The term *dentigerous cyst* has been misused often in the veterinary literature. In the author's experience dentigerous cysts are rare and are found only in dogs and cats.[3]

B

Fig. 8.6. **A.** Large fibromatous epulis of periodontal ligament origin in the rostral maxilla of a dog. **B.** Photomicrograph of view A showing periodontal ligament stroma and collagenous matrix.

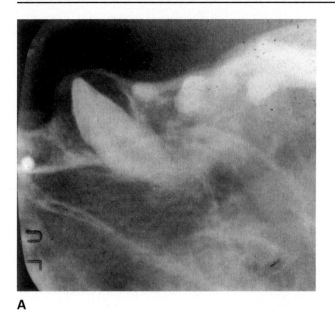

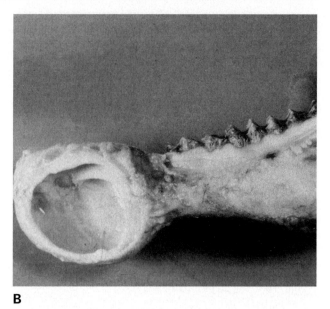

A   B

Fig. 8.7. **A.** Radiograph of a dentigerous cyst in the maxilla of a dog. The cyst forms around a developing tooth and attaches at the crown. **B.** Ovine odontogenic cyst at rostral mandible in a sheep. [Courtesy Drs. R. Fairley and M. Orr.]

Radicular Cysts

Radicular cysts are squamous epithelium lined cysts adjacent to the tooth root of affected species. These are reactive lesions associated with inflammatory oral disease. The cyst probably originates secondary to inflammatory activation of the cell rests of Malassez adjacent to the tooth root in the periodontal ligament.[2] Histologically, they are characterized by stratified squamous epithelium and have an inflammatory component. The characteristic features are the location adjacent to the roots and the association with inflammation. The author has found examples of these cysts in horses, cats, and rabbits.

Ovine Odontogenic Cysts

Ovine odontogenic cysts are characterized as radiolucent cystic lesions of the mandibular incisor region of mature ewes seen in New Zealand and reported in parts of Scotland and England. Characteristically, they occur in association with advanced wear of this incisor tooth and with periodontitis (fig. 8.7B). Histologically, they are characterized by stratified squamous epithelium, and they may or may not contain dental elements, most particularly cementum. These lesions have not been reported in the United States.[4-6]

Temporal Teratoma in Horses

Temporal teratomas are rare lesions that present as open mass-like lesions or cystic tumors of the temporal bone occurring inferior to the ear canal in horses. They contain abnormal tooth-like structures and are lined by stratified squamous epithelium.[3,7-9]

REFERENCES

1. Poulet, F.M., Valentine, B.A., and Summers, B.A. (1992) A survey of epithelial odontogenic tumors and cysts in dogs and cats. *Vet Pathol* 29:369–380.
2. Kramer, I.R.H., Pinborg, J.J., and Shear, M. (1992) *Histological Typing of Odontogenic Tumors,* 2nd ed. Springer-Verlag, Berlin.
3. Gardner, D.G. (1993) Dentigerous cysts in animals oral surgery. *Oral Surg Oral Med Oral Pathol* 75:348–352.
4. Orr, M.B., O'Callaghan, M.W., West, D.M., and Bravere, A.N. (1979) A syndrome of dental abnormalities of sheep: II. The pathology and radiology. *New Zealand Vet J* 27:276–278.
5. Dyson, D.A. (1979) A cystic jaw lesion in sheep. *Vet Record* 105:467–468.
6. Gardner, D.G. (1990) Dentigerous cysts (ovine odontogenic cysts) in sheep. *New Zealand Vet J* 38:148–150.
7. Mason, J.E. (1974) Temporal teratomas in the horse. *Vet Rec* 95:226–228.
8. Fessler, J.F. (1988) Heterotopic polyodontia in horses: Nine cases (1969–1986). *J Amer Vet Med Assoc* 192:535–538.
9. Lindsaw, W.A., and Beck, K.A. (1986) Temporal teratoma in a horse. *Comp Contin Educ Pract Vet* 8:168–171.

OTHER TUMORS OF THE ALIMENTARY TRACT

K.W. Head and R.W. Else

TUMORS OF THE SALIVARY GLANDS

The anatomical nomenclature of salivary glands is based on their size, that is, major and minor glands. The major glands are large encapsulated organs (parotid, mandibular, zygomatic, and compact sublingual) or diffuse nonencapsulated masses (dorsal, middle, and ventral buccal and diffuse sublingual). The minor glands are the scattered small glands not usually visible to the naked eye and named according to their location (labial, buccal, gingival palatine, lingual, etc.). This anatomical subdivision leads to interspecies differences in classification; for example, the bovine upper nasolabial glands form a 1.5 cm thick sheet unlike the discrete labial glands of the dog, whereas the compact zygomatic gland of the dog is probably equivalent to the diffuse dorsal buccal gland of the ox. Similarly, differences exist between species and between glands in their histological composition. The glands are tubuloalveolar, but the acinar cells can be simple (all serous or all mucous) or mixed (serous and mucous, or mucous with serous demilunes). These differences in anatomy and histology reflect variations in physiology.[1,2]

Species Distribution

The majority of salivary gland tumors occur in old animals. Most carcasses examined by meat inspectors are from young animals; it is not surprising, then, that a survey of suspected tumor samples from British abattoirs found no salivary gland tumors in 4.5 million sheep or in 3.7 million pigs examined by meat inspectors and only two carcinomas and one pleomorphic adenoma in 1.3 million slaughtered cattle.[3] Salivary tumors do occur in older sheep: four cases were listed among 891 sheep tumors found in a 35 year abattoir survey.[4]

Horses are often kept until well into maturity, but salivary gland neoplasia is uncommon; for example, two carcinomas and one salivary cystadenoma were found in 687 necropsies and 635 biopsies.[5] In a review of 1148 equine tumors, two adenocarcinomas of major salivary glands were found, and in a collection of 124 tumors in horses, a single case in the soft palate was recorded.[6,7]

The number of cases per 100,000 dogs was calculated to be 1.6 for benign mixed salivary gland tumors (one case) and 3.1 for adenocarcinoma (two cases); for feline adenocarcinoma the estimate was 8.4.[8] In a study of 35,451 canine neoplasms from all sites, the following salivary gland tumor types were diagnosed: 4 adenomas, 4 mixed tumors, 26 adenocarcinomas, and 1 carcinoma. In cats, 30 salivary gland tumors were found among 4762 tumors of all types.[9-11] Other surveys reported 1043 canine oropharyngeal tumors with 14 adenocarcinomas.[12-14] Nine adenocarcinomas of minor glands in the cheek and gum were recorded among 395 feline oropharyngeal neoplasms; another study postulated that 9 palatine adenocarcinomas may have origins in nasal glands.[15,16]

A review of the diagnoses made on 245 specimens of salivary glands reported 41 of 160 salivary glands from dogs had a malignant primary neoplasm (38 adenocarcinoma/carcinoma and 3 malignant mixed tumors); whereas 36 of 85 glands from cats had primary neoplasms (1 papillary adenoma, 2 adenoma/cystadenoma, and 33 adenocarcinoma/carcinoma).[17] Secondary neoplasia was seen in one cat (fibrosarcoma) and six dogs (lymphoma). The salivary gland of origin could not be determined for all these tumors, but the mandibular gland was most commonly involved, then the parotid, and least commonly the dispersed salivary tissue of the oropharynx, including the minor glands of the tongue. A survey of the literature reported 72 salivary gland tumors in dogs, 48 in cats, 16 in horses, 10 in cattle and 4 in sheep.[19]

Salivary gland tumors are usually unilateral, although the major glands are paired. In the benign form the organ of origin is easily located, the tumor being surrounded by the surviving normal salivary gland; but malignant tumors may obliterate the gland of origin and even extend to involve other adjacent salivary glands, making their origin problematic.

Despite the fact that there are differences in the morphology and physiology of salivary glands in males and females, no bias in the sex distribution of salivary tumors has been demonstrated. One study indicated that many dogs of British ancestry, particularly spaniels, are affected, but locally popular breeds such as boxer, dachshund, and German shepherds were not.[20] Other authors have not confirmed this suggestion.

Classification

The classification used here is similar to that used in the second edition of the WHO sponsored *International Histological Classification of Salivary Gland Tumors*.[21,22] The main changes from the first edition are that Primary Benign Epithelial Tumors have expanded from Pleomorphic and Monomorphic Adenomas to a list of nine headings; the list for Malignant Epithelial Tumors has expanded from 5 to 18 headings, or even 24 headings if low, intermediate, and high grade tumors are separated; the nomenclature for Mucoepidermoid and Acinic cell neoplasms has been changed from *tumor* to *carcinoma* since these tumors are potentially malignant; the term *adenolymphoma* has been dropped in favor of *Warthin tumor* as the lymphoid tissue is not malignant.[23]

Salivary gland tumors mimic the cell type and cell patterns seen in normal salivary glands. This could be because differentiated neoplastic cells still express some of the characters of their parent cell type or because tumors arise from the pluripotential reserve or stem cells located between the intercalated ducts and the acini.[24] The tumor cells differentiate to resemble the secretary alveolar cells of the type present normally in that gland (serous acinic cell or mucinous cell tumor), into duct-like structures (adenoma basal cell tumor or adenocarcinoma), or into epithelium and myoepithelium (pleomorphic tumors); or the epithelium may show metaplasia (mucoepidermoid tumors).

Cytochemistry and immmocytochemistry should clarify the histogenesis of each tumor type, however their use has been limited in veterinary pathology. Antikeratin monoclonal antibodies have been used to demonstrate epithelium and myoepithelium in normal and neoplastic salivary glands of dogs and cats with varying degrees of success.[25,26] Surface carbohydrate antigen and lectin binding histochemistry have also been employed in studies of normal and neoplastic dog and cat salivary tissues.[26,27]

Most tumors of salivary glands in domestic animals are malignant at the time they are first detected. There are few well documented cases of benign salivary gland tumors in the veterinary literature, especially of cases that have had long-term follow-up after treatment.

Primary Benign Epithelial Tumors

Pleomorphic Adenoma

This tumor is also known as a mixed tumor because it is composed of several types of cell (epithelial, myoepithelial, and stromal). The epithelium can be in the form of ducts or more solid masses of cells with intercellular bridges or even keratinization. The myoepithelial cells are polygonal or spindle shaped with eosinophilic or sometimes clear cytoplasm; they can form a ring around the duct-like epithelium or form sheets with mucoid or myxoid ground substances, which may differentiate into cartilage. Endochondral or membranous ossification may be seen. There is not a distinct separation between epithelial, myoepithelial, and stromal areas.

This is the most common human salivary tumor, but it is rare in animals. Scattered cases in horse, ox, dog, and cat are found in the literature.[18,19,28] The fact that there are only a few cases of mixed salivary gland tumors recorded in canines is surprising considering the frequency of mixed mammary tumors.

The size of the tumor usually causes the presenting signs, but the duration and rate of growth of the tumor is seldom known. Growth by expansion may lead to a bosselated surface with a compression capsule of varying thickness. A wide excision margin is difficult and recurrence is common. Because of the variable tumor pattern and the fact that some previously benign tumors developed malignant foci, several blocks should be examined histologically to make a correct diagnosis.

Oncocytoma (Oxyphil or Oncocytic Adenoma)

The neoplastic cells have a characteristic granular cytoplasm and are believed to be derived by metaplasia from epithelial cells. Other cells with nearly identical eosinophilic granular cytoplasm have been shown by electron microscopy and immunohistochemistry to be of muscle origin.[29] It is a rare tumor in humans and animals. A case with two postsurgical recurrences in the parotid region of a 5-year-old male cat has been recorded.[30]

The tumor is composed of solid masses, trabeculae, or even tubules set in a delicate stroma and has a thin, sometimes incomplete, capsule. The capsule differentiates it from multifocal oncocytic adenomatous hyperplasia. Neoplastic cells are large, round, closely packed and therefore polyhedral, with intensely granular eosinophilic cytoplasm and distinct cell borders. The granularity is due to numerous mitochondria filling the cytoplasm. The centrally located nuclei are usually small and dark, but sometimes chromatin granules and a nucleolus may be seen. Scattered throughout the tumors are cells with an eccentric nucleus and vacuolated cytoplasm, so-called clear cells. These cells still have traces of granular cytoplasm, thus allowing the diagnosis of clear cell oncocytoma to be made when they form the bulk of the tumor.

Canalicular Adenoma

An encapsulated tumor composed of tubules or anastomosing strands of epithelial cells set in a delicate, loose connective tissue stroma. The cells range from low cuboidal to columnar and sometimes form bilayered structures. The nuclei are basal and the cytoplasm granular or vacuolated due to secretion products. A 1.5 cm diameter tumor of this type has been reported in the right submandibular and caudal sublingual glands of a 9-year-old female cat.[31]

Sebaceous Adenoma

Sebaceous glands are present in the epithelium of the mouth and the lining of the major ducts of salivary glands in humans and may on rare occasions give rise to sebaceous neoplasms. A sebaceous adenoma on the alveolus of a 5-year-old female cat, and sebaceous nests in a squamous papilloma of the gum of a 7-year-old male cat have been reported, but there was no evidence of salivary gland origin in either case.[32]

Ductal Papilloma

Both projecting and inverted papilloma have been recorded in the human, but they are rare. Cases in the parotid duct of dogs have been reported.[18,33]

Cystadenoma

These tumors form a multicystic mass lined by well-differentiated cuboidal to columnar mucus-producing epithelium. A feline case has been recorded in the parotid gland of a 6-year-old male.[31]

Other Patterns of Benign Epithelial Tumors

There are some rare tumors in the classification system used in human medicine that have not yet been recorded in the veterinary literature.

Myoepithelioma (Myoepithelial Adenoma)

This tumor is composed of spindle shaped, plasmacytoid or epithelioid, myoepithelial cells that are positive for S-100 protein, actin, and myosin. Unlike in pleomorphic adenoma, there are no epithelial duct-like structures.

Basal Cell Adenoma

This tumor is composed of monomorphic small cells with indistinct cell borders and little cytoplasm that resemble basal cells of the lobular and lobar ducts. Unlike in pleomorphic adenomas, the various patterns of epithelial cells are separated from the stroma by a distinct PAS positive basement membrane, and there is no mucoid or myxoid tissue.

Warthin Tumor

The previously used term *adenolymphoma* is inappropriate because the lymphoid tissue is not neoplastic. It could be called a *papillary cystic adenoma lymphomatosum* because the cysts formed by a double layer of epithelium are set in stroma containing variable amounts of lymphoid tissue. The embryology of the cranial lymph nodes and the salivary glands in dogs explains why Warthin tumors have not been seen in this species.[34] Although the developing tubules of the submandibular and sublingual glands are close to the developing lymph nodes during the early stages of growth, these salivary glands are encapsulated, so lymphoid tissue can not be incorporated into the salivary gland. The lymph nodes adjacent to the parotid salivary gland sprouts are encapsulated, and the nodal hylus faces away from the salivary gland, so again a mixture of lymphoid and salivary tissue is unlikely.

Primary Malignant Epithelial Tumor

These are the most common tumors of salivary glands in dogs and cats, and the two tumors seen most frequently are acinic cell carcinomas and adenocarcinomas.

Acinic Cell Carcinoma

Some cells resembling normal acinar salivary gland cells must be found in a tumor before a diagnosis of acinic cell carcinoma can be made. This tumor is usually unicentric but may be multicentric. It has a capsule, but histologically the capsule may be incomplete, and localized infiltrative growth may be seen, hence the change in nomenclature from acinic cell tumor to acinic cell carcinoma. It is of low grade malignancy and cellular atypia, and mitotic figures are uncommon. Metastases are rare and occur late in the disease. There are five cell types, and each of these cell types can be distributed in the form of one of four growth patterns. Usually one growth pattern is dominant.

Cell Types

The five cell types seen in acinar cell carcinoma are as follows:

1. *Acinar cells.* These cells are large and round or polygonal and are arranged in small nests surrounded by a basement membrane. The cytoplasm is finely granular and basophilic or amphophilic when stained with H&E. The granules are PAS positive, diastase resistant, and do not stain with mucicarmine or alcian blue. The nuclei are round, uniform in size, small, dark, and usually eccentric. This is the most common cell type in acinic cell carcinoma.
2. *Intercalated duct-like cells.* These cells are smaller than acinar cells and are cuboidal, often being arranged around a small lumen. The cytoplasm is amphophilic to acidophilic when stained with H&E. The nuclei are similar to those in an acinar cell.
3. *Vacuolated cells.* These cells resemble acinar cells, but in the cytoplasm there are one or more vacuoles that do not stain for lipid or glycogen but may stain for mucopolysaccharide.
4. *Clear cells.* These cells have the morphology of acinar or intercalated duct-like cells, but the cytoplasm does not stain with H&E, and special stains do not reveal fat, mucus, or glycogen.
5. *Nonspecific glandular cells.* These pleuripotential stem cells appear to form a syncytium because they have no distinct cell borders. The cytoplasm is amphophilic when stained with H&E, and the nuclei are larger than those of the other cell types and are vesicular and pleomorphic.

Growth Patterns

Acinic cell carcinoma exhibits four growth patterns:

1. *Solid.* This is the most common growth pattern. It consists of a uniform field of tumor cells supported by a sparse vascular stroma, sometimes grouping the cells in an organoid pattern.
2. *Microcystic.* The tumor cells surround cysts 3–10 times the size of acinar cells. The cysts contain proteinaceous or mucinous material.
3. *Papillary cystic.* The tumor cells surround larger cysts and extend as fingers and papillary projections into the lumen.
4. *Follicular.* Cuboidal to low columnar cells line cysts of varying size resembling the appearance of the thyroid. Between the cysts there may be packets of tumor cells.

Of 72 salivary gland tumors reported in dogs, 21 were acinic cell carcinomas.[19] The age of the dogs ranged from 3 to 15 years (mean 9.5), and the site distribution was 10 in parotid gland, 3 in sublingual gland, 2 each in the mandibular gland and gum, and 1 each in lip, tongue, and larynx. In all cases there was local invasive growth, and two had pulmonary metastases. No breed or sex predisposition was apparent. The majority were of acinar cell, solid pattern, but one case was almost exclusively composed of clear cells of the hypernephroma type,[18] and a 1 cm tumor on the tongue was a microcystic clear cell variant.[35] The size of the tumor at diagnosis varied, the largest was 5–8 cm and was in the parotid and mandibular glands, while those in the mouth were only 1–2 cm when first noticed.

Three of 48 salivary gland tumors in cats were acinic cell carcinoma; 2 were in the parotid, and 1 in the mandibular gland. Three of 10 salivary gland tumors recorded in cattle were acinic cell carcinoma. Two were in the parotid gland and had metastasized to the drainage lymph node, and another had invaded the mandible from the gum. Single, locally invasive, cases have been reported in the parotid gland of a horse and a sheep.

Mucoepidermoid Carcinoma

This tumor is a mixture of squamous epidermoid cells, mucus-producing cells, and intermediate type cells. Since these cell types occur in different proportions in the one tumor, several sections may have to be examined before all three components are found.

There is a range in the degree of malignancy expressed by mucoepidermoid tumors from low grade (well differentiated) to high grade (poorly differentiated). This behavioral classification is based on the number of well-differentiated mucous cells, the degree of differentiation of the epidermoid cells, anaplasia, and the growth pattern (all are poorly encapsulated, but the margins vary from broad "pushing" invasion to infiltrative growth). Those with infiltrative growth frequently metastasize and often recur after incomplete removal.

Both the mucous and the epidermoid cells occur as solid masses or form the lining of cysts and may protrude as papillae into the cyst lumen. If the cysts rupture, they provoke a granulomatous inflammatory reaction with foreign body giant cells and cholesterol clefts. The vacuoles seen in the mucous cells with H&E staining react positively with mucicarmine, alcian blue, or PAS. The epidermoid cells rarely keratinize, and there are therefore few epithelial pearls; but intercellular bridges should be demonstrable, and the cells are positive for epithelial membrane antigen. Some clear cells do not stain for mucus, and these represent hydropic change in epidermoid cells. The intermediate cells are smaller than the other two types with hyperchromic nuclei and form solid masses or strata several cells thick under the lining of the cysts.

In a review of salivary gland tumors in animals, 6 of 72 canine cases were mucoepidermoid carcinoma, 4 in the parotid gland, and 1 each in the mandibular gland and palate.[19] The age at diagnosis ranged from 5 to 14 years (mean 9.2). In four dogs, there was local invasive growth, with metastasis to the drainage lymph node in three and to distant organs in two. A parotid mucoepidermoid carcinoma in a 12-year-old cat had metastatic foci in the lung.[20]

Cystadenocarcinoma

These are rare adenocarcinomas in which cysts are a dominant feature. Many of the cysts are filled with papillae. Infiltrative growth, nuclear pleomorphism, and numerous mitoses differentiate it from cystadenoma.

A possible case has been described as a cystic mass arising from the zygomatic gland or duct of an 8-year-old Labrador male.[36] There were large areas of necrosis and, in the loose stroma, foci of hyalin and mineralized collagen; some cells were ciliated, and no metastases were found at necropsy.

Mucinous adenocarcinoma is another recently categorized entity in human medicine. Mucus production is the main feature, such that some of the cysts have a flattened lining, and pools of mucin appear to lie in the fibrous stroma.

Adenocarcinoma

This is a tumor with a variety of glandular patterns that exhibit cytological features of malignancy and have infiltrative borders. The predominant pattern may be acinar, ductular, trabecular (small strands), or solid masses, but usually examples of each growth pattern can be found. The term is used for those tumors that do not have the diagnostic criteria of the subtypes of glandular tumors detailed elsewhere in this classification.

There are 74 published records of salivary gland tumors in dogs for which the type, site, age, breed, and sex has been specified, and of these 23 proved to be adenocarcinoma, 11 in the parotid, 5 mandibular, 3 sublingual, 2 pharynx, and 1 involving both parotid and mandibular glands. The age range was 3–15 years (mean 10 years). No breed or sex predisposition was apparent. All 23 were locally invasive, 5 had spread to the local lymph node, and 2 to both draining lymph nodes and lung. There are reports of these tumors metastasizing to bone and eye.[37,38] A TNM staging system was applied to three canine cases of parotid adenocarcinoma that were given orthovoltage radiation therapy.[39]

Thirty-three of 48 salivary gland tumors in cats were adenocarcinoma,[19] and the site distribution was 12 parotid, 13 mandibular, 3 cheek, 2 pharynx, and 1 each in lip, larynx, and sublingual gland. There was no sex or breed predisposition, and the age range was 8–15 years (mean 12.3 years). All had a locally invasive growth pattern, 11 had spread to the local lymph node, and in 7 there were widespread metastases. These findings are similar to those in a previous report on diseases of the salivary glands: 31 of 36 tumors were adenocarcinoma/carcinoma; the mandibular gland was involved most often and then the parotid.[17] It is important in cats with an adenocarcinoma involving the parotid region to check the external auditory meatus as this may be the site of a primary tumor that has invaded the salivary gland. A case report of a tumor in the mandible of a 13-year-old domestic shorthair cat detailed how transmission electron microscopy and immunocytochemistry (positive reaction for cytokeratin and negative for vimentin and actin) established that the tumor was of ductular rather than myoepithelial origin.[40]

A few cases have been recorded in other species.[19] Six of 14 equine salivary gland tumors were adenocarcinomas, and the sites, where known, were three in the parotid and one in the mandibular gland, and the age range was 7–18 years (mean 11.8). One adenocarcinoma of the sublingual gland in an adult cow was found in 10 cattle salivary gland tumors.[42]

Malignant Myoepithelioma (Myoepithelial Carcinoma)

This is a rare tumor in humans. It has similar cell types to those seen in myoepithelioma, but the cells have features of malignancy, and there is an infiltrative growth pattern. There is one report in a dog.[33]

Carcinoma in Pleomorphic Adenoma (Malignant Mixed Tumor)

This is a salivary gland tumor that has developed a malignant epithelial component in a previously benign pleomorphic adenoma. It is rare for this to be a carcinosarcoma; most cases are examples of adenocarcinoma, mucoepidermoid carcinoma, squamous cell carcinoma, or malignant myoepithelioma developing in a pleomorphic adenoma. The longer a pleomorphic adenoma is left untreated, the greater the chance of malignancy developing, and if the new clone of cells grows rapidly, there may be difficulty in finding the benign mixed component. Reports in the veterinary literature note the mixed nature of the tumor cells and the malignant behavior of the tumor rather than whether it arose in a benign pleomorphic adenoma.

Three of 72 canine salivary gland tumors fall into this category.[19] They occurred in dogs 4–13 years old; one involved both zygomatic and parotid glands, the other two were located in the mandibular gland and in the pharynx. All were locally invasive, one recurred three times after surgery, and one metastasized to the draining lymph node.

Two cases have been reported in 49 cat tumors.[19] A tumor in the submandibular salivary gland of a 12-year-old cat was a true carcinosarcoma having sarcomatous and adenocarcinomatous elements as well as cartilage and bone.[28] The second tumor was in the submandibular gland of a 6-year-old cat; the tumor had myoepithelium, bone, cartilage, and areas showing a mucoepidermoid pattern.[41]

Of the 10 well-documented bovine salivary gland tumors, 3 were malignant mixed tumors.[19] All were in the parotid gland of old cows, and all spread to local and dis-tant lymph nodes. Electron microscopy of two other cases confirmed the presence of myoepithelial and serous-secreting epithelial cells.[42]

Squamous Cell Carcinoma

The tumor pattern may range from masses of squamous epidermoid cells with intercellular bridges to desmoplastic well-differentiated squamous cell carcinoma with keratin pearls. There are few unequivocal cases of primary salivary gland squamous cell carcinoma in the veterinary literature.[1,18,20,42] The presence of salivary gland tissue in a squamous cell carcinoma does not prove salivary origin; the salivary gland may have been infiltrated by an adjacent primary tumor in the eye or lingual glands in the tongue (cats) or pharyngeal glands from the tonsil (dogs). Mucoepidermoid carcinoma must be excluded by careful search of several slides stained for mucus. Care must be taken to recognize nonneoplastic reactive ductal change. Patchy hyperplasia and squamous metaplasia of interlobular ducts may be induced by vitamin A deficiency and highly chlorinated naphthalene poisoning. Similar changes are seen in ducts at the periphery of necrotic tissue in salivary gland infarction in dogs and cats.[17,48]

Undifferentiated Carcinoma

This diagnostic category should be reserved for those tumors that, after careful search of several slides, have no areas of recognizable differentiation except that of being of epithelial origin. Of the 72 canine salivary gland tumors in one review, 8 were undifferentiated carcinomas; the age range was 7–13 years.[19] Three occurred in the mandibular gland and one each in the parotid, buccal, gingival, lingual, and pharyngeal glands. In one there was extensive invasion into the mandible causing osteolysis, four metastasized to the drainage lymph nodes, and in two there was widespread metastasis. An unusual case in a 5-year-old dog metastasized widely and extended into the brain by local invasive growth, replacing the pituitary and leading to adrenocortical, testicular, and thyroid atrophy.[43]

Three of the 14 equine cases, 2 of the 10 bovine cases, and 2 of the 4 tumors in sheep were classified as undifferentiated carcinomas[19].

Other Patterns of Carcinoma

There are some malignant epithelial tumors that have been characterized in human medicine but have not yet been described in the veterinary literature.

Adenoid Cystic Carcinoma

This neoplasm resembles a basal cell tumor with an infiltrative edge, that is, it is a basal cell carcinoma with some glandular differentiation. Each tumor is predominantly formed by either solid (basaloid) masses or by glandular or tubular structures, and areas of all three growth patterns may be found in one tumor.

Polymorphous Low-Grade Adenocarcinoma

The characteristic feature of this tumor is various growth patterns in one tumor, namely, solid lobular, papillary cystic, cribriform trabecular, and tubular.

Epithelial-Myoepithelial Carcinoma

This is a rare tumor composed of duct-like structures of small dark cuboidal cells set in lobules of clear myoepithelial cells. Peripheral invasive growth can give rise to metastases and recurrence.

Basal Cell Adenocarcinoma

Like the basal cell adenoma the tumor masses are composed of small round cells with little cytoplasm and small dark nuclei; sometimes the peripheral cells form a palisade. This rare tumor, unlike the basal cell adenoma, exhibits many mitoses and is locally infiltrative; therefore, recurrence is common, but metastases are rare.

Sebaceous Carcinoma, Oncocytic Carcinoma, and Salivary Duct Carcinoma

These rare tumors are differentiated from sebaceous adenoma, oncocytoma, and ductal papilloma by infiltrative growth and the presence of cellular atypia and mitotic figures.

Small Cell Carcinoma

Like the small cell carcinoma of the lung, this tumor is composed of sheets of small darkly staining cells with little cytoplasm that may contain neuroendocrine granules.

Other Tumors and Tumor-Like Lesions

Lipomatosis

The stroma of salivary glands contains many cell lineages each of which can theoretically give rise to a tumor, but only a few such tumors have been reported in the veterinary literature. There are no records of salivary gland liposarcoma in animals, and it is probable that cases reported as lipoma were examples of lipomatosis. *Lipomatosis* (fatty infiltration or lipomatous infiltration) is a progressive, slowly growing, unilateral mass, sometimes with a thin capsule separating it from the surviving normal gland. Histologically the lesion differs from a lipoma in that the lobules of well-differentiated fat cells are interspersed with groups of normal salivary glands. Seven cases have been described in dogs, three in the parotid and four in the submandibular glands.[44,45] The age at surgery ranged from 4 to 14 years (mean 8 years). Two dogs were followed for 6 years without evidence of recurrence. In none of these cases were lipomatous masses found elsewhere in the body.

Postinflammatory lipomatosis (parenchymatous atrophy) should be distinguished from lipoma and lipomatosis. The acute phase of sialadenitis is unlikely to be confused with these conditions; however, for unknown reasons, in the healing phase there is lobule for lobule replacement of the gland by adipose tissue, leading to gland enlargement. Such cases can be recognized histologically by the presence of atrophic acini, foci of inflammatory cells, and areas of fibrosis.

Lymphoma

Salivary glands may contain lymphoma due to direct extension from an adjacent neoplastic lymph node or from neoplastic transformation of the lymphocytes of the mucosal associated lymphoid tissue normally scattered through the stroma and in the epithelium.

Mast Cell Tumor

A mast cell tumor nodule was found in the mandibular salivary gland of a 9-year-old English setter that had, in addition, three subcutaneous mast cell tumors and a tumor cell in the retropharyngeal lymph node.[46]

Melanomas

Melanomas occur in salivary glands due to extension from a local melanotic tumor, as part of a widespread systemic disease (often seen in the parotid gland of old gray horses with melanomas), or the salivary gland may be the primary site.[18]

Sialadenosis

Sialadenosis describes a noninflammatory, nonneoplastic usually bilateral, enlargement of salivary glands. The enlargement is due to serous acinar hypertrophy, with the nuclei displaced to the basal part of the cells. Although there may be interstitial edema and slight compression atrophy of the ducts, there are no other signs of past or present inflammation. It has been reported in the parotid of a sheep.[19]

Hyperplastic Lesions

Hyperplastic foci may not cause enlargement of the gland. The cells resemble normal cells, and the lesion is not encapsulated. Microscopic ductal hyperplasia has been described in an apparently normal parotid salivary gland of a 10-year-old bull.[1] Larger masses may interfere with swallowing, as in the case of a pendulous hyperplastic mass hanging between the tonsils of a 3-year-old collie.[47]

Salivary Gland Infarction

Necrotizing sialometaplasia is the term used in human medicine for this condition to stress the marked squamous metaplasia of the ducts, which might be mistaken for a well-differentiated squamous cell carcinoma (fig. 8.8) except that there is no cellular atypia, no kera-

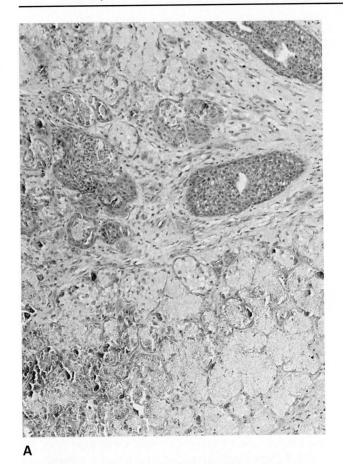

A

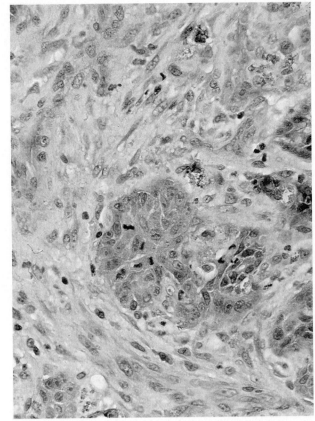

B

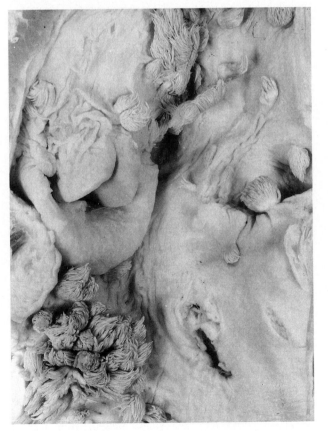

C

Fig. 8.8. **A.** Salivary gland infarction in an 11-month-old dog with areas of necrosis and ductular hyperplasia. **B.** Higher magnification of ducts lined by multiple layers of squamous epithelium. **C.** Infectious papillomas in the oropharynx of a young dog.

tinization, and no infiltration of tissues.[48] Retrospective reviews of cases of salivary squamous cell carcinoma and mucoepidermoid carcinoma indicated they were actually infarcts of the salivary gland with marked squamous metaplasia of salivary ducts. Twenty cases of salivary gland infarction were reported in a review of 245 salivary gland lesions examined over 41 months.[17] Eleven of these were from 85 cat specimens and 9 from 160 dog samples. All were in the mandibular gland except one in the sublingual gland. There was no obvious sex or age predisposition.

The condition is unilateral. An incisional biopsy of the enlarged hardened gland is needed to ensure a correct diagnosis. There is extensive coagulation necrosis in the gland, and in this necrotic tissue are arteries with fibrinoid necrosis and thrombosis. Between the necrotic and viable tissue there is a zone of edematous, congested, and hemorrhagic connective tissue infiltrated by neutrophils and macrophages. Most cases have some fibroblasts, and the surviving ducts are lined by up to six layers of hyperplastic cells, or cells that have undergone metaplasia to nonkeratinized squamous cells (fig. 8.8). Unlike in epithelial tumors, the ducts in salivary gland necrosis remain as distinct isolated structures and do not proliferate into a coalescing mass. Uneventful recovery follows complete excision of the gland; alternatively, the condition is said to respond to antiinflammatory drug therapy. It is not known whether the thrombosed vessels are the cause or the result of the necrosis.[48] The etiology of salivary gland necrosis is unknown; some authors have suggested that the vascular damage and necrosis is initiated by trauma,[17] while others believe that afferent vagal reflex may be involved.[49]

Salivary Gland Cysts

Salivary gland cysts are formed when the rate of secretion exceeds the rate of drainage and reabsorption. Aspiration of the cyst may yield a fluid that resembles the secretion from the mucus glands, hence the term for a mucus-containing cyst is *mucocoele*. When the fluid is similar to the secretion from the serous glands, one can use the term *serocoele*. However, the fluid may be unlike normal saliva because of the altered gland secretion or because of autodigestion, so the term sialocoele can be used to cover all examples of salivary gland cysts. Clinically, the anatomical location is appended to this term, for example, labial, palatine, parotid, zygomatic, cervical, or sublingual (also called a ranula because it resembles the belly of a small frog). The only way to differentiate with certainty between a true cyst, a pseudocyst, and a cystic tumor is by histological examination of the excised specimen.

Extravasated Pseudocyst (Sialocoele)

Extravasated pseudocyst is a fluid-filled structure lined by granulation tissue infiltrated by lymphocytes, plasma cells, macrophages, and giant cells. In dogs and cats it is usually unilateral and unilocular. It is seldom the result of rupture of the main duct; usually the rupture occurs in small ducts or in lobules of glands that do not have a thick capsule.[19] Leakage of saliva into adjacent tissues stimulates inflammation and fibrosis. In dogs both cervical and sublingual sialocoeles arise from damage to lobules of the diffuse (anterior) sublingual gland. Cats also develop extravasated cysts, but less commonly than dogs. In cattle, these cysts are found along the sides of the tongue, possible causes being trauma, calculi, and foreign bodies such as grass seeds.

True Salivary Cysts

True salivary cysts are less frequent than pseudocysts, and the critical distinction is that the fluid filled cavity is lined by epithelium, which grows to keep pace with the accumulation of the secretion. The cysts can range in size from a small retention cyst lined by a single layer of cells to larger cysts that may be lined by bistratified epithelium of interlobular duct type or by nonkeratinized stratified squamous epithelium, as in excretory ducts. Cystic dilation to the whole gland system, caused by atresia of the opening of the parotid duct, has been recorded in a 1-year-old horse.[50] Likewise, developmental defects were thought to be the cause of unilateral cysts extending to the parotid

glands of five Anglo-Nubian goats, 7 weeks to 15 months old.[51] Cystic dilatation of occluded ducts may be acquired later in life and has been associated with oral necrosis caused by chronic renal failure that subsequently blocked the submandibular duct, and with scar tissue that constricted the parotid duct following caudal maxillectomy.[52]

Branchial Cysts

Branchial cysts are not derived from salivary glands, but from remnants of the fetal pharyngeal pouches that persist as cysts lined by nonkeratinizing stratified squamous or columnar ciliated epithelium. These cysts may be associated with lymphoid tissue since their precursor structures are concerned in the formation of tonsil and thymus. Branchial cysts have been described in a 10-year-old dog[53] and in an 8-month-old heifer.[54]

TNM Classification

Neoplasia of the minor salivary glands is classified as for tumors of the lip and oropharynx. There are no published articles dealing with the staging of major salivary gland tumors of domestic animals, presumably because there are too few case history follow-up studies. The rules for the staging of carcinoma of the major salivary glands in the human have been published,[22] and these were used in three dogs treated with radiation therapy.[39]

T_0 represents an occult primary, the presence of which is detected because of secondary tumors. N_0 implies no nodal metastases, that is, the drainage lymph nodes are not enlarged or fixed. M_0 indicates no distant metastases detected. When the T,N, or M status can not be assessed, the symbols $T_x N_x$ and M_x are used.

The categories T_1 to T_4 are based on tumor size and degree of local extension. The presence of tumor extension is judged firstly on the loss of mobility of the tumor both on the underlying soft tissue or bone and on the overlying soft tissue and skin. Secondly, extension is suspected if there is loss of function of the adjacent nerves.

In humans there are 12 named cervical regional lymph node sites with multiple nodes at most sites, so the N_1 to N_3 categories are based on the number and size of the nodes that are involved as well as the location of the affected nodes (ipsilateral, contralateral, or bilateral). The anatomy of the nodes and the drainage pattern of the lymphatic system in domestic animals differs from that of humans. In the horse and pig, groups of nodes occur, whereas in the ox, sheep, dog, and cat there are usually from one to four discrete structures at each site. In the horse the mandibular, parapharyngeal, and suprapharyngeal lymph node groups should be considered as sites of metastases; in the other species the mandibular, parotid, and suprapharyngeal lymph nodes; and in ruminants the atlantal.

The extent of the tumor is expressed by grouping the TNM categories into four stages ranging from stage I (T_1, N_0, M_0) to Stage IV (Any T, Any N, M_1).

REFERENCES

1. Head, K.W. (1976) International histological classification of tumors of domesticated animals. XI. Tumors of the upper alimentary tract. *Bull WHO* 53:145–166.

2. Reifel, C.W., and Travill, A.A. (1972) Structure and carbohydrate histochemistry of postnatal canine salivary glands. *Amer J Anat* 134:377–393.

3. Anderson, L.J., Sandison, T.A., and Jarrett, W.F.H. (1969) A British abattoir survey of tumors in cattle, sheep and pigs. *Vet Rec* 84:547–551.

4. Head, K.W. (1990) Tumors in sheep. *Practice* 12:68–80.

5. Sundberg, J.P., Bumstein, T., et al. (1977) Neoplasms of Equidae. *J Amer Vet Med Assoc* 170:150–152.

6. Stackhouse, L.L., Moore, J.J., and Hylton, W.E. (1978) Salivary gland carcinoma in a mare. *J Amer Vet Med Assoc* 172:271–273.

7. Baker, J.R., and Leyland, A. (1975) Histological survey of tumours of the horse, with particular reference to those of the skin. *Vet Rec* 96:419–422.

8. MacVean, D.W., Moulux, A.W., et al. (1978) Frequency of canine and feline tumors in a defined population. *Vet Pathol* 15:700–715.

9. Bastianello, S.S. (1983) A survey of neoplasia in domestic species over a 40 year period from 1935 to 1974 in the Republic of South Africa. V. Tumors occurring in the cat. *Onderstepoort J Vet Res* 50:105–110.

10. Bastianello, S.S. (1983) A survey on neoplasia in domestic species over a 40 year period from 1935 to 1974 in the Republic of South Africa. VI. Tumors occurring in dogs. *Onderstepoort J Vet Res* 50:199–220.

11. Carberry, C.A., Flanders, J.A., Harvey, H.J., and Ryan, A.M. (1988) Salivary gland tumours in dogs and cats: A literature and case review. *J Amer Anim Hosp Assoc* 24:561–567.

12. Brodey, R.S. (1970) The Biological behavior of canine oral and pharyngeal neoplasm. *J Small Anim Pract* 11:45–53.

13. Dorn, C.R., and Priester, W.A. (1976) Epidemiologic analysis of oral and pharyngeal cancer in dogs, cats, horses and cattle. *J Amer Vet Med Assoc* 169:1202–1206.

14. Vos, J.H., and van der Gaag, I. (1987) Canine and feline oral-pharyngeal tumors. *J Amer Vet Med Assoc* 34:420–427.

15. Kapatkin, A.S., Marretta, S.M., et al. (1991) Mandibular swellings in cats: Prospective study of 24 cats. *J Amer Anim Hosp Assoc* 27:575–580.

16. Stebbins, K.E., Morse, C.C. and Goldschmidt, M.H. (1989) Feline oral neoplasia: A ten-year survey. *Vet Pathol* 26:121–128.

17. Spangler, W.L., and Culbertson, M.R. (1991) Salivary gland disease in dogs and cats: 245 cases (1985–1988) *J Amer Vet Med Assoc* 198:465–469.

18. Koestner, A., and Buerger, L. (1965) Primary neoplasms of the salivary glands in animals compared to similar tumors in man. *Pathol Vet* 2:201–226.

19. Head, KW. (1995) Salivary gland disease in domestic animals. In de Burgh Norman, J.E., and McGurk, M. (eds.) *Salivary Glands: Color Atlas & Text,* Ch. 17. Mosby-Wolfe, pp. 367–389.

20. Karbe, E., and Schiefer, B. (1967) Primary salivary gland tumors in carnivores. *Can Vet J* 8:212–215.

21. Thackray, A.C., and Sobin, L.H. (1972) Histological Typing of Salivary Gland Tumors. International Histological Classification of Tumors No. 7. World Health Organization, Geneva.

22. Seifert, G. (1991) *Histological Typing of Salivary Gland Tumours,* 2nd ed. SpringerVerlag, London.

23. Seifert, G,, Brocheriou, C., Cardesa, A., and Eveson, J.W. (1990) WHO international histological classification of tumours. Tentative histological classification of salivary gland tumours. *Pathol Res Pract* 186:555–581.

24. Chaudhry, A.P., Cutler, L.S., et al. (1986) Histogenesis of acinic cell carcinoma of the major and minor salivary glands: An ultrastructural study. *J Pathol* 148:307–320.

25. Desnoyers, M.M., Haines, D.M., and Searcy, G.P. (1990) Immunohistochemical detection of intermediate filament proteins in formalin fixed normal and neoplastic canine tissues. *Can J Vet Res* 54:360–365.

26. Sozmen, M., Brown, P.J., Eveson, J.W., and Scott, H.W. (1998) Epithelial-myoepithelial carcinoma of the salivary gland in two cats. *Eur J Vet Pathol* 4:93–96.

27. Haines, D.M., Matte, G., et al. (1989) Immunohistochemical staining and radionuclide imaging of canine tumors, using a monoclonal antibody recognizing a synthetic carbohydrate antigen. *Amer J Vet Res* 50:875–881.

28. Wells, G.A.H., and Robinson, M. (1975) Mixed tumour of salivary gland showing histological evidence of malignancy in a cat. *J Comp Pathol* 85:77–85.

29. Tang, K.N., Mansell, J.L., Herron, A.J., and Sangster, L.T. (1994) The histologic, ultrastructural and immunohistological characteristics of a thyroid oncocytoma in a dog. *Vet Pathol* 31:269–271.

30. Case, M.T., and Simon, J. (1966) Oncocytomas in a cat and a dog. *Vet Med* 61:41–43.

31. Holzworth, J. (1987) Tumours of salivary glands. In Holzworth, J. (ed.), *Diseases of the Cat: Medicine and Surgery,* Vol. 1. W.B. Saunders, Philadelphia, pp. 489–492.

32. Levene, A. (1984) Sebaceous gland differentiation in tumours of the feline oral mucosa. *Vet Rec* 114:69.

33. Gorlin, R.J., Barron, C.N., et al. (1959) The oral and pharyngeal pathology of domestic animals: A study of 487 cases. *Amer J Vet Res* 20:1032–1061.

34. Karbe, E. (1965) Lateral neck cysts in the dog. *Amer J Vet Res* 36:717–722.

35. Brunnert, S.R., and Altman, N.H. (1990) Canine lingual acinic cell carcinoma (clear cell variant) of minor salivary gland. *Vet Pathol* 27:203–205.

36. Buynkmihci, N., Rubin, L.F., and Harvey, C.E. (1975) Exophthalmos secondary to zygomatic adenocarcinoma in a dog. *J Amer Vet Med Assoc* 167:162–165.

37. Grevel, V., Schmidt, S., and Mettler, F. (1978) Multiple bone metastases of a salivary gland carcinoma in the dog. *Schweiz Arch Tierheilk* 120:13–22.

38. Habin, D.J., and Else, R.W. (1995) Parotid salivary gland adenocarcinoma with bilateral ocular and osseous metastases in a dog. *J Small Anim Pract* 36:445–449.

39. Evans, S.M., and Thrall, E.D. (1983) Postoperative orthovoltage radiation therapy of parotid salivary gland adenocarcinoma in three dogs. *J Amer Vet Med Assoc* 182:993–994.

40. Burek, K.A., Munn, R.J., and Madewell, B.R. (1994) Metastatic adenocarcinoma of a minor salivary gland in a cat. *J Amer Vet Med Assoc* 41:485–490.

41. Carpenter, J.L., and Bernstein, M. (1991) Malignant mixed (pleomorphic) mandibular salivary gland tumor in a cat. *J Amer Anim Hosp Assoc* 27:581–583.

42. Bundza, A. (1983) Primary salivary gland neoplasia in three cows. *J Comp Pathol* 93:629–632.

43. Bright, J. McI., Bright, R.M., and Mays, M.C. (1983) Parotid carcinoma with multiple endocrinopathies in a dog. *Compend Contin Educ* 5:728–734.

44. Brown, P.J., Lucke, V.M., et al. (1997) Lipomatous infiltration of the canine salivary gland. *J Small Anim Pract* 38:234–236.

45. Bindseil, E., and Madsen, J.S. (1997) Lipomatosis causing tumorlike swelling of a mandibular salivary gland in a dog. *Vet Rec* 140:583–584.

46. Carberry, C.A., Flanders, J.A., Anderson, W.I., and Harvey, H.J. (1987) Mast cell tumor in the mandibular salivary gland in a dog. *Cornell Vet* 77:362–366.

47. Borthwick, R., Else, R.W., and Head, K.W. (1982) Neoplasia and allied conditions of the canine oropharynx. In Grunsell, C.S.G., and Hill, F.W.G. (eds.), *The Veterinary Annual,* 22nd ed. Scientechnia, Bristol, pp. 248–269.

48. Kelly, D.F., Lucke, V.M., Denny, H.R., and Lane, J.G. (1979) His-

tology of salivary gland infarction in the dog. *Vet Pathol* 16:438–443.

49. Schroeder, H., and Berry, W.L. (1998) Salivary gland necrosis in dogs: A retrospective study of 19 cases. *J Small Anim Pract* 39:121–125.

50. Fowler, M.E. (1965) Congenital atresia of the parotid duct in a horse. *J Amer Vet Med Assoc* 146:1403–1404.

51. Brown, P.J., Lance, J.G., and Lucke V.M. (1989) Developmental cysts in the upper neck of Anglo-Nubian goats. *Vet Rec* 125:256–258.

52. Muir, P., and Rosin, E. (1995) Parotid duct obstruction after caudal maxillectomy in a dog. *Vet Rec* 136:46.

53. Karbe, E., and Nielsen, S.W. (1965) Branchial cyst in a dog. *J Amer Vet Med Assoc* 147:637–640.

54. Smith, D.F., and Gunson, D.E. (1977) Branchial cyst in a heifer. *J Amer Vet Med Assoc* 171:64–65.

TUMORS OF THE MOUTH AND PHARYNX

General Considerations

Prevalence

Tumors of the mouth and pharynx have rarely been reported in the pig, and only sporadic cases have been described in the horse. In cattle and sheep there is a geographic variation in prevalence. All surveys show that they are moderately common in dogs and cats, but the frequency varies dependant on the population from which the cases are drawn. Analysis of data from a defined population of healthy and sick dogs demonstrated a frequency of 20 tumors per 100,000 dogs per year.[1] In contrast a prevalence rate of 335 for dogs and 230 for cats per 100,000 was found in a clinic population, presumably of mainly sick animals.[2] Analysis of data from 13 North American clinic populations gave an estimate for the crude rates of occurrence per 100,000 patient years at risk as 130 for dogs, 45 for cats, 28 for horses and 3 for oxen.[3]

Most authorities agree that squamous cell carcinoma, malignant melanoma, and fibrosarcoma are the most common malignancies found in the mouth and pharynx of dogs, but there is a variation in the order of precedence of squamous cell carcinoma and malignant melanoma.[4] Thus in the United States there was an estimate of frequency of 12.7 per 100,000 for malignant melanoma, 6.4 for squamous cell carcinoma, and 5.8 for fibrosarcoma,[5] while in the United Kingdom 41 percent of cases were squamous cell carcinoma, 26 percent fibrosarcoma, and 6 percent malignant melanoma.[6] These differences could be due to a true geographical variation in distribution or a bias in the method of recording. It has been suggested that malignant melanomas are usually advanced when first recognized and are not referred to a treatment center; therefore they would not figure in clinic records.[6] Alternatively, the explanation could lie in differences in exposure to carcinogens in different geographical areas or at different times. It has been shown that tonsillar squamous cell carcinoma was 4 times more common in southeastern England than in Melbourne, Australia, in 1984, and that it was 15 times more common in London, United Kingdom, in 1950 than in Melbourne in 1984. These differences might be due to smoke from solid fuel fires in urban areas, but there were no such differences demonstrable for squamous cell carcinoma at other sites in the mouth or for malignant melanoma, fibrosarcoma, or other malignant neoplasms.[7]

Diagnosis and Clinical Staging

The presenting signs include ptyalism, dysphagia, halitosis, hemorrhage, displacement or loss of teeth, and facial swelling. Most animals with oral tumors have a short history of illness (less than 3 months), and other tumors are incidental findings. Adequate sampling often requires a general anesthetic and deep wedge biopsies that penetrate below the surface ulceration, where reaction to secondary infection can mask the true nature of the tumor. Radiography should indicate any bone involvement and all except early lung metastases (under 0.5 cm).[8]

In order to compare the results of various treatment regimes, it is important to ensure that each case in a series is at a similar clinical stage in the progress of the disease. A WHO committee set out the rules for the TNM staging of some tumors in domestic animals, and this system has been used in an increasing number of articles and has been reproduced for the mouth and pharynx.[6,9] The mouth and pharynx are dealt with by three protocols, one each for the lips (upper and lower labia), the oral cavity, and the oropharynx. The oral cavity covers the cheeks (buccae), gums (gingiva), hard palate, floor of the mouth, and anterior two-thirds of the tongue; because the problems in treatment of tumors in soft tissues differ from those in bone, the T categories are divided into those with and without bone invasion. The oropharynx extends from the level of the junction of the hard and soft palate to the larynx and esophagus, and unlike the other two protocols, it is designed for equine as well as canine and feline tumors. This third protocol includes the tonsil as well as the posterior third of the tongue and accordingly has a separate category for "tumor with invasion of the tonsil only."

Treatment

Treatments for oral and pharyngeal malignancy include surgery, cryosurgery, chemotherapy, radiotherapy, hyperthermia, immunotherapy, and photodynamic therapy, either alone or in combination.[10] The method of treatment appropriate in a particular case depends on the patient, the tumor site, the tumor type, and the owner. The value of palliative therapy in old dogs with extensive tumors of low metastatic potential should not be overlooked.[11]

Complete success of surgical excision depends on total removal of the primary tumor before metastasis has occurred. The margins of the excised lesion should therefore be examined histologically to ensure that they are free of tumor because microscopic infiltrative growth beyond the point of removal is the main cause of local recurrence.

Enlarged drainage lymph nodes should be biopsied to differentiate between metastasis and reactive hyperplasia. Maxillectomy and mandibulectomy with and without adjuvant or preceding chemotherapy/radiation therapy in dogs and cats has been summarized.[12] These authors point out that the anatomy of the tumor in the host influences the outcome more than the type of neoplasm; thus, rostral tumors have a better prognosis than caudal ones (especially if the palate is involved), dogs are better candidates than cats, and dolichocephalic/mesaticephalic breeds are better than brachycephalic.

Chemotherapy has been used more often in conjunction with surgery than as the sole method of treatment.[13] Old dogs frequently have periodontal disease, and a risk with chemotherapy is the mobilization of bacterial infection from such sites.[14] In addition, there may be damage to hematopoietic tissue.[15] The use of radiation therapy in the treatment of oral neoplasia has been described[16] both in general and for more localized sites,[17,18] as has its value with and without hyperthermia.[19] The oral complications following local radiotherapy are mucosal atrophy with subsequent bacterial infection of areas of ulceration, osteonecrosis, xerostomia (dry mouth), and caries.[14] The principles of hyperthermia as a treatment as well as mean survival times for the main oral malignancies after radiation/hyperthermia contrasted with those following radiation alone, surgery alone, and no therapy have been recorded.

Tumors of Squamous Epithelium

Tumors of Cattle, Sheep, Horses, and Pigs

The location and type of squamous epithelial tumors in the upper alimentary tract vary between species. In cattle benign and malignant epithelial tumors are found at all sites from mouth to rumen, but most occur in the esophagus and forestomachs (9 upper alimentary tract epithelial tumors, all in the esophagus and rumen, were found in a series of 606 cattle neoplasms[20]). These tumors are less common in sheep. From 129,981 sheep samples examined in United Kingdom investigation centers, 75 tumors were confirmed. Thirteen of these were in the upper alimentary tract, including one squamous cell carcinoma of the gum, one pharyngeal SSC, and two papillomas in the rumen.[21]

Squamous papillomas of the upper alimentary tract in horses are rare and are found on the lips. Eight oropharyngeal squamous cell carcinomas of 141 squamous cell carcinomas involved the oropharynx.[22] They have been reported on the tongue,[23] hard palate, gingiva, soft palate, pharynx, and guttural pouches.[24] Squamous cell carcinoma occurs in old horses in the form of a nodular ulcerated mass that is locally invasive and sometimes metastizes to the local lymph node. Tumors of the paranasal sinuses can

extend into the mouth in the molar teeth region and vice versa, making the site of origin difficult to ascertain. Once large enough to be diagnosed, squamous cell carcinomas in horses have seldom been treated.

Most pigs are slaughtered when young, so squamous cell carcinomas are unlikely to be seen. Only a few tumors of all types have been recorded in the mouth of pigs; for example, in 15,782 porcine necropsy and biopsy diagnoses only three oral tumors were seen: one ameloblastoma, one oral papilloma of a 1-week-old piglet, and one melanoma in a 2-week-old black pig that involved the tonsil and pharynx as well as many other sites.[25] Some papillary lesions are chronic inflammatory hyperplasia rather than true tumors.

REFERENCES

1. Dorn, C.R., Taylor, D.O.N., Schneider, R., Hibbard, H.H., and Klauber, M.R. (1968) Survey of animal neoplasms in Alameda and Contra Costa Counties, California. II Cancer morbidity in dogs and cats from Alameda County. *J Natl Cancer Inst* 40:307–318.
2. Brodey, R.S. (1966) Alimentary tract neoplasms in the cat: A clinicopathologic survey of 46 cats. *Amer J Vet Res* 27:74–80.
3. Dorn, C.R., and Priester, W.A. (1976) Epidemiologic analysis of oral and pharyngeal cancer in dogs, cats, horses and cattle. *J Amer Vet Med Assoc* 169:1202–1206.
4. Vos, J.H., and van der Gaag, I. (1987) Canine and feline oral-pharyngeal tumors. *J Vet Med* 34:420–427.
5. Cohen, D., Brodey, R.S., and Chen, S.M. (1964) Epidemiologic aspects of oral and pharyngeal neoplasms of the dog. *Amer J Vet Res* 25:1776–1779.
6. White, R.A.S., Jefferies, A.R., and Freedman, L.S. (1985) Clinical staging for oropharyngeal malignancies in the dog. *J Small Anim Pract* 26:581–594.
7. Bostock, D.E., and Curtis, R. (1984) Comparison of canine oropharyngeal malignancy in various geographical locations. *Vet Rec* 114:341–342.
8. Frew, D.G., and Dobson, J.M. (1992) Radiological assessment of 50 cases of incisive or maxillary neoplasia in the dog. *J Small Anim Pract* 33:11–18.
9. Hoyt, R.F., and Withrow, S.J. (1984) Oral malignancy in the dog. *J Amer Anim Hosp Assoc* 20:83–90.
10. Oakes, M.G., Lewis, D.D., Hedlund, C.S., and Hosgood, G. (1993) Canine oral neoplasia. *Comp Cont Edu Pract Vet* 15:15–30.
11. Harvey, H.J. (1985) Oral Tumors. *Vet Clin N Amer Small Anim Pract* 15:493–500.
12. Jeglum, K.A., and Sadanaga, K. (1996) Oral tumors: The surgeon and the medical oncologist. *Vet Clin N Amer Small Anim Pract* 26:145–153.
13. Hammer, A.S., and Conto, C.G. (1990) Adjuvant chemotherapy for sarcomas and carcinomas. *Vet Clin N Amer Small Anim Pract* 20:1015–1036.
14. Spodnick, G.J. (1993) Oral complications of cancer therapy and their management. *Semin Vet Med Surg (Small Anim)* 8:213–220.
15. Henry, C.J., Brewer, W.F., and Stutler, S.A. (1993) Early-onset leukopenia and severe thrombocytopenia following doxorubicin chemotherapy for tonsillar squamous cell carcinoma in a dog. *Cornell Vet* 83:163–168.
16. Burke, R.L. (1996) Radiation therapy in the treatment of oral neoplasia. *Vet Clin N Amer Small Anim Pract* 26:155–163.
17. Evans, S.M., and Shofer, F. (1988) Canine oral nontonsillar squamous cell carcinoma. *Vet Radiol* 29:133–137.

18. LaDue-Miller, T., Price, G.S., Page, R.L. and Thrall, D.E. (1996) Radiotherapy of canine non-tonsillar squamous cell carcinoma. *Vet Radiol Ultrasound* 37:74–77.
19. Page, R.L., and Thrall, D.E. (1990) Clinical indications and applications of radiotherapy and hyperthermia in veterinary oncology. *Vet Clin N Amer Small Anim Pract* 20:1075–1092.
20. Bastianello, S.S. (1982) A Survey on Neoplasia in Domestic Species over a 40 year period from 1935 to 1974 in the Republic of South Africa. I. Tumors occurring in cattle. *Onderstepoort J Vet Res* 49:195–204.
21. Ross, A.D., and Williams, P.A. (1983) Neoplasms of sheep in Great Britain. *Vet Rec* 113:598–599.
22. Schuh, J.C. (1986) Squamous cell carcinoma of the oral, pharyngeal and nasal mucosa in the horse. *Vet Pathol* 23:205–207.
23. Henson, W.R. (1939) Carcinoma of the tongue in a horse. *J Amer Vet Med Assoc* 94:124.
24. Hance, S.R., and Bertone, A.L. (1993) The equine head: Neoplasia. *Vet Clin N Amer Equine Pract* 9:213–234.
25. Fisher, L.F., and Olander, H.J. (1978) Spontaneous neoplasms of Pigs—A study of 31 cases. *J Comp Pathol* 88:505–517.

Oral Papilloma of the Dog

Age, Breed, Sex, and Sites

These tumors mainly affect young dogs (mean age of 1 year), and there is no breed or sex prevalence. Oral papillomas are almost always multiple. They affect the buccal mucosa, tongue, palate, pharynx, and epiglottis, but not the esophagus. Papillomas of the lip ordinarily grow more slowly than those of the mouth. The prevalence of oral papilloma seems to vary in some districts with time, but this may be because the lesions are easily recognized and are self-limiting, so they are not recorded.[1]

Gross Morphology and Histological Features

These neoplasms vary from white flattened smooth firm nodules a few millimeters in diameter to lesions that are gray or pink in color, up to 2 cm in diameter, and pedunculate or sessile with a cauliflower-like surface (see fig 8.8C). They grow outward (exophilic), are never inverted, and on cut surfaces have a fibrovascular core.

The pathogenesis of experimental canine oral papilloma has been described.[2] The initial change is simple hyperplasia of the epithelium. The cells of the basal layer remain normal in size, but there are increased mitotic figures here and in the thickened stratum spinosum, where the cytoplasm and nuclei of the cells increase in size. The overlying stratum corneum becomes thickened. With the epithelial proliferation the surface of the tumor is thrown into folds that contain connective tissue cores. No virus is seen at this stage, but in the next stage cells are diverted from growth into virus production. The stratum granulosum becomes more prominent, with many basophilic keratohyaline granules of varying size. Some large cells in the stratum granulosum lose their nucleoli and develop amphophilic, irregular, intranuclear inclusions that can be a single mass or multiple bodies. The cytoplasm of these cells may have an open, nonstaining appearance (balloon-ing degeneration) because of mitochondrial swelling, disruption of the endoplasmic reticulum, and failure of tonofibril and keratohyaline granules. Such cells are called koilocytes.

At this stage transmission electron microscopy shows that the intranuclear masses are packed with virions. These particles are first seen in the cells of the upper stratum spinosum. Virus soon spreads throughout the nuclei of the more superficial cells of the stratum corneum where the cells are undergoing degenerative change prior to desquamation.

Behavior

The experimental neoplasms first appear as pale smooth elevations along the lines of the scarification. In about a month the tumor reaches full size, persists for about a month, then regresses. Macroscopically, the regressing tumor darkens in color and becomes dryer, the "fingers" of the papilloma open, and the lesion shrinks; complete regression takes several weeks. Histologically, regressing papillomas lose the surface epithelium, and the central connective tissue cores become more prominent so that the lesion may resemble a fibropapilloma. This fibrovascular core becomes infiltrated with lymphocytes. Healing occurs without scar formation. Dogs in which papillomas have regressed are solidly immune to further experimental transmission. Regression is enhanced by passage of "immune" lymphocytes from dogs in which the tumor has regressed. Progression of oral papillomatosis to squamous cell carcinoma is a rare event.[3]

Etiology and Transmission

Tumors can be transmitted to scarified oral mucous membranes using whole cells or cell-free filtrates.[4,5] The incubation period of the experimental disease, 30 to 33 days, may be shorter in malnourished or sickly puppies. Canine oral papilloma virus multiplies only in the oral or pharyngeal mucosa of the domestic dog. Papillomas fail to develop when the virus is scarified into the hairy skin or vagina of the dog. The virus has been demonstrated in oral papilloma of other species in the genus *Canis* (coyotes and wolves).

Studies using immunohistochemistry and in situ hybridization to investigate canine oral papillomatosis have been summarized.[6] Immunoperoxidase techniques have been used to demonstrate papilloma group–specific antigens and papilloma virus–specific epitopes in the nuclei of the stratum granulosum in some oral papilloma and fibropapilloma. The genome of the canine oral papilloma virus has been cloned and characterized. It is one of a group of at least four papilloma viruses, each with a high degree of tissue specificity.

IgA deficiency in beagle dogs has been associated with the development of extensive oral papillomatosis. An 8-month-old Chinese shar-pei dog, which may have had a similar hereditary immunodeficiency and which had been treated with corticosteroids for demodectic mange, developed papillomata in the mouth and on the skin of the trunk and limbs.[7] The virus in the skin lesions was shown to be identical to the canine oral papillomatosis virus. The papillomas at both sites regressed after an autogenous vaccine was administered. These reports suggest immune suppression may mobilize latent papilloma virus infection and break the tissue tropism of the virus.[7]

Treatment

Live virus vaccine is very effective in protecting against natural and experimental infection, as are formalin inactivated vaccines. Some dogs developed cutaneous squamous cell carcinoma at the injection site of the live virus vaccine. It should be noted, however, that although papilloma viral antigens have been detected in canine oral papilloma and in some canine cutaneous and vulval/vaginal squamous cell carcinoma, so far they have not been found in canine oral squamous cell carcinoma.

Other Oral Papilloma

Oral papilloma in older dogs that histologically have no koilocytes and no inclusion bodies have been described.[1] Although there were many cells in mitosis, they did not exhibit cellular atypicism. Newer techniques to demonstrate papilloma virus have not yet been applied to such rare lesions.

A similar old-age squamous papilloma removed from the maxillary gum of a 7-year-old cat has been described, and this lesion was of special interest because sebaceous glands were demonstrated to be developing in the papillary epithelium.[8]

Canine Oral and Pharyngeal Squamous Cell Carcinoma

Prevalence and Site

Squamous cell carcinomas in different sites in the mouth have different behavior patterns and require different clinical management. From several sources nontonsillar squamous cell carcinoma has a prevalence rate of between 6.4 and 7.3 per 100,000. Whereas in the city of London a prevalence for tonsillar squamous cell carcinoma of 120 cases per 100,000 has been reported,[9] and in Philadelphia it was 91 per 100,000, in rural Pullman, Washington, only 2 cases were seen in 10 years in a population similar in age, breed, and sex to the Philadelphia series.[10] It is interesting that these two cases were referred from large industrial cities. The possible influence of air pollution on the high prevalence of tonsillar carcinoma in an urban environment has been discussed.

The frequency distribution at different nontonsillar sites shows that the gingiva are more often affected than the other soft tissue sites (e.g., gingivae 35–42 percent, lips 4.9–7.3 percent, tongue 1.2–4.3 percent,

palate 1.9–3.1 percent, and pharynx 1.2–1.9 percent).[12] The distribution in the upper and lower jaw and to a location rostral or caudal to the canine tooth varies between authors, but many agree that the maxilla is most frequently affected[11]; for example, one study reported 16 maxillary cases (8 rostral, 7 caudal, 1 both) and 8 mandibular (6 rostral, 2 both). Lingual squamous cell carcinomas have been reported to be distributed mainly in the mid-third (9 cases).[13]

Age, Breed, and Sex

There is a rising mean age distribution for oral malignancies as follows: squamous cell carcinoma, 8 years old; fibrosarcoma, 9 years old; osteosarcoma, 10 years old; and melanoma, 12 years old. Nontonsillar squamous cell carcinoma has a reported mean age of 8 years (range 0.4 to 14.5 years); tonsillar squamous cell carcinoma, 9.6 years (range 4 to 13 years); and tongue squamous cell carcinoma, 9.5 years (range 7 to 13 years).[13]

Although several series suggest a breed predisposition for nontonsillar squamous cell carcinoma, it seems probable that the breeds listed are those that are popular locally.[12] German shepherd dogs are high on the list of dogs with tonsillar squamous cell carcinoma, and it has been suggested that large dogs (≥ 23 kg) are twice as likely to develop nontonsillar squamous cell carcinoma than smaller dogs.[11] Dogs with a white coat color, particularly poodles, seem to be predisposed to squamous cell carcinoma of the tongue.[13,14]

No sex bias is reported in some collections of oral tumors, other reports indicate a strong male predisposition for tonsillar squamous cell carcinoma, and a few record a slight male bias for nontonsillar squamous cell carcinoma.

Gross Morphology

The early stage of tonsillar squamous cell carcinoma is rarely detected since it appears as a small granular lesion on the tonsillar surface. Later the tonsil is replaced by neoplastic tissue that occupies the entire tonsillar fossa. The tumor is gray and firm in contrast to the soft, smooth pink enlargement caused by lymphoma. The tumor forms a plaque that is sometimes ulcerated and in the form of a cauliflower-like mass. The lesion may spread to the pharyngeal wall, soft palate, and root of the tongue. The neoplasm usually involves only one tonsil but can be bilateral.

The early lesions of gingival squamous cell carcinoma are white or pink nodular masses measuring 0.5 to 1 cm in diameter along the dental arcade, and as they extend they may form either fleshy masses around the teeth, or ulcerated plaque-like lesions. Some tumors around the carnasial teeth extend onto the palate, making it difficult to decide whether the lesion originated in the gingiva or the palate. This neoplasm invades locally, destroys periodontal structures causing loosening of the teeth, and possibly stimulates osteoclasts to erode bone in front of the advancing tumor. Ulceration is often exacerbated by secondary infection. Primary tumors invading the maxilla may extend into the nasal cavity and periorbital tissue. In a frequency ranking of the various tumors that involve bones in the head of dogs, 48 squamous cell carcinomas in the maxilla and 54 in the mandible were recorded.[15]

Most lingual squamous cell carcinomas are bilaterally symetrical and variable in size: less than 2 cm to more than 4 cm.[13] In another series, 5 of the tumors were located on the ventral surface, 5 on the dorsal surface, and 11 extended through the whole thickness of the tongue.[14] This spread to involve the whole organ may be due to movement of the tongue massaging the lymphatic drainage. Labial and buccal squamous cell carcinomas are usually in the form of ulcerated plaques with slow growth and low metastatic potential.

Histological Features

Tonsillar squamous cell carcinoma arises from the epithelium of the tonsillar fossa. Cords of squamous cells invade the underlying lymphoid tissue and are accompanied by proliferation of connective tissue stroma. "Epithelial pearls" are common, and degeneration in the centers of these keratinizing invading columns may result in a pseudoglandular appearance. There are no studies on precancerous lesions to determine whether squamous metaplasia of the crypts precedes neoplasia.

Gingival squamous cell carcinoma often causes bone destruction as the tumor invades the mandible or maxilla. On the basis of radiographs it has been shown that whereas all melanomas and fibrosarcomas are osteolytic, a few squamous cell carcinomas are osteoblastic.[11]

When the growth in culture of normal canine oral keratinocytes was compared with that of neoplastic canine keratinocytes derived from a spontaneous oral squamous cell carcinoma, the squamous cell carcinoma cells grew and differentiated faster than the normal epithelium, even when the normal cells were stimulated by epidermal growth factor. Interestingly, when the squamous cell carcinoma cells grew submerged in medium they showed anisocytosis and binucleate cells, but when grown in an air-liquid interface they differentiated into well-organized, stratified squamous epithelium like normal keratinocytes, with only 5–10 percent showing whorls of basal cells as in squamous cell carcinoma.[16]

Human oral squamous cell carcinoma consists of heterogeneous cell populations with different behavior patterns, depending on the location of the tumor cells either on the deep invasive margins or in the superficial areas of the tumor.[17] When histological features were used to grade these tumors, the deep invasive margins gave better prognostic values than examination of the superficial areas. The features scored were decrease in keratinization, increase in nuclear polymorphism, change from pushing to infiltrative growth, decrease in lymphocyte/plasma cell infiltration, and increase in mitotic rate. Using a similar grading system to score 10 cases of canine lingual squamous cell carcinoma on

an increasing malignancy scale of I to III, the superficial area scored grade I and the deep layers grade III.[13]

A variant reported in the maxilla of an 18-week-old dog had normal oral mucosa merging into papillary outgrowths with thin fibrovascular cores (verrucous hyperplasia), which in turn became an "invasive carcinoma" with a low mitotic index.[18] Six months after surgery, there was no clinical or radiographic evidence of recurrence. Three other cases occurred in dogs 2 to 5 months old with "papillary squamous cell carcinoma" in the region of the canine and premolar teeth. Two exhibited invasion of the bone with osteolysis, and one had a history of an oral papilloma having been removed 2 months earlier.[19] Although invasive, the epithelium had hyperplastic features and an absence of keratin pearls. The tumors were surgically removed, and after radiotherapy the dogs remained disease free for 10, 32, and 39 months. Papilloma virus, virions, antigen, and DNA were not detected in the tumors, but this may be due to the use of an inappropriate probe.[19]

Growth and Metastasis

Tonsillar squamous cell carcinoma metastasizes early in the disease; 98 percent spread to the regional lymph nodes, and 63 percent have distant metastases.[20] Metastasis occurs first in the ipsilateral retropharyngeal lymph node, and then, when this is replaced, in the contralateral node. In the late stages, mandibular, precapsular, and parotid lymph nodes may be affected because of altered lymph flow. Contiguous spread often occurs to the anterior pole of the adjacent thyroid. The large regional lymph nodes may be misdiagnosed as the primary lesion since they are much larger than the primary tumor in the tonsil. Bloodborne metastases of tonsillar squamous cell carcinoma in the dog have been reported in the lung, liver, and spleen and, more rarely, in the pericardium, heart, kidney, adrenal, and pituitary. Involvement of bone may be extensive. The lungs may not have macroscopically visible lesions even when the large metastases in other organs indicate that tumor emboli must have passed through them.[1,11]

Surgical removal of gingival squamous cell carcinoma is often followed by recurrence, probably because of incomplete removal of tongues of tumor tissue penetrating deeply between bone spicules of the jaw. Such recurrences may develop as soon as 3 weeks after apparent complete ablation by cryosurgery. Only 5–10 percent of gingival squamous cell carcinomas metastasize to regional lymph nodes, usually ipsilateral nodes, and only 3 percent spread to distant sites.[20,22] This may be because these tumors are less malignant in the gum than in the tonsil; alternatively, the lymphatic drainage from the gum may be more restricted than that from the tonsil. In a series of nontonsillar squamous cell carcinomas, 23 of 32 cases had bone involvement, but only 3 had nodal metastases, and none had distant metastases. The actuarial survival rate at 12 months after treatment was 44 percent, compared with 22 percent for tonsillar squamous cell carcinoma.

Lingual squamous cell carcinoma grows between the muscle bundles, and foci of tumor are present some distance from the main tumor. Some of these cells are in thin walled veins and lymphatics, resulting in local recurrence in approximately 50 percent of cases even with apparently adequate surgical removal.[14] Despite removing a 2 cm margin of healthy tissue beyond the macroscopically visible edge of the tumor, one series found resection was incomplete in four of eight cases.[13] Regional lymph nodes usually have metastases, but distant metastases after treatment are rare.[14]

Etiology

Mobilization of a latent papilloma virus may be part of the etiology of squamous cell carcinoma at any site in the mouth and pharynx. Squamous cell carcinoma has occurred in the gluteal region of two beagles 45 and 51 months after vaccination with live unattenuated canine oral papilloma virus,[23] and a squamous cell carcinoma developed in a dog exhibiting oral papillomatosis.[3] Trauma and infection initiating an inflammatory reaction leading to squamous metaplasia and subsequent promotion to neoplasia by carcinogens could account for some squamous cell carcinomas.[24]

The development of three squamous cell carcinomas among 32 dogs that had previously been irradiated for acanthomatosus epulis has been recorded,[25] and a puppy irradiated 2 days postpartum developed a squamous cell carcinoma in the rostral mandible at 4 months of age.[26]

REFERENCES

1. Borthwick, R., Else, R.W., and Head, K.W. (1982) Neoplasia and allied conditions of the canine oropharynx. Vet Ann 22:248–269.
2. Chambers, V.C., Evans, C.A., and Weiser, R.S. (1960) Canine oral papillomatosis. II. Immunologic aspects of the disease. Cancer Res 20:1083–1093.
3. Watrach, A.M., Small, E., and Case, M.T. (1970) Canine papilloma: Progression of oral papilloma to carcinoma. J Natl Cancer Inst 45:915–920.
4. McFadyean, J., and Hobday, F. (1898) Note on the experimental transmission of warts in the dog. J Comp Pathol Therap 11:341–344.
5. Koniski, S., Tokita, H., and Ogata, H. (1972) Studies on canine oral papillomatosis. I. Transmission and characterisation of the virus. Jpn J Vet Sci 34:263–268.
6. Sundberg, J.P. (1995) Mucosotropic papilloma virus infections. Comp Pathol Bull 27(4): 4–6.
7. Sundberg, J.P., Smith, E.K., Herron, A.J., Jenson, A.B., Burk, R.D., and Van Ranst, M. (1994) Involvement of canine oral papilloma virus in generalised oral and cutaneous verrucosis in a Chinese sharpei dog. Vet Pathol 31:183–187.
8. Levene, A. (1984) Sebaceous gland differentiation in tumors of the feline oral mucosa. Vet Rec 114:69.
9. Withers, F.W. (1938) Squamous-cell carcinoma of the tonsil in the dog. J Pathol Bacteriol 49:429–432.
10. Ragland, W.L., and Gorham, J.R. (1967) Tonsillar carcinoma in rural dogs. Nature 214:925–926.
11. Todoroff, R.I., and Brodey, R.S. (1979) Oral and pharyngeal neoplasia in the dog: A retrospective study of 361 cases. J Amer Vet Med Assoc 175:567–571.
12. Hoyt, R.F., and Withrow, S.J. (1984) Oral malignancy in the dog. J Amer Anim Hosp Assoc 20:83–90.
13. Carpenter, L.G., Withrow, S.J., Powers, B.E., Ogilvie, G.K., et al. (1993) Squamous cell carcinoma of the tongue in 10 dogs. J Amer Anim Hosp Assoc 29:17–24.
14. Beck, E.R., Withrow, S.J., McChesney, A.E., et al. (1986) Canine tongue tumors: A retrospective review of 57 cases. J Amer Anim Hosp Assoc 22:525–532.
15. Knecht, C.D., and Priester, W.A. (1978) Musculoskeletal tumors in dogs. J Amer Vet Med Assoc 172:72–74.
16. Suter, M.M., Pantano, D.M., Flanders, J.A., Augustin-Voss, H.G., Dougherty, E.P., and Varvayanis, M. (1991) Comparison of growth and differentiation of normal and neoplastic canine keratinocyte cultures. Vet Pathol 28:131–138.
17. Bryne, M., Koppang, H.S., Lilleng, R., and Kjoerheim, A. (1992) Malignancy grading of the deep invasive margins of oral squamous cell carcinomas has high prognostic value. J Pathol 166:375–381.
18. Lownie, J.F., Altini, M., Austin, J.C., and Le Roux, P.L. (1981) Verrucous carcinoma presenting in the maxilla of a dog. J Amer Anim Hosp Assoc 17:315–319.
19. Ogilvie, G.K., Sundberg, J.P.,O'Banion, M.K., et al. (1988) Papillary squamous cell carcinoma in three young dogs. J Amer Vet Med Assoc 192:933–936.
20. Brodey, R.S. (1970) The biological behaviour of canine oral and pharyngeal neoplasms. J Small Anim Pract 11:45–53.
21. Werner, R.E., Jr. (1981) Canine and neoplasia: A review of 19 cases. J Amer Anim Hosp Assoc 17:67–70.
22. Brodey, R.S. (1960) A clinical and pathologic study of 130 neoplasms of the mouth and pharynx of the dog. Amer J Vet Res 21:787–812.
23. Meunier, L.D. (1990) Squamous cell carcinoma in beagles subsequent to canine oral papilloma virus vaccine. Lab Anim Sci 40:568 (Abstract).
24. Madsen, C. (1989) Squamous cell carcinoma and oral, pharyngeal and nasal lesions caused by foreign bodies in feed. Cases from a long term study in rats. Lab Anim 23:241–247.
25. Thrall, D.E., Goldschmidt, M.H., and Biery, D.N. (1981) Malignant tumor formation at the site of previously irradiated acanthomatous epulides in four dogs. J Amer Vet Med Assoc 178:127–139.
26. Benjamin, S.A., Lee, A.C., et al. (1986) Neoplasms in young dogs after perinatal irradiation. J Natl Cancer Inst 77:563–571.

Feline Oral and Pharyngeal Tumors of Squamous Epithelium

Prevalence and Site

Oral tumors form 10 percent of all feline neoplasia; 89 percent of these are malignant, and 75 percent of oral tumors in cats are squamous cell carcinoma.[1] Although single cases of papilloma have been listed in collections of neoplasms, no details of these oral tumors have been given[1-3]. Two cases of multiple, oral, fibropapillomata in cats less than 2 years of age have been reported.[4] Histologically these lesions resembled a sarcoid, being composed of hyperplastic epithelium and active immature fibrosis of the underlying connective tissue. Fibrogingival hyperplasia may also be associated with periodontal disease in cats. Other lesions that may mimic neoplasia on macroscopic inspection but are clearly different on histological examination are eosinophilic granuloma and the plasma cell/lymphocyte ulcerative proliferative stomatitis, which is often associated with feline immunodeficiency virus and/or feline calicivirus infection.[5]

Whereas in the dog, squamous cell carcinoma (SCC), fibrosarcoma, and malignant melanoma (MM) were the three most common malignant oral tumors, in the cat squamous cell carcinomas are by far the most common tumor to be encountered; for example, when data from five studies are added together, they show 272 squamous cell carcinomas, 61 fibrosarcomas, 23 adenocarcinomas, 15 lymphomas, and 12 malignant melanomas.[1,3,6,7,17]

Oral squamous cell carcinoma in cats is most common in the tongue and gingiva; of 33 oral squamous cell carcinomas, half were from the tongue; of 55 oral squamous cell carcinomas, 23 were from the gingiva, 22 the tongue, 5 the tonsils, 3 the palate, and 2 the pharynx[3]; of 37 oral squamous cell carcinomas, 19 were from the tongue, 10 the gingiva, 3 the lip, 3 the pharynx, 1 the cheek, and 1 the tonsil. It has been suggested that tonsillar squamous cell carcinomas are rare in North America but more common in the United Kingdom[2,8]; in a series of 71 cases, 27 percent were in the tongue and 17 percent in the tonsil.[9,10] Lingual squamous cell carcinoma is rare in Australia.[11] This data suggests that there may be geographical and temporal differences in the site distribution of oral squamous cell carcinoma. All workers agree that squamous cell carcinomas in the tongue of cats are infralingual and in the midline near the frenulum; this contrasts with the situation in the human and the dog, where they are said to be lateral.[3] There is no clear-cut pattern of distribution of gingival squamous cell carcinoma in the cat; for example, one study found 7 mandibular and 4 maxillary cases,[8] and another found 16 cases between the canine and last molar (10 maxillary and 6 mandibular).[12]

Age, Breed, and Sex

Almost all cats affected with oral squamous cell carcinoma are adult or aged, and although the range is 0.4 to 21 years the median age is between 11.6 and 12.5 years.[6,7,12,13] No breed predisposition has been recorded. Most authors could show no sex bias, but all 11 gingival cases reported in one series[8] were in females, although as these authors point out the United Kingdom cases[10] suggested that castrated males were predisposed.

Clinical Considerations

The presenting signs, in decreasing order of frequency, are a facial mass, excessive salivation, anorexia, loose teeth, bone loss, dysphagia, weight loss, bad breath, and fractured mandible.[6,12,14,15] Although these signs may only have been seen for 1 to 12 weeks (median 3 weeks), the tumor is usually in an advanced state.[13] Two of seven cats with mandibular squamous cell carcinoma had hypercalcemia (12.6 mg/dl), which resolved after surgical removal of the tumor and radiotherapy.[13]

Gross Morphology

The usual location for lingual squamous cell carcinoma in the cat is infralingual, near the ventrolateral to midline surface at about the level of the reflection of the frenulum.[16] The extent of the tumor visible on the mucosa of the tongue is often small, appearing as a white nodular lesion; however, palpation or dissection reveals a more extensive involvement. A few neoplasms extend out from the surface as a finely nodular mass.

Gingival squamous cell carcinomas rapidly become ulcerated, and it has been suggested that morbidity and mortality are the result of local disease rather than distant metastases.[18] Dysphagia and aspiration pneumonia may lead to euthanasia of the animal before the full metastatic potential of the tumor is realized.[2] The mandible is often infiltrated, and one group of authors found that they were unable to distinguish between malignant neoplastic and nonneoplastic disease except on the basis of histological examination of a bone and soft tissue biopsy.[6]

Tonsillar squamous cell carcinomas are rare in cats and are usually unilateral, but rapid infiltrative growth causes extension from the crypt to the surrounding pharyngeal region.[5]

Histological Features, Growth, and Metastasis

Lingual tumors are typical squamous cell carcinomas with well-differentiated squamous epithelium, keratin pearls, many mitoses, and hyperchromatic nuclei. Invasion of soft tissues and muscle by the tumor elicits connective tissue proliferation and atrophy of the muscle. Muscle bundles at right angles to the infiltrating tumor columns act as a barrier, whereas bundles that are parallel to the line of tumor become infiltrated. Metastases occur by lymphatics to the regional mandibular and retropharyngeal lymph nodes and are seen in many cases.

Gingival squamous cell carcinomas infiltrate the jaw bone in the form of keratinizing tumor masses and trabeculae with a low to moderate mitotic rate and only few acellular keratin pearls.[13] There is remodeling of bone by osteolysis and replacement with large amounts of reactive connective tissue infiltrated by tumor. The tumor and the osteolysis extend farther than the macroscopic examination would suggest, but regional lymph node or organ metastases are uncommon.[12,13] In one series, 15 of 52 oral squamous cell carcinomas had enlarged mandibular lymph nodes and/or retropharyngeal lymph nodes, but only 7 of these had squamous cell carcinoma metastases in them when examined by fine needle aspiration cytology.[12] In another series of seven cases, the ipsilateral submandibular lymph nodes were removed; only two nodes were enlarged and neither contained tumor, but one node that was not enlarged had a metastatic focus.[13] No vascular invasion was recorded, but in two of the seven cats perineural infiltration was observed in the primary tumor.

Treatment

Surgical excision of oral squamous cell carcinoma is followed by a 1 year survival rate of less than 20 percent, most cats being euthanized within 6 months of diagnosis. Mandibulectomy followed by radiation of the primary site and the regional lymph nodes extended the median survival time to 14 months (3 to 36 months), despite the fact that the tumors were WHO stage 3 (> 4 cm).[13] Others have considered that radiotherapy and mitoxantrone treatment were better than radiation or chemotherapy (with mitoxantrone, cyclophosphamide, or doxorubicin) alone.[19] Among 11 oral squamous cell carcinomas, 8 cases showed complete disappearance of the tumor for a median time of 170 days, and 1 case showed a partial remission of 60 days duration. The choice among surgery, radiotherapy, radiotherapy and chemotherapy, or radiotherapy with local hyperthermia for the treatment of oral squamous cell carcinoma did not affect the survival time in one series.[12] Staging the tumor at the time of diagnosis may be predictive; for example, 38 cases in stages I, II, and III had a survival time of 2.5 to 3 months, whereas for nine cats at stage IV the survival time was 0.8 month.

Etiology

The distribution of the tumor in the ventrolateral areas of the tongue may be due to prolonged contact of a carcinogen at this site.[20] Alternatively, it would be interesting to know the cell tumor rate of the epithelium in different areas of the oral cavity in relation to the penetration of chemicals and to the varying degrees of keratinization.

In a survey of the literature, it was noted that oral squamous cell carcinoma has an increased incidence in feline immunodeficiency virus (FIV) infected cats and that there is synergism between feline leukemia virus (FeLV), FIV, and feline sarcoma virus.[21] Virus infection can only be one factor in carcinogenesis since in one series of 12 mandibular squamous cell carcinomas all were FeLV positive but FIV negative,[6] and in another series of 40 oral squamous cell carcinomas only 2 were FeLV positive.[12] Impaction of foreign material, infection, and trauma probably play a part in induction of gingival squamous cell carcinoma.

REFERENCES

1. Bastianello, S.S. (1983) A survey of neoplasia in domestic species over a 40 year period from 1935 to 1974 in the Republic of South Africa. V. Tumors occurring in the cat. *Onderstepoort J Vet Res* 50:105–110.
2. Bradley, R.L. (1984) Selected oral, pharyngeal and upper respiratory conditions in the cat. *Vet Clin N Amer Small Anim Pract* 14:1173–1194.
3. Levene, A. (1984) Upper digestive tract neoplasia in the cat. *J Laryn Otol* 98:1221–1223.
4. Rest, J.R., Gumbrell, R.C., Heim, P., and Rushton-Taylor, P. (1997) Oral fibropapillomas in young cats. *Vet Rec* 141:528.
5. Willoughby, K., and Coutts, A. (1995) Differential diagnosis of throat and ear disease in cats. *Practice* (May): 206–214.
6. Kapatkin, A.S., Marretta, S.M., Patnaik, A.K., et al. (1991) Mandibular swelling in cats: Prospective study of 24 cats. *J Amer Anim Hosp Assoc* 27:575–580.
7. Stebbins, K.E., Morse, C.C., and Goldschmidt, M.H. (1989) Feline oral neoplasia: A ten year Study. *Vet Pathol* 26:121–128.
8. Patnaik, A.K., Liu, S.-K., Hurvitz, A.I., and McClelland, A.J. (1975) Nonhematopoietic neoplasms in cats. *J Natl Cancer Inst* 54:855–860.
9. Dorn, C.R., Taylor, D.O.N., and Schneider, R. (1971) Sunlight exposure and risk of developing cutaneous and oral squamous cell carcinoma in cats. *J Natl Cancer Inst* 46:1072–1078.
10. Cotchin, E. (1957) Neoplasia in the cat. *Vet Rec* 69:1–10.
11. Young, P.L. (1978) Squamous cell carcinoma of the tongue of the cat. *Austral Vet J* 54:133–134.
12. Posterino Reeves, N.C., Turrel, J.M., and Withrow, S.J. (1993) Oral squamous cell carcinoma in the cat. *J Amer Anim Hosp Assoc* 29:438–441.
13. Hutson, C.A., Willaner, C.C., Walder, E.J., Stone, J.L., and Klein, M.K. (1992) Treatment of mandibular squamous cell carcinoma in cats by use of mandibulectomy and radiotherapy: Seven cases (1987–1989). *J Amer Vet Med Assoc* 201:777–781.
14. Quigley, P.J., Leedale, A., and Daason, I.M.P. (1972) Carcinoma of mandible of cat and dog simulating osteosarcoma. *J Comp Pathol* 82:15–18.
15. Miller, A.S., McCrea, M.W., and Rhodes, W.H. (1969) Mandibular epidermoid carcinoma with reactive bone proliferation in a cat. *Amer J Vet Res* 30:1465–1468.
16. Bond, E., and Dorfman, H.D. (1969) Squamous cell carcinoma of the tongue in cats. *J Amer Vet Med Assoc* 154:786–789.
17. Carpenter, J.L., Andrews, L.K., and Holzworth, J. (1987) Tumors and tumor-like lesions. In Holzworth, J. (ed.), *Diseases of the Cat: Medicine and Surgery*, Vol. 1. W.B. Saunders, Philadelphia, pp. 406–496.
18. Cotter, S.M. (1981) Oral pharyngeal neoplasms in the cat. *J Amer Anim Hosp Assoc* 17:917–920.
19. Ogilvie, G.K., Moore, A.S., Obradovich, J.E., et al. (1993) Toxicoses and efficacy associated with administration of mitoxantrone to cats with malignant tumors. *J Amer Vet Med Assoc* 202:1839–1844.
20. Cotchin, E. (1966) Some aetiological aspects of tumors in domesticated animals. *Ann Roy Coll Surg England* 38:92–116.
21. Hutson, C.A., Rideout, B.A., and Pederson, N.C. (1991) Neoplasia associated with feline immunodeficiency virus infection in cats of Southern California. *J Amer Vet Med Assoc* 199:1357–1362.

Malignant Melanoma in Dogs

Prevalence

Oral malignant melanoma is seen often in dogs, and some consider it to be the most common malignant oral tumor. A prevalence figure of 12.7 per 10,000 has been given, alternatively expressed as 6 percent of all oral tumors.[1,2]

Age, Breed, and Sex

The relative risk of developing tumors increases with age more markedly in malignant melanoma than in either squamous cell carcinoma or fibrosarcoma.[1] Different series have remarkably similar age distributions: 11.4, 11.9, and 11.7 years, with a range from 1 to 17 years.[1,32] Amelanotic melanomas are reported with an average age of 10.4 years.[5]

An increased risk for oral melanoma in five breeds including cocker spaniels has been demonstrated and these authors discussed the mapping of oral pigmentation to explain breed predisposition[1]. A cocker spaniel breed predisposition was suggested in the United States, but this was not confirmed in the United Kingdom. It was suggested that breeds weighing less than 23 kg had a ratio of malignant melanoma of 1.8:1 compared with breeds weighing more than 23 kg.[5] Twenty-one cases were recorded in dachshunds and 15 in poodles among 51 oral malignant melanomas[4]; others found that the top three breeds were poodle, cocker spaniel, and dachshund. A recent study indicated chow chow, golden retriever, and Pekingese/poodle mix breeds were overrepresented, and boxer and German shepherds were underrepresented.[32] Twelve of 14 oral malignant melanomas were found in black miniature poodles.[3] In contrast, in a series of seven malignant melanomas of the tongue, only two cocker spaniels were reported, and others could not demonstrate a breed distribution governed by breed or weight.[7]

Some authors report that males are overrepresented, ranging from 1.6:1 to 6:1, male to female[8]; others have not identified a gender predisposition.[7,32]

Site and Clinical Features

Gingiva and labia are the two most common sites.[5,7,32] A summary of two European series gives a site distribution of 60 gum, 21 lip, 8 cheek, 7 tongue, 6 palate, and 2 tonsil and pharynx; for the United States, the distribution is 42–63 percent gum, 15–33 percent cheek and lip, 10–16 percent soft and hard palate, and 1–3 percent tongue.[5] Almost any site on the gingiva can be affected; for example, one study showed 25 maxillary sites (19 rostral, 6 caudal) and 14 mandibular sites (7 rostral, 7 caudal).[7] Hypoglycemia has been reported in a dog with malignant melanoma and pulmonary metastases.[9]

Gross Morphology

The tumors are solitary, and there is seldom a problem determining whether a lesion is a recurrence or a new tumor focus. Occasionally asymptomatic nodules less than 1 cm in size are found during dentistry. Usually the lesions are 3 to 4 cm in maximum dimension when they first cause clinical signs. They are sessile and often have an ulcerated surface, and gingival tumors tend to be oval in shape, molded by the anatomy of the jaw. The deep surface is usually irregular, making them immobile. The surface may be black in color, but white mucosa can overlie pigmented tumors, and a red granulation tissue reaction to ulceration may mask melanin pigment. The tumor consistency is firm unless necrosis and secondary infection have led to softening. Some tumors are uniformly black on cut surfaces, but more often there are foci of varying sizes with less pigment, and these areas are brown, gray, or white (amelanotic). Amelanotic tumors may give rise to pigmented secondaries and vice versa.

Histological Features

Although the tumors are solitary, on histological examination small foci of up to 20 heavily pigmented cells may be found in the basal levels of the epithelium of the adjacent mucosa. When bleached, the cells of this junctional change are uniformly round or polygonal with uniformly round or oval central nuclei. Unlike in this junctional change, the cells in intraepithelial tumors show variation in the size and shape of both cytoplasm and nuclei. Most oral melanotic tumors have infiltrated into the submucosa, and some also spread upward into the epithelium. The tumor is divided into lobules, and the cells are supported by the minimum of collagenous stroma.

The melanin content and the mitotic index may vary in different areas of a tumor and between tumors. Pigment granules may obscure the nucleus unless sections are bleached with 1 percent potassium permanganate. Melanophages in the stroma concentrate melanin granules released from tumor cells and so may help in the diagnosis of poorly pigmented tumors. Amelanotic tumor cells may be made to reveal their true nature by Masson Fontana silver stain, but this also reacts with lipofuscin and argentaffin granules. If tissue is available for frozen sections, dihydroxyphenylalanine oxidase (DOPA) can be demonstrated. Two monoclonal antibodies that recognize melanoma associated antigens in human tissues were used to stain sections of 14 canine tumors and metastases.[10] The amelanotic cells that had not developed melanin were visualized better than the heavily pigmented cells.[10] Electron microscopy has been used to visualize premelanosomes in amelanotic tumors.[11,12]

Three patterns of cells have been described in canine oral malignant melanoma. The epithelial type (20 percent) consisted of closely packed round or polyhedral cells with abundant pigmented eosinophilic cytoplasm that have well-defined borders and large central nuclei with one or more prominent nucleoli. In the spindle cell type (35 percent) the outline of the cells can be seen in unbleached sections because of the pigment; the nuclei are ovoid or elongated and have small nucleoli. The third type is mixed (40 percent) and has areas of epithelioid and spindloid patterns. This combined type is common in the oral cavity; for example, two studies report 43 combined, 30 epithelioid, and 10 spindloid.[4,7] Clear cell and adenoid/papillary patterns are uncommon.[32] Chondroid differentiation is rare.[32]

It is generally agreed that virtually all canine oral melanomas are malignant, but benign forms have been diagnosed.[13] The histological classification of 54 oral malignant melanomas, 9 of which were amelanotic, were compared with their biological behavior.[3] Researchers found that 4 histologically benign tumors had a postoperative malignant clinical course, and of the 50 histologically malignant tumors 2 had a benign clinical course. Flow cytometric analysis of DNA content was performed on 26 of these oral malignant melanomas and on 5 metastases from them. Of the primary tumors that were considered histologically malignant, two were incorrectly classified as benign using flow cytometry. In four of the five metastases the ploidy was similar in the primary and secondary tumors. The author's conclusion was that histology and flow cytometry did not differ in ability to predict behavior, and because of expense and technical difficulties, histopathology remains the preferred method.[3]

Immunohistochemistry may be needed to establish the diagnosis in a poorly pigmented tumor. If immunohistochemistry is applied to oral melanomas the following results are expected: vimentin, 100 percent positive; melan A, 93 percent; NSE, 90 percent; and S100, 76 percent.[32] A recent study concluded that melan A was a highly sensitive and specific marker for melanocytic tumors.[32] These investigators reported that canine oral melanomas and melanocytes reacted positively to melan A, but melanophages did not.

Growth and Metastasis

Approximately 70 percent metastasize to regional lymph nodes and 67 percent to distant sites, the lung being the most common site. Lung metastases are often miliary, so they may be found at necropsy but not detected in chest radiographs. Moreover, the widespread location of metastases in organs throughout the body may merely reflect the ease with which pigmented secondary tumors can be seen. The primary tumor grows rapidly, and in as many as 57 percent of gingival malignant melanomas the underlying bone is invaded. Because of this invasive growth, recurrences post-surgery and/or metastases are frequent. In one series with follow-up data after surgery, 23 of 54 tumors metastasized to regional lymph nodes; 13 of these spread to other lymph nodes, and in 9 of these 13 there also were distant metastases, mainly in brain and lung.[3] In a series of 67 tumors, 11 spread to local lymph nodes, 8 to lung, 5 to kidney. Sometimes there is evidence of tumor extension to the retrobulbar region,[14,15] which may be due to perineural spread. The size of the primary tumor does not govern its invasiveness.[6]

Staging and Treatment

The survival time following surgery for malignant oral melanoma is short because of recurrence and metastasis. A mean survival time of 3 months after operation has been reported; the death rate was 73 percent at 6 months, 84 percent at 1 year, and 86 percent at 2 years in a series of 51 dogs.[4] The data for 42 dogs are similar, with a death rate of 90 percent at the age of 2 years and a median post-surgery survival of 14 weeks.[13] However, if one selects patients with no detectable involvement in the adjacent bone or regional lymph node and with normal thoracic radiographs, then the median survival time of dogs with surgical excision is better than in those with no operation (242 days versus 65 days).[16]

A tumor-free period of 3 to 44 months can be achieved by maxillectomy and mandibulectomy, but 20 percent local recurrences and 80 percent metastases usually lead to death or euthanasia within 1 year.[7,19] Partial mandibulectomy may provide better results for local tumor treatment than conventional surgery, but the problem of metastases remains.[20] The survival of dogs with lingual malignant melanoma after a variety of treatments is similarly poor because of recurrence and metastasis. The results of more radical surgery and alternative therapies, either alone or as adjuvants to surgery, have been summarized.[15] A median survival of 228 days for 47 dogs treated by surgery alone was extended to 370 days for 42 dogs when surgery was combined with *C. parvum* adjuvant therapy.[17] When broken down by stage, dogs with stage II and III disease (< 2 cm diameter) were the ones that benefited from this therapy. However, another worker found that all eight dogs in which debulking of the oral malignant melanoma was followed by a single intralesional *C. parvum* injection had to be euthanized within 6 months because of recurrence and/or metastasis.[18]

Repeated intralesional implants of chemotherapeutic agents resulted in destruction of the primary tumor in 55 percent of dogs, with a mean survival of 54.2 weeks, but 6 of these 11 animals developed metastasis.[15] In this study mandibular tumors and small early lesions (4 ± 1 cm² initial tumor volume) responded better than large non-mandibular tumors (e.g., lingual).

In attempts to find some feature on which an improved prognosis could be based, several workers have analyzed the influence of a variety of factors on the course of the disease.[4,7,13,15,16] No significant differences were found for remission length or survival time for the following clinical parameters: age, breed, body weight, tumor duration and previous treatments, soft tissue only or with bone involvement, normal or ulcerated tumor surface, or circumscribed or infiltrative tumor margin. Likewise, none of the following histological features predicted tumor behavior: junctional activity, pigmentation, histological type, size of nucleoli, polymorphism, degree of lymphocyte infiltration, or tumor infiltration into lymphatic vessels. These authors found that when considered individually the tumor volume at the start of treatment, tumor location, tumor mitotic index, and the metastatic status of the dog had no influence on the remission length or survival time when the animal was followed to death or for 3 years from diagnosis and treatment. Other workers agreed, but they found that where combined these factors had a predictive value, and they suggested an alternative staging system.[7]

A recent study on over 300 canine oral melanomas did not find statistically significant differences in survival among different sites or mitotic indices.[32] The prognosis for oral melanomas is poor and is apparently unrelated to sex, site, mitotic index, histological type, amount of pigment, or volume of tumor.

Etiology

Little is known about the causative factors of oral malignant melanoma, but fetal irradiation 55 days postcoitus was followed by oral malignant melanoma development at 3.2 years.[21] One year after a lingual squamous cell carcinoma in a 9-year-old dog was treated by surgery and radiotherapy with hyperthermia, an amelanotic melanoma appeared in the radiation field. This tumor was resected, but the dog died 16 months after the squamous cell carcinoma operation because of gastrointestinal lymphoma.

Melanotic Tumors in Cats

Malignant melanotic tumors are rare in the mouths of cats. Over periods ranging from 10 to 40 years authors have recorded a prevalence of 1 in 243 neoplasms,[22] 4 in 3248,[23] and 3 in 1285.[24] When dealing with only oropharyngeal tumors the figures are 3 in 371,[25] 4 in 169,[26] and 1 in 50.[1] There does not seem to be a sex or breed predisposition, and the age range is 8 to 16 years (mean 12 years).[25,27] The tumor sites include gum, lip, palate, and tongue. The histological appearance resembles the combined epithelioid/spindloid pattern seen in dogs, and highly pigmented and pleomorphic tumors are uncommon.[27] Most cats had to be euthanized because of metastases in 1 to 135 days (mean 61 days).

Melanotic Tumors in Ox, Sheep, Horse, and Pig

Occasionally, melanomas are found in the ramus of the mandible of ox and sheep at the abattoir. Although this tumor may grow sufficiently large to cause fracture of the ramus, metastases do not develop. Melanocytes can be demonstrated in the fat and connective tissue around the mandibular nerve of the other ramus, and these may be the source of such tumors. Melanomas were observed in the ramus of the mandible and surrounding structures in two calves; one was 14 months old and the other 9 months old.[28] In the latter, the tumor had been observed since birth. Histologically this neoplasm resembled the human melanotic neuroepidermal tumor of infancy, that is, there are epithelium-like melanin-containing cells and small lymphocyte-like cells set in a fibrous stroma. A 7-month-old steer with a mandibular melanoma had light and electron microscopic features consistent with a congenital fibrotic melanoma.[29]

One series mentioned 5 melanomas in 29 equine oropharyngeal malignancies. A 25 × 10 cm melanotic tumor involving the ventral aspect of both guttural pouches of a 13-year-old gray gelding was controlled by a histamine antagonist which restored cell mediated and humoral immunity.[30]

A 2-week-old black pig that was paralyzed from birth because melanotic skeletal muscle tumors had extended into the thoracic vertebral canal also had multicentric tumor foci in pharynx, tonsil, esophagus, stomach, intestine, heart, lung, liver, kidney and spleen.[31]

REFERENCES

1. Dorn, C.R., and Priester, W.A. (1976) Epidemiologic analysis of oral and pharyngeal cancer in dogs, cats, horses and cattle. *J Amer Vet Med Assoc* 169:1202–1206.
2. Cohen, D., Brodey, R.S., and Chen, S.M. (1964) Epidemiologic aspects of oral and pharyngeal neoplasms of the dog. *Amer J Vet Res* 25:1776–1779.
3. Bolon, B., Calderwood Mays, M.B., and Hall, B.J. (1990) Characteristics of canine melanomas and comparison of histology and DNA ploidy to their biologic behavior. *Vet Pathol* 27: 96–102 and 1991 28 453–456.
4. Frese, K. (1978) Verlaufsuntersuchungen bei Melanomen der Haut und der Mundschleimhaut des Hundes. *Vet Pathol* 15:461–473.
5. Birchard, S., and Carothers, M. (1990) Aggressive surgery in the management of oral neoplasia. *Vet Clin N Amer Small Anim Pract* 20:1117–1140.
6. Bradley, R.L., MacEwen, E.G., and Loar, A.S. (1984) Mandibular resection for removal of oral tumors in 30 dogs and 6 cats. *J Amer Vet Med Assoc* 184:460–463.
7. Hahn, K.A., DeNicola, D.B., Richardson, R.C., and Hahn, E.A. (1994) Canine oral malignant melanoma: Prognostic utility of an alternative staging system. *J Small Anim Pract* 35:251–256.
8. Hoyt, R.F., and Withrow, S.J. (1984) Oral malignancy in the dog. *J Amer Anim Hosp Assoc* 20:83–90.
9. Leifer, L.E., Peterson, M.E., Matus, R.E., and Patnaik, A.K. (1985) Hypoglycemia associated with non islet tumors in 13 dogs. *J Amer Vet Med Assoc* 186:53–55.
10. Berrington, A.J., Jimbow, K., and Haines, D.M. (1994) Immunohistochemical Detection of Melanoma-associated antigens on formalin-fixed, paraffin-embedded canine tumors. *Vet Pathol* 31:445–461.
11. Carpenter, J.W., Novilla, M.N., and Griffing, W.J. (1980) Metastasis of a malignant, amelanotic lingual melanoma in a dog. *J Amer Anim Hosp Assoc* 16:685–689.
12. Turk, J.R., and Leathers, C.W. (1981) Light and electron microscopic study of the large pale cell in a canine malignant melanoma. *Vet Pathol* 18:829–832.
13. Bostock, D.E. (1979) Prognosis after surgical excision of canine melanomas. *Vet Pathol* 16:32–40.
14. De Haan, C.E., Papageorges, M., and Kraft, S.L. (1991) Radiographic diagnosis. *Vet Radiol* 32:75–77.
15. Kitchell, B.E., Brown, D.M., Luck, E.E., Woods, L.L., Orenberg, E.W., and Block, D.A. (1994) Intralesional implant for treatment of primary oral malignant melanoma in dogs. *J Amer Vet Med Assoc* 204:229–246.
16. Harvey, H.J., MacEwen, E.G., Braun, D., Patnaik, A.K., Withrow, S.J., and Jongeward, S. (1981) Prognostic criteria for dogs with oral melanoma. *J Amer Vet Med Assoc* 178:580–582.
17. MacEwan, E.G., Patnaik, A.K., Harvey, H.J., Hayes, A.A., and Matus, R. (1986) Canine oral melanoma: Comparison of surgery versus surgery plus *Corynebacterium parvum*. *Cancer Invest* 4:397–402.
18. Misdorp, W. (1987) Incomplete surgery, local immunostimulation and recurrence of some tumor types in dogs and cats. *Vet Quarterly* 9:279–286.
19. White, R.A.S. (1991) Mandibulectomy and maxillectomy in the dog: Long term survival in 100 cases. *J Small Anim Pract* 32:69–74.

20. Salisbury, S.K., and Lantz, G.C. (1988) Long-term results of partial mandibulectomy for treatment of oral tumors in 30 dogs. *J Amer Anim Hosp Assoc* 24:285–294.

21. Benjamin, S.A., Lee, A.C., et al. (1986) Neoplasms in young dogs after perinatal irradiation. *J Natl Cancer Inst* 77:563–571.

22. Bastianello, S.S. (1983) A survey of neoplasia in domestic species over a 40 year period from 1935 to 1974 in the Republic of South Africa. V. Tumors occurring in the cat. *Onderstepoort J Vet Res* 50:105–110.

23. Carpenter, J.L., Andrews, L.K., and Holzworth, J. (1987) Tumors and tumor-like lesions. In Holzworth, J. (ed.), *Diseases of the Cat: Medicine and Surgery*, Vol. 1. W.B. Saunders, Philadelphia, pp. 406–496.

24. Levene, A. (1984) Upper digestive tract neoplasia in the cat. *J Laryn Otol* 98:1221–1223.

25. Stebbins, K.E., Morse, C.C., and Goldschmidt, M.H. (1989) Feline oral neoplasia: A ten year Study. *Vet Pathol* 26:121–128.

26. Cotter, S.M. (1981) Oral pharyngeal neoplasms in the cat. *J Amer Anim Hosp Assoc* 17:917–920.

27. Patnaik, A.K., and Mooney, S. (1988) Feline melanoma: A comparative study of ocular, oral and dermal neoplasms. *Vet Pathol* 25:105–112.

28. Wiseman, A., Breeze, R.G., and Pirie, H.M. (1977) Melanotic neuroectodermal tumor of infancy (melanotic progonoma) in two calves. *Vet Rec* 101:264–266.

29. Long, G.G., Leathers, C.W., Parish, S.M., and Breeze, R.G. (1981) Fibrotic melanoma in a calf. *Vet Pathol* 18:402–404.

30. Hance, S.R., and Bertone, A.L. (1993) The equine head: neoplasia. *Vet Clin N Amer Equine Pract* 9:213–234.

31. Fisher, L.F., and Olander, H.J. (1978) Spontaneous neoplasms of Pigs—A study of 31 cases. *J Comp Pathol* 88:505–517.

32. Remus-Vara, J.A., Beissenherz, M.E., Miller, M.A., et al. (2000) Retrospective study of 338 canine oral melanomas with clinical, histologic and immunohistochemical review of 129 cases. *Vet Pathol* 37:597–608.

Tumors of Mesenchymal Tissue

Benign mesenchymal tumors can often be diagnosed on their histological appearance in H&E stained sections, but undifferentiated tumors may require histochemistry, immunochemistry, or electron microscopy to establish their origin. This often requires more than one marker because the neoplastic cells may not have differentiated sufficiently to express the characters of the normal parent cell type. Sometimes this is not possible, and the diagnosis should remain anaplastic sarcoma or undifferentiated tumor; for example, in one series of canine oral tumors, 94 had specific diagnoses, 3 were categorized as anaplastic sarcoma, and another 3 as carcinoma.[1]

Fibroma and Fibrosarcoma in Dogs

Prevalence

Transitional forms exist between histologically well-differentiated fibroma durum, fibroma molle, and fibrosarcoma. Even nonencapsulated, invasively growing tumors with many mitotic figures do not often metastasize, but recurrence following treatment is common. Most published series of tumors list few benign fibromas in the oropharynx; for example, in a series of 396 oral tumors, 56 were fibrosarcoma and 11 were fibroma.[3] Fibrosarcoma is common in the dog but less frequent than malignant melanoma or squamous cell carcinoma. Prevalence has been estimated at 5.8 cases per 100,000 dogs.[4] The frequency in a series of oral tumors varies between 17 percent and 26 percent.[1]

Age, Breed, and Sex

Fibrosarcomas occur in younger dogs than do malignant melanoma and squamous cell carcinoma, although the age range of 6 months to 16 years is wide. Animals less than 5 years old account for 25 percent of fibrosarcoma cases,[7] and the mean age is 7.2 ± 1.7 years.[1]

The weight of the patient may be more predictive than breed; that is, there is a weight predisposition for large breeds over small breeds of 2.3 to 1.[5] This observation has been born out by other workers; for example, dogs weighing 23 kg or more are at greater risk.[7,14,15] Males are affected more often than females: 1.4 to 1, to 2.8 to 1,[6] and 4.2 to 1.[1]

Well-differentiated fibrosarcoma is described in the maxilla (72 percent of cases) and mandibles (28 percent of cases) of large purebred dogs.[90] The median age was 8 years, median weight was 28 kg, and sexes were equally represented; however, 13 of 25 dogs (52 percent) were golden retrievers.

Well-differentiated fibrosarcomas in the golden retriever and other large breeds have a characteristically benign histologic appearance but are biologically high-grade.[90] The tumors have a haphazard proliferation of fibrous tissue with abundant stroma, moderately low to low cellularity, minimal nuclear pleomorphism, and a low mitotic index (0–1 mitoses/400X field). The tumors are invasive and some contain foci of mononuclear cells. Initial histologic diagnoses in 25 dogs were nodular fasciitis (n = 10), low-grade fibrosarcoma (n = 11), and chronic inflammation with granulation tissue (n = 4). Nearly 75 percent of the dogs had radiographic evidence of bone destruction, and none had detectable pulmonary metastasis at presentation. Pulmonary metastasis was eventually detected in 3 dogs (12 percent), and lymph node metastasis in 5 dogs (20 percent). Metastatic lesions and recurrent primary lesions resembled high-grade fibrosarcomas (increased cellularity, nuclear pleomorphism, and a higher mitotic rate). Recognition and appropriate treatment of these histologically benign but biologically malignant tumors are important for patient care.

Gross Morphology

The site distribution is reported as 56–87 percent on the gum, 7–17 percent hard and soft palate, lip more often than cheek 4–22 percent, and tongue 1.3–2 percent.[6] Gingival fibrosarcomas probably occur in equal numbers in the mandible[9] or maxilla.[13,14,16] It was suggested that most cases in the maxilla develop between canine and carnassial teeth and extend onto the hard palate.[7]

These tumors are usually unicentric and unilateral, firm, gray white to pink in color, smooth surfaced, and sessile, except on rare occasions when they are nodular and even pedunculate. The surface is ulcerated less often than in squamous cell carcinoma and malignant melanoma, and the ulcers are not cratiform. Gingival and palatine fibrosarcomas are usually fixed to the underlying bone. The cut surface may show a faint striated pattern. They are usually over 4 cm in longest dimension when diagnosed.[9,15,16]

Histological Features

Fibromas are rare and should not be confused with fibrous overgrowth (fibromatosis), the result of prolonged irritation due to foreign bodies or trauma. Fibromatosis is often characterized by large amounts of collagen with only a few fibrocytes scattered throughout. Fibrosarcomas have numerous uniform to pleomorphic spindle cells separated by small amounts of collagen or surrounded by reticulin fibers in silver stained sections. The tumor is composed of interlacing bundles, some cut longitudinally (elongated cells) and others tangentially or at right angles (round cells). Highly malignant tumors have numerous mitotic figures, infiltrative borders, pleomorphic cells, and even multinucleate giant cells.[14]

Growth and Metastasis

Fibrosarcomas infiltrate extensively, and a high proportion recur after conventional surgery.[17] Infiltration into the jaw bone by gingival fibrosarcoma can be demonstrated in 50 percent of cases at the time of diagnosis and in up to 92 percent at necropsy or when mandibulectomy/maxillectomy samples are examined.[1,2,7,14,15] Approximately 20 percent of cases have enlarged local lymph nodes with metastatic foci.[7,15] Distant metastases to the lungs can be demonstrated by radiographs in 10–20 percent of cases at the time of diagnosis, and this increases to 27 percent at necropsy.[7,15] Spread beyond the lung is rare, possibly because local recurrence influences the owner to request euthanasia of the patient before further secondaries develop; for example, 1 of 19 spread to the kidney.[2]

Treatment

Tumor free survival after local excision can be as short as 1 month before recurrence necessitates euthanasia.[7] Cryosurgery achieved a 7 percent survival at 1 year,[18] radiotherapy alone 12 percent at 1 year, radiotherapy and hyperthermia 32–50 percent at 1 year.[8] Radiotherapy combined with a radiosensitizer resulted in a median time to recurrence of 5.6 months,[16] suggesting an improvement over the 3.5 months achieved with radiotherapy alone,[15] but this was not statistically significant. Radical surgery can result in a tumor free survival time as long as 32 months, but the median survival time is only 7 months, and the survival at 1 year remains at 50 percent.[8,13,14]

Fibroma and Fibrosarcoma in Cats

Although oral fibrosarcomas are second in frequency to squamous cell carcinomas,[11] they are not common,[60] being recorded only once in 243 neoplasms over a 40 year period[12] and five times in 3248 tumors in 35 years.[19] Neither are they common among collections of oral tumors; for example, studies showed 5 fibrosarcomas in 95 oral tumors,[19] 6 in 93,[20] and 48 in 371.[25] These figures are lower than the 16–20 percent given elsewhere.[22] Fibromas are even less common than fibrosarcomas.[2]

Taking the data from all the references in this section, the average age of affected cats is 13.6 years (range 1 to 21). There is no breed or sex predilection. The sites of tumors in decreasing order of frequency are gingival, palatine, labial, pharyngeal, and lingual.[2,22] The maxilla and mandible appear to be equally affected, and the lesions are rostral more than caudal.[13,14]

Local invasive growth and lack of widespread metastases resemble the pattern in the dog. The histological pattern, like that in the dog, is of densely packed pleomorphic fibroblasts in interwoven fascicles with variable amounts of collagen. The tumors have up to five mitoses per high power field, and 3 of 43 cases exhibited a few multinucleate cells.[21,23] Fibromatous polyps in the pharynx of cats under 3 years of age should be investigated carefully since they may be nonneoplastic.[24]

Survival times for cats treated with combined immunotherapy, chemotherapy, and cryosurgery are 382 and 1205 days for fibrosarcoma of the mandible and hard palate, respectively, compared with 49 and 59 days for squamous cell carcinoma.[25] Mandibulectomy and maxillectomy has been followed by recurrence in periods from 2 to 3.5 months.[14]

Cats with neoplasms of the skin induced by feline sarcoma virus (FeSV) may also have lesions on the lips. Such fibrosarcomas are usually in cats less than 5 years old and are usually multicentric rather than solitary.[26] From present evidence it appears that oral fibrosarcomas are not examples of the relatively rare FeSV induced multicentric tumor, but FeLV may contribute to their development.

Fibrosarcoma in Other Species

In a survey of tumors reported by Veterinary Investigation Centers in the United Kingdom, 9 fibrosarcomas were found among 75 tumors of sheep, 3 in the maxilla and 6 in the mandible.[27] Some of these had already been reported in a paper dealing with a high prevalence of tumors in sheep grazing on bracken (*Pteris aquilina*).[28] The tumors appear to originate around the roots of mandibular or maxillary molar teeth (fig. 8.9). They grew to a very large size, eroding the adjacent bones, but metastases were few in number and only arose in the regional lymph nodes. One of eight lambs, when examined after 34

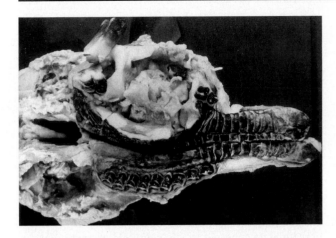

Fig. 8.9. Fibrosarcoma in the jaw of a 5-year-old ewe. Tumor replacing much of the right maxilla. Note displacement of molar teeth, extension to the hard palate, and the ulcerated necrotic center of the tumor.

months of bracken feeding, had a moderately sized fibrosarcoma associated with the left molar maxillary teeth and a small fibrous tissue tumor in the fat around the left mandibular nerve.[29] The relationship between these jaw fibrosarcomas and the ingestion of bracken fern remains to be elucidated. A fibroma with a 2.5 cm long nail embedded in it was reported in the incisor region of a heifer.[30]

Searches of the older literature revealed examples of myxosarcoma, fibroma, and sarcoma of the mandible of young horses, one fibrosarcoma in the tongue of a 3-year-old mare.[2] In contrast a fibroma was found in the guttural pouch of a 13-year-old mare. The proliferating fibro-osseous lesions of the mandible and premaxilla were probably what are now classified as ossifying fibroma.[31]

Granular Cell Tumors

Although with H&E staining and light microscopy granular cell tumors form a morphologically similar group, immunocytochemistry using a panel of antisera indicates that they have a varied histogenesis.[33,34] The majority are of primitive neuroectodermal precursor origin; they are positive for vimentin, S-100, and neuron specific enolase and negative for cytokeratin. Some tumors are vimentin, antitrypsin, and lysozyme positive, suggesting histocytic cell origin.[34] Other tumors, with a histological pattern characteristic of basal cell tumors but with a granular cytoplasm, are cytokeratin positive and neuron specific enolase (NSE) negative.[33] If immunocytochemical results are to be relied on, the tumor samples must have optimal fixation and should contain control structures.[35]

Site, Age, Breed, and Sex

Granular cell tumors are more common in the tongue (7 of 57 lingual tumors[39]) than elsewhere in the oral cavity (1 in 30 mandibular tumors[10]). Of the 17 canine lingual cases in the literature, the mean age is 9.4 years (range 2.5 to 15 years)[33-35]; for 5 labial cases, 8.2 years (4 to

14 years)[33,34,36]; for 3 gingival tumors, 6 months, 5, and 5.5 years[34]; and for 2 palatine cases, 4 years and unknown age. The lingual tumors are more often dorsolateral than ventral and are equally distributed along the length of the tongue. Many of the dogs were of mixed breed, and the remainder were of different pure breeds. There was no sex bias. Four cases in the cat were distributed as follows, one each in the tongue,[34] gum,[36] palate,[33] and tonsil.[35]

Gross Morphology and Histological Features

The tumors are firm and white and have a distinct edge, but there is no fibrous capsule. The usual size at diagnosis is between 0.5 and 2.0 cm, but they can be up to 7 cm diameter. Those on the tongue have a smooth surface in contrast to the pseudoepitheliomatous hyperplasia of the overlying epithelium recorded in the human. Labial lesions are more often ulcerated than are lingual tumors.

The uniformly sized benign tumor cells are large, rounded, or polygonal and are set in a delicate fibrovascular stroma. In more malignant tumors, the cells vary in size and have shapes ranging from spindloid to ovoid. Although the tumors are not invasive there may be some trapped muscle fibers at the edges. In some cases the cells have indistinct borders and are in ill-defined sheets (syncytial pattern), while in other cases groups of 10–20 cells are surrounded by reticulin fibers (organoid pattern); the collagenous stroma or vascular component can be marked.[34]

These tumors have a large amount of pale, eosinophilic, finely granular cytoplasm, and the nuclei are central or eccentric, small, and dense, with one or two nucleoli and few mitoses. The granules are PAS positive and diastase resistant; they are not metachromatic with toluidine blue or acid fast stains. In one series luxol fast blue did not stain all the granules,[34] but the PAS counterstain, because it stains myelin breakdown products, may have masked the blue-green of myelin-like material.[38]

Ultrastructurally, the irregular deeply indented nuclear membrane is said to be characteristic, and three types of cells have been described.[36] Granular cells have small, membrane bound granules composed of vesicular, granular, or amorphous subunits. Interstitial cells are fusiform with little cytoplasm. Angulate body cells appear to be intermediate between granular and interstitial cells and contain membrane bound angulate bodies with microtubular subunits. The interstitial cells are believed to be the multipotent precursors of Schwann cells and granular cell tumors.

Growth and Metastases

Most of the tumors are slow growing, some having been present for 1 to 5 years before removal.[39] No recurrences have been recorded following removal, and only one case developed metastases in lung, heart, and diaphragm 10 months after surgery.[39]

Tumors of Muscle Tissue

Smooth Muscle Tumors

Occasional examples of oral leiomyosarcoma are listed in tumor surveys; for example, 1 in 393 canine mouth tumors,[89] 1 in 95 feline oral tumors,[19] and 1 in 57 canine lingual tumors.[39]

Striated Muscle Tumors

Prevalence, Site, Age, Breed, and Sex

They are rare; for example, studies show 1 in 93 feline tongue tumors,[40] 1 in 30 canine oral tumors,[9] and 1 in the tongue in 124 equine tumors. Striated muscle tumors may arise in skeletal muscle or from undifferentiated mesenchyme in areas where there is no skeletal muscle. They have been recorded in the base of the tongue, in a 5-year-old horse (rhabdomyosarcoma)[41] and in a 9-year-old dog (rhabdomyoma).[42] Of five canine rhabdomyosarcomas involving the jaws, only one was in an old dog (13 years old), and the other four were so-called juvenile rhabdomyosarcomas in animals between 11 and 24 months of age.[43,44] There is no evidence of breed or sex predisposition.

Gross Morphology and Histological Features

The tumors are circumscribed but not encapsulated, are firm in consistency, and on cut surface are lobulated due to fibrous septa; they are white to tan in color with focal areas of necrosis and hemorrhage.

These tumors range from benign, well-differentiated rhabdomyoma to highly malignant anaplastic rhabdomyosarcoma with few recognizable features of striated muscle. Indisputable rhabdomyomas are composed of large, finely granular, deeply acidophilic, round to strap shaped cells exhibiting moderately numerous cross striations and few mitotic figures.[45] The oral tumors described in animals have been poorly differentiated, so careful search and the use of special techniques have been required to find differentiated cells. Tumors that metastasize are clearly sarcoma, but when there are no metastases it becomes a matter of the pathologist's judgment as to whether to designate such a tumor a rhabdomyoma or a low grade rhabdomyosarcoma.[42,44]

Immunohistochemistry has helped in the recognition of striated muscle tumors, and it has been shown that a positive reaction is more intense when the antibody used is from the same species as the tumor bearing animal.[46]

Growth and Metastases

It has been suggested that small round cells no longer divide but differentiate to develop contractile protein when subjected to inadequate nutrition. This may explain how the cells of an undifferentiated bovine serosal tumor differentiated when they metastasized to solid organs and after serial transplantation in nude mice.[46]

Metastases occur via lymphatics to the draining lymph nodes of the head and neck and via the bloodstream to the lungs and other organs.[9,43,44]

Tumors and Tumor-Like Lesions of Vascular Tissue

Vascular tumors in the oropharynx are rare, and most are of blood vessel origin. The terms *angiomatosis, disseminated hemangioma,* and *multifocal hemangiosarcoma* have been used when describing a lesion that might be a multicentric malformation or a tumor with multiple primary sites. Most cases in animals are of unknown etiology. In the human exposure to vinyl chloride, thorium dioxide, arsenic, and radiation are causative factors. In veterinary medicine, vascular tumors have been produced by inhalation of radioisotopes in dogs, and C type virus particles have been demonstrated in cutaneous angioma of cats.

Factor VIII related antigen can be used in formalin fixed, paraffin processed sections as a marker for normal and neoplastic endothelial cells as well as for reactive and tumor neovascularizations; the majority of canine cutaneous hemangioma cells have been shown to contain intracytoplasmic positive granules.[47,48]

Hemangiomas have been recorded in cattle and horses, but it is only in cats and dogs that frequency of occurrence has been estimated; for example, studies have shown frequency as 1.75 percent of canine lingual tumors,[39] 0.5 percent of canine maxillary tumors,[3] and 1.1 percent of feline lingual tumors.[40]

In dogs the frequency of hemangiosarcoma in oral tumors ranges from 0.5 percent[89] to 1.28 percent,[5] and for lingual tumors the figure for dogs is 5.26 percent[39] and for cats 1.1 percent.[40]

Hemangiopericytoms rarely occur as oral tumors; they have characteristic whorls of round to spindle shaped cells surrounding a central vascular space.[9,39]

A pedunculate lymphangioma in the roof of the nasopharynx of a 7-year-old German shepherd has been described,[49] and three lymphangiomas of the tongue in cats have been listed.[40]

Bovine Blood Vessel Tumors

Nine hemangiomas involving one site have been recorded, all involving calves 6 months old or younger.[50-53] In two other cases, multiple tumor sites were involved, raising the problem of differentiating between multifocal hemangioma and hemangiosarcoma with metastasis.[54]

The single site tumors were usually noticed at birth or within 3 days of birth. More females than males were affected, and there was no breed predisposition. All the cases involved the mandible, eight in the region of the incisors. The tumors formed plaques or nodules; the surface was pink to red, and when ulcerated it bled. Histologically the lesions exhibited capillary, cavernous, and solid patterns. Because these masses were found in young animals, the question arises as to whether they are hamartomas or hemangiomas, but in some cases the vessel linings had two or more layers of cuboidal endothelium, suggesting neoplasia. No metastases were seen. An 8-month-old male holstein fetus was found with a pedunculated $1.5 \times 6 \times 1$ cm hemangioma on the tongue and similar tumors in the placenta and skin of the corpus.[54] A 2-week-old Angus calf had tumors in the skin of the head, the skeletal and heart muscles, and the nasal cavity extending into the hard palate and gums, and at all these sites the histological pattern was of a hemangiosarcoma.

It seems that there is a range of lesions from hamartoma through benign tumor to malignant neoplasia, and it may be that all cases start as a malformation and some progress to become true neoplasms.

Equine Blood Vessel Tumors

A hemangioma was present in the roof of the medial compartment of the guttural pouch of a 16-year-old thoroughbred,[55] and hemangiosarcomas have been reported in the mandible and the maxilla.[31,55]

Canine Blood Vessel Tumors

Hemangiomas have been recorded in the jaw[3] and tongue.[39,57] In one case the lesion had been present for 4 years, and there was no recurrence 2 years after removal. Hemangiosarcoma has been reported in the tongue and the mandibular incisor region.[39] Hemangiosarcoma of the skin was identified in 13 of 800 beagles, and the tumors were first seen at an average age of 12.6 years.[58] In 3 of these 13 dogs, discrete red tumors less than 0.5 cm diameter were present in the anterior free portion of the tongue, and 2 of the 3 also had internal hemangiosarcoma.

Feline Blood Vessel Tumors

Hemangiosarcomas have been recorded in the gum (twice), palate (once), and tongue (once).[40] Multiple hemangiomas on the anterolateral edges of the tongue in a 2.5-year-old Siamese were treated by resection but recurred at the surgical margins.[59] Cyclophosphamide and prednisolone, along with irradiation, controlled but did not abolish the lesions, and no metastases were detected 18 months after the first diagnosis.

Other Tumors

Four oral neuroendocrine tumors, three gingival and one labial, that consisted of round and polygonal cells in an organoid pattern have been described in dogs.[61] The pale basophilic cytoplasm with H&E may stain with Gremelius argyrophilic stain, but does not stain with PAS or toluidine blue. With transmission electron microscopy neuroendocrine membrane bound granules can be demonstrated. The pleomorphic oval nuclei have convoluted indentations of the nuclear membrane, and a few multinucleate cells are present.

There are scattered references to histiocytoma in surveys of canine tumors affecting the lip: of 8 histiocytomas

in 393 oral tumors, 7 were labial cases.[89] Myeloma and two lipomas have been reported in the tongue of older dogs.[39] Between 2 percent and 8 percent of oral tumors defied classification and were recorded as anaplastic or undifferentiated sarcomas.[8,14,39]

A diagnosis of mandibular fibrous histiocytoma was made in a 10.5-year-old dog and an 11.7-year-old cat.[10] Myxoma and myxosarcoma may be seen in the mouth of older dogs[8,39] and cats.[21,89]

Tumors of perineural fibroblasts and Schwann cells occur in adult and aged cattle, dogs, and cats. Benign and malignant schwannomas form 1 percent of all canine oral tumors[1] and 4 percent of canine maxillary and mandibular tumors.[8] They are also occasionally recorded in the cat[3,7] and in the tongue of cattle.[62]

Bone tumors form 1.5–4 percent of canine oral tumors[1,2] and 3.5 percent of feline oral tumors.[21] The figure given for mandibular and maxillary bone tumors in the dog is between 3 percent and 10 percent[9,10,13] and for the mandible in the cat is 7.7 percent.[64] Benign proliferative fibro-osseous lesions (possibly hamartomas) have been reported occasionally in all species but have received most attention in horses. Some tumors are a mixture of osteogenic, chondrogenic, fibroblastic and unidentified mesenchymal cells.[63]

Lymphomas

Canine Lymphoma

Lymphoid tumors account for approximately 5 percent of all oral tumors.[1] Tonsillar enlargement may be unilateral or bilateral; when bilateral, the disease may be part of multicentric lymphoma. Other cases have been designated T cell–like lymphoma (epitheliotropic lymphoma; mycosis fungoides) even when there are no accompanying chronic skin lesions.[66]

Dogs with lymphoid tumors in the mouth also have lymphoma in other sites along the alimentary tract, drainage lymph nodes, liver, and the mantle zone of the spleen. These are believed to be examples of mucosal associated B cell lymphoma.[67]

Extragenital canine transmissible venereal tumor can sometimes give rise to tumors of the lip and buccal mucosa even when there are no genital lesions. Immunophenotyping suggests that at least some are of histiocytic origin.[68]

Feline Lymphoma

Three percent of all oral tumors are lymphoid.[21] The gingiva are involved more often than the tonsil and pharynx.[2,21,64] Cats as young as 1 year old have developed tumors, but the tumors are mostly seen in adult animals, mean age 9.5 years.[2,21] Some gingival cases are T cell–like lymphoma.[21] Oral extranodal lymphomas are more common in cats infected with FeLV and FIV[64]; however, lymphoma tumorigenesis is multifactorial, involving inactivation of tumor suppressor genes and activation of oncogenes.[69]

Ruminant Lymphoma

Bovine lymphomas are divided into enzootic cases found in adult cattle (4 to 8 years old) associated with BLV, and sporadic cases in young animals with no virus infection. Enzootic cases do not appear to involve the mandible, but lymphoma causing enlargement of the mandible and osteolysis, macroscopically resembling actinomycosis, have been recorded in three heifers 19 to 24 months old.[70,71] In two of these cases there was lymphoma in the mandibular lymph nodes, and in the third case there were multiple lesions in the alimentary tract and widespread tumors in other viscera as well as a leukemia.

Lymphomas of the jaws have occasionally been reported in adult goats.[72]

Equine Lymphoma

There have been five recorded cases of lesions that caused thickening of the mucosa between the hard and soft palate.[73-75] These cases were considered to be lymphoma on the basis of disruption of normal tissue architecture by large lymphocytes with many mitotic figures. Moreover, the drainage lymph nodes were involved in three cases, and in one case there was neoplasia in the turbinates, pharynx, and subcutaneous lymph nodes.

Oral Extramedullary Plasmacytoma

Prevalence

It is difficult to assess the prevalence of these tumors because they can be easily misdiagnosed. One retrospective study in which cases of round cell tumors were reviewed found that the initial diagnosis of 50 of 75 plasmacytoma cases was incorrect[76]; 22 of the 75 cases were located in the mouth region, and a common "misdiagnosis" was "reticulum cell sarcoma."

Clinical Features and Gross Morphology

The mean age at diagnosis is approximately 10 years in dogs, with a range of 3 to 22 years.[76,77] There is no clear breed predisposition, but males appear to be affected more often than females. The lips and gums (mucotaneous) are the most commonly affected sites, but cases have been recorded on the tongue and pharynx. The tumors on the lips are usually sessile and 1 to 2 cm in diameter, while those at other sites tend to be larger and ulcerated and may be pedunculated. Solid tumors are usually solitary and have distinct borders but are not encapsulated.

Histological Features

Examination of cytological preparations indicates a round cell tumor with some multinucleate giant cells; there are anisocytosis, anisokaryosis, and variable numbers of mitotic figures. H&E stained sections contain almost uniform fields of round to oval plasmacytoid cells set in a sparse fibrovascular stroma. There often is a range of undifferentiated round cells with binucleation and anisokaryosis admixed with more differentiated cells that have plasma cell characteristics: eccentric clock faced nuclei and a clear perinuclear crescent. The cytoplasm is basophilic in H&E staining; it is pyroninophilic and may contain PAS positive, diastase sensitive, granules of glycogen. In poorly differentiated cells transmission electron microscopy reveals that the abundant rough endoplasmic reticulum is seldom in parallel stacks. Multinucleate giant cells are sometimes found, as are cells with Russell bodies, and infrequently there are areas of amyloid. The amyloid reacts to lambda light chain probes but not to IgG; the giant cells are negative, suggesting that they are reacting to the amyloid rather than processing it.[78] Immunoglobulin staining shows that the neoplasms are monoclonal reacting to dog heavy chain classes IgG or IgA (usually IgG) and human light chain types lambda or kappa.[77,78]

Growth and Metastases

The rate of growth is slow, and infiltration into surrounding tissue has only been recorded in some tumors of the gum and pharynx. No metastases to regional lymph nodes have been recorded, even in tumors with numerous mitoses. None of the reported solitary oral plasmacytoma have gone on to develop multiple plasma cell myeloma, although a tumor in the tongue and pharynx proved to be part of a systemic disease with widespread multiple lesions. Probably because the tumors have been solitary, small, and localized, abnormal levels of serum and urinary proteins have not been noted.

Treatment

Local surgical removal provides a cure in most cases. Even when tumors had invaded the underlying bone, no recurrences were observed after partial mandibulectomy and chemotherapy, even though some cases were followed for up to one year.[9,13,76]

Mast Cell Tumors

Mast cell tumors form 6 percent of oral tumors in dogs.[1] They have been reported in animals 2 to 15 years old (mean 7.3 years) and are more common in males than females at a 2:1 ratio.[1] Unlike in cutaneous mast cell tumors, there is no breed predisposition. Mast cell tumors occur most frequently in the lip[79] but also in the gum,[9,10,37] tongue,[39] and hard palate.[37] The tumors are not encapsulated and can be up to 4 cm in diameter. Histological diagnosis is confirmed by metachromatic staining with toluidine blue or a Romanosky stain. Cell pleomorphism, mitotic index, size and number of granules, number of eosinophils, and infiltration at the periphery do not predict their metastatic potential. It has been suggested that AgNOR frequency is more reliable than histological grading in predicting mast cell behavior.[80] Some tumors are part of a systemic disease, and therefore evaluation of the drainage lymph nodes and bone marrow by exfoliative cytology as well as radiographs of the lung may be warranted before surgical removal of the tumor.[79] One series had an actuarial survival rate at 12 months of 17 percent,[1] but longer survival periods are recorded.[79]

A few cases have been reported in the lip and soft palate of adult cats[21] and in the tongue of young cattle.[81]

Tumors Arising in Developmental Anomalies

Ectopic Thyroid Carcinoma

These tumors have been described in mature and old dogs in the ventral wall of the pharynx at the base of the tongue. Cystic neoplasms are thought to develop in the wall of thyroglossal duct cysts; solid tumors probably arise from remnants of the thyroid isthmus or central thyroid plate.[82]

Branchioma

This is the name given to squamous cell carcinomas that form in vestiges of the branchial apparatus. At least some examples in the older literature may have been metastases from small undetected primary tumors located elsewhere in the head and neck.[2]

Nonneoplastic Oropharyngeal Masses

Calcinosis circumscripta (calcium gout) has been reported in the tongue of the dog and cat and in the submandibular salivary gland of a dog.[83,84] Macroscopically the nodular lesion is composed of multiple locules of chalky white friable material separated by connective tissue stroma with variable amounts of granulomatous inflammation. The etiology of these lesions is unknown; some have been termed *apocrine cystic calcinosis* on the basis that trauma causes cystic dilatation and abnormal secretion, which then becomes calcified; others are associated with advanced renal disease, secondary hyperparathyroidism, and metastatic visceral calcification. It has been suggested that the calcinosis nodules in the tongue originate in minor salivary glands.

Nasopharyngeal Polyp in the Cat

Unilateral or, rarely, bilateral polyps up to 2.5 cm in size have been observed in the pharynx. They have been associated with increased respiratory sounds and dyspnea in kittens as young as 4 months old and may be congenital. The pedicle of such polyps extends to the pharyngeal opening of the auditory (eustachian) tube. The evidence is conflicting as to whether these polyps arise exclusively from one site, namely, the auditory tube, the middle ear, or the distal external auditory canal. Histologically stratified squamous epithelium, with mucous glands, covers bone and fibrous tissue that contains many blood vessels. There are variable numbers of inflammatory cells associated with ulceration of the surface. The etiology is unknown, but postinfection and aberrant growth from branchial arch remnants have been suggested.[85]

Eosinophilic Granuloma

The eosinophilic granuloma complex in cats is divided into eosinophilic (rodent) ulcers involving the lip and skin, eosinophilic plaques of the oral cavity, and linear granulomas usually seen in the skin of the thigh.[86] The degree of infiltration of mature eosinophils into the lesion is variable, as is the granulomatous reaction around foci of lytic collagen, both being most marked in linear granuloma. There is no clear-cut breed, age, or sex predisposition.

Oral eosinophilic granuloma in Siberian husky dogs produces multiple raised yellow brown plaques that are sometimes ulcerated and found in animals under 4 years old on the tongue and soft palate, with males being affected more often than females.[87,88] Histologically, the lesions resembled feline linear granuloma. Eosinophilic granulomas are the result of primary hypersensitivity to an antigen or of a secondary hypersensitivity to degeneration of collagen. The lesions usually respond to corticosteroid therapy, but recurrence or spontaneous regression may be seen.

REFERENCES

1. White, R.A.S., Jefferies, A.R., and Freedman, L.S. (1985) Clinical staging for oropharyngeal malignancies in the dog. *J Small Anim Pract* 26:581–594.
2. Cotchin, E. (1956) Neoplasms of the Domesticated Mammals, A Review Series. No. 4. Commonwealth Bureau of Animal Health, Commonwealth Agricultural Bureaux, Farnham Royal, Bucks, England.
3. Frew, D.G., and Dobson, J.M. (1992) Radiological assessment of 50 cases of incisive or maxillary neoplasia in the dog. *J Small Anim Pract* 33:11–18.
4. Cohen, D., Brodey, R.S., and Chen, S.M. (1964) Epidemiologic aspects of oral and pharyngeal neoplasms of the dog. *Amer J Vet Res* 25:1776–1779.
5. Dorn, C.R., and Priester, W.A. (1976) Epidemiologic analysis of oral and pharyngeal cancer in dogs, cats, horses and cattle. *J Amer Vet Med Assoc* 169:1202–1206.
6. Hoyt, R.F., and Withrow, S.J. (1984) Oral malignancy in the dog. *J Amer Anim Hosp Assoc* 20:83–90.
7. Todoroff, R.I., and Brodey, R.S. (1979) Oral and pharyngeal neoplasia in the dog: A retrospective study of 361 cases. *J Amer Vet Med Assoc* 175:567–571.
8. White, R.A.S. (1991) Mandibulectomy and maxillectomy in the dog: Long term survival in 100 cases. *J Small Anim Pract* 32:69–74.
9. Salisbury, S.K., and Lantz, G.C. (1988) Long-term results of partial mandibulectomy for treatment of oral tumors in 30 dogs. *J Amer Anim Hosp Assoc* 24:285–294.
10. Bradley, R.L., MacEwen, E.G., and Loar, A.S. (1984) Mandibular resection for removal of oral tumors in 30 dogs and 6 cats. *J Amer Vet Med Assoc* 184:460–463.
11. Brodey, R.S. (1970) The biological behavior of canine oral and pharyngeal neoplasms. *J Small Anim Pract* 11:45–53.
12. Bastianello, S.S. (1983) A survey of neoplasia in domestic species over a 40 year period from 1935 to 1974 in the Republic of South

Africa. V. Tumors occurring in the cat. *Onderstepoort J Vet Res* 50:105–110.

13. Salisbury, S.K., Richardson, D.C., and Lantz, G.C. (1986) Partial maxillectomy and premaxillectomy in the treatment of oral neoplasia in the dog and cat. *Vet Surg* 15:16–26.

14. Emms, S.G., and Harvey, C.E. (1986) Preliminary results of maxillectomy in the dog and cat. *J Small Anim Pract* 27:291–306.

15. Thrall, D.E. (1981) Orthovoltage radiotherapy of oral fibrosarcomas in dogs. *J Amer Vet Med Assoc* 179:159–162.

16. Creasey, W.A., and Thrall, D.E. (1982) Pharmacokinetic and antitumor studies with radiosensitizer misonidazole in dogs with spontaneous fibrosarcomas. *Amer J Vet Res* 43:1015–1018.

17. Smeak, D.D. (1992) Lower labial pedicle rotation flap for reconstruction of large upper lip defects in two dogs. *J Amer Anim Hosp Assoc* 28:565–569.

18. Harvey, H.J. (1980) Cryosurgery of oral tumors in dogs and cats. *Vet Clin North Amer* 10:821–830.

19. Carpenter, J.L., Andrews, L.K., and Holzworth, J. (1987) Tumors and tumor-like lesions. In Holzworth, J. (ed.), *Diseases of the Cat: Medicine and Surgery*, Vol. 1. W.B. Saunders, Philadelphia, pp. 406–496.

20. Levene, A. (1984) Upper digestive tract neoplasia in the cat. *J Laryn Otol* 98:1221–1223.

21. Stebbins, K.E., Morse, C.C., and Goldschmidt, M.H. (1989) Feline oral neoplasia: A ten year study. *Vet Pathol* 26:121–128.

22. Cotter, S.M. (1981) Oral pharyngeal neoplasms in the cat. *J Amer Anim Hosp Assoc* 17:917–920.

23. Kemp, W.B., Abbey, L.M., and Taylor, L.A. (1976) Pseudosarcomatous fasciitis of the upper lip in a cat. *Vet Med Small Anim Clin* 71:923–925.

24. Bedford, P.G.C. (1982) Origin of the nasopharyngeal polyp in the cat. *Vet Rec* 110:541–542.

25. Brown, N.O., Hayes, A.A., et al. (1980) Combined modality therapy in the treatment of solid tumors in cats. *J Amer Anim Hosp Assoc* 16:719–722.

26. Hardy, W.D. (1981) The feline sarcoma viruses. *J Amer Anim Hosp Assoc* 17:891–997.

27. Ross, A.D., and Williams, P.A. (1983) Neoplasms of sheep in Great Britain. *Vet Rec* 113:598–599.

28. McCrea, C.T., and Head, K.W. (1978) Sheep tumors in north east Yorkshire. I. Prevalence on seven moorland farms. *Brit Vet J* 134:454–461.

29. McCrea, C.T., and Head, K.W. (1981) II. Experimental production of tumors. *Brit Vet J* 137:21–30.

30. Nair, N.R., Tiwari, S.K., and Katoch, R.S. (1988) Fibroma of the lower jaw in a heifer with involvement of gum and teeth and its surgical treatment. *Indian Vet J* 65:817–818.

31. Richardson, D.W., Evans, L.H., and Tulleners, E.P. (1991) Rostral mandibulectomy in five horses. *J Amer Vet Med Assoc* 199:1179–1182.

32. Merriam, J.G. (1972) Guttural pouch fibroma in a mare. *J Amer Vet Med Assoc* 161:487–489.

33. Geyer, C., Hafner, A., Pfleghaar, S., and Hermanns, W. (1992) Immunohistochemical and ultrastructural investigation of granular cell tumors in dog, cat and horse. *J Vet Med* 39:485–494.

34. Patnaik, A.K. (1993) Histologic and immunohistochemical studies of granular cell tumors in seven dogs, three cats, one horse, and one bird. *Vet Pathol* 30:176–185.

35. Wilson, R.B., Holscher, M.A., et al. (1989) Tonsillar granular cell tumor in a cat. *J Comp Pathol* 102:109–112.

36. Turk, M.A.M., Johnson, G.C., Gallina, A.M., and Trigo, F.J. (1983) Canine granular cell tumor (myoblastoma): A report of four cases and review of the literature. *J Small Anim Pract* 24:637–645.

37. Gorlin, R.J., Barron, C.N., Chaudhry, A.P., and Clark, J.J. (1959) The oral and pharyngeal pathology of domestic animals: A study of 487 Cases. *Amer J Vet Res* 20:1032–1061.

38. Kelley, L.C., Hill, J.E., et al. (1995) Spontaneous equine pulmonary granular cell tumors: morphologic, histochemical, and immunohistochemical characterization. *Vet Pathol* 32:101–106.

39. Beck, E.R., Withrow, S.J., McChesney, A.E., et al. (1986) Canine tongue tumors: A Retrospective Review of 57 Cases. *J Amer Anim Hosp Assoc* 22:525–532.

40. Levene, A. (1984) Upper digestive tract neoplasia in the cat. *J Laryn Otol* 98:1221–1223.

41. Hansen, P.D., Frisbie, D.D., Dubielzig, R.R., and Markel, M.D. (1993) Rhabdomyosarcoma of the tongue in a horse. *J Amer Vet Med Assoc* 202:1281–1284.

42. Reams Rivera, R.Y., and Carlton, W.W. (1992) Lingual rhabdomyoma in a dog. *J Comp Pathol* 106:83–87.

43. Kim, D-Y., Hodgin, E.C., Cho, D-Y., and Varnado, J.E. (1996) Juvenile rhabdomyosarcomas in two dogs. *Vet Pathol* 33:447–450.

44. Seibold, H.R. (1974) juvenile alveolar rhabdomyosarcoma in a dog. *Vet Pathol* 11:558–560.

45. Meuten, D.J., Calderwood Mays, M.B., Dillman, R.C., Cooper, B.J., Valentine, B.A., Kuhajda, F.P., and Pass, D.A. (1985) Canine laryngeal rhabdomyoma. *Vet Pathol* 22:533–539.

46. Matsui, T., Imai, T., Han, J.S., et al. (1991) Bovine undifferentiated alveolar rhabdomyosarcoma and its differentiation in xenotransplanted tumors. *Vet Pathol* 28:438–445.

47. Augustin-Voss, H.G., Smith, C.A., and Lewis, R.M. (1990) Phenotypic characterization of normal and neoplastic canine endothelial cells by lectin histochemistry. *Vet Pathol* 27:103–109.

48. Von Beust, B.R., Suter, M.M., and Summers, B.A. (1988) Factor VII-related antigen in canine endothelial neoplasms: An immunohistochemical study. *Vet Pathol* 25:251–255.

49. Stambaugh, J.E., Harvey, C.E., and Goldschmidt, M.H. (1978) Lymphangioma in four dogs. *J Amer Vet Med Assoc* 173:759–761.

50. Sheahan, B.J., and Donnelly, W.J.C. (1981) Vascular hamartomas in the gingiva of two calves. *Vet Pathol* 18:562–564.

51. Stanton, M.E., Meunier, P.C., and Smith, D.F. (1984) Vascular hamartoma in the gingiva of two neonatal calves. *J Amer Vet Med Assoc* 184:205–206.

52. Gaag, I. Van der, Vos, J.H., and Goedegebaure, S.A. (1988) Lobular capillary haemangiomas in two calves. *J Comp Pathol* 99:353–356.

53. Richard, V., Drolet, R., and Fortin, M. (1995) Juvenile bovine angiomatosis in the mandible. *Can Vet J* 36:113–114.

54. Kirkbride, C.A., Bicknell, E.J., and Robb, M.G. (1973) Haemangiomas of a bovine fetus with a chorioangioma of the placenta. *Vet Pathol* 10:238–240.

55. Green, H.J., and O'Connor, J.P. (1986) Haemangioma of the guttural pouch of a 16 year old thoroughbred mare: Clinical and pathological findings. *Vet Rec* 118:445–446.

56. Sweigard, K.D., and Hattel, A.L. (1993) Oral hemangiosarcoma in a horse. *Equine Prac* 15:10–13.

57. Gaag, I. Van der, Voss, J.H., Linde-Sipman, et al. (1989) Canine capillary and combined capillary-cavernous haemangioma. *J Comp Pathol* 101:69–74.

58. Culbertson, M.R. (1982) Hemangiosarcoma of the canine skin and tongue. *Vet Pathol* 19:556–558.

59. Crow, S.E., Pulley, L.T., and Wittenbrock, T.P. (1981) Lingual haemangioma in a cat. *J Amer Anim Hosp Assoc* 17:71–74.

60. Brodey, R.S. (1966) Alimentary tract neoplasms in the cat: A clinicopathologic survey of 46 cats. *Amer J Vet Res* 27:74–80.

61. Whiteley, L.O., and Leininger, J.R. (1987) Neuroendocrine (Merkel) cell tumors of the canine oral cavity. *Vet Pathol* 24:570–572.

62. Monlux, A.W., Anderson, W.A., and Davis, C.L. (1956) A survey of tumors occurring in cattle, sheep and swine. *Amer J Vet Res* 17:646–677.

63. Di Bartola, S.P., Cockerell, G.L., Minor, R.R., and Hoffer, R.E. (1978) A mixed mesenchymal sarcoma in the soft palate of a dog: Light and electron microscopic findings. *Cornell Vet* 68:396–410.

64. Kapatkin, A.S., Marretta, S.M., Patnaik, A.K., et al. (1991) Mandibular swelling in cats: Prospective study of 24 cats. *J Amer Anim Hosp Assoc* 27:575–580.

65. Lucke, V.M., Pearson, G.R., Gregory, S.P., and Whitbread, T.J. (1988) Tonsillar polyps in the dog. *J Small Anim Pract* 29:373–379.

66. Ackerman, L. (1984) Oral T cell-like lymphoma in a dog. *J Amer Anim Hosp Assoc* 20:955–958.

67. Da Silva Curiel, J.M.A., McCaw, D.L., Turk, M.A.M., and Schmidt, D.A. (1988) Multiple mucocutaneous lymphosarcoma in a dog. *Can Vet J* 29:1001–1002.

68. Mozos, E., Méney, A., et al. (1996) Immunohistochemical characterisation of canine transmissible venereal tumor. *Vet Pathol* 33:257–263.

69. Okuda, M., Umeda, A., et al. (1994) Cloning of feline p53 tumor-suppressor gene and its aberration in hematopoietic tumors. *Intl J Cancer* 58:602–607.

70. Kritchevsky, J.E., and Usenik, E.A. (1983) Lymphosarcoma and fracture of the mandible in a cow. *J Amer Vet Med Assoc* 183:803–804.

71. Hamir, A.N., Perkins, C., and Jones, C. (1989) Bovine mandibular lymphosarcoma. *Vet Rec* 125:238.

72. Guedes, R.M.C., Facury Filho, E.J., and Lago, L.A. (1998) Mandibular lymphosarcoma in a goat. *Vet Rec* 143:51–52.

73. Meaghar, D.M., and Brown, M.P. (1978) Lymphoid masses in the pharynx of a thoroughbred filly. *Vet Med/Small Anim Clin* 73:171–174.

74. Adams, R., Calderwood, M.M., and Peyton, L.C. (1988) Malignant lymphoma in three horses with ulcerative pharyngitis. *J Amer Vet Med Assoc* 193:674–676.

75. Lane, J.G. (1985) Palatine lymphosarcoma in two horses. *Equine Vet J* 17:465–467.

76. Rakich, P.M., Latimer, K.S., Weiss, R., and Steffens, W.L. (1989) Mucocutaneous plasmacytomas in dogs: 75 cases (1980–1987) *J Amer Vet Med Assoc* 194:803–810.

77. Kyriazidou, A., Brown, P.J., and Lucke, V.M. (1989) An immuno-histochemical study of canine extramedullary plasma cell tumors. *J Comp Pathol* 100:259–266.

78. Rowland, P.H., and Linke, R.P. (1994) Immunohistochemical characterisation of lambda light-chain-derived amyloid in one feline and five canine plasma cell tumors. *Vet Pathol* 31:390–393.

79. Smeak, D.D. (1992) Lower labial pedicle rotation flap for reconstruction of large upper lip defects in two dogs. *J Amer Anim Hosp Assoc* 28:565–569.

80. Kravis, L.D., Vail, D.M., et al. (1996) Frequency of agyrophilic nucleolar organiser regions in fine needle aspirates and biopsy specimens from mast cell tumor in dogs. *J Amer Vet Med Assoc* 209:1418–1420.

81. Hill, J.E., Langheinrich, K.A., and Kelley, L.C. (1991) Prevalence and location of mast cell tumors in slaughter cattle. *Vet Pathol* 28:449–450.

82. Lantz, G.C., and Salisbury, S.K. (1989) Surgical excision of ectopic thyroid carcinoma involving the base of the tongue in dogs. *J Amer Vet Med Assoc* 195:1606–1608.

83. Anderson, W.I., Cline, J.M., and Scott, D.W. (1988) Calcinosis circumscripta of the tongue in a cat. *Cornell Vet* 78:381–384.

84. Movassaghi, A.R. (1999) Calcinosis circumscripta in the salivary gland of a dog. *Vet Rec* 144:52.

85. Stanton, M.E., Wheaton, L.G., Rander, J.A., and Bjevins, W.E. (1985) Pharyngeal polyps in two feline siblings. *J Amer Vet Med Assoc* 186:1311–1313.

86. Scott, D.W. (1975) Observations on the eosinophilic granuloma complex in cats. *J Amer Anim Hosp Assoc* 11:261–270.

87. Madewell, B.R., Stannard, A.A., Pulley, L.T., and Nelson, V.G. (1980) Oral eosinophilic granuloma in siberian husky dogs. *J Amer Vet Med Assoc* 177:701–703.

88. Potter, K.A., Tucker, R.D., and Carpenter, J.L. (1980) Oral eosinophilic granuloma of Siberian huskies. *J Amer Anim Hosp Assoc* 16:595–600.

89. Vos, J.H., and van der Gaag, I. (1987) Canine and feline oral-pharyngeal tumors. *J. Vet. Med.* 34:420–427.

90. Ciekot, P.A., Powers, B.E., et al. (1994) Histologically low-grade, yet biologically high-grade, fibrosarcomas of the mandible and maxilla in dogs: 25 cases (1982–1991). *J Amer Vet Med Assoc* 204:610–615.

TUMORS OF THE ESOPHAGUS AND ESOPHAGEAL REGION OF THE STOMACH

Epithelial Tumors in the Dog and Cat

Papilloma

The viral oropharyngeal papillomas of young dogs rarely extend into the esophagus, and when they do it is into the pharyngeal region. True benign papillomas have not been reported in the cat, although there is one description of multiple papillomatous lesions in a 1-year-old domestic shorthair cat[1] that was interpreted as a hyperplastic reaction secondary to chronic esophagitis.

Squamous Cell Carcinoma

Prevalence

Primary tumors in the esophagus of the dog are rare. One review reported four squamous cell carcinomas, four undifferentiated carcinomas, one each of scirrhous carcinoma and adenocarcinoma, and five leiomyomas.[6] Only eight esophageal tumors were observed in 49,229 dogs over an 11 year period; two of these were primary (leiomyoma and squamous cell carcinoma), and six were secondary (three thyroid, two respiratory tract, and one gastric).[6] In the London area of the United Kingdom carcinoma of the esophagus was reported as rare in the dog (1 in 117 alimentary carcinomas) but common in the cat (21 squamous cell carcinomas in 97 alimentary tract carcinomas collected over a period of 18 years).[2] This contrasts with the figures for the Edinburgh area of the United Kingdom over the same period, in which there were 4 feline esophageal squamous cell carcinomas in 54 alimentary carcinomas. This geographical variation in frequency of occurrence was further emphasized by the observation of only 2 cases in 494 cats necropsied in Utrecht,[3] and 4 esophageal squamous cell carcinomas in 3248 feline tumors and tumor-like lesions collected in the United States over a 35 year period.[4]

Age, Breed, and Sex

Tumor bearing cats in all geographical locations are elderly; in the United Kingdom the mean age was 10.5 years and in the United States 12 years (range 6 to 20 years).[4,5,7] Castrated males were overrepresented, but there was no breed predisposition. Dogs with esophageal tumors had no breed or sex bias, but most were old, ranging from 6 to 11 years of age.

Site and Clinical Characteristics

In both dogs and cats the most frequently reported site is in the middle third of the esophagus at the level of the first two ribs, cranial to the aortic arch; primary squamous cell carcinoma was reported at this site in 24 of 29 feline cases in one series.[7] Clinical signs include progressive weight loss, salivation, and regurgitation of food and fluid. If the mucosal surface has become ulcerated, hematemesis may be seen. The difference between regurgitation and vomiting is important because vomiting only occurs with gastric carcinoma that has extended into the esophagus.[6]

Morphology

The lesion tends to be an ulcerated plaque with rolled edges that forms a single annular thickening completely encircling the esophagus and extending for a length of up to 8 cm by the time the tumor is diagnosed. The neoplasm spreads circumferentially and longitudinally by the submucosal lymphatic vessels. On endoscopy the epithelial surface appears as a white nodularity with areas of ulceration and hemorrhage.[8] There are no special histological features, the pattern ranging from a noncornifying to a well-differentiated tumor with keratin pearls. Inflammatory reaction may be extensive due to infection of the ulcerated surface. Endoscopic biopsies should be interpreted with care, since the inflammatory reaction is superficial, above the recognizable tumor cells.[5]

Growth and Metastasis

The tumor grows by infiltration of tissue spaces and lymphatic vessels. Direct extension by local infiltration is often extensive, even invading the wall of the trachea.[8] Tumors in this region will spread to the caudal cervical, mediastinal, and even bronchial lymph nodes. Distant blood borne metastases have been reported in lung, kidney, thyroid, and spleen, but the onset of clinical signs forestalls extensive metastases.

Etiology

In human beings the localized geographical distribution has indicated some etiological factors apart from alcohol, tobacco, and gastric reflux; dietary deficiencies of vitamins and zinc as well as the ingestion of mycotoxins and nitrosamines have been incriminated.[9,10]

Extracts from cultures of *Fusarium* spp. when given by stomach tube to rats and mice are immunosuppressive and cause hyperplasia of the squamous epithelium of the esophagus and esophageal region of the stomach, and such mycotoxins could be carcinogenic.[9] Many nitrosamine compounds when ingested can induce esophageal papillomas and squamous cell carcinomas in rats. A nitrosamine compound injected intraperitoneally will also produce multicentric tumors at all levels of the esophagus.[10] Since there were no tumors at the site of injection, the chemical need not act during swallowing, but needs enzymatic activation to become carcinogenic; one site for this may be the esophagus.

Esophageal tumors in cats may be due to ingestion of a carcinogen (possibly licked from the fur during self-grooming), the location of the tumor in the esophagus cranial to the aortic arch being due to delayed passage of ingesta.[7]

Adenocarcinoma

Glandular tumors of the esophagus have rarely been reported in the dog and cat. In people squamous cell carcinomas are more common than adenocarcinoma except at the gastroesophageal junction, where adenocarcinoma may originate from the submucosal esophageal glands or by extension from a gastric carcinoma. Alternatively, glandular tumors may arise from heterotopic foci of gastric-type epithelium, retained areas of fetal-type columnar epithelium, or metaplastic epithelium resulting from gastric secretion reflux and ulceration. Esophageal carcinomas show multidirectional differentiation, that is, squamous cell carcinomas have focal glandular areas, adenocarcinomas have foci of squamous differentiation, and neurosecretory granules are found in cells of both squamous cell carcinoma and adenocarcinoma,[12] which may mean that esophageal epithelial tumors arise from totipotential stem cells. An adenocarcinoma occurred in the cranial esophagus of a cat, but there are no glands in the esophagus at this point.[4] Scirrhous adenocarcinoma of the esophageal glands of an 8-year-old Irish setter extended into a caudal lung lobe, the diaphragm, and the gastric cardia and was associated with hypertrophic osteopathy.[11]

Neuroendocrine Carcinoma

Although neuroendocrine cells are present in the esophagus, there is only one report of a tumor arising from these cells in the literature. The reported case was in a 9-year-old domestic shorthair castrated cat that had a $3 \times 2 \times 1.5$ cm intraluminal sessile mass removed from the midthoracic esophagus.[13] No other primary tumors were documented, but a necropsy was not permitted. The tumor had characteristic light microscopic features of a neuroendocrine tumor, there were numerous granules that stained with a modified Grimelius stain, and transmission electron microscopy revealed only a few dense core neurosecretory type granules. Some cells stained immunocytochemically for calcitonin and somatostatin but did not stain for ACTH, glucagon, gastrin, insulin, or serotonin.

Mesenchymal Tumors

Smooth Muscle Tumors

There are only a few published reports of esophageal smooth muscle tumors.[14,15] In a survey of 15,215 canine accessions over a 15 year period, only two such cases were found, and they were grouped with tumors of the stomach.[15] Leiomyomas in the dog are usually nodular masses situated at the gastroesophageal junction in animals over 8 years old. An intramural leiomyoma in a 2.5-year-old dog[16] resembled leiomyomatosis, which is a malformation or hamartoma characterized as a diffuse hyperplasia of the smooth muscle of the esophagus seen in young adult human beings.[17]

The older literature states that leiomyoma was common in the thoracic esophagus of horses.[21] There are no recent reports of equine esophageal leiomyoma, but in one case both distal esophagus and cranial stomach were involved in a leiomyosarcoma, and the stomach was recorded as the primary.[18]

Other Tumors

A large multinodular plasma cell tumor was detected in the caudal esophagus of a 14-year-old dog.[19] Among a battery of immunohistochemical reagents, only those for vimentin, IgM, and lambda light chains were positive, and transmission electron microscopy revealed that the cells had the character of plasma cells.

A 10-year-old dog had a 10 cm diameter osteosarcoma removed from the wall of the cranial cervical region of the esophagus.[20] The tumor was composed of sarcomatous chondromatous, osteoid, and osseous areas. There was no radiographic evidence of an occult primary osteosarcoma and no evidence of spirocercosis, hence the authors concluded this was a primary extraskeletal osteosarcoma.

REFERENCES

1. Wilkinson, G.T. (1970) Chronic papillomatous oesophagitis in a young cat. *Vet Rec* 87:355–356.
2. Cotchin, E. (1959) Some tumors of dogs and cats of comparative veterinary and human interest. *Vet Rec* 71:1040–1054.
3. Happé, R.P., van den Gaag, I., et al. (1978) Esophageal squamous cell carcinoma in two cats. *Tijdschr Diergeneesk* 103:1080–1086.
4. Carpenter, J.L., Andrews, L.K., and Holzworth, J. (1987) Tumors and tumor-like lesions. In Holzworth, J. (ed.), *Diseases of the Cat: Medicine and Surgery*, Vol. 1. W.B. Saunders Co., Philadelphia, pp. 406–596.
5. Fernandes, F.H., Hawe, R.S., and Loeb, W.F. (1987) Primary squamous cell carcinoma of the esophagus in a cat. *Comp Anim Pract* 1:16–22.
6. Ridgway, R.L., and Suter, P.F. (1979) Clinical and radiographic signs in primary and metastatic esophageal neoplasms of the dog. *J Amer Vet Med Assoc* 174:700–704.
7. Cotchin, E. (1966) Some etiological aspects of tumors in domesticated animals. *Ann Roy Coll Surg England* 38:92–116.
8. McCaw, D., Pratt, M., and Walshaw, R. (1980) Squamous cell carcinoma of the esophagus in a dog. *J Amer Vet Med Assoc* 16:561–563.
9. Schoental, R., and Joffe, A.Z. (1974) Lesions induced in rodents by extracts from cultures of *Fusarium pooe* and *F. sporotrichioides*. *J Pathol* 112:37–42.
10. Levison, D.A., et al. (1979) Esophageal neoplasia in male wistar rats due to parenteral D; (2-hydroxypropyl)-nitrosamine. *J Pathol* 129:31–36.
11. Randolph, J.F., Centre, S.A., et al. (1984) Hypertrophic osteopathy associated with adenocarcinoma of the esophageal glands in a dog. *J Amer Vet Med Assoc* 184:98–99.
12. Newman, J., Antanakopoulous, G.N., et al. (1992) The ultrastructure of esophageal carcinomas: Multidirectional differentiation. A transmission electron microscopic study of 43 cases. *J Pathol* 167:193–198.
13. Patnaik, A.K., Erlandson, R.A., and Lieberman, P.H. (1990) Esophageal neuroendocrine carcinoma in a cat. *Vet Pathol* 27:128–130.
14. Rajurkar, S.R., Rajurmer, R.R., and Moregaonker, S.D. (1995) Leiomyoma of esophagus in a non-descript bullock: A case report. *Indian Vet J* 72:511–513.
15. Hayden, D.W., and Nielsen, S.W. (1973) Canine alimentary neoplasia. *Zbl Vet Med* 20A:1–22.
16. Rolfe, D.S., Twedt, D.C., and Seim, H.B. (1994) Chronic regurgitation or vomiting caused by esophageal leiomyoma in three dogs. *J Amer Anim Hosp Assoc* 30:425–430.
17. Watanabe, H., Jass, J.R., and Sobin, L.H. (1990) *Histopathological Typing of Esophageal and Gastric Tumors*. Springer-Verlag Berlin, Heidelberg, p. 17.
18. Boy, M.G., Palmer, J.E., Heyer, G., and Hamir, A.N. (1992) Gastric leiomyosarcoma in a horse. *J Amer Vet Med Assoc* 200:1363–1364.
19. Hamilton, T.A., and Carpenter, J.L. (1994) Esophageal plasmacytoma in a dog. *J Amer Vet Med Assoc* 204:1210–1211.
20. Wilson, R.B., Holscher, M.A., and Laney, P.S. (1991) Esophageal osteosarcoma in a dog. *J Amer Vet Med Assoc* 27:361–363.
21. Cotchin, E. (1956) Neoplasms of the Domesticated Mammals, A Review Series. No. 4. Commonwealth Bureau of Animal Health, Commonwealth Agricultural Bureaux, Farnham Royal, Bucks, England.

TUMORS ASSOCIATED WITH *SPIROCERCA LUPI*

Spirocercosis is widely but unevenly distributed in tropical and subtropical countries, the variation in incidence probably reflecting the management of the population studied, for example, it is common in stray rural dogs and uncommon in urban, pedigreed, well cared for dogs.[1-3]

The life cycle of the parasite starts with the intermediate host, one of several species of coprophagous beetles (dung beetle) eating the feces of the definitive host that contains the embryonated eggs of *Spirocerca lupi*. The larvae migrate via the walls of the arteries from the stomach to the thoracic aorta, reaching the wall of the lower esophagus in about 3 months. During this passage they cause exostosis of the ventral surface of vertebrae T6 to T12 and nodular lesions in the aortic adventitia (fig. 8.10A). In the esophageal wall, the larvae become adults in about 3 months, copulate, and discharge eggs to be passed in the feces to restart the cycle. Nonneoplastic lesions are found in the esophagus in 15–40 percent of dogs (fig. 8.10B, C), in the esophagus and aorta in 23–86 percent, and in the aorta alone, in dogs less than 1 year old, in 7–30 percent.[2,4] The characteristic aortic scars and spondylitis persist at least 5–8 years after the adults in the esophagus have died.

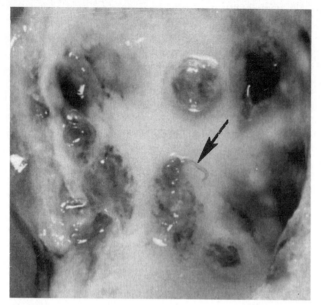

A

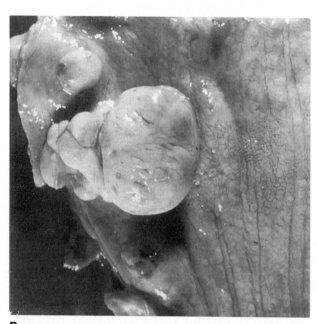

B

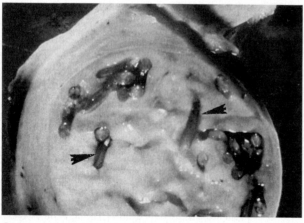

C

The percentage of infected dogs that develop tumors, although low, is variable; in Sierra Leone, one tumor was found in 235 infected dogs, whereas in Kenya 43 sarcomas were found in 206 infected dogs.[2,5] Not all these neoplasms have worms in or adjacent to them: 13 of 17 fibrosarcomas and 11 of 25 osteosarcomas had worms in the tumor mass.[2] Dogs with esophageal tumors but no worms usually had nonneoplastic lesions, indicating a previous patent spirocercosis. There are a few reports of tumors arising in the aortic and vertebral lesions.[2] It has been suggested that spirocerca acts as a cocarcinogen, with oncogenesis being enhanced by unknown promoting agent(s). Worms in aberrant sites can induce tumors as in a pulmonary fibrosarcoma containing several *S. lupi*.[6]

Nonneoplastic lesions are most common in the thoracic aorta and in the first few centimeters of the abdominal aorta. The aortic lesion consists of an adventitial mass of granulation tissue surrounding necrotic material that contains worms in about 5 percent of cases (fig. 8.10). The loss of elastic fibers in the wall of the aorta, atrophy of muscle, and fibrosis lead to aneurysms or aneurysmal scars.[7] About 85 percent of the esophageal nodules are located between the aortic arch and the diaphragm, often 1–2 inches from the hiatus of the esophagus. The nodules consist of a central cavity that contains tightly entwined parasites in a pool of greenish yellow exudate. The lesions in the esophagus can cause pleuritis, reflux esophagitis, ulceration, and perforation.[7]

Histologically the initial lesion in the esophagus consists of loose, highly vascular fibroblastic proliferation (fig. 8.10). Macrophages, mast cells, and numerous neutrophils, but not eosinophils, are found in the center of the lesion. Plasma cells are especially prominent in the fibrous capsule. Subendothelial collagenous plaques that almost occlude the lumen may be seen in the arteries in the wall of the esophagus, and they may also contain metaplastic cartilage and bone.[8]

Clinical Characteristics, Age, Breed, and Sex

Most nonmalignant cases do not exhibit clinical signs. In one series only 30 of 206 infected dogs had clinical signs of spirocercosis, and of these, 29 had definite tumors; in 4 others the esophageal nodules were classed as "parasarcoma."[2] The average age of dogs with esophageal tumors associated with this parasite is 7 years.

Because of the time necessary for migration of the parasite and for development to the adult stage, dogs under

Fig. 8.10. *Spirocerca lupi* lesions of the dog. **A.** Intimal surface of aorta with part of an immature worm (arrow) protruding into the lumen. **B.** Nonneoplastic pedunculated lesion of the esophagus. **C.** Cross section of esophageal wall with nonneoplastic mass containing adult worms (arrowheads). [Courtesy Dr. W.S. Bailey.]

6 months of age are unlikely to have an established lesion.[7] There is no known breed predilection; the lesions are seen most often in indigenous scavenger dogs, especially in developing countries; and the incidence in these countries is much lower in dogs cared for and fed adequately by their owners.[5] Sexes of dogs are affected about equally.

Gross Morphology and Histological Features

The tumors that arise in the esophageal nodules may contain parasites (fig. 8.10 C). The tumors are pedunculated, nodular, or fungiform and project into the lumen of the esophagus (fig. 8.11). The tumors measure up to 10 cm in diameter and are fibrous or bony in consistency. The color is generally grayish white, and the surface is commonly ulcerated.

Histological examination of some of these esophageal nodules shows that there are areas with active fibroblastic tissue and a high mitotic rate (fig. 8.11). With continued proliferation, the fibroblasts form small neoplastic foci that eventually combine to form a typical invasive fibrosarcoma. The borderline cases of encapsulated chronic inflammatory granuloma with foci of fibroma and fibrosarcoma have been called "parasarcoma."[2]

Some of these tumors display metaplastic transformation of fibroblastic tissue into osteoid and cartilage with numerous osteoblasts and osteoclasts.[8] Several sections need to be taken from the nodule as there may be considerable variation in the histological pattern in a single lesion. The sarcomas exhibiting osteoid, cartilage, and bone tend to occur in older dogs, for example, dogs with fibrosarcoma had an age range of 1–11 years (mean, 5 years), and those with oestosarcoma had an age range of 3–15 years (mean, 7.5 years).[2] Moreover, the fibrosarcomas tended to be smaller (< 5 cm in diameter) than osteosarcomas.

Growth, Metastases, and Paraneoplastic Syndromes

Immature worms may be found in the esophagus of animals as young as 6 months old, but they take 5 months or more to mature. When induced, the sarcoma must be able to grow rapidly since tumors have been reported in 1-year-old animals. Sarcomas may show infiltrative growth into both tissue spaces and blood vessels. Established metastases are observed in 10–50 percent of tumor cases (2 of 17 fibrosarcomas and 12 of 25 osteosarcomas had metastasized[2]). Lungs and bronchial lymph nodes are the most common sites for metastasis; myocardium, pleura, diaphragm, kidney, liver, spleen, adrenal, and parietal pleura are less commonly affected. Hypertrophic osteopathy has been seen associated with esophageal tumors with and without metastasis to the lungs.[4,6]

REFERENCES

1. Bailey, W.S. (1972) *Spirocerca lupi*. A continuing inquiry. *J Parasitol* 58:3–22.
2. Wandera, J.G. (1976) Further observations on canine spirocercosis in Kenya. *Vet Rec* 99:348–351.
3. Campbell, J.R., Pirie, H.M., and Weiper, W.L.W. (1964) Osteogenic sarcoma of the esophagus in a dog. *Vet Rec* 76:244–246.
4. Fox, S.M., Burns, J., and Hawkins, J. (1988) Spirocercosis in dogs. *Comp Cont Educ* 10:807–822.
5. Kamara, J.A. (1964) The incidence of canine spirocercosis in the freetown area of Sierra Leone. *Bull Epiz Dis Afr* 12:465–468.
6. Stephens, L.C., Gleiser, C.A., and Jardine, J.H. (1983) Primary pulmonary fibrosarcoma associated with *Spirocerca lupi* infection in a dog with hypertrophic pulmonary osteoarthropathy. *J Amer Vet Med Assoc* 182:496–498.
7. Hamir, A.N. (1986) Oesophageal perforation and pyothorax associated with *Spirocerca lupi* infestation in a dog. *Vet Rec* 119:276.
8. Murray, M. (1986) Incidence and pathology of *Spirocerca lupi* in Kenya. *J Comp Pathol* 78:401–405.

TUMORS OF UPPER ALIMENTARY TRACT IN RUMINANTS

Papilloma and Squamous Cell Carcinoma in Cattle

Tumors of the upper alimentary tract in cattle have been reported throughout the world, but it is difficult to compare the prevalence in different countries because of variations in collecting the data. Tumors that cause clinical signs may be overrepresented in records from clinics, for examples, one author reports two fibroma/fibropapillomas in eight tumors causing ruminal tympany.[1] In contrast, rumen carcinomas are rare in apparently healthy cattle in abattoir statistics; studies show 0 in 1000 in United States,[2] 1 in 447 in Canada,[3] and 1 in 208 in the Netherlands.[4] Although these tumors may be this uncommon, it is also possible that small easily recognizable lesions such as papilloma may not be submitted by a meat inspector to a pathologist, that the processor may trim off such small lesions when dressing parts of the carcass and viscera that are not used for human food, or that viscera that look normal externally may not be opened at the slaughterhouse. One squamous cell carcinoma of the rumen but no papillomas was reported in 1.3 million cattle submitted by United Kingdom meat inspectors,[5] but 19 percent of 7746 healthy lowland cattle had papillomas in a United Kingdom abattoir survey, in which, contrary to the usual practice, the esophagus and rumen were opened.[6] Similarly, the prevalence of papilloma of the palate in an Australian abattoir survey may have been underestimated.[7]

Alimentary carcinomas are so common in some regions that the disease is recognized as an entity by farmers and veterinarians, who clinically diagnosed upper ali-

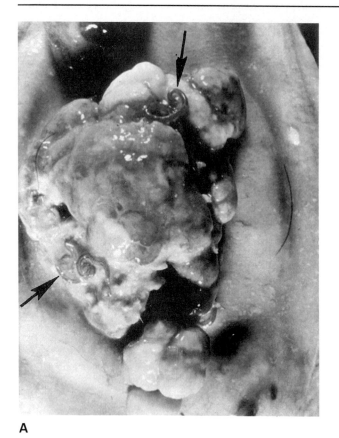

A

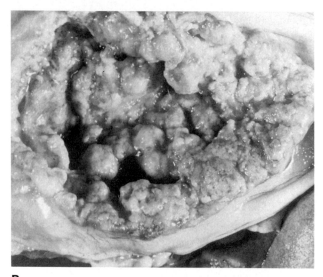

B

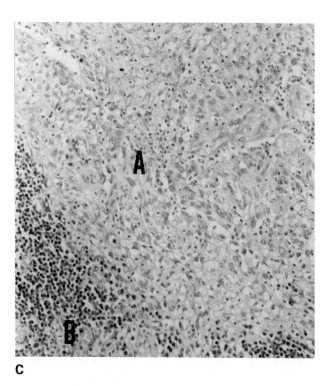

C

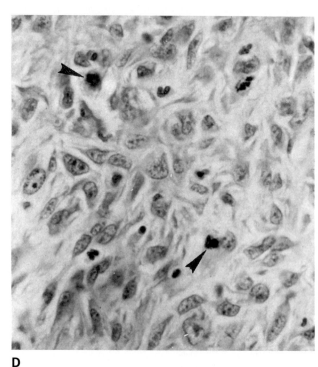

D

Fig. 8.11. Neoplasms of the esophagus associated with *Spirocerca lupi* infection. **A.** Pedunculated masses protruding into the lumen; adult worms (arrows) embedded in neoplasm. **B.** Cavitated multinodular sarcoma. [Courtesy of Dr. W.S. Bailey.] **C.** Active fibroblastic proliferation (*A*) surrounded by masses of plasma cells (*B*). **D.** Transitional stage between fibroblastic proliferation and sarcoma; mitotic figures (arrowheads).

mentary tract neoplasia in 80 cattle from Scottish Highland "cancer farms" and on necropsy confirmed 169 squamous cell carcinomas.[6] In the Nasampolai valley in Kenya the disease is a ruminal carcinoma,[8] in Brazil it is a pharyngeal carcinoma linked with enzootic hematuria,[9] and in

the west of Scotland 96 percent of cattle with squamous cell carcinoma had papilloma in the upper alimentary tract, while 56 percent of them also had intestinal adenomas and adenocarcinomas and 30 percent bladder tumors.[6]

Squamous Papilloma and Fibropapilloma

Clinical Characteristics

Papillomas are found at all ages. The age distribution in one series was 55 percent in cattle less than 2 years old, 9 percent in cattle between 2 and 3 years, and 36 percent in cattle more than 3 years old[6]; in another study, 16 percent of 940 cattle, mostly over 3.5 years old, had papilloma on the palate, but there were none in 100 calves under 3 months of age, and only 5 percent in 170 yearlings.[7] The breed and sex of affected animals reflected the predominant breed and sex of the cattle kept in the region.

Squamous papillomas are frequently asymptomatic but in large numbers may lead to salivation and interference with suckling or chewing. The larger fibropapillomas in the forestomachs are often associated with recurrent ruminal tympany especially if they are in the region of the cardia and esophageal groove.

Gross Morphology and Sites

Squamous papillomas are seldom solitary and usually occur in groups at several sites along the tract. They may be found at any site from mouth to rumen, but the esophagus and rumen have the highest percentage of lesions.[6,8] Squamous papillomas range in size from 1 to 10 mm in diameter but sometimes reach 20 to 30 mm in the oropharynx. The smaller tumors tend to be sessile, flattened, and white with a pitted surface. Larger papillomas are pedunculate and brown-white in color; they resemble a large oat seed when the papilloma is "closed," and the finger-like "leaves" are only seen on cut surfaces (see fig. 8.13 D). Unlike squamous cell carcinoma these lesions are mobile over the underlying tissue.

Fibropapillomas also tend to be multiple and occur in groups, particularly in the esophagus, the rumenoreticular groove, and the rumen. They range in size from 1 mm to 30 cm. The larger tumors in the rumen tend to be in the form of a nodular pedunculate mass like a bunch of grapes, each nodule from 1 to 4 cm in diameter, whereas those in the esophagus are more often elongated and plaque-like. There may be shallow ulceration of the surface, and tumors remain mobile. On cut surface there is a narrow white epithelial covering to the fibrous appearance of the bulk of the lesion. Occasionally the fibrous moiety has a mucoid quality, and there is a record of a 5 kg chondrofibroma developing in a longstanding fibropapilloma of the rumen wall.[10]

Histological Features

Squamous papillomas are composed of long fronds of epithelium (filiform pattern) with narrow fibrous cores. A few mitoses are present in the stratum basale. Most of the epithelium is formed by stratum spinosum and stratum granulosum, with only a moderately thick covering of stratum corneum. In the layers just below the keratinized cells some intranuclear inclusion bodies may be found, and some cells have nonstaining cytoplasm (koilocytes). With electron microscopy, intranuclear virions can be demonstrated in the cells of this layer.[11] In situ hybridization has revealed viral DNA in the deeper layers where virions are not visible ultrastructurally.[12]

Fibropapillomas have two components: the surface epithelium and a fibromatous core with interlacing bundles of fibrous tissue, many fibroblasts, but few mitoses. The surface epithelium shows no cytopathologic change under the stratum corneum but has branching and anastomosing exaggerated rete peg–like structures (plexiform acanthosis). In the larger lesions the fibroma-like tissue forms the bulk of the lesion, with only a thin rim of epithelium, so that if this epithelium had eroded the mass may have been recorded as a fibroma.

Behavior

Untreated papilloma will normally regress, but this may take months. This regression is the result of cell mediated immunity, so if this response is deficient or depressed, the papillomas may persist or even increase in number and in size. In some squamous papillomas with typical papillomatous fronds, there is a breakdown of the basement membrane between the epithelium and the fibrous tissue, allowing invasion of the underlying connective tissue and muscle, indicating transformation of the papilloma to a carcinoma. No transformation from fibropapilloma to squamous cell carcinoma has been observed.

Treatment

Surgical removal of localized fibropapilloma/fibroma of the rumen can be successful, but removal of multiple papillomas distributed along widespread regions of the tract is not possible.[1] Established papilloma may respond to vaccine therapy in as short a time as 7–10 days, but it should be noted that infection by one virus type does not always protect from infection by a different type.

Squamous Cell Carcinoma

Clinical Characteristics

Carcinomas are found in cattle more than 4 years of age and usually between 6 and 12 years old. The breeds affected reflect those predominant in the region. There are more females with carcinoma simply because more mature cows are kept than adult bulls.

Animals with carcinomas present with pain or difficulty on swallowing and rumination. Regurgitation of watery ruminal contents from mouth and nostril may be encountered. Recurrent ruminal tympany so frequently accompanies the tumor that in Kenya the Masai name *embonget*, meaning tympany or bloating, was given to the disease. In advanced cases abdominal pain and loss of condition result in death or slaughter in extremis. The whole course of the condition can be as short as 1 month or as long as 36 months, but is usually between 6 and 9 months from the onset of signs.

Sites

In the high geographical incidence areas, the site distribution of squamous cell carcinoma is 7 percent lingual, 4 percent palatine, 8 percent pharyngeal, 51 percent esophageal, and 30 percent ruminal, with 96 percent of all cattle also having multiple papillomas at these sites.[6] The distribution of ruminal carcinoma is mainly on the anterior wall of the dorsal sac of the rumen where there are no distinct papillae, but some are present on the esophageal opening, esophageal groove, and on the pillars.[8] Sporadic tumor cases occur in the same site distribution pattern, but they tend to be solitary.

Gross Morphology and Histological Features

Sporadic examples of carcinoma tend to form large tumor masses. Those in the esophagus form annular stenosing thickenings of the wall up to 2 cm thick and as long as 12 cm in length (fig. 8.12). Those in the rumen can be up to 60 cm in diameter and often become ulcerated with secondary infection of the surface, causing a foul smell (fig. 8.13). The cut surface has white or yellow flecks through a fibrous stroma. The lesions grow by infiltration into the muscle coat and sometimes into the surrounding

tissue, and plugs of tumor thrombus may be seen in blood vessels. In high carcinoma areas the cases are probably recognized early, so although there may be large lesions, there are also multiple small lesions, some resembling papillomas, and others that are ill-defined, brown, roughened lesions that prove to be carcinoma in situ.[8] Large squamous cell carcinomas have no unique features and are typical of squamous cell carcinomas seen elsewhere.

Growth and Metastasis

Despite infiltration, the metastatic rate is 20–40 percent, even in cattle with large lesions, and the most common site is the drainage lymph node. Transcoelomic spread of esophageal tumors to pleura or from rumen to peritoneum and hence to pleura is sometimes seen. Blood borne spread occurs from the rumen to the liver, and the lung is sometimes affected by hematogenous or lymphohematogenous routes.

Etiology

In Brazil, carcinomas of the pharynx and esophagus, enzootic hematuria, and hemangioma of the urinary bladder were all linked to bracken fern (*Pteridium aquilinum*) grazing.[9] Although enzootic hematuria is recognized in parts of Kenya, it is absent in the Nasampoli valley, where there is a high incidence of ruminal carcinoma (2.5 percent of all cattle and 5 percent of adult cattle).[8]

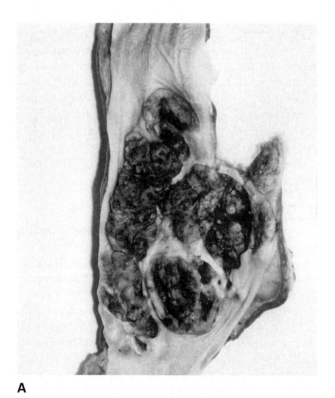

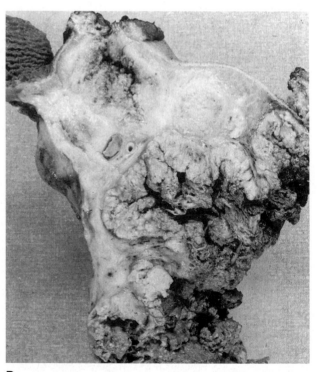

A   **B**

Fig. 8.12.   **A.** Squamous cell carcinoma in the esophagus of a cow from an area of high incidence of esophageal and rumen carcinoma in Kenya. [Courtesy Dr. W. Plowright.] **B.** Cut surface of a squamous cell carcinoma in the rumen of an aged Highland cow from Scotland. Fungating tumor growing into lumen of rumen has distinct edges in some regions, but elsewhere it has infiltrating borders. Tumor thrombi are present in blood vessels.

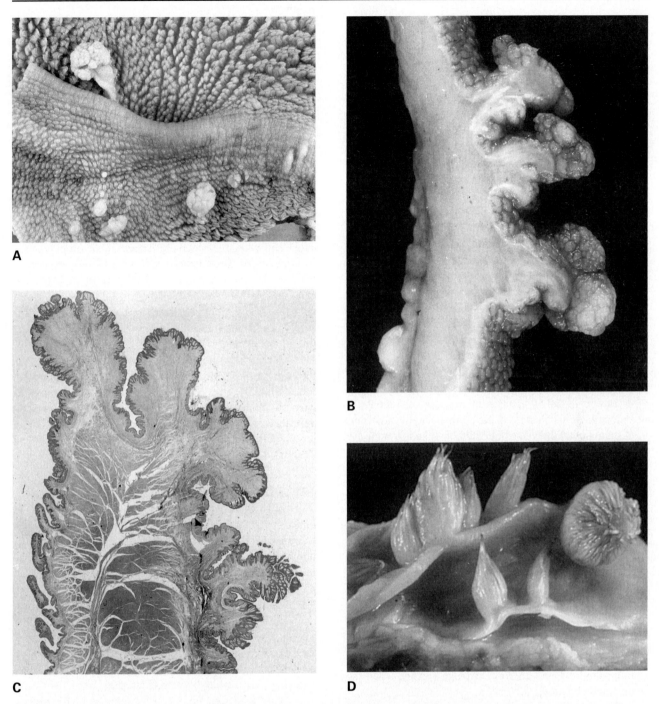

Fig. 8.13. Papilloma in the rumen of sheep. **A.** Pedunculate and sessile, nodular, and linear papilloma on ruminal pillar. **B.** Cut surface of rumen fibropapilloma. **C.** Rumen pillar showing normal rumen papillae on left and fibropapilloma at the top and right. **D.** Multiple pedunculate papillomas in the esophagus of a 2-year-old female cow. Note that in some of the older lesions the tumor fronds are beginning to separate.

Various pieces of epidemiological data, including the observation that the cattle did not eat the bracken fern, suggested that there might be nitrate in the forest plants that could be converted into nitrite in the rumen, and hence nitrosamines could be formed from secondary amines.[8] It was found that 6.1 percent of slaughtered Kenyan cattle usually had less than 3 and no more than 21 esophageal papillomas, but in Nasampolai, 100 or more papillomas were present in cattle with squamous cell car-

cinoma.[13] Some farms had a high carcinoma incidence: 85 percent of cattle on high tumor incidence farms had more than 5 papillomas, and the tumors were spread over more than one site in 65 percent of cases; in contrast, on low tumor incidence farms 90 percent of cattle had less than 5 papillomas, and they were confined to one site in 95 percent of cases. These types of observations led to investigations that demonstrated a link between bovine papilloma virus (BPV) and alimentary cancer.[6]

Squamous papillomas of the upper alimentary tract are caused by and can be experimentally reproduced using BPV-4, the genome of which has been sequenced. Large amounts of mature virus can be demonstrated in the nuclei of the stratum corneum of the papilloma by electron microscopy, and structural antigen expression is shown by immunohistochemistry. However, when transformation of a squamous papilloma into a squamous cell carcinoma occurs, no virus genome can be demonstrated. Moreover, intestinal adenomas and adenocarcinomas and their metastases are similarly devoid of viral DNA.[12] This indicates that the viral genome of BPV-4 is not needed for the maintenance of malignancy once it has been initiated. Immunosuppressive agents in bracken allow the papilloma virus to spread more widely and persist for longer periods than in immunocompetent animals, and cocarcinogens in the bracken may stimulate full malignant transformation.[15] The site specificity of BPV-4 may not be absolute as the virus also has been observed in a skin papilloma.[17]

Fibropapillomas of the upper alimentary tract are associated with BPV-2. Unlike in squamous papillomas, no structural antigen can be revealed in epithelial or fibromatous cells by immunohistochemistry, no replicating virus can be shown by electron microscopy, and there are no cytopathogenic changes in the epithelial cells; however, viral genomes of BPV-2 can be demonstrated in both the epithelial and the fibromatous cells. The probable explanation for these observations is that in the skin BPV-2 proliferates in the stratum granulosum but not in the fibrous moiety of fibropapilloma, whereas in the alimentary tract, since there is no stratum granulosum, the virus can transform cells but not produce infectious virus.[14] There is no evidence for malignant transformation of fibropapilloma of the upper alimentary tract even after immunosuppression or cocarcinogen stimulation. Infective virus in the saliva may be the mode of transmission of oral papilloma between cattle.[7] Experiments indicate that BPV-1 and BPV-2 can exist in a latent form both in epithelium and in circulating lymphocytes in clinically normal animals but can be activated by changes in intrinsic factors, such as immunosuppression, and/or extrinsic factors, such as trauma and chemicals.[16]

The work of many years of testing bracken extracts indicated that bracken fern contains a "chemical cocktail" that has different effects in different species at different dosages.[18] The multifactorial etiology of bovine alimentary tract neoplasia has four components: an oncogenic virus that initiates the transformation of cells, an environmental carcinogen or cocarcinogen (such as quercetin in bracken) that promotes the cells to full neoplastic potential, immunosuppression that allows the altered cells to grow, and lastly activation of the cell proliferation genes of the host and an increase in the number of epidermal growth factor receptors.[15] These components may act in sequence or individually or in a series of combinations to produce a variety of end results.

Papilloma and Squamous Cell Carcinoma in Sheep

Prevalence

There are few references to upper alimentary tumors in the literature. Esophageal tumors in South African sheep dosed with nicotine and copper sulphate have been described,[19] and one case of esophageal papilloma was noted in an abattoir survey of 4.5 million sheep,[5] but no histological details were given. Among 86 ewes with tumors in England there were 13 fibropapillomas of the rumen, 1 ruminal squamous papilloma, 3 squamous cell carcinomas of the rumen (with papilloma present in each case), and 3 squamous cell carcinomas in the oropharynx.[20] In a survey of forestomachs that were being prepared as tripe for human consumption, 12.5 percent of 200 adult ewes and a smaller number of 1-year-old lambs had ruminal papilloma.[21] Meat inspectors on a line slaughter system would not see these lesions, because the alimentary tract is not yet open.

A large squamous cell carcinoma of the reticulum is the only carcinoma in the forestomach of sheep reported in Iceland in 35 years.[22] This paper mentioned the only other case in the literature as a carcinoma of the omasum described in South Africa in 1936. Two ovine oral squamous cell carcinomas have been recorded in New Zealand.[23]

Sites and Gross Morphology

In sheep, in contrast to cattle, benign and malignant tumors occur in the forestomachs and not in the esophagus. Ruminal papillomas are usually multiple, from 1 to 5 in number, but sometimes as many as 30 are seen (fig. 8.13). In nearly 90 percent of cases they are found in linear groupings on the ruminal pillars where there are signs of active ruminitis or scars of previous damage. Less frequently, the tumors are located in the adjacent rumen sacs. These papillomas range from 2 to 30 mm in size; the smaller ones are sessile, and the larger ones are often pedunculate. On cut surface they have a 1 mm epithelial covering over a white branching stroma.

The large squamous cell carcinomas of the mouth, reticulum, and omasum noted above are at sites where papillomas have not been recorded. The ruminal squamous cell carcinomas we have found in the United Kingdom associated with ruminal papillomas resemble the larger sessile papillomas macroscopically and can be up to 25 mm in diameter.

Histological Features

Fibropapillomas have a normal thickness of covering epithelium from which an exaggerated rete peg formation extends into a mass of mature fibrous tissue that has some areas of fibroblasts (fig. 8.13). The epithelium has few mitotic figures, and some cells have large nucleoli. No intranuclear inclusion bodies are found. The cytoplasm of some cells, especially in the keratinized zone, are hydropic, and eosinophilic inclusions may be found in over 30 percent of these vacuoles.

In a series of 500 ruminal papillomas examined histologically 3 were squamous papillomas and 1 was a squamous cell carcinoma; all the rest were fibropapillomas.[21] The squamous papillomas coexisted with fibropapillomas in the same rumens and did not have eosinophilic inclusions or mitotic figures. The squamous cell carcinomas we have seen in the rumen, alongside the fibropapillomas, were well differentiated and did not penetrate far into the underlying tissue.

Etiology

Unlike ruminal papillomas, cutaneous papillomas are rare in the United Kingdom. Papilloma and squamous cell carcinomas on the skin of the head and perianal region of sheep in many arid tropical and subtropical countries are believed to be the result of solar radiation activating latent viral papilloma infection. Virions can be seen ultrastructurally, and papilloma virus-like DNA has been demonstrated in the lesions.

In Edinburgh we have been unable to find virus particles in electron microscopic examination of sections of 30 rumen papillomas or in disaggregated material. Viral DNA was not detected, but when an antiserum raised against the putative ovine rumen papilloma virus was used in an immunoperoxidase test, 6 out of 10 papillomas had occasional cells reacting positively in the stratum corneum.[21] The differences between the cutaneous ovine papilloma and the ruminal ovine papilloma may mean that there is little mature virus present at any one time because the cells are shed rapidly. Perhaps the situation is similar to that seen in cattle with fibropapilloma associated with BPV-2, where infectious virus is not produced because there is no stratum granulosum in the ruminal epithelium.

There is evidence that there are several papillomaviruses in sheep, as there are in cattle,[24] but much more work is needed to unravel the possible role of such viruses in the production of tumors. If an oncogenic virus is responsible for the initiation of neoplasia but requires both a carcinogen/cocarcinogen (as a promoter of malignancy) and immunosuppression (to allow growth of the neoplastic clone of cells) for tumor development, then papilloma virus and solar radiation may operate in the skin, but papillomavirus (possibly latent) activated by trauma and bracken may be the combination needed in the alimentary tract.

One small rumen papilloma was found in one of eight wether lambs fed dried bracken fern for 5 years.[25] The dried bracken was active, since one sheep died of acute bracken poisoning, another developed blindness, and seven had bladder tumors. This contrasts with the increase in esophageal papillomas reported in cattle; however, the virus infection status of these sheep was not known.

Growth and Metastasis

Rumen papillomas and upper alimentary tract carcinomas we have encountered have been small, clinically silent, nonmetastazing tumors recorded either as incidental findings in healthy slaughtered animals or found in animals killed because of the presence of large tumors in other sites. This indicates an interesting species difference between sheep and cattle. No reported survey has been able to establish a correlation between rumen papilloma frequency, adenocarcinoma of the intestine, and bracken in the pasture of sheep, as there is in cattle.

REFERENCES

1. Bertone, A.L., Roth, L., and O'Krepky, J. (1985) Forestomach neoplasia in cattle: A report of eight cases. *Comp Cont Educ* 7:585–590.
2. Brandley, P.J., and Migaki, G. (1963) Types of tumors found by federal meat inspection in an eight year survey. *Ann NY Acad Sci* 108:872–879.
3. Plummer, P.J.G. (1956) A survey of six hundred and thirty-six tumors from domesticated animals. *Can J Comp Med* 20:239–251.
4. Misdorp, W. (1967) Tumors in large domestic animals in the Netherlands. *J Comp Pathol Therap* 77:211–216.
5. Anderson, L.J., Sandison, A.T., and Jarrett, W.F.H. (1969) A british abattoir survey of tumors in cattle, sheep and pigs. *Vet Rec* 84:547–551.
6. Jarrett, W.F.H. (1980) Bracken fern and papilloma virus in bovine alimentary cancer. *Brit Med Bull* 36:79–81.
7. Samuel, J.L., Spradbrow, P.B., Wood, A.L., and Kelly, W.R. (1985) Oral papillomas in cattle. *Zbl Vet Med B* 32:706–714.
8. Plowright, W., Linsell, C.A., and Peers, F.G. (1971) A focus of rumenal cancer in Kenyan cattle. *Brit J Cancer* 25:72–80.
9. Döbereiner, J., Tokarnia, C.H., and Canella, C.F.C. (1967) Ocorrencia da hematuria enzootica e de carcinomas epidemoide no trato digestivo superior em bovinos no brasil. *Pesquisa Agropec Bras* 2:489–504.
10. Salunke, V.M., et al. (1995) Ruminal tumor in a bullock—A case report. *Indian Vet J* 72:273–274.
11. Hamada, M., Oyamada, T., Yoshikawa, H., and Yoshikawa, T. (1989) Morphological studies of esophageal papilloma naturally occurring in cattle. *Jpn J Vet Sci* 51:345–351.
12. Campo, M.S., Moar, M.H., et al. (1985) The presence of bovine papillomavirus type 4 DNA is not required for the progression to, or the maintenance of, the malignant state in cancers of the alimentary canal in cattle. *EMBO J* 4:1819–1825.
13. Thorsen, J., Cooper, J.E., and Warwick, G.P. (1974) Esophageal papillomata in cattle in Kenya. *Trop Anim Hlth Prod* 6:95–98.
14. Jarrett, W.F.H., Campo, M.S., et al. (1984) Alimentary fibropapilloma in cattle: A spontaneous tumor, nonpermissive for papillomavirus replication. *J Natl Cancer Inst* 73:499–504.
15. Campo, M.S. (1987) Papillomas and cancer in cattle. *Cancer Surv* 6:39–54.
16. Campo, M.S., Jarrett, W.F.H., et al. (1994) Latent papillomavirus infection in cattle. *Res Vet Sci* 56:151–157.
17. Bloch, N., Breen, M., et al. (1996) Bovine papillomavirus type 4 DNA isolated from a skin lesion in a steer. *Vet Rec* 138:414–416.
18. Evans, I.A., Prorok, J.H., et al. (1992) The carcinogenic, mutagenic and teratogenic toxicity of bracken. *Proc Roy Soc Edinburgh* 81B:65–77.
19. Schütte, K.H. (1968) Esophageal tumors in sheep: Some ecological observations. *J Natl Cancer Inst* 41:821–824.
20. McCrea, C.T., and Head, K.W. (1978) Sheep tumors in north east Yorkshire. I. Prevalence on Seven Moorland Farms. *Brit Vet J* 134:454–461.

21. Norval, M., Michie, J.R., et al. (1985) Rumen papillomas in sheep. *Vet Microbiol* 10:219–229.

22. Georgsson, G. (1973) Carcinoma of the reticulum of a sheep. *Vet Pathol* 10:530–533.

23. Cordes, D.O., and Shortridge, E.H. (1971) Neoplasms of sheep: A survey of 256 cases recorded at Ruakura Animal Health Laboratory. *N Z Vet J* 19:55–64.

24. Tilbrook, P.A., Sterrett, G., and Kulski, J.K. (1992) Detection of papillomaviral-like DNA sequences in premalignant and malignant perineal lesions of sheep. *Vet Microbiol* 31:327–341.

25. McCrea, C.T. and Head, K.W. (1981) Sheep tumors in north east Yorkshire. II. Experimental production of tumors. *Brit Vet J* 137:21–30.

SQUAMOUS CELL CARCINOMA IN MONOGASTRIC DOMESTIC ANIMALS

Prevalence

Among monogastric domestic animals, only pigs and horses have a moderately extensive stratified squamous epithelium-lined esophageal region to the stomach. Sporadic cases of carcinoma of the esophageal region of the horse stomach have been reported from many parts of the world,[1] but at any one center they are rare; in 687 necropsies and 635 biopsies, only two squamous cell carcinomas of the stomach and one papilloma of the esophagus were found.[2] In a survey in 1952 only 21 of the 50 gastric carcinomas reported in the older literature (going back a hundred years) were thought acceptable; 18 of these cases were squamous cell carcinomas of the esophageal region of the stomach, and 3 were adenocarcinomas of the glandular region of the stomach.[3] The majority of cases described in the United States and Canada are thought to have been observed since 1970,[4] and in Denmark 12 cases have been described since 1977.[1,4] It is not known whether this represents an increasing frequency of occurrence or an improvement in diagnostic techniques.

Ulceration of the esophageal region in the stomach of the domestic pig is common, but squamous cell carcinoma has not been recorded. Two squamous cell carcinomas in this region of the stomach were reported in Kenyan giant forest hogs that grazed the forest clearings where cattle with ruminal carcinoma were herded.[5]

Age, Sex, and Breed

Gastric squamous cell carcinoma is a disease of adult horses; the age range is 6 to 18 years, and the mean age in three series was 10.7, 12.6, and 12.8 years, respectively.[1,4,6] Although one series had a male to female ratio of 4:1, other workers have not been able to establish such a sex bias.[1,4,7] There appears to be no breed prediliction.

Clinical Characteristics

The clinical signs are vague, but the presenting signs and the laboratory diagnostic data have been described.[1,8] Intermittent anorexia leads to progressive weight loss and even emaciation. As the tumor enlarges, there may be persistent ptyalism, dysphagia, and recurrent esophageal obstruction with regurgitation that may result in inhalation pneumonia. Colic is not a common sign. Anemia may develop due to gastric hemorrhage from the ulcerated tumor and/or to depression of erythropoiesis. If there has been metastatic spread, enlarged lymph nodes near the root of the mesentery and nodules on the serosal surfaces of other viscera may be palpated on rectal examination. At this time up to 25 or even 60 liters of ascitic fluid may have accumulated, causing distention of the abdomen. By the time the diagnosis is made, the tumor is inoperable.

Esophageal carcinoma can be confirmed by endoscopic examination,[9] but either lesions in the stomach are not easily reached or the tumor growth within the wall of the terminal esophagus prevents the passage of the instrument to the observably abnormal stomach lining.[10] The problem of the length of the endoscope may be overcome by employing midcervical esophagoscopy[10] or midthoracic pleuroscopy,[11] and this also allows biopsy samples to be taken.

Clinical Laboratory Findings

Exfoliative cytology of pleural and ascitic fluid may reveal isolated squamous epithelial cells and cell nests in addition to numerous neutrophils.[1,4] Keratinized cells stained by the Papanicolaou method and examined by polarizing microscopy may be birefringent.[7] In a series of nine squamous cell carcinomas, only five were positive for tumor cells in ascitic fluid, and one of the four negative cases had a "normal" peritoneal fluid analysis.[8] Hematological examination often reveals a mature neutrophilia, normochromic, normocytic anemia (hemorrhage from the ulcerated tumor surface), massive melena, hyperfibrinogenemia, hypoalbuminemia, and hyperglobulinemia.[4,9]

A gastric squamous cell carcinoma in an 11-year-old Arabian stallion was associated with weakness and gastrointestinal hypomotility due to cancer associated hypercalcemia (serum calcium 18.2–19.3 mg/dl).[12]

Sites and Gross Morphology

Lesions usually cover extensive areas of the esophageal region, which in the horse forms the greater part of the left sac of the stomach and may extend to involve the distal third of the esophagus.[11] Small growths have also been reported near the margo plicatus. Some tumors apparently arise from areas of squamous differentiation from multipotent cells in the base of the crypts in the glandular region of the stomach. Squamous cell carcinoma of the equine esophagus is rare if one excludes the few cases where there has been extension from a primary carcinoma in the stomach.[13] Most of the gastric tumors form a large, roughly nodular, cauliflower-like mass 10–30 cm in diameter bulging into the lumen. The luminal surface exhibits ulcers 1–3 cm in diameter, hemorrhage, and areas that are secondarily infected and necrotic (yellow). The muscular wall becomes infiltrated and thickened as much as 10 cm by the tumor and its characteristic fibrous reaction. Although there is usually a sharp border to the tumor on the mucosal surface, infiltration in the gastric wall may extend under the normal epithelium.

Esophageal squamous cell carcinoma can appear as a thickening of the wall with areas of ulceration or papilliform and verrucose elevation of the epithelium or as a feed filled diverticulum that must be washed out before the ulcerated tumor can be seen.[9]

Histological Features

These tumors have no unique features and are typically well-differentiated squamous cell carcinomas with keratin pearls, intercellular bridges, and desmoplasia (fig. 8.14). The large amount of collagen rich stroma in the neoplasm may extend into adjacent areas. Degenerating cells in the centers of the neoplastic cords become liquefied and attract neutrophils, and cyst-like structures form. At the periphery of the neoplasm the tumor cells may infiltrate into lymphatics and blood vessels, where they may be seen some distance beyond the main border of the tumor.

Growth and Metastasis

The tumors grow by infiltration of tissue spaces, lymphatic vessels, and small blood vessels. Metastases to drainage lymph nodes of the stomach and esophagus are common. Infiltrative growth in the stomach leads to direct extension of the carcinoma to contiguous organs and viscera, diaphragm, liver, and spleen. Nodular deposits may then form on the surface of more distant abdominal structures, and the neoplasm may metastasize from the peritoneum to the pleural surfaces via lymphatics coursing through the diaphragm. The latter growths are seldom as advanced as in the abdomen and therefore rarely cause clinical signs. Blood borne metastases are rare but can be found in the liver and, less commonly, in the lung, kidney, and adrenal gland.

Although some workers suggest that gastric squamous cell carcinomas are directly or indirectly related to damage caused by *Gasterophilus intestinalis* larvae,[6] there is little data to support this.

REFERENCES

1. Olsen, S.N. (1992) Squamous cell carcinoma of the equine stomach: A report of five cases. *Vet Rec* 131:171–173.
2. Sundberg, J.P., Burnstein, T., et al. (1977) Neoplasms of Equidae. *J Amer Vet Med Assoc* 170:150–152.
3. Krahnert, R. (1952) Zum magenkrebs des Pferdes. *Mh Vet Med* 7:399–404.
4. Tennant, B., Keirn, D.R., et al. (1982) Six cases of squamous cell carcinoma of the stomach of the horse. *Equine Vet J* 14:238–243.
5. Plowright, W., Linsell, C.A., and Peers, F.G. (1971) A focus of rumenal cancer in Kenyan cattle. *Brit J Cancer* 25:72–80.
6. Cotchin, E. (1977) A general survey of tumors in the horse. *Equine Vet J* 9:16–21.
7. Wester, P.W., Franken, P., and Hani, H.I. (1980) Squamous cell carcinoma of the equine stomach. A report of 7 cases. *Vet Quarterly* 2:95–103.
8. Zicker, S.C., Wilson, D., and Medearis, I. (1990) Differentiation between intra-abdominal neoplasms and abscesses in horses, using clinical and laboratory data: 40 cases (1973–1988). *J Amer Vet Med Assoc* 196:1130–1134.
9. Campbell-Beggs, C.L., Kiper, M.L., MacAllister, C., Henry, G., and Roszel, J.F. (1993) Use of esophagoscopy in the diagnosis of esophageal squamous cell carcinoma in a horse. *J Amer Vet Med Asso* 202: 617–618.
10. Keirn, D.P., White, K.K., et al. (1982) Endoscopic diagnosis of squamous cell carcinoma of the equine stomach. *J Amer Vet Med Assoc* 180:940–942.
11. Ford, T.S., Vaala, W.E., et al. (1987) Pleuroscopic diagnosis of gastroesophageal squamous cell carcinoma in a horse. *J Amer Vet Med Assoc* 190:1556–1558.
12. Meuten, D.J., Price, S.M., Seiler, R.M., and Krook, L. (1978) Gastric carcinoma with pseudohyperparathyroidism in a horse. *Cornell Vet* 68:179–195.
13. Green, S., Green, E.M., and Aronson, E. (1986) Squamous cell carcinoma: An unusual cause of choke in a horse. *Mod Vet Pract* 65:870–875.

TUMORS OF THE GLANDULAR STOMACH

In domestic animals neoplasia of the glandular stomach is not common and primarily affects the dog. In many

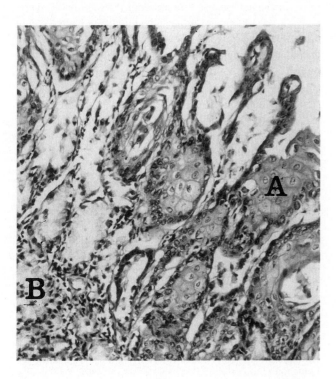

Fig. 8.14. Squamous cell carcinoma in the stomach of the horse. Superficial mucosa from the fundic region of the stomach showing metaplastic change to squamous epithelial cells (*A*) from columnar cells (*B*).

cases, clinical presentation is often late, with a large tumor or extensive involvement of the gastric mucosa and deeper layers. The use of diagnostic aids such as radiological or ultrasonic imaging in concert with endoscopic sampling of early neoplasms or suspicious lesions has led to improved prognosis in humans, with 5 year survival rates of more than 90 percent when lesions are detected early.[1]

Classification

The World Health Organization's (WHO) system of classification of gastric neoplasia in animals is similar to the human classification system.[2,3] A modified system of classification has been reported, and some studies have tended to use a combination of both systems.[4-6] One of these studies involved TNM grading as an additional parameter.[5] The system of classifying gastric neoplasms in this chapter is based on the histopathologic identification of the principal cell type (table 8.2).

Comparative Aspects

In human patients the main types are adenoma, adenocarcinoma, and carcinoids.[3] An alternative classification system divides carcinomas into intestinal types (i.e., the tumor cells have intestinal epithelium–like morphology) and diffuse types, the latter referring to a combination of tubular or acinar pattern with infiltrative growth.[4] Adenomas and high grade dysplasia are recognized as precancerous lesions, and high grade dysplasia often coexists with carcinoma.[7] There is considerable evidence indicating progression from chronic atrophic gastritis, through gastric intestinal metaplasia and dysplasia, to carcinoma.[8,9] Intestinal metaplasia was initially thought to be a reliable indicator of precancerous gastric change, but it is now known to occur in association with both benign and malignant tumors and also in nonneoplastic lesions. Panels of immunohistochemical markers are useful in detecting the histogenesis of early primary neoplastic foci. Markers of cellular proliferation (Ki-67) are being used for the identification of early malignant change.[10]

Incidence

The highest incidence of gastric tumors is in the dog, but even in dogs, gastric tumors are uncommon compared to their incidence in man.[25] One review of gastric tumors reported in 61 cases in dogs (0.18 percent in 10,179 dogs), 4 in cats, 4 in horses, and 1 each in a pig and an ox.[11] Although gastric tumors are rare in horses,[12] squamous cell carcinoma is more common than adenocarcinoma. The lack of reports of gastric neoplasia in the pig is likely due to their use for food production and death at an early ("preneoplastic") age. High dietary levels of polychlorinated biphenyl compounds induce gastric hypertrophy, hyperplasia, and ulceration in pigs, and the majority of intensely reared pigs have gastric ulcers.[13] In humans there are links between chronic gastritis and ulceration, leading to intestinal metaplasia and carcinoma.[1]

Epithelial neoplasms of the ovine abomasum are rare, and this is probably related to the relatively young age at slaughter.[14] Solitary or multiple pedunculated papillomas are seen on the ruminal pillars in abattoir slaughtered sheep, but similar tumors in the abomasum are rare. Abomasal adenocarcinomas, with and without widespread metastases, have been reported in cattle,[15,16] but a survey of 1.3 million cattle processed at an abattoir found only 1 cow with abomasal carcinoma.[15] There is one reported case of a bovine abomasal mastocytoma.[17]

In the cat, gastric tumors other than lymphoid types are rare. An adenocarcinoma and an undifferentiated carcinoma were the only gastric tumors found in a series of 44 cats identified with gastrointestinal neoplasia in a 14 year period,[18] and 1 undifferentiated gastric carcinoma was identified in a retrospective series of 11 feline gastrointestinal tumors.[19]

As shown in table 8.3, carcinomas (of all histological types) are the most frequently reported primary tumor, followed by smooth muscle tumors (leiomyomas and leiomyosarcomas). According to the WHO survey, lymphoid tumors are common, but they may not be primary gastric tumors.[2]

TABLE 8.2. Classification of tumors of the glandular stomach

Primary Epithelial (Glandular Tumors)
Adenoma: papillary, tubular, papillotubular
Adenocarcinoma: tubular or acinar signet-ring cell type, mucinous
Undifferentiated carcinoma

Primary Nonepithelial (Nonglandular) Tumors
Leiomyoma/leiomyosarcoma
Lymphoma
Lipoma/liposarcoma
Fibroma/fibrosarcoma
Hemangioma
Carcinoid

Secondary Tumors
Metastatic carcinoma
Mesothelioma

Tumor-Like Lesions
Polyps (inflammatory or regenerative)
Scirrhous eosinophilic gastritis
Hypertrophic gastritis
Acquired pyloric stenosis

TABLE 8.3. Types of canine gastric neoplasms reported in the literature

Tumor Type	Number of Cases Reported	
	Literature	WHO
Carcinoma	223	35*
Adenoma	6	
Leiomyoma	30	19*
Leiomyosarcoma	4	
Lymphoid	6	79
Carcinoid	1	1

*No differentiation between 35 carcinomas and adenomas or 19 leiomyomas and leiomyosarcomas [Head, K.W. (1976) Tumors of the lower alimentary tract. *Bull WHO* 53:167-186].

Benign glandular tumors in the canine stomach are much less common than carcinomas.[20,21] The benign tumors described are often solitary, polypoid lesions, 0.5–1 cm in diameter, found in the pyloric region as incidental lesions at necropsy. Some authors have classified these lesions as adenomatous polyps and have described hyperplastic epithelium on the polyp, with both atrophy and patchy hyperplasia of the adjacent gastric mucosa.[22] Others have described focal or early malignant change in gastric polyps or concurrent diffuse scirrhous adenocarcinoma.[28,29] Adenomas in human beings may be premalignant.

Carcinoid tumors[30,31] of the stomach are rare, and only two canine cases are recorded in the literature.[2,27] Carcinoids of the intestines occur rarely in old animals and are located in the colon, rectum, and duodenum.[32]

Age, Breed, and Sex

Affected dogs range in age from 3 to 16 years, with an average of 7.5–10.2 years.[4,5,20,21] Although only a few adenomas have been reported, the average age for these dogs was 9.5 years.[20] The reported male to female ratio in one study was 1:5 for adenomas and 17:7 for adenocarcinomas.[20] Another study found a ratio of 6 males to 1 female,[22] and the predisposition for males in carcinoma formation has been demonstrated in other reports.[4,24] In contrast, in a series of 13 dogs with gastric neoplasia diagnosed by ultrasonography, there was a greater number of females (9) than males (4).[6] Taken together, these figures may reflect a true sex bias, but they need to be compared with the sex distribution of the source population.

Many authors have failed to demonstrate significant breed predispositions for gastric carcinomas, but one report suggested that small terriers (cairn and West Highland white) were overrepresented.[33] Rough collies and Staffordshire bull terriers also have a significant proportion of gastric carcinomas.[24] A familial pattern of occurrence has been reported in Belgian shepherd dogs.[5] There is little accurate information available for the cat, but an average age of occurrence of 10.6 years has been reported.[18,19]

Clinical Characteristics

Clinical signs in the dog are initially nonspecific disturbances of the gastrointestinal tract and include progressive loss of weight, anorexia, diarrhea, melena, hematemesis, and dullness.[23] Duration of symptoms can be as short as 2 weeks, with 56 percent of dogs having a history lasting 8 weeks or less.[24] Vomiting, often not related to food intake, is associated with gastric neoplasia and has been reported in as many as 97 percent of cases.[24] Hematological and biochemical parameters are usually within reference ranges, although nonregenerative and regenerative anemias have been reported in dogs with ulcerated carcinomas.[28]

Characteristic radiographic features are the absence of normal gastric shape, filling defects in the pyloric and lesser curvature areas, and delayed emptying with residual barium staining.[28] Visualization of the gastric lesions, together with lesional sampling by means of endoscopes, is the best technique to establish a positive diagnosis.[6,24,34]

Sites

The most common site in dogs is the pyloric antrum, with extension into the body region, usually along the lesser curvature.[4,5,24] The body region is the next most common, with involvement of the lesser curvature more frequent than that of the greater curvature.[4,21] Tumors in the fundic region of the canine stomach are rare. Tumors located in the lesser curvature tend to infiltrate widely within the stomach wall, while pyloric carcinomas are reported to be less invasive and to tend to involve the antrum, forming an annular stricture. Interestingly, all the tumors localized on the lesser curvature were found in Belgian shepherd dogs.[5]

Most gastric tumors in horses are squamous cell carcinomas and arise in the stratified squamous portion of the stomach. The gastric adenocarcinomas reported in horses have involved the glandular body or antral region.[12] The few gastric carcinomas reported in cattle were located in the abomasum.[15,16]

Gross Morphology

In order of frequency, the three main patterns of carcinoma in the dog are a plaque-like thickening, often ulcerated; a diffuse, nonulcerated thickening; and a raised sessile polyp. Tumors are usually gray or white, firm and fibrous, with replacement of normal gastric wall structure. Some tumors exude mucinous fluid from the cut surface.

Ulceration is common, and often the ulcers are deep and crateriform (fig. 8.15) because of thickened raised margins that are a mixture of tumor and scirrhous reaction.[35] Ulcer diameter may be as large as 10 cm, and some ulcers cause perforation of the stomach. Ulceration of the primary tumor may follow occlusion of local blood and lymphatic vessels by tumor emboli. Ulcers may also be secondary to tumors such as malignant mast cell tumors, pancreatic islet cell tumors (Zollinger-Ellison syndrome), or severe liver disease.

Omental adhesions to the gastric serosa are common, irrespective of gastric perforation. Adhesions seem to develop before actual perforation, and therefore peritonitis following perforation of an ulcerated tumor is infrequent. Omental and mesenteric sclerosis have been recorded and are associated with metastasis.[23] It is common to see prominent "corded" or arborescent lymphatic vessels on the serosal surface of the thickened gastric wall, and these are the result either of lymphatic blockage by tumor emboli or metastatic involvement of the drainage lymph node. When most of the stomach wall is neoplastic, as is the case in the diffuse type of carcinoma, the stomach develops a stiffened wall and is referred to as "leather bottle" or *linitis plastica*. In the regions adjacent to the neoplastic mucosa, the normal rugal pattern is lost.

Histological Features

Adenocarcinomas form tubular structures but may be subdivided according to a predominant growth pattern (see table 8.2). The classic pattern is one of branching tubules or acini embedded in a fibrous stroma. Occasionally, papillary development may occur, in which finger-like fibrous cores are clothed with neoplastic epithelium-like cells and form a polypoid growth. This type of formation may be mistaken for an adenoma, but careful examination usually reveals its true carcinomatous nature with invasion of carcinoma cells below the muscularis mucosa. Infiltration of the gastric wall by tumor cells is a common feature and often induces excessive fibrosis (scirrhous reaction), which may mask the presence of scattered tumor acini. The term *carcinoma in situ* is used when carcinoma is present, but it has not penetrated the muscularis mucosa.

When more than half of a gastric adenocarcinoma produces mucin, it is classified as a mucinous adenocarcinoma. Mucin production is often marked and may appear as intracytoplasmic vacuoles containing acid mucin, as granules of acid mucin filling the cytoplasm (akin to normal goblet cells), or as eosinophilic cytoplasmic granules of neutral mucin. Excessive mucin production may cause cells to rupture and form "lakes" of mucin, which may be visible macroscopically. The third subtype of adenocarcinoma is the signet ring cell type, so-called because the tumor cells have eccentric nuclei and distended cytoplasm filled with mucin. Gastric carcinomas that have no glandular structure are classified as undifferentiated; an alternative term is *solid carcinoma* (fig. 8.15).

The presence of intestinal metaplasia in the tumor and in nonneoplastic gastric mucosa adjacent to tumors has been described.[11,35] The cells form tubules and resemble intestinal columnar epithelial cells with prominent brush borders. This may be an important feature since evidence in human studies indicates that intestinal metaplasia is linked to both gastric carcinoma and atrophic gastritis, the latter caused by *Helicobacter pylori* infection.[9,38]

Although one series of canine gastric adenocarcinomas was typed using the human intestinal and diffuse typing system,[35] it is considered inappropriate by the present authors since it is related to the geographic prevalence of human gastric cancer. Histologically, most gastric carcinomas in the dog are tubular or poorly differentiated, with excessive fibrosis, ulceration, and invasive growth. The well-differentiated tumors tend to have tubular or acinar arrangements with columnar mucus secreting cells near the surface of the tumor. More diffuse types have poorly differentiated cells with poorly developed tubular growth patterns. They tend to have a highly infiltrative growth and invade the deeper layers of the mucosa and even the submucosa, muscularis, and serosa. A prominent feature of the diffuse type of gastric carcinoma is the pronounced fibrous reaction (scirrhous reaction). Often small packets or irregular acini are seen embedded in the proliferating fibrous tissue. Many of the carcinoma cells adopt a signet-cell morphology, with eccentrically placed nuclei and cytoplasm distended with mucin. It may be difficult on some occasions to differentiate solitary signet cells from macrophages, but immunocytochemical markers are help-

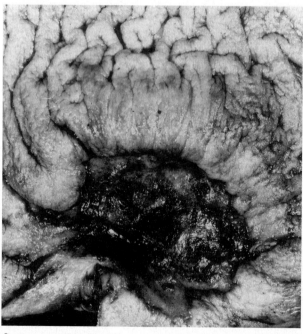

A

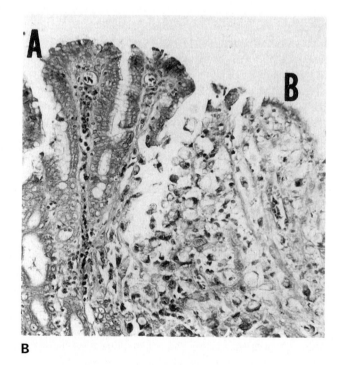

B

Fig. 8.15. Carcinoma in the stomach of a dog. **A.** Mucosal ulcer on lesser curvature distal to cardia of stomach. Microscopic examination of the stomach wall revealed an adenocarcinoma. **B.** Histological section from margin of this ulcer. Normal mucosa (*A*) is partially replaced by a diffuse infiltration of undifferentiated carcinoma cells (*B*). (Courtesy Dr. C.H. Lingeman).

ful. Some reports indicate that there are small numbers of argyrophilic cells scattered within the primary tumor and metastases. The significance of these cells is not certain.

The use of immunohistochemical stains is beneficial where carcinomas are poorly differentiated or where there is doubt about the histogenesis. Broad spectrum and more specific cytokeratin monoclonal antibodies are useful in identifying carcinoma cells. Other markers such as epithelial membrane antigen (EMA), carcinoembryonic antigen (CEA), and factor VIII antigen (to rule out vascular origin tumors) are less specific. One report has described staining of gastric carcinoma cells in dogs using a monoclonal antibody, B72.3, that is reactive with a broad spectrum of human epithelial malignancies.[36] In man, CD antibodies are used to identify lymphomas, but relatively little information is currently available for the dog.[37] Some of the human monoclonal antibodies do not cross-react with canine or feline tissue.

Benign polyps or true adenomas are usually confined to the pyloric stomach in dogs. Histologically, it may be difficult to differentiate between hyperplasia and adenoma. In hyperplastic polypoid growths there are usually well-differentiated columnar cells supported by fibrous cores of tissue and well-differentiated, sometimes cystic, glandular structures below. Smooth muscle branches extend up from the underlying muscularis mucosa. The lesions are often pedunculate, but may be sessile. Infiltrations of mononuclear inflammatory cells may be present, and some polyps may have foci of lymphocytes.

Adenomas may also be sessile or pedunculated, but they have more cellular atypia than polyps, with a higher mitotic index than adjacent normal mucosa. The glands in adenomas have irregularly thickened, multilayered, cellular linings with greater cellular atypia. Papillary type adenomas are composed of finger-like processes covered by well-differentiated but multilayered benign tumorous epithelial cells. Tubular adenomas (sometimes referred to as adenomatous polyps) tend to be pedunculate with branching tubules of well-differentiated benign neoplastic epithelial cells.

Etiology

There is no definitive etiology for gastric neoplasia in the dog or other domestic species. In man, epidemiological factors have been examined; these include gastric achlorhydria associated with pernicious anemia, exposure to environmental carcinogens such as polycyclic hydrocarbons formed in preservation of meat and fish by smoking, or exposure to mycotoxins such as aflatoxin.[11] The relative rarity of gastric carcinoma in dogs, even in parts of the world where there is a high incidence of human gastric tumors (such as Japan), suggests that domestic animals are not exposed to the same agents, are not exposed for a long enough period, or have a species resistance.

N-nitrosamines are potent carcinogens in rodent experiments, and it has been suggested that nitrates ingested in plants or contaminated water supplies could be reduced to nitrites by gastric and bladder bacteria. Under normal conditions, the low gastric pH, with relatively few bacteria present, prevents high concentrations of nitrite, the precursors of N-nitrosamines, from developing. By contrast, in the achlorhydric or hypochlorhydric stomach there is bacterial growth, resulting in increased levels of bacterial nitrate reductase, which allows production of nitrites and increased N-nitrosamine accumulation. In human populations in the western hemisphere, gastric anacidity is a natural consequence of aging, and hypochlorhydria is a precursor stage in gastric carcinogenesis. The mechanism may involve nitrosamine compounds operating on atrophic gastric mucosa, with resultant intestinal metaplasia and eventually carcinogenesis. Whether such a mechanism operates in the dog is not known.

Adenocarcinomas in the stomach of four dogs were induced by oral administration of N-methyl-N′-nitro-N-nitrosoguanidine starting at 3 months of age and continuing for 14 months.[39] All four dogs had multiple gastric adenocarcinomas when euthanized between 18 and 36 months of age. The tumors occurred in areas of histologically atrophic but macroscopically normal mucosa. The carcinomas were never more than 1 cm in diameter and were superficial or intramucosal in growth pattern. Histologically, the tumors were papillary, tubular, or signet ring cell in type. No metastases were found. In a similar canine experiment using the same compound with the addition of Tween-60 solution, the dogs developed intermittent hematemesis, melena, and vomiting.[40] At necropsy examination, gastric lesions ranged from mucosal atrophy with microscopic intramural carcinomas to obvious carcinomas measuring up to 55 mm in diameter. The carcinoma types were tubular, papillotubular, or signet ring cell, and in two cases they were transmural. The tumors were sited in the subcardiac and antrum regions of the stomach. In one dog (the longest survivor) there was metastasis to the pancreatic and thoracic lymph nodes.

Swine given high doses of dietary polychlorinated biphenyls postweaning develop gastric epithelial hypertrophy with mucin production and hyperplasia and ulcers in the fundic and pyloric gastric regions.[13] Miniature swine fed methylnitrosourea for 4.5 years were clinically normal but had multiple small gastric adenomatous polyps with early malignant change at necropsy examination.[41]

Helicobacter pylori (formerly *Campylobacter pylori*) plays a role in human duodenal and peptic ulceration, gastritis, and gastric cancer.[38] H. pylori was initially regarded as a benign commensal organism; however, where the mucosa becomes heavily colonized, a chronic active enteritis in the duodenum and/or a gastritis develops, and chronic or recurrent ulceration often ensues.[42] In addition, chronic *Helicobacter* gastritis leads to mucosal atrophy, sometimes with progression to intestinal metaplasia.[38] There is increasing evidence that the intestinal metaplasia state is associated with intestinal type gastric cancer, and the infection carries a three- to six-fold increased risk of developing gastric cancer in man.[38] It has been suggested that the mode of action of the bacterium is as a long-term promoter agent rather than as an initiator.[42] Other than nonhuman primates, gnotobiotic pigs and dogs are the only animals to have been successfully infected with *H. pylori*. There are no data to suggest *H. pylori* is associated with gastric tumors in dogs.[42]

Helicobacter felis is commonly found in the stomachs of cats and dogs without gastric lesions. Although a lymphoid gastritis is sometimes present, there are no studies indicating that this lesion is caused by *H. felis*. A hyperplastic gastritis has been associated with a *Campylobacter*-like infection in a beagle dog, but to date there is no convincing correlation between gastric cancer and *Campylobacter*-like bacterial infection.[43]

Although there is some evidence for oncogene involvement in the genesis of colorectal cancer in man, little work has been done on gastric neoplasia.[44] Oncogenes such as c-*myc* and c-*ras,* together with inactivation of *p53* tumor suppressor gene, may be as important as in other tumor systems.

Growth and Metastasis

Dogs with gastric carcinoma are usually presented with advanced disease, often with local spread of carcinoma to adjacent abdominal organs and/or with disseminated metastases. Surgical excision is difficult and often only gives remission of signs for 3–6 months before recurrence necessitates euthanasia.[25,26] More recent reports have given longer median postsurgical survival times of 12 months and 35 months.[4,24]

Most carcinomas start as carcinoma in situ in the gastric glands. Invasion through the basement membrane of the glands into the lamina propria but not as far as submocusa signals the next phase; it is then intramucosal carcinoma growth. Both in situ and intramucosal growth patterns alone are rarely seen; by the time most canine patients are presented clinically or examined postmortem, the primary gastric tumor is advanced. It is likely, however, that the most aggressive carcinomas commence metastatic spread at the intramucosal stage because of the close proximity of lymphatics and blood vessels. The next stage is marked by lateral spread into the lamina propria and through the muscularis mucosa into the underlying submucosa. Thereafter, tumor spread into the outer muscular layers and serosa usually occurs via blood vessels and lymphatics. Tumor cells may provoke an intense fibrosis ("scirrhous reaction") as a result of growth factor secretion.

Metastasis from primary canine gastric carcinomas should be expected because the diagnosis is made relatively late in the progression of the tumor. There is one report, however, that found no metastases in 11 of 14 cases despite the presence of tumor cells in gastric lymphatics and venules.[21] Most reports indicate that metastasis to regional lymph nodes (gastric, gastroduodenal, splenic) via lymphatics is the most common; omental, mesenteric, and peritoneal carcinomatosis is next most frequent[2,4,5,23,24];

and metastases to the liver and spleen are least frequent.[4,5] The visceral surface of the diaphragm is often studded with multiple small metastases. Peritoneal and omental involvement usually produces multinodular sclerotic foci or larger adhesions of omentum and mesentery with abundant fibrosis that contain small nests of carcinoma cells.[23] Widespread systemic metastasis is unusual, and the lungs are rarely involved. Peritoneal carcinomatosis arises as a result of direct "seeding" of tumor from the primary gastric lesion. Ascites may develop as a result of blockage of lymphatics in carcinomatosis.

In the abomasal adenocarcinomas described in cattle, only one case had metastatic lesions.[15,16] The metastases formed a "carcinomatosis" pattern in the peritoneum and pleura, and there was involvement of one adrenal gland.[16]

Diagnostic Problems in Gastric Carcinoma

1. It may be difficult to differentiate severe glandular dysplasia and early tubular adenocarcinoma. In such situations it is essential to obtain a resection specimen rather than an endoscopic or incisional biopsy in order that the presence or absence of invasion of the lamina propria may be assessed. Once the basement membrane has been disrupted and tumor cells are in the lamina propria, the preferred diagnosis is carcinoma in situ. Differentiation of dysplasia, adenoma, and carcinoma is made on a careful assessment of cellular atypia, loss of cellular microarchitecture, and mitotic index.

2. Distinguishing poorly differentiated carcinoma from lymphoma or neuroendocrine tumors may be difficult. In cases of poorly differentiated carcinomas, a panel of monoclonal antibodies can be used, that is, cytokeratins, EMA, CEA, and CAM 5.2 epithelial markers versus leukocyte common antigen (LCA) and lymphoid markers (CD3, CD79a, BLA). The chromogranin reaction and S-100 antigen stain are useful for identifying neuroendocrine tumors.

3. Individual or poorly differentiated signet ring cells may be mistaken for macrophages in lamina propria. Cytokeratin and lysozyme antibodies are useful, together with periodic acid Schiff and alcian blue stains for mucin identification.

4. Giving a prognosis for very early carcinomas or carcinoma in situ may be difficult, and there are no studies to date that have correlated survival times with growth mode or spread of the primary tumor, although grading the degree of differentiation and level of microanatomical spread within the gastric wall have been indicated as useful criteria.[2] A proper sample is needed to determine the level of invasion as intramucosal or submucosal or beyond, and the degree of expansion laterally within mucosa or submucosa.

REFERENCES

1. Stevens, A., and Lowe, J. (1995) Alimentary tract. In *Pathology,* Ch. 11. Mosby, London, pp. 218–241.

2. Head, K.W. (1976) Tumors of the lower alimentary tract. *Bull WHO* 53:167–186.

3. Watanabe, H., Jass, J.R., and Sobin, L.H. (1990) *Histological Typing of Esophageal and Gastric Tumors,* 2nd ed. Springer-Verlag, Berlin.

4. Fonda, D., Gualtieri, M., and Scanziani, E. (1989) Gastric carcinoma in the dog: A clinicopathological study of 11 cases. *J Small Anim Pract* 30:353–360.

5. Scanziani, E., Giusti, A.M., Gualtieri, M., and Fonda, D. (1991) Gastric carcinoma in the Belgian shepherd dog. *J Small Anim Pract* 32:465–469.

6. Kaser-Hotz, B., Hauser, B., and Arnold, P. (1996) Ultrasonographic findings in canine gastric neoplasia in 13 patients. *Vet Radiol Ultrasound* 37:51–56.

7. Ming, S-C., Bajtai, A., Correa, P., et al. (1984) Gastric dysplasia significance and pathologic criteria. *Cancer* 54:1794–1801.

8. Porrea, P. (1988) A human model of gastric carcinogenesis. *Cancer Res* 48:3554–3560.

9. Tosi, P., Filipe, M.I., Baak, et al. (1990) Morphometric definition and grading of gastric intestinal metaplasia. *J Pathol* 161:201–208.

10. Filipe, M.I., Rosa, J., et al. (1991) Is DNA ploidy and proliferative activity of prognostic value in advanced gastric carcinoma? *Human Pathol* 22:373–378.

11. Lingeman, C.H., Garner, F.M., and Taylor, D.O.N. (1971) Spontaneous gastric adenocarcinomas of dogs: A review. *J Natl Cancer Inst* 47:137–153.

12. Sundberg, J.P., Burnstein, T., et al. (1977) Neoplasms of Equidae. *J Amer Vet Med Assoc* 170:150–152.

13. Hansen, L.G., Wilson, D.W., and Byerly, C.S. (1976) Effects on growing swine and sheep of two polychlorinated biphenyls. *Amer J Vet Res* 37:1021–1025.

14. Ross, A.D., and Williams, R.A. (1983) Neoplasms of sheep in Great Britain. *Vet Rec* 113:598–599.

15. Anderson, L.J., Sandison, A.T., and Jarret, W.F.H. (1969) A British abattoir survey of tumors in cattle, sheep and pigs. *Vet Rec* 84:547–551.

16. Ritchey, J.W., Marshall, C., David, C., and Brown, T.T. (1996) Mucinous adenocarcinoma in the abomasum of a cow. *Vet Pathol* 33:454–456.

17. Groth, A.H., Bailey, W.S. and Walker, D.F. (1960) Bovine mastocytoma. *J Amer Vet Med Assoc* 137:242–244.

18. Turke, M.A.M., Galina, A.M., and Russell, T.S. (1981) Nonhematopoietic gastrointestinal neoplasia in cats: A retrospective study of 44 cases. *Vet Pathol* 18:614–620.

19. Cribb, A.E. (1988) Feline gastrointestinal adenocarcinoma: A review and retrospective study. *Can Vet J* 29:709–712.

20. Patnaik, A.K., Hurvitz, A.I., and Johnson, G.F. (1977) Canine gastrointestinal neoplasms. *Vet Pathol* 14:547–555.

21. Sautter, J.H. and Hanlon, G.F. (1975) Gastric neoplasms in the dog: A report of 20 cases. *J Amer Vet Med Assoc* 166:691–696.

22. Hayden, D.W., and Nielsen, S.W. (1973) Canine alimentary neoplasia. *Zbl Vet Med* 20A:1–22.

23. Roth, L., and King, J.M. (1990) Mesenteric and omental sclerosis associated with metastases from gastrointestinal neoplasia in the dog. *J Small Anim Pract* 31:28–31.

24. Sullivan, M., Lee, R., et al. (1987) A study of 31 cases of gastric carcinoma in dogs. *Vet Rec* 120:79–83.

25. Dorn, A.S., Anderson, N.V., et al. (1996) Gastric carcinoma in a dog. *J Small Anim Pract* 17:109–117.

26. Olivieri, M., Gosselin, Y., and Sauvageau, R. (1984) Gastric adenocarcinoma in a dog: Six and one-half month survival following partial gastrectomy and gastroduodeostomy. *J Amer Anim Hosp Assoc* 20:78–82.

27. Albers, T.M., Alroy, J., et al. (1998) A poorly differentiated gastric carcinoid in a dog. *J Vet Diag Invest* 10:116–118.

28. Murray, M., Robinson, P.B., et al. (1972) Primary gastric neoplasia in the dog: A clinicopathological study. *Vet Rec* 91:474–479.

29. Conroy, J.D. (1969) Multiple gastric adenomatous polyps in a dog. *J Comp Pathol* 79:465–469.

30. Waldum, H.L., Aase, S., et al. (1998) Neuroendocrine differentiation in human gastric carcinoma. *Cancer* 83:435–444.

31. Wright, N.A. (1999) The origin of gut and pancreatic neuroendocrine (APUD) cells. *J Pathol* 189:439–440.

32. Patnaik, A.K., Hurvitz, A.I., and Johnson, G.F. (1980) Canine intestinal adenocarcinoma and carcinoid. *Vet Pathol* 17:149–163.

33. Else, R.W., and Head, K.W. (1980) Some pathological conditions of the canine stomach. *Vet Ann* 20:66–81.

34. Simpson, J.W. (1996) Gastrointestinal endoscopy. In Thomas, D.A., Simpson, J.W., and Hall, E.J. (eds.), *Manual of Canine and Feline Gastroenterology.* British Small Animal Veterinary Association, Cheltenham, pp. 20–36.

35. Patnaik, A.K., Hurvitz, A.I., and Johnson, G.F. (1978) Canine gastric adenocarcinoma. *Vet Pathol* 15:600–607.

36. Clemo, F.A.S., Di Nicola, D.B., et al. (1995) Immunoreactivity of canine epithelial and non-epithelial neoplasms with monoclonal antibody B72.3. *Vet Pathol* 32:147–154.

37. Cobbold, S., and Metcalfe, S. (1994) Monoclonal antibodies that define canine homologues of human CD antigens. *Tissue Antigens* 43:137–154.

38. Axon, A.T.R. (1993) *Helicobacter pylori* infection. *J Antimicro Chemo* 32(Suppl. A): 61–68.

39. Shimasato, Y., Tanaka, N., et al. (1971) Histopathology of tumors of canine alimentary tract produced by N-methyl-N′-Nitro-N-nitrosoguanidine. *J Natl Cancer Inst* 47:1053–1070.

40. Kurihara, M., Shirakabe, H., et al. (1974) A new method for producing adenocarcinomas in the stomach of dogs with N-ethyl-N-mitro-N-nitrosuguanidine. *Gann* 65:163–177.

41. Stavrou, D., Dahme, E., and Kalich, J. (1976) Induction of tumors of the stomach in miniature swine by the administration of methylnitrosourrea. *Res Exp Med* 169:33–43.

42. Skirrow, M.B. (1994) Diseases due to *Campylobacter, Helicobacter* and related bacteria. *J Comp Pathol* 111:113–149.

43. Leblanc, B., Fox, J.G., et al. (1993) Hyperplastic gastritis with intraepithelial *Campylobacter*-like organisms in a beagle dog. *Vet Pathol* 30:391–394.

44. Talbot, I.C. (1988) Phenotypes and genotypes in colorectal neoplasia. *J Pathol* 156:185–186.

SMOOTH MUSCLE TUMORS OF THE STOMACH

Classification and Histology

Well-differentiated leiomyomas present no problem in recognition, and highly malignant muscle tumors are obviously sarcomas, but they may be difficult to categorize as leiomyosarcomas. It may be impossible to predict the future behavior of smooth muscle tumors that have a histological pattern lying between these two extremes.[1] Small benign tumors usually arise in the outer muscle coats, not the muscularis mucosa, but the site of origin of larger malignant tumors is usually lost.

Leiomyomas are composed of bundles of spindloid cells running in various directions and merging with one another at sharp angles. Longitudinally cut cells have abundant eosinophilic spindle shaped cytoplasms and elongated nuclei with rounded ends. The cytoplasm stains positive for muscle with van Gieson's stain and with Masson's trichrome. Where possible, the section should include some normal gut muscle to act as a control. Nonstriated myofibrils can be demonstrated with phosphotungstic acid hematoxylin stain. The nuclei have stippled chromatin with few small nucleoli, and there are few if any mitotic figures. The stroma is minimal, and leiomyomas of the gut seldom become fibrotic or calcified. Indisputable benign tumors are usually small and are often multiple. They grow by expansion but often do not have a complete or distinct capsule.

In leiomyosarcomas, there is a high nuclear to cytoplasmic ratio, so the bundles appear more cellular than in leiomyomas. The cells vary from spindle shaped to round and are pleomorphic, independent of the plane of section. The nuclei also vary in size and some are hyperchromic, and there are many typical and atypical mitotic figures. Giant nuclei and multinucleate giant cells may be seen, especially in leiomyosarcoma of the rectum. An increased mitotic rate in human specimens is set at 10 mitoses per 59 high power fields.[1] These tumors are usually large and solitary. They often have hemorrhage, coagulative necrosis, and pseudocystic formation, and they may be ulcerated if they extend to the mucosal surface. The growth rate is slow, and the periphery may show infiltrative as well as "pushing" invasive growth. Metastases occur late in the disease and may be seen when no invasive growth has been detected. The growth rate of the metastasis is also slow, and the secondary tumor may appear some time after the primary has been removed.[2] When judging the degree of malignancy of a biopsy specimen, in view of the unpredictability of the behavior of leiomyosarcoma, it is probably best to give a guarded prognosis, with the proviso that invasive growth is limited and spread occurs late in the disease.

Immunohistochemistry may be used on formalin fixed tissues to distinguish among tumors of muscle, fibrous tumors, and spindle cell carcinoma. Desmin demonstrates smooth, striated, and heart muscle, but all fibrous tissue tumors are negative. Myoglobin is found in rhabdomyosarcomas but not in leiomyosarcomas. Smooth muscle tumors of the gut may stain with desmin, vimentin, both, or neither.[4] Fixation is important since antigenicity is reduced if tissues are left unfixed for more than 12 hours or are left in fixative for more than 24 hours. It is now possible to "unmask" some antigens in fixed tissue by use of microwave techniques.[5] Electron microscopy may be used to demonstrate the difference in the myofibrils in smooth and striated muscle tumors and to reveal the true nature of anaplastic leiomyosarcoma when myofibrils are sparse.[6]

In humans, a subset of smooth muscle tumors has been designated "epithelial leiomyosarcoma" or leiomyoblastoma. Such tumors have a high proportion of round and polygonal cells with eosinophilic cytoplasm, in which there is a clear space around the nucleus.

Canine Gastric Smooth Muscle Tumors

Incidence

Carcinomas of the stomach are more common than smooth muscle tumors[7] (see table 8.3), and benign and malignant smooth muscle tumors are more common in the intestine than in the stomach.[2,7-9] The best example of a series of leiomyomas that did not cause illness and were recorded as incidental findings is from a beagle colony used in a lifetime radionucleoid study.[10] Seventy of the 306 dogs necropsied when they were between 8 and 18 years old had one or more leiomyomas.

Age, Breed, and Sex

Smooth muscle tumors are found in dogs over 8 years old and increase in frequency with increasing in age.[11] Large malignant tumors cause clinical signs because of their size and position, but small benign tumors may remain undetected until the dog dies from some other lesion. This may explain the observation that dogs with leiomyosarcomas had a mean age of 7 years, but dogs with leiomyomas had a mean age of 16 years.[11] In the same series, the male to female ratio for leiomyoma was 12:3 and for leiomyosarcoma 2:1; as details of more cases accumulate, no breed or sex predisposition seems to be emerging.

Sites and Gross Morphology

Leiomyomas may be found at all sites in the stomach, they may be multiple, and the most frequent site is the gastroesophageal junction; the tumor site was the gastroesophageal junction in 66 of 70 dogs, the fundus in 2, and the cardia and pylorus in 1 each.[10] This contrasts with gastric carcinomas, which have a site bias toward the pylorus. In 49 other dogs the leiomyomas were multiple, and in 21 they were solitary. Sometimes the benign tumors were identified as microscopic foci adjacent to macroscopically visible tumors.[12] Tumors range in size from 0.5 to 24 cm in diameter, are round or oval with a thin capsule, and bulge out of the serosal surface so the overlying mucosa is intact. The cut surface is pink to white and has a slightly whorled pattern of fibers, in contrast to the more homogeneous granular cut surface of carcinoma.

Tumors in the cardia region may restrict entry of food into the stomach, leading to dilatation of the esophagus and regurgitation of food; or they may act as a ball valve, leading to gastric distention.[15,16] When the mass protrudes into the lumen of the stomach, the overlying mucosa may become ulcerated and can be detected by ultrasonography. Such tumors can give rise to hemorrhage and iron deficiency anemia.[14,16] On cut surface there may be necrosis, hemorrhage, and less obvious patterns of fibers than in the small lesions. The larger tumor masses are sometimes accompanied by smaller tumors distant from the main mass, and these polypoid lesions may be adenomatous hyperplasia rather than leiomyomas.[14,15]

Growth and Metastasis

Although small tumors may have a thin capsule, the larger ones often have an indistinct border. Nevertheless, excision of the tumor and partial gastroectomy or removal by gastrotomy and submucosal resection usually results in a successful outcome, with postoperative survivals from 8 to 24 months.[14-16] Even tumors shown histologically to have indistinct borders have not recurred or metastasized.

The rate of growth in most cases is unknown. Tumors in the region of the cardia have a history of clinical signs of 3–6 weeks before the nature of the illness is diagnosed, while those in the fundus may have caused intermittent signs for up to 8 months. No evidence has been presented to prove that leiomyosarcoma develops from leiomyoma.

Hypoglycemia

Hypoglycemia has been recorded in association with gastrointestinal smooth muscle tumors.[3,13] Possible mechanisms are hypersecretion of insulin or an insulin-like substance, excessive glucose utilization by a large tumor, or low caloric intake due to tumor size and vomiting. Immunocytochemistry and in situ hybridization techniques on a 20 cm diameter mass in the wall of the pyloric antrum showed that the hypoglycemia was due to overproduction of an insulin-like growth factor (IGF-II).[13] The seizures and hypoglycemia, which had begun 5 months before the removal of this tumor, were not seen in the ensuing 2 years. Other clinical problems reported with leiomyomas and leiomyosarcomas include polydipsia, polyuria, seizures, and hind limb weakness. One of the dogs with a leiomyosarcoma redeveloped signs 28 months after removal of the primary tumor; two pulmonary metastases were found and removed, and the dog became normal again within 2 months.

Smooth Muscle Tumors in Other Species

Reports of smooth muscle tumors in species other than the dog are rare: one feline gastric leiomyoma in a series of 5000 feline necropsies[17]. A 30 cm leiomyosarcoma involving the distal esophagus, cranial two-thirds of the stomach, and the visceral surface of the liver was diagnosed in a 12-year-old thoroughbred.[18] A 10 cm diameter ulcerated mass within the pyloric wall was described in a 1-year-old gilt in association with esophageal and gastric ulceration.[19]

Some gastrointestinal tumors that were originally classified as of smooth muscle histogenesis (i.e., leiomyoma and leiomyosarcoma) are, in fact, of different lineage. Several studies using neurogenic markers such as S-100 and neuron specific enolase (NSE) in tandem with vimentin, actin, and myosin immunocytochemistry have demonstrated that some of the tumors probably originate from autonomic neural or stromal elements, while others are truly of muscle origin.[20-22] On the basis of more complex histogenesis or differentiation than was originally anticipated, this group of tumors should be designated gastrointestinal stromal tumors pending immunohistological characterization. Smooth muscle tumors are a specific type of gastrointestinal stromal cell tumor.[22]

Gastric Lymphoma

Alimentary forms of lymphoma commonly affect the stomach of cats and dogs, the bovine abomasum, and to a much lesser extent, the stomach of the horse. In the monogastric species gastric lymphoma can form a diffuse infiltration of tumor cells that uniformly expands the mucosa and sometimes the deeper layer, or it can appear as multiple pale to white plaques on the mucosa that may extend transmurally onto the serosal surface. Ulceration of the mucosa may occur, but the ulcers are not as crateriform as in carcinoma and tend to be multiple, small, and shallow.

Lymphoma is usually found in animals older than 10 years, although in cats young individuals are also affected. Primary gastric lymphoma is extremely rare in dogs.[23] Male dogs are twice as frequently affected as females. Although alimentary lymphoma (involving stomach, intestine, or mesenteric lymph nodes) is the most common anatomic form of this neoplasm in cats, gastric involvement in this species is less common than intestinal tumors.[24]

Most alimentary lymphomas in cats are of B cell origin.[25] This is probably true for other species as well. The neoplastic lymphocytes are thought to arise from mucosal lymphoid tissue. At least 50 percent of cats with tumors have negative FeLV test results, but this is consistent with integrated virus causing neoplastic transformation.[24]

Histologically, neoplastic infiltration is often transmural but can be confined to the mucosa. The muscles frequently atrophy, leaving irregular layers of lymphoid neoplasia supported by surviving reticulum meshwork. The characteristic monotonous cellular appearance of lymphoid neoplasia may be seen, although more primitive cell forms occur, and plasmacytic differentiation also occurs. Plasmacytomas of the stomach have been described in the dog.[26] Adjacent regional lymph nodes (gastric, hepatic, and pancreatic) are usually neoplastic, especially in the cat. An unusual form of gastrointestinal lymphoma with epitheliotropism has been described in dogs.[23] These lymphomas were of probable T cell origin, as judged by immunohistochemical evaluation.

In the bovine abomasum, lymphoma shows as cream-colored, soft, homogeneous masses that include thickened mucosal folds. The thickened rugae may become ulcerated, and regional abomasal lymph nodes are often involved. Generally the lymphoma is widespread and is found in other characteristic locations: heart, uterus, and lymph nodes.[27]

Immunocytochemical staining using CD markers is useful in identifying the lymphoid nature of the tumors and delineating T or B cell origin. However, there are few CD reagents, with the exception of CD3 and CD79a, that work in formalin fixed tissue. Furthermore, lymphomas may vary in their expression of membrane or cytoplasmic markers, and because of this it may not be possible to define the lymphoma histogenesis.

Nonneoplastic Lesions

Polyps

Nonneoplastic polyps can be differentiated from true adenomas only by histology. Polyps have a branching core of lamina propria in which smooth muscle extends upward from the muscularis mucosa. This core of stroma is covered by epithelium that resembles the adjacent normal epithelium in cell type, mitotic index, and relatively low number of cell layers. Polyps have been seen most often in dogs. They are solitary or multiple, sessile or polypoid, and are seldom more than 1.5 cm in diameter[28,29]; however, a large (20 cm) pedunculated gastric polyp has been described in the pylorus of a 13-year-old horse.[30] The microarchitecture of adenomas is more dysplastic than in benign hyperplasia, with a more sessile, nonpedunculated lesion without branching of the stroma in the case of adenomas. Carcinomatous transformation has been reported in an average of 50 percent of polypoid adenomas in humans,[31] but there is no corresponding information for the veterinary species. Immunohistochemical studies on human fundic gland polyps[32] indicate an augmented cell proliferation with an immature mucin expression (positive for the epitope sialyl-Tn, which is expressed only by fetal gastric mucosa), consistent with a benign hyperplastic proliferation.

Some polyps have varying inflammatory components (macrophages, plasmacytes), and some contain eosinophils. The latter are termed eosinophilic granulomatous polyps. Benign lymphoid hyperplastic polyps have been described in dogs. These are solitary or multiple polyps that are probably central lymphoid nodules covered by normal or regenerating gastric epithelium. The lymphoid nodules often have germinal centers, but there is little epithelial or lymphoid cell atypia.

Scirrhous Eosinophilic Gastritis

These lesions resemble diffuse lymphoma or scirrhous carcinoma macroscopically, but histologically the thickened tissue is composed of nonneoplastic granulation tissue heavily infiltrated by eosinophils.[33] In addition, many of the gastric arteries exhibit changes ranging from fibrinoid necrosis to panarteritis.

Acquired Pyloric Stenosis

Acquired pyloric stenosis is seen in old dogs and is characterized macroscopically by fibrosing stricture with annular hypertrophy of pyloric musculature. These lesions can mimic scirrhous carcinoma, but histological examination shows the nonneoplastic nature of the changes.[34] The etiology of these lesions is unknown.

Similar lesions have been reported in the horse, but they are usually regarded as being of congenital origin.[35] Cases of acquired pyloric stenosis associated with large fibrous masses[36] and/or granulation tissue have been described.[37] The fibrosis may be a sequel to ulceration, and gastric ulceration may predispose to the acquisition of varying degrees of pyloric stenosis.

Chronic Hypertrophic Gastropathy

Canine chronic hypertrophic gastropathy, resembling Ménétrier's disease in humans, produces plaque-like, usually rugal, thickening of the mucosa over a portion of the greater curvature.[38] Areas of atrophic gastritis may be adjacent to the hypertrophic lesions, and there is often a low grade lymphocytic-plasmacystic gastritis and enteritis. Multiple polyps, gastritis, and antral hypertrophy may also occur.[39] The etiology of the condition is unknown. It is nonneoplastic in the dog, but in human beings it is thought to be a precancerous lesion.

REFERENCES

1. Watanabe, H., Jass, J.R., and Sobin, L.H. (1990) *Histological Typing of Oesophageal and Gastric Tumors,* 2nd ed. Springer-Verlag, Berlin.
2. Gibbons, G.C., and Murtaugh, R.J. (1989) Cecal smooth muscle neoplasia in the dog. Report of 11 cases and literature review. *J Amer Anim Hosp Assoc* 25:191–197.
3. Bagley, R.S., Levy, J.K., and Malarkey, D.E. (1996) Hypoglycemia associated with intra-abdominal leiomyoma and leiomyosarcoma in six dogs. *J Amer Vet Med Assoc* 208:69–71.
4. Andreasen, C.B., and Mahaffey, E.A. (1987) Immunohistochemical demonstration of desmin in canine smooth muscle tumors. *Vet Pathol* 24:211–215.
5. Shi, S.R., Cote, R.J., and Taylor, C.R. (1997) Antigen retrieval immunohistochemistry: Past, present and future. *J Histochem Cytochem* 45:327–343.
6. Livesey, M.A., Hulland, T.J., and Yovich, J.V. (1986) Colic in two horses associated with smooth muscle intestinal tumors. *Equine Vet J* 18:334–337.
7. Kaser-Hotz, B., Hauser, B., and Arnold, P. (1996) Ultrasonographic findings in canine gastric neoplasia in 13 patients. *Vet Radiol Ultrasound* 37:51–56.
8. Kapatkin, A.S., Mullen, H.S., et al. (1992) Leiomyosarcoma in dogs: 44 cases (1983–1988) *J Amer Vet Med Assoc* 201:1077–1079.
9. Myers, N.C., and Penninck, D.G. (1994) Ultrasonographic diagnosis of gastrointestinal smooth muscle tumors in the dog. *Vet Radiol Ultrasound* 35:391–397.
10. Culbertson, R., Branan, J.E., and Rosenblatt, L.S. (1983) Esophageal/gastric leiomyoma in the laboratory beagle. *J Amer Vet Med Assoc* 183:1168–1171.
11. Patnaik, A.K., Hurvitz, A.I., and Johnson, G.F. (1977) Canine gastrointestinal neoplasms. *Vet Pathol* 14:547–555.

12. Head, K.W. (1976) Tumors of the lower alimentary tract. *Bull WHO* 53:167–186.

13. Boari, A., Barreca, A., et al. (1995) Hypoglycemia in a dog with a leiomyoma of the gastric well producing an insulin-like growth factor II-like peptide. *Eur J Endocrinol* 132:744–50.

14. Kerpsack, S.J., and Birchard, S.J. (1994) Removal of leiomyomas and other non-invasive masses from the cardia region of the canine stomach. *J Amer Anim Hosp Assoc* 30:500–504.

15. Rolfe, D.S., Twedt, D.C., and Sein, H.B. (1994) Chronic regurgitation or vomiting caused by esophageal leiomyoma in three dogs. *J Amer Anim Hosp Assoc* 30:425–430.

16. Grooters, A.M., and Johnson, S.E. (1995) canine gastric leiomyoma. *Comp Cont Educ Small Anim* 17:1485–1491.

17. Turke, M.A.M., Galina, A.M., and Russell, T.S. (1981) Non-hematopoietic gastrointestinal neoplasms in cats: A retrospective study of 44 cases. *Vet Pathol* 18:614–620.

18. Boy, M.G., Palmer, J.E., et al. (1992) Gastric leiomyosarcoma in a horse. *J Amer Vet Med Assoc* 200:1363–1364.

19. Fisher, L.F., and Olander, H.J. (1978) Spontaneous neoplasms of pigs—A study of 31 cases. *J Comp Pathol* 88:505–517.

20. Ueyama, T., Guo, K.J., et al. (1991) A clinicopathologic and immunohistochemical study of gastrointestinal stromal tumors. *Cancer* 69:947–955.

21. Ma, C.K., Amin, M.B., et al. (1993) Immunohistologic characterization of gastrointestinal stromal tumors. *Mod Pathol* 6:139–144.

22. La Rock, R.G., and Ginn, P.E. (1997) Immunohistochemical staining characteristics of canine gastrointestinal stromal tumors. *Vet Pathol* 34:303–311.

23. Steinberg, H., Dubielzig, R.R., et al. (1995) Primary gastrointestinal lymphosarcoma with epitheliotropism in three shar-pei and one boxer dog. *Vet Pathol* 32:423–426.

24. Mahony, O.M., Moore, A.S., et al. (1995) Alimentary lymphoma in cats: 28 cases (1988–1993). *J Amer Vet Med Assoc* 207:1593–1598.

25. Holmberg, C.A., Manning, J.S., and Osburn, B.I. (1976) Feline malignant lymphomas: Comparison of morphologic and immunologic characteristics. *Amer J Vet Res* 37:1455–1460.

26. Brunner, S.R., Dee, L.A., et al. (1992) Gastric extramedullary plasmacytoma in a dog. *J Amer Vet Med Assoc* 200:1501–1502.

27. Bertone, A.L., Roth, L., and O'Krepky, J. (1985) Forestomach neoplasia in cattle: A report of eight cases. *Comp Cont Educ* 7:585–590.

28. Conroy, J.D. (1969) Multiple gastric adenomatous polyps in a dog. *J Comp Pathol* 79:465–467.

29. Happé, R.P., Van Der Gaag, I., et al. (1977) Multiple polyps of the gastric mucosa in two dogs. *J Small Anim Pract* 18:179–189.

30. Morse, C.C., and Richardson, D.W. (1988) Gastric hyperplastic polyp in a horse. *J Comp Pathol* 99:337–342.

31. Tomasulo, J. (1971) Gastric polyps: Histologic types and their relationships to gastric carcinoma. *Cancer* 27:1346–1355.

32. Odze, R.D. (1996) Gastric fundic polyps: A morphological study including mucin histochemistry, stereometry, and M1B-1 immunohistochemistry. *Hum Pathol* 27:896–903.

33. Hayden, D.W., and Fleischman, R.W. (1977) Scirrhous eosinophilic gastritis in dogs with gastric arteritis. *Vet Pathol* 14:441–448.

34. Else, R.W., and Head, K.W. (1980) Some pathological conditions of the canine stomach. *Vet Ann* 20:66–81.

35. Barth, A.D., Barber, S.M., and McKenzie, N.T. (1980) Pyloric stenosis in a foal. *Can Vet J* 21:234–236.

36. McGill, C.A., and Bolton, J.R. (1984) Gastric retention associated with a pyloric mass in two horses. *Aust Vet J* 61:190–195.

37. Church, S., Baker, J.R., and May, S.A. (1996) Gastric retention associated with acquired pyloric stenosis in a gelding. *Equine Vet J* 18:332–334.

38. Bellinger, C.R., Maddison, J.E., Macpherson, G.C., and Ilkiw, J.E. (1990) Chronic hypertrophic pyloric gastropathy in 14 dogs. *Aust Vet J* 67:317–320.

39. Happé, R.P., Van Der Gaag, I., Woverkamp, W.T.C., and Van-Toorenburg, J. (1977) Multiple polyps of the gastric mucosa in two dogs. *J Small Anim Pract* 18:179–189.

TUMORS OF THE INTESTINES

Epithelial Tumors

Classification and Nomenclature

A polyp is a sessile or pedunculate growth from a mucous surface. It may be the result of hyperplasia or neoplasia. Adenomas are differentiated from nonneoplastic lesions because they show degrees of dysplasia.[1] The shape of the gland is altered, and some glands have a single luminal opening but more than one base (i.e., crypt fission). Cells of the diffuse endocrine system and mitotic figures are scattered along the length of the gland, not just at the base. The presence of a few residual endocrine cells does not indicate a carcinoid tumor. Dysplastic nuclei are hyperchromatic, change from elongated to rounded, lie in the center of the cell, not at the base, and occupy a large area. More than one layer of cells develops along the length of the gland. There are three terms to describe the histological pattern of these benign tumors. *Tubular* or *adenomatous* refers to a lesion in which more than 80 percent of the tumor is composed of tubules set in lamina propria. A *villous* or *papillary adenoma* is the diagnosis for a lesion in which more than 80 percent of the tumor is formed by finger-like lamina propria covered by dysplastic epithelium. *Tubulovillous* or *papillotubular* is the term used to describe lesions where both patterns are present in equal amounts. *Familial adenomatous polyposis* is a term used in human medicine for a dominantly inherited precancerous condition associated with deletion of the adenomatous polyposis coli gene that results in the development of more than 100 polyps in the colon and rectum. The disease has not been described in animals. Another precancerous epithelial abnormality in humans is found in flat mucosa of normal thickness and consists of dysplastic, undifferentiated, proliferating columnar cells on the surface of the mucosa overlying normal crypts. This type of lesion has been recorded in animals.

There are four categories of malignant epithelial tumor. *Adenocarcinoma* must have some glands forming tubules or acini and some mucin production. The term *mucinous adenocarcinoma* is reserved for lesions in which mucin forms more than 50 percent of the tumor, either in cysts or as extracellular pools. In contrast, a diagnosis of *signet ring cell carcinoma* implies that more than 50 percent of the tumor is composed of isolated cells with intracellular mucin. In *undifferentiated* or *solid carcinoma*, neither glands nor mucin can be identified. Neutral mucin is demonstrated by the PAS technique and acid mucin by the high iron–diamine–alcian blue reagent, where sulphomucin stains black and sialomucin stains blue. When more than one pattern is present in a single tumor, the dominant feature is used to classify the lesion. The four terms can be qualified by using a grading system, low grade carcinomas being well or moderately differentiated and high grade tumors poorly differentiated or undifferentiated. If more than one grade is present within one tumor, the most severe change is used for classification. Furthermore, the degree of fibroblastic stromal reaction can be indicated by the terms *medullary* and *scirrhotic*. The amount of peritumoral lymphocyte infiltration and the type of marginal growth, well circumscribed expanding or diffusely infiltrating, should be mentioned since these have a prognostic significance. The rate of cell turnover is less in carcinoma that have a pushing expansive border than in those with an infiltrating border. Trauma to an adenoma may result in pseudocarcinomatous changes; namely, cystic glands may rupture, releasing mucin and displaced glands into the submucosa, but the presence of hemorrhage or hemosiderin and the retention of lamina propria without fibrosis indicate that this is not a carcinoma.

There are four tumor-like lesions that may be confused with true tumors. *Hamartomas* are composed of normal nondysplastic epithelium; in humans, the Peutz-Jeghers polyp has a branching central core of smooth muscle. *Heteropia* refers to the presence of normal epithelium in an abnormal site and may be seen as gastric heteropia in the intestine. *Hyperplastic inflammatory polyps* represent a nonneoplastic regenerative change; they are characterized by lengthened tubules lined by nondysplastic columnar cells with little mucin production, mitoses confined to the base of the glands, and the presence of inflammatory cells in the lamina propria. *Lymphoid hyperplastic polyps* have normal epithelium covering the lymphocyte reaction.

Gross Morphology

The tumors may be solitary or multiple. Localized circumscribed lesions may be intramural or intraluminal.[2] Intramural tumors may form a nodule or be circumferential. The stalk of intraluminal polyps may become elongated as the tumor is dragged along by the traction of intestinal movement. Infiltrating tumors in human patients have lost the ability to produce cell adhesion molecules, and the inhibitor protein to protease normally found in the serum is reduced; this circumstance allows the breakdown of extracellular protein so that the nonadherent carcinoma cells can invade. Localized infiltrating tumors may form a plaque or be circumferential. Plaque-like tumors do not spread longitudinally but extend deeply toward the serosa and become ulcerated with a depressed center. Lymphatic vessels are distributed radially so that when they are invaded an annular, often stenosing, tumor is produced. Diffuse circumferential intramural tumors produce a thickened segment of intestine with corrugated mucosa.

Species and Site Distribution
Horses

Glandular tumors of the intestinal tract are rare in horses; intestinal lymphoma and gastric squamous cell

carcinomas are more common.[3] Too few cases have been recorded to suggest a breed or sex predisposition, but all cases were in horses over 8 years old (mean 16 years). The common presenting signs were inappetance, weight loss and intermittent colic.[3] The cecum and large colon were involved three times more often than the small intestine.[4-6] Reports in the early literature of multiple adenomatous polyps appear from the histological descriptions to be hyperplastic inflammatory polyps. All of the more recent cases have been solitary, well-differentiated adenocarcinoma, often with ulceration of the mucosal surface. The tumors were in the form of a nodule or plaque rather than an annular stenosing lesion. By the time the tumor was diagnosed, it had usually extended to the serosa. Metastases to the liver, spleen, lungs, and peritoneal surfaces occurred in about a third of the cases.[4,5] Only horses that had extensive secondary carcinomatosis were diagnosed on the basis of cytological examination of peritoneal fluid. Most of the tumors had fibroplasia, and some had osteoid or cartilage spicules between the neoplastic glands.[4-6] Necrotic tumors with osseous metaplasia may break free and be found as concretions in the colonic lumen.[6] The adenocarcinoma cells were positive for S-100 and cytokeratin and negative for vimentin, unlike mesothelioma cells.[4]

REFERENCES

1. Jass, J.R., and Sobin, L.H. (1989) *Histological Typing of Intestinal Tumors,* 2nd ed. Springer-Verlag, Berlin.
2. Head, K.W., and Else, R.W. (1981) Neoplasia and allied conditions of the canine and feline intestine. *Vet Ann* 21:190–208.
3. Zicker, S.C., Wilson, W.D., and Medearis, I. (1990) Differentiation between intra-abdominal neoplasms and abscesses in horses, using clinical and laboratory data: 40 cases (1973–1988). *J Amer Vet Med Assoc* 196:1130–1134.
4. Kiupel, M., Van Alstine, W.G., and Ritmeester, A. (1998) Small intestinal adenocarcinoma in a horse. *Eur J Vet Pathol* 4:39–42.
5. Rottman, J.B., Roberts, M.C., and Cullen, J.M. (1991) Colonic adenocarcinoma with osseous metaplasia in a horse. *J Amer Vet Med Assoc* 98:657–659.
6. Kirchhof, N., Steinhauer, D., and Fey, K. (1996) Equine adenocarcinomas of the large intestine with osseous metaplasia. *J Comp Pathol* 114:451–456.

Cattle

The prevalence of epithelial neoplasms of the lower intestinal tract varies in different areas of the world.[1] In some areas such tumors are relatively common and are associated with BPV-4 infection combined with ingestion of Bracken fern. In these areas an animal may have multiple lesions, ranging from sessile plaques of hyperchromatic epithelium through adenomatous polyps to carcinoma, at all levels of the intestine, including the duodenum.[2] In other geographic regions rare cases of solitary adenocarcinoma were located in the jejunum, less commonly in the duodenum, cecum, and rectum, and the least commonly in the ileum and colon.[3,4] The age distribution was from 6 to 12 years, but one rectal case was in a 3-year-old.[5] Some lesions are in the form of a mass that protrudes into the lumen and has a cauliflower-like or villous surface; others form an annular stenosing tumor, with the tubular carcinoma pattern invading the wall. By the time the tumor has been diagnosed, most cases have extended onto the serosa, producing extensive transcoelomic metastases and often binding loops of the intestine together. In the majority of cases widespread metastases occur to the drainage lymph nodes, liver, lungs, ovaries, and adrenals. "Apparently successful" removal of the neoplastic segment of intestine was followed by recurrence and metastases in 8 and 12 months.[4,6] The histological pattern is of a moderately well differentiated adenocarcinoma with some PAS positive mucus production and even some mucin containing cysts, but not enough for a diagnosis of mucinous adenocarcinoma. There is less fibrous tissue than in the sheep tumors.[1] There can be peritumoral lymphocytic infiltration and mesenteric nodules of fat necrosis.[3] Hyperplastic polyps may be seen in chronic enteric conditions as recorded in the ileum of a holstein homozygous for the bovine leukocyte adhesion deficiency allele.[7]

Sheep and Goats

The reports of ovine intestinal epithelial tumors in the literature have all been adenocarcinoma. They are moderately common in New Zealand, Australia, United Kingdom, Norway, and Iceland, but fewer cases have been recorded in North America, mainland Europe, Africa, and India.[8,9] This variation may be due to management systems since in some countries ewes culled at about 7 years old are not worth the cost of transport to an abattoir. The incidence can be expressed as between 2 and 42 percent of all sheep tumors or between 0.2 and 3 percent of sheep over 1 year old inspected at abattoirs. The age range is from 1 to 13 years, with a mean of 6 years; most cases are in ewes except where castrated males are kept for wool production. The presenting clinical signs include progressive loss of appetite, weight loss, and ascites (1–35 L).[10] The ascitic and thoracic fluid may contain isolated neoplastic cells or tumor acini. The tumors are usually solitary and are mainly located in the midjejunum, but some are found in the ileum and a few in the duodenum and spiral colon. The primary tumor is a 1–2 cm annular stenosing lesion (sometimes with an intralumenal polyp) that extends from the mucosal surface transmurally to the serosa (fig. 8.16). Tumors that are on the serosa and grow into muscle layers but do not enter the mucosa are considered secondary. The extensive fibrous transcoelomic secondary deposits on peritoneal surfaces may be more dramatic than the primary tumor and are associated with dilated rigid loops of intestine fused into a mass proximal to the primary tumor (fig. 8.16). This is probably because extension into the mesentery via the lymphatics to the mesenteric lymph nodes promotes retro-

grade lymph flow. Lymphogenous spread to the diaphragm can cause a neoplastic pleurisy, and lymphohematogenous dissemination occasionally results in deposits in the lung and kidney. Unlike in the bovine, hematogenous metastases to the liver are rarely seen in sheep, but can be seen in goats (fig. 8.17). In pregnant ewes deposits may be found in the ovaries and oviducts, probably because the altered position of the gravid uterus allows transcoelomic deposits in these organs.[11] Histologically the tumor in the intestine is a tubular adenocarcinoma with some PAS positive mucin production, but the serosal deposits are mainly composed of fibrous tissue in which there are a few signet ring cells and gland formations. Areas of osseous metaplasia are sometimes found. This histological picture and the fact that the serosal secondaries are more obvious than the primary has often led to misdiagnosis of the condition as chronic peritonitis or a mesothelioma. Transmission electron microscopy studies have shown that the tumors are composed of polygonal undifferentiated cells, (presumably arising from the crypt cells) and more differentiated absorptive epithelial cells and goblet cells.[8] Masson-Fontana stain reveals some endocrine cells in both the primary and secondary tumors. The etiology of adenocarcinoma of the intestine of sheep is unknown. There is no evidence of a viral etiology. Ingestion of bracken fern might be one of a complex of causal factors, but the tumor is common in some areas where there is no bracken.[12] The use of herbicides has been associated with a significant increase in tumor rates.[10,13]

A similar annular stenosing tumor to that seen in sheep has been reported in a 5-year-old Toggenburg female goat.[14]

REFERENCES

1. Johnstone, A.C., Alley, M.R., and Jolly, R.D. (1983) Small Intestinal carcinoma in cattle. *N Z Vet J* 31:147–149.
2. Jarrett, W.F.H. (1980) Bracken fern and papilloma virus in bovine alimentary cancer. *Brit Med Bull* 36:79–81.
3. Bristol, D.G., Baum, K.H., and Messa, L.E. (1984) Adenocarcinoma of the jejunum in two cows. *J Amer Vet Med Assoc* 185:551–553.
4. Tontis, A., Schatzmann, H., and Luginbuhl, H. (1976) Colloid carcinoma in the jejunum of a cow. *Schweiz Arch Tierheilk* 118:535–537 and 543–545.
5. Suzuki, T., and Ohshima, K. (1993) Scirrhous adenocarcinoma of the rectum in a cow. *J Vet Med Sci* 55:1063–1065.
6. Archer, R.M., Cooley, A.J., et al. (1988) Jejunojejunal intussusception associated with a transmural adenocarcinoma in an aged cow. *J Amer Vet Med Assoc* 192:209–211.
7. Ackermann, M.R., Kehrli, M.E., et al. (1996) Alimentary and respiratory tract lesions in eight medically fragile holstein cattle with bovine leukocyte adhesion deficiency (BLAD). *Vet Pathol* 33:273–281.
8. Ross, A.D., and Day, W.A. (1985) An ultrastructural study of adenocarcinoma of the small intestine in sheep. *Vet Pathol* 22:552–560.
9. Pérez, V., Corpa, J.M., and García Marín, J.F. (1999) Intestinal adenocarcinoma in sheep in Spain. *Vet Rec* 144:76–77.
10. Ulvund, M.J. (1983) Occurrence of intestinal adenocarcinomas in sheep in the south western part of Norway. *NZ Vet J* 31:177–178.

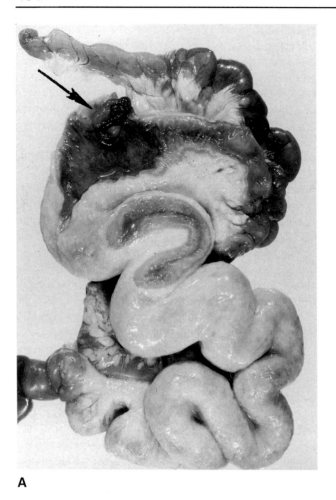

A

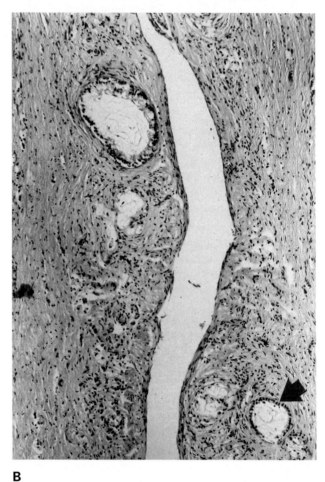

B

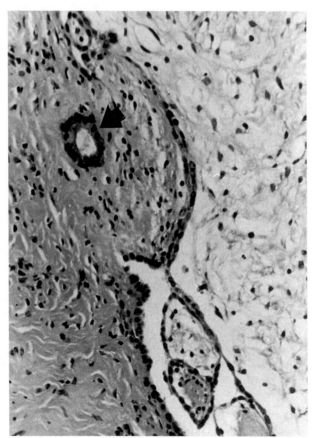

C

Fig. 8.16. Adenocarcinoma in the small intestine of an aged ewe. **A.** Proximal intestinal loops (bottom) are dilated, thick walled, and show serosal fibrosis. The primary annular stenosing tumor is marked by a polypoid mass (arrow). Beyond this the intestine rapidly narrows and becomes normal. **B.** Section of fibrosed mesentery at the level of the primary tumor showing a plexus of lymphatics plugged with mucin-producing tumor cells (arrowhead); note valve on one end of lymphatic vein. **C.** Peritoneal surface of the diaphragm of the ewe with transcoelomic metastases of an intestinal adenocarcinoma. Single, well-differentiated acinus embedded in dense fibrous tissue (arrowhead). Infoldings of the serosa lined by cuboidal, activated mesothelial cells can produce acinar-like structures.

11. Pearson, G.R., and Cawthorne, R.J.G. (1978) Intestinal adenocarcinoma in a ewe. *Vet Rec* 103:409–477.
12. McCrea, C.T., and Head, K.W. (1978) Sheep tumors in north east Yorkshire. II. Experimental production of tumors. *Brit Vet J* 137:21–30.
13. Newell, K.W., Ross, A.D., and Renner, R.M. (1984) Phenoxy and picolinic acid herbicides and small intestinal adenocarcinoma in sheep. *Lancet* 2:1301–1305.
14. Haibel, G.K. (1990) Intestinal adenocarcinoma in a goat. *J Amer Vet Med Assoc* 196:326–328.

Dogs

Epithelial tumors of the canine intestine are not common and form about 0.3 percent of all canine necropsy and biopsy submissions. Up to 60 percent of all intestinal

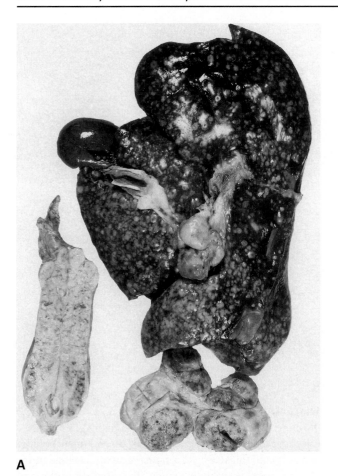

A

tumors are located in the colon and rectum, but many of these are lymphomas. The majority of cases are in old animals, the mean age being 9 years, with a range from 1 to 14 years. Rectoanal polyps are seen in slightly younger dogs (mean age 7 years). Although some series showed a bias to collies and German shepherds, other workers could not demonstrate a breed predisposition. There is general agreement that males are affected more often than females. Adenomas in the colorectum occur and may be multiple, but they are rare in the small intestine. Adenocarcinomas are usually solitary, and they are slightly more common in the colorectum than in the small intestine. Colorectal tumors are often polypoid when benign but more extensive and plaque-like when malignant (fig. 8.18). Occasionally they are diffuse, with circumferential thickening of considerable lengths of the colon. Adenocarcinoma of the small intestine are nearly always annular stenosing and may occur at any level from duodenum to ileum. Animals with small-intestinal tumors have a wide range of signs including weight loss, anorexia, vomiting, diarrhea, melena, and anemia. An abdominal mass may be palpable, and radiography may demonstrate a mass or an obstruction, but laparotomy and biopsy are usually needed to establish a diagnosis.[1,2] Rectal tumors may cause prolapse and can be diagnosed by endoscopic biopsy; they are associated with weight loss, anorexia, and mucus and fresh blood in the feces.[3,4] Constipation may occur if the tumor is stenosing or very large.

Intestinal tumors in dogs are predominantly the tubular adenocarcinoma type, with some mucin production (intracellular or extracellular), signet ring cells, or mucinous cysts (fig. 8.19). The tumor in the mucosa is seldom

B

Fig. 8.17. **A.** Metastasis of colon carcinoma to liver and lymph nodes in a goat. **B.** Metastatic nodule in the cortex of the lymph node from a dog with jejunal adenocarcinoma. Note desmoplasia around the poorly formed tubules.

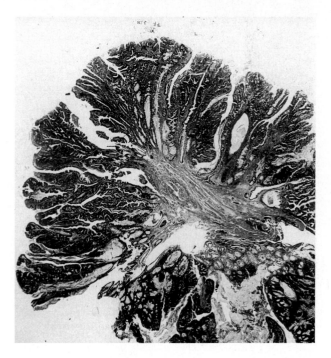

Fig. 8.18. Papillotubular adenoma in the rectum of the dog.

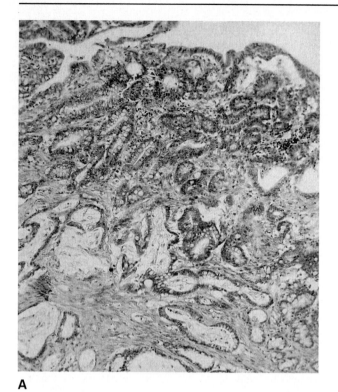

A

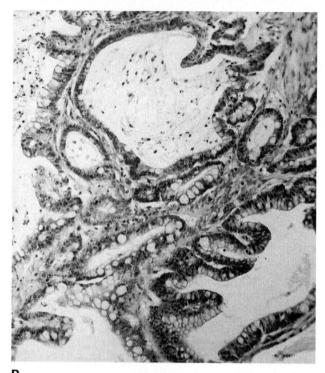

B

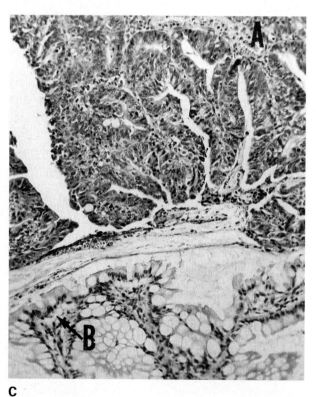

C

Fig. 8.19.   Adenocarcinoma in the large intestine. **A.** Tubular adeno-carcinoma in the colon of the cat showing irregular branching tubules embedded in a moderate amount of fibrous stroma. **B.** Higher magnification showing tubules lined by columnar, cuboidal, and flattened cells, some of which form cysts that contain mucin. **C.** Papillary adenocarcinoma in the rectum of the dog. Contrast non–mucin-containing neoplastic columnar cells (*A*) with goblet cells in the normal epithelium (*B*).

scirrhotic but the serosal extension usually shows marked desmoplasia. Most polyps are either adenoma or regenerative hyperplasia, but two examples of ulcerated nodular and polypoid thickening of lengths of small intestine (up to 25 cm long) resembling human Peutz-Jeghers polyps of normal, well-differentiated epithelium have been reported.[5] A small tumor plaque in the jejunum proved to be an adenocarcinoma arising in heterotopic gastric mucosa: the cells lining the acini were parietal, chief, and mucous cells resembling those in the pylorus.[6] Adenocarcinoma of the small intestine rapidly extends by permeation of tissue spaces and lymphatics into the serosa and mesentery and by lymphatics to the mesenteric lymph node. Transcoelomic peritoneal carcinomatosis and hematogenous spread to the liver is less common, and lymphohematogenous metastasis to the lung and other organs is rare.[2] Adenocarcinomas in the rectum spread in the lymphatics to lymph nodes and sometimes produce peritoneal seeding.[4] It is difficult to explain the metastatic pathway in some cases of colorectal cancer, as for example, in metastases to the leptomeninges extending from L6 to T10, causing paralysis,[7] or to the skin of the ventral abdomen and hind leg.[8] Colorectal adenomatous polyps are mainly papillotubular in pattern and may only involve the superficial mucosa over normal crypts, but some have marked cellular atypia and limited invasion of the submucosa. This malignant transformation of polypoid tumors should be considered in light of the observations that the mucosa adjacent to the polyp may show early tumor formation and that some dogs develop a second polyp in from 1 to 18 months after an initial polypectomy. It is obvious, then, that polyps need careful histological examination before prognosis is made.

A suggested TNM classification is T_1, tumor in mucosa and submucosa only; T_2, extension to muscle and serosa; T_3, extension to contiguous structures; N_0, nodes normal; N_1, regional nodal metastases; N_2, distal nodal involvement; M_0, no widespread metastases; and M_1, distal metastases present. Using this system to identify $T_1N_0M_0$ rectoanal adenocarcinoma cases, single high dose radiotherapy resulted in an apparent cure in about half the cases.[9] Radiation therapy may be followed by a recurrence because hypoxic cells are radioresistant; this was shown in one series of tumors where groups of adenocarcinoma cells situated in extensive intercellular connective tissue were hypoxic but not necrotic on histological examination.[10] Chemotherapy may not be beneficial since both normal and neoplastic intestinal epithelium reacts for P-glycoprotein, a factor in tumor cell multidrug resistance.[12] Following polypectomy, a proportion of dogs develop a carcinomatous recurrence. Removal of the tumor and a segment of small intestine may be followed by recurrence at the site of anastomosis or by the appearance of metastases in organs that looked normal previously. Histological evaluation of a biopsy that determines invasion is the best method of predicting behavior. Tests, such as the detection of overexpression of p53 protein are of little value since intestinal adenocarcinomas are known to have a low prevalence of positivity.[11]

Cats

Hematopoietic tumors (lymphoma and mast cell tumors) are the most common type of neoplasia seen in the feline intestine, and adenocarcinomas are next most frequent at about 7 percent of cases. Up to 90 percent of reported epithelial intestinal tumors are malignant. Adenomatous polyps are far less common, and at least one, an adenoma of the cecum, was reclassified as a hyperplastic polyp on subsequent histological examination. Duodenal polyps up to 1.5 cm in size can cause acute or chronic vomiting, hematemesis, and anemia.[13] Surgical resection of polyps is usually curative; unlike the situation in dogs, there does not seem to be a progression from colorectal adenomatous polyp to adenocarcinoma. Intestinal adenocarcinoma is seen more in males than females, the mean is 11 years (range 2 to 17 years), and Siamese appear overrepresented. Affected cats have a history of weight loss, anorexia, diarrhea, vomiting, ascites with tumor cells, and anemia. Diagnosis is aided in about 50 percent of cases by abdominal palpation of a mass and contrast radiography to show obstruction.

About 90 percent of the tumors are in the small intestine, with the number in the jejunum and ileum exceeding those at the ileocecocolic junction and the duodenum being rarely affected. Annular stenosing tumors are the usual gross finding. Histologically, most of the tumors are tubular with some acid and neutral mucin production and some signet ring cells; about a third of the cases have areas of osseous or cartilagenous metaplasia. By the time the primary tumor has been diagnosed there are metastases in the mesenteric lymph node and on the peritoneal surfaces, with associated ascites in about half the cases. Metastases to the lungs and other organs, including the skeleton, are rare, and hematogenous spread to the liver is seldom seen. Resection of the affected segment of the small-intestine has resulted in an average survival time of 15 months (range 2 days to 2 years), but most of the cats were old, and many died from other geriatric diseases. It has been noted that following surgical removal of the primary tumor, cats can survive for up to 28 months with mesenteric lymph node metastases and carcinomatosis.[14] An unusual duodenal tubular adenocarcinoma has been described occurring in the hepatopancreatic ampulla at the confluence of biliary, duodenal, and pancreatic epithelium and producing concurrent obstruction to bile and pancreatic ducts.[15] The etiology of all these types of intestinal epithelial tumors is unknown. All the cats tested have been negative for FeLV and FIV.

Pigs

Intestinal epithelial tumors are very rare, probably because few sows and even fewer boars reach old age, when adenocarcinomas are likely to develop. Five cases of annular stenosing, mucus producing, scirrhotic tubular adenocarcinoma have been described in the middle or distal third of the jejunum of mature and old sows.[16] In three of these cases metastases were present in the mesenteric lymph node, and in one metastases were also in the lungs. There is a report of a mucinous adenocarcinoma in the cecum that had metastasized to the regional lymph nodes and lungs.[16]

REFERENCES

1. Gibbs, C., and Pearson (1986) Localised tumors of the canine small intestine: A report of twenty cases. *J Small Anim Pract* 27:507–519.
2. Birchard, S.J., Couto, C.G., and Johnson, S. (1986) Nonlymphoid intestinal neoplasia in 32 dogs and 14 cats. *J Amer Anim Hosp Assoc* 22:533–537.
3. Holt, P.E., and Lucke, V.M. (1985) Rectal neoplasia in the dog: A clinicopathological review of 31 cases. *Vet Rec* 116:400–405.
4. Brunnert, S.R., Deel, L.A., et al. (1993) Primary linitis plastica (signet ring) carcinoma of the colon in a dog. *J Amer Anim Hosp Assoc* 29:75–77.
5. Brown, P.J., Adam, S.M., et al. (1994) Hamartomatous polyps in the intestine of two dogs. *J Comp Pathol* 110:97–102.
6. Panigrati, D., Johnson, A.N., and Wosu, N.J. (1994) Adenocarcinoma arising from gastric heterotopia in the jejunal mucosa of a beagle dog. *Vet Pathol* 31:278–280.
7. Stampley, A.R., Swayne, D.E., and Prasse, K.W. (1987) Meningeal carcinomatosis secondary to a colonic signet-ring cell carcinoma in a dog. *J Amer Anim Hosp Assoc* 23:655–658.

8. Hampson, E.C.G.M., Wilkinson, G.T., et al. (1990) Cutaneous metastasis of a colonic carcinoma in a dog. *J Small Anim Pract* 31:155–158.

9. Turrel, J.M., and Theon, A.P. (1986) Single high-dose irradiation for selected canine rectal carcinomas. *Vet Radiol* 27:141–145.

10. Cline, J.M., Thrall, D.E., et al. (1990) Immunohistochemical detection of a hypoxia marker in spontaneous canine tumors. *Brit J Cancer* 62:925–931.

11. Gamblin, R.M., Sagartz, J.E., and Couto, C.G. (1997) Overexpression of p53 tumor suppressor protein in spontaneously arising neoplasms of dogs. *Amer J Vet Med* 58:857–863.

12. Ginn, P.E. (1996) Immunohistochemical detection of P-glycoprotein in formalin-fixed and paraffin-embedded normal and neoplastic canine tissues. *Vet Pathol* 33:533–541.

13. MacDonald, J.M., Mullen, H.S., and Moroff, S.D. (1993) Adenomatous polyps of the duodenum in cats: 18 cases (1985–1990). *J Amer Vet Med Assoc* 202:647–651.

14. Kosovsky, J.E., Matthiesen, D.T., and Patnaik, A.K. (1988) Small intestinal adenocarcinoma in cats: 32 cases (1978–1985). *J Amer Vet Med Assoc* 192:233–235.

15. Haines, V.L., Brown, P.R., et al. (1996) Adenocarcinoma of the hepatopancreatic ampulla in a domestic cat. *Vet Pathol* 33:439–441.

16. Vitovec, J. (1977) Carcinomas of the intestine in cattle and pigs. *Zbl Vet Med* 24A:413–421.

Carcinoids

Tumors derived from the neuroendocrine cells of the gastrointestinal mucosa are known as carcinoids because, histologically, they closely resemble carcinomas of intestinal epithelial origin, but they have a different histogenesis. The cells, originally termed *argentaffin* or *Kulchitsky cells,* contain cytoplasmic granules that contain 5-hydroxytryptamine (5-HT, serotonin) and related neurosecretory substances that react to argentaffin, argyrophil, and diazonium staining techniques.[1] In addition to 5-HT, the cells contain enteroglucagon, secretin, somatostatin, bombesin, motilin, and gastrin.[2] Each cell type synthesizes and stores a single hormone, with the active secretion being either short chain polypeptides and/or biologically active amines. It has been shown that not all neuroendocrine cells can decarboxylate an amine precursor, and the APUD (amine precursor uptake and decarboxylation) system concept has been modified and renamed the diffuse endocrine system.

Ideally, diagnosis should be made on freshly collected and fixed material rather than postmortem tissue since the active cell secretions rapidly degenerate, unlike their inactive precursors. Frozen tissue for histochemical staining and, ideally, small blocks fixed in glutaraldehyde and processed for electron microscopy should be collected where the presence of a carcinoid is suspected. Reprocessing of formalin fixed tissue for retrospective electron microscopy examination can be performed as neurosecretory granules tend to preserve, while details of other organelles are less than optimal with formalin fixation.

Classification

Tumors of the diffuse endocrine system in humans have been broadly categorized as carcinoids, mucocarcinoids, and mixed carcinoid-adenocarcinomas.[1] The mixed type of tumor has areas that are clearly carcinoid (packets of granule-containing epithelium-like cells) and others that are adenocarcinoma without granules. Mucocarcinoids resemble well-differentiated adenocarcinomas with differentiation to both mucus secreting, epithelium-like, tumor cells and more overtly endocrine cells. Occasional endocrine cells may be found in tumors classified as adenocarcinomas of intestinal epithelial origin. The presence of argyrophilic neuroendocrine cells in carcinomas is explained by the fact the gut epithelial cell and the neuroendocrine cells develop from the same endodermal progenitor cells.[2] The origin of intestinal neuroendocrine cells is debatable, but endodermal progenitors, rather than the neural crest, are the most likely cells of origin.[3]

Incidence

Most reports of gastrointestinal carcinoids in the veterinary literature are of single cases: 1 horse,[4] 3 cows,[5,6] 4 cats,[7,8] and 13 dogs.[9-13] One study reported a frequency distribution of 4 carcinoids out of 64 intestinal tumors from 10,270 canine necropsies.[10]

Age, Breed, and Sex

In the dog, carcinoids have been reported in both sexes, several different breeds, and over an age range of 9 to 13 years. The cats were 9 to 13 years old and were castrated males. The bovine tumors were all from adult cows with a median age of 5 years.

Clinical Characteristics

Theoretically, tumors of the diffuse neuroendocrine system should invoke a recognizable clinical syndrome related to their secretory products, but this is not consistently observed. Vasoactive amines released from the tumors may result in diarrhea, skin flushing or cyanosis, hypertension, bronchoconstriction, pulmonary valvular stenosis, and right heart failure. Carcinoids that secrete gastrin (G cell tumors) are responsible for the Zollinger-Ellison syndrome, characterized by severe gastric hypersecretion and peptic ulceration, with watery diarrhea.[14] The syndrome has been reported in dogs and cats, usually associated with a non–beta cell pancreatic islet cell tumor rather than a gastrointestinal tumor.[15-17] The typical carcinoid syndrome, as seen in humans, has not been reported in domestic animals, although skin abnormalities associated with pancreatic islet cell tumors have been reported in the dog.[18] Diarrhea and weight loss may be associated with noncarcinoid intestinal tumors, and anemia or episodic intestinal hemorrhage in dogs with carcinoids may be due to ulceration of the mucosa.[11] Weakness and ataxia without obvious muscle wasting have also been observed.[13]

Tumor Sites

Carcinoids in humans occur most frequently in the appendix and ileum and less often in the rectum, colon, and stomach. In animals there are insufficient data to give definitive locations, but in dogs there seems to be a predilection for the large intestine: rectum (five cases),[11] colon (two cases),[9] cecocolic junction (three cases),[11,12] one gastric carcinoid,[13] and two duodenal carcinoids.[9] In contrast, feline carcinoids are most often in the ileum.[7] One cat had a duodenal lesion closely associated with a pancreatic mass, and this may have been a primary pancreatic carcinoid with spread to the adjacent bowel.[8] The proximal jejunum was the site of the only equine intestinal carcinoid reported in the literature,[4] and in the bovine one was located in the proximal colon[5] and two in the small intestine.[6]

Gross Morphology

In humans some carcinoids are reported as yellow, orange, or tan-colored on cut surface, and others are gray but may turn yellow on formalin fixation. This latter event has not been described in animals, and intestinal carcinoids are yellowish or tan on cut surface.[5,10] There is no characteristic shape to the tumors, and they range from annular stenosing thickenings to nodular masses, approximately 5 cm in diameter in dogs or up to a 10-cm diameter in cattle. In the rectum the tumors are nodular, intraluminal fungating masses, or they may form pedunculated nodules that protrude at the anus.[11] The tumors may be ulcerated or eroded, with secondary superficial inflammation. Multiple primary lesions are seen in about 25 percent of human cases. This feature has not been reported in animals, although metastatic and transcoelomic spread of carcinoids occurs.[13]

Histological Features

Carcinoid tumors consist of nests and cords of small, uniform round cells separated by vascular channels or thin fibrous trabeculae. Tumor cells form solid islands of uniform cells with eosinophilic granular cytoplasm and poorly defined cell boundaries. There may be palisading of peripherally located cells. Stromal content is variable but may be marked by tumor cells forming cords of cells within the connective tissue. In humans, two other patterns are seen: ribbon-like anastomosing loops of cells that resemble the garland form of basal cell tumors in the skin; or irregular cell aggregates, sometimes forming acini or rosettes with accumulations of periodic acid-Schiff positive material. Some carcinoids may have mucous droplets in the cells. Other tumors may be poorly differentiated, with only small areas of the tumor exhibiting recognizable patterns.

Histological diagnosis of carcinoid is confirmed by examining the affinity of tumor cells for silver stains (argentaffin and argyrophil reactions), immunocytochemistry staining for neuroendocrine substances, and ultrastructural examination for membrane bound neurosecretory granules in the cytoplasm.[1,13] The use of high and low molecular weight cytokeratin, neuron specific enolase, synaptophysin, and chromagranin reactions are the most useful, with most carcinoids staining positively with synaptophysin and chromagranin. The use of immunohistological markers is particularly helpful since gastrointestinal adenomas and carcinomas may contain sufficiently

significant numbers of argyrophilic cells to be potentially confusing in carcinoid diagnosis.[2]

Carcinoid cells examined by electron microscopy contain small, dense-core, neurosecretory granules that are membrane bound in the cytoplasm.

Growth and Metastasis

Carcinoids in all species arise deep in the mucosa and invade the submucosa, initially producing a larger mass than in the mucosa itself. Growth occurs in all planes, with eventual ulceration of the mucosal surface and penetration of the outer muscle coat and serosa of the bowel. In domestic animals carcinoids are generally regarded as malignant, slow growing neoplasms that metastasize in a similar manner to adenocarcinomas, through lymphatic and hematogenous routes. In many of the reported cases there is local spread to the adjacent mesentery, with adhesion and tumor growth.[4] Microscopically, plugs of tumor cells are common in portal veins in the liver. In cats, metastatic deposits occur in the mesentery, omentum, and lymph nodes.[7] In dogs the small intestinal carcinoids spread to lung and pleura, liver, local lymph nodes, and pancreas.[9,10] The involvement of the pancreas in the cat and dog might be misleading since this organ may be the site of a primary neuroendocrine tumor of islet cells.[15,17]

Although reported canine rectal and cecal carcinoids had a high mitotic index and there was spread to the adjacent colonic mesentery or vascular tumor embolism, there was no associated widespread metastatic disease in these cases.[11,12] One report of a colonic tumor, however, cited involvement of multiple body organs,[13] and in another canine case, the gastric carcinoid metastasized widely.[19] In the reported equine and bovine cases, the carcinoids caused localized adhesions, and tumor cells were found in drainage lymph nodes, but there were no metastases to organs.

REFERENCES

1. Solcia, E., Kloppel, G., and Sobin, L.H. (1999) *Histological Typing of Endocrine Tumors,* 2nd ed. Springer, New York.
2. Scanziani, E., Rippa, L., Giusti, A.M., Gualtieri, M., and Mandelli, G. (1993) Argyrophil cells in gastrointestinal epithelial tumors of the dog. *J Comp Pathol* 108:405–409.
3. Wright, M.A. (1999) The origin of gut and pancreatic neuroendocrine (APUD) cells. *J Pathol* 198:439–440.
4. Orsini, J.A., Orsini, P.G., Sepesy, L., Acland, H., and Gillette, D. (1988) Intestinal carcinoid in a mare: An etiologic consideration for chronic colic in horses. *J Amer Vet Med Assoc* 193:87–88.
5. Cho, D.-Y., and Archibald, L.F. (1985) Carcinoid tumor in the colon of a cow. *Vet Pathol* 22:639–641.
6. Anjiki, T., Ishikawa, Y., Kadota, K., and Ishino, S. (1996) Tubular adenocarcinoma with neuroendocrine type secretory granules and Paneth cell granules in a cow. *J Nihon Univ Vet Sci* 42:1–16.
7. Patnaik, A.K., Liu, S.-K., and Johnson, G.F. (1976) Feline intestinal adenocarcinoma. A clinicopathologic study of 22 cases. *Vet Pathol* 13:1–10.
8. Carakostas, M.C., Kennedy, G.A., Kittleston, M.D., and Cook, J.E. (1979) Malignant foregut carcinoid tumor in a domestic cat. *Vet Pathol* 16:607–609.

9. Patnaik, A.K., Hurvitz, A.I., and Johnson, G.F. (1977) Canine gastrointestinal neoplasms. *Vet Pathol* 14:547–555.

10. Patnaik, A.K., Hurvitz, A.I., and Johnson, G.F. (1980) Canine intestinal adenocarcinoma and carcinoid. *Vet Pathol* 17:149–163.

11. Sykes, G.P., and Cooper, B.J. (1982) Canine intestinal carcinoids. *Vet Pathol* 19:120–131.

12. Couglin, A.S. (1992) Carcinoid in canine large intestine. *Vet Rec* 130:499–500.

13. Albers, T.M., Alroy, J., McDonnell, J.J., and Moore, A.S. (1988) A poorly differentiated gastric carcinoid in a dog. *J Vet Diag Invest* 10:116–118.

14. Zollinger, R.M., and Ellison, E.H. (1955) Primary peptic ulcerations of the jejunum associated with islet cell tumors of the pancreas. *Ann Surg* 142:709–728.

15. Shaw, D. (1988) Gastrinoma (Zollinger-Ellison syndrome) in the dog and cat. *Can Vet J* 29:448–452.

16. English, R.V., Breitschwerdt, E.B., Grindem, C.B., Thrall, D.E., and Gainsburg, L.A. (1988) Zollinger-Ellison syndrome and myelofibrosis in a dog. *J Amer Vet Med Assoc* 192:1430–1434.

17. Van der Gaag, I., vanden Ingh, T.S.G.A.M., Lamers, C.B.H.W., and Lindeman, J. (1988) Zollinger-Ellison syndrome in a cat. *Vet Quarterly* 10:151–155.

18. Gross, T.L. (1990) Glucagon-producing pancreatic endocrine tumors in two dogs with superficial necrolytic dermatitis. *J Amer Vet Med Assoc* 197:1619–1622.

19. Patnaik, A.K., and Lieberman, P.H. (1981) Canine goblet cell carcinoid. *Vet Pathol* 18:410–413.

Mesenchymal Tumors

Vascular Tumors and Malformations

In the dog, metastases to the intestine and mesentery from a primary hemangiosarcoma at another site is common, but primary tumors in the intestine, mesentery, or omentum are rare.[1] Vascular tumors in cats are rare at any site. Four primary hemangiosarcomas in the mesentery of old cats were found to be locally invasive into the duodenum, pancreas, and colon, and they produced metastases in the liver, spleen, and heart.[2] Cavernous angiomatous malformations produce plaque-like lesions in the muscle coat of the small colon and have been described in foals as young as 4 months.[3] Diffuse lymphangiosarcoma produced multicystic fluid filled masses in the root of the mesentery, omentum, and cranial mediastinum in an 11-year-old cat.[4] As in the case of blood vascular lesions, it may be difficult to separate true tumors from congenital lymphangectasia.[5]

Tumors of Fibrous Tissue, Bone, and Cartilage

Fibrosarcomas originating in the intestinal tract have been described rarely, and separation from leiomyosarcomas requires histochemical and/or immunohistochemical confirmation.[6-8] Intestinal myxosarcoma has been reported; one produced a large broadly pedunculate mass in the smooth muscle, and consisted of atypical fibroblastic cells with an Alcian blue positive mucinous stroma. This myxosarcoma was similar to two previous cases, all of which had metastasized to the regional lymph node.[9]

Primary extraskeletal osteosarcomas in dogs have ranged in size from 4 to 27 cm and were found in the jejunum, ileum, gastric ligament, and perianal region, and all had metastasized within the abdomen.[10] Examination of multiple sections may be necessary to find islands of osteoid tissue between pleomorphic mesenchymal cells. In one case the osteosarcoma was associated with a gauze swab left in the abdomen during an ovariohysterectomy 6 years previously.[11] Some osteosarcomas had areas of chondroplastic differentiation, and in one case only chondrosarcomatous differentiation was found.[10]

Neurogenic Tumors

Peripheral nerve sheath tumors of the abdominal autonomic ganglia and the myenteric plexuses are rare, but examples have been recorded in cattle, horses, and dogs.[12,13] In cattle, the hepatic plexus was involved as one of a series of multiple lesions of bovine schwannomatosis.[12] Solitary large tumors have been found in the duodenum and cecum of dogs and in the colon of horses. Multiple subserosal and intramuscular neurofibromas and schwannomas in association with hyperplasia of the myenteric plexus have been reported in the horse.[13] All these tumors were benign, being composed of interlacing bundles of spindloid cells showing little atypia and few if any mitoses. The neurofibroma pattern of mature perineural cells can be differentiated from leiomyoma with H&E, histochemistry, and or immunohistochemistry. Sometimes these tumors trap normal nonneoplastic ganglionic neurons and their surrounding satellite cells, and such lesions must be differentiated from ganglioneuromas.

Proliferation of the ganglionated plexuses of the intestinal wall may produce hyperplastic or neoplastic lesions, both of which are described in domestic animals.[14-17] Ganglioneuroma is the term used for solitary, well-demarcated neoplasms that show limited local invasiveness, have few or no mitoses, and have a low metastatic potential. Ganglioneuromatosis represents a hyperplasia involving all the layers of the wall from the lamina propria to the serosa; it is probably a congenital malformation that continues to grow from birth until maturity.[15,17] Both conditions are composed of variable sized ganglion cells, either singly or in groups, and interlacing bundles of nerve fibers with their perineural sheaths. Transmission electron microscopy can be used to identify these cell types: silver stains can be used to demonstrate the axons and luxol fast blue to show that the nerves are nonmyelinated.[14,15] Immunocytochemically the Schwann cells are S-100 and vimentin positive, the nerve fascicles positive for neurofilament protein, and the ganglion cells positive for neuron specific enolase.[16] Both types of lesions are rare. Ganglioneuromas have been described in the distal common bile duct and ampulla of Vater of a 5-year-old dog, and in the jejunum of an 18-month-old dog, a 5-week-old cat, and a 7-year-old horse; ganglioneuromatosis affected a 12-month-old dog and a 7-month-old steer.[17]

Tumors of Adipose Tissue

In older horses lipomas are common, but in other species they are rare.[18] We have only seen one liposarcoma, and it was in an 18-month-old cat; it originated in the ileum and had metastases in the mesenteric lymph node and kidney. Liposarcomas have distinct nuclei and are cellular, and the cells have abundant cytoplasm with one or more droplets of fat, in contrast to the cells of a lipoma, which have inconspicuous nuclei and cytoplasm that resembles normal fat. It is accepted practice to refer to a pedunculate mass of fat surrounded by a connective tissue capsule and attached to the mesentery as a lipoma, especially in horses. Whether there are neoplastic cells in these tumors is debatable and unproven. Histologically, these lesions often have fat necrosis and dystrophic calcification, especially if the blood vessels are compressed by the peduncle becoming twisted. Solitary and multiple mesenteric pedunculate lipomas have been recorded in pigs, dogs, and horses. The peduncle may strangulate a segment of intestine,[18] and such lesions are commonly associated with colic in old horses.[19] The lesions start as a localized plaque of fat in the mesentery, and they develop a peduncle as the mass grows.[19] Asymptomatic pedunculate lipomas have a median weight of 21 g. Horses over 12 years old are affected (mean age 17.6 years), and more lesions are reported in geldings than in mares or stallions. One large series showed that ponies had lipomas more often than thoroughbreds, and it was suggested that this was because ponies had a different lipid metabolism from other horses and that they were kept fat for show purposes in contrast to lean thoroughbreds. Unlike dogs and horses, cattle with lipomatosis and fibrolipomatosis of the abdominal fat do not seem to develop pedunculate lipoma.

REFERENCES

1. Brown, N.O., Patnaik, A.K., and MacEwen, E.G. (1985) Canine haemangiosarcoma. Retrospective analysis of 104 cases. *J Amer Vet Med Assoc* 186:56–58.
2. Patnaik, A.K., and Liu, S.-K. (1977) Angiosarcoma in cats. *J Small Anim Pract* 18:191–198.
3. Platt, H. (1987) Vascular malformations and angiomatous lesions in horses: A review of 10 cases. *Equine Vet J* 19:500–504.
4. Stobie, D., and Carpenter, J.L. (1993) Lymphangiosarcoma of the mediastinum, mesentery, and omentum in a cat with chylothorax. *J Amer Anim Hosp Assoc* 29:78–80.
5. Milne, E.M., Woodman, M.P., et al. (1994) Intestinal lymphangiectasia as a cause of chronic diarrhoea in a horse. *Vet Rec* 134:603–604.
6. Brody, R.S., and Cohen, D. (1964) An epizootiologic and clinicopathologic study of 95 cases of gastrointestinal neoplasms in the dog. In Scientific Proceedings of the 101st Annual Meeting of the AVMA, Chicago, pp. 167–179.
7. Turk, M.A.M., Gallina, A.M., and Russell, T.S. (1981) Nonhematopoietic gastrointestinal neoplasia in cats: A retrospective study of 44 cases. *Vet Pathol* 18:614–620.
8. Hayden, D.W., and Nielsen, S.W. (1973) Canine alimentary neoplasia. *Zbl Vet Med* 20A:1–22.
9. Edens, L.M., Taylor, D.D., et al. (1992) Intestinal myxosarcoma in a thoroughbred mare. *Cornell Vet* 82:163–167.
10. Patnaik, A.K. (1990) Canine extraskeletal osteosarcoma and chondrosarcoma: A Clinicopathologic study of 14 cases. *Vet Pathol* 27:46–55.
11. Pardo, A.D., Adams, W.H., et al. (1990) Primary jejunal osteosarcoma associated with a surgical sponge in a dog. *J Amer Vet Med Assoc* 195:935–938.
12. Canfield, P. (1978) A light microscopic study of bovine peripheral nerve sheath tumors. *Vet Pathol* 15:283–291.
13. Kirchhoff, N., Scheidemann, W., and Baumgärtner, W. (1996) Multiple peripheral nerve sheath tumors in the small intestine of a horse. *Vet Pathol* 33:727–730.
14. Ribas, J.L., Kwapien, R.P., and Pope, E.R. (1990) Immunohistochemistry and ultrastructure of intestinal ganglioneuroma in a dog. *Vet Pathol* 27:376–379.
15. Fairley, R.A., and McEntee, M.F. (1990) Colorectal ganglioneuromatosis in a young female dog (Lhasa apso). *Vet Pathol* 27:206–207.
16. Allen, D., Swayne, D., and Belknap, J.K. (1989) Ganglioneuroma as a cause of small intestinal obstruction in the horse: A case report. *Cornell Vet* 79:133–141.
17. Cole, D.E., Migaki, G., and Leipold, H.W. (1990) Colonic ganglioneuromatosis in a steer. *Vet Pathol* 27:461–462.
18. McLaughlin, R., and Kuzma, A.B. (1991) Intestinal strangulation caused by intra-abdominal lipomas in a dog. *J Amer Vet Med Assoc* 199:1610–1611.
19. Edward, G.B., and Proudman, C.J. (1994) An analysis of 75 cases of intestinal obstruction caused by pedunculated lipomas. *Equine Vet J* 26:18–2!.

Lymphoid Tumors

Anatomical Patterns

The mucosa associated lymphoid tissue (MALT) of the gastrointestinal tract can be the primary site of lymphoma, and such tumors rarely coexist with carcinomas or leiomyomas. There is no possibility of confusion between thymic or cutaneous forms of lymphoma and the primary alimentary (AL) form of the disease. AL is differentiated from a widespread multicentric lymphoma (ML) on the basis that the peripheral lymph nodes are not involved in AL tumors. Localized lymphoma involving the mesenteric lymph node but not the intestinal tract occurs, and such cases should be classified with the miscellaneous group of lymphomas.

AL may be diffuse or localized; when localized, the lesion can bulge intraluminally or be intramural. The tumors may be restricted to one site in the intestinal tract, or multiple tumors may occur at various levels. The tumors can be plaque-like, nodular, or fusiform (circumferential) in shape. Fusiform intramural or transmural lesions frequently balloon outward because the invaded muscle atrophies, leaving rows of lymphocytes supported only by parallel bands of delicate reticulum fibers. Diffuse lesions present as thickened rigid mucosal folds in the stomach, and in intestinal cases the mucosal surface has a granular, or cobblestone appearance. T cell tumors exhibit epitheliotropism, exemplified by early lesions in which tumor infiltration is intraepithelial and in the periglandular lamina propria, whereas B cell tumors start in germinal centers in the submucosa.

Cats

The original definition of AL indicated that the main lesion was in either one or both of the intestinal tract and the drainage lymph nodes.[1] This raises the problem of where solitary lymphoma of the mesenteric lymph node should be classified; it should probably be in the unclassified (miscellaneous) category since this covers tumors in individual nodes as well as those in extranodal sites. AL in the cat is more common than adenocarcinoma or leiomyomatous tumors. ALs are usually seen in cats over 5 years of age (modal age about 10 years), whereas multicentric cases have a wider age range, being seen in cats from 1 to 18 years old. There is no consistently reported breed or sex predisposition. Cats are seldom leukemic or hypercalcemic.[1] The sites of AL, in decreasing order of frequency, are the jejunum, ileocecocolic junction, duodenum, colon, and stomach.[2] Multiple tumors can affect any combination of these sites. All forms of the tumor may be seen, but intramural fusiform tumor is the most common pattern in the intestines.[3] When ML affects the gut, any of the tumor patterns may be seen, but a diffuse lesion is the most common. Diffuse thickening of the intestine in a cat with a localized tumor may indicate a coexistent lymphoplasmacytic enteritis rather than a diffuse lymphoma.[1] In AL the tumor is usually of the B cell type, and is first seen in the germinal centers of the gut, MALT, and drainage lymph nodes, but this origin is quickly obliterated by local invasive growth. In contrast, the primary site of ML is the paracortical or thymic dependent areas of the lymph node, and the tumor is of T cell type. The B cells are usually polyclonal because FeLV transforms a multipotent precursor cell, but monoclonal gammopathy with Bence-Jones protein in the urine has been recorded.[4] In the late stages of ML, there are macroscopic lesions in many sites, and in addition, histological examination usually reveals that most organs contain neoplastic lymphocytes. By the time AL is diagnosed, tumor nodules may also be present in the spleen, liver, kidney, abdominal serosal surfaces, many abdominal lymph nodes, and even sternal nodes, making distinction between AL and ML difficult.

At least half of the cases of AL are FeLV negative, as are many of the MLs in older cats. This may mean that the virus is integrated without replication or, alternatively, that there are other etiological agents operating. Feline immunodeficiency virus infection (FIV) may reactivate nonexpressed latent FeLV infection, or FIV may be oncogenic.[5] FIV may induce a large pool of proliferating B cells from which malignant cells emerge. Certainly AL can develop in cats with no exposure to FeLV.[6]

Dogs

AL is less common than the multicentric form of the disease, but it is the most frequent form of lymphoma to affect the intestinal tract. According to most reports, carcinoma occurs more often than AL.[7] There is a wide age range, from puppies upward, but most cases are in middle-aged dogs.[7,8] There is no consistent breed predisposition,

but there may be breeds with a high incidence of lymphocytic-plasmacytic enteritis, where mutations in reactive lymphocytes can result in the formation of a tumor clone.[9] The most common site for a single focal tumor is the small intestine, followed by the stomach and then the large intestine.[10] Multifocal tumors, which are less common than single tumors, may involve various combinations of different sites, for example, stomach and small intestine or stomach and rectum. Usually the earliest lesions are seen in the submucosa and are considered to be of B cell origin; however, epitheliotropic T cell types have been reported.[9,10]

Horses

Lymphoreticular tumors are moderately common, and ML is more common than AL. Only a few cases of the multicentric tumor have lesions in the gastrointestinal tract. Tumors of the gut associated lymphoid tissue are usually seen in horses over 5 years old, but all ages can be affected, and a case has been recorded in a newborn foal in which virus-like particles were recorded. There is no breed or sex predisposition. The lesions appear as a nodular mass, as a diffuse thickening of the wall, or as a combination of the two patterns.[11] Sites that contain lymphoma, in decreasing order of frequency, are small intestine, colon, stomach, and rectum.[11,12] Spread to other sites may occur late in the disease; these sites include liver, kidney, spleen, other lymph nodes, and heart. The observation that the tumor arises in Peyers patches and is composed of centrocytes in a nodular pattern, sometimes with plasmacytoid differentiation, suggests these tumors are of B cell origin.[11] Leukemia is rarely seen, but tumor cells can be found in the ascitic fluid because the tumor has spread transmurally to form serosal nodules. It is difficult to distinguish lymphoma from granulomatous enteritis via clinical, gross, or even histological features because some lymphomas have many epithelioid and giant cells.[11] Grossly, these two diseases may be indistinguishable. Recurrent colic, diarrhea, malabsorption, and weight loss result from colonic and small intestinal tumors.[13]

Cattle

Bovine ML is characterized by widespread but not always bilaterally symetrical enlargement of lymph nodes and tumor nodules in other organs. Multicentric disease is more common than the AL. The pyloric region of the abomasum is the favored site; tumors in the forestomachs and intestines are less common either alone or in combination with abomasal lymphoma.[14] Sometimes only the abomasum is involved in a solitary or atypical lymphoid tumor.[15] Sporadic cases of solitary alimentary and juvenile ML (under 1 year old) are usually composed of null cells. Adult multicentric disease (animals over 3 years old) may be seen as sporadic cases in a herd or as multiple cases designated *enzootic bovine leukemia*. The lymphocytes in sporadic cases are null cells, but in the enzootic cases they are B cells. Enzootic bovine leukemia is associated with the bovine leukemia virus, but no antibody to the virus can be detected by ELISA, and no viral nucleic acids are recovered by polymerase chain reaction in the sporadic form of the disease.[16]

Sheep

The intestinal tract of sheep is involved in about one-third of ML cases. Localized AL cases are seen less often than ML, and in AL although there is no peripheral lymphadenopathy, other organs in the abdomen and thorax may be affected.[17] MLs are mainly T cell in type, but ALs are mainly of B cell type.[18] The Peyers patches of the jejunum and ileum are more often the site of the tumor than the rumen, reticulum, or abomasum. In multiple incidence flocks, a retrovirus is believed to be involved, and bovine leukemia virus can be transmitted to sheep either iatrogenically or experimentally. The cause is unknown in flocks where only sporadic cases are seen. All ages of animals may be affected, but it is most common in adult sheep (over 2 years old) and therefore is mainly seen in ewes.

Pigs

ML is more common than primary AL, which occurs as multiple plaques or annular fusiform thickenings of the stomach or intestine, either alone or in combination with involvement of the drainage lymph nodes.[19] Another alimentary pattern is of a single ileal nodule with spread to the drainage lymph node and to the serosa of abdominal organs.[20] This form arises in large noncleaved B cells of the germinal centers and is monoclonal for IgM.[20] Localized involvement of the abdominal lymphoid tissue but with few if any intestinal tract lesions occurs in two forms: (1) massive enlargement of gastric and mesenteric lymph nodes with late spread to all organs, sometimes including the gut, and (2) enlargement of the para-aortic and iliac lymph nodes, which may spread to other abdominal organs but not the intestinal tract. Most pigs are slaughtered under 1 year of age, and most cases of lymphoma are recorded in 6-month-old animals, but a few cases are seen in sows. The etiology of lymphoma on farms with sporadic cases is unknown, but in some multiple incidence herds the disease is associated with an autosomal recessive gene.[21]

REFERENCES

1. Mahony, O.M., Moore, A.S., et al. (1995) Alimentary lymphoma in cats: 28 cases (1988–1993) *J Amer Vet Med Assoc* 207:1593–1598.
2. Mackey, L.J., and Jarrett, W.F.H. (1972) Pathogenesis of lymphoid neoplasia in cats and its relationship to immunologic cell pathways. 1. Morphologic Aspects. *J Natl Cancer Inst* 49: 853–865.
3. Head, K.W., and Else, R.W. (1981) Neoplasia and allied conditions of the canine and feline intestine. *Vet Ann* 21:190–208.
4. Rosenberg, M.P., Hohenhaus, A.E., and Matus, R.E. (1991) Monoclonal gammopathy and lymphoma in a cat infected with feline immunodeficiency virus. *J Amer Anim Hosp Assoc* 27:335–337.
5. Callanan, J.J., McCandlish, I.A.P., et al. (1992) Lymphosarcoma in experimentally induced feline immunodeficiency virus infection. *Vet Rec* 130:293–295.
6. Jarrett, O., Edney, A.T.B., Toth, S., and Hay, D. (1984) Feline

leukaemia virus-free lymphosarcoma in a specific pathogen free cat. *Vet Rec* 115:249–250.
7. Patnaik, A.K., Hurvits, A.I., and Johnson, G.F. (1977) Canine gastrointestinal neoplasms. *Vet Pathol* 14:547–555.
8. Cuoto, C.G., Rutgers, H.C., Scherding, R.G., and Rojko, J. (1989) Gastrointestinal lymphoma in 20 dogs. A retrospective study. *J Vet Intern Med* 3:73–78.
9. French, R.A., Seitz, S.E., and Valli, V.E.O. (1996) Primary epitheliotropic alimentary T-cell lymphoma with hepatic involvement in a dog. *Vet Pathol* 33:349–352.
10. Steinberg, H., Dubielzig, R.R., et al. (1995) Primary gastrointestinal lymphosarcoma with epitheliotropism in three shar-pei and one boxer dog. *Vet Pathol* 32:423–426.
11. Platt, H. (1987) Alimentary lymphomas in the horse. *J Comp Pathol* 97:1–10.
12. Dabareiner, R.M., Sullins, K.E., and Goodrich, L.R. (1996) Large colon resection for treatment of lymphosarcoma in two horses. *J Amer Vet Med Assoc* 208:895–897.
13. Roberts, M.C., and Pinsent, P.J.N. (1975) Malabsorption in the horse associated with alimentary lymphosarcoma. *Equine Vet J* 7:166–172.
14. Bertone, A.L., Roth, L., and O'Krepky, J. (1985) Forestomach neoplasia in cattle: A Report of eight Cases. *Comp Cont Educ* 7:585–590.
15. Bertone, A.L. (1990) Neoplasms of the bovine gastrointestinal tract. *Vet Clin N Amer Food Anim Pract* 6:515–524.
16. Klinteval, K., Berg, A., et al. (1993) Differentiation between enzootic and sporadic bovine leukosis by use of serological and virological methods. *Vet Rec* 133:272.
17. Head, K.W. (1990) Tumors in sheep. *Practice* 12:68–80.
18. Dixon, R.J., Moriarty, K.M., and Johnstone, A.C. (1984) An immunological classification of ovine lymphomas. *J Comp Pathol* 94:107–113.
19. Marcato, P.S. (1987) Swine lymphoid and myeloid neoplasms in Italy. *Vet Res Comm* 11:325–337.
20. Tanimoto, T., Minami, A., Yano, S., and Ohtsuki, Y. (1994) Ileal lymphoma in swine. *Vet Pathol* 31:629–636.
21. Head, K.W., Campbell, J.G., et al. (1974) Hereditary lymphosarcoma in a herd of pigs. *Vet Rec* 95:523–527.

Plasma Cell Tumors

Primary extramedullary plasma cell tumors (EMPT) of the intestinal tract are seen occasionally in dogs and less commonly in cats. They are one type of round cell tumor, and when they are undifferentiated, it may be difficult to distinguish them from other round cell tumors, especially from lymphoma.[1] Prior to the use of immunohistochemistry and other techniques, they were incorrectly categorized as reticulum cell sarcomas, poorly differentiated sarcomas, lymphomas, or various other tumors.[1] EMPTs are differentiated from multiple myelomas, which may have extramedullary tumor foci but are characterized by bone and bone marrow involvement. All reported cases of EMPT have been in animals over 3 years old, but there are too few cases to establish age, breed, or sex distribution patterns. The few cases that have been seen in the stomach and ileum macroscopically resembled lymphoma. Most cases occur in the colon and rectum, where grossly they are in the form of nodules up to 4 cm in size; coexistent cutaneous plasmacytoma was present in one case.

Histologically, EMPTs are composed of round to oval cells with varying degrees of differentiation from plasmablasts to plasmacytes. The most differentiated cells have basophilic cytoplasm with indistinct cell borders, a perinuclear Golgi apparatus and condensed nuclei, central or eccentric, some of which may have a "clockface" pattern. Sometimes the cytoplasm is eosinophilic and granular, and occasional intracytoplasmic aggregates of immunoglobulin are seen (Russel bodies). Binucleate and multinucleate cells are observed, and when the latter are associated with amyloid they are thought to be reacting to the amyloid and not processing it.[2] A fine stroma supports the cells, sometimes forming packets reminiscent of a carcinoid, and although argentaffin staining may be positive, argyrophil staining is negative, and no neurosecretory substance can be demonstrated.[3] Mast cell tumors are eliminated on the basis of toluidine blue and Giemsa stains, and the cytoplasm of the more differentiated cells stain with methyl-green pyronin.[5] Ultrastructural studies demonstrate large profiles of rough endoplasmic reticulum.[1,4] Submucosal, perivascular, and intracellular amyloid may be demonstrated with thioflavin T or Congo red stains,[5] and it is of light chain origin.[2] Immunohistochemistry indicates the tumor cells are monoclonal for IgG, IgM, or IgA and for either lamda or kappa light chain; IgG is the immunoglobulin most commonly expressed.[6] Monoclonal gammopathies are infrequent,[3] and if present, the serum concentrations will return to normal ranges after removal of the tumor.[5] Urinary Bence-Jones protein has not been found in these solitary intestinal tumors. They are circumscribed but not encapsulated, only have a moderate number of cells in mitosis, and are of low grade malignancy. Metastases to the drainage lymph node and even to the spleen have been reported in a few cases; bone marrow was examined in these cases, and no tumor was found.[3,5,6] One year after excision of a rectal tumor, necropsy revealed tumor in the bone marrow, liver, spleen, and some lymph nodes.[4] Chemotherapy after surgery is recommended, and staging of EMPT into primary site alone, primary site and drainage lymph node, and widespread metastasis (but not involving bone marrow) has been proposed.[5]

Mast Cell Tumors

Mast cell tumors involving the intestinal tract have been reported most often in the cat, but occasional cases have been seen in cattle and dogs.[7,11] In all these species, mast cell tumors are much less common than lymphoma or adenocarcinoma. They present diagnostic problems for several reasons: cytoplasmic granules may not stain because either the cells are anaplastic or they have degranulated; there is evidence that mucosal mast cells are not the same as mesenchymal mast cells and require special fixation to enhance metachromasia; because mast cells release eosinophil chemotactic substance, some degranulated mast cell tumors may have more eosinophils than mast cells and may be mistakenly diagnosed as examples of the hypereosinophilic complex of diseases.[8,9] Some "mast cell tumors" may actually be large granular lymphomas (glob-

ular leukocyte tumors), and unless sections are stained with PTAH the diagnosis is missed.

All cases have been in adult animals; in the cat the mean age is 13 years. There is no breed or sex predisposition. Intestinal mast cell tumors may be diffuse, solitary, or multiple; nodular, plaque-like or fusiform; intraluminal or intramural; confined to the intestinal tract or part of a multicentric disease. In most cases there are no circulating mast cells in the blood. There are usually eosinophils in the tumor, but only in a few cases is there a peripheral blood eosinophilia.[9]

The site of the tumor in cats is usually in the distal small intestine and colon.[7,10] In primary intestinal mast cell tumor, only the drainage lymph nodes are enlarged, unlike in cases in which there is gut involvement as part of a multicentric mast cell tumor. The size of the tumor in the drainage lymph nodes may be greater than the tumor in the gut,[8,9] and in some cases, particularly in the dog, only the mesenteric lymph node is affected by the tumor. In cattle the lesions resemble lymphoma of the abomasum, forestomachs, and duodenum.[11,12]

On histological examination, the localized lesions are well demarcated but not encapsulated. The main mass of the tumor is in the submucosa and muscle coat, but the mucosa may eventually be involved. In most cases the cells are supported by a fine stroma, and they may be grouped in packets resembling a carcinoid.[7] Mitoses are few. The mast cells have a finely granulated cytoplasm with indistinct borders when stained with H&E. The granules are metachromatic with acid toluidine blue (pH 2.5), red with aldehyde fuschin, and PAS positive, and in cats Bismark brown is considered a reliable stain.[7] Touch imprints stained with Wright-Giemsa usually reveal cytoplasmic granules, but Diff Quik stained mast cell tumors are sometimes negative, especially in cats.

Surgical removal of the tumor is sometimes feasible, but chemotherapy seldom produces true remission. The etiology of mass cell tumors is unknown; antibody to bovine leukemia virus has been reported in some cases of bovine mast cell tumors, but not in others.[12]

Tumors of Globule Leukocytes

Globule leukocytes are round cells of uncertain histogenesis that are found between intestinal epithelial cells. Some investigators suggest that they are transformed mast cells and others that they are of lymphoid origin.

Tumors of globule leukocytes are rare and have only been described in cats.[13-15] They are located most frequently in the ileum and may extend into the mesentery.[13] The tumor cells are round, uniform, and have fewer and larger eosinophilic granules than mast cells when stained with H&E (8–30 in number). The granules are indistinct with H&E and do not stain with alcian blue, Giemsa, or PAS, but they are brown or black with PTAH. The nonlobulated nuclei are round to pleomorphic, often eccentric, and have dense chromatin. There are few, if any, mitoses. Mesenteric lymph nodes may contain tumor cells, and metastases to the thymus, tracheobronchial lymph nodes, and liver have been described. Incomplete removal was followed by recurrence in 13.5 months despite chemotherapy.[14]

One report compared "granulated round cell tumors" in five cats with two "globular leukocyte tumors," one large granular lymphoma, one intestinal mass cell tumor, and samples of normal feline intestine.[15] The authors could detect no significant differences in the morphology, histochemistry, immunohistochemistry, or transmission electron microscopy among the granulated tumors, globular leukocyte tumors, and the large granular lymphoma and concluded that these tumors probably had a common cellular origin. The distribution of tumors in the five cases of "granulated cell tumors" was also compatible with lymphoma.

REFERENCES

1. Rakich, P.M., Latimer, K.S., et al. (1989) Mucocutaneous plasmacytomas in dogs: 75 cases (1980–1987). *J Amer Vet Med Assoc* 194:803–810.

2. Rowland, P.H., and Linke, R.P. (1994) Immunohistochemical characterization of lambda light-chain-derived amyloid in one feline and five canine plasma cell tumors. *Vet Pathol* 31:390–393.

3. Jackson, M.W., Helfand, S.C., et al. (1994) Primary IgG secreting plasma cell tumor in the gastrointestinal tract of a dog. *J Amer Vet Med Assoc* 204:404–406.

4. Lester, S.J., and Mesfin, G.M. (1980) A solitary plasmacytoma in a dog with progression to a disseminated myeloma. *Can Vet J* 21:284–286.

5. Trevor, P.B., Saunders, G.K., et al. (1993) Metastatic extramedullary plasmacytoma of the colon and rectum in a dog. *J Amer Vet Med Assoc* 203:406–409.

6. Kyriazidou, A., Brown, P.J., and Lucke, V.M. (1989) An immunohistochemical study of canine extramedullary plasma cell tumors. *J Comp Pathol* 100:259–266.

7. Alroy, J., Lear, L., DeLellis, R., and Weinstein, R.S. (1975) Distinctive intestinal mast cell neoplasms of domestic cats. *Lab Invest* 33:159–167.

8. Howl, J.H., and Petersen, M.G. (1995) Intestinal mast cell tumor in a cat: Presentation as eosinophilic enteritis. *J Amer Anim Hosp Assoc* 31:457–461.

9. Bartnowski, H.B., and Rosenthal, R.C. (1992) Gastrointestinal mast cell tumors and eosinophilia in two cats. *J Amer Anim Hosp Assoc* 28:271–275.

10. Garner, F.M., and Lingeman, C.H. (1970) Mast cell neoplasms of the domestic cat. *Vet Pathol* 7:517–530.

11. Groth, A.H., Bailey, W.S., and Walker, D.F. (1960) Bovine mastocytoma. *J Amer Vet Med Assoc* 137:241–244.

12. Shaw, D.P., Buoen, L.C., and Weiss, D.J. (1991) Multicentric mast cell tumor in a cow. *Vet Pathol* 28:450–452.

13. Finn, J.P., and Schwartz, L.W. (1972) A neoplasm of globule leukocytes in the intestine of a cat. *J Comp Pathol* 82:323–329.

14. McPherron, M.A., Chauvin, M.J., et al. (1994) Globule leukocyte tumor involving the small intestine in a cat. *J Amer Vet Med Assoc* 204:241–245.

15. McEntee, M.F., Horton, S., Blue, J., and Meuten, D.J. (1993) Granulated round cell tumor of cats. *Vet Pathol* 30:195–203.

Smooth Muscle Tumors

Gastrointestinal tumors that have a mesenchymal morphology and that stain immunohistochemically with markers for smooth muscle should be classified as leiomyoma or leiomyosarcoma. There are also mesenchymal tumors in the intestine and cecum of dogs, horses, nonhuman primates, and human beings that are morphologically similar to smooth muscle tumors but that are negative or have variable results for immunohistochemical markers of smooth muscle.[25,26] These tumors are classified as gastrointestinal stromal cell tumors (GIST). Although the lesions are similar histologically, they are a heterogenous group of tumors via immunohistochemistry. GIST are discussed in more detail in chapter 6.

Horses
Clinical Characteristics

These tumors are rare; only 15 cases of intestinal smooth muscle tumors were found in the literature.[1-7] The animals ranged in age from 2 to 22 years (average 11.6 years old), and no sex or breed predisposition was apparent. Three tumors were in the duodenum, eight in the small intestine, one in the large colon, two in the small colon, and one in the rectum. Most were associated with colic.

Gross and Histological Features

The tumors ranged in size from 3 cm long annular thickenings to a 10 cm diameter mass.[1,5] They may be pedunculated and protrude into the lumen of the gut or remain intramural.[3,6]

The separation of leiomyoma from leiomyosarcoma is difficult, and descriptions in the literature are not clear. An absence of mitotic figures, sharply delineated borders, and well-differentiated cells favor leiomyoma. Although reports have identified leiomyosarcoma based on numerous mitotic figures, no metastases were observed in any of the cases. In light of "intestinal stromal tumors," it is interesting that several authors mention fibrous and granulation tissue mixed with the smooth muscle tumor cells.[2,5,6] Despite limited invasive growth, the prognosis in these cases is good, providing the devitalization of the gut is not too advanced.[3,4,6]

Dogs
Incidence

One series found seven leiomyomas in 15,215 canine necropsies.[8] Another series reported 19 intestinal tumors, all of which were leiomyosarcomas.[9] Because of the difficulty in predicting the behavior of smooth muscle tumors and because there is no consistent difference in distribution along the intestinal tract between benign and malignant tumors, they are considered here as one group, showing a continuous spectrum of degrees of malignancy.

Clinical Characteristics

Reported cases have an age range from 4 to 16 years (average 10 years); one exception is a well-differentiated leiomyosarcoma in a 17-month-old dog.[14] Some series found intestinal leiomyosarcomas to be more common in females than males,[9,14] but others have not.[15-17] No breed appears to be predisposed, although some authors have noted that medium to large dogs are more often affected.[11,12,17] Most tumors caused clinical signs of gastrointestinal disease, but approximately one-third exhibited only subtle signs or were found during examination of the dog for other reasons.[10,12,17]

Clinical problems include anemia, melena, hypoglycemia, tenesmus, obstruction, weight loss, and perforation of the gut.[8,12,13,18] Peritonitis developed in up to half the cases,[11,16,19] and sometimes the tumor was found within an intussusception.[17,18] Diagnostic imaging by radiography and ultrasonography is useful because abdominal palpation is often unrewarding.[12]

Gross Morphology

The literature cited includes over 100 smooth muscle tumors, and the locations of the tumors were the duodenum (13 cases), jejunum (32 cases), ileum (5 cases), cecum (37 cases), colon (2 cases), and rectum (14 cases). All tumors were solitary, and they ranged in size from 1 to 17 cm in diameter. Small tumors that were encountered as incidental findings at necropsy clearly arose in the outer muscle coats and not in the muscularis mucosa. In the larger tumors that cause clinical signs, the site of origin is usually lost, and there may be ulceration of the mucosa and even sinus formation from the mucosa to the peritoneal cavity, leading to peritonitis. Most of the tumors in the small intestine occurred as an eccentric nodular mass, often on the antemesenteric side. Such nodules could either bulge extramurally or grow into the lumen of the bowel. A few cases, particularly in the duodenum and ileum, were fusiform and caused stenosis. In the rectoanal region, the tumors were usually plaque-like.

Growth and Metastasis

The rate of growth, even of malignant tumors, seems to be slow, and the formation of metastases occurs late in the disease. Designation of a tumor as either leiomyoma or leiomyosarcoma is difficult. Reports in the literature describe a change in the diagnosis of leiomyoma to leiomyosarcoma when histological examination was repeated due to the development of multiple smooth muscle tumors 28 months after removal of a leiomyoma.[11]

Metastases to the mesenteric lymph node and/or liver are uncommon:[20] 1 of 11 leiomyosarcomas had spread to the mesenteric lymph nodes and/or liver; 2 of 6 tumors spread to the mesenteric lymph node;[10] in 11 cases, 1 tumor spread to the liver and 1 to the lung.[19] Tumors in the rectoanal region spread to the iliac lymph node, but one dog had metastases in the sternal and bronchial lymph nodes, lung, pleura, heart, liver, and kidney.[16] Metastases have been detected up to 3 years after removal of the primary tumor.[11,19] Surgical resection is usually worth attempting,[13] and survival after surgery can be as long as 7 years (mean 10 months).[11,17,19]

Staging and Grading

TNM staging and grading has been used for intestinal smooth muscle tumors.[10] The tumor status was represented by T_0, for an occult tumor where only the metastases were identified; T_1, where tumor was not invading the serosa; T_2, where tumor was invading the serosa; and T_3, where tumor was invading neighboring structures; N_0 and M_0 indicated no metastases. Regional lymph node metastases were symbolized by N_1 and distant metastases by N_2 and M_1. Histological grades were given a score of 1 for least affected, 3 for most affected, and 2 for intermediate grade. The features graded were cellularity/necrosis, nuclear pleomorphism, and giant nuclei, and to the sum of these scores the mitotic index was added.

Other Species

Cats do not develop smooth muscle tumors as often as dogs. In one series, one leiomyosarcoma was found in 2494 feline accessions,[21] and in another one leiomyoma was found in 171 tumors and tumor-like lesions of the intestine collected over a 35 year period.[22] In Edinburgh, 67 feline intestinal tumors were collected over a period of 30 years, and 2 of these were of smooth muscle origin.[23] The gross and microscopic features are similar to the more common canine tumors.

Cases of bovine intestinal leiomyoma are rare: a 20 cm diameter leiomyoma in the spiral colon of a 10-year-old cow was associated with ruminal stasis and melena[24]; another was reported in the rectum of a cow. See chapter 6 for additional information.

REFERENCES

1. Haven, M.L., Rottman, J.B., and Bowman, K.F. (1991) Leiomyoma of the small colon in a horse. *Vet Surg* 20:320–322.
2. Kasper, C., and Doran, R. (1993) Duodenal leiomyoma associated with colic in a two year old horse. *J Amer Vet Med Assoc* 202: 769–770.
3. Livesey, M.A., Hulland, T.J., and Yovich, J.V. (1986) Colic in two horses associated with smooth muscle intestinal tumors. *Equine Vet J* 18:334–337.
4. Clem, M.F., deBowes, R.M., and Leipold, H.W. (1987) Rectal leiomyosarcoma in a horse. *J Amer Vet Med Assoc* 191:229–230.
5. Mair, T.S., Taylor, F.G.R., and Brown, P.J. (1990) Leiomyosarcoma of the duodenum in two horses. *J Comp Pathol* 102:119–123.
6. Mair, T.S., Davies, E.V., and Lucke, V.M. (1992) Small colon intussusception associated with an intraluminal leiomyoma in a pony. *Vet Rec* 130:403–404.
7. Collier, M.A., and Trent, A.M. (1983) Jejunal intussusception with leiomyoma in an aged horse. *J Amer Vet Med Assoc* 182:819–821.
8. Hayden, D.W., and Nielsen, S.W. (1973) Canine alimentary neoplasia. *Zbl Vet Med* 20A:1–22.
9. Patnaik, A.K., Hurvitz, A.I., and Johnson, G.F. (1977) Canine Gastrointestinal Neoplasms. *Vet Pathol* 14:547–555.
10. Bruecker, K.A., and Withrow, S.J. (1988) Intestinal leiomyosarcomas in six dogs. *J Amer Anim Hosp Assoc* 24:281–284.
11. Gibbons, G.C., and Murtaugh, R.J. (1989) Cecal smooth muscle

neoplasia in the dog: Report of 11 cases and literature review. *J Amer Anim Hosp Assoc* 25:191–197.

12. McPherron, M.A., Withrow, S.J., et al. (1992) Colorectal leiomyomas in seven dogs. *J Amer Anim Hosp Assoc* 28:43–46.

13. Davies, J.V., and Read, H.M. (1990) Sagittal pubic osteotomy in the investigation and treatment of intrapelvic neoplasia in the dog. *J Small Anim Pract* 31:123–130.

14. Laratta, L.J., Center, S.A., et al. (1983) Leiomyosarcoma in the duodenum of a dog. *J Amer Vet Med Assoc* 183:1096–1097.

15. Andreasen, C.B., and Mahaffey, E.A. (1987) Immunohistochemical demonstration of desmin in canine smooth muscle tumors. *Vet Pathol* 24:211–215.

16. Head, K.W., and Else, R.W. (1981) Neoplasia and allied conditions of the canine and feline intestine. *Vet Ann* 21:190–208.

17. Myers, N.C., and Penninck, D.G. (1994) Ultrasonographic diagnosis of gastrointestinal smooth muscle tumors in the dog. *Vet Radiol Ultrasound* 35:391–397.

18. Comer, K.M. (1990) Anemia as a feature of primary gastrointestinal neoplasia. *Comp Cont Educ Pract Vet* 12:13–19.

19. Kapatki, A.S., Mullen, H.S., et al. (1992) Leiomyosarcoma in dogs: 44 cases (1983–1988). *J Amer Vet Med Assoc* 201:1077–1079.

20. Chen, H.H.C., Parris, L.S., and Parris, R.G. (1984) Duodenal leiomyosarcoma with multiple hepatic metastases in a dog. *J Amer Vet Med Assoc* 184:1506.

21. Turk, M.A.M., Gallina, A.M., and Russell, T.S. (1981) Nonhematopoietic gastrointestinal neoplasia in cats: A retrospective study of 44 cases. *Vet Pathol* 18:614–620.

22. Carpenter, J.L., Andrews, L.K., and Holzworth, J. (1987) Tumor and tumor-like lesions. In Holzworth, J. (ed.), *Diseases of the Cat: Medicine and Surgery*, Vol. 1. W.B. Saunders Coy, Philadelphia, pp. 406–596.

23. Head, K.W., and Else, R.W. (1981) Neoplasia and allied conditions of the canine and feline intestine. *Vet Ann* 21:190–208.

24. Saidu, S.N.A., and Chineme, C.N. (1978) Intestinal leiomyoma in a cow. *Vet Rec* 104:495–496.

25. Del Piero, F., Summers, B.A., Credille, K.M., Cummings, J.F., and Mandelli, G. (1996) Gastrointestinal stromal tumors in *Equidae*. *Vet Pathol* 33:611.

26. Hafner, S., Harmon, B.G., and King, T. (2001) Gastrointestinal stromal tumors of the equine cecum. *Vet Pathol* 38:242–246.

TUMORS OF SEROSAL SURFACES

Prevalence

Primary tumors arising from the mesothelial cells lining the peritoneal cavity, mesothelioma, have been recorded in the abdominal cavity of cattle,[1,2] horses,[3,4] dogs,[5,6,7] and cats.[8,9] Primary tumors derived from the submesothelial fibrous tissue, muscle, fat, and lymphatic vessels are even less common but have been described in cattle, dogs, and cats. Mesothelioma must be differentiated from activated or reactive mesothelium and from carcinomatosis.

Histological and Growth Features

The flattened normal mesothelial cells react to inflammatory stimuli by becoming cuboidal or even columnar. The cytoplasm is then easily seen and may contain glycogen. The nuclei have an increased number of nucleolar organizer regions. The peritoneal lining may develop papillary outgrowths, but these papillae remain lined by a single layer of activated or reactive mesothelial cells. Electron microscopy reveals microvilli similar to those in normal mesothelium but there are fewer of them, and they are of variable length.[10] Sometimes activated cells are desquamated and become trapped in organizing inflammatory exudate giving rise to an appearance superficially resembling transcoelomic carcinoma metastases.

No single feature can be used to differentiate between activated and neoplastic mesothelium. Mesothelioma can be papillary epithelioid, or sarcomatoid, or most commonly biphasic in pattern. The epithelioid cells vary in size but are larger than reactive cells. The central nuclei are larger, hyperchromatic, pleomorphic, have nucleolar organizer regions, and some cells may be binucleate. Mitotic figures are rare even in metastatic tumors. The cells lining the papillae form several layers. Histochemistry and immunocytochemistry are not helpful in differentiating reactive from neoplastic mesothelium but can be used to recognize adenocarcinoma cells.[11] Mesothelioma are of low grade malignancy so there is limited invasive growth. The invasive tongues of tumor can produce pseudoacini that are recognizable because the cells are pleomorphic and there is no lumen. Metastases to drainage lymph nodes are rare and distant metastases very rare. It is not always possible to determine whether widespread involvement of the peritoneal cavity and tunica vaginalis is the result of secondary spread or of multicentric origin.

To eliminate a diagnosis of transcoelomic carcinoma metastasis, a careful examination of the genitalia and intestines for small malignant primary tumors must be undertaken. It is often possible to show that the tumor emboli are in subserosal lymphatic vessels unlike mesotheliomatous foci. Adenocarcinoma acini have uniform cells with basal nuclei set around an acinus. The cells may contain mucin but little or no glycogen.[1] Ultrastructurally, the cells have short fat microvilli on the apical pole whereas in mesothelioma, the long thin villi are present on all surfaces.[10,12,13]

Ascitic fluid arising from a variety of causes, including mesothelioma, often contains many desquamated normal and activated mesothelial cells as well as macrophages.[14] In smears or in sections of cell pellets, activated cells are larger than normal, slightly anisocytotic with deep blue cytoplasm, and are found both singly and in clumps of up to 10–80 cells. They often appear as flat sheets with distinct cell to cell contact and no nuclear crowding. The large nuclei are central, round, and uniform with few small nucleoli; some cells are binucleate. In contrast, mesothelioma cells are up to 10 times the size of normal cells. The long slender microvilli, which have a length to diameter ratio of 12 to 1, may be seen in light microscopy. In addition to single cells, clumps of up to 50 cells and even fragments of papillae, but not acini, are found. Anisocytosis and anisokaryosis are more marked than in activated cells, the nucleoli are larger, and there are more multinucleate cells with up to four nuclei.

REFERENCES

1. Stober, M., Tammen, F.C., Veltmann, P., Stockhofe-Zurwieden, N., and Pohlenz, J. (1990) Mesothelioma in cattle: Clinical, post-mortem, and environmental findings. *Wien. Tierarzt. Monatsh.* 77:78–93.
2. Wolfe, D.F., Casson, R.L., Hudson, R.S., Boosinger, T.R., Mysinger, P.W., Pow, T.A., Clayton, M.S., and Angel, K.I. (1991) Mesothelioma in cattle: Eight cases (1970–1988). *J. Amer. Vet. Med. Assoc.* 199:486–491.
3. Colbourne, C.M., Bolton, J.R., Mills, J.N., Whitaker, D., Yovich, J.V., and Howell, J.Mc.M. (1992) Mesothelioma in horses. *Aust. Vet. J.* 69:275–278.
4. Hinrichs, U., Brugmann, M., Harps, O., and Wohlstein, P. (1997) Malignant biphasic peritoneal mesothelioma in a horse. *Eur. J. Vet. Pathol.* 3:95–97.
5. Thrall, D.E., and Goldschmidt, M.H. (1978) Mesothelioma in the dog: Six case reports. *J. Amer. Vet. Radiol. Soc.* 19:107–115.
6. Dubielzig, R.R. (1979) Sclerosing mesothelioma in five dogs. *J. Amer. Anim. Hosp. Asoc.* 15:745–748.
7. Harbison, M.L., and Godleski, J.J. (1983) Malignant mesothelioma in urban dogs. *Vet. Pathol.* 20:531–540.
8. Tilley, L.P., Owens, J.M., Wilkins, R.J., and Patnaik, A.K. (1975) Pericardial mesothelioma with effusion in a cat. *J. Amer. Anim. Hosp. Assoc.* 11:60–65.
9. Umphlet, R.C., and Bertoy, R.W. (1988) Abdominal mesothelioma in a cat. *Mod. Vet. Pract.* 69:71–73.
10. Trigo, F.J., Morrison, W.B., and Breeze, R.G. (1981) An ultrastructural study of canine mesothelioma. *J. Comp. Pathol.* 98:531–537.
11. Pizarro, M. Brandau, C., Sanchez, M.A., and Flores, J.M. (1992) Immunocytochemical identification of a bovine peritoneal mesothelioma. *J. Vet. Med.* 39:476–480.
12. Vitellozzi, G., Rueca, F., Mariotti, F., Porciello, F., Mandera, M.T., and Spaterna, A. (1988) Equine peritoneal mesothelioma: Clinical, anatomo-histopathological, and ultrastructural studies. *Eur. J. Vet. Pathol.* 4:29–36.
13. Hashimoto, N., Oda, T., and Kadota, K. (1989) An unltrastructural study of malignant mesotheliomas in two cows. *Jpn. J. Vet. Sci.* 51:327–336.
14. Van Ooijen, P.J. (1978) Exfoliative cytology in the diagnosis of diffuse mesothelioma in the dog. *Tijdschr. Diergeneesk.* 103:1116–1120.

TUMORS OF THE EXOCRINE PANCREAS

Tumors of the exocrine pancreas have been reported infrequently in carnivores and rarely in other domestic animals. It is common in older cats and dogs to observe multiple tumor-like nodules of hyperplasia (fig. 8.20A). Neoplasms of the exocrine pancreas are broadly divided into adenomas and carcinomas, but such a rigid division may be incorrect, and it may be more realistic to view some tumors as "transitional" or of "uncertain malignant potential," as described in human beings.[1]

Exocrine Adenoma

Incidence and Clinical Features

Exocrine adenomas are rare and are less common than their malignant counterparts. A progression of hyperplasia through adenoma to carcinoma has not been demonstrated. They have been found in canine and bovine pancreas.[2] These benign lesions are often small and may be confused with hyperplastic nodules on macroscopic examination. They cause no clinical or biochemical signs and are incidental lesions found at necropsy or during exploratory coeliotomy.

Gross and Histological Features

Tumors are small, singular, rarely more than 0.5 cm in diameter, and protrude slightly from the organal surface. They may be white or fawn and are usually clearly encapsulated. Occasionally they are cystic, but more often the nodules are solid and resemble hyperplastic foci (fig. 8.20B).

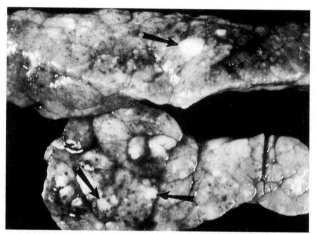

A

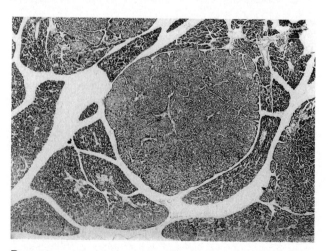

B

Fig. 8.20. **A.** Multiple foci of nodular hyperplasia (arrows) appear as small pale nodules on the surface of the pancreas in a dog. **B.** Single, discrete, lightly encapsulated pancreatic adenoma.

Adenomas are invariably surrounded by a thin fibrous capsule. They may compress adjacent normal acini and resemble benign hyperplastic nodules in this respect. They have tubular and acinar patterns supported by thin collagenous trabeculae.[16] Sometimes the cystic spaces are lined by tumor cells with papillary projections into the cystic lumen. This type of formation suggests a possible ductular origin, but this is not proven. Solid acini resemble benign nodular hyperplasia and consist of well-differentiated acinar epithelial cells with eosinophilic, granular cytoplasm. Zymogen granules are less obvious than in normal acinar cells. Nuclei are round and mitoses are rare.

It may be difficult to distinguish adenoma from nodular hyperplasia. Adenomas are solitary lesions, are rare, and are partially or totally encapsulated (see fig. 8.21). Nodular hyperplasia produces multiple macroscopic or microscopic foci, is common and not encapsulated, and compresses adjacent parenchyma less than adenoma. Immunostaining for cytokeratins is not helpful in distinguishing adenoma from other tumors or hyperplastic nodules. If needed, immunohistochemical staining with neuron specific enolase and chromogranin A is helpful in distinguishing islet cell tumors (positive reaction for both reagents with endocrine tumors).

Growth and Metastasis

Metastasis does not occur, but local compressive growth patterns may result in atrophy of adjacent acini. There is no good evidence that primary benign adenomas convert to carcinomas.

Exocrine Carcinoma

Incidence

This is the most common tumor of the exocrine pancreas. There are numerous reports in the dog[2-5,8,10] and fewer in the cat,[4,6,7] and it is rare in horses,[2,5,9] cattle,[2,5,10] and swine.[10] Older animals are more often affected, although dogs as young as 3 years of age have been recorded.[5,18] There are apparently no sex differences in the incidence of the tumor; however, in human beings there is a predominance in males.[1] Breed risk is not obvious; some figures indicate a higher risk for Airedale and boxer breeds.[5]

Clinical Characteristics

Common clinical signs are abdominal pain, vomiting, and weight loss. There is usually a palpable and painful anterior abdominal mass.[3,11] Jaundice and cholestasis are often features of well-established tumors, resulting from obstruction of the bile duct by the tumor and/or secondary liver disease.[12] Ascites may occur as a result of transcoelomic spread of neoplasia or as a consequence of compression of the portal vein or its major branches.[12,13] The corrosive effects of leakage of proteolytic enzymes from carcinomas of the pancreas may result in cystic change in the primary tumor[11] and necrotizing steatitis in the omental and peritoneal fat.[14]

Gross Morphology

In dogs these tumors produce a mass, often in the midportion of the pancreas, but in cats pancreatic carcinomas are more diffuse and can resemble chronic pancreatitis or nodular hyperplasia.[2,3] Some tumors are discrete and nodular (fig. 8.21), but more often they are poorly circumscribed irregular masses with variable consistency, are friable, and infiltrate adjacent normal pancreatic stroma. Areas of softening and necrosis may be apparent and focal or diffuse hemorrhagic zones are common, particularly in the cat.[7,15]

Individual nodules are white or fawn in color. It can be difficult to differentiate infiltrating neoplasia from normal pancreas. Calcification is sometimes a feature, with or without concurrent necrosis, and can be appreciated readily on gross sectioning as small irregular white calcified foci. Inflammation or necrosis of adjacent omental or mesenteric fat creates firm nodules (2–4 mm diameter), and it is important to differentiate this reaction from transcoelomic metastasis.[14]

Histological Features

Exocrine carcinomas have a tremendous range of differentiation: some tumors are well-differentiated tubular adenocarcinomas (fig. 8.21A,B,C) with acinar structures lined by irregular cuboidal or more differentiated columnar cells, or they may form more solid sheets of poorly differentiated cells that no longer resemble pancreatic acini.[3,7,15,16] Individual cells have eosinophilic cytoplasm that is often vacuolated, but zymogen granules (eosinophilic) are only seen in well-differentiated carcinomas. Nuclei are uniform, oval, with sparse chromatin and are basally sited in columnar cells lining acini. In poorly differentiated tumors, cell borders are not easily discerned, and nuclei are crowded together and tend to be more irregular in shape and variable in size, with variable amounts of coarse chromatin. Nuclear to cytoplasmic ratio depends on the relative degree of differentiation of the tumors. Well-differentiated carcinomas with acinar formations usually have uniform cells with regular polarity and low nuclear to cytoplasmic ratio. Mitotic index reflects the level of differentiation: poorly differentiated tumors have more numerous mitoses per high power microscopic field (e.g., 5–6 mitoses per 400×) than well-differentiated tubular adenocarcinomas (2–3 mitoses per 400× field). Mitoses are numerous in solid type, poorly differentiated carcinomas.

Supporting stroma is usually dense in poorly differentiated tumors, with a resultant scirrhous reaction (fig. 8.21D). In tubular adenocarcinomas the tubules are supported by a thin but regular fine collagenous trabecular structure. Large tumors often have relatively more stromal components, but encapsulation of the whole tumor is uncommon. Hemorrhage and necrosis often induces an inflammatory reaction comprising moderate numbers of neutrophils, macrophages, and lymphocytes. Focal aggregates of lymphocytes, usually of T cell origin, are some-

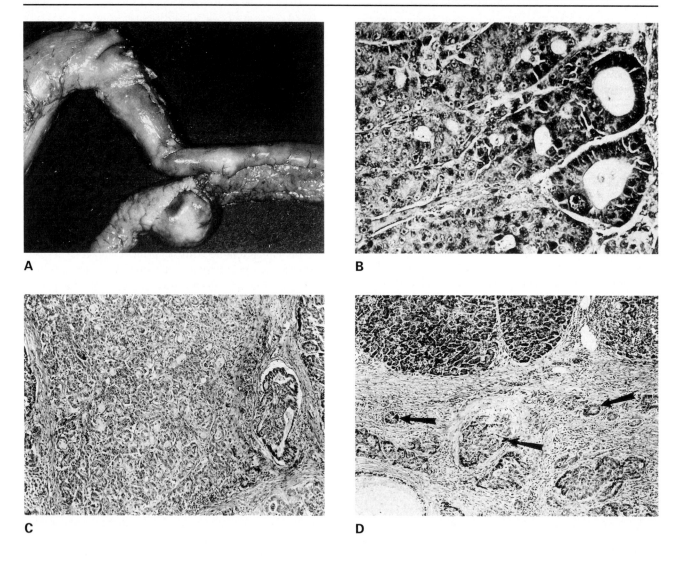

Fig. 8.21. **A.** Exocrine carcinoma in the middle portion of the pancreas in a cat. **B.** Adenocarcinoma of pancreas with acinar and tubular differentiation merging from poorly differentiated region. (Courtesy Dr. J. Alroy, *Amer J Path*) **C.** Pancreatic carcinoma forming acini and tubules with minimal desmoplasia. **D.** Exocrine pancreatic carcinoma with packets of neoplastic foci (arrows) encased by scirrhous stroma. [With permission from reference 17.]

times seen. These foci are usually peripheral, but they may also occur in the neoplastic stroma.

Distinction between exocrine carcinomas and tumors of islet cell (endocrine) origin may be difficult in poorly differentiated carcinomas. If histopathology is indeterminant, immunohistological identification using antibodies to insulin, glucagon, or somatostatin can be useful in making the diagnosis. Metastases or transcoelomic spread of pancreatic carcinoma can be difficult to distinguish from other malignant carcinomas (e.g., gastrointestinal, renal, or ovarian carcinomas).

The histogenesis of exocrine carcinomas remains uncertain. A ductular origin is anticipated from the tubular architecture, but ultrastructural analysis indicates that acinar cells may be the originator cell type.[17]

Growth and Metastasis

Local destructive infiltration, widespread contiguous growth, and transcoelomic metastasis are hallmarks of exocrine pancreatic carcinoma. In addition, widespread metastases to distant sites are common and are often established by the time of clinical presentation.[3,16] Local infiltrative growth may destroy the common bile duct, causing icterus and marked increases in serum hepatic enzymes.[14] The most frequent sites for metastasis are the peritoneum, mesentery, and adjacent gastrointestinal organs, followed by lungs and liver and, less frequently, spleen, kidney, and diaphragm.[2-4,7,15] The combination of rapid local growth, early metastasis, and proteolytic side effects makes pancreatic exocrine carcinomas aggressive and painful neoplasms.[1,10]

Nonepithelial Tumors

Primary nonepithelial tumors that are not of pancreatic acinar origin have been reported infrequently.[16,18] They are usually mesenchymal and include fibromas, fibrosarcomas, lymphomas, nerve sheath tumors, liposarcomas, and hemangiosarcomas. Hemangiosarcoma in the dog is usually part of a generalized aggressive metastatic or multifocal neoplasia with similar tumors in spleen, liver, and/or skeletal muscles.

Tumor-Like Lesions

Cystic changes may be associated with rapidly growing carcinomas, but true cysts are relatively well defined and obviously thin walled.[11] They may be solitary or multiple, are probably of ductular origin, and may be the result of congenital malformation. Alternatively, obstruction to ductular drainage in adult animals may create cysts.[13] A number of reports have cited pseudocyst development associated with pancreatitis in cats and dogs.[19,20]

Benign nodular hyperplasia is very commonly encountered in older dogs and cats as an incidental necropsy finding or at laparotomy and occurs in the pancreas of adult cattle. There are no associated clinical problems. In animals younger than 5 years of age, such nodular changes should be treated as indicative of inflammation or scarring rather than neoplasia or hyperplasia. Nodular hyperplasia is not generally regarded as a preneoplastic lesion.[1,16]

Hyperplasia may be manifested as solitary nodular lesions, but more commonly it produces multiple small nodules ranging from a few millimeters to a maximum of about 1 cm diameter. The nodules are often white or fawn and well circumscribed, and they may, if of the larger size, protrude slightly from the pancreatic surface (fig. 8.21A).

Microscopically, the lesions are not encapsulated and do not compress adjacent pancreatic tissue. The affected lobules are larger than adjacent nonaffected lobules and are composed of a mixture of larger or smaller than normal pancreatic acinar cells. There is increased intensity of staining of cells; the cytoplasm is more eosinophilic but may be vacuolated as well, and there is no cellular atypia. In some cases the pancreas has areas of atrophy or chronic pancreatitis.

Ductular hyperplasia is an uncommon lesion in the pancreas. The finding is usually histological but may accompany acinar hyperplasia as described above. In these ducts there is variable hyperplasia of ductular epithelium that can form epithelial folds and obstructions. The latter in turn can lead to cystic ductular dilatation.

REFERENCES

1. Klöppel, G., Solcia, E., et al. (1996) *Histological Typing of Tumors of the Exocrine Pancreas,* 2nd ed. WHO International Histological Classification of Tumors. Springer, Berlin.
2. Rowlatt, U. (1967) Spontaneous epithelial tumors of the pancreas of mammals. *Brit J Cancer* 21:82–107.
3. Anderson, N.V., and Johnson, K.H. (1967) Pancreatic carcinoma in the dog. *J Amer Vet Med Assoc* 150:286–295.
4. Hänichen, T., and Minkus, G. (1990) Retrospective study of diseases of the exocrine pancrease in dogs and cats. *Tierärztliche-Umschau* 45:363–368.
5. Priester, W.A. (1974) Data from eleven United States and Canadian Colleges of Veterinary Medicine on pancreatic carcinoma in domestic animals. *Cancer Res* 34:1372–1375.
6. Banner, B.F., Alroy, J., and Kipnis, R.M. (1979) Acinar cell carcinoma of the pancreas in a cat. *Vet Pathol* 16:543–547.
7. Dill-Macky, E. (1993) Pancreatic diseases of cats. *Comp Cont Educ Pract Vet* 15:589–598.
8. Rabanal, R., et al. (1992) Immunocytochemical detection of amylase activity in carcinoma of the exocrine pancreas of the dog. *Res Vet Sci* 52:217–223.
9. Carrick, J.B., et al. (1992) Hematuria and weight loss in a mare with pancreatic adenocarcinoma. *Cornell Vet* 82:91–97.
10. Monlux, A.W., et al. (1956) A survey of tumors occurring in cattle, sheep and swine. *Amer J Vet Res* 17:646–677.
11. Edwards, D.F., et al. (1990) Pancreatic masses in seven dogs following acute pancreatitis. *J Amer Anim Hosp Assoc* 26:189–198.
12. Pastor, J., et al. (1997) Sclerosing adenocarcinoma of the extrahepatic bile duct in a cat. *Vet Rec* 140:367–368.
13. King, J.M. (1995) Obstructive perilobular fibrosis of the pancreas. *Vet Med* 90:533.
14. Brown, P.J., et al. (1994) Multifocal necrotizing steatitis associated with pancreatic carcinoma in three dogs. *J Small Anim Pract* 35:129–132.
15. Munster, M., and Reusch, C. (1988) Tumors of the exocrine pancreas in the cat. *Tierärztliche-Praxis,* 16:317–320.
16. Kircher, C.H., and Nielsen, S.W. (1976) Tumors of the pancreas. *Bull WHO* 53:195–202.
17. Banner, B.F., Alroy, J., et al. (1978) An ultrastructural study of acinic cell carcinomas of the canine pancreas. *Amer J Pathol* 93:165–182.
18. Cotchin, E. (1975) Spontaneous tumors in young animals. *Proc Roy Soc Med* 68:653–655.
19. Hines, B.L., et al. (1996) Pancreatic pseudocyst associated with chronic-active necrotizing pancreatitis in a cat. *J Amer Anim Hosp Assoc* 32:147–152.
20. Wolfsheimer, K.J. (1991) Pancreatic pseudocyst in a dog with chronic pancreatitis. *Canine Pract* 16:6–9.

9 Tumors of the Liver and Gall Bladder

J. M. Cullen and J. A. Popp

EPITHELIAL NEOPLASMS OF THE LIVER

Nodular Hyperplasia

Incidence

Nodular hyperplasia of the liver occurs quite frequently in older dogs, has been reported in swine, and is rare in other domestic species.[1-4] In dogs, age is the major determinant for the occurrence of nodular hyperplasia since there is no sex or breed predisposition. Nodular hyperplasia can be found in dogs by the time they are 6 to 8 years old, and 70 to 100 percent of dogs have nodular hyperplasia by 14 years of age.[1,2,5] The incidence in swine has been reported to be 4 per 100,000 animals, but this is probably a low estimate since the data is derived from a slaughterhouse study conducted in young pigs.[3] There is no data to suggest nodular hyperplasia is a preneoplastic lesion in domestic animals or that it is associated with hepatic regeneration.

Clinical Characteristics

No clinical signs or adverse effects on liver function have been documented as a result of nodular hyperplasia. Although the lesions are expansile and compress adjacent parenchyma, the extent of liver involvement is insufficent to affect liver function. Consequently, nodular hyperplasia of the liver is most often found as an incidental lesion during postmortem examinations. The cytologic appearance of hepatocytes obtained by fine needle aspirates from areas of nodular hyperplasia is virtually identical to that of normal hepatocytes.[6] Hepatocytes from areas of nodular hyperplasia may contain abundant vacuoles of glycogen or lipid, but this is not distinctive since such vacuoles can be found in normal hepatocytes. Nodular hyperplasia presents a diagnostic challenge for the ultrasonographer; it is difficult to distinguish these lesions from primary hepatic malignancies and from metastatic masses.[7]

Gross Morphology

Nodular hyperplasia of the liver is characterized by distinct masses that are randomly distributed throughout the lobes of the liver.[1,2,8] In most circumstances, the liver is otherwise normal. Often the nodules bulge from the capsular surface of the liver. The nodules on the capsular surface tend to blend smoothly with the adjacent liver tissue. Other nodules may be completely within the liver parenchyma. They are usually spherical to ovoid and well circumscribed, but without a fibrous capsule (fig. 9.1). There is no increase in fibrosis within the nodules, and their consistency is usually softer than normal parenchyma. On the cut surface the nodules are usually well demarcated from the normal parenchyma. Nodules are usually multiple and may be too numerous to count. The size of nodules of hyperplasia ranges from 2 mm to 3 cm in diameter. They may be paler than normal hepatic parenchyma, darker than normal hepatic parenchyma, or difficult to detect because of their similarity to normal parenchyma. Some nodules are pale yellow to a pinkish tan due to a relative lack of blood and an increase in lipid or glycogen or a combination of both. Other nodules are dark red due to an accumulation of blood. Nodules of sev-

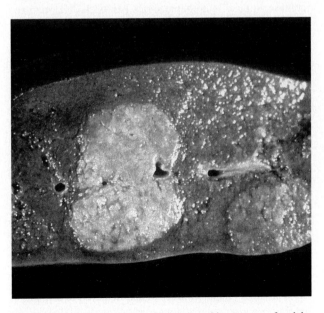

Fig. 9.1. Cut surface of a liver from a dog with two areas of nodular hyperplasia. Nodular hyperplasia is well circumscribed, but unencapsulated, and may bulge from the cut surface. The uninvolved liver is usually normal.

483

eral different appearances may be found in a single liver. During routine postmortem examination nodular hyperplasia may be underestimated, since the areas of nodular hyperplasia that have a color similar to the normal liver may only be apparent when liver slices are rinsed.

Since nodular hyperplasia is a symmetrical, expansile lesion, it cannot be distinguished from hepatocellular adenoma on the basis of gross pathological appearance alone.

Histological Features

There is considerable confusion and frequent overlap in the literature regarding the histological descriptions of nodular hyperplasia (common lesion in dogs) and hepatocellular adenomas (apparently rare in most species) in domestic species. The term nodular hyperplasia should be reserved for those nodular lesions that have an increased number of cells, yet retain normal liver architecture.[2,5] The characteristic histological appearance of nodular hyperplasia includes the retention of relatively normal lobular arrangement, but central veins and portal triads are more separated than normal.[1,2] The nodules are never encapsulated, although they often compress adjacent normal tissue, and there may be a relative increase in stroma of the unaffected liver. There is never an increase in fibrous tissue within the nodule, even when fibrosis is a primary feature of the surrounding liver. Hepatocytes are arranged into plates one to two cells wide. Within the nodule, vacuolization, when present, can be diffuse or focal. Vacuolated hepatocytes contain lipid or glycogen, alone or in combination. Generally, hepatocytes in nodules of hyperplasia are enlarged because of increased cytoplasm or because of extensive vacuolization.[1] Usually, nuclei have a normal appearance, but nucleoli are occasionally enlarged. An increase in binucleate hepatocytes has been described for nodular hyperplasia.[2] Mitotic figures are uncommon, but may be more frequent than those found in normal liver.

A variant of nodular hyperplasia has been termed the *micronodule* because the nodules are smaller than a lobule and are not visible to the unaided eye.[1] Micronodules, like nodular hyperplasia, expand and compress adjacent parenchyma and are composed of thickened plates of hepatocytes. An association with congestive heart failure has been noted in a large proportion of the cases. Therefore, micronodules may be generated in response to the atrophy or loss of centrolobular hepatocytes that can occur in right-sided heart failure.

Another type of nodular hepatic lesion results from hyperplasia of hepatocytes in damaged, usually fibrotic, livers. These *regenerative nodules* arise from viable hepatocytes in response to the destruction of hepatic parenchyma. This process can result from chronic exposure to various hepatotoxins. Often the insult is unknown, but the response of some dogs to anticonvulsant drugs such as phenobarbital or phenytoin serves as an example.[9,10] Regenerative nodules are unlikely to be related to nodular hyperplasia since regenerative nodules arise from the pro-

liferation of hepatocytes in response to hepatocyte loss and the incidence is not related to age. Regenerative nodules are readily distinguished from nodular hyperplasia since the process occurs in the presence of significant fibrosis and disruption of normal hepatic parenchymal architecture (fig. 9.2). Since these lesions result from the outgrowth of surviving hepatocytes, there is usually only a single portal tract within the regenerative nodules. Regenerative nodules can be difficult to distinguish from hepatocellular adenomas on the basis of histology alone, although there are a few distinguishing features. Regenerative nodules are composed of hepatic plates that are no more than two cells thick, and adenomas may have thicker hepatic plates. Hepatocellular adenomas are more likely to be solitary lesions and usually do not arise in a background of hepatic injury and fibrosis.

Etiology

The cause of nodular hyperplasia is unknown. Idiopathic, age related hyperplasia is not limited to the liver; it occurs in other glands such as the prostate, exocrine pancreas, and adrenal cortex. This type of hyperplasia has been speculatively attributed to a local dysregulation of growth factors.[11] Nodular hyperplasia in dogs does not seem to be induced by treatment with experimental carcinogens and does not appear to be a preneoplastic lesion.[2,12,13]

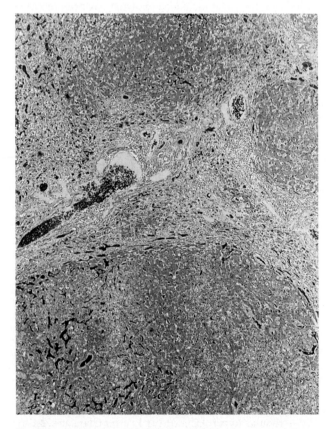

Fig. 9.2. Regenerative nodules in the liver. Fibrosis or condensed stromal elements that are retained following hepatocyte loss frequently surround these lesions.

Hepatocellular Adenoma

Incidence

Hepatocellular adenomas have been described in dogs,[12,14,15] cattle,[16,17] sheep,[16,18,19] cats,[20,21] and pigs.[16,22,23] In most of these reports, the diagnostic criteria that distinguish hepatocellular adenomas from nodular hyperplasia and malignant hepatocellular neoplasms have not been well characterized. It is clear that hepatocellular tumors are uncommon. Although benign hepatocellular neoplasms are described in most domestic animal species, they represent a minor proportion of neoplasms in each of the species. Based on several tumor surveys in dogs, the species that has been studied most extensively, benign hepatocellular neoplasms appear to occur less frequently, or are diagnosed less often, than their malignant counterpart.[15,24] In one study in which hepatocellular adenomas were diagnosed, hepatocellular carcinomas were more common (1 percent) than hepatocellular adenomas (0.4 percent).[15] There were no benign hepatocellular neoplasms reported in other surveys of canine neoplasms.[24-26] Most hepatocellular adenomas are reported in older dogs. Due to their infrequent occurrence and the lack of clear diagnostic criteria, there is insufficient data to determine if there is a sex or breed predisposition for hepatocellular adenomas. Consequently, the age of onset and the incidence of these lesions are similarly difficult to determine from the literature. However, surveys of food animals conducted in slaughterhouses have found hepatocellular adenomas in young pigs and sheep.[16]

Clinical Characteristics

There are no recognized clinical signs or characteristic clinical pathology patterns associated with hepatocellular adenomas. Compression of adjacent structures could conceivably disrupt blood or bile flow through the affected region of the liver, but there are no reports of hepatic injury associated with hepatocellular adenomas. Given the significant functional reserve of the liver, these lesions would be unlikely to alter hepatic function or produce detectable hepatic injury. They are most frequently detected as incidental lesions at necropsy.

Gross Morphology

Hepatocellular adenomas are most often solitary, but they can be multiple. They range from 2 to 8 cm in diameter and are usually roughly spherical masses due to their uniform expanding growth pattern. Typically, they are well demarcated due to compression of adjacent parenchyma, but they are not encapsulated. The color of hepatocellular adenomas varies from yellowish-brown to the dark mahogany red of normal liver parenchyma. Lipid or glycogen accumulation imparts the lighter color to the paler lesions, which often have a soft and friable consistency compared to normal liver. Hepatocellular adenomas are never firmer than normal liver since they do not contain increased fibrous tissue. Usually, hepatocellular adenomas

have a uniform color and consistency on the cut surface without evidence of hemorrhage or necrosis. Depending on their position, hepatocellular adenomas may bulge from the capsular surface or only be evident on the cut surface of the liver. They are indistinguishable from nodular hyperplasia on gross examination.

Histological Features

Hepatocellular adenomas usually have a circular outline and are well demarcated from adjacent parenchyma by a circumferential zone of compression (fig. 9.3). Although there may be an accumulation of connective tissue (the so-called reticulin fibers) at the interface of the adenoma and the normal liver, fibrosis is not a feature of hepatocellular adenomas. Within the circumferential zone of normal hepatocytes, compression and atrophy disrupt the normal hepatic lobular architecture. These atrophic hepatocytes may contain cytoplasmic vacuoles of lipid or glycogen as well as an increase in lipofuscin.

The hepatocytes within an adenoma have a uniform appearance. They tend to be identical in size, may be larger than normal hepatocytes, and may be vacuolated. The cytoplasm of the hepatocytes may contain abundant glycogen, lipid, or a combination of the two. The nuclei are similar to those in normal hepatocytes, but nucleoli may be

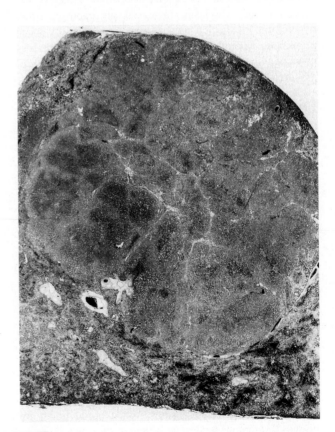

Fig. 9.3. Hepatocellular adenoma in the liver of a dog. Histologically, hepatocellular adenomas can be recognized by circumferential compression of adjacent liver tissue and the lack of normal hepatic lobular architecture. Usually, only a single portal tract is present within the mass.

more prominent. Mitotic figures are rare. Usually, all the cells in a particular adenoma have a similar appearance, but hepatocytes from other adenomas within the same liver may differ in their characteristics.

Hepatocellular adenomas usually have a trabecular or an acinar pattern. A mixture of trabecular and acinar patterns can also occur. In trabecular adenomas the hepatocytes are arranged in typical plates, but their orientation is often distinctly different than the normal lobular orientation. In place of lobular orientation, the hepatic plates tend to be arranged in a radial orientation that intersects the normal hepatic plates at right angles, accentuating the margins of the adenoma. The hepatocytes are arranged into plates or trabeculae that may be two to three cells thick, but usually thinner than the significantly larger trabeculae of hepatocellular carcinomas. The trabeculae of adenomas tend to be consistent in their thickness in contrast to the varying thickness of trabeculae in hepatocellular carcinoma. Consistent features of adenomas are the absence of a central vein and the lack of more than one portal triad, while both features are preserved in nodular hyperplasia. Any additional portal tracts probably result from entrapment of normal hepatic parenchyma in the mass of proliferating hepatocytes.

The cytological characteristics of hepatocytes from hepatocellular adenomas are quite similar to normal hepatocytes, but there are subtle differences: mild anisocytosis, basophilia of cytoplasm, increased glycogen or lipid, hyperchromatic nuclei, anisokaryosis, and slightly more prominent nucleoli.[6] However, these changes are less prominent in adenomas than in carcinomas. Mitotic figures are uncommon.

Differential Diagnosis

Because of their close resemblance to normal hepatocytes, adenomatous hepatocytes are always readily recognized, while the hepatocytic origin of malignant hepatocytes may not be obvious. Hepatocellular adenomas have a symmetrical and expansile pattern of growth that distinguishes them from the invasive carcinomas that may extend into adjacent parenchyma or vasculature. The architecture of the hepatic plates consists of plates that are usually no more than three cells in thickness, while the irregular trabeculae in carcinomas may be many cells thick. The absence of hemorrhage and necrosis are also typical of adenomas.

Hepatocellular adenomas can be difficult to distinguish from nodular hyperplasia of the liver. Some direction can be obtained from the gross pathological appearance: hepatocellular adenomas are usually individual lesions, and nodular hyperplasia occurs more often as multiple lesions. Lobular architecture is the best single criterion to distinguish the different lesions. When portal tracts are present throughout the lesion (although they may be separated to a greater degree than in the normal parenchyma) and hepatic plates retain normal arrangement, nodular hyperplasia is the appropriate diagnosis. Hepatocellular adenomas generally have an abnormal lobular architecture and a single portal tract or none at all. The presence of extensive hepatic damage and associated fibrosis in adjacent liver should support the diagnosis of regenerative nodules. These criteria can pose a particular diagnostic dilemma when evaluating needle biopsies, in particular, since lobular architecture and the degree of fibrosis can not be thoroughly evaluated.

Growth and Metastasis

Hepatocellular adenomas grow by symmetrical expansion. They typically have a spherical shape and compress adjacent parenchyma uniformly. Because hepatocellular adenomas are benign lesions, their growth is limited to the site of origin. Neither local invasion nor metastasis occurs.

Etiology

There is no known etiology for hepatocellular adenomas of domestic animals, although it is possible that chemical carcinogens may have a role in the production of these lesions. The liver is a frequent target of numerous man-made as well as naturally occurring chemical carcinogens.[12,13,22,23,27] Several naturally occurring carcinogens, most notably aflatoxins and nitrosamines, have the ability to produce hepatocellular carcinomas in experimental settings, and these substances are food contaminants for large and small animals.

Hepatocellular Carcinoma

Incidence

Hepatocellular carcinoma occurs in numerous species, including cats,[28-32] dogs,[4,15,24-26,33-35] cows,[16,17,36] sheep,[18,19,37] pigs,[16,38] and the horse.[39,40] The precise incidence in the various species is unclear because the incidence data reported are based on selected populations, usually from a small geographic area. Comparisons of the incidence of hepatocellular carcinomas among species are unavailable for similar reasons. The failure to distinguish benign from malignant hepatocellular neoplasms in many reports creates another challenge in estimating tumor incidence. However, information from abattoirs in the United Kingdom indicates that hepatocellular and biliary neoplasms are 4 times more common in cattle than sheep and nearly 18 times more common in cattle than pigs.[16] These authors also reported that hepatic and biliary neoplasms account for 10 percent of all neoplasms in cattle, 31 percent in sheep, and 4 percent in pigs. The dog may have a higher incidence of hepatocellular carcinomas than other species, based on several studies, but such reports may simply reflect a disproportionate interest in neoplasms of dogs.[5,24,34,41,42] The incidence of hepatocellular carcinoma in dogs has been reported to be from 0.52 to 1.6 per 100,000[25,35] and less than 1 percent of all neoplasms.[24] In dogs, hepatocellular carcinomas occur in 4.6-6.3 per 1000 necropsies.[33,35]

Results from more recent studies indicate that hepatocellular carcinomas are more common in dogs than cholangiocellular tumors,[26,15] but there are contradictory studies.[24,34] Hepatocellular carcinomas arise less often than cholangiocarcinomas in cats,[20,30,43,44] although there has been one study with contradictory results.[28] In most reports cattle had hepatocellular malignancies more often than cholangiocarcinomas,[17,19,45] although there has been one study with the opposite conclusion.[16] Hepatocellular tumors were more frequent than biliary neoplasms in sheep in several studies.[16,18,19,45]

The age distribution of animals with hepatocellular carcinoma varies among species. The average age of affected dogs is 10 to 11 years, although they have been reported in dogs as young as 4 years of age.[26,34] Affected cats range from 2 to 18 years of age.[29] Sheep and pigs can develop hepatocellular carcinomas at an early age. Sheep less than 1 year of age[16,18,19] and pigs less than 6 months old have developed hepatocellular carcinomas.[16] Hepatocellular carcinoma in cattle is also reported at an early age, but this can be attributed to the fact that the incidence data comes from abattoir surveys.[16,17] It is not known if the incidence of these tumors would increase with age in cattle, pigs, and sheep since most data is derived from abattoir studies, and relatively few animals at the later stages of their life expectancy have been studied. In dogs, this neoplasm is more frequent in males than in females, but no breed predisposition has been identified.[26,33] There is no breed or sex predisposition recognized for other domestic species.

Clinical Characteristics

In dogs and cats, the clinical signs associated with hepatocellular carcinoma are nonspecific. They include anorexia, vomiting, ascites, lethargy, and weakness.[5,15,26,29,35] Other, less common, signs include jaundice, diarrhea, and weight loss. Some affected dogs may have seizures, presumably due to hepatoencephalopathy or hypoglycemia, since hepatic metastases to the brain are rare.[35,46] During the physical examination of cats and dogs, hepatomegaly causing abdominal enlargement and a palpable mass in the cranial abdomen is often evident.[15,29]

Dogs with hepatocellular carcinoma frequently have increased serum activities of alkaline phosphatase, aspartate aminotransferase, alanine aminotransferase, and gamma glutamyltransferase.[15,26,35,47] Increased levels of fasting bile acids alone or in combination with increased levels of serum alkaline phosphatase have been shown to be indicative of hepatic neoplasia, but did not distinguish primary neoplasia from metastatic disease or other hepatobiliary disease.[47,48] Less often, other markers of hepatic damage such as serum lactate dehydrogenase and bilirubin may be increased. Hypoglycemia, reported in dogs and a horse, is an uncommon consequence of hepatocellular carcinoma.[33,40,46,49] The mechanism by which hepatocellular carcinomas affect this change in blood glucose levels has been attributed to the release of an insulin-like substance.[46]

TABLE 9.1. Hepatic neoplasia

Epithelial
  Nodular hyperplasia
    Micronodules
    Regenerative nodules
  Hepatocellular adenoma
  Hepatocellular carcinoma
    Trabecular
    Adenoid
    Solid
  Hepatoblastoma
  Cholangioma/biliary cystadenoma
  Cholangiocarcinoma/bile duct cystadenocarcinoma
  Adenoma of the gall bladder
  Adenocarcinoma of the gall bladder
  Carcinoids
Mesenchymal
  Hemangiosarcoma
  Myelolipoma
  Other sarcomas

Since all of these laboratory test results may be altered in a variety of hepatic diseases, they cannot separate hepatocellular carcinoma from other primary hepatic or metastatic neoplasms in the liver. Slightly over half of the dogs with hepatocellular carcinoma have nonspecific hematological abnormalities such as leukocytosis and anemia.[26]

Serum alpha-fetoprotein has been used as a marker for hepatocellular carcinoma in cattle and dogs.[37,50,51] Although alpha-fetoprotein is increased in a proportion of animals with hepatocellular carcinoma, it is not increased in all affected animals. Other neoplasms, such as cholangiocarcinoma, and inflammatory conditions of the liver also increase concentrations of serum alpha-fetoprotein.[50]

Radiographic signs of hepatocellular carcinoma are also nonspecific. The most frequently observed change in abdominal radiographs of dogs with hepatocellular carcinoma is displacement of the stomach to the right ventral aspect of the abdomen.[52] This change is not specific for hepatocellular carcinoma and can be seen with other space occupying lesions of the liver. Hepatocellular carcinomas are reported to have a characteristic hyperechoic pattern; however, while ultrasound examination of the liver can readily detect masses within the liver, the technique cannot identify specific tumor types or separate hyperplastic lesions from neoplastic lesions.[7,53]

Gross Morphology

Hepatocellular carcinomas can be massive, nodular, or diffuse. Massive hepatocellular carcinomas are usually a single neoplasm that involves one or contiguous liver lobes (fig. 9.4). Nodular hepatocellular carcinoma forms scattered nodules, often within multiple liver lobes. Diffuse hepatocellular carcinomas are characterized by minute indistinct masses spread throughout the liver parenchyma. The massive form is more common in dogs than the other forms.[15,33] Hepatocellular carcinoma can be found in all lobes of the liver, but the left lateral lobe is reported to be affected most often.[33] Why one lobe of the

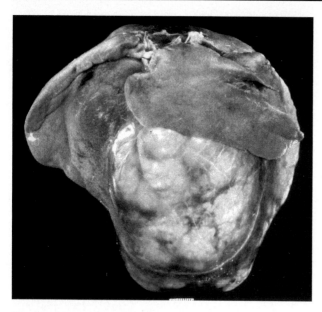

Fig. 9.4. A massive hepatocellular carcinoma from a dog. The left lateral lobe is nearly replaced by the tumor.

liver would be affected more often than the others is not clear. Given the fact that the left lobe is one-third to one-half of the total mass of the liver, its greater volume compared to other liver lobes may account for the increased frequency of involvement if tumor development is a random event.[54] Multiple hepatocellular carcinomas within the liver may arise from intrahepatic metastasis or multiple individual points of origin, but it is not currently possible to distinguish between these possibilities.

Hepatocellular carcinomas have a considerable range of appearances. They vary from small, round, discrete lesions a few centimeters in diameter to large, diffuse masses that may be greater than 10 cm in diameter.[4,5,19,33,34] Smaller lesions tend to be spherical or oval with a smooth surface and resemble benign hepatocellular neoplasms. The larger masses usually have an uneven to multinodular surface and an irregular shape. Umbilication is not a feature of hepatocellular carcinomas. Carcinomas often protrude from the liver capsule and distort the profile of the liver. Hepatocellular carcinomas usually have a discrete border, and they can be distinguished from the adjacent normal liver parenchyma even in multinodular masses. Adhesions between the neoplasm and adjacent structures such as the diaphragm or body wall may be found, but are not common.[15]

The color and the consistency of hepatocellular carcinomas vary considerably from one neoplasm to another, and often regions within a single mass have different characteristics.[34] The smaller neoplasms are more likely to be uniform and to resemble normal liver. Larger neoplasms frequently have a mottled appearance, with some areas resembling normal liver, while other sites are light gray to tan. In some instances, lipidosis of the neo-

plastic lesion imparts a light tan to yellow appearance to the entire lesion. Focal areas of dark red discoloration caused by hemorrhage and necrosis are common in larger tumors. Light gray to white areas, usually found within the central regions of the neoplasm, are caused by necrosis without associated hemorrhage. The friable and soft consistency of hepatocellular carcinomas is a useful diagnostic feature that distinguishes this neoplasm from the firm consistency of cholangiocarcinomas. Since hepatocellular carcinomas are friable, rupture of the tumor with resultant hemoperitoneum or blood clots on the capsule is fairly common. However, hemoperitoneum would be more commonly associated with hemangiosarcoma of the liver or spleen.

Histological Features

The histological appearance of hepatocellular carcinomas varies considerably, depending on the degree of differentiation of the individual hepatocytes and the histological arrangement of the cells.[8,15,33] This wide spectrum of histological appearance has led to different classification systems for the carcinoma.[8,33] Some systems are complex, while others have fewer categories. The term *hepatoma* should be avoided as a diagnostic term for hepatic malignancies because it is confusing. Although hepatoma has been used for many years and is still in use in human hepatic malignancies, the suffix -*oma* suggests a benign neoplasm. We favor the simplified categorization of hepatocellular carcinomas since individual masses frequently contain different histological patterns within different areas. The three major diagnostic categories are *trabecular, adenoid,* and *solid.* In the more differentiated *trabecular hepatocellular carcinomas,* the histological arrangement and cytology bear a close resemblance to normal liver. The neoplastic cells can form thin plates in some sites, but thickened trabeculae are a frequent component of the neoplasm (fig. 9.5). It is characteristic to find a plate of neoplastic hepatocytes that is 5 to 10 cells thick and occasionally as much as 20 cells thick. Variability in hepatocellular plate thickness is one of the criteria used to differentiate a well-differentiated trabecular hepatocellular carcinoma from a hepatocellular adenoma. Little or no connective tissue stroma occurs in the trabeculae. Necrosis may be found in the center of the wide trabeculae. In other cases, the neoplasm has widely dilated sinusoids, occasionally forming blood filled cavernous spaces that separate trabeculae and irregular clusters of tumor cells.

Although the trabecular pattern is the most common histological form of the tumor in domestic animals, other patterns have been recognized.[33,34] The *adenoid hepatocellular carcinoma* is characterized by crude acini formed by neoplastic hepatocytes (fig. 9.6). The lumens may vary in size, and some may contain proteinaceous material. Solid sheets of neoplastic hepatocytes with no apparent pattern (fig. 9.7) characterize the *solid hepatocellular carcinoma.* The cells that compose this form of hepatocellular carcinoma are often poorly differentiated and pleomorphic. The

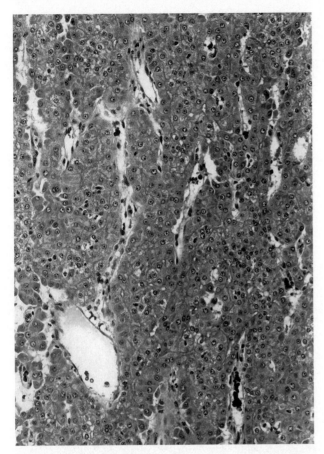

Fig. 9.5. Hepatocellular carcinoma from a dog: trabecular. Hepatocellular carcinomas often form characteristic trabeculae composed of hepatocytes from 3 to more than 20 cells thick. Hepatocytes may possess cytologic features of malignancy.

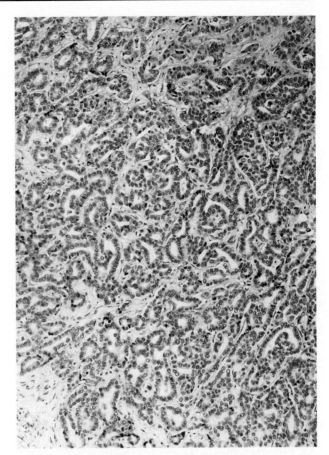

Fig. 9.6. Hepatocellular carcinoma from a dog: adenoid. Adenoid forms of hepatocellular carcinomas are characterized by formation of acini lined with well-differentiated hepatocytes and scant connective tissue stroma between acini. (Courtesy of A.K. Patnaik) [Canine hepatocellular carcinoma. Patnaik, A.K., et al. *Vet Pathol* (1981) 18:427–438; with permission.]

amount of stroma within this tumor is variable. Large vascular spaces, frequently filled with blood and occasionally associated with foci of necrotic neoplastic hepatocytes, may be found within all types hepatocellular carcinomas. In a minority of hepatocellular carcinomas, thin strands of connective tissue separate clusters of neoplastic cells. These histological patterns are not mutually exclusive; several different patterns may be identified within a single neoplasm.

The cytologic features of hepatocytes in hepatocellular carcinomas are variable.[8,15,33,34] Hepatocytes in well-differentiated carcinomas strongly resemble normal hepatocytes, with central, round nuclei and usually moderately eosinophilic cytoplasm. The cytoplasm, however, may be pale staining or even vacuolated if filled with glycogen or lipid. Some hepatocellular carcinomas may be entirely composed of vacuolated cells. At the other end of the spectrum, poorly differentiated hepatocellular carcinomas have very pleomorphic cells that may not be readily recognized as hepatocytic in origin (fig. 9.8). The nuclei of these cells are variable in both size and shape; it is not unusual for the nuclei of different cells to vary in diameter by threefold, and tumor giant cells can be found. The cytoplasm of the cells is generally basophilic and greatly

reduced in volume, resulting in an obviously increased nuclear to cytoplasmic ratio. The neoplastic cell often lacks the square shape of the sectioned normal hepatocyte. The cells may assume a round or, rarely, spindle shape. Nucleoli tend to be enlarged in most cells, irrespective of the general state of differentiation. Individual giant cells are sometimes found in the poorly differentiated neoplasms. Mitotic figures occur more often in the carcinomas than in adenomas, but they are relatively rare in well-differentiated carcinomas.

Some rare carcinomas have the histological and cytological characteristics of both hepatocellular carcinoma and biliary carcinoma.[33,55] In some cases, these carcinomas appear to have arisen as a single mass, but others may result from mutual invasion causing the convergence of two independent masses. In either case, such tumors with clear hepatocellular and bile ductular components are best designated as *hepatocholangiocarcinomas,* although they are also referred to as *combined hepatocellular and cholangiocarcinoma.*

Ultrastructural study suggests that the sinusoidal lining cells in hepatocellular carcinomas of dogs differ from those found in normal liver. The typical fenestration of the

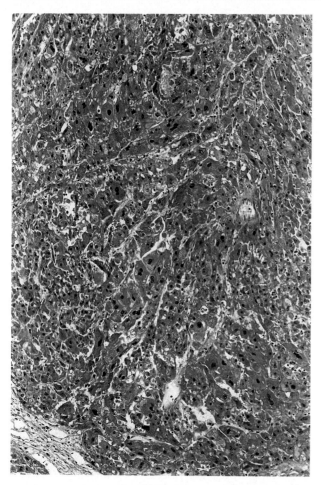

Fig. 9.7. Hepatocellular carcinoma from a dog: solid. Sheets of neoplastic hepatocytes that do not form sinusoids or contain significant fibrosis characterize the solid pattern of hepatocellular carcinomas.

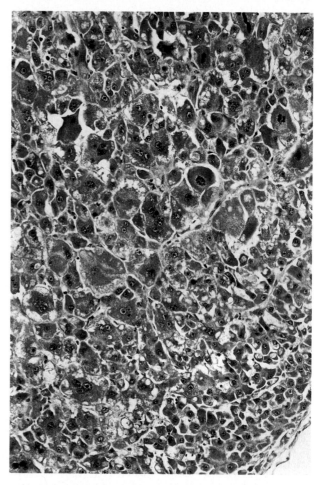

Fig. 9.8. Hepatocellular carcinoma from a dog: solid, poorly differentiated. These types of hepatocellular carcinomas are composed of pleomorphic cells that may have little residual resemblance to hepatocytes.

normal sinusoidal endothelial cells is lost. Also, unlike the normal pattern for sinusoidal endothelial cells, there is deposition of basement membrane material beneath the endothelial cells in hepatocellular carcinomas.[56] Another change in the vessels in hepatocellular carcinomas that is consistent with their conversion from sinusoids to a capillary-like structure is the appearance of factor VIII–related antigen in the endothelial cytoplasm. This protein is usually expressed in the endothelial cells of most vessels, but not in normal hepatic sinusoids. Other changes in the sinusoids of hepatocellular carcinomas include increased alpha–smooth muscle actin staining and/or a decrease in desmin staining of hepatic stellate cells (lipocytes or Ito cells). In contrast to these changes in endothelial cells, ultrastructural studies of hepatocytes in hepatocellular tumors from pigs have not been helpful in distinguishing these lesions from other liver conditions.[57]

The nonneoplastic liver parenchyma is usually histologically normal in animals with hepatocellular carcinoma. This is in contrast to the situation in humans, in which cirrhosis is a frequent prelude to hepatocellular carcinoma. Dogs, cats, and cattle rarely have evidence of cirrhosis in

cases with hepatocellular carcinoma, although chemically induced liver cancer in pigs has been associated with hepatic fibrosis.[16,22,23,33]

Touch imprints have limited utility in the diagnosis of well-differentiated hepatocellular carcinoma. Hepatocytes from well-differentiated hepatocellular carcinomas may resemble normal hepatocytes or hepatocytes from hepatocellular adenomas and nodular hyperplasia.[6] Cells with a recognizable hepatocytic origin and with marked atypia, such as altered nuclear to cytoplasmic ratios, staining alterations, and variation in the size of cells and nuclei, support a diagnosis of hepatocellular malignancy. The possibility of metastatic epithelial neoplasms must always be considered when poorly differentiated cells are encountered in aspirates or imprints.

Differential Diagnosis

A diagnosis of this carcinoma is based on first finding histological evidence that the neoplasm is of hepatocellular origin. While hepatocellular characteristics are easy to recognize in more differentiated neoplasms, this distinction is often difficult in poorly differentiated tumors.

Fortunately, most neoplasms will have at least some areas with hepatocellular characteristics. The distinction between well-differentiated hepatocellular carcinoma and hepatocellular adenoma is also difficult.[8] When tumor cell invasion is lacking, the diagnosis is based on the overall size of the tumor, the degree of cytological alteration, and the variable thickness of hepatocellular plates. Invasion into adjacent hepatic parenchyma is the most certain way to identify a carcinoma. Vascular invasion is rarely seen, but when present, it clearly identifies the malignant varieties.

Difficulty may arise in distinguishing hepatocellular carcinoma with an adenoid pattern from cholangiocarcinoma. In this case, a distinction can be made by examining the cytological characteristics as well as the general histological pattern. The neoplastic acini of adenoid hepatocellular carcinomas may contain proteinaceous material, while cholangiocarcinomas are more likely to have PAS positive mucin within neoplastic acini.[33,58] In addition, the cholangiocarcinoma usually has an extensive collagenous stroma compared to the modest or absent stromal elements in adenoid hepatocellular carcinomas. At the ultrastructural level, biliary epithelial cells can be recognized by the presence of a basement membrane, a feature that is absent in hepatocytes.

Special techniques have been used to characterize hepatocellular carcinoma in animals. Immunohistochemistry may be useful to distinguish adenoid hepatocellular carcinomas from biliary malignancies. In cats, neoplastic biliary epithelial cells may be distinguished from hepatocytes because most biliary epithelial cells contain a population of cytokeratins, while normal, and presumably neoplastic, hepatocytes do not.[30,59] Although hepatocellular carcinomas and cholangiocarcinomas in dogs contained similar cytokeratins, this approach may be useful in other species. Hepatocellular carcinomas in dogs have been separated from cholangiocarcinomas on the basis of their immunohistochemical staining patterns for oncofetal antigens in one report.[51] The hepatocellular carcinomas could be stained for the presence of alpha-fetoprotein, and the cholangiocarcinomas contained carcinoembryonic antigen. However this observation may require clarification, since other authors report increases in serum alpha-fetoprotein for both hepatocellular carcinoma and cholangiocarcinoma in dogs.[50]

Hepatocellular carcinoma must also be distinguished from primary hepatic carcinoid on the basis of histological appearance and the use of silver impregnation stains that demonstrate secretory granules in carcinoid cells.[8,60] Immunohistochemical detection of neurosecretory products in the cytoplasm of carcinoids is also a useful technique for identification of these tumors.

Growth and Metastasis

Hepatocellular carcinoma progressively invades the adjacent hepatic tissue. Invasion tends to occur by clusters of neoplastic cells and, rarely, as individual neoplastic cells; it does not occur uniformly around the periphery of the neoplasm and may occur only in a few areas. This feature necessitates examining multiple sections of questionably malignant tumors. Invasion of blood vessels and lymphatics occurs but is rarely obvious within a single section; thus, it should not be considered a necessary requirement for diagnosis of malignancy. Vascular invasion is more common than lymphatic invasion.

Metastasis occurs most commonly in the lung and hepatic lymph nodes.[8,16,26,29,33] While the local lymph nodes may contain metastatic neoplastic cells, they are rarely massively enlarged. When present, metastatic sites in the lung are usually numerous and relatively small. The earliest metastatic foci are located in the capillaries of the alveolar wall, indicating a hematogenous spread. Hepatocellular carcinoma is also known to occasionally metastasize to a variety of other organs.[16,33] The neoplasm also spreads by direct extension to the omentum and peritoneum.[15,23,34] This occurs when neoplastic cells from a friable neoplasm are dispersed within the peritoneal cavity after rupture of the primary tumor. Anaplastic and pleomorphic neoplasms tend to metastasize more often than the more differentiated neoplasms.[33] The metastatic rate for hepatocellular carcinomas in dogs was reported to be less than 25 percent in one study[15] and 61 percent in another.[33] The rate of metastasis was reported to be 28 percent for cats.[29] These rates may be variable, depending on the time of diagnosis in relation to the stage of tumor development and on the effort expended to search for evidence of metastasis. Metastatic rate in cattle is reported to be 39 percent, but data for other species are unavailable.[36]

Metastasis generally occurs late in the course of neoplastic development. In general, the primary neoplasm is large, while the metastases are small. Therefore, the resulting devitalization of the affected animal is usually due to the primary neoplasm and not to the metastasis. Hence, the prognosis is considered favorable for dogs with hepatocellular carcinoma that involves only one or two lobes. Surgical resection of affected lobes can prolong life by about 1 year in the majority of dogs, and reoccurrence of the neoplasm is uncommon.[61,62]

Etiology

The etiology of the spontaneously occurring hepatocellular carcinoma in domestic animals is unknown, but chronic infections or chemical ingestion may play a role in tumor development. Some clues to the cause of liver cancer in domestic species may be provided by studies in humans and laboratory animals. Chronic viral infections of the liver caused by hepatitis B virus and hepatitis C virus are clearly associated with an increased risk of liver cancer in humans.[63,64] More compelling evidence of the carcinogenicity of members of the hepatitis B virus family, Hepadnaviridae, is provided by studies in woodchucks.[65] Woodchucks chronically infected with woodchuck hepatitis virus have a 100 percent risk of developing hepatocellular carcinoma. However, chronic hepatic infections with similar viruses have not been identified in domestic animals. The role of chronic infections with bacteria, such as the *Helicobacter* spp. that have been shown to cause liver cancer in some strains of mice, has not been evaluated in domestic animals.[66]

There is a comprehensive body of information concerning chemical carcinogenesis of the liver. A variety of chemicals are known to cause hepatocellular carcinoma in domestic animals.[2,13,22,23,27] There are numerous other examples of chemical hepatocarcinogens in laboratory rodents that may also be carcinogenic in domestic animals. Domestic animals are unlikely to be exposed to these chemicals because their use is restricted to industrial or experimental settings. Naturally occurring carcinogens such as aflatoxins, pyrrolizidines, and nitrosamines may play a role in liver cancer in domestic animals. Dietary aflatoxins can cause liver cancer in pigs when fed at a concentration of 1 ppm.[23] Experimental administration of diethylnitrosamine leads to liver cancer in dogs and swine.[13,22]

Hepatoblastoma

Hepatoblastomas are benign neoplasms that are composed of cells resembling fetal hepatocytes.[8] They are rare in domestic species, and there is no information available concerning incidence or clinical characteristics. Most hepatoblastomas have been reported in lambs,[67] although individual reports for an equine fetus[68] and a dog[69] are in the literature.

Hepatoblastomas can form firm, lobulated, yellowish white masses with areas of necrosis and hemorrhage. In sheep the nodules range from 0.5 to 20 cm in diameter. Histologically, the masses compress adjacent liver parenchyma, but there is no evidence of invasion. Tumor cells are arranged in irregular cords or trabeculae and may form acini. Tumor cells tend to be smaller than normal hepatocytes and have a granular cytoplasm. Extramedullary hematopoiesis is frequently found within the mass. Portal tracts are absent, although there is a fine fibrous septation supporting the mass. Mitotic figures are uncommon.

REFERENCES

1. Bergman, J.R. 1985. Nodular hyperplasia in the liver of the dog: An association with changes in the Ito cell population. *Vet Pathol* 22:427-438.
2. Fabry, A., Benjamin, S.A., and Angleton, G.M. (1982) Nodular hyperplasia of the liver in the beagle dog. *Vet Pathol* 19:109-119.
3. Hayashi, M.A., Tsuda, H., and Ito, N. (1983) Histopathological classification of spontaneous hyperplastic liver nodules in slaughtered swine. *J Comp Pathol* 93:603-612.
4. Mulligan, R.M. (1949) In Mulligan, R.M. (ed.) *Neoplasms of the Dog.* Williams and Wilkins Co., Baltimore. pp. 111-114.
5. Mulligan, R.M. (1949) Primary liver-cell carcinoma (hepatoma) in the dog. *Cancer Res* 9:76-81.
6. Blue, J.T., French, T.W., and Meyer, D.J. (1999) The liver. In Cow-

ell, R., Tyler, R.L., and Meinkoth, J.M. (eds.), *Diagnostic Cytology and Hematology of the Dog and Cat.* Mosby, St. Louis, pp. 183-194.
7. Nyland, T.G., and Park, R.D. (1983) Hepatic ultrasonography in the dog. *Vet Radiol* 24:74-84.
8. Ponomarkov, V., and Mackey, L.J. (1976) Tumours of the liver and biliary system. *Bull WHO* 53:187-194.
9. Bunch, S.E., Castleman, W.L., Hornbuckle, W.E., and Tennant, B.C. (1982) Hepatic cirrhosis associated with long-term anticonvulsant drug therapy in dogs. *J Amer Vet Med Assoc* 181:357-362.
10. Dayrell-Hart, B., Steinberg, S.A., VanWinkle, T.J., and Farnbach, G.C. (1991) Hepatotoxicity of phenobarbital in dogs: 18 cases (1985-1989). *J Amer Vet Med Assoc* 199:1060-1066.
11. Cotran, R.S., Kumar, V., and Collins, T. (1999) Neoplasia. In Cotran, R.S., Kumar, V., and Collins, T. (eds.), *Pathologic Basis of Disease.* W.B. Saunders, Philadelphia , pp. 260-327.
12. Allison, J.B., Wase, A.W., Leathem, J.H., and Wainio, W.W. (1950) Some effects of 2-acetylaminofluorene on the dog. *Cancer Res* 10:266-271.
13. Hirao, K., Matsumura, K., Imagawa, A., Enomoto, Y., Hosogi, Y., Kani, T., Fujikawa, K., and Ito, N. (1974) Primary neoplasms in dog liver induced by diethylnitrosamine. *Cancer Res* 34:1870-1882.
14. Dagle, G.E., Bristline, R.W., Lebel, J.L., and Watters, R.L. (1984) Plutonium-induced wounds in beagles. *Health Phys* 47:73-84.
15. Trigo, F.J., Thompson, H., Breeze, R.G., and Nash, A.S. (1982) The pathology of liver tumours in the dog. *J Comp Pathol* 92:21-39.
16. Anderson, L.J., and Sandison, A.T. (1967) Tumors of the liver in cattle, sheep and pigs. *Cancer* 21:289-301.
17. Bastianello, S.S. (1982) A survey on neoplasia in domestic species over a 40-year period from 1935 to 1974 in the Republic of South Africa. I. Tumours occurring in cattle. *Onderstepoort J Vet Res* 49:195-204.
18. Bastianello, S.S. (1982) A survey on neoplasia in domestic species over a 40-year period from 1935 to 1974 in the Republic of South Africa. II. Tumours occurring in sheep. *Onderstepoort J Vet Res* 49:205-209.
19. Monlux, A.W., Anderson, W.A., and Davis, C.L. (1956) A survey of tumors occurring in cattle, sheep and swine. *Amer J Vet Res* 17:646-677.
20. Lawrence, H.J., Erb, H.N., and Harvey, H.J. (1994) Nonlymphomatous hepatobiliary masses in cats: 41 cases (1972 to 1991). *Vet Surg* 23:365-368.
21. Messow, C. 1952. Die Lebertumoren unserer Haussaugetiere. *Wiss Z Humbolt-Univ Berlin* 2:121-152.
22. Graw, J.J., and Berg, H. 1977. Hepatocarcinogenetic effect of DENA in pigs. *Z Krebsforch* 89:137-143.
23. Shalkop, W.T., and Armbrecht, B.H. (1974) Carcinogenic response of brood sows fed aflatoxin for 28 to 30 months. *Amer J Vet Res* 35:623-627.
24. Bastianello, S.S. 1983. A survey on neoplasia in domestic species over a 40-year period from 1935 to 1974 in the Republic of South Africa. VI. Tumours occurring in dogs. *Onerstepoort J Vet Res* 50:199-220.
25. MacVean, D.W., Monlux, A.W., Anderson, P.S., Jr., Silberg, S.L., and Rozel, J.F. 1978. Frequency of canine and feline tumors in a defined population. *Vet Pathol* 15:700-715.
26. Patnaik, A.K., Hurvitz, A.I., and Lieberman, P.H. 1980. Canine hepatic neoplasms: a clinicopathologic study. *Vet Pathol* 17:553-564.
27. Stula, E.F., Barnes, J.R., Sherman, H., Reinhardt, C.F., and Zapp, J.A., Jr. (1978) Liver and urinary bladder tumors in dogs from 3,3'-dichlorobenzidine. *J Environ Pathol Toxicol* 1:475-490.
28. Bastianello, S.S. (1983) A survey on neoplasia in domestic species over a 40-year period from 1935 to 1974 in the Republic of South Africa. V. Tumours occurring in the cat. *Onderstepoort J Vet Res* 50:105-110.
29. Carpenter, J.L., Andrews, L.K., and Holzworth, J. (1987) Tumors and tumor-like lesions, In Holzworth, J. (ed.), *Diseases of the Cat.* W.B. Saunders, Philadelphia, pp. 406-596.

30. Patnaik, A.K.(1992) A morphologic and immunocytochemical study of hepatic neoplasms in cats. *Vet Pathol* 29:405-415.

31. Patnaik, A.K., and Liu. S.-K.H.A.I.M.A.J. (1975) Nonhematopoietic neoplasms in cats. *J Natl Cancer Inst* 54:855-860.

32. Priester, W.A., and McKay, F.W. (1980) The occurence of tumors in domestic animals. *J Natl Cancer Inst Monog* 54:210-216.

33. Patnaik, A.K., Hurvitz, A.I., Lieberman, P.H., and Johnson, G.F. (1981) Canine hepatocellular carcinoma. *Vet Pathol* 18:427-438.

34. Rooney, J.R. (1959) Liver carcinoma in the dog. *Acta Pathol Microbiol Scand* 45:321-330.

35. Strombeck, D.R. (1978) Clinicopathologic features of primary and metastatic neoplastic disease of the liver in dogs. *J Amer Vet Med Assoc* 173:267-269.

36. Vitovec, J. 1974. Hepatozelluare Karzinome beim Rind und ihre Beziehung zur Biliaren Zirrhose Fasziolaren Ursprungs. *Vet Pathol* 548-557.

37. Kithier, K., Al-Sarraf, M., Belamaric, J., Radl, J., Valenta, Z., Zizkovsky, V., and Masopust, J. (1974) Alpha-fetoprotein in bovine hepatocellular carcinoma. *J Comp Pathol* 84:133-141.

38. Ramachandran, K.M., Rajan, A., Mony, G., and Maryamma, K.I. (1970) Hepatocellular carcinoma in a pig. *Indian Vet* 47:304-306.

39. Bastianello, S.S. (1983) A survey on neoplasia in domestic species over a 40-year period from 1935 to 1974 in the Republic of South Africa. IV. Tumours occurring in equidae. *Onderstepoort J Vet Res* 50:91-96.

40. Roby, K.A., Beech, J., Bloom, J.C., and Black, M. 1990. Hepatocellular carcinoma associated with erythrocytosis and hypoglycemia in a yearling filly. *J Amer Vet Med Assoc* 196:465-467.

41. Dorn, C.R., Taylor, D.O.N., Frye, F.L., and Hibbard, H.H. (1968) Survey of animal neoplasms in Alameda and Contra Costa Counties, California. I. Methodology and description of cases. *J Natl Cancer Inst* 40:295-303.

42. Dorn, C.R., Taylor, D.O.N., Schneider, R., Hibbard, H.H., and Klauber, M.R. (1968) Survey of animal neoplasms in Alameda and Contra Costa Counties, California, II. Cancer morbidity in dogs and cats from Alameda County. *J Natl Cancer Inst* 40:307-318.

43. Post, G., and Patnaik, A.K. 1992. Nonhematopoietic hepatic neoplasms in cats: 21 cases (1983-1988). *J Amer Vet Med Assoc* 201:1080-1082.

44. Schmidt, R.E., and R.F. Langham, R.F. (1967) A survey of feline neoplasms. *J Amer Vet Med Assoc* 151:1325-1328.

45. Cotchin, E. (1960) Tumours of farm animals: A survey of tumours examined at the Royal Veterinary College, London, during 1950-60's. *Vet Rec* 72:816-823.

46. Strombeck, D.R., Krum, S., Meyer, D., and Kappesser, R.M. (1976) Hypoglycemia and hypoinsulinemia associated with hepatoma in a dog. *J Amer Vet Med Assoc* 169:811-812.

47. Center, S.A., Slater, M.R., Manwarren, T., and Prymak, K. 1992. Diagnostic efficacy of serum alkaline phosphatase and gamma-glutamyltranferase in dogs with histologically confirmed hepatobiliary disease: 270 cases (1980-1990. *J Amer Vet Med Assoc* 201:1258-1264.

48. Center, S.A., Baldwin, B.H., Erb, H.N., and Tennant, B.C. 1985. Bile acid concentrations in the diagnosis of hepatobiliary disease in the dog. *J Amer Vet Med Assoc* 187:935-940.

49. Leifer, C.E., Peterson, M.E., Matus, R.E., and Patnaik, A.K. (1985) Hypoglycemia associated with nonislet cell tumor in 13 dogs. *J Amer Vet Med Assoc* 186:53-55.

50. Lowseth, L.A., Gillett, N.A., Chang, I.Y., Muggenburg, B.A., and Boecker, B.B. 1991. Detection of serum alpha-fetoprotein in dogs with hepatic tumors. *J Amer Vet Med Assoc* 199:735-741.

51. Martin de las Mulas, J., Gomez-Villamandos, J.C., Perez, J., Mozos, E., Estrado, M., and Mendez, A. (1995) Immunohistochemical evaluation of canine primary liver carcinomas: Distribution of alpha-fetoprotein, carcinoembryonic antigen, keratins and vimentin. *Res Vet Sci* 59:124-127.

52. Evans, S.M. (1999) The radiographic appearance of primary liver neoplasia in dogs. *Vet Radiol* 28:192-196.

53. Whiteley, M.B., Feeney, D.A., Whiteley, L.O., and Hardy, R.M. (1989) Ultrasonographic appearance of primary and metastatic canine hepatic tumors: A review of 48 cases. *J Ultrasound Med* 8:621-630.

54. Miller, M.E., Christensen, G.C., and Evans, H.E. (1964) The digestive system and abdomen, In Miller, M.E., Christensen, G.C., and Evans, H.E. (eds.), *Anatomy of the Dog.* W.B. Saunders, Philadelphia, pp. 645-712.

55. Kato, M., Higuchi, T., Orita, Y., Ishikawa, Y., and Kakinoki, M. (1997) Combined hepatocellular carcinoma and cholangiocarcinoma in a mare. *J Comp Pathol* 116:409-413.

56. Shiga, A., Shirota, K., and Nomura, Y. (1996) Immunohistochemical and ultrastructural studies on the sinusoidal lining cells of canine hepatocellular carcinoma. *J Vet Med Sci* 58:909-914.

57. Ito, T., Miura, S., Ohshima, K., and Numakunai, S. (1972) Fine structure of hepatocellular carcinoma in swine. *Jap J Vet Sci* 34:33-37.

58. Patnaik, A.K., Hurvitz, A.I., Lieberman, P.H., and Johnson, G.F. (1981) Canine bile duct carcinoma. *Vet Pathol* 18:439-444.

59. Adler, R., and Wilson, D.W. 1995. Biliary cystadenoma of cats. *Vet Pathol* 32:415-418.

60. Patnaik, A.K., Lieberman, P.H., Hurvitz, A.I., and Johnson, G.F. (1981) Canine hepatic carcinoids. *Vet Pathol* 18:445-453.

61. Fry, P.D., and Rest, J.R. (1993) Partial hepatectomy in two dogs. *J Small Anim Pract* 34:192-195.

62. Kosovsky, J.E., Manfra-Marretta, S., Matthiesen, D.T., and Patnaik, A.K. (1989) Results of partial hepatectomy in 18 dogs with hepatocellular carcinoma. *J Amer Anim Hosp Assoc* 25:203-206.

63. Beasely, R.P. (1988) Hepatitis B virus, the major etiology of hepatocellular carcinoma. *Cancer* 61:1942-1956.

64. Reid, A.E., Koziel, M.J., Aiza, I., Jeffers, L., Reddy, R., Schiff, E., Lau, J.Y., Dienstag, J.L., and Liang, T.J. (1999) Hepatitis C virus genotypes and viremia and hepatocellular carcinoma in the United States. *Amer J Gastroenterol* 94:1619-1626.

65. Popper, H., Shih, J.W.K., Gerin, J.L., Wong, D.C., Hoyer, B.H., London, W.T., Sly, D.L., and Purcell, R.H. (1981) Woodchuck hepatitis and hepatocellular carcinoma: Correlation of histologic with virologic observations. *Hepatology* 1:91-98.

66. Sipowicz, M.A., Chomarat, P., Diwan, B.A.A.M.A., Awasthi, Y.C., Ward, J.M., Rice, J.M., Kasprzak, K.S., Wild, C.P., and Anderson, L.M. (1999) Increased oxidative DNA damage and hepatocyte overexpression of specific cytochrome P450 isoforms in hepatitis of mice infected with *Helicobacter hepaticus. Amer J Pathol* 151:933-941.

67. Manktelow, B.W. (1965) Hepatoblastomas in sheep. *J Pathol Bact* 89:711-714.

68. Neu, S.M. (1993) Hepatoblastoma in an equine fetus. *J Vet Diag Invest* 5:634-637.

69. Shiga, A., Shirota, K., Shida, T., Yamada, T., and Nomura, Y. (1997) Hepatoblastoma in a dog. *J Vet Med Sci* 59:1167-1170.

Biliary Neoplasms

Cholangioma and Biliary Cystadenoma

Incidence

Cholangiomas are reported in dogs,[1] cats,[2-6] sheep,[7-9] and pigs.[10,11] There are individual reports of cholangiomas in cows.[9,12] These benign neoplasms of biliary epithelium appear to be uncommon in all species based on the limited number of reported cases and their absence in some surveys of neoplasms.[8,11,13-15] Cholangiomas have been reported to occur less frequently than cholangiocarcinomas in dogs,[15] but cholangiomas were reported to be the most common hepatobiliary neoplasm in cats in two case series.[5,6] The rarity of these lesions makes it difficult to obtain an accurate incidence rate for individual species or to compare the relative frequency among species. Cholangiomas appear to arise most frequently within the hepatic parenchyma. In most species extrahepatic cholangiomas are rare, with the possible exception of cats.[6]

Clinical Characteristics

The clinical impact of cholangiomas has not been reported in any species except the cat, and even in this species there are no characteristic signs.[3,5] In one study, all the clinical signs in cats with benign biliary neoplasms were attributed to concurrent disease processes.[3] Anorexia was observed in another study, but concurrent problems with these cats were not discussed.[16] It is not likely that cholangiomas cause appreciable problems in most circumstances. Hepatic enlargement was detected in more than 60 percent of cats with cholangiomas.[5] Cholangiomas develop in geriatric cats (greater than 10-12 years of age), and there is no clear sex predilection.[3,5,6] These tumors may not be detected earlier because they are clinically silent and are not noticed until the affected animal is examined for another reason.

Gross Morphology

Cholangiomas are usually solitary, well circumscribed, solid masses that may contain a small area of small caliber cysts (fig. 9.9). Tumors with larger, multilocular cysts are a subtype designated as biliary cystadenomas. Both are benign tumors derived from biliary epithelium and simply differ in the sizes of their cystic structures.[3] Cholangiomas and cystadenomas can be single or multiple. Solid cholangiomas are pale white to pale gray. Biliary cystadenomas vary from a spongy consistency to multicystic. Cystic tumors vary from 2 to 8 cm in diameter, although some tumors can be larger and involve the majority of individual liver lobes.[4] Cysts contain a clear gray to green fluid that has a watery to viscous or mucinous consistency. Benign biliary neoplasms grow by expansion and are roughly spherical masses that tend to expand and bulge past the normal outline of the liver, although they can occur as intrahepatic masses.

Histological Features

Cholangiomas are gland-like structures formed by tubules lined with cuboidal epithelium and moderate amounts of stroma.[17] The tubules may have narrow lumens or be distended by fluid-forming cystic structures of variable sizes. Biliary cystadenomas typically have a nonencapsulated, multilocular cystic structure (fig. 9.10). Hepatocytes are usually compressed at the margins, but they may be entrapped by expanding cysts and form islands of normal appearing hepatocytes. The stroma of the cyst wall consists of fibrovascular tissue with moderate amounts of

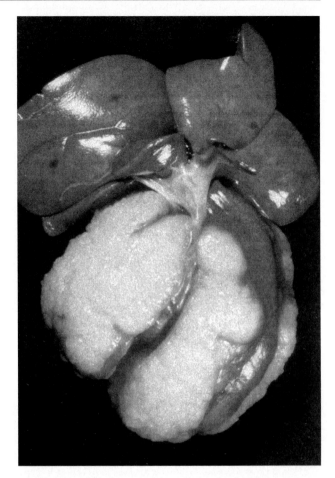

Fig. 9.9. Cholangioma in the liver of a cat. Cholangiomas are well demarcated from the adjacent parenchyma. The natural surface has a fine lobular appearance or may contain multiple, fine, cystic spaces.

collagen. Cysts are lined with benign biliary epithelium, simple cuboidal to flattened. The lining epithelium tends to be more flattened in the biliary cystadenomas, presumably due to compression. Cuboidal biliary epithelial cells have a moderate amount of pale eosinophilic cytoplasm. Nuclei are round to oval, vesicular, and oriented centrally. Nucleoli are small or inapparent. Biliary epithelial cells occasionally line the cystic spaces in multiple layers and may form papillary projections extending into the cystic spaces.

In cats, the lining epithelial cells of biliary cystadenomas have been immunostained with a cocktail of antibodies that recognizes cytokeratins 8,18, and 19, which is typical of normal biliary epithelium, but not of hepatocytes or sinusoidal lining cells of this species.[3]

Differential Diagnosis

Usually, cholangiomas are readily diagnosed on the basis of their well-differentiated appearance, with typical biliary epithelium lining the tubular or cystic structures. They can be distinguished from cholangiocarcinoma on the basis of the degree of differentiation of the lining epithelium and the absence of an invasive pattern of

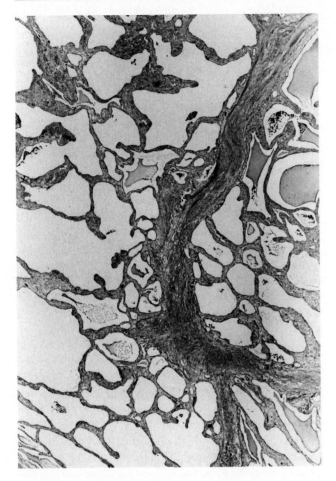

Fig. 9.10. Biliary cystadenoma in the liver of a cat. Biliary cystadenomas are composed of multilocular cystic spaces lined by flattened to cuboidal biliary epithelium. The cyst walls contain variable amounts of fibrous tissue and vascular structures.

growth. Cholangiomas grow by expansion and may compress surrounding parenchyma. There is no local invasion into adjacent hepatic parenchyma or vascular structures.

Some confusion exists concerning the distinction between biliary cysts and biliary cystadenomas. Biliary cysts are usually solitary, with scant supporting stroma. Biliary cystadenomas are typically multicystic and have moderate amounts of stroma.

Growth and Metastasis

Cholangiomas do not metastasize. Progressive expansion of these masses, particularly the cystic variants, can cause significant compression of adjacent hepatic parenchyma. The prognosis for cats with benign biliary tract neoplasia is good following surgical resection.[18]

Etiology

The etiology of cholangiomas is unknown. Certain chemical carcinogens such as nitrosamines can produce this tumor type in dogs[19] and swine.[10]

Cholangiocarcinoma

Incidence

Cholangiocarcinoma (bile duct carcinoma) has been reported in dogs,[1,13,20-23] cats,[2,4,14,24,25] sheep,[9] cattle,[9,12,26] horses,[27] and a goat.[28] Cholangiocarcinomas have not been reported in swine.[9,11,29] These neoplasms are relatively uncommon in all domestic species. Cholangiocarcinomas comprise less than 1 percent of all neoplasms found in dogs and cats, sheep, and horses, but may be more frequent in cattle. The frequency of cholangiocarcinomas in cattle was not consistent in two large surveys conducted at abattoirs. Of 302 neoplasms from cattle in one survey, 22 were cholangiocarcinomas,[9] but only one cholangiocarcinoma was detected among 908 primary bovine neoplasms in another study.[26] Because of their scarcity in most species, estimates of their incidence vary considerably. Consequently, it is not possible to obtain an accurate estimate of the relative frequency of cholangiocarcinoma in these species. The incidence of cholangiocarcinoma in dogs has been estimated to be 1.6 per 100,000 dogs[20] and 0.36 percent of all neoplasms.[23]

There is more information available regarding cholangiocarcinoma in cats and dogs than in other species. Even in these better studied species there are conflicts in the data. The relative frequencies of cholangiocarcinoma and hepatocellular carcinoma in dogs remain uncertain and may vary with the location in which the survey is conducted. In dogs, hepatocellular carcinomas have been reported to be more frequent than cholangiocarcinomas in surveys conducted in the United States[30] and less frequent in other studies from Scandinavia and South Africa.[1,13,15,22] These neoplasms arise within the intrahepatic biliary system much more frequently than in extrahepatic ducts or the gall bladder. Malignant biliary neoplasms are more common than benign neoplasms in dogs.[1] Sixty-five percent of dogs with cholangiocarcinomas are greater than 10 years of age, and a greater number of female than male dogs have been reported with cholangiocarcinoma.[15] However, other studies observed different patterns.[1] Comparison of intact female dogs with male dogs revealed no sex predisposition, although spayed female dogs had a 1.5 times greater risk than intact females.[31]

In cats, cholangiocarcinomas are reported to be the most frequent primary hepatic malignancy in some studies,[4-6,16,25,32] although not all surveys have borne this out.[2,14] As in dogs, cholangiocarcinomas of intrahepatic origin are much more common than those that arise in the extrahepatic bile ducts or gall bladder.[4,16,33-35] Cholangiomas may be as frequent as or more frequent than cholangiocarcinomas in cats, unlike dogs.[5,6,16] Female cats are reported to be at a higher risk for this neoplasm.[2,4] There is no clear breed predilection for cholangiocarcinoma in cats. The age of cats with cholangiocarcinomas is usually greater than 9 to 10 years.[4-6]

There is little information available regarding the incidence of cholangiocarcinomas in food producing animals. Most information comes from studies performed in abattoirs, and younger animals are disproportionately represented. Consequently, the age at which cholangiocarcinomas occur in these species is not clear. A review of cholangiocarcinomas indicates that the age range for affected cattle is 3 to 12 years, with a large proportion occurring in animals around 3 years of age.[9] Cholangiocarcinomas were less frequent than hepatocellular carcinomas in surveys of cattle and sheep, but the overall number of neoplasms were small in both studies.[8,12] Sheep less than 1 year of age can develop cholangiocarcinoma.[36] Tumor-bearing horses generally ranged from 12 to 23 years of age in a series of nine cases.[29]

Clinical Characteristics

The clinical signs for cholangiocarcinoma are nonspecific and are similar for cats and dogs. There is considerable overlap in the clinical signs and laboratory data for cholangiocarcinoma and hepatocellular carcinoma. Lethargy, anorexia, vomiting, weight loss, and dyspnea are most frequently reported. Polydipsia and polyuria occur in some cats.[4] Ascites and hypoalbuminemia are less common than the previously mentioned signs in cats and dogs. A hepatic mass or hepatomegaly can often be palpated.

Clinical chemistry, like the clinical signs, is indicative of liver damage, but does not distinguish among primary hepatic malignancies or distinguish primary from metastatic neoplasms. Alkaline phosphatase was increased in the majority of dogs with cholangiocarcinoma in several reports.[1,15] Aspartate transaminase and alanine transaminase were increased in the majority of dogs in one series[1] but not in another.[15] In cats aspartate transaminase and alanine transaminase can be increased, but serum alkaline phosphatase is only increased rarely, probably due to its shorter half-life in cats compared to dogs.[4-6] Alpha-fetoprotein and bile acids may be increased in dogs with cholangiocarcinoma, but cholangiocarcinoma can not be distinguished from hepatocellular carcinoma by these assays.[37,38] Approximately 10-40 percent of cats and dogs with cholangiocarcinoma are jaundiced.[1,5,6,15,16,21] There is insufficient information available regarding clinical chemistry alterations in cholangiocarcinoma for other species to draw conclusions.

Cholangiocarcinomas can be detected by ultrasonography in dogs.[6,39] In some circumstances canine cholangiocellular carcinomas were distinguished from primary hepatocellular carcinoma because the hepatocellular carcinomas tended to have a focal pattern while cholangiocarcinomas were multifocal.[39] Echogenicity was not particularly helpful because cholangiocellular carcinomas can be hyperechoic, hypoechoic, or have a mixed pattern and are difficult to distinguish from hepatocellular carcinoma or metastatic lesions in the liver.

There is little information available regarding the prognosis for animals with cholangiocarcinoma following chemotherapy or surgery, but the outlook is generally poor.

Isolated masses can be resected, but these neoplasms tend to be multifocal and are frequently spread throughout the liver, making complete resection impossible.

Gross Morphology

Cholangiocarcinomas can have a massive or multinodular appearance.[1,21] Massive lesions can replace an entire liver lobe and extend into adjacent lobes as well (fig. 9.11). In the multinodular form, tumors range from 0.5 to 4 cm in diameter and tend to be scattered throughout all lobes of the liver. Tumors often have an umbilicated appearance, particularly when they protrude above the capsule of the surrounding liver. Larger tumors and massive cholangiocarcinomas are frequently lobulated. The cut surface of the tumors varies from white to gray-white to yellow-brown. The borders of the lesions are generally well delineated from the adjacent hepatic parenchyma, although the border is frequently irregular. Texture is an important gross pathological feature of cholangiocarcinomas. Characteristically, most tumors are firm because of abundant connective tissue that is typical of these neoplasms. This firm texture distinguishes cholangiocarcinoma from hepatocellular carcinomas that are typically soft and friable. Cystic areas containing yellow-brown viscous fluid may be randomly distributed throughout the cholangiocarcinoma. Variant neoplasms that are composed of a high proportion of cystic areas are termed biliary cystadenocarcinomas. Areas of necrosis, characterized by softening of the tissue and reddish discoloration, can be found in the central regions of nodular tumors as well as in focal areas of large single neoplasms.

Although multiple lobes are often affected, there is no evidence that a particular lobe is affected more frequently than any other. It has not been determined if multiple nodules arise from intrahepatic metastasis from one primary lesion or represent multiple sites of independent tumor formation.

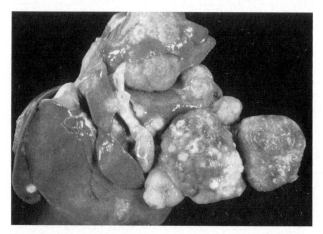

Fig. 9.11. Cholangiocarcinoma in the liver of a cat. Several liver lobes are entirely involved, and nodules of variable size are found scattered in several liver lobes.

Histological Features

The histological features of cholangiocarcinomas are similar in all species.[1,4,17,21,23,36,40] The tumors are composed of cells that retain a resemblance to biliary epithelium. Characteristically, well-differentiated carcinomas are organized into a tubular or acinar arrangement. In less differentiated neoplasms some acinar arrangements can be detected among solid masses of neoplastic cells (fig. 9.12). Poorly differentiated carcinomas are composed of packets, islands, or cords, and areas of squamous differentiation can occur.[17,21] The epithelial components of the neoplasms are usually separated by fibrous connective tissue. The abundance of the connective tissue varies among tumors, but a florid deposition of collagen, termed a *scirrhous response,* is relatively common and is responsible for the firm texture of these neoplasms. The presence of mucin within the lumen of the neoplastic tubules or acini is frequently observed.[1,17,21] The mucin is eosinophilic to weakly basophilic by standard hematoxylin and eosin staining and is readily stained with alcian blue–periodic acid Schiff stain at pH 2.5, indicative of its acidic nature. Bile plugs, occasionally observed in hepatocellular carcinomas, are rare in cholangiocarcinomas.[1,17]

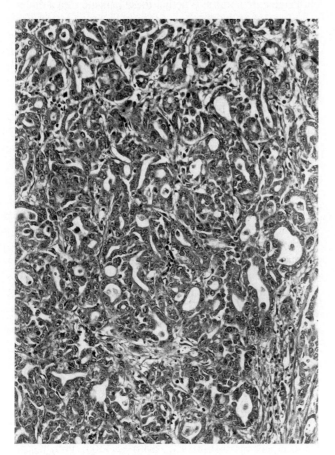

Fig. 9.12. Cholangiocarcinoma from a cat. These neoplasms are composed of small, irregular, gland-like structures or packets of neoplastic cells embedded in connective tissue stroma.

The margins of cholangiocarcinomas are characterized by multiple sites of local invasion by tumor cells of surrounding hepatic parenchyma. Multiple sites of hepatic necrosis are also common in the adjacent parenchyma. Fibrosis produced by the deposition of abundant collagen by activated fibroblasts is an attendant feature of the interface of cholangiocarcinomas with normal hepatic parenchyma.

Similar to its benign counterpart, if there are numerous or large cysts within the neoplasm, these tumors can be designated as bile duct cystadenocarcinomas. The histological characteristics of this variant include the formation of cysts of variable volume lined with single to multiple layers of neoplastic biliary epithelium. The cysts frequently contain an abundant mucinous secretion. Papillary projections extend into the lumen of the cysts. The significance of this histological subdivision of cholangiocarcinomas is probably slight in view of the fact that the biological behavior of the bile duct cystadenocarcinoma is the same as the biological behavior of cholangiocarcinomas.

Histological characteristics of cholangiocarcinomas vary with the degree of differentiation of the neoplasm. Well-differentiated cholangiocarcinomas are composed of cells that retain the characteristics of biliary epithelium. The neoplastic cells, like the normal ductual lining cells, have a moderate amount of clear to pale eosinophilic cytoplasm and are cuboidal to columnar. Tubules or acinar structures may be present. Nuclei are round to oval and vesicular, with a fine reticular pattern to the chromatin. Nucleoli are often inapparent. In less differentiated neoplasms the cells are more pleomorphic. Anaplastic cells are characteristic of the least differentiated cholangiocarcinomas. It is not uncommon to encounter areas that appear benign or well differentiated at the periphery or scattered among anaplastic areas within a neoplasm.[21] Multinuclear tumor giant cells and karyomegaly are not features of this neoplasm. An abundance of mitotic figures is a distinctive feature of cholangiocarcinomas and assists in distinguishing these neoplasms from hepatocellular carcinoma.[1]

Differential Diagnosis

Cholangiocarcinomas are readily distinguished from hepatocellular carcinomas histologically. The typical acinar or tubular composition of the neoplasms and the cuboidal to columnar lining epithelium are usually not difficult to distinguish from hepatocellular carcinomas. The adenoid variant of hepatocellular carcinoma is the most difficult to distinguish from cholangiocarcinoma. However, the presence of desmoplasia, the abundance of mitotic figures, and mucin production by biliary epithelium are additional features that can be used to separate cholangiocarcinomas from adenoid hepatocellular carcinomas. Although the adenoid variant can form acinar structures, the acini are relatively rudimentary, and the lumens of these acini rarely contain a secreted product.

Immunohistochemistry can assist in the identification of poorly differentiated cholangiocarcinoma that occurs within the hepatic parenchyma of cats. Neoplastic biliary epithelial cells, but not hepatocytes, can be stained immunohistochemically with broadly reactive antibody mixtures that recognize high and low molecular weight cytokeratins.[3,16]

Hepatic carcinoids have a distinct histological appearance characterized by alveolar formations with rosettes, ribbons, or solid areas. Because they are neuroendocrine cells, they can be identified by the presence of argyrophilic cytoplasmic granules. Immunohistochemical stains using antibodies that bind to neuron specific enolase in carcinoids can be useful, although this stain may lack the desired specificity. Additional stains to detect neurosecretory products in the cytoplasm of carcinoids can be useful in tumor identification.

Cholangiomas can be distinguished from cholangiocarcinomas on the basis of the well-differentiated appearance of the cells that form cholangiomas. Associated features of cholangiocarcinomas such as local invasion, fibrosis, and increased mitotic index are not found in benign biliary neoplasms.

A greater diagnostic challenge arises when cholangiocarcinomas are to be distinguished from metastatic adenocarcinomas in the liver. The histological characteristics of many gland-forming malignancies overlap, and it can be very difficult to identify the specific tissue of origin. It is possible that at some time in the future, reliable markers, such as tissue-specific cytokeratins, will become available to specifically identify biliary epithelium. Until such markers are available, it is imperative that a thorough postmortem examination be performed to eliminate the possibility of a primary neoplasm in another site before a diagnosis of primary cholangiocarcinoma is made. The patient's record should be reviewed, as well, to determine if there have been previous surgeries, such as removal of mammary masses, that could remove the primary mass and leave only metastatic lesions in the liver and other tissues.

The cytologic characteristics of cholangiocarcinomas can be used to differentiate them from cholangiomas or hepatocellular carcinomas. The typical hallmarks of cholangiocarcinomas include a tendency to exfoliate in dense clusters, a thin rim of cytoplasm, smaller size than neoplastic hepatocytes, and variation in size of cells and nuclei.[41]

Growth and Metastasis

Cholangiocarcinomas have a highly invasive pattern of growth and metastasize frequently. The rate of extrahepatic metastasis in dogs has been reported to be from 60 to 88 percent.[1,42,43] The more frequent sites of metastasis include lymph nodes, lungs, and peritoneal cavity. In cats the rate of metastasis is also high; 11 of 14 cholangiocarcinomas (78 percent) were metastatic in one survey.[4] The lungs, hepatic lymph nodes, and abdominal serosa were the most common sites affected. Metastasis is also common in cattle and sheep,[9,40] and the common sites of metas-

tasis are the same as those in dogs and cats.[29] In all species cholangiocarcinomas can be disseminated throughout the body, and virtually any organ can be affected.[1,21,22,27,29] Cholangiocarcinomas may metastasize within the liver; however, it is not possible to distinguish multiple primary sites of origin from metastasis.

Etiology

Cholangiocarcinomas do not have a recognized cause in domestic animals. Ovariohysterectomized dogs are reported to have a higher risk for cholangiocarcinoma than intact female dogs or male dogs.[31] There is an association between biliary intraductular parasitism and cholangiocellular carcinoma in humans; infection with flukes that inhabit the biliary tract such as *Clonorchis sinensis* is linked to biliary carcinoma.[44] The mechanism by which this parasite may promote tumor development is unknown. In two studies with small numbers of dogs and cats, *Clonorchis sinensis* infection was associated with cholangiocarcinoma in dogs and cats.[24,25] However, the limited nature of these studies makes it difficult to draw clear conclusions regarding the role of parasitism in the pathogenesis of spontaneously occurring cholangiocarcinoma. Intestinal parasites such as *Ancylostoma* sp. and *Trichuris vulpis* have been associated with an increased risk for cholangiocarcinoma.[31] Whether these parasites are a direct cause of neoplasia or serve as a marker for exposure to other agents is not known. Chronic inflammation, regardless of cause, may provoke increased replication of biliary epithelial cells that could facilitate tumor development. For example, adenomatous hyperplasia of biliary epithelium in dogs has been demonstrated in experimentally induced bile stasis and chronic bacterial infection of the bile ducts.[46] Conceivably, neoplasms could arise when similar conditions occur spontaneously and persist.

Carcinogenic chemicals may play a role in the etiology of cholangiocarcinomas. There are several chemicals, such as furans, that can cause malignant transformation of biliary epithelium in rodents.[47] Dogs are susceptible to chemically induced carcinogenesis of the biliary epithelium. When dogs were exposed to nitrosamine and other chemicals such as *o*-aminoazotoluine and aramite, neoplasms of the biliary epithelium developed.[48-50] Data for other species are not available.

REFERENCES

1. Trigo, F.J., Thompson, H., Breeze, R.G., and Nash, A.S. (1982) The pathology of liver tumours in the dog. *J Comp Pathol* 92:21-39.
2. Patnaik, A.K., and Liu, S.-K.H.A.I.M.A.J. (1975) Nonhematopoietic neoplasms in cats. *J Natl Cancer Inst* 54:855-860.
3. Adler, R., and Wilson, D.W. 1995. Biliary cystadenoma of cats. *Vet Pathol* 32:415-418.
4. Carpenter, J.L., Andrews, L.K., and Holzworth, J. (1987) Tumors and tumor-like lesions. In Holzworth, J. (ed.), *Diseases of the Cat*. W.B. Saunders, Philadelphia, p. 406-596.
5. Post, G., and Patnaik, A.K. (1992) Nonhematopoietic hepatic neoplasms in cats: 21 cases (1983-1988). *J Amer Vet Med Assoc* 201:1080-1082.

6. Lawrence, H.J., Erb, H.N., and Harvey, H.J. (1994)) Nonlymphomatous hepatobiliary masses in cats: 41 cases (1972 to 1991). *Vet Surg* 23:365-368.

7. Watt, D.A. (1970) A hepatocholangioma in a sheep. *Aust Vet J* 46:552.

8. Bastianello, S.S. (1982) A survey on neoplasia in domestic species over a 40-year period from 1935 to 1974 in the Republic of South Africa. II. Tumours occurring in sheep. *Onderstepoort J Vet Res* 49:205-209.

9. Anderson, L.J., and Sandison, A.T. (1967) Tumors of the liver in cattle, sheep and pigs. *Cancer* 21:289-301.

10. Graw, J.J., and Berg, H. 1977. Hepatocarcinogenetic effect of DENA in pigs. *Z Krebsforch* 89:137-143.

11. Bastianello, S.S. (1983) A survey on neoplasia in domestic species over a 40-year period from 1935 to 1974 in the Republic of South Africa. III. Tumours occurring in pigs and goats. *Onderstepoort J Vet Res* 50:25-28.

12. Bastianello, S.S. (1982) A survey on neoplasia in domestic species over a 40-year period from 1935 to 1974 in the Republic of South Africa. I. Tumours occurring in cattle. *Onderstepoort J Vet Res* 49:195-204.

13. Bastianello, S.S. (1983) A survey on neoplasia in domestic species over a 40-year period from 1935 to 1974 in the Republic of South Africa. VI. Tumours occurring in dogs. *Onderstepoort J Vet Res* 50:199-220.

14. Bastianello, S.S. (1983) A survey on neoplasia in domestic species over a 40-year period from 1935 to 1974 in the Republic of South Africa. V. Tumours occurring in the cat. *Onderstepoort J Vet Res* 50:105-110.

15. Patnaik, A.K., Hurvitz, A.I., and Lieberman, P.H. (1980) Canine hepatic neoplasms: A clinicopathologic study. *Vet Pathol* 17:553-564.

16. Patnaik, A.K. (1992) A morphologic and immunocytochemical study of hepatic neoplasms in cats. *Vet Pathol* 29:405-415.

17. Ponomarkov, V., and Mackey , L.J. (1976) Tumours of the liver and biliary system. *Bull WHO* 53:187-194.

18. Trout, N.J., Berg, J., McMillan, M.C., Schelling, S.H., and Ullman, S.L. (1995) Surgical treatment of hepatobiliary cystadenomas in cats: Five cases (1988-1993). *J Amer Vet Med Assoc* 206:505-507.

19. Allison, J.B., Wase, A.W., Leathem, J.H., and Wainio, W.W. 1950. Some effects of 2-acetylaminofluorene on the dog. *Cancer Res* 10:266-271.

20. MacVean, D.W., Monlux, A.W., Anderson, P.S., Jr., Silberg, S.L., and Rozel, J.F. 1978. Frequency of canine and feline tumors in a defined population. *Vet Pathol* 15:700-715.

21. Patnaik, A.K., Hurvitz, A.I., Lieberman, P.H., and Johnson, G.F. (1981) Canine bile duct carcinoma. *Vet Pathol* 18:439-444.

22. Rooney, J.R. (1959) Liver carcinoma in the dog. *Acta Pathol Microbiol Scand* 45:321-330.

23. Strafuss, A.C. (1976) Bile duct carcinoma in dogs. *J Amer Vet Med Assoc* 169:429.

24. Hou, P.C. (1964) Primary carcinoma of bile duct of the liver of the cat infested with *Clonorchis sinensis*. *J Pathol Bactiol* 87:239-244.

25. Schmidt, R.E., and Langham,. R.F. (1967) A survey of feline neoplasms. *J Amer Vet Med Assoc* 151:1325-1328.

26. Monlux, A.W., Anderson, W.A., and Davis, C.L. (1956) A survey of tumors occurring in cattle, sheep and swine. *Amer J Vet Res* 17:646-677.

27. Messow, C. (1952) Die Lebertumoren unserer Haussäugetiere. *Wiss Z Humbolt-Univ Berlin* 2:121-152.

28. Chauhan, H.V.S., and Singh , C.M. (1969) Bile duct carcinoma in a goat with metastasis in the lungs. *Indian Vet J* 46:945-946.

29. Rehmtulla, A.J. (1974.) Occurrence of carcinoma of the bile ducts: A brief review. *Can Vet J* 15:289-291.

30. Mulligan, R.M. (1949) In Mulligan, R.M. (ed.), *Neoplasms of the Dog*. Williams and Wilkins Co., Baltimore, pp. 111-114.

31. Hayes, H.M., Morin, M.M., and Rubenstein, D.A. 1983. Canine biliary carcinoma: Epidemiological comparisons with man. *J Comp Pathol* 93:99-107.

32. Whitehead, J.E. (1967) Neoplasia in the cat. *Vet Med Small Anim Clin* 62:357-358.

33. Feldman, B.F., Strafuss, A.C., and Gabbert, N. (1976) Bile duct carcinoma in the cat: Three case reports. *Feline Prac* (Jan):33-39.

34. Barsanti, J.A., Higgins, R.J., Spano, J.S., and Jones, B.D. (1976) Adenocarcinoma of the extrahepatic bile duct in a cat. *J Small Anim Pract* 17:599-605.

35. Haines, V.L., Brown, P.R., Hruban, R.H., and Huso, D.L. (1996) Adenocarcinoma of the hepatopancreatic ampulla in a domestic cat. *Vet Pathol* 33:439-441.

36. Cordes, D.O., and Shortridge, E.H. (1971) Neoplasms of sheep: A survey of 256 cases recorded at Ruakura Animal Health Laboratory. *N Z Vet J* 19:55-64.

37. Lowseth, L.A., Gillett, N.A., Chang, I.Y., Muggenburg, B.A., and Boecker, B.B. (1991) Detection of serum alpha-fetoprotein in dogs with hepatic tumors. *J Amer Vet Med Assoc* 199:735-741.

38. Center, S.A., Baldwin, B.H., Erb, H.N., and Tennant, B.C. (1985) Bile acid concentrations in the diagnosis of hepatobiliary disease in the dog. *J Amer Vet Med Assoc* 187:935-940.

39. Whiteley, M.B., Feeney, D.A., Whiteley, L.O., and Hardy, R.M. (1989) Ultrasonographic appearance of primary and metastatic canine hepatic tumors: A review of 48 cases. *J Ultrasound Med* 8:621-630.

40. Strafuss, A.C., Vestweber, J.G.E., Njoku, C.O., and Ivoghli, B. 1973. Bile duct carcinoma in cattle. *Amer J Vet Res* 34:1203-1205.

41. Blue, J.T., French, T.W., and Meyer, D.J. 1999. The liver. In Cowell, R., Tyler, R.L., and Meinkoth, J.M. (eds.), *Diagnostic Cytology and Hematology of the Dog and Cat*. Mosby, St. Louis, pp. 183-194.

42. Patnaik, A.K., Hurvitz, A.I., Lieberman, P.H., and Johnson, G.F. (1981) Canine hepatocellular carcinoma. *Vet Pathol* 18:427-438.

43. Montali, R.J., Hoopes, P.J., and Bush, M. (1981) Extra-hepatic biliary carcinomas in asiatic bears. *J Natl Cancer Inst* 66:603-608.

44. Hou, P.C. (1956) The relationship between primary carcinoma of the liver and infestation with *Clonorchis sinensis*. *J Pathol Bactiol* 72:239-246.

45. Hou, P.C. (1965) Hepatic clonorchiasis and carcinoma of the bile duct in a dog. *J Pathol Bacteriol* 89:365-367.

46. Ohta, T., Nagakawa, T., Ueda, N., Nakamura, T., Kayahara, M., Ueno, K., Miyazaki, I., Terada, T., and Nakanuma, Y. (1991) Adenomatous hyperplasia of the bile duct epithelium of the canine liver, caused by bacterial infection. *Scan J Gastroenterol* 26:1107-1114.

47. Maronpot, R.R., Giles, H.D., Dykes, D.J., and Irwin, R.D. 1991. Furan-induced hepatic cholangiocarcinomas in Fischer F344 rats. *Toxicol Pathol* 19:561-570.

48. Hirao, K., Matsumura, K., Imagawa, A., Enomoto, Y., Hosogi, Y., Kani, T., Fujikawa, K., and Ito, N. (1974) Primary neoplasms in dog liver induced by diethylnitrosamine. *Cancer Res* 34:1870-1882.

49. Nelson, A.A., and Woodward, G. (1953) Tumors of the urinary bladder, gall bladder and liver in dogs fed *o*-aminoazotoluine and *p*-dimethylaminoazobenzene. *J Natl Cancer Inst* 13:1479-1509.

50. Sternberg, S.S., Popper, H., Oser, B.L., and Oser, M. (1966) Gallbladder and bile duct adenocarcinomas in dogs after long term feeding of aramite. *Cancer* 13:780-789.

Adenomas and Carcinomas of the Gall Bladder

Incidence

Adenomas of the gall bladder are rare in all species with the exception of cattle. Gall bladder adenomas were one of the more common epithelial neoplasms of the liver found in surveys of cattle conducted at abattoirs.[1-3] There are a few reports of gall bladder adenomas in cats and dogs,[5-7] but not in other species. Carcinomas of the gall bladder may occur more often than adenomas, but they are, none the less, very[5,8-10] uncommon. Carcinomas of the gall bladder are reported in dogs,[9,16] cats,[4,11,12] and cattle.[3,13] There are individual reports describing gall bladder carcinomas in swine.[1,14] A neuroendocrine carcinoma has been reported in the gall bladder of a dog.[15]

Failure to carefully inspect the gall bladder as part of routine necropsies may partially account for the small number of tumors of this structure, but it seems likely that the limited number of cases described derives from the rarity of tumor development in this site. In a 40-year retrospective study of canine neoplasia, a single gall bladder carcinoma was reported.[9] Cattle with gall bladder adenomas and carcinomas were all young, but this would be expected in a survey conducted at an abattoir.[3] There is insufficient information to ascribe any breed, age, or sex predilection for neoplasms of the gall bladder.

Clinical Characteristics

There is little information available concerning the clinical effects of gall bladder carcinomas because they are uncommon. Nonspecific signs such as weakness, abdominal distention, and anorexia are reported in cats.[4]

Gross Morphology

Most benign and some malignant neoplasms of the gall bladder extend into the lumen, and may distend it, but do not alter the serosal surface. These neoplasms can only be detected by palpating or incising the gall bladder at necropsy. Gross pathological descriptions of gall bladder adenoma in cats and cattle are similar.[3,4,13] They are often pedunculated and attached to the fundic portion of the gall bladder by a thick stalk. The masses are yellow to red or gray. They are often firm, with a rugose surface containing numerous infoldings or cystic spaces. In cattle they are about 5-7 cm in diameter, and at this size they can distort the gall bladder.

Carcinomas of the gall bladder are more likely to disrupt the structure of the gall bladder and are more apparent from the serosal surface. Carcinomas are firm and white and may have numerous convolutions. They have an aggressive growth pattern that typically invades the wall of the gall bladder and may extend into the adjacent liver parenchyma.[3,4,12,13] Intramural mineralization of the gall bladder has been associated with gall bladder carcinoma in the dog.[16]

Histological Features

These tumors are essentially extrahepatic biliary adenomas and cholangiocarcinomas, and the histological features are similar to those described earlier for those tumors.[3,13,17] Some adenomas have papillary projections that extend into the lumen of the gall bladder (fig. 9.13). Cystic variants of these neoplasms, termed *papillary cystadenomas,* occur. The lining cells of the acini have a tall

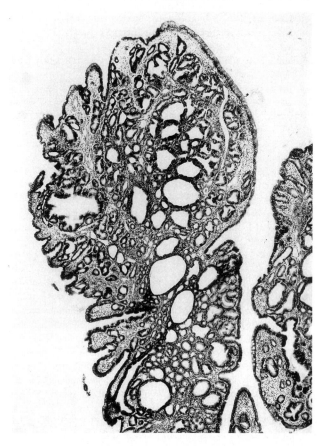

Fig. 9.13. Papillary adenoma of the gall bladder in a cat. The papillary structures are covered by columnar epithelium resembling normal gall bladder epithelium. (Courtesy of Dr. R.C. Cattley and Auburn University, Alabama)

columnar profile typical of normal gall bladder epithelium, and they may contain abundant apical mucin, which imparts a clear appearance to the cytoplasm in hematoxylin and eosin stained sections. Nuclei are basal, and mitotic figures are rare. Unlike the malignant counterpart of this neoplasm, the tumor stroma is not abundant, and when present, it is composed of loose, often edematous, connective tissue. Small numbers of infiltrating lymphocytes may be present, but significant inflammation is not a component of this neoplasm.

Gall bladder adenocarcinomas are composed of acinar and tubular structures that are separated by thin fibrous stroma. Some areas of the neoplasm may contain abundant fibrous tissue typical of the scirrhous response that can be provoked by biliary neoplasia within the liver. Within the glandular areas of the tumor there may be accumulations of mucus. The lining cells are similar to those in other areas of the biliary tract, cuboidal to columnar with moderate amounts of eosinophilic cytoplasm, but more pleomorphic than benign biliary neoplasms. Cytoplasmic and extracellular mucin can be abundant. Nuclei are basally oriented and vesicular and have a single prominent nucleoli. Necrosis can be scattered within the mass.[4,10] Despite the aggressive behavior of these neoplasms, the mitotic index is typically low[10,17] Necrosis within the neoplasm is common. The growth of these neoplasms is invasive; the neoplastic cells penetrate the wall of the gall bladder and invade adjacent hepatic parenchyma. Adenomatous hyperplasia of adjacent regions of the gall bladder mucosa has been described in cats.[4,12]

Growth and Metastasis

Gall bladder adenomas grow by expansion and are often pedunculated. Growth usually occurs into the lumen of the gall bladder with little effect on other tissues.

Carcinomas of the gall bladder have an invasive pattern of growth. They invade the wall of the gall bladder and can extend into the nearby hepatic parenchyma. Metastasis is common and frequently affects the serosal surfaces of the abdominal cavity, lymph nodes, lungs, and liver.[4,10,12,13]

Etiology

The cause of gall bladder neoplasia is unknown. The gall bladder epithelium of dogs, like intrahepatic biliary epithelium, is susceptible to several carcinogenic chemicals such as *o*-aminoazotoluine, methylcholanthrene, aramite, and others, but none of the recognized carcinogens of the biliary tract are likely to be encountered outside of experimental settings.[3] Cholelithiasis has been associated with gall bladder carcinoma in humans, but there is no support for this pathogenesis of gall bladder carcinoma in animals.

Cystic Hyperplasia of the Gall Bladder

Incidence and Clinical Characteristics

Cystic hyperplasia of the gall bladder mucosa has only been reported in dogs and sheep. It is an age-associated lesion in dogs and occurs in response to progestational compounds.[18,19] There is an association with pregnancy and these lesions in sheep.[20] The average age of dogs with spontaneous cystic hyperplasia is 10.5 years.[18] Although age has been established as a significant factor for the development of this lesion in dogs, there is insufficient information available to establish the incidence of this lesion or to determine any breed or sex predilections.

Cystic hyperplasia of the gall bladder is an incidental lesion, and there are no clinical signs in affected dogs or sheep.

Gross Morphology

In all likelihood, cystic hyperplasia of the gall bladder frequently goes undetected. There are no apparent abnormalities evident from the exterior of the gall bladder, and the features of cystic hyperplasia can only be appreciated by opening the gall bladder and draining residual bile that may obscure the mucosa. Affected mucosa is gray-white when the bile is rinsed away and has a diffusely

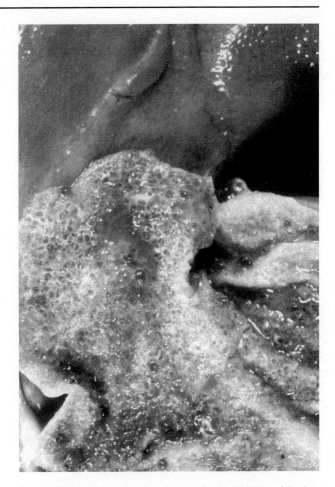

Fig. 9.14. Cystic mucinous hyperplasia of the gall bladder of the dog. This process creates a thickened gall bladder mucosa with a characteristic honeycombed appearance.

thickened, sponge-like consistency (fig. 9.14). Numerous 1 to 3 mm cysts within the hyperplastic mucosa impart the characteristic appearance. Occasionally, large cysts occur, and they are evident as papillary projections into the lumen of the gall bladder.

Histological Features

The hallmark of cystic hyperplasia of the gall bladder is the abundance of variably sized cystic spaces that distort and thicken the entire mucosa of the gall bladder.[18] The cysts are lined with a single layer of epithelial cells (fig. 9.15). Most of the cysts contain a copious amount of mucus. The majority of the lining epithelial cells are typical of the normal gall bladder epithelium, tall columnar with abundant apical cytoplasmic mucus. However, epithelial cells that face the lumen of the gall bladder may be cuboidal, and in uncommon instances, foci of squamous metaplasia can be identified. The mucus in the cells and in the cysts is easily detected with a PAS stain. Hyperplastic epithelium may form papillary projections that extend from the mucosa into the lumen of the gall bladder. Mitotic figures are rare and have a normal appearance when they are

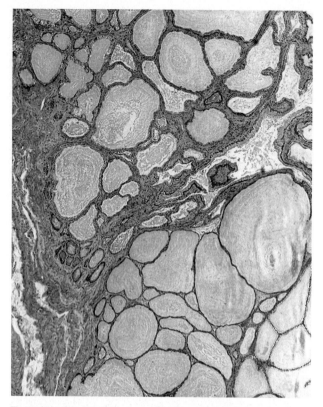

Fig. 9.15. The histologic appearance of cystic mucinous hyperplasia of the gall bladder is characterized by numerous mucus filled, variably sized, cystic spaces lined with gall bladder epithelium.

found. The mucosa may have a scant lymphoid infiltrate, or there may be no evidence of inflammation.[17,18] The stroma may be thickened by hypertrophy of smooth muscle cells.

Etiology

The cause of cystic hyperplasia of the gall bladder is not known. This lesion, like many other idiopathic hyperplastic lesions (nodular hyperplasia of the liver, exocrine pancreas, adrenal cortex, and perianal hepatoid glands) is age related. An abundance or dysregulation of growth factors has been proposed as a possible common thread in the pathogenesis of age-related hyperplastic lesion, but definitive work is needed in this area.[21] Hormonal factors may play a role in this lesion. Cystic hyperplasia of the gall bladder in sheep is associated with pregnancy and may be related to prolonged exposure to progesterone or its metabolites.[20] Some support for this theory is derived from a case report of a dog that had cystic hyperplasia of the gall bladder and was receiving progestational compounds.[19] However, due to the clinically silent nature of cystic hyperplasia, it may have been present prior to drug administration and was a spontaneous change.[5]

REFERENCES

1. Anderson, L.J., and Sandison, A.T. (1967) Tumors of the liver in cattle, sheep and pigs. *Cancer* 21:289-301.

2. Rao, P.R., Christopher, J., and Sastry, G.A. (1964) Cholangiocellular carcinoma in an ewe. *Indian Vet J* 41:197-199.

3. Anderson, W.A., Monlux, A.W., and Davis, C.L. 1958. Epithelial tumors of the bovine gall bladder: A report of eighteen cases. *Amer J Vet Res* 19:58-65.

4. Carpenter, J.L., Andrews, L.K., and Holzworth, J. (1987) Tumors and tumor-like lesions,. In Holzworth, J. (ed.), *Diseases of the Cat.* W.B. Saunders, Philadelphia, pp. 406-596.

5. Hayes, H.M., Morin, M.M., and Rubenstein, D.A. (1983) Canine biliary carcinoma: Epidemiological comparisons with man. *J Comp Pathol* 93:99-107.

6. Goodpasture, E.W. (1918) An anatomical study of senescence in dogs, with especial reference to the relation of cellular changes of age to tumors. *J Med Res* 38:127-190.

7. Stalker, L.K., and Schlotthauer, C.F. (1936) Papillary adenoma of the gall-bladder in two dogs: Intrahepatic gall-bladder in one. *J Amer Vet Med Assoc* 89:207-212.

8. Trigo, F.J., Thompson, H., Breeze, R.G., and Nash, A.S. (1982) The pathology of liver tumours in the dog. *J Comp Pathol* 92:21-39.

9. Bastianello, S.S. (1983) A survey on neoplasia in domestic species over a 40-year period from 1935 to 1974 in the Republic of South Africa. VI. Tumours occurring in dogs. *Onderstepoort J Vet Res* 50:199-220.

10. Patnaik, A.K., Hurvitz, A.I., Lieberman, P.H., and Johnson, G.F. 1981. Canine bile duct carcinoma. *Vet Pathol* 18:439-444.

11. Patnaik, A.K., and Liu, S.-K.H.A.I.M.A.J. (1975) Nonhematopoietic neoplasms in cats. *J Natl Cancer Inst* 54:855-860.

12. Patnaik, A.K. (1992) A morphologic and immunocytochemical study of hepatic neoplasms in cats. *Vet Pathol* 29:405-415.

13. Monlux, A.W., Anderson, W.A., and Davis, C.L. (1956) A survey of tumors occurring in cattle, sheep and swine. *Amer J Vet Res* 17:646-677.

14. Ito, T., Miura, S., Ohshima, K., and Numakunai, S. (1972)) Fine structure of hepatocellular carcinoma in swine. *Jpn J Vet Sci* 34:33-37.

15. Willard, M.D., Dunstan, R.W., and Faulkner, J. (1988) Neuroendocrine carcinoma of the gallbladder in a dog. *J Amer Vet Med Assoc* 192:926-928.

16. Bromel, C., Smeak, D.D., and Leveille, R. (1998) Porcelain gallbladder associated with primary biliary adenocarcinoma in a dog. *J Amer Vet Med Assoc* 213:1137-1139.

17. Ponomarkov, V., and Mackey, L.J. (1976) Tumours of the liver and biliary system. *Bull WHO* 53:187-194.

18. Kovatch, R.M., Hildebrandt, P.K., and Marcus, L.C. (1965) Cystic mucinous hypertrophy of the mucosa of the gallbladder in the dog. *Vet Pathol* 2:574-584.

19. Mawdesley-Thomas, L.E., and Noel, P.R.B. (1967) Cystic hyperplasia of the gall bladder in the beagle associated with administration of progestational compounds. *Vet Rec* 80:658-659.

20. Fell, B.F., Robinson, J.J., and Watson, M. (1983) Cystic hyperplasia of the gall bladder in breeding ewes. *J Comp Pathol* 93:171-178.

21. Cotran, R.S., Kumar, V., and Collins, T. (1999) Neoplasia. In Cotran, R.S., Kumar, V., and Collins, T. (eds.), *Pathologic Basis of Disease.* W.B. Saunders, Philadelphia, pp. 260-327.

Hepatic Carcinoids

Incidence and Clinical Characteristics

Carcinoids of the liver, extrahepatic bile ducts, and the gall bladder are rare neoplasms in domestic animals, but have been reported in dogs,[1,2] cats,[3] and one cow.[4] Because they are so uncommon, there is insufficient information to make determinations on age, breed, or sex predilections. In dogs, carcinoids appear to occur at a younger age than other primary hepatic neoplasms.[1]

Clinical signs associated with hepatic carcinoids

have only been reported for dogs. The signs are nonspecific and include anorexia, ascites, weight loss, diarrhea, and jaundice.[1] In dogs, hepatomegaly is seen less often in cases of carcinoid than with hepatocellular carcinoma or cholangiocarcinoma.[1] Increased activity of liver related enzymes in the serum occurs in dogs with carcinoids, but there is no specific pattern of enzyme change.

Gross Morphology

In the dog, hepatic carcinoids can form large masses or multiple nodules scattered throughout the liver, and most of the lobes of the liver tend to be involved. Generally, they are firm gray to tan masses with areas of necrosis and hemorrhage scattered throughout. A carcinoid that arose in the gall bladder formed a papillary mass within the lumen.[2] There are no distinguishing gross features to definitively identify this tumor.

Histological Features and Differential Diagnosis

The tumors are presumed to originate from neuroendocrine cells that reside in the bile ducts or gall bladder. The neoplasms are composed of uniform oval to spindle shaped cells with hyperchromatic round or oval nuclei[4] and abundant granular eosinophilic cytoplasm.[1] Hepatic carcinoids, like other endocrine cell neoplasms, form small aggregates or nests of cells that are separated by fine fibrovascular stroma (fig. 9.16). Cells tend to be oriented toward their basement membrane, forming a rosette or pseudolobular pattern. Areas of abundant fibrosis, often containing areas of hyalinized collagen or foci of mineralization, may be scattered throughout the tumors. Mitotic figures are usually frequent. Suspected carcinoid tumors should be stained by silver impregnation to detect typical argyrophilic cytoplasmic granules. When carcinoids are stained by immunohistochemical methods they are usually negative for cytokeratin and typically contain neuron specific enolase.[3] Other cell types may also stain with antibodies to neuron specific enolase, so more precise identification of carcinoids can be obtained by detecting neurosecretory products, such as glucagon or serotonin, in their cytoplasmic granules. However, suspect tumors have to be examined for more than one type of neurosecretory product since these cells may express any of several types of products.

Hepatic carcinoids can be confused with other primary neoplasms of the liver. Cholangiocarcinomas pose the greatest challenge in this regard, since these two neoplasms can have a similar gross pathological appearance. While cholangiocarcinomas form massive lesions more frequently than carcinoids, and carcinoids are often diffuse, both neoplasms can have a multinodular pattern.[1] Both hepatic carcinoids and cholangiocarcinomas form firm nodules that may have central necrosis with umbilication. Areas of hemorrhage and necrosis, however, are more frequent in carcinoids than in cholangiocarcinomas. Cystic spaces containing mucinous to gelatinous material are

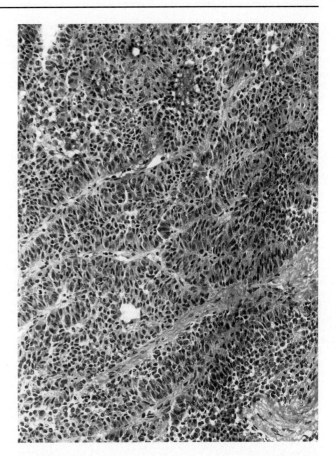

Fig. 9.16. Hepatic carcinoid from the liver of a cat. Hepatic carcinoids form nests of cells separated by fine fibrovascular stroma. Cells can form a pseudolobular pattern due to their orientation toward their basement membrane.

another gross pathological feature characteristic of cholangiocarcinomas that may help distinguish them from carcinoids, since this lesion is not typical of carcinoids.

There can be some overlap in the histological morphology of carcinoids and cholangiocarcinoma, although the features are usually distinct. Variants of carcinoids can form rosettes with a central lumen that can resemble the tubules of cholangiocarcinoma. In cases that can not be resolved by histology alone, special stains can be helpful. Mucin, demonstrated by the PAS stain, is common in cholangiocarcinomas but is not a feature of carcinoids. In carcinoids that lack abundant granules, immunohistochemical stains can be used. Neuron specific enolase is typically present in carcinoids, but it can also be found in cholangiocarcinomas and in a variety of other tissues, limiting the value of this antigen.[3] Preliminary work in cats suggests that cytokeratins are absent in carcinoids and present in cholangiocarcinomas and therefore may serve to distinguish carcinoids from cholangiocarcinoma.[3]

Hepatocellular and biliary neoplasms can be readily distinguished from carcinoids based on histological, histochemical, and if needed, immunohistochemical staining characteristics. However, distinguishing a primary hepatic carcinoid from a metastatic endocrine neoplasm is a difficult task. A thorough postmortem examination is necessary to determine if there are other sites affected and if these sites are the primary neoplasm.

Growth and Metastasis

Hepatic carcinoids are aggressive neoplasms with an invasive pattern of growth that is characterized by extension into the peritoneum. Virtually all carcinoids have metastasized by the time of necropsy.[3] Intrahepatic spread is frequent, and most tumors have a diffuse pattern of distribution within the liver. Metastasis to local lymph nodes occurs in the majority of cases. Diffuse peritoneal involvement is frequent, and spread to the lungs and other organs occurs less often.

REFERENCES

1. Patnaik, A.K., Lieberman, P.H., Hurvitz, A.I., and Johnson, G.F. (1981) Canine hepatic carcinoids. *Vet Pathol* 18:445-453.
2. Willard, M.D., Dunstan, R.W., and Faulkner, J. (1988) Neuroendocrine carcinoma of the gallbladder in a dog. *J Amer Vet Med Assoc* 192:926-928.
3. Patnaik, A.K. (1992) A morphologic and immunocytochemical study of hepatic neoplasms in cats. *Vet Pathol* 29:405-415.
4. Ponomarkov, V., and Mackey, L.J. (1976) Tumours of the liver and biliary system. *Bull WHO* 53:187-194.

MESENCHYMAL TUMORS OF THE LIVER

Hemangiosarcoma

Incidence and Clinical Characteristics

Primary hemangiosarcoma has been reported in the liver of dogs[1-6] and cats.[7-9] There is a single report of a hemangiosarcoma in a sheep[10] and an individual report of a vascular neoplasm, probably benign, in a pig.[11] Fewer than 5 percent of primary hepatic neoplasms in dogs are hemangiosarcomas.[1,5] In cats, hemangiosarcomas are estimated to comprise from 0[12] to 6-12 percent of primary hepatic neoplasms.[7,13,14] The variability may result from two factors: the low incidence of these neoplasms making an accurate estimation difficult to obtain, and the difficult task of determining the primary site of the hemangiosarcoma when more than one organ is involved. It is the third most frequent primary hepatic neoplasm in the liver of dogs and cats in several surveys[1,5,7,13,14] and the most common metastatic tumor in dogs in another.[15] Primary hemangiosarcoma in the liver of other species is very rare.

Most dogs with primary hepatic hemangiosarcomas are more than 10 years old.[16] There are too few primary hepatic hemangiosarcomas reported to determine a breed predilection, but German shepherds are the breed most commonly affected with hemangiosarcomas when all primary sites are considered, and they may, therefore, be at

the greatest risk for primary hepatic hemangiosarcoma.[4]

There is limited information available on the clinical course of primary hepatic hemangiosarcoma. Rapid clinical deterioration has been reported in two affected dogs.[5] Hepatic and/or splenic hemangiosarcomas may bleed intermittently, and degrees of anemia may range from mild to severe. They are also associated with massive hemoperitoneum, fatal blood loss, and sudden death. Other than these presentations, clinical signs are nonspecific and include dullness, anorexia, and abdominal enlargement.

Gross Morphology

Primary hepatic hemangiosarcomas have the same gross pathological characteristics of hemangiosarcomas that arise in other sites[2,5] (fig. 9.17). The color of the masses is determined by the amount of perfusion, since it is blood that imparts the dark red hue. Some hemangiosarcomas are white to light yellow and may have a mottled appearance on cut surfaces. Other masses with a greater blood supply or areas of necrosis are dark red and fluctuant, or contain cystic structures. Blood or blood tinged fluid runs freely

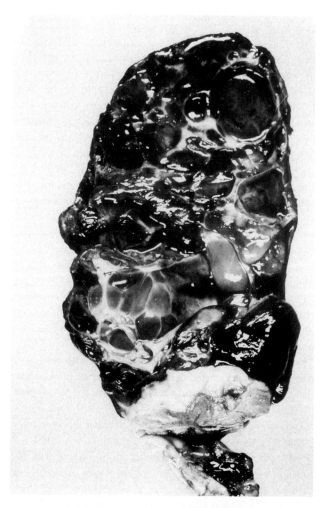

Fig. 9.17. Hemangiosarcoma in the liver of a dog. This lesion contains numerous large, blood filled, cystic spaces. (Courtesy of Dr. B.G. Short.)

from the cut surface of these masses. Tumors range from 1 mm to 10 cm in diameter. They may occur as large single masses within the liver or as multiple masses throughout the liver. The multiple sites may arise from multiple primary sites or as the result of intrahepatic metastasis.

Histological Features and Differential Diagnosis

Hemangiosarcomas are composed of neoplastic endothelial cells. The endothelial cells may line large, cystic, vascular spaces; form numerous small caliber capillary-like spaces; or form solid masses that may contain only small clefts. Each of these patterns may be found within an individual neoplasm. The vascular spaces formed by these cells are fragile and prone to hemorrhage, necrosis, and thrombus formation. The cells may resemble normal endothelial cells with a spindle shaped outline, but more often they tend to be hyperchromatic and large, with a plump cellular profile that bulges into the vascular lumen. Pleomorphism is common. The nuclear to cytoplasmic ratio is higher than that of normal endothelial cells, and mitotic figures are frequent.

Distinguishing primary hepatic hemangiosarcoma from metastatic lesions is a diagnostic challenge. There are no clear guidelines to determine the primary site of origin for hemangiosarcomas that have multiple organ involvement. The histological appearance of the neoplasms is rarely, if ever, a useful guide to determining which of several masses is the primary neoplasm. Frequently, the largest mass is presumed to be the oldest, and therefore the primary, lesion. This assumption may not be correct in all circumstances since limits on tumor growth may vary from site to site. For example, growth conditions in the liver or spleen may be more supportive for tumor cells than the right atrial appendage of the heart or subcutaneous sites. These issues await clarification by advances in tumor biology. The possibility of multicentric origin of hemangiosarcomas should also be considered when confronted with multiple organ involvement.

Solid hemangiosarcomas can often be distinguished from other types of sarcomas by the presence of the endothelial cell marker factor VIII–related antigen.[17] Staining can be detected in the large majority of hemangiosarcomas as well as in virtually all normal and benign endothelial cells, but not in other mesenchymal neoplasms. Hemangiosarcomas can be distinguished from hemangiomas by the same criteria used to identify malignant endothelial cells in other sites.

In cattle, vascular hamartomas, a developmental anomaly characterized by abnormal proportions or mixing of normal tissue, have been described as entities distinct from hemangiomas.[18] The hamartomas were characterized by the presence of abundant stroma, aberrant blood vessels with papillary infoldings, the presence of arteries and veins, and the loss of hepatic parenchyma in affected sites. Areas of telangiectasia can be distinguished from vascular neoplasms by the well-differentiated appearance of the endothelial cells.

Growth and Metastasis

Primary hepatic hemangiosarcomas in cats and dogs are aggressive neoplasms with a markedly invasive growth pattern.[5,7] The borders of tumor masses extend into adjacent parenchyma along the interface with the normal tissue. Because these tumors are composed of endothelial cells, it seems intuitive that they can more readily enter the blood stream than other tumor types that have to penetrate blood or lymph vessels to gain access to the circulation. This fact may account for the frequent dissemination of this neoplasm to many tissues within the body. The lungs, kidney, and abdominal lymph nodes are common sites of tumor spread in dogs.[5] Spread to the peritoneum can also occur.

Sarcomas and Other Mesenchymal Tumors

Other than hemangiosarcomas, primary sarcomas of the liver are rare. Leiomyosarcomas and fibrosarcomas of the liver have been reported in dogs[5,16,19] and cats.[7,13,20] Experimental administration of diethylnitrosamine to dogs has produced primary fibrosarcomas.[19] Rare cases of primary osteosarcoma[16,21] and a malignant mesenchymoma have been reported in dogs.[22] Dogs with primary hepatic sarcomas are usually greater than 10 years of age.[5,16] No sex or breed predilection has been determined for any of these sarcomas because of their rarity. Single cases of primary hepatic rhabdomyosarcoma, hepatic lymphangioma, and hepatic plasmacytoma have also been reported in cats.[23-25] Individual cases of fibrosarcoma[26] and a hemangiopericytoma[11] have been reported in cattle. There are no characteristic clinical signs associated with primary sarcomas of the liver, other than hemangiosarcomas, due to the limited number of reported cases.

Primary sarcomas of the liver have the same gross characteristics as other sarcomas that arise in more frequently affected sites. With the exception of primary osteosarcoma in the dog[21] and rhabdomyosarcoma in the cat,[25] primary hepatic sarcomas tend to be firm and pale white on the natural and cut surface. These neoplasms may be aggressive and involve adjacent structures in the gastrointestinal tract. The histological appearance of primary sarcomas of the liver is typical of the cell of origin.

Differential Diagnosis, Growth, and Metastasis

The key issue in the diagnosis of primary sarcomas of the liver is distinguishing metastatic lesions from primary neoplasms. Without a thorough postmortem examination it is impossible to be certain if a given neoplasm within the liver is a primary lesion. Histology alone is insufficient to determine if a given neoplasm is primary or metastatic. In general, the presence of multiple neoplasms within the liver suggests a metastatic origin, since neither multiple primary neoplasms nor intrahepatic spread of a rare hepatic sarcoma are likely. As discussed earlier with regard to hemangiosarcomas, multicentric origin can not be discounted as an explanation for tumors found in several organs or in multiple sites within a single organ.

Primary hepatic sarcomas tend to have an invasive pattern of growth that is typical for mesenchymal malignancies. Invasion of local tissue and metastasis has been reported for these tumors. The spleen appears to be a frequent site of metastasis in the dog.[16]

Myelolipoma

Myelolipoma of the liver is rare and has only been reported in domestic and wild cats.[7,27-31] Cheetahs appear to develop this neoplasm more often than other wild felids based on the limited literature on myelolipomas.[30]

There are no specific clinical signs that would suggest the presence of myelolipomas. They are only detectable as an incidental lesion during laparotomy or necropsy.

Gross Morphology and Histological Features

Myelolipomas are usually found as multiple growths that may be located in more that one lobe of the liver. They frequently protrude above the surface of the liver, but they also may be found deep in the hepatic parenchyma. They vary in size from several millimeters to several centimeters in diameter; their shape is often spherical. The surface is usually irregular and nodular. Myelolipomas are generally light yellowish gray or light orange. Portions of the tumors may be dark red due to hemorrhage, and they usually have a soft and friable consistency.

The neoplasm is composed of mature and normal appearing adipose and myeloid tissue (figs. 9.18 and 9.19). The edge of the mass is frequently irregular, with the adipose cells interdigitating with relatively normal hepatocytes. In other growths, a fine fibrous capsule may be observed. Focal areas of hemorrhage are sometimes found throughout the tumor.

The relative proportion of adipose and myeloid tissue is extremely variable between tumors or even between different areas within the same tumor. However, there is usually more myeloid tissue than adipose tissue in the growth. Mature and immature cells of the granulocytic, erythrocytic, and megakaryocytic series are found within the myeloid component. The proportion of the various cell types is variable.

There is no differential diagnostic problem with this neoplasm because the histology is characteristic. It is considered to be neoplastic on the basis of its expansile characteristics. Myelolipomas must be differentiated from areas of hepatic lipidosis, particularly if there is extramedullary hematopoiesis present. Little information is available on the biological characteristics of hepatic myelolipomas. The well-differentiated histological pattern of the tumor suggests that multiple sites of tumor within the same liver rep-

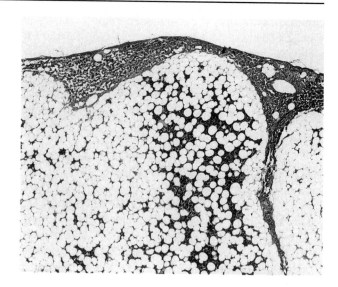

Fig. 9.18. Myelolipoma in the liver of a cat. The lesion resembles normal bone marrow.

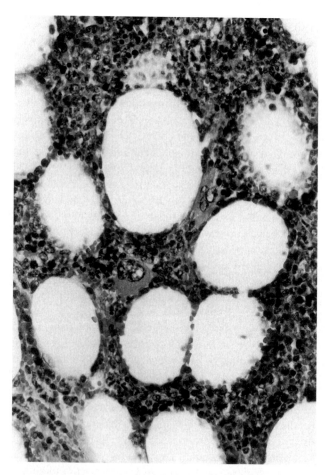

Fig. 9.19. Myelolipoma from the liver of a cat. Myelolipomas are characterized by the presence of focal aggregates of adipocytes admixed with myeloid elements. (Courtesy of Dr. D.P. Shaw.)

resent separate primary neoplasms rather than intrahepatic metastases. The irregular borders of the tumor have been interpreted as evidence of invasive potential. Metastasis to other organs has not been reported.

REFERENCES

1. Bastianello, S.S. (1983) A survey on neoplasia in domestic species over a 40-year period from 1935 to 1974 in the Republic of South Africa. VI. Tumours occurring in dogs. *Onderstepoort J Vet Res* 50:199-220.

2. Benjamin, S.A., Hahn, F.F., Chiffelle, T.L., Boecker, B.B., Hobbs, C.H., Jones, R.K., McClellan, R.O., and Snipes, M.B. (1975) Occurrence of hemangiosarcomas in beagles with internally deposited radionuclides. *Cancer Res* 35:1745-1755.

3. Brown, N.O., Patnaik, A.K., and MacEwen, E.G. (1985) Canine hemangiosarcoma: Retrospective analysis of 104 cases. *J Amer Vet Med Assoc* 186:56-58.

4. Priester, W.A. (1976) Brief communication: Hepatic angiosarcomas in dogs: An excessive frequency as compared with man. *J Natl Cancer Inst* 57:451-454.

5. Trigo, F.J., Thompson, H., Breeze, R.G., and Nash, A.S. (1982) The pathology of liver tumours in the dog. *J Comp Pathol* 92:21-39.

6. Waller, T., and Rubarth, S. (1967) Haemangioendothelioma in domestic animals. *Acta Vet Scand* 8:234-261.

7. Carpenter, J.L., Andrews, L.K., and Holzworth, J. (1987) Tumors and tumor-like lesions, p. 406-596. In Holzworth, J. (ed.), *Diseases of the Cat*. W.B. Saunders, Philadelphia.

8. Messow, C. (1952) Die Lebertumoren unserer Haussaugetiere. *Wiss Z Humbolt-Univ Berlin* 2:121-152.

9. Patnaik, A.K. and S.-K.H.A.I.M.A.J. Liu. (1975) Nonhematopoietic neoplasms in cats. *J Natl Cancer Inst* 54:855-860.

10. Bastianello, S.S. (1982) A survey on neoplasia in domestic species over a 40-year period from 1935 to 1974 in the Republic of South Africa. II. Tumours occurring in sheep. *Onderstepoort J Vet Res* 49:205-209.

11. Anderson, L.J., and A.T. Sandison. (1967) Tumors of the liver in cattle, sheep and pigs. *Cancer* 21:289-301.

12. Bastianello, S.S. (1983) A survey on neoplasia in domestic species over a 40-year period from 1935 to 1974 in the Republic of South Africa. V. Tumours occurring in the cat. *Onderstepoort J Vet Res* 50:105-110.

13. Patnaik, A.K. (1992) A morphologic and immunocytochemical study of hepatic neoplasms in cats. *Vet Pathol* 29:405-415.

14. Post, G., and A.K. Patnaik. (1992) Nonhematopoietic hepatic neoplasms in cats: 21 cases (1983-1988). *J Amer Vet Med Assoc* 201:1080-1082.

15. Strombeck, D.R., and W.G. Guilford. (1996) Hepatic neoplasms. In Guilford, W.G., Center, S.A., Strombeck, D.R., Williams, D.A., and Meyer, D.J. (eds.), *Small Animal Gastroenterology*. W.B. Saunders Co., Philadelphia, pp. 847-859.

16. Patnaik, A.K., Hurvitz, A.I., and Lieberman, P.H. (1980) Canine hepatic neoplasms: A clinicopathologic study. *Vet Pathol* 17:553-564.

17. Von Beust, B.R., Suter, M.M., and Summers, B.A. (1988) Factor VIII-related antigen in canine endothelial neoplasms: An immuno-histochemical study. *Vet Pathol* 25:251-255.

18. Ladds, P.W. (1983) Vascular hamartomas of the liver of cattle. *Vet Pathol* 20:764-767.

19. Hirao, K., Matsumura, K., Imagawa, A., Enomoto, Y., Hosogi, Y., Kani, T., Fujikawa, K., and Ito, N. (1974) Primary neoplasms in dog liver induced by diethylnitrosamine. *Cancer Res* 34:1870-1882.

20. Lawrence, H.J., Erb, H.N., and Harvey, H.J. (1994) Nonlymphomatous hepatobiliary masses in cats: 41 cases (1972 to 1991). *Vet Surg* 23:365-368.

21. Jeraj, K., Yano, B., Osborne, C.A., Wallace, L.J., and Stevens, J.B. (1981) Primary hepatic osteosarcoma in a dog. *J Amer Vet Med Assoc* 179:1000-1003.

22. McDonald, R.K., and Helman, R.G. (1986) Hepatic malignant mesenchymoma in a dog. *J Amer Vet Med Assoc* 188:1052-1053.

23. Larsen, A.E., and Carpenter, J.L. (1994) Hepatic plasmacytoma and biclonal gammopathy in a cat. *J Amer Vet Med Assoc* 205:708-710.

24. Lawler, D.F., and Evans, R.H. (1993) Multiple hepatic cavernous lymphangioma in an aged male cat. *J Comp Pathol* 109:83-87.

25. Minkus, G., and Hillemanns, M. (1997) Botryoid-type embryonal rhabdomyosarcoma of liver in a young cat. *Vet Pathol* 34:618-621.

26. Bastianello, S.S. (1982) A survey on neoplasia in domestic species over a 40-year period from 1935 to 1974 in the Republic of South Africa. I. Tumours occurring in cattle. *Onderstepoort J Vet Res* 49:195-204.

27. Schuh, J.C.L. (1987) Hepatic nodular myelolipomatosis (myelolipomas) associated with a peritoneo-pericardial diaphragmatic hernia in a cat. *J Comp Pathol* 97:231-235.

28. Gourley, M., Popp, J.A., and Park, R.D. (1971) Myelolipomas of the liver in a domestic cat. *J Amer Vet Med Assoc* 158:2053-2056.

29. Ikede, B.O., and Downey, R.S. (1972) Multiple hepatic myelolipomas in a cat. *Can Vet J* 13:160-163.

30. Lombard, L.S., Fortna, H.M., Garner, F.M., and Brynjolfsson, G. (1968) Myelolipomas of the liver in captive wild felidae. *Vet Pathol* 5:127-134.

31. McCaw, D.L., da Silva Curiel, J.M.A., and Shaw, D.P. (1990) Hepatic myelolipomas in a cat. *J Amer Vet Med Assoc* 197:243-244.

METASTATIC NEOPLASIA

Metastatic tumors in the liver are more common than primary neoplasms in most species, except sheep.[1] In the dog, metastatic neoplasms are approximately three times more common than primary liver tumors.[2] In dogs, and probably most other species, the liver is the most common organ to be involved in metastasis, exceeding the lung and lymph nodes by a small margin.[3] Hepatic metastasis was reported to occur in over 30 percent of malignant neoplasms in dogs.[3] Lymphoma is the most common type of neoplasm to metastasize to the liver in dogs,[3] (table 9.2),

TABLE 9.2. Classification of metastatic tumors of the canine liver

Tumors	Number of Cases
Hematopoietic	
Lymphoma	71
Myeloid leukemia	7
Malignant mastocytosis	2
Monocytic leukemia	1
Total	81
Carcinomas	
Pancreatic	9
Adrenal	3
Thyroid	3
Gastric	2
Mammary	2
Ovarian	2
Squamous cell	2
Other carcinomas	4
Total	27
Sarcomas	
Hemangiosarcoma	15
Fibrosarcoma	4
Melanosarcoma	1
Osteosarcoma	1
Total	21

Number of animals
Modified from Trigo, F.J., Thompson, H., Breeze, R.G., and Nash, A.S. (1982) The pathology of liver tumours in the dog. *J Comp Pathol* 92:21-39.

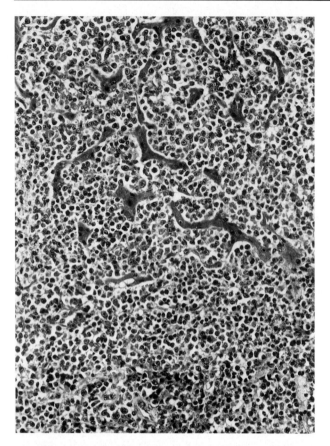

Fig. 9.20. Myeloid malignancy of the liver of a dog. These neoplasms typically infiltrate the sinusoids of the liver. Their presence is associated with local atrophy of hepatocytes.

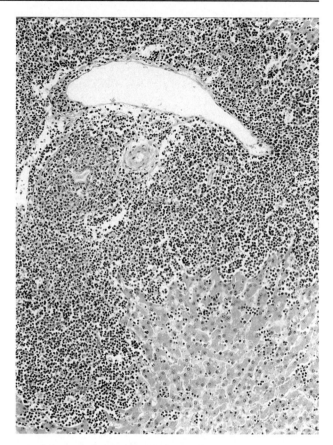

Fig. 9.21. Lymphoma in the liver of a cat. Neoplastic lymphocytes accumulate in the portal areas and often expand into adjacent hepatic parenchyma. Central vein areas may also be infiltrated.

TABLE 9.3.   Metastatic tumors of the liver of cattle, sheep, and pigs

Animals	Total No. of Tumors	Primary Hepatic Tumors	Metastatic Hepatic Tumors	Proportion of Lymphomas
Cattle	302	36	50	19/50
Sheep	107	32	18	10/18
Pigs	139	6	46	42/46

Number of animals examined: cattle, 1.3 million; sheep, 4.5 million; pigs, 3.7 million.

Modified from *Cancer* (1967) 21:289–301. © Am Cancer Soc. Reprinted with permission, Wiley-Liss, Inc., subsidiary of John Wiley & Sons, Inc.

cattle, sheep, and pigs (table 9.3).[1] There is one report that indicates that hemangiosarcoma is the most common metastatic lesion in the liver of dogs, although this may reflect the difficult task of distinguishing primary and metastatic forms of hemangiosarcoma.[4] In dogs, pancreatic carcinoma is the most common metastatic epithelial malignancy in the liver.[3]

The histological appearance of metastatic epithelial neoplasms usually corresponds to the tumor of origin. Spindle cell sarcomas and matrix producing sarcomas such as osteosarcomas that metastasize to the liver also resemble the cells of origin. The gross appearance of metastatic round cell sarcomas such as lymphomas and myeloid malignancies is characterized by uniform expansion of the liver, although nodular forms of these neoplasms can also occur. Despite the similar gross appearance of these neoplasms in the liver, there is a typical histological appearance for each. Neoplastic myeloid cells are usually distributed along the sinusoids of affected livers and can compress hepatocytes, thereby causing atrophy (fig. 9.20). When lymphoma involves the liver, the neoplastic lymphocytes are usually found within the portal tracts or within the connective tissue surrounding the central vein (fig. 9.21). Neoplastic lymphocytes may considerably expand the borders of affected portal tracts.

REFERENCES

1. Anderson, L.J., and Sandison, A.T. (1967) Tumors of the liver in cattle, sheep and pigs. *Cancer* 21:289-301.
2. Strombeck, D.R. (1978) Clinicopathologic features of primary and metastatic neoplastic disease of the liver in dogs. *J Amer Vet Med Assoc* 173:267-269.
3. Trigo, F.J., Thompson, H., Breeze, R.G., and Nash, A.S. (1982) The pathology of liver tumours in the dog. *J Comp Pathol* 92:21-39.
4. Strombeck, D.R., and Guilford, W.G. (1996) Hepatic neoplasms. In Guilford, W.G., Center, S.A., Strombeck, D.R., Williams, D.A., and Meyer, D.J. (eds.), *Small Animal Gastroenterology.* W.B. Saunders Co., Philadelphia. pp. 847-859.

10 Tumors of the Urinary System

D. J. Meuten

RENAL NEOPLASMS

Primary renal neoplasms are uncommon in domestic animals. The two most common primary neoplasms are renal cell carcinoma and embryonal nephroma (nephroblastoma). Primary renal tumors may be multiple or bilateral and have a multicentric origin in cattle and dogs. The most common neoplasm in the kidneys of domestic animals is lymphoma, due to the common occurrence of this systemic tumor. There is a unique tumor in the thoracolumbar segments of the spinal cord in young dogs (primarily German shepherds) that is interpreted as nephroblastoma and arises from rests of renal anlage. Nodular dermatofibrosis occurs as a familial disease in German shepherds and is associated with renal cell adenocarcinomas.

An immunohistochemical marker that has been used to diagnose and study renal tumors in animals and people is uromodulin (Tamm-Horsfall protein), which is a unique protein synthesized exclusively in the kidney.[1] Antibodies directed against various epitopes of tumor associated glycoprotein (TAG-72) have been used to identify a variety of carcinomas in humans, including those of urothelial origin. In dogs, greater than 50 percent of pulmonary, nasal, mammary, and transitional cell carcinomas stain positively to one of the epitopes of TAG (Mab B72.3).[2] This antibody did not stain normal or hyperplastic transitional epithelium, which is in contrast to results in people. Urine concentration of basic fibroblast growth factor has been used in dogs as a noninvasive indicator of transitional cell carcinoma.[3] This is a proangiogenic peptide used to detect tumor progression and is in high concentrations in urine from humans with urinary and nonurinary tumors.[4]

Epithelial Tumors

Approximately 75-90 percent of primary renal neoplasms in dogs are of epithelial origin,[5,6] which is similar to the archival material from North Carolina State University and cases retrieved through the Purdue Veterinary Medical Data Base (table 10.1). Although 90 percent of the epithelial neoplasms are classified as malignant based on light microscopy or gross size (greater than 2 cm), this distinction is difficult and arbitrary and may have led to overclassification of carcinomas. Regardless, reported metastatic rates of approximately 60 percent in dogs indicates that metastases occur, and much more frequently than is reported in cattle with renal cell tumors. Most renal cell tumors in cattle are greater than 2 cm in diameter, but only 5 percent metastasize.[7] Renal cell tumors are considered malignant in horses and cats; however, relatively few cases have been studied. The cells of origin are considered to be the proximal convoluted tubular epithelium and the collecting duct.[14,26]

The combined data from four sources totaled 464 primary renal neoplasms in dogs (table 10.2), and indicated 76 percent of which were epithelial, 16 percent mesenchymal, and 8 percent mixed; 91 percent were classified malignant, and 9 percent benign.[5,6,8]

From the archival material in the Veterinary Medical Data Base (VMDB) 579 canine and 252 feline renal tumor

TABLE 10.1. Renal neoplasia

| | Total | Primary (%) | Primary | | Both | Secondary |
			Epithelial	Mesenchymal		
Canine	579	181 (32) Benign Malignant	141 (75) 5 (3) 136 (97)	40 (21) 12 (30) 28 (70)	6 (4)	392 (68)
Feline	252	30 (12) Benign Malignant	23 (77) 0 23	7 (23) 0 7		222 (88)

181 primary canine neoplasms, 164 (91%) classified malignant.
30 primary feline neoplasms, 100% classified malignant.
392 secondary neoplasms in dogs: 91 lymphoma, 120 adenocarcinoma, 121 hemangiosarcoma.
222 secondary neoplasms in cats: 196 lymphoma.

diagnoses were retrieved. For dogs, 181 (32 percent) were primary renal neoplasms; 91 percent were classified as malignant, 124 as carcinoma (adenocarcinoma was the most common diagnosis), and 6 as nephroblastomas (tables 10.1 and 10.2). There were twice as many secondary tumors in dogs, 392 (68 percent); 121 were hemangiosarcoma, 120 were carcinoma, and 91 were lymphoma. In cats, 30 of 252 (12 percent) were primary tumors and 222 (88 percent) were secondary, of which 196 were lymphoma (table 10.1). The canine population base for this study was approximately 467,000, and the feline population was 144,900, for incidences of 0.16 percent and 0.2215 percent in dogs and cats, respectively, which is similar to published rates. Two reports summarizing 73 cases in cats reported renal carcinomas were the most common tumor (28), followed by nephroblastomas (18) and sarcomas (15).[8,9] Archival material from the VMDB indicated that 23 of 30 primary renal tumors in cats were epithelial (77 percent), and all of these were malignant; 7 of 30 were mesenchymal (23 percent). There were 252 diagnoses of feline renal tumors, and 99 percent of all tumors were classified as malignant. A report of relatively few cases in cats indicates renal cell tumors are 4.5 times more frequent than in dogs.[10]

Renal cell tumors are rare in other species. Most primary tumors are epithelial, and they are considered benign in cattle and malignant in horses. Twenty-nine tumor diagnoses were retrieved through the VMDB from a population base of 134,268 horses; 11 were primary and 18 secondary. The population base was 73,195 cattle, with 16 tumor diagnoses, 3 primary and 13 secondary; 7265 sheep with 2 tumors, both secondary; and 7764 goats with two tumors, one each primary and secondary.

Most articles that summarize renal tumors list the different morphological diagnoses but generally do not separate clinical information for each histological diagnosis. Those that provide this information by tumor diagnosis indicate the differences are slight or none, and the number of animals in each group is small. The information on clinical characteristics and incidence in this section is more reflective of renal tumors in general, than of a specific histological type of tumor.

Adenoma

Incidence

This is a rare tumor in domestic animals, and when found it usually is an incidental lesion at necropsy or slaughter because these tumors are clinically silent.[7,11,18] Of 464 primary renal cancers in dogs, there were 13 (3 percent) classified as adenoma (see table 10.2). There are no studies on actual incidence, age, breed, or sex predilection for renal adenomas, although there is some data for renal tumors in food animals. Over an 11 year period, 20 renal cell tumors were identified in approximately 13,500 cattle processed for slaughter.[7] All 20 cows were adults, 2-20 years of age. Nineteen of 20 cows had multiple tumors; 11 of these were visualized grossly, and 8 others were microscopic. Only one tumor metastasized, and one tumor was classified as an adenoma (8 x 10 mm single lesion in one kidney). The authors discussed the difficulties of distinguishing adenoma from carcinoma. They suggested the renal tumors in these cattle were carcinomas, based on the multiplicity of tumors, and indicated they may develop in multiple sites within the kidneys. The occurrence of metastases in only one cow was a clearly different biological behavior from the high rate of metastases seen in renal carcinomas in humans, dogs, and horses.

TABLE 10.2.   Primary renal neoplasia in dogs

	1	2	3	4	Total (%)
Tumors, n	181	175	54	48	464
Carcinoma, n(%)	124 (66)	113 (65)	35 (65)	31 (65)	303 (65)
Adenoma	4	3	1	5	13 (3)
TCC	12	0	5	4	21 (5)
Papilloma	1	0	3	2	6 (1)
Undifferentiated CA	0	0	2	0	2 (0.4)
Nephroblastoma	6	26	2	2	36 (8)
SCC	0	9	0	0	9 (2)
Fibroma	9	2	1	0	12 (3)
Fibrosarcoma	5	2	0	2	9 (2)
Hemangioma/sarcoma	0	10	1	1	12 (3)
Lymphoma	0	0	1	1	2 (0.4)
Undifferentiated SA	22	4	3	0	29 (6)
Leiomyoma	3	1	0	0	4 (1)
Rhabdomyosarcoma	1	1	0	0	1 (0.2)
Epithelial	141 (75)	125 (71)	46 (85)	42 (88)	355 (76)
Mesenchymal	40 (21)	23 (13)	6 (11)	4 (8)	72 (16)
Mixed	6 (4)	27 (15)	2 (4)	2 (4)	37 (8)
Benign	17 (9)		5 (9)	8 (16)	37 (9)
Malignant	170 (91)		49 (91)	40 (84)	398 (91)

1 = VMDB - Veterinary Medical Data Base.
2 = *Current Veterinary Therapy VIII* 1980:1203; 1 each - leiomyosarcoma, lipoma, reticulum cell sarcoma, teratoma.
3 = *J Amer Anim Hosp Assoc* 24:443, 1988.
4 = *Vet Pathol* 14:591, 1977.

Gross Morphology and Histological Features

Adenomas are discrete, solitary, tan to white tumors located in the renal cortex (fig. 10.1 A). In dogs and cats they are small (usually < 2 cm), but in horses and cattle tumors may be large (> 6 cm) and have central areas of hemorrhage and necrosis. Tumors may only be found if the kidneys are sliced in multiple areas. On cut surface they are well demarcated and bulge, and only larger neoplasms have discolored necrotic centers. Bilateral and/or multiple adenomas occur, especially in dogs[12] and cows.[7] A distinct entity is associated with dermatofibrosis in German shepherds; the renal adenomas in these dogs are almost always multiple, and there is concurrent renal adenocarcinoma.[12]

Tumors are nonencapsulated but sharply demarcated from the adjacent cortex. They are composed of well-differentiated tubules and acini that may be subclassified as tubular, papillary, or solid based on the major histological pattern: central or elongated lumens (tubular type); papillary growths of varying sizes that project into lumens (papil-lary) (see fig. 10.2 A); or solid sheets. Mixtures of all three types can occur, but this is seen more frequently with renal carcinoma. Cytological and nuclear features are uniform and benign. A single layer of cubodial epithelial cells with

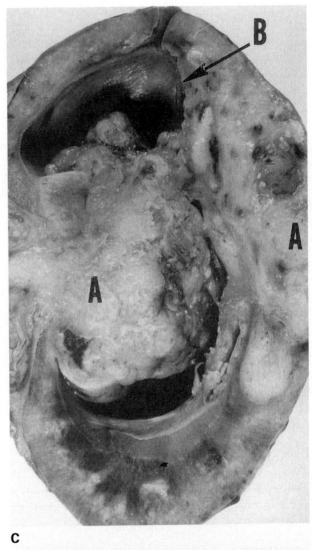

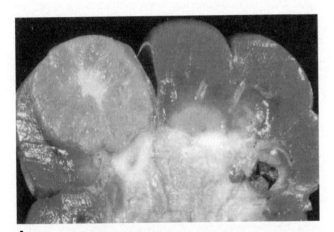

A

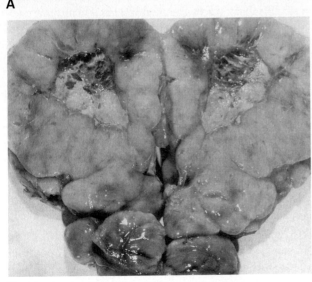

B

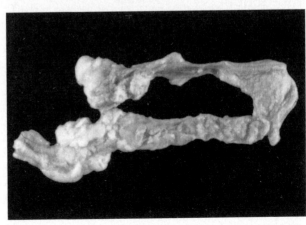

C

D

Fig. 10.1. A. Renal adenoma in a cow is singular, has expanded one lobule, is well demarcated, and is paler than unaffected lobules. **B.** Effacement of the kidney by a renal cell carcinoma in a dog. **C.** Renal carcinoma in the cortex and pelvis *(A)* associated with hydronephrosis *(B)*. **D.** Ureter with implantation metastasis in a dog with transitional cell carcinoma, hydroureter, and hydronephrosis.

ample eosinophilic cytoplasm lines tubules or papillary projections. Nuclei are single, placed centrally or basally, and have a single nucleolus; mitotic figures are not observed or found rarely. There is a paucity of supporting stroma, usually thin strands at the base of tubules. Corpora amylacea are common in renal cell tumors of cattle.

Growth and Metastases

The histological distinction of renal adenoma from carcinoma is difficult, because carcinomas may be well differentiated. Some pathologists use an arbitrary cutoff of 2 cm as a criterion of malignancy: less than 2 cm adenoma, greater than 2 cm carcinoma. In dogs and cats this may be useful, but in cattle many tumors are greater than 2 cm in diameter, yet in a report of 20 renal cell tumors only one metastasized. The criterion of size is based on older information in renal tumors in humans.[13] Renal adenomas and carcinomas have not been studied with techniques that identify rapid cell turn over. Neither adenomas nor carcinomas have a capsule. Multiplicity of tumors suggests a malignant classification or metastases from a nonrenal organ, lung, prostate, or mammary. However, 19 of 20 bovine renal cell tumors were multiple, and only one of these metastasized. Carcinomas that are large and infiltrative and have cellular and nuclear atypia are easy to classify. They are distinguished from adenomas that are smaller, sharply demarcated, noninvasive, and composed of well-differentiated epithelium with no to few mitoses. Gradations of the two can make clear distinction difficult, and whether these are true features of adenoma or can be present in well-differentiated carcinomas needs to be proven.

Carcinoma

General Considerations

These are malignant epithelial tumors without any embryonal differentiation. They have also been classified as renal cell carcinoma, malignant nephroma, clear cell carcinoma, hypernephroma, and Grawit's tumor.[14]

Incidence

Renal carcinoma is an uncommon tumor in domestic animals, but it is the most common primary renal tumor in dogs, cats, and horses. The reported incidence for dogs is 1.5 in 100,000 and for cats 0.7 in 100,000.[15] Other reported incidences include 0.3-1.5 percent for dogs[5] and 0.2-0.5 percent for cats.[9] A retrospective study found 4 (0.05 percent) in 8149 canine tumors and 3 (0.23 percent) in 1299 feline neoplasms, suggesting that in this limited number of cases renal carcinoma was 4.5 times more frequent in cats than in dogs.[10] Table 10.2 summarizes four studies, and of 464 canine neoplasms, 303 were classified as renal cell carcinoma (65 percent), 21 as transitional cell carcinoma (TCC), and 2 as undifferentiated carcinoma. The percentage of renal carcinomas in these four studies is remarkably similar. Two studies report 73 renal neoplasms in cats that consisted of 28 renal carcinomas, 18 nephroblastomas,

15 sarcomas, 5 transitional cell carcinomas, 2 each adenoma, squamous cell carcinoma, and leiomyosarcoma, and 1 undifferentiated carcinoma.[8,9]

There are several case reports and a few summaries of renal carcinoma in horses.[16-20] In archival material only four tumors were identified in the kidneys of 3633 horses (0.11 percent), two renal cell carcinoma (0.055 percent), one renal adenoma, and one mesenchymal tumor.[18] The reported incidence of 0.11 percent (4/3633) for renal tumors and 0.055 percent for renal cell carcinoma is similar to citations in the older literature of 62 in 40,000 necropsies.[18] Abattoir surveys report rates of 8.5, 4.3, and 0.9 renal tumors per million animals in cattle, pigs, and sheep, respectively.[21] Over an 11 year period, 20 renal cell tumors were identified in 13,500 cattle processed for slaughter. One tumor was classified as an adenoma, a single 8 x 10 mm mass in one kidney, and the other 19 were considered carcinomas even though only one tumor metastasized.[7] The diagnosis of carcinoma was based on multiplicity of tumors.

Age, Breed, and Sex

Primary renal tumors are reported to occur in middle aged male dogs (mean age 8-9 years), and there are no breed predilections.[5,6] Nearly all reports suggest a male predominance in dogs, approximately 2:1. In humans the incidence of renal tumors is two to five times greater in males.[14] In cats renal tumors (all types) tend to occur in the 8-year-old age group (range 2-13 years) and in males.[8] A summary of 15 cases in horses reported they ranged in ages from 4 to 20 years, with seven cases in horses less than 10 years old.[16] There were no breed or sex predilections. Twenty cows with renal cell tumors ranged in age from 2 to 20 years.[7]

Clinical Characteristics

In ruminants the tumors are usually asymptomatic or at least they are undetected antemortem. In horses they may be asymptomatic or associated with colic, weight loss, hematuria (most common lab abnormality), ascites/hemoperitoneum, and edema.[16-20] A mass can be palpated per rectum in approximately half of the equine cases. In dogs and cats the most common clinical problems are an abdominal mass (50 percent), weight loss, hematuria (50-100 percent), pollakiuria, and proteinuria (75 percent), often associated with other nonspecific problems such as lethargy, vomiting, and anorexia.[5,6,8] Azotemia is a common finding but probably involves superimposed prerenal (dehydration) or renal (concurrent disease) components.[6] One report provides information on clinical characteristics, laboratory data, and diagnostic evaluation by histologic groups.[6] Most results are similar across groups; notable differences were that hematuria was more common with TCC than with renal tubular cell tumors, and none of the eight dogs with TCC had detectable metastases at the time of initial diagnosis.

By the time these tumors produce clinically detectable problems in dogs, cats, and horses the tumor is advanced and malignant. Metastatic disease can be detected with thoracic radiographs in approximately 50 percent of dogs with renal carcinomas at initial presentation. Ultrasound or intravenous pyelograms are reported to correctly detect a mass in 80-100 percent of the cases, depending on the host and location of the tumor.[6] Abdominal radiographs will detect a mass in 80 percent of the cases, and in 50 percent of these the mass can be identified in a kidney.[6,8] Searching for tumor cells in urine is generally futile.

Secondary absolute polycythemia has been reported infrequently with renal tumors.[22,23] The increased red blood cell mass is due to the production and secretion of erythropoietin or erythropoietin-like peptide from the tumor. Packed cell volume will be increased in the range of 60-70 percent in dogs and will return to reference range post tumor removal. This syndrome is associated with renal adenoma, carcinoma, nephroblastoma, transitional cell carcinoma, fibrosarcoma, and lymphoma as well as nonneoplastic lesions such as cysts and hydronephrosis.

Gross Morphology

Most carcinomas are unilateral, but they can be bilateral, and neither kidney is more predisposed.[7,12,24,27] They are well-demarcated masses, yellow, tan-brown to cream colored, often located at one pole, and they vary considerably in size, from 2 cm in diameter to occupying greater than 80 percent of one kidney (see fig. 10.1 B). The smaller the tumor is, the more difficult it is to differentiate from adenoma. Large masses have expected areas of necrosis and hemorrhage and are friable due to little supporting stroma. Larger neoplasms invade the renal pelvis and enter blood vessels and may infiltrate perinephric tissues (see fig. 10.1 C). Rarely, they infiltrate through the retroperitoneal space and spread by implantation metastasis through the abdomen. Multiplicity of tumors is a feature of dogs, cattle, and humans; however, some tumors are only found during microscopic examination. Nineteen of 20 cows with renal cell neoplasia had multiple tumors; 11 of these were visualized grossly, and 8 others were microscopic. Canine tumors can be cystic, and the cysts contain variable amounts of clear or red-brown fluid.

Histological Features

Although these tumors are subdivided into histological and cytological types, there is no known difference in their biological behavior. The terms *papillary, tubular,* and *solid* refer to the predominant type of histological organization, but mixtures of these types can be present in one tumor (see fig. 10.2 A-D). The most common variety seen in domestic animals is tubular. Each of these histological types can be further classified as chromophobic, eosinophilic, or clear cell, and mixtures of all three are usually present. When present, foci of clear cells aid in the identity of renal cell origin. Perhaps the only classification worthy of effort is to differentiate renal adenocarcinoma from transitional carcinoma of the pelvis. The distinguishing histological features are the formation of elongated,

irregular, tubules with lumens. Variations on this produce round acini with lumens, solid acini, sheets, and lobules. Interstitial stroma ranges from mild, with just enough stroma for tubules to rest on, to marked desmoplastic reactions. If present, a capsule is not complete. Tumors tend to grow by pushing at the edges more than by infiltrating. Cellular morphology has a range of patterns depending on the degree of differentiation. The more differentiated varieties resemble adenoma and have one or two layers of well differentiated eosinophilic cells lining tubules (fig. 10.2 D). Metastases may be as fully differentiated as the primary tumor. Less differentiated varieties have the expected features of reduced cytoplasmic area, indistinct cell borders, nuclear crowding, multiple cells piled together, various sizes and shapes of nuclei, mitoses, and vesicular chromatin (fig. 10.2 C). Hemosiderin, proteinaceous secretions, and corpora amylacea are features of renal cell tumors in cattle. Cysts of various sizes are features of these tumors. Cysts may be empty or contain a lightly stained homogenous product.

Clear cell variants are seen more frequently in laboratory animals and human beings but are observed rarely in cattle and dogs as the predominant cellular constituent. The distinctive feature is a "clear" cytoplasm in H&E stained sections, due to their high glycogen and lipid content (fig. 10.2 E,F). They tend to be solid rather than tubular. Cell borders are usually distinct, cytoplasm is abundant, and nuclei are round and dense, providing the appearance of a well-differentiated tumor. The clear cytoplasm and solid growth that resembles adrenal cortical tissue led to the name *hypernephroma*. Foci of clear cells can be found in many renal cell tumors if they are searched for.

The eosinophilic cell type is a variant of a chromophobe renal carcinoma in which the cytoplasm is intensely eosinophilic. Both have abundant, granular, lightly or intensely eosinophilic cytoplasm with cuboidal shaped cells that form trabeculae of various widths, usually without lumens. This is the most common variant in cattle (19/20 cattle tumors eosinophilic, clear cell 1/20). The eosinophilic variant and oncocytomas look similar with H&E. Oncocytomas have numerous mitochondria and an absence of cytoplasmic vesicles, and they are positive to cytokeratin but negative to vimentin.[24] Renal cell carcinomas in humans are reported to be cytokeratin and vimentin positive.[14,24] Human tumors stain light blue with histochemical stains for colloidal iron.[14] Occasional renal carcinomas in animals have a marked desmoplastic reaction in which tumor cells may be encased in connective tissue. Differentiation from sarcoma requires immunohistochemical staining positive for vimentin and negative for cytokeratin; if both are positive the diagnosis is renal carcinoma.

Growth and Metastases

Ninety percent of renal epithelial tumors in dogs are classified as malignant; metastases are detected in 50–60 percent of canine cases; and in one report 37 of

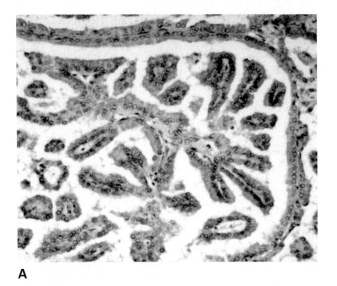

A

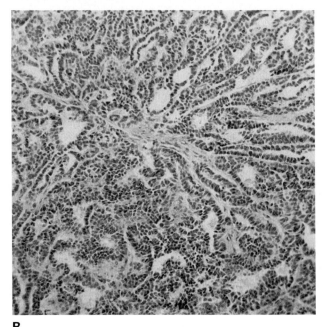

B

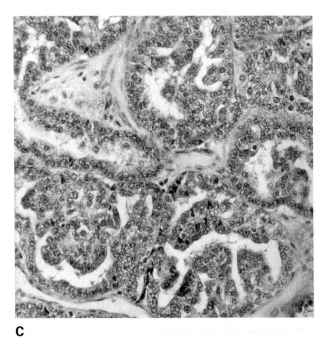

C

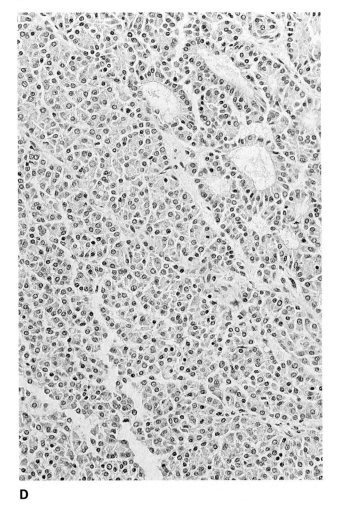

D

Fig. 10.2. **A.** Renal adenoma in a horse, papillary cell type. Papillae and tubules are lined by a single layer of well-differentiated epithelium. **B.** Renal carcinoma in a dog, papillary type with long ribbons and tubules lined by epithelial cells with little cytoplasm. **C.** Renal carcinoma with tubular formation and small papillary ingrowths of neoplastic cells. **D.** Renal carcinoma in a dog with areas of solid and tubular differentiation. Cells in both areas are well differentiated with small amounts of lightly eosinophilic cytoplasm, uniform nuclei, and no mitoses. Mixtures of solid, tubular, and papillary types, as well as eosinophilic and clear cells, are often present in the same tumor.

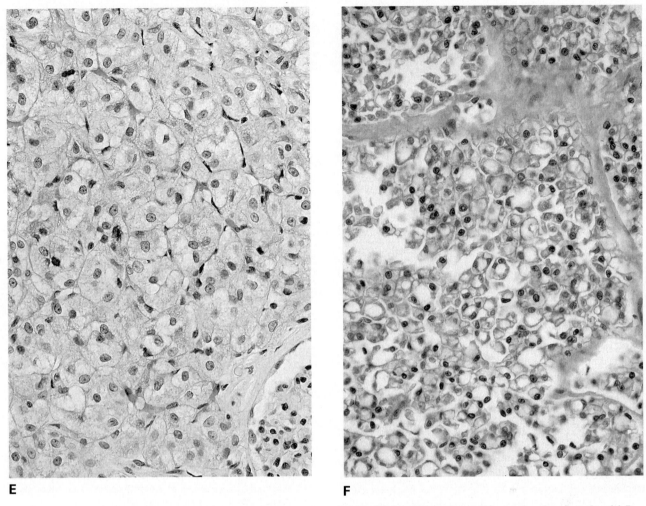

E

F

Fig. 10.2. (continued)   **E.** Solid, clear cell type is characterized by large cells with abundant, light to clear cytoplasm and uniform central nuclei. Portion of glomerulus at edge of tumor. **F.** Solid, clear cell type with large cytoplasmic vacuoles and eccentric nuclei.

54 dogs with renal tumors survived less than 21 days.[6] Some dogs survived 8-24 months.[6] It can be difficult to decide if a small tumor is benign or malignant. Large tumors are often easy to classify because the tumor has already metastasized or invaded the renal pelvis, capsule, or vessels. In the absence of an obvious criterion such as invasion of adjacent parenchyma or blood vessels, then gross size, necrosis, mitoses, and degree of anaplasia are used. Although tumor size has been stated to be a criterion (< 2 cm adenoma, > 2 cm favors carcinoma), this is an oversimplification from the older literature[13] and is probably only useful in dogs and cats since tumors in cattle[7] behave in a benign fashion even though tumors can be as large as 60 cm. Only 1 of 20 renal cell tumors studied in cattle metastasized; most had minimal cellular atypia yet were classified as carcinoma based on their multiplicity. Two of the 20 had marked cellular pleomorphism; one metastasized and one did not. The one tumor classified as an adenoma was 8 x 10 mm and was confined to one kidney. In dogs variations of cellular and histological morphology seem to be acceptable predictors of malignancy. A high mitotic index, necrosis, invasion, and cellular atypia

are characteristics of carcinoma, not adenoma, but metastasis from well-differentiated tumors occurs. Characteristics that favor carcinoma are large size, large areas of necrosis, infiltration, invasion of parenchyma or vessels, mitoses, and cellular atypia. None of these are definitive or correlated with long term follow-up studies. Classification by histological or cytological subtype is not predictive of biological behavior in domestic animals. Multiplicity of primary renal cell tumors occurs in 33 percent of canine and in 95 percent of bovine cases. If a renal tumor metastasizes to the opposite kidney, there are invariably metastases in other organs.

Perhaps the best indicator is to know the biological behavior of renal cell tumors for the different species: in dogs 50-60 percent metastasize,[5,6] in cows 5 percent,[7] in horses 70 percent,[16-20] and in other species too few cases have been studied. In dogs the most likely sites are lung, regional lymph node, liver, serosal surfaces, and ipsilateral adrenal gland.[5,6] Metastases are usually widespread and occur in any organ; however, although the skin is an unusual site for metastases in general, this site has been reported with renal tumors in dogs. Metastases are common in horses and are widely disseminated, with lungs and liver being the two most frequent sites.[16,17]

In German shepherds there is progression from renal cell hyperplasia to adenoma and carcinoma.

Diagnostic Considerations

Determination of a primary renal versus metastatic neoplasm and benign versus malignant can be challenging. Adenoma and adenocarcinoma of renal cell origin resemble similar tumors that originate in lung, mammary, and prostate glands. If lesions are confined to the kidney, especially the cortex, and/or regional lymph nodes, a diagnosis of primary renal carcinoma is warranted. Renal tumors that are multiple and bilateral yet do not metastasize are most likely to be primary renal cell tumors of multicentric origin. If a renal tumor metastasizes to the opposite kidney, there are metastases in other organs. When metastases are widespread, the distinction is less easy and the criterion more subjective: location of the largest tumor suggests that organ as the primary site, and metastases to the kidney are multiple, often involve the medulla, and are accompanied by metastases elsewhere. Renal carcinomas invariably arise in the cortex, and lesions in the medulla favor a metastatic tumor. Foci of clear cells are consistent with renal origin. Corpora amylacea are features of bovine renal cell tumors. Uromodulin, a unique protein synthesized by the kidney,[1] has been a useful immunohistochemical marker for studying renal cell tumors. In one study positive immunoreactivity was present in all renal cell tumors in cattle.[7] Tumor associated glycoprotein antigen (TAG-72) has been used on transitional cell carcinoma (TCC), but it has not been used on renal cell tumors.[2] Renal carcinomas in humans stain positively for both cytokeratin and vimentin, but comparable studies in animals have not been done.[14]

Oncocytoma

This is a rare, usually benign, tumor composed of oncocytes. The histogenesis is not clear, but these tumors may arise from the intercalated cells of collecting ducts.[14,24] It is a variant of renal epithelial cell tumors and has been described in a dog.[24] Microscopically, these neoplasms consist of solid areas, nests, or cords and tubules of closely packed, round to polygonal, monomorphic cells with intensely eosinophilic, granular cytoplasm. Nuclei are round to oval with coarsely stippled chromatin and a prominent nucleolus. There may be anisocytosis and anisokaryosis and bi- or multinucleate tumor cells. The diagnosis of renal oncocytoma is based on distinctive granular, eosinophilic cytoplasm; a positive periodic acid Schiff (PAS) reaction; immunoexpression of cytoplasmic cytokeratin, but not vimentin; abundant mitochondria; and an absence of ultrastructural vesicles. The main differential consideration is the eosinophilic variant of a chromophobe renal cell carcinoma, which has ultrastructural cytoplasmic vesicles and otherwise is similar to an oncocytoma. The case reported in the dog was bilateral and invaded adjacent

muscles; there were no clinically detectable metastases, but a necropsy was not performed.[24] There is one other report of an oncocyte-like renal cell carcinoma in a German shepherd with dermatofibrosis.[25] In humans oncocytomas are considered benign.[14]

REFERENCES

1. Hession, C., Decker, J.M., Sherblom, A.P., et al. (1987) Uromodulin (Tamm-Horsfall glycoprotein): A renal ligand for lymphokines. *Science* 237:1479-1484.
2. Clemo, F.A.S., DeNicola, D.B., Carolton, W.W., et al. (1995) Immunoreactivity of canine transitional cell carcinoma of the urinary bladder with monoclonal antibodies to tumor-associated glycoprotein 72. *Vet Pathol* 32:155-161.
3. Allen, D.K., Waters, D.J., Knapp, D.W., et al. (1996) High urine concentrations of basic fibroblast growth factor in dogs with bladder cancer. *J Vet Intern Med* 10:231-234.
4. Ross, J.S., and Cohen. M.B. (1999) Ancillary methods for the detection of recurrent urothelial neoplasia. *Cancer Cytopathology* 90:75-86.
5. Baskin, G.B., Paoli, A.D. (1977) Primary renal neoplasms of the dog. *Vet Pathol* 14:591-605.
6. Klein, M.K., Cockerell, G.L., Harris, C.K., et al. (1988) Canine primary renal neoplasms: A retrospective review of 54 cases. *J Amer Anim Hosp Assoc* 24:443-452.
7. Kelley, L.C., Crowell, W.A., et al. (1996) A retrospective study of multicentric bovine renal cell tumors. *Vet Pathol* 33:133-141.
8. Caywood, D.D., Osborne, C.A., Johnston, G.R. (1980) Neoplasms of the canine and feline urinary tracts. *Current Veterinary Therapy VIII.* W.B. Saunders Co., Philadelphia, pp. 1203-1212.
9. Osborne, C.A., Quast, J.F., et al. (1971) Renal pelvic carcinoma in a cat. *J Amer Vet Med Assoc* 159:1238-1241.
10. Wimberely, H.C., Lewis, R.M. (1979) Transitional cell carcinoma in the domestic cat. *Vet Pathol* 16:223-228.
11. Clark, W.R., Wilson, R.B. (1988) Renal adenoma in a cat. *J Amer Vet Med Assoc* 193:1557-1559.
12. Lium, B., and Moe, L. (1985) Hereditary multifocal renal cystadenocarcinomas and nodular dermatofibrosis in the German shepherd dog: Macroscopic and histopathologic changes. *Vet Pathol* 22:447-455.
13. Bell, E.T. (1938) A classification of renal tumors with observations of the frequency of the various types. *J Urol* 39:238-243.
14. Eble, J.N., and Young, R.H. (2000) Tumors of the urinary tract. In Christopher Fletcher, *Diagnostic Histopathology of Tumors,* 2nd ed. Churchill Livingstone, Inc. pp. 475-565.
15. Nielsen, S.W., Moulton, J.E. (1990) Tumors of the urinary system. *Tumors in Domestic Animals,* 3rd ed. University of Calif Press, Berkely, pp. 458-478.
16. Traub-Dargatz JL. Urinary tract neoplasia. Vet Clin N Am:Eq Pract. 14:495-504 1998
17. West, H.J., Kelly, D.F., and Ritchie, H.E. (1987) Renal carcinomatosis in a horse. *Equine Vet J* 19:548-551.
18. Haschek, W.M., King, J.M., et al. (1981) Primary renal cell carcinoma in two horses. *J Amer Vet Med Assoc* 179:992-994.
19. Owen, R.H., Haywood, S., and Kelly, D.F. (1986) Clinical course of renal adenocarcinoma associated with hypercupraemia in a horse. *Vet Rec* 119:291-294.
20. Baker, J.L., Aleman, M., and Madigan, J. (2001) Intermittent hypoglycemia in a horse with anaplastic carcinoma of the kidney. *J Amer Vet Med Assoc* 218:235-237.
21. Sandison, A.T., Anderson, L.J. (1968) Tumors of the kidney in cattle, sheep and pigs. *Cancer* 21:727-742.
22. Crow, S.E., Allen, D.P., et al. (1995) Concurrent renal adenocarcinoma and polycythemia in a dog. *J Amer Anim Hosp Assoc* 31:29-33.

23. Gorse, MJ. (1988) Polycythemia associated with renal fibrosarcoma in a dog. *J Amer Vet Med Assoc* 192:793-794.

24. Buergelt, C.D., and Adjiri-Awere, A. (2000) Bilateral renal oncocytoma in a greyhound dog. *Vet Pathol* 37:188-192.

25. Vilafranca, M., Fondevila, D., et al. (1994) Chromophilic-eosinophilic (oncocyte-like) renal cell carcinoma in a dog with nodular dermatofibrosis. *Vet Pathol* 31:713-716.

26. Wolf, D.C., Whiteley, H.E. et al. (1995) Preneoplastic and neoplastic lesions of rat hereditary renal cell tumors express markers of proximal and distal nephron. *Vet Pathol* 32:379-386.

27. Steinberg, H., Thomson, J. (1994) Bilateral renal carcinoma in a cat. *Vet Pathol* 31:704–705.

Nodular Dermatofibrosis and Renal Cell Tumors

This unique syndrome is hereditary in German shepherd dogs and produces multiple subcutaneous fibrous nodules, uterine leiomyomas, and multiple renal adenocarcinomas/adenomas.[1-4] It appears to have an autosomal dominant mode of inheritance, associated with an as yet unidentified gene localized to chromosome 53. One study could link the heritage of 43 dogs with this syndrome to one male. It has also been reported in the golden retriever, boxer, and mongrels and is seen more frequently in females. The average age of affected dogs is 8.5 years, with a range of 5-11 years.

Gross Morphology and Histological Features

The subcutaneous nodules vary from a few millimeters in diameter to large masses greater than 5 cm in diameter. They are well delineated nonencapsulated nodules of benign fibroblasts and associated collagen. The dermal portions tend to blend in with adjacent collagen, and the subcutaneous portions are well circumscribed. They can be found anywhere on the body but are most frequently seen along the limbs, back, and head. They produce a distinct bulging, palpable, mass in the subcutis, but larger masses may have an ulcerated surface. Ten of 11 German shepherd bitches with this disease had multiple uterine leiomyomas.[1]

In the kidneys the epithelial tumors are bilateral, multiple, and cystic (43 of 45 dogs with renal tumors). They are sharply delineated, bulge on cross section, and vary from tan-white to gray. Sizes range from a few millimeters to greater than 10 cm for the solid tumors and greater than 25 cm for the cystic portions. Cysts contain gelatinous, clear to red-brown fluid and may rupture into the peritoneal space.

There is a range of microscopic lesions from hyperplasia to adenoma and progressing to adenocarcinoma. Some lesions may only be microscopic, and the smaller gross lesions consist of well differentiated epithelial cells that line tubules or cysts with occasional papillary projections into lumenal spaces. Cysts are such a characteristic component of these tumors that they are often referred to as cystadenocarcinomas. Like other primary renal adenocarcinomas these tumors have areas of tubular, papillary, or solid growth patterns, often admixed in one tumor. An oncocyte-like variety has also been described.[4] The solid areas tend to be more anaplastic; the cells are pleomorphic, ranging from cuboidal to spindle shaped, with bizarre nuclei and numerous mitotic figures.

Metastases resemble the primary tumor, and they were detected in 10 of 23 dogs necropsied; most common locations of metastases were sternal and renal lymph nodes, but metastases were also found in the peritoneum, liver, spleen, lung, pleura, and bone.[1,2,4]

Transitional Cell Papilloma and Carcinoma, Squamous Cell Carcinoma, and Undifferentiated Carcinoma

All these tumors occur rarely in the kidneys and when present usually arise from urothelium in the pelvis.[16] Urothelium retains the embryonic potential to differentiate into glandular epithelium (secreting mucus) and squamous and transitional epithelium. In the urinary bladder TCC are subclassified using combinations of papillary and infiltrating and qualifiers of metaplasia, but these variants have not been applied to renal TCC. *Undifferentiated carcinoma* is a term used when the tumor cells are so poorly differentiated that the cell of origin can not be determined. It is not applied to renal cell cancers that can be classified but are anaplastic.

Histological Features

Papillomas are rare (1 percent), and they consist of papillae lined by one or a few layers of well differentiated cuboidal or columnar epithelial cells that form a thin covering of transitional epithelium on small fibrous septa. These structures are of various lengths and project into the lumen of the pelvis. Papillary growths may occasionally be seen macroscopically in the pelvis.

Transitional cell carcinomas (5 percent; table 10.2) usually originate in the pelvis or ureter and have identical histological features to TCC in the urinary bladder. Squamous cell carcinomas (2 percent) occur in the pelvis, and they have intercellular bridges and keratinization sufficiently developed to justify this diagnosis. Undifferentiated carcinomas are located in the cortex and are invasive. They are epithelial neoplasms that do not differentiate into recognizable tubular, transitional, or squamous epithelium. Confirmation of their epithelial origin may require immunohistochemical staining. This term should not be used for anaplastic neoplasms that can still be classified. Of the 464 renal cell tumors in dogs only 2 (0.4 percent) were classified as undifferentiated carcinoma. This probably reflects the histology of these tumors, in that nearly every renal carcinoma has a focus of clear cells, tubules, or other identifying characteristics that help define renal cell origin; or it may be that poorly differentiated tumors that lack these features were considered sarcoma. Some carcinomas can be so poorly differentiated and produce such a desmoplastic response that they can only be differentiated from a sarcoma with the use of cytokeratin and vimentin. Renal cell carcinomas can stain positively for both or only with cytokeratin, and sarcomas are only positive with vimentin. Table 10.2 indicates that undifferentiated sarcomas accounted for 6 percent of primary renal cell tumors in dogs. However, these diagnoses were not based on the results of immunohistochemistry. Desmoplasia and single cells encased by connective tissue can be features of renal carcinomas.

Embryonal Tumors

Nephroblastoma (Embryonal Nephroma)

General Considerations

Names for this neoplasm include Wilm's tumor, embryonal adenosarcoma, embryonal nephroma, and nephroblastoma.[5-8] A variety of studies indicate the tissue of origin is the metanephric blastema and that the stromal cells and blastema develop from a common stem cell.[5] The tumor is a mixture of embryonic renal tissue with immature glomerular-like buds, tubules, and myxomatous mesenchyme in various amounts. They can also contain nonepithelial tissues such as muscle (smooth and striated), cartilage, bone, and fat. The tumors arise from neoplastic transformation during nephrogenesis or from nephrogenic rests that persist postnatally. The latter has been reported in a dog with nephroblastoma and polycythemia.[5] In people the Wilms' tumor gene (*WT1* on chromosome 11) is a causative factor, and there are strains of rats that develop nephroblastoma.[12]

Age, Breed, and Sex

This is a congenital neoplasm, and many develop during fetal life but are not detected until later in life when a clinical problem is obvious. They have been reported in the bovine fetus. Approximately 92 percent of nephroblastomas are present in swine less than 2 years of age, and 77 percent are present at 1 year of age, suggesting that some do develop later in life.[7] Most of these animals are asymptomatic, and the tumor is discovered at necropsy/slaughter. The tumors appear to be more common in males by a 2:1 ratio of males to females (although no difference was reported in another study of swine). Case reports in dogs also indicate a male predominance.[5-8,10]

Incidence

This is the most common primary renal neoplasm in swine and chickens and is the second most common tumor in dogs [36/464 tumors (8 percent), table 10.2) and cats [18/73 tumors (25 percent)].[9,10] Whether this reflects a true incidence for dogs and cats or the propensity to report an interesting tumor is not clear. Estimates of these tumors are 4.4 to 20 per 100,000 pigs in the United States and 0.35 per

100,000 in the United Kingdom.[7] Authors speculated that the incidence would be even higher in abattoir surveys of swine if all suspected lesions had been submitted for microscopic confirmation. They have been reported in all the other domestic animals.[6,9,10]

Gross Morphology

Characteristically, the neoplasms are unilateral, single, and at one pole and are located in the cortex and extending through the capsule, where they adhere to the body wall or mesentery. Exceptions to this appear as bilateral tumors, multiple tumors, and invasion into the pelvis. They usually occupy a large proportion of the affected kidney (fig. 10.3 A) and may be large enough to compress abdominal viscera. Tumors greater than 50 cm in diameter and weighing over 34 kg are reported in breeding age sows.[7] The natural and cut surfaces are lobulated, meaty to firm, white to tan with cystic areas and other areas discolored yellow, gray, or red. Rarely, fat, muscle, cartilage, and bone may be present. The presence of these tissues has led to the terms *adenosarcoma, mixed tumor,* and *sarcocarcinoma.*

Histological Features

The critical feature is a disorganized mixture of embryonal epithelial and mesenchymal tissues (fig.10.3 B-D), the most impressive of which are embryonic glomeruli formed by tufts of epithelium that invaginate into a lumen that is lined by epithelial cells with little cytoplasm (see fig. 10.4 A). These structures will be in various stages of differentiation. Embryonic glomeruli are surrounded by irregular, branching tubules that have lumens of various sizes; some form small acini or tubules, and others are elongated and dilated into a collecting drainage-like system. A classic pattern is a proliferation of epithelial cells in the center of which are partially developed tubules and glomeruli, and all of these structures are encompassed by variable amounts of loose mesenchymal stroma (fig.10.3 B). Foci of undifferentiated, proliferating blast-like cells, with no visible cytoplasm will be scattered through the tumor. They can contain a few open spaces and appear to form lumens. In lesser numbers there are cystic structures lined by cuboidal epithelium or squamous epithelium with or without the presence of mucus, sloughed epithelial cells, or keratin.

The mesenchyme is loose, areolar, and myxomatous, has a light basophilic hue, and is rarely dense enough to be birefringent. In ruminants the mesenchymal elements tend to be equally as developed as the epithelial components. There can be regions with herringbone patterns and dense fibrous proliferation similar to a fibrosarcoma. Differentiation and or metaplasia into muscle may be present, and less frequently there is formation of cartilage and/or bone. Tumors in people are reported to be positive for desmin but negative for other markers of muscle. The blastemal and stromal elements are positive for vimentin, and the epithelial components are cytokeratin positive.[4]

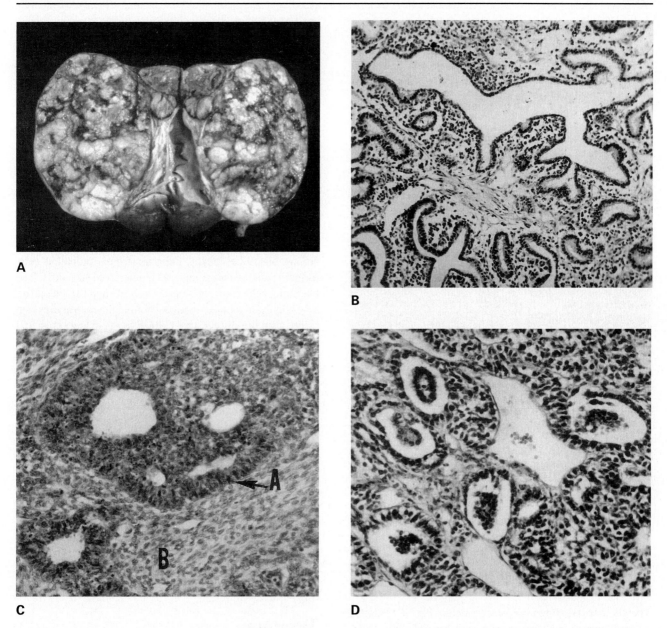

Fig. 10.3. **A.** Embryonal nephroma in a dog has replaced most of the renal parenchyma. **B.** Embryonal nephroma in a pig has irregularly shaped tubular structures and abundant myxomatous stroma. **C.** Embryonal nephroma in a dog with neoplastic epithelial cells *(A)* adjacent to highly cellular mesenchymal stroma *(B).* **D.** Embryonal nephroma with primitive tubules and tuft-like invaginations into a central lumen.

Growth and Metastasis

In swine and poultry metastases are rare, but in dogs and cats metastasis is expected (> 50 percent). The epithelial and mesenchymal components may be present in metastases. Histological and cytological criteria for estimating the biological behavior are not well established. Tubular and glomerular differentiation may indicate a less aggressive growth, and sarcomatous, anaplastic differentiation an increased likelihood of metastases. If the host is a species other than swine, metastases are anticipated. Likely sites are regional sublumbar and mesenteric lymph nodes; lungs, liver, and the contralateral kidney are other sites of metastasis.

Spinal Cord Tumor (Nephroblastoma) of Young Dogs

General Considerations

This unique tumor occurs in the spinal cord of young dogs, and the histogenesis of the tumor has been debated. It is present in the thoracolumbar junction and is seen most frequently in German shepherds.[11-15] The two most likely tissues of origin and tumors are neural rests/neuroblastoma or ectopic renal blastema/nephroblastoma. Light microscopically, the tumors are clearly identifiable and are not confused with ependymoma or choroid plexus tumors.

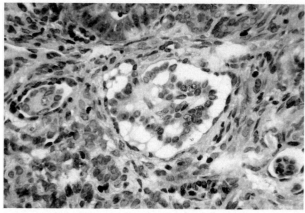

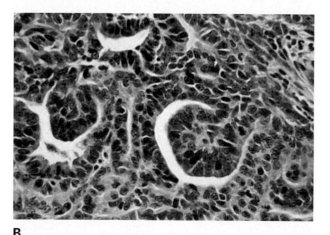

Fig. 10.4. **A.** Embryonal nephroma in dog with invaginations of epithelial cells that resemble embryonic glomeruli. **B.** Spinal cord nephroblastoma in an 11-month-old dog with tubules and glomeruloid structures that resemble embryonic glomeruli.

They do not stain immunohistochemically for GFAP, NSE, neurofilament, or chromogranin, and four of six stained positively for cytokeratin; therefore, neural origin is ruled out.[11,13,14] The tumors form structures that resemble embryonic glomeruli, react positively to polysialic acid (present in embryonic renal cells and nephroblastomas in humans), stain for Wilm's tumor gene product[12] (WT1), and are best interpreted as nephroblastomas. There is ample gross, histological and immunohistochemical data to conclude these tumors are nephroblastomas. These tumors likely develop from remnants of renal rests trapped between the dura and developing spinal cord.

Clinical Characteristics

These are rare tumors and so far have only been reported in dogs. Reported ages of the dogs have ranged from 5 months to 7 years, but the majority are between 6 months and 3 years.[11,13,15] Although too few cases are documented, it appears the German shepherd breed is predisposed.

Dogs present for hind limb paresis or ataxia and have signs of upper motor neuron disease. The lesion is usually localized to the thoracolumbar region, intervertebral disc disease is not present, and special radiographic studies often indicate an extramedullary space–occupying mass.

Gross Morphology and Histological Features

At surgery or necropsy there is an intradural, extramedullary, nonencapsulated mass of variable size in the thoracolumbar segments (T10–L2) of the spinal cord, with or without associated hyperemia and/or hemorrhage. Occasionally fronds of proliferating tissue are visible in the dural space. Characteristic histological features are proliferating blast-like cells, a delicate stroma, epithelial cells forming tubules and acini, and glomeruloid-like tufts. The blastemal cells form solid nests or sheets and can line primitive tubular structures with a central lumen. Tubules and rosettes are usually present. Critical to the diagnosis are the presence of embryonic glomeruli formed by tufts of epithelial cells projecting from an epithelial lining into a small lumen (see fig.10.4 B). When the tufts are cut in cross section there is a solid ball of cells in the center of the lumen, and cells lining the space have little to no visible cytoplasm and create a rim of "naked nuclei." Supporting stroma is sparse and loose, and often has a light basophilic hue. Primitive tubules and acini can be found in different regions. Mitotic figures are variable in number: they can be numerous or rare. The mesenchymal component is vimentin positive, and the epithelial structures are cytokeratin positive.

Although surgeons often report that the tumor "shelled out" easily, the tumor may also have villous projections that invade the subarachnoid space, adjacent parenchyma, and nerve roots, making recurrence in the first 6 months postsurgery likely. There is one report of multifocal and/or metastatic disease.[14]

Teratoma

These are rare tumors in the kidneys of domestic animals that contain cellular components from all three germ layers. Most mixed tumors are classified as nephroblastomas. The presence of gut, lymphoid, sweat glands, and hair favor a germ cell neoplasm over nephroblastoma.

REFERENCES

1. Lium, B., and Moe, L. (1985) Hereditary multifocal renal cystadenocarcinomas and nodular dermatofibrosis in the German shepherd dog: Macroscopic and histopathologic changes. *Vet Pathol* 22:447-455.

2. Cosenza, S.F., and Seely, J.C. (1986) Generalized nodular dermatofibrosis and renal cystadenocarcinomas in a German shepherd dog. *J Amer Vet Med Assoc* 189:1587-1590.

3. Jonasdottir, T.J., Mellersh, C.S., et al. (2000) Genetic mapping of a naturally occurring hereditary renal cancer syndrome in dogs. *Proc Natl Acad Sci USA* 97:4132-4137.

4. Vilafranca, M., Fondevila, D., et al. (1994) Chromophilic-eosinophilic (oncocyte-like) renal cell carcinoma in a dog with nodular dermatofibrosis. *Vet Pathol* 31: 713-716.

5. Simpson, R.M., Gliatto, J.M., Casey, H.W., et al. (1992) The histologic, ultrastructural, and immunohistochemical features of a blastema-predominant canine nephroblastoma. *Vet Pathol* 29:250-253.

6. Nielsen, S.W., and Moulton, J.E. (1990) Tumors of the urinary system. *Tumors in Domestic Animals*, 3rd ed. University of Califonia Press, Berkely, pp. 458-478.

7. Migaki, G., Nelson, L.W., and Todd, G.C. (1971) Prevalence of embryonal nephroma in slaughtered swine. *J Amer Vet Med Assoc* 159:441-442.

8. Takeda, T., et al. (1989) Congenital mesoblastic nephroma in a dog: Benign variant of nephroblastoma. *Vet Pathol* 26:281-282.

9. Caywood, D.D., Osborne, C.A., and Johnston, G.R. (1980) Neoplasms of the canine and feline urinary tracts. *Current Veterinary Therapy VIII*. W.B. Saunders Co., Philadelphia, pp. 1203-1212.

10. Osborne, C.A., Low, D.G., Perman, V., et al. (1968) Neoplasms of the canine and feline urinary bladder: incidence, etiologic factors, occurrence and pathologic features. *Amer J Vet Res* 29:2041-2053.

11. Baumbartner, W., and Peixoto, P.V. (1987) Immunohistochemical demonstration of keratin in canine neuroepithelioma. *Vet Pathol* 24:500-503.

12. Pearson, G.R., Gregory, S.P., and Charles, A.K. (1997) Immunohistochemical demonstration of Wilms' tumor gene product WT1 in canine "neuroepithelioma" providing evidence for its classification as an extrarenal nephroblastoma. *J Comp Pathol* 116:321-327.

13. Summer, B.A., deLahunta, A., McEntee, M., et al. (1988) A novel extramedullary spinal cord tumor in young dogs. *Acta Neuropathol* 75:402-410.

14. Terrell, S.F., Platt, S.R., et al. (2000) Possible intraspinal metastasis of a canine spinal cord nephroblastoma. *Vet Pathol* 37:94-97.

15. Neel, J., and Dean, G.A. (2000) What is your diagnosis? A Mass in the spinal column of a dog. *Vet Clin Pathol* 29:87-89.

16. Goldsmid, S.E., Bellenger, C.R., Watson, A.D.J., et al (1992) Renal transitional cell carcinoma in a dog. *J Amer Anim Hosp Assoc* 28:241-244.

Mesenchymal Tumors

General Considerations

Primary neoplasms may arise from mesenchymal tissues in the kidney. The most common tumors are undifferentiated sarcoma, fibroma/fibrosarcoma, and hemangioma/hemangiosarcoma; however, rare examples of leiomyomas and lipomas or their malignant counterparts are reported.[1-3]

Undifferentiated Sarcoma

Undifferentiated sarcoma was the most frequently diagnosed sarcoma in dogs (6 percent, table 10.2). These diagnoses were primarily made on H&E stained sections, and whether they would remain sarcomas after the application of immunohistochemistry is speculative. Mesenchymal neoplasms that can not be classified otherwise are placed in this group, and confirmation can be obtained by negative cytokeratin and positive vimentin staining characteristics. These tumors have variable amounts of stroma, which can be abundant and can isolate tumor cells.

Hemangioma and Hemangiosarcoma

Hemangioma and hemangiosarcoma may be solitary. When they are widely disseminated, it is difficult to impossible to distinguish multicentric origin from metastatic lesions, but the latter is much more likely. When present they usually grow through the renal capsule and cause considerable hemorrhage, and a large proportion of the total mass is nonneoplastic. Histologically, they appear as blood vessel tumors and stain with antibodies against factor VIII. They are seen in dogs most frequently and are rare in other species.

Fibroma and Fibrosarcoma

Fibroma and fibrosarcoma account for approximately 5 percent of primary renal cell tumors in dogs. They appear as their counterparts in other locations.[1-3] A spindle cell neoplasm with pointed nuclei, no visible cell borders, birefringent matrix, collagen that stains appropriately histochemically (Masson's or Van Gieson), and if applied, positive immunoreactivity to vimentin are some of the salient features. A report on four cases of fibroma in dogs indicated they are well demarcated, singular or multiple, and usually located at the corticomedullary junction.[1]

Renal Interstitial Cell Tumors

Renal interstitial cell tumors have all the characteristics described for fibroma, and the distinguishing feature is the presence of cytoplasmic lipid droplets that may require ultrastructural study to document.[4,5] They are also located at the corticomedullary junction, tend to be multiple, and are believed to arise from renal interstitial cells that contain prostaglandin, arachidonic acid, and a neutral antihypertensive lipid that may lower arterial blood pressure. Macroscopically and microscopically they are indistinguishable from fibroma. In human tumors there is controversy as to whether these are neoplastic or hyperplastic lesions.[5]

REFERENCES

1. Picut, C.A., and Valentine, B.A. (1985) Brief communications: Renal fibroma in four dogs. *Vet Pathol* 22:422-423.

2. Rudd, R.G., Whitehair, J.G., and Leipold, H.W. (1991) Spindle cell sarcoma in the kidney of a dog. *J Amer Vet Med Assoc* 198:1023-1024.

3. Gorse, M.J. (1988) Polycythemia associated with renal fibrosarcoma in a dog. *J Amer Vet Med Assoc* 192:793-794.

4. Diter, R.W., and Wells, M. (1986) Brief communications: Renal interstitial cell tumors in the dog. *Vet Pathol* 23:74-76.

5. Eble, J.N., and Young, R.H. (2000) Tumors of the urinary tract. In Christopher Fletcher, *Diagnostic Histopathology of Tumors*, 2nd ed. Churchill Livingstone, Inc., pp. 475-565.

Etiology

Chemical, physical, and viral etiologies are associated with renal cell tumors in animals and humans.[1-17] Chemical carcinogens known to induce renal cell tumors in animals include nitrosamines,[8,17] aromatic amines[1] (dyes, rubber, coal, gas industries), nitrosureas,[8] triphosphates,[1] cadmium,[3] aflatoxin,[4] and lead.[7] Estrogen administration is reported to cause renal carcinoma in the Syrian hamster.[10] Compounds associated with renal carcinomas in human beings are asbestos,[1] cigarette smoke,[9] coffee,[1,9] phenacetin,[9] diuretics,[9] hydroquinone,[20] and analgesic abuse.[11] Viruses are a cause of renal cell tumors in chickens (avian leukosis oncornavirus), leopard frogs (Lucke adenocarcinoma—herpes virus), and gray squirrels (pox virus).[12-14] Renal tumors are common in budgerigars: up to 25 percent of all tumors in this host are of renal cell origin, and retrovirus sequences have been detected in these tumors.[15] There is an association between nephrotoxicity and nephrocarcinogenicity in laboratory animals,[20] and there is a higher incidence of renal cell tumors in human beings with end stage renal disease and cysts.[1,17] An important factor in renal cell neoplasia is gender; males have a higher incidence in humans (two- to five-fold greater in males) and laboratory animal models, and nearly all reports suggest a male predominance in dogs, approximately 2:1.[1,2,16]

Wistar rats have familial renal adenomas,[18,19] as do German shepherds with renal cystadenocarcinoma and nodular dermatofibrosis.[21] The Eker rat is a model for hereditary renal carcinoma in which a single suppressor gene, the *Tsc-2* gene on chromosome 10q12 has been identified and is responsible for cancer induction.[19,20] Heterozygote animals develop multicentric renal cell adenomas and carcinomas by 1 year of age. The trait is autosomal dominant, and homozygotes are lethal, with death of the fetus at approximately 13 days of gestation.[19] Familial renal cell carcinoma in people is associated with suppressor genes *VHL* (von-Hippel Lindau) on chromosome 3p25 and *RCC* on 3p141.[22,23] The tumor suppressor gene *WT1*, on chromosome 11p13 is the "Wilm's tumor" gene and is associated with nephroblastoma.[1,24] Chromosome 3 translocations are associated with clear cell tumors in human beings, and the short arm of chromosome 3 (3p) is associated with nonpapillary renal carcinoma, while trisomy of chromosome 17 is associated with papillary renal carcinoma.[1] The *ras* oncogene family is associated with nephroblastomas and N-nitrosoethylurea induced renal carcinomas in rats but is not critical in the genesis of renal cell carcinomas in humans.[1,25] Mutations of the *p53* gene are more important in the progression step of renal carcinogenesis than initiation but are not common alterations in renal neoplasia. In humans there are multiple cytogenetic and molecular alterations associated with phenotypic variants of renal epithelial tumors.[1,22,23] Comparable studies in domestic animals have not been done.

There are two isoforms of cyclooxygenase (COX), COX-1 functions in normal cell physiology and COX-2 functions in inflammatory diseases and is a regulator of cell growth.[26] COX-2 is present in low levels in normal canine kidney and is expressed in several-fold higher levels in fetal kidneys.[26] COX-2 may play a role in normal nephrogenesis, and its expression in canine renal cell carcinomas may indicate it modulates tumor cell growth. The response of urinary and colorectal cancers to NSAIDs is likely due to inhibition of COX enzymes.

REFERENCES

1. Eble, J.N., and Young, R.H. (2000) Tumors of the urinary tract. In Christopher Fletcher, *Diagnostic Histopathology of Tumors,* 2nd ed. Churchill Livingstone, Inc., pp. 475-565.
2. Osborne, C.A., Low, D.G., Perman, V. et al. (1968) Neoplasms of the canine and feline urinary bladder: Incidence, etiologic factors, occurrence and pathologic features. *Amer J Vet Res* 29:2041-2053.
3. Kolonel, L.N. (1976) Association of cadmium with renal cancer. *Cancer* 137:1782-1787.
4. Epstein, S,M,, Bartus, B., and Farber, E. (1969) Renal epithelial neoplasms induced in male Wistar rats by oral aflatoxin. *Blood Cancer Res* 29:1045-1050.
5. MacLure, M. (1987) Asbestos and renal adenocarcinoma: A case control study. *Environ Res* 42:353-361.
6. Arison, R.N., and Feudale, E.L. (1967) Induction of renal tumor by streptozotocin in rats. *Nature* 214:1254-1255.
7. Boyland, E., Dukes, C.E., et al. (1962) The induction of renal tumors by feeding lead acetate to rats. *Br J Cancer* 16:283-288.
8. Dees, H., Heatfield, B.M., et al. (1980) Adenocarcinoma of the kidney. *J Natl Cancer Inst* 64:1537-1541.
9. Yu, M.C., Mack, T., and Hanisch, R.(1986) Cigarette smoking, obesity, diuretic use and coffee consumption as risk factors for renal cell carcinoma. *J Natl Cancer Inst* 77:351-356.
10. Kirkman, H. (1959) Estrogen-induced tumors of the kidney in the Syrian hamster. *Natl Cancer Inst Monogr* 1:1-139.
11. Palvio, D.H.B., Andersen, J.C., et al. (1987) Transitional cell carcinoma of the renal pelvis and ureter associated with capillarosclerosis indicating analgesic drug abuse. *Cancer* 59:972-976.
12. Lucke, B. Kidney carcinoma in the leopard frog: A virus tumor. *Ann NY Acad Sci* 54:1093-1109.
13. Ackerman, N., Hager, D.A., et al. (1990) Ultrasound appearance and early detection of VX2 carcinoma in the rabbit kidney. *Vet Radiol* 30:88-96.
14. O'Connor, D.J., Diters, R.W., and Nielsen, S.W. (1980) Poxvirus and multiple tumors in an eastern gray squirrel. *J Amer Vet Med Assoc* 177:792-795.
15. Gould, W.J., O'Connell, P.H., et al. (1993) Detection of retrovirus sequences in budgerigars with tumors. *Avian Pathol* 22:33-45.
16. Hayes, H.M., and Fraumeni, J.F. (1977) Epidemiological features of canine renal neoplasms. *Caner Res* 37:2553-2556.
17. Newsome, G.D., and Vugrin, D. (1987) Etiologic factors in renal cell adenocarcinoma. *Semin Nephrol* 7:109-116.
18. Eker, R. (1954) Familial renal adenomas in Wistar rats. A preliminary report. *Acta Pathol Microbiol Scand* 34:554-562.
19. Everitt, J.I., Goldsworthy, T.L., et al. (1992) Hereditary renal cell carcinoma in the Eker rat. *J Urol* 146:1932-1936.
20. Lau, S.S., Monks, T.J., Everitt, J.I., et al. (2001) Carcinogenicity of a nephrototoxic metabolite of the "nongenotoxic" carcinogen hydroquinone. *Chem Res Toxicol* 14:25-33.

21. Lium, B., and Moe, L. (1985) Hereditary multifocal renal cystadeno-carcinomas and nodular dermatofibrosis in the German shepherd dog: Macroscopic and histopathologic changes. *Vet Pathol* 22:447-455.

22. Melmon, K.L., and Rosen, S.W. (1964) Lindau's disease. Review of the literature and study of a large kindred. *Amer J Med* 36:595-617.

23. Pathak, S., Strong, L.C., Ferrell, R.E., Trindale, A. (1982) Familial renal cell carcinoma with a 3;11 chromosome translocation limited to tumor cells. *Science* 217:939-941.

24. Pearson, G.R., Gregory. S.P., and Charles, A.K. (1997) Immunohistochemical demonstration of Wilms' tumor gene product WT1 in canine "neuroepithelioma" providing evidence for its classification as an extrarenal nephroblastoma. *J Comp Pathol* 116:321-327.

25. Gamblin, R.M., and Couto, C.G. (1997) Overexpression of p53 tumor suppressor protein in spontaneously arising neoplasms of dogs *Amer J Vet Res* 58:857-863.

26. Khan, K.N.M., Stanfield, K.M., et al. (2001) Expression of cyclooxygenase-2 in canine renal cell carcinoma. *Vet Pathol* 38:116-119.

Metastatic Tumors

General Considerations

Metastatic neoplasms are two times as common as primary neoplasms in dogs and seven times as frequent in cats (see table 10.1). The most common metastases in dogs are hemangiosarcoma, adenocarcinoma (unspecified primary), and lymphoma; in cats the most common tumor by a wide margin is lymphoma (some of these may be myeloproliferative tumors). Most neoplasms metastatic to the kidneys also have metastases in the lungs. An exception to this is lymphoma, in which pulmonary tumors are rare and renal metastases common. If lesions in the kidney(s) are metastatic, then there are metastases elsewhere. Problematic tumors are metastatic prostate, mammary, and pulmonary neoplasms, which can be difficult to distinguish from primary renal cell tumors. Size of the tumors, locations of tumors, histology, regional lymph nodes involved, and the low prevalence of primary renal cell tumors are usually the deciding factors. Immunohistochemical markers may help identify suspected metastases, and uromodulin has been used to confirm renal cell origin.

Lymphoma

Lymphoma is the most common tumor in the kidneys of cats and is one of the most common tumors in kidneys of all species.[1] Lymphoma is not confined to the kidneys, and tumor tissue will be located in lymph nodes and other lymphoid tissues. The neoplasm can cause azotemia by destroying over 75 percent of the parenchyma or by a unique location in the excretory pathway obstructing the outflow of urine. They can be associated with nonregenerative anemia, polycythemia, or hypercalcemia.

Tumors form multiple, bulging, soft, white-tan masses of varying sizes that can be confluent (fig. 10.5 A). Histologically they are "typical" lymphoma, characterized

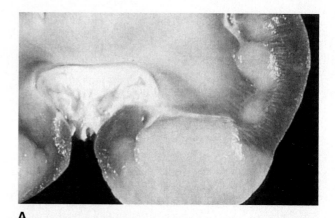

A

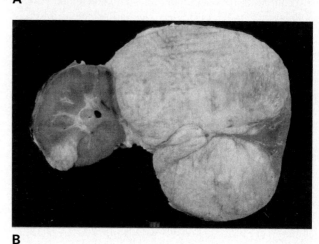

B

Fig. 10.5. **A.** Lymphoma, multicentric, forming discrete soft, white tumors in the renal cortex of a dog. Polycythemia from production of erythropoietin-like peptides is associated with various renal lesions including lymphoma. **B.** Cut surface of a kidney from a horse with tumor-like masses from marked granulomatous nephritis due to *Halocephalobus deletrix.*

by round, blastic nuclei, little visible cytoplasm, and no supporting stroma, dissecting through the interstitium. They could be confused with other poorly differentiated neoplasms, histiocytic tumors, or myeloproliferative disease, but usually the distribution in lymph nodes, histology/cytology, and if needed, immunohistochemistry are sufficient to establish a diagnosis.

Adrenal Tumors

Adrenal cortical carcinomas or pheochromocytomas occur with frequency in the kidneys from circulatory metastasis or direct extension.

Tumor-like Lesions

Hamartoma

Hamartoma has been described in an 8-month-old heifer with a 0.5 cm mass at the corticomedullary junction.[2]

The lesion was a mixture of tubules, spindle cells, collagen, glomerular-like structures, and blood vessels.

Telangiectasia

Telangiectasia is described in Welsh corgi dogs and consists of nonneoplastic proliferations of blood vessels in both kidneys and other organs, including duodenum, brain, vertebrae, subcutaneous tissue, and spleen.[3] In the kidney they produce multiple bulging red nodules that grossly look like hemangiomas or hemangiosarcomas. The distinction from hemangioma is that the blood-filled spaces in telangiectasia are lined by simple endothelium, and there is no proliferation of endothelial cells along the blood vessels or between thin trabeculae separating the cavernous spaces. They congregate at the corticomedullary area. They probably represent malformations and have been compared to hemangiomatous syndromes in humans.

Granulomas

Granulomatous interstitial nephritis can produce gross lesions that resemble neoplastic nodules. Diseases that mimic this appearance are feline infectious peritonitis, white spotted kidney disease and hairy vetch in cattle, and *Halocephalobus (Micronema) deletrix* in horses. Distribution of other lesions and histology usually make the identification of these diseases easy. *Halocephalobus deletrix* is more common in Europe but occurs worldwide and may produce large renal granulomas that are grossly indistinguishable from neoplasms (fig. 10.5 B). There are concurrent microscopic lesions in the nervous system. Histologically the lesions are typical granulomas with intralesional larvae.

Cysts

Solitary or multiple (polycystic) congenital cysts may be confused with cystic tumors grossly, but microscopic assessment clearly distinguishes them. Cysts contain transparent, amber to yellow fluid and are lined by a single layer of epithelial cells that are usually compressed and elongated. There is no proliferation of lining or papillary projections. In West Highland white terriers a polycystic renal and hepatic disease is reported to be autosomally recessive.[4] The cysts arise from the collecting ducts. Acquired cysts are part of inflammatory or neoplastic renal diseases that form due to obstruction of outflow of the glomerular filtrate. Cysts are often present in nephroblastomas and primary adenocarcinomas.

REFERENCES

1. Mooney, S.C., Hayes, A.A., Matus, R.E., et al. (1987) Renal lymphoma in cats: 28 cases (1977-1984). *J Amer Vet Med Assoc* 191:1473.
2. Hodgin, E.C. (1985) Meningeal hemangioma and renal hamartoma in a heifer. *Vet Pathol* 22:420-421.
3. Moore, F.M., and Thornton, G.W. (1983) Telangiectasia of pembroke Welsh corgi dogs. *Vet Pathol* 20:203-208.
4. McAloose, D., Casal, M., et al. (1998) Polycystic kidney and liver disease in two related West Highland white terrier litters. *Vet Pathol* 35:77–81.

TUMORS OF THE RENAL PELVIS AND URETER

Tumors of the renal pelvis and ureter are rare; when present, they are invariably a TCC or the same with squamous differentiation. When in either location they are likely to cause hydronephrosis and spread to the lower urinary tract by implantation metastases (see fig. 10.1 C). Occasionally they can disseminate throughout a ureter as plaques or small raised nodules (see fig. 10.1 D). In the pelvis they invade the medullary crest and start to ascend to the medulla while eroding lateroventrally through the capsule and into the perirenal tissues. Metastases are usually present by the time a diagnosis is established or a necropsy is performed. Other primary or metastatic tumors can localize in these regions, but they are uncommon.

Papillomas are rare, occur in the pelvis, and are characterized by papillae lined by one to five layers of mature transitional epithelium that covers a thin fibrous septum. They are of variable length and some may be macroscopically visible.

Hemangiomas are reported to occur in the renal pelvis and ureter of cattle with enzootic hematuria. Leiomyosarcoma has been reported in the ureter of a dog.[15] Archival material in files at NCSU contained rare examples of leiomyosarcoma and TCC in dogs and lymphoma in a cow ureter.

TUMORS OF THE URINARY BLADDER AND URETHRA

Neoplasia of the urinary bladder is common in dogs, relatively frequent in cats, and rare in all other species. An exception is cattle in endemic areas where bracken fern (*Pteridium* spp.) grows and is reported to produce bladder tumors in as high as 25 percent of cattle. Outside these geographic niches, the incidence of bladder cancer is much lower, 0.01-0.1 percent of cattle in abattoirs.[1,2]

Tumors of the bladder and urethra account for approximately 0.5-1.0 percent of all canine neoplasms and 2 percent of all malignant canine neoplasms.[3,4] Approximately 90 percent of urinary bladder neoplasms in dogs are of epithelial origin and are malignant (tables 10.3 and 10.4); 50-90 percent of these will have metastases, and approximately 75-90 percent of primary epithelial urinary bladder tumors are TCC. Only 10 percent are of mesenchymal origin, and they are split 50:50, benign and malignant (table 10.3). Smooth muscle tumor is the most common primary mesenchymal bladder neoplasms in dogs, and hemangioma is reported to be in cattle, at least those that are exposed to bracken fern. Benign epithelial tumors are rarely

TABLE 10.3. Urinary bladder neoplasia

		Total	Primary (%)	Primary Epithelial	Primary Mesenchymal	Secondary
Canine			807 (96)	752 (93)	55 (7)	
		845	Benign	0	35 (58)	38 (4)
			Malignant	752 (100)	20 (42)	
	Polyp	28				
Feline			56 (89)	52 (93) *	4 (7)	
		63	Benign	0	0	7 (11)
			Malignant	52	4	
	Polyp	3				

*45 TCC, 7 undifferentiated carcinoma.
807 primary canine tumors, 752 (96%) classified malignant.
56 primary feline neoplasms, 100% classified malignant.
Polyps were not classified as neoplasms.

TABLE 10.4. Canine primary urinary bladder tumors

	1	2	3	4	5	6	Total
Tumors, n	807	297	124	115	110	94	1547
TCC, n (%)	656 (81)	143 (48)	43 (35)	100 (87)	100 (91)	81 (87)	1124 (73)
Undiff. carcinoma	83	42	15	2	1	3	146 (9)
Adenocarcinoma	7	15	6	7	6	2	43 (3)
SCC	6	19	11	2	0	3	43 (3)
Adenoma	0	0	0	1	0	0	1
Papilloma	0	7	22	0	0	0	29 (2)
Leiomyoma	29	12	8*	2	3	2	57 (4)
Leiomyosarcoma	0	12	4	1	0	1	18 (1)
Fibroma	4	12	5	0	0	0	21 (1)
Fibrosarcoma	2	8	4	0	0	0	16 (1)
Hemangioma	2	2**	1	0	0	0	5 (0.3)
Rhabdomyosarcoma	9	11	1	0	0	2	23 (1)
Sarcoma	14	7	6	0	0	0	27 (2)
Lymphoma, secondary	9	0	2	0	0	2	13
Carcinoma, secondary	24	0	2	0	0	3	29

1 = VMDB: Veterinary Medical Data Base, 845 tumors, 807 primary.
2 = *Current Veterinary Therapy VII* 1980:1203; **6 Hemangiosarcoma not included in this table.
3 = *Amer J Vet Res* 29:2041, 1968; 130 tumors, 124 primary; *5 leiomyoma, 3 fibroleiomyoma.
4 = *J Vet Int Med* 6:145, 1992.
5 = *J Comp Pathol* 113:113, 1995.
6 = NCSU: North Carolina State University; 99 tumors, 94 primary and 5 secondary.

found as incidental lesions at necropsy, and by the time a neoplasm produces sufficient problems to be diagnosed clinically, the tumor is advanced and 20 percent will have clinically detectable metastases. Necropsy data shows that the rate of metastasis increases to 50-90 percent, the majority of these go to lungs and regional lymph nodes.[5] Nonpapillary (flat/sessile) and infiltrating TCC are the most likely to metastasize (100 percent), and papillary noninfiltrating are the least likely to spread.

Primary tumors of the bladder are much more common than secondary tumors, and metastasis to the urinary bladder is a rare occurrence. In material retrieved from the Veterinary Medical Data Base, 807 of 845 canine urinary bladder tumors were primary (96 percent) and 38 were secondary (table 10.3); in cats there were only 63 tumors, of which 56 were primary (89 percent) and 7 were secondary. Literature reviews indicate that cats[3,6,7] have neoplasms in the bladder comparable to those in dogs, with relatively similar percentages: TCC, 55 percent;, squamous cell carcinoma, 8 percent; adenocarcinoma, 5 percent; undifferen-

tiated carcinoma, 3 percent; leiomyoma, 6 percent; leiomyosarcoma, 5 percent; and examples of papilloma, hemangiosarcoma, fibroma, rhabdomyosarcoma, myxosarcoma, and cystadenoma.[3,6,7,9]

Paraneoplastic diseases associated with bladder or urethral tumors include hypercalcemia, cachexia, hyperestrogenism, hypertrophic osteopathy, and polycythemia. There are not many examples of bladder cancer reported in horses, and squamous cell carcinoma is the most common, although TCC, fibromatous polyp, rhabdomyosarcoma, and lymphoma also occur.

Clinical Pathology

Most of the clinical information available is for tumors in the urinary bladder of dogs, and observations are usually not separated for specific types of tumor. Some of the clinical signs are nonspecific (weight loss, weakness, lameness, dyspnea, etc.), and some are at least referable to the urinary system: dysuria [95/115 (84 percent)], pollakiuria (37 percent), abdominal pain (10 percent), and incontinence (9 percent) were reported in dogs with bladder or urethral tumors.[4]

Urinalysis

Approximately 90 percent of dogs with epithelial or mesenchymal tumors of the urinary bladder or urethra have one or more abnormalities detected on urinalysis.[3-6.] The most common are hematuria (76 percent of 100 dogs), pyuria (53 percent), proteinuria (31 percent), and bacteriuria (28 percent). Hematuria is due to physical disruption of blood vessels, either in the tumor or from contact and/or invasion of the tumor into adjacent parenchyma.

Chemistry

Hypercalcemia has been reported with a few tumors of the lower urinary tract.[4] Increased liver enzymes (ALP 27 percent, ALT 17 percent) are reported with tumors of the bladder and urethra in dogs.[4] The mechanism is not known but may be secondary to corticosteroid induced stress or concurrent hepatic problems. Azotemia is present in approximately 15 percent of dogs with bladder or urethra tumors and is most likely due to obstruction of the outflow of urine, resulting in postrenal azotemia.[3,4] Invasion through the wall of the bladder by the tumor or rupture of the bladder and production of uroabdomen is extremely rare. The expected changes are azotemia, creatinine and urea nitrogen concentrations greater in the abdominal fluid than serum, hyperphosphatemia, hyponatremia, hypochloremia, and hyperkalemia.

Anemia

If present, the anemia is nonregenerative, and there are multiple mechanisms superimposed. The most important of these are the anemia of chronic inflammatory disease and blood loss in the urine. Hypereosinophilia has been reported in one 14-year-old cat with a TCC.[8]

Cytology

Cytological confirmation of tumor cells in the urine seems a logical diagnostic aid but must be interpreted cautiously in suspected bladder tumors. Inflammation of the urinary tract stimulates hyperplasia of transitional epithelium, making the distinction of hyperplasia from dysplasia or neoplasia difficult. In dogs, approximately 30 percent (29/96) of transitional cell tumors can be diagnosed from urine cytologic examination, 77 percent (10/13) from prostatic or urethral washes, and 90 percent (20/22) from percutaneous fine needle aspirational cytology.[4] Ultrasound guided sampling and aspiration of the mass are critical to an accurate diagnosis. Relying on neoplastic cells that slough into the urine and can then be retrieved in cytologic preparations is insufficient. The diagnosis of a urinary bladder tumor is based on the recovery of numerous, large, anaplastic epithelial cells in clusters and/or individually

with little or no inflammation. Most tumors will evoke some inflammation, and it is preferable to examine a second sample when the urinalysis is devoid of, or shows minimal, inflammation. The best method for examining suspected cells in a urine sample is to collect a fresh sample, prepare a concentrated preparation, make a film of the sediment, and stain with a Diff-Quik type stain (do not diagnose from a wet mount, sedi-stain preparation). A cell-block of the sediment can also be processed and stained with H&E. Tumor cells will be in clusters or individual,[7] will be extremely large (> 40 μm diameter), and will have marked cytologic and nuclear variability (various sizes and shapes to cells, nuclei, and nucleoli), and some cells will contain large cytoplasmic vacuoles (see fig. 10.9 B). The more numerous these abnormalities and the less evidence of inflammation, the more likely the cells are neoplastic. If only a few of these cytologic abnormalities are identified and there is inflammation, then the cellular atypia more likely is due to dysplasia or hyperplasia of transitional epithelium than to neoplasia. Correlate results with other data, such as a mass in the trigone region of the bladder.

Markers

Basic fibroblast growth factor (bFGF) is a proangiogenic peptide used as a marker for urologic and nonurologic tumors in human beings and has been detected in high concentrations in the urine of dogs with bladder cancer.[10] Although the numbers of dogs were small, one study demonstrated significantly higher concentrations of bFGF in dogs with bladder cancer than in normal dogs or dogs with urinary tract infection (UTI).[10] Results are expressed as ng/g creatinine, and the median concentration of bFGF was 2.23 in normal dogs, 2.45 in dogs with UTI, and 9.86 in dogs with bladder cancer. One dog with bladder cancer did not have increased concentrations of bFGF, and one dog with UTI had concentrations of bFGF comparable to dogs with cancer; 86 percent of dogs with cancer could be correctly identified by increased concentrations of bFGF, and 90 percent of dogs with UTI did not have increased concentrations. The commercially available ELISA test kit uses a monoclonal antibody to recognize natural and recombinant human bFGF.[10,12,13]

Another commercially available test is the bladder tumor associated antigen (BTA). The assay detects a glycoprotein antigen complex that is of host basement origin and partly of tumor origin.[11-13] The dipstick test was used on 65 dogs, 20 with TCC, 19 healthy controls, and 26 urologic controls; the specificity (dogs with cancer have positive results) was reported to be 78 percent, and the sensitivity (dogs without cancer have negative results) 90 percent.[11] Results are not quantified: they are either positive or negative. False positive results can be seen with pyuria, hematuria, proteinuria, and glucosuria.[11] When these abnormalities are present the utility of the dipstick test is greatly limited, and if used, the test should be performed in conjunction with cytology and other ancillary tests. The dipstick test may be more appropriately applied as a screening test in older dogs for bladder cancer; however, cost and index of suspicion may limit its usefulness. Second generation BTA stat tests use a monoclonal antibody to recognize a human complement complex that is secreted into the urine of humans with bladder cancer. When applied to dogs with TCC the results have been negative, and they were attributed to the lack of cross reactivity of the monoclonal antibody to canine TCC generated antigens.[11]

An accurate noninvasive marker to detect bladder cancer is needed in veterinary medicine to help identify tumors as early as possible. Presently most cases of bladder cancer in domestic animals are recognized when the tumor is advanced, and therefore the prognosis is uniformly poor. There are a variety of substances secreted into the urine of human patients with bladder cancer, and there are assays to detect these substances.[12-14] However, there is no clear answer as to which is best. Future studies should be designed to evaluate some of these markers in animals and determine which are noninvasive, reliable, rapid, inexpensive, and accurate, with high sensitivity and specificity.

REFERENCES

1. Borzacchiello, G., Ambrosio, V., Galati, P., et al. (2001) The pagetoid variant of urothelial carcinoma in situ of urinary bladder in a cow. *Vet Pathol* 38:113-116.

2. Monlux, A.W., Anderson, W.A., and Davis, C.L. (1956) A survey of tumors occurring in cattle, sheep, and swine. *Amer J Vet Res* 17:646-677.

3. Osborne, C.A., Low,D.G., Perman, V., et al. (1968) Neoplasms of the canine and feline urinary bladder: Incidence, etiologic factors, occurrence and pathologic features. *Amer J Vet Res* 29:2041-2053.

4. Norris, A.M., Laing, E.J., Valli, V.E.O., et al. (1992) Canine bladder and urethral tumors: A retrospective study of 115 cases (1980-1985). *J Vet Intern Med* 6:145-153.

5. Valli, V.E., Norris, A., Jacobs, R.M., et al. (1995) Pathology of canine bladder and urethral cancer and correlation with tumor progression and survival. *J Comp Pathol* 113:113-130.

6. Caywood, D.D., Osborne, C.A., and Johnston, G.R. (1980) Neoplasms of the canine and feline urinary tracts. *Current Veterinary Therapy VIII*, W.B. Saunders Co., Philadelphia, pp. 1203-1212.

7. Walker, D.B., Cowell, R.L., et al. (1993) Carcinoma in the urinary bladder of a cat: Cytologic findings and a review of the literature. *Vet Clin Pathol* 22:103-108.

8. Sellon, R.K., Rottman, J.B., et al. (1992) Hypereosinophilia associated with transitional cell carcinoma in a cat. *J Amer Vet Med Assoc* 201:591-593.

9. Patnaik, A.K., Schwarz, P.D., and Greene, R.W. (1986) A histopathologic study of twenty urinary bladder neoplasms in the cat. *J Sm Anim Pract* 27:433-445.

10. Allen, D.K., Waters, D.J., Knapp, D.W., et al. (1996) High urine concentrations of basic fibroblast growth factor in dogs with bladder cancer *J Vet Intern Med* 10:231-234.

11. Borjesson, D.L., Christopher, M.M., et al. (1999) Detection of canine transitional cell carcinoma using a bladder tumor antigen

urine dipstick test. *Vet Clin Pathol* 28:33-38.

12. Ross, J.S., and Cohen, M.B. (1999) Ancillary methods for the detection of recurrent urothelial neoplasia. *Cancer Cytopathol* 90:75-86.

13. Sawczuk, I.S., Burchardt, T., et al. (2000) Bladder cancer markers: Current availability and the future standard of care. *Mod Lab Observ* (March): 30-41.

14. Pode, D., Shapiro, A., et al. (1999) Noninvasive detection of bladder cancer with the BTA stat test. *J Urol* 161:443-446.

15. Berzon, J.L. (1978) Primary leiomyosarcoma of the ureter in a dog. *J Amer Vet Med Assoc* 172:1427-1429.

Epithelial Tumors

Ninety percent of urinary bladder neoplasms in dogs are epithelial (see table 10.3), 85-98 percent of these are classified histologically as malignant, and 50-90 percent of these will have metastases. Benign epithelial neoplasms are rarely found, but polyps are relatively frequent. Urinary bladder carcinomas are classified as transitional carcinoma (75-90 percent of canine and 55-90 percent of feline tumors), squamous cell carcinoma (most common bladder tumor in horses), adenocarcinoma, or undifferentiated carcinoma, based on the predominant type of cell or organization in the tumor. Transitional cell carcinomas are further divided based on their patterns of growth as papillary (project into the lumen), nonpapillary (sessile or flat) and infiltrating (90 percent in dogs), or noninfiltrating (10 percent in dogs).

Most studies on domestic animals do not separate the clinical characteristics for each of the types of tumor, and therefore most of the reported data is for bladder neoplasms in general or bladder carcinomas. In this chapter information is provided for bladder carcinoma, primarily transitional cell carcinoma, and limited information is specific for other tumors of the bladder.

Papilloma

Incidence

In this author's experience papillomas are rare; however, 14 percent of the bladder tumors in cattle grazing bracken may be classified as papilloma,[1] and one report classified 17 percent of canine bladder tumors as papilloma.[2] Others have not reported such a high prevalence of papilloma in dogs, and the distinction of papilloma, polyp, and TCC in situ is subjective. Polyps and polypoid cystitis are relatively common, and some polyps may have been misclassified as papilloma, or vice versa. Of 1547 canine bladder tumors, 29 were classified as papilloma, and 22 of these were from one report (see table 10.4); the VMDB cases had no lesions classified as papilloma, however, there were 28 polyps in dogs and 3 in cats. In cattle papillomas are associated with bracken fern and/or bovine papilloma virus. Experimentally they will progress into carcinoma, and it is logical that the same is true for spontaneous lesions, but this has not been demonstrated. Experimentally induced lesions in dogs by 2-naphthylamine[3] tend to be flatter (fig. 10.6 A-C) than the papillae seen in spontaneous lesions.

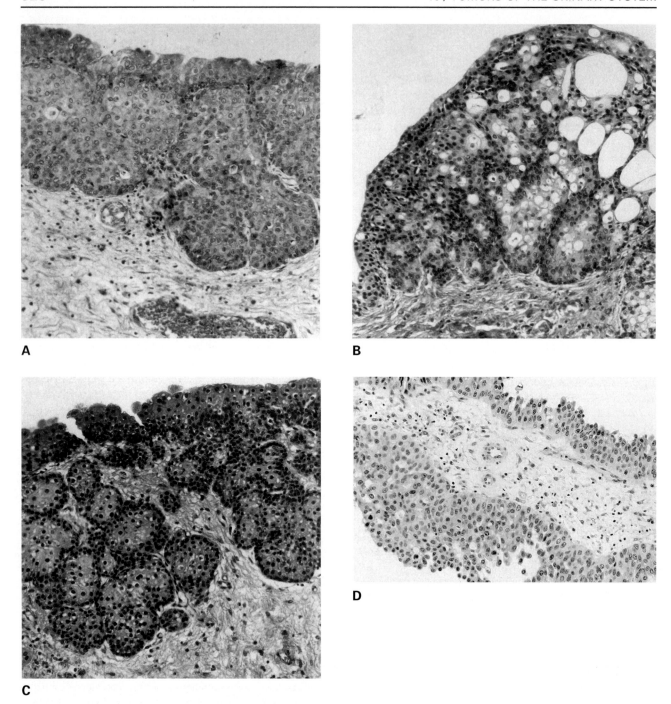

Fig. 10.6. Neoplasia of the urinary bladder of dogs, experimentally induced with 2-naphthylamine. **A.** Preneoplastic epithelial hyperplasia has multiple layers of transitional epithelium and invaginations projecting toward the lamina propria. (Courtesy of *J Natl Cancer Inst*) **B.** Early papilloma has formed a bulging nodule of transitional cells with considerable squamous metaplasia. Tumor has not yet organized into papillae with connective tissue stalks. (Courtesy of *J Natl Cancer Inst*) **C.** Nodular thickening composed of transitional cells in early papillomatous change. Continued growth could be either luminal or downward, penetrating the basement membrane and forming an invasive transitional cell carcinoma. (Courtesy of *J Natl Cancer Inst*) **D.** Papillary TCC versus papilloma. The central stalk is thin and not infiltrated by tumor cells. One side is covered with relatively few cells (top); the opposite side has multiple layers of cells. Dysplasia and anaplasia are minimal, the basement membrane appears intact, and the lesion was interpreted as a papilloma. This lesion was adjacent to areas of invasive, papillary TCC. [A,B,C. *J Natl Cancer Inst* (1972) 49(3):193–205; with permission.]

Histological Features

Papillomas are characterized by focal papillary projections of transitional epithelium (urothelium) covering a thin central fibrous stalk devoid of inflammation. The covering cells are one to five layers thick, they appear as normal urothelium, and mitoses are not present. The epithelial cells do not penetrate the stalk or the substantia propria at the base of the papilloma.

Differential Diagnoses

Polyps are broader based, and the core of the stalk contains inflammatory cells and blood vessels. The overlying urothelium is hyperplastic, usually with more cell layers than in papilloma, and there often is local erosion or ulceration. There may be concurrent cystitis glandularis or Brunn's nests. Granulation tissue, neovascularization, and inflammation in the submucosa usually make the distinction from papilloma easy. Some polyps contain a proliferative mass of fibrous tissue. Size, orientation, and selection of the specimen are factors that should be considered when differentiating a papilloma from a noninvasive papillary TCC. If the specimen is obtained at necropsy the pathologist can be certain the lesion is singular and benign. A lesion interpreted as a papilloma or benign epithelial tumor in a surgical specimen should be done so cautiously because size, orientation, and site of sample may influence the diagnosis. Benign lesions and carcinoma in situ may lie adjacent to invasive carcinoma (fig. 10.6 D). Reorientation or cutting through the entire block may reveal foci of invasion or cellular atypia.

The differentiation of a papilloma from a papillary noninfiltrating TCC is subjective and is based on the size of the lesion, cellular atypia, and branching in the lesion. Characteristics that favor TCC are small branches from the larger main growth, cellular atypia, greater than seven cell layers of epithelium, and fusion of stalks at the base of the lesion. Preference to classify lesions as papillary noninfiltrating TCC would help explain the discrepancies between the relatively high incidence of papilloma previously reported in dogs and the apparently low incidence in more recent surveys.[2,7,9,11] In one study papillomas were reported to be several millimeters to several centimeters in size, sometimes involved a considerable portion of the mucosa, and were most common in the trigone, and as they increased in size they tended to become necrotic.[2] It seems likely some of these could be classified as early TCC.

Distinction of papilloma from Brunn's nests or cystitis glandularis is of no clinical consequence. The latter two lesions do not form papillae, lie beneath hyperplastic urothelium, often are associated with an ulcer or inflammation, and have cellular features of squamous or glandular differentiation.

Adenoma

This is either a very rare tumor or at least is rarely diagnosed: 1 in 1547 canine tumors (see table 10.4). As pathologists our preference is to recognize a clearly benign epithelial growth as papilloma or polyp, but when invasion or cellular atypia is present to any degree, carcinoma is the preferred diagnosis. Adenomas are reported in cattle grazing on bracken. The most likely origin for these tumors, and adenocarcinoma is metaplasia of the transitional epithelium. Less likely, but diagnosed in humans, is urachal origin.[4]

Grossly, they are identical to a papilloma. The distinguishing feature is the formation of glands and histological infiltration into the substantia propria, but not deeper muscle layers (adenocarcinoma or transitional carcinoma). The tumors consist of well differentiated columnar epithelium devoid of anaplastic features. There will be areas of transitional epithelium, and there may be squamous metaplasia. Glands, or cystic spaces lined by a single layer of epithelium and containing variable amounts of mucin are present. There may be sloughed epithelial cells admixed with the mucin. Adenomas in humans can resemble villous adenomas of intestinal origin.[4] Mitotic figures are not visualized. Progression to TCC is possible based on observations in chemical carcinogenesis studies. If located in the dome (anterior region) of the bladder, they may be of urachal origin.[4]

Transitional Cell Carcinoma

General Considerations

This is the most commonly diagnosed tumor in the urinary bladder of domestic animals by a wide margin. Bladder neoplasms of any type are rare in horses, sheep, goats, and pigs.[3,5,6] Cattle rarely develop carcinomas spontaneously but have a high prevalence in geographic regions where enzootic hematuria exists.[5] There is a similar association in sheep that grazed on related ferns in Australia (5-8 percent of sheep developed TCC).

Incidence, Age, Breed, and Sex

Of the 1547 canine tumors summarized in table 10.4, 1124 (73 percent) were TCC. The report with the greatest number of papillomas also had the fewest TCC.[2] This is a neoplasm of older dogs (average age 9-11 years).[2,7-11] Despite an approximate 2:1 ratio of female to male for bladder neoplasms in numerous studies,[7-10] there is not always a statistically significant difference. Studies that linked bladder tumors to females suggested that the decreased frequency of urination in females, as compared to males, would result in a longer contact time of potential carcinogens with the bladder epithelium. This would not seem applicable to dogs housed inside since both males and females might only be allowed to urinate two to three times per day. The greater prevalence of bladder tumors in men is attributed to increased exposure of factory workers to industrial carcinogens.[11,12] Neutered dogs seem to be predisposed to bladder neoplasms, and breeds that may have a greater risk are Airedales, beagles, and Scottish terriers, while German shepherds are under-represented.[8,11]

Urinary bladder carcinomas may be underdiagnosed in cats since they occur in geriatric pets with concurrent diseases.[13-17] Forty-three cases in the literature and 56 listed in table 10.3 produce 99 cases in cats of which 84 were epithelial (60 TCC, 12 undifferentiated carcinoma, 5 squamous cell carcinoma, 4 adenocarcinoma, 2 papilloma, and 1 cystadenoma), and 15 were mesenchymal (7 smooth muscle, 4 vascular, 2 undifferentiated sarcoma, 1 rhabdomyosarcoma, and 1 myxosarcoma).[13-17] TCCs are reported infrequently in the cat, and reports suggest they are rare, citing frequencies of 0.07 percent.[3,15] Archival material from pathology reports over a 10 year period produced 4393 accessions, 1299 neoplasms, and 8 TCCs in cats for a frequency of 0.18 percent of all accessions and 0.38 percent of all tumors.[17] In dogs the frequency of blad-

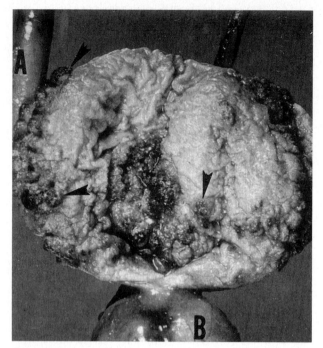

A

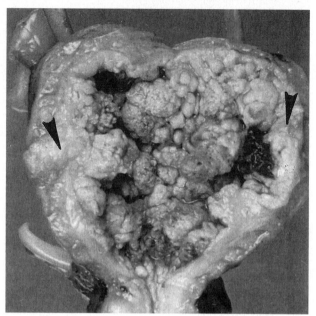

B

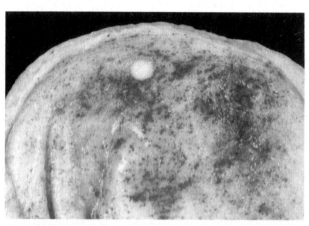

C

Fig. 10.7. Urinary bladder neoplasms in dogs given 2-naphthylamine daily for periods of 18 to 25 months. Bladders opened on ventral surfaces. **A.** Clusters of papillomatous to carcinomatous growths (arrowheads) in trigone and ventral surfaces; ureter *(A)* is dilated (hydronephrosis) and part of prostate is visible *(B)*. **B.** Nodular masses of an invasive carcinoma on the mucosal surfaces and infiltration into the muscle layers (arrowheads). Microscopic infiltration is the single most important predictor of metastasis. (Courtesy of *J. Natl Cancer Inst*) **C.** Small papilloma in a dog found as an incidental lesion at necropsy. [B. *J Natl Cancer Inst* (1972) 49(3):193–205; with permission.]

Nearly 90 percent of dogs present for clinical problems referable to the urinary system: hematuria, pollakiuria, or dysuria.[7,10,23] The other 10 percent present for signs unrelated to the urinary system: lameness due to bone metastases or dyspnea from pulmonary metastases.[7]

Gross Morphology

The most common location of this tumor in dogs is in the trigone area of the urinary bladder. Radiographic studies that demonstrate a filling defect and/or a mass in the trigone region of a dog with hematuria are helpful in the clinical diagnosis of this tumor. Contrast cystograms/urethrograms indicated a mass or filling defect in 87 of 91 dogs (96 percent).[7] Prostatic and lower urinary tract urethra are other common sites in dogs. In cats the carcinomas are usually located in the fundus or ventral wall rather than the neck of the bladder.[13,14]

Most tumors are solitary and only rarely are multiple on gross examination, although they may cover a large portion of the bladder mucosa (fig. 10.7). When tumors are multiple, it is difficult to distinguish multicentric origin from implantation metastases. They form papillary growths that project into the lumen of the bladder or bulge from the mucosa as nonpapillary, flat plaques or masses.

der tumors was 0.36 percent, and the data was interpreted to indicate that TCCs in the cat were not rare and that they occur as frequently as in the dog.[17] No sex or breed predilections could be obtained from the data.

Cattle with enzootic hematuria and bladder neoplasms are older, 4-12 years of age.[1,5,18,19] In endemic areas urinary bladder tumors are common, 15 percent in 5567 cattle in Turkey and up to 25 percent in some regions where bracken grows.[5,18,19] Related ferns in Australia produce similar lesions in sheep and cattle.[3] Outside of these geographic niches bladder cancer is rare in cattle, and little is known about the clinical characteristics.[5,6]

Too few cases have been reported in horses for reliable estimates. Of six horses with bladder tumors, one was 3 years old and had a fibromatous polyp, the other five were 13-23 years of age, and all six had a palpable mass in the urinary bladder.[20-22]

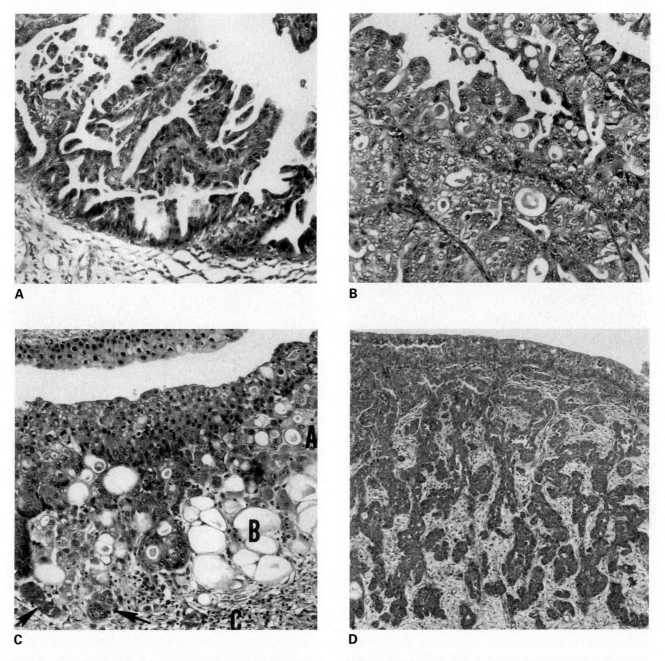

Fig. 10.8. **A.** Papillary noninfiltrating transitional cell carcinoma growing outward from surface has not penetrated the basement membrane. Foci of carcinoma in situ may be adjacent to invasive carcinomas and the size and orientation of biopsy specimens are critical to correct diagnosis. **B.** Papillary noninfiltrating carcinoma with fronds covered by anaplastic epithelium forming signet ring cells and microcysts. **C.** Squamous metaplasia *(A)* in basilar layers of epithelium with early invasion (arrows); marked vacuolation of cells *(B)* is a dysplastic feature seen in spontaneous hyperplasia and in experimentally induced preneoplastic and neoplastic squamous cells. Intracytoplasmic vacuoles produce characteristic signet ring cells and appearance of acini. Inflammatory reaction is present *(C)* in basilar stroma. **D.** Nonpapillary and invasive transitional cell carcinoma with prominent stromal fibrosis. This variant is the most likely to metastasize.

The base of nonpapillary types is broad, and most infiltrate into the muscle layers, producing a thick bladder wall (see fig. 10.9 A,D). When advanced, transmural extension is present, and there are tumors on the external surface of the bladder and in pelvic tissues. Carcinomatosis is not usually present grossly, but widespread peritoneal and distant metastases are often present on microscopic examination. The bladder wall is thickened and sclerotic in the region of

the tumor. Bilateral hydronephrosis develops secondarily to obstruction of outflow.

Histological Features

Transitional cell carcinomas are divided based on their patterns of growth (fig. 10.8) as papillary (project into the lumen, approximately 50 percent of cases) or nonpapillary (sessile or flat, 50 percent) and infiltrating

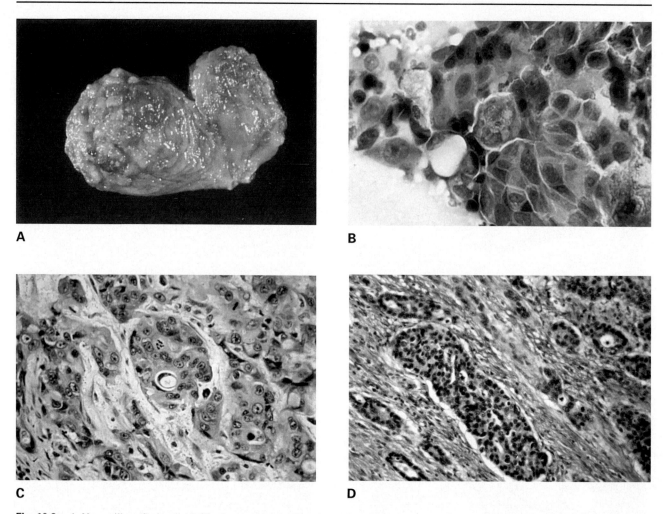

Fig. 10.9. **A.** Nonpapillary (flat/sessile) infiltrative transitional cell carcinoma that covers approximately one-third of the mucosa. By the time these carcinomas produce clinical problems they are advanced, 20 percent will have radiographically detectable pulmonary metastases at initial presentation. **B.** Cytologic preparation of TCC is devoid of inflammatory cells and is characterized by aggregates and morulae of transitional cells with cell-cell adhesion, moderate to marked nuclear and cytoplasmic variability, and signet ring formation. Approximately 30 percent of TCC can be diagnosed by cytologic examination of urine and 75-90 percent by cytologic examination of an ultrasound guided fine needle aspiration. **C.** Histologic section of TCC that mimics the cytologic pattern in view B. **D.** Infiltrative TCC; moderate desmoplasia, tumor is organized into solid nests and acini and tubules.

(90 percent) or noninfiltrating (10 percent). The reported prevalence of papillary versus nonpapillary varies widely in the literature; some indicate that papillary was the most common variant (80 percent),[11] and others that nonpapillary was (66 percent).[9] The consistent observation is that invasion is present in the majority of the samples, 90 percent, and that carcinoma in situ is rarely found.

Papillary and infiltrating is one of the most common variants of TCC; as the name implies, they form papillary or cauliflower growths that project into the lumen of the bladder (see fig. 10.7 A,B). They are often multiple. The papillary growths are tall and have branches. The papillae are covered by multiple layers of neoplastic urothelium that has mild to marked cellular atypia. Tumor cells infiltrate into the stalk of the tumor, substantia propria, and muscle layers and may be transmural. Metastases are expected.

Papillary and noninfiltrating TCCs have a similar luminal growth pattern but do not invade the stroma of their own stalk, or go beyond the substantia propria (fig. 10.8 A,B). Metastases are not likely with this variant. Differentiation from papilloma is subjective and is based on cellular atypia, small branches off the main lesion, greater than seven cell layers, and fusion of the growths at their base (see 10.6 D).

Nonpapillary and infiltrating transitional carcinomas form plaques, flat nodules, and masses that are often ulcerated and infiltrate into deeper muscle layers (fig. 10.9 A,D). The thickness of the bladder wall depends on the degree of invasion. There is marked histological and cytological variability. This variant is the most likely to metastasize. Depending on the study, this is either the second or the most common variant.[7,9,11]

Nonpapillary and noninfiltrating is the least common

type, and such tumors are confined to the surface epithelium, do not form papillae, and are synonymous with carcinoma in situ. They may be found adjacent to invasive carcinoma. If no other tumors are identified, paraffin blocks with carcinoma in situ should be cut deeper to determine if invasion is present. The neoplastic epithelium is more intensely eosinophilic, and cells can range from dysplastic to anaplastic. Loss of intercellular cohesion is a feature.

Qualifiers that can be used are *with squamous metaplasia; with glandular metaplasia;* and *with both squamous and glandular metaplasia.*[9] The degree of desmoplasia and inflammation can also be evaluated. The single most important observation to be examined for is invasion. Pathologists should report the morphological diagnosis, atypia, level of muscle invasion and presence of vascular or lymphatic invasion.

All variants consist of transitional cell epithelium in various degrees of differentiation (fig. 10.9). Carcinoma in situ is the most well differentiated; tumor cells remain within the surface epithelium and when seen are usually an incidental finding at necropsy or, more commonly, are adjacent to a larger malignant mass, as small lesions do not cause clinical problems. In biopsy specimens multiple samples are necessary to determine if all lesions are confined to the mucosa or if some infiltrate. The increase in cytoplasmic eosinophilia of tumor cells produces a sharp contrast with adjacent, more lightly colored nonneoplastic epithelium. The neoplastic cells have varying degrees of dysplasia and anaplasia. A 10-year-old cow that grazed on bracken fern and had enzootic hematuria for 5 years had a carcinoma in situ at necropsy. The carcinoma did not penetrate the basement membrane and had anaplastic cells with pleomorphic nuclei that sometimes formed nests and that resembled pagetoid cells.[1] The tumor cells were positive for cytokeratin; normal and neoplastic cells expressed fragile histidine triad (FHIT) protein, and some of the pagetoid cells did not. *FHIT* is a tumor suppressor gene that is inactivated in the majority of bladder TCC in humans.

The other variants of TCC are more anaplastic and invasive. The amount of cytoplasm is variable, some tumors have nuclei closely apposed, and others have abundant eosinophilic cytoplasm with sharp cell borders. Nuclei are large and vesicular, and nucleoli are prominent. Syncytial cells, atypical nuclei, and mitotic figures are common. Bizarre mitoses can be seen in cytological and histological preparations. There can be regions with squamous and/or glandular metaplasia, but these should not change the diagnosis from the predominant cellular proliferation, transitional cell epithelium. Cystic degeneration of the neoplastic epithelium gives the appearance of acini with lumens. Large cytoplasmic vacuoles ("signet rings") add to this appearance and are highly characteristic of TCC (fig. 10.9 B,C). Some spaces contain amphophilic to mucinous material that is PAS positive. A few tumors will have foci of glandular differentiation.

Tumors may stimulate a marked desmoplastic reaction in the primary and metastatic lesions. The primary lesions are associated with various degrees of lymphoid inflammation. Vascular invasion is seen in approximately 40 percent of the canine cases, and metastases may occur with or without the observation of vascular invasion in the primary neoplasm.

The papillary varieties have a central stalk covered by multiple layers of neoplastic epithelial cells that form a thick confluent mat. Invariably the tumors invade the stalk as well as the subjacent wall of the bladder.

Growth and Metastases

These are one of the most malignant neoplasms in domestic animals. By the time they are diagnosed clinically they have radiographically detectable pulmonary metastases in approximately 20 percent of the dogs, enlarged sublumbar lymph nodes in 9 percent, and metastases to lumbar or pelvis bones in 6 percent.[7,9,11] Metastases are present in the majority (50-90 percent) of dogs at necropsy[7,9,23]; lungs and lymph nodes are the two most common sites, but bones[24] are frequently involved, and most organs will have microscopic metastases. In dogs, reported rates for regional lymph nodes are 48 percent (36/75) and for distant sites 51 percent (38/75).[7,9] The anaplastic, nonpapillary, and infiltrating variants are highly prone to metastasize and readily spread to regional lymph nodes, lungs, and internal organs, and in some cases nearly every tissue will contain microscopic foci of TCC.

Using the classification outlined above, noninfiltrating TCC did not metastasize, papillary infiltrating TCC metastasized in 8 of 14 cases, and nonpapillary infiltrating TCC had metastases in 26 of 26 cases, for which necropsy slides were reviewed.[9] Histological classification was a predictor of metastases. Whether infiltration is an early event in TCC or develops late in the disease is not known. There was considerable histological variation in these tumors; foci of carcinoma in situ could be observed adjacent to infiltrating areas, and grades of the tumor would vary from one region to the next.[9] The most aggressive regions of tumor growth should be used to classify cells and the degree of infiltration. A recent study in dogs reported that histological criterion and immunohistochemical characteristics did not correlate with prognosis.[25] These investigators used immunohistochemical markers that may be important in drug resistance (P-glycoprotein, glutathione-S-transferase) and tumor angiogenesis (factor VIII–related antigen).[25]

Some investigators assess the extent of infiltration, character of invasion, and vessel invasion and grade the cancer as 1, 2, or 3.[9] Grade 1 tumors (22 percent) were well differentiated, and cells had normal volume, regular nuclear placement, round nuclei, and small or unapparent nucleoli. Grade 2 tumors (57 percent) were moderately differentiated; there was moderate variation in cytoplasmic volume, nuclear placement, and nuclear size and shape;

and nuclei were hyperchromatic with a single nucleolus. Grade 3 tumors (21 percent) were anaplastic; there was marked variation in cell, nuclear, and nucleolar size and shape, nuclear placement, and nuclear crowding. There was a correlation between grade and survival; however, survival was short for all dogs with TCC, even with therapy. Dogs with Grade 1 tumors survived longer than dogs with Grade 2 or 3 tumors, but survival was poor in any group, with notable exceptions: 12 of 18 dogs with Grade 1 survived less than 6 months; 54 of 60 dogs with Grade 2 survived less than 6 months; and 17 of 20 dogs with Grade 3 tumors survived less than 1 month. Others have not observed a statistically significant correlation between grade and prognosis, but there was a tendency toward decreased survival for dogs with higher grade tumors.[25]

Vascular invasion is a logical predictor of metastases, but the correlation was not consistent in the few cases studied. The results of two separate studies[9,25] show vascular invasion present in 42 percent (5/12) of biopsies from dogs that developed lymph node metastases and in 10 percent (5/48) that did not. Vascular invasion was present in 10 percent (4/40) of biopsies from dogs that developed distant metastases and in 32 percent (6/19) that did not; of the dogs that were necropsied, tumor emboli were seen in 38 percent (14/37) that had metastases, and tumor emboli were not seen in 62 percent (23/37) that had metastases.[9] Although lymphatic invasion did not correlate significantly with survival, the median survival of dogs with microscopic invasion of lymphatics was 145 days versus 349 days for dogs without lymphatic invasion. The number of dogs in this study was small, and the specimens evaluated were biopsy samples.[25]

Involvement of the urethra by the TCC is reported to be associated with distant metastases, but the difference is not large; urethral involvement was present in 76 percent of 25 dogs with metastases and in 50 percent of 54 dogs without metastases.[7] However, concurrent TCC in the bladder and urethra is associated with the shortest survival times. The number one organ for metastases is the lung (30-50 percent), followed by regional lymph nodes (25-40 percent), liver (10-20 percent), and muscle (20 percent), with lesser percentages for gastrointestinal, adrenal, bone, prostate, and uterus.[7,9,11] Microscopic examination can sometimes demonstrate metastases in nearly every organ examined.

The observation of squamous or glandular metaplasia in TCC may be important in the prediction of metastases; however, the number of cases studied is too few to be certain.[9] TCCs without either subtype had 100 percent metastases (n = 12), and two dogs with squamous or glandular metaplasia were free of metastases. Similarly, desmoplasia appeared to be a predictor of metastases in that all dogs with desmoplasia that were necropsied had metastases; however, only 10 dogs were evaluated, and in that study 90 percent of dogs necropsied had metastases.[9] Desmoplasia was present in 41 (38 percent) dogs, absent in 69 (62 percent), but the majority of these dogs were not necropsied. The degree of lymphoid infiltration also

TABLE 10.5.   TNM (clinical stage) of canine bladder cancer

Stage	Description
Primary tumors (T)	
T_0	No evidence of primary tumor
Tis	Carcinoma in situ
T_1	Superficial papillary tumor
T_2	Tumor invading the bladder wall
T_3	Tumor invading adjacent organs
Regional lymph node (RLN), internal and external iliac lymph node (N)	
N_0	No RLN involved
N_1	RLN involved
N_2	RLN and juxta-RLN involved
Distant metastases (M)	
M_0	No evidence of metastasis
M_1	Distant metastasis present—specify size

appeared to help predict metastases; tumors with minimum lymphoid inflammation tended to metastasize, and tumors with marked inflammation had fewer metastases.[9]

In summary, the following features were associated with metastases: nonpapillary, infiltrating, Grade 2 or 3, desmoplasia, minimum lymphoid inflammation, and urethral involvement. The first two of these are the most reliable. The following features were associated with survival: sex (spayed females survived 358 days versus 145 days for castrated males) and treatment selection (358 days for one protocol versus 132 days).[25]

Bladder carcinomas are also staged in human beings via the TNM system or as A-D based on degree of invasion: A, tumor in mucosa and submucosa; B, tumor in muscularis; C, tumor in pervesicular fat or peritoneum; D, organ (distant) metastases.[4,11] Staging criteria have been applied to dogs with bladder cancer (see table 10.5).[7] In veterinary medicine we need earlier diagnostic techniques to detect the tumors more than we need classification systems after a tumor is recognized.

An interesting characteristic is the ability of these tumors to proliferate within an abdominal incision. If tumor cells are "spilled" or "seeded" during surgical celiotomy for biopsy/excision of the neoplasm, they will readily proliferate and form macroscopic and microscopic growths of implantation metastases in the abdominal wall muscles.[26] Most cases are recognized within the first 3 months postsurgery as swellings or nodules at the incision site. In one case there was no evidence of the primary TCC in the bladder 131 weeks after the initial surgery and chemotherapy, but tumor was still present in the abdominal incision despite prior resection of the abdominal wall mass (no adjuvant therapy).[26]

Metastases are expected in approximately 50 percent of cats with TCC, although as in dogs nearly 100 percent have microscopic evidence of malignancy, local invasion, and/or intralymphatic nests of neoplastic cells.[13,14,16] The prognosis for horses with bladder cancer is equally poor as the tumor recurs and/or metastasizes.[20] Bladder tumors in the horse are reported to extend transmurally and produce carcinomatosis, but spread via lymphatics to regional nodes or distant organs did not occur in six horses with bladder tumors.[22]

Approximately 20 percent of the dogs with bladder cancer will have a second primary tumor.[7,9,11] Although this could be related to a defect(s) in growth regulation or exposure to a carcinogen(s), there are no data to confirm this.

Presently bladder cancers in dogs and cats are recognized so late in the stage of their progression that any ancillary techniques used to predict survival, metastases, or treatment protocols are biased. Whether histological features, immunohistochemical markers, or other techniques can be correlated with survival, metastatic predictions, or treatment protocols need to be determined on lesions in their earlier stages of development. The prognosis for dogs with neoplasms in the bladder or urethra is uniformly poor, with only 16 percent of treated dogs surviving for 1 year or more.[7]

Markers

Antibodies directed against epitopes of tumor associated glycoprotein 72 (TAG-72) have been shown to be positive in 53 percent of TCC from dogs.[10] This antigen is not unique to urothelium, and a variety of carcinomas in humans will stain positively. In dogs, greater than 50 percent of pulmonary, nasal, mammary, and transitional cell carcinomas were reported to stain positively to one of the epitopes of TAG (Mab B72.3). This antibody did not stain normal for hyperplastic canine transitional epithelium, which is in contrast to results in people. It was negative when used on a TCC from a horse.[21]

Antibodies to cytokeratin can be employed, but seem to be of limited utility in identifying tissue of origin since other epithelial tumors will stain positively. Positive staining has been demonstrated in canine and equine TCC.[21] In humans, cytokeratin stains positively in approximately 80 percent of the cases of TCC.[4,27] The basal layer of transitional epithelium expresses a greater variety of cytokeratin types than do the mature superficial cells. In addition to prostate specific antigen (PSA), the coordinate expression of cytokeratins 7 and 20 have been used to differentiate prostate adenocarcinoma and bladder urothelial carcinoma in men.[28] As expected, all urothelial tumors were negative for PSA, and 49 of 50 prostatic tumors were positive. Only 1 of 59 prostate tumors was positive for both cytokeratins 7 and 20, while 17 of 28 urothelial tumors were copositive. Coordinate expression of cytokeratins as a means to differentiate origins of unknown primary neoplasms may prove helpful in tumors of domestic animals. The majority of human TCCs will stain positive for epithelial membrane antigen and carcinoembryonic antigen, and they, along with epidermal growth factor receptors, have been correlated with grade, stage, and prognosis in human beings.[4,27] Whether immunohistochemical markers in dogs can be

correlated with survival predictions, metastatic predictions, or treatment protocols remain to be determined.

Urine concentration of basic fibroblast growth factor (bFGF) was significantly higher in dogs with bladder cancer than in normal dogs or dogs with bacterial cystitis. In a relatively small number of dogs it was determined that 86 percent of dogs with cancer could be correctly identified by increased concentrations of bFGF, and 90 percent of dogs with UTI did not have increased concentrations (see clinical pathology section).

The majority (79 percent) of canine TCCs are aneuploid, and normal or hyperplastic urinary bladders are diploid. There is no correlation, however, between DNA aneuploidy and numerous clinical and pathological features, including survival time, histological grade, clinical stage, growth pattern, and individual morphological features.[30] Fifty percent of the samples were tetraploid, 47 percent were hyperdiploid, and 3 percent were hypertetraploid.[30]

Argyrophilic nucleolar organizing regions (AgNOR) are not useful in distinguishing hyperplastic or polypoid cystitis from TCC in dogs and led to misclassifications of these lesions.[29] There was also no correlation between AgNORs and mitotic index in these same lesions. Mitotic index correctly identified all hyperplastic lesions (n = 7) but was less specific, identifying 70 percent of 12 malignancies.[29] The authors concluded that mitotic index was a useful means to separate hyperplastic from malignant urothelium but that AgNOR counts were not useful. Subjective criterion of invasion and atypia are equal to or better than mitotic index.

There are no ancillary techniques that effectively predict survival or metastases or influence treatment protocols for urinary bladder carcinomas in dogs and cats.

Squamous Cell Carcinoma

Clinical Features

Of the 1547 canine tumors, 3 percent were classified as squamous cell carcinoma (SCC). There are no unique clinical features in dogs with SCC versus other tumors of the urinary bladder. Of the 99 cases in cats, 5 were SCC.[2,13-15]

In horses squamous cell carcinoma is the most common primary tumor of the bladder, but very few cases have been reported.[20-22] Relatively small foci of squamous cell epithelium are present in the equine urinary bladder, and it is postulated that SCCs arise from these foci, although metaplasia of transitional cell epithelium is another source. In horses hematuria is the most frequent lab abnormality, and the majority of horses are older (13-23 years of age). Of six horses with primary bladder tumors four had SCC, one TCC, and one a fibromatous polyp. A mass was palpable in the urinary bladder of all six horses.[20,22] Distant metastases are not present, but there tends to be transmural spread into adjacent pelvic cavity and peritoneal carcinomatosis.[21,22]

Gross Morphology and Histological Features

Grossly they are nonpapillary and infiltrative and indistinguishable from TCC. Distinction from TCC is based on keratinization of cytoplasm, intercellular bridges, and keratin pearl formation. The majority of the neoplasms should have these features before this diagnosis is assigned. Areas of squamous cell differentiation in a TCC should be classified as TCC. Desmoplasia is more characteristic of SCC than of TCC.

Adenocarcinoma

The most likely origin of these tumors is metaplasia of transitional cell epithelium, but urachal remnants are another source.[4,31,32] There are few studies that describe transition from either glandular metaplasia or urachal remnants. Adenocarcinomas in human beings are divided into urachal and nonurachal origin because of different clinical data, prognoses, histological subtypes, and treatment regimens.[31,32] Urachal origin is suggested based on anterior location (dome), sharp demarcation between cancer and surface epithelium, absence of cystitis glandularis or intestinal metaplasia, and absence of a primary adenocarcinoma elsewhere.[4,31,32] Whether adenocarcinoma in animals is preceded by cystitis glandularis or inflammatory diseases of the bladder is not known.

Gross Morphology and Histological Features

Adenocarcinoma compromise approximately 3-5 percent of primary bladder cancers in dogs, cats, and cattle. Similarly to TCC, they grow as papillary or nonpapillary, and they infiltrate the bladder wall to various depths, but all have the same malignant behavior. The critical histological feature is the formation of acini, tubules, and/or glands with lumens and a secretory product. Lining epithelium is columnar, cuboidal, goblet cell with some transitional cells, but the majority of the tumor must have glandular features to justify this diagnosis. If limited areas of an otherwise TCC have glandular differentiation, then the tumor is classified as TCC with glandular metaplasia. Mucin production can be evident with H&E and can be demonstrated more clearly with stains for mucin.

Differential Diagnoses

The diagnostic dilemma is to determine if the tumor is a primary bladder adenocarcinoma or metastases or direct extension from prostate, uterus or rectum. Any diagnosis of a bladder adenocarcinoma in a male dog should be done after or on the premise that there is not a concurrent prostatic adenocarcinoma. Prostatic carcinomas will seed the mucosal surface of the bladder, as well as spread to the wall. In dogs prostate adenocarcinoma is more common than bladder adenocarcinoma. Immunohistochemistry to differentiate prostatic epithelium (prostate specific antigen, prostate acid phosphatase) from urothelium is not available in domestic animals, and to rule out an adenocarcinoma of prostate origin on histologic criteria is difficult. Even in human tumors multiple markers for prostate epithelium and combinations of cytokeratins are needed to distinguish these two tumors, and a percentage of these will not be clear cut.[4,28]

Criteria to suggest an adenocarcinoma is primary in the bladder are (1) no tumors in other sites of possible primary origin, (2) transition of nonneoplastic epithelium to neoplastic epithelium (versus abrupt delineation), (3) carcinoma in situ in adjacent area(s), and (4) regions of transitional epithelium in the adenocarcinoma. Tumors in the trigone and tumors confined to the mucosal surface are more likely of bladder origin. Tumors only in the wall or serosa should be considered metastases, and concurrent location in mucosa and wall are problematic and require the criteria outlined above. If a tumor is metastatic to the bladder, there are metastases in other organs.

Undifferentiated Carcinoma

Most primary urinary bladder tumors are well differentiated enough to classify; however, if a cell type can not be recognized then this classification is appropriate. It is not to be applied to primary bladder tumors that can be recognized as a histological type but are highly anaplastic. It was the second most common classification in the 1547 canine tumors summarized in table 10.4 (146 or 9 percent). It was also the second most common primary tumor of the bladder in cats (12/99).[2,13-15] Undifferentiated carcinoma cells form solid sheets with no architectural or cytological patterns. The cytoplasm is indistinct, nuclei oval to round and crowded close together. Immunohistochemical stains to identify some cytokeratin positive cells is generally needed. Metastases are expected.

REFERENCES

1. Borzacchiello, G., Ambrosio, V., Galati, P., et al. (2001) The pagetoid variant of urothelial carcinoma in situ of urinary bladder in a cow. *Vet Pathol* 38:113-116.
2. Osborne, C.A., Low, D.G., Perman, V., et al. (1968) Neoplasms of the canine and feline urinary bladder: Incidence, etiologic factors, occurrence and pathologic features. *Amer J Vet Res* 29:2041-2053.
3. Nielsen, S.W., and Moulton, J.E. (1990) Tumors of the urinary system. *Tumors in Domestic Animals,* 3rd ed. University of California Press, Berkely, pp. 458-478.
4. Eble, J.N., and Young, R.H. (2000) Tumors of the urinary tract. In Christopher Fletcher, *Diagnostic Histopathology of Tumors,* 2nd ed. Churchill Livingstone, Inc. pp. 475-565.
5. Ozkul, I.A., and Aydin, Y. (1996) Tumours of the urinary bladder in cattle and water buffalo in the Black Sea region of Turkey. *Br Vet J* 152:473-475.
6. Monlux, A.W., Anderson, W.A., and Davis, C.L. (1956) A survey of tumors occurring in cattle, sheep, and swine. *Amer J Vet Res* 17:646-677.
7. Norris, A.M., Laing, E.J., Valli, V.E.O., et al. (1992) Canine bladder

and urethral tumors: A retrospective study of 115 cases (1980-1985). *J Vet Intern Med* 6:145-153.

8. Hayes, H.M. (1976) Canine bladder cancer: Epidemiological features. *Amer J Epidemiol* 104:673-677.

9. Valli, V.E., Norris, A., Jacobs, R.M., et al. (1995) Pathology of canine bladder and urethral cancer and correlation with tumor progression and survival. *J Comp Pathol* 113:113-130.

10. Clemo, F.A.S., DeNicola, D.B., Carolton, W.W., et al. (1995) Immunoreactivity of canine transitional cell carcinoma of the urinary bladder with monoclonal antibodies to tumor-associated glycoprotein 72. *Vet Pathol* 32:155-161.

11. Knapp, D.W., Glickman, N.W., et al. (2000) Naturally occurring canine transitional cell carcinoma of the urinary bladder. *Urologic Oncol* 5:47-59.

12. Friedell, G.H., Gopal, C.P., et al. (1980) The pathology of human bladder cancer. *Cancer* 45:1823-1831.

13. Walker, D.B., Cowell, R.L., et al. (1993) Carcinoma in the urinary bladder of a cat: Cytologic findings and a review of the literature. *Vet Clin Pathol* 22:103-108.

14. Caywood, D.D., Osborne, C.A., and Johnston, G.R. Neoplasms of the canine and feline urinary tracts. (1980) *Current Veterinary Therapy VIII*, W.B. Saunders Co., Philadelphia, pp. 1203-1212.

15. Patnaik, A.K., Schwarz, P.D., and Greene, R.W. (1986) A histopathologic study of twenty urinary bladder neoplasms in the cat. *J Sm Anim Pract* 27:433-445.

16. Engle, G.C., Brodery, R.S., et al. (1969) A retrospective study of 395 feline neoplasms. *J Amer Anim Hosp Assoc* 5:21-31.

17. Wimberly, H.C., and Lewis, R.M. (1979) Transitional cell carcinoma in the domestic cat. *Vet Pathol* 16:223-228.

18. Pamukcu, A.M., Price, J.M., and Bryan, G.T. (1976) Naturally occurring and bracken-fern-induced bovine urinary bladder tumors. *Vet Pathol* 13:110-122.

19. Campo, M.S., Jarrett, W.F.H., et al. (1992) Association of bovine papillomavirus type 2 and bracken fern with bladder cancer in cattle. *Cancer Res* 52:6898-6904.

20. Traub-Dargatz, J.L. (1998) Urinary tract neoplasia. *Vet Clin N Amer: Equine Pract* 14:495-504.

21. Patterson-Kane, J.C., Tramontin, R.R., Giles, R.C., and Harrison, L.R. (2000) Transitional cell carcinoma of the urinary bladder in a thoroughbred, with intra-abdominal dissemination. *Vet Pathol* 37:692-695.

22. Fischer, A.T., Spier, S., Carlson, G.P., et al. (1985) Neoplasia of the equine urinary bladder as a cause of hematuria. *J Amer Vet Med Assoc* 186:1294-1296.

23. Strafuss, A.C., and Dean, M.J. (1975) Neoplasms of the canine urinary bladder. *J Amer Vet Med Assoc* 166:1161-1163.

24. McCaw, D.L., Hogan, P.M., and Shaw, D.P. (1988) Canine urinary bladder transitional cell carcinoma with skull metastasis and unusual pulmonary metastases. *Can Vet J* 29:386-388.

25. Rocha, T.A., Nel Mauldin, G. et al. (2000) Prognostic factors in dogs with urinary bladder carcinoma. *J Vet Intern Med* 14:486-490.

26. Gilson, S.D., and Stone, E.A. (1990) Surgically induced tumor seeding in eight dogs and two cats. *J Amer Vet Med Assoc* 196(11): 1811-1815.

27. Nakopoulou, L., Zervas, A., et al. (1995) Epithelial antigens and epidermal growth factor receptors in transitional cell bladder carcinoma: Correlation with prognosis. *Urol Int* 54:191-197.

28. Bassily, N.H., Vallorosi, C.J., Akdas, G., et al. (2000) Coordinate expression of cytokeratins 7 and 20 in prostate adenocarcinoma and bladder urothelial carcinoma. *Amer J Clin Pathol* 113:383-388.

29. Johnson, G.C., Miller, M.A., and Ramos-Vara, J.A. (1995) Comparison of argyrophilic nucleolar organizer regions (AgNORs) and mitotic index in distinguishing benign from malignant canine smooth muscle tumors and in separating inflammatory hyperplasia from neoplastic lesions of the urinary bladder mucosa. *J Vet Diagn Invest* 7:127-136.

30. Clemo, F.A.S., DeNicola, D.B., Carlton, W.W., et al. (1994) Flow cytometric DNA ploidy analysis in canine transitional cell carcinoma. *Vet Pathol* 31:207-215.

31. Grignon, D.J., Ro, J.Y., et al. (1991) Primary adenocarcinoma of the urinary bladder. *Cancer* 67:2165-2172.

32. Miller, D.C., Gang, D.L., et al. (1983) Villous adenoma of the urinary bladder: A morphologic or biologic entity? *Amer J Clin Pathol* 79:728-731.

Treatment and Survival

The prognosis for dogs with neoplasms in the bladder or urethra is uniformly poor, with only 16 percent of treated dogs surviving for 1 year or more. Neoplasia in both the bladder and urethra is associated with the shortest survival times. In dogs with no clinically detectable metastases, the complete surgical excision of bladder tumors yielded the longest median survival, 365 days.[1]

There are no consistent treatments for TCC that will produce a cure, and until the tumors can be recognized early, survival times and/or cures will be limited. The "late" diagnosis is attributable to mild clinical manifestations (dysuria, pollakiuria, hematuria) that delay presentation and to the difficulty of clinically distinguishing neoplastic from nonneoplastic diseases of the lower urinary tract. Superficial bladder cancer is a rare event in dogs or is recognized infrequently, yet it represents up to 80 percent of bladder cancers in humans.[2] This may be due to the clinically silent nature of the cancer in dogs, to inherent differences in the oncogenesis of bladder cancer between dogs and humans, or to the use of screening tests for early detection of bladder cancer in human patients. In any event, by the time cancer of the urinary bladder is recognized in dogs, the neoplasm has infiltrated the wall of the bladder (80-90 percent) and is in an advanced stage of the tumor's life, with clinically detectable metastases already present in 20 percent of the dogs at initial presentation.[1,3,4]

Generally, by the time a tumor is identified, it is large, invasive, and nonresectable. The nonresectable nature of the tumor (trigone, large, infiltrative) greatly reduces successful treatment.[5] Critical to improved treatment and survival will be an earlier diagnosis. Cytological evaluation of the urine identifies neoplastic cells in only 30 percent of dogs with advanced bladder cancer. Potential markers for bladder cancer that can be measured in the urine, such as basic fibroblast growth factor or BTA, may help establish an earlier diagnosis.

Factors associated with an unfavorable outcome are the advanced stage of the cancer at the time of diagnosis, size and/or location of the tumor such that resection is not feasible, tumor presence in bladder and urethra, and limited responses of bladder cancer to chemotherapy or radiation therapy.[1,6,7] Features associated with metastases are nonpapillary, infiltration, Grade 2 or 3, and urethral involvement.[3] A report on 25 dogs with bladder cancer indicated that histological diagnosis and immunohistochemical characteristics did not correlate with prognosis.[6] Factors associated with a favorable outcome are tumor size and location that permit resection and restriction of tumor to bladder or urethra. The following features were associated with survival: sex (spayed females survived 358 days versus 145 days for castrated males) and treatment selection (358 days for one protocol versus 132 days).[6] Anatomic and hormonal differences may contribute to longer survival in females. Although the number of dogs studied was small and there were multiple treatment variables, the dogs that received an anthracycline drug in addition to a platinum compound survived almost three times as long as dogs treated with only a platinum compound.[6]

Alone or in various combinations, treatments include surgical removal,[5] partial cystectomy, ureterocolonic anastomosis,[9] radiation, systemic chemotherapy regimens, platinum compounds, intravesical chemotherapy, and non-steroidal anti-inflammatory drugs (NSAID).[5-14] Depending on the report, the median and mean survival times are 180 to 270 days, with ranges of 3 days to complete remission.[1,12] One of the most common strategies is chemotherapy with or without the NSAID piroxicam. Piroxicam has been used in dogs with TCC, and responses include complete remission in two dogs and partial remission or stable disease in many others.[7] It has also been used as a chemo-preventative in rodent models of bladder cancer.[13] Prostaglandin E2 has multiple roles in promoting tumor growth and is found in increased concentrations in TCC of dogs, and the enzymes that produce prostaglandins, cyclooxygenase-2, and cyclooxygenase-1, are expressed in canine TCC, while only cyclooxygenase-1 is expressed by normal canine bladder epithelium.[7,12,14] Cyclooxygenase-1 (COX-1) functions in normal physiology, and COX-2 functions in inflammatory diseases and is a regulator of cell growth.[14] The response of urinary and colorectal cancers to NSAIDs is likely due to inhibition of COX enzymes and decreased prostaglandin production.

Etiology

Although there are a variety of chemicals that can induce urinary bladder neoplasms experimentally, there are few known spontaneous carcinogens other than bracken fern. Tryptophan, an essential amino acid, is metabolized to orthoaminophenol metabolites (aromatic amines), and the excretion of these through the urinary system results in high concentrations of these carcinogenic metabolites in the urine.[15-17] These intermediate metabolites of tryptophan induce bladder neoplasms in experimental animals and are implicated as an etiology in spontaneous bladder neoplasms in dogs and human beings. The greater prevalence of neoplasms in the bladder than in the rest of the urinary system is attributed to retention of urine in the bladder and longer exposure of transitional epithelium to carcinogens. Cats process tryptophan differently than do dogs, rats, and humans and have near zero concentrations of orthoaminophenol metabolites in their urine.[16,17]

Administration of cyclophosphamide has been associated with hemorrhagic cystitis and TCC of the bladder in dogs,[18] and cyclophosphamide increases the risk of bladder cancer nearly ten-fold in humans.[2] Risk factors associated with bladder cancer in dogs include topical insecticides, exposure to marshes sprayed with chemicals for mosquito control, female gender (nearly 2:1), obesity, and breed.[7,19] The Scottish terrier has a 19-fold increased risk compared to mixed breeds.[7,19] No specific chemical in topical insecticides could account for the increased risk, and therefore the inert ingredients, which may be 95 percent of the total product, were considered the probable carcinogen.[19] Inert ingredients include solvents such as benzene, toluene, xylene, and petroleum distillates. Benzene is associated with bladder cancer in human beings.[2,19]

Chemical carcinogens in the nitrosamine family can induce bladder cancer in dogs, rats, and mice.[20-22] Chemically induced tumors progress through an "orderly" series of cellular and histological stages. The earliest visible changes are focal hyperplasia of transitional epithelium and squamous metaplasia. These hyperplastic "foci" progress into dysplastic changes, carcinoma in situ, papilloma, adenoma, and carcinoma (transitional, squamous, adeno-).[21,22] Although it is logical that spontaneous tumors would also progress through these steps, there are no studies documenting this sequence. Vascular endothelial growth factor promotes tumor angiogenesis, and it appears to play a more important role in nirosamine induced bladder cancers in rats then does basic fibroblast growth factor.[22] Three primary aromatic amines (2-naphthylamine, benzidine, and 4-aminodiphenyl) associated with bladder cancer in men induce urinary bladder carcinoma in dogs following prolonged systemic administration.[2,7,23] Metabolites of these compounds can be 200 times greater in the urine then in the blood. There is a correlation between the occurrence of canine and human bladder cancers and the level of industrial activity, suggesting roles for environmental factors.[23,24] Smoking cigarettes is linked to bladder cancers in humans, but the role of sidestream smoke is less clear, and it is unrelated to bladder cancer in dogs.[2,19,22] *Schistosoma hematobium* excretes free nitrites, nitrosamines, in the urine and is associated with bladder tumors.[25]

Immunoreactivity for p53 was not prominent in one study,[26] but others have suggested it was observed in canine tissue samples and in a canine TCC cell line.[7] The tumor suppressor gene *FHIT* (fragile histidine triad) is located at chromosomal region 3p14.2 in humans, and inactivation of this gene by deletions occurs in many primary tumors. It has been demonstrated that *FHIT* is inactivated in the majority of TCC in bladder tumors of humans.[27] A recent report of a 10-year-old cow with enzootic hematuria and carcinoma in situ had nests of anaplastic cells (pagetoid cells) that did not express FHIT protein, although adjacent normal and neoplastic urothelium did.[28]

Hematuria, anemia, hemorrhage, and/or neoplasms in the lower urinary tract characterize a syndrome in cattle associated with the ingestion of bracken (*Pteridium aquil-*

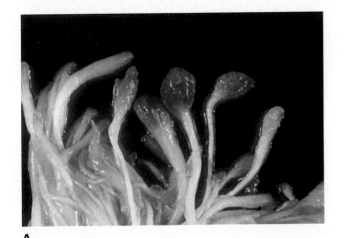

A

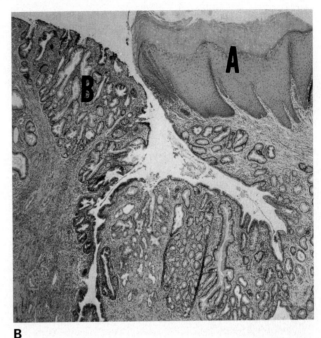

B

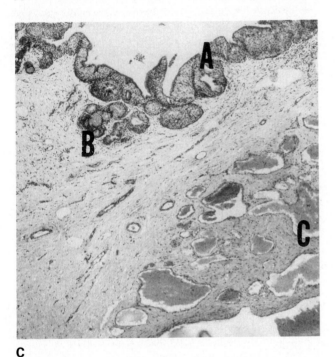

C

Fig. 10.10. **A.** Marked papillary hyperplasia of the urinary bladder epithelium in a cow with cystitis; no history of bracken fern ingestion in North Carolina. Views B and C are early and/or preneoplastic lesions in the urinary bladder of a cow that had chronic hematuria and that had ingested bracken fern for a long period. **B.** Marked squamous cell *(A)* and glandular *(B)* metaplasia of the mucosal epithelium. **C.** Atypical and hyperplastic transitional uothelium *(A)* overlying small nests of transitional cells, Brunn's nests *(B)*. Hemangiomatous tissue *(C)* in submucosa. (Courtesy of Dr. Carl Olson.)

inum) or other ferns (*Cheilantres sieberi*), termed *enzootic hematuria.*[28-32] A primary feature of bracken fern poisoning is multiple hemorrhages in the urinary system, subcutis, alimentary and nasal mucosa, heart, and lungs. Bladder histological changes (fig. 10.10 B,C) occurring before or in conjunction with neoplasms include congestion, edema, hemorrhage, ulceration, endarteritis obliterans, and detachment of endothelium. In over 90 percent of the cases, urinary bladder tumors are reported as the cause of the hematuria, but enzootic hematuria may occur in cattle without neoplasms. Young animals are usually not involved, and a long period of residence in an affected area is required before an animal develops hematuria. Urinary bladder tumors are common, 15 percent in 5567 cattle, in 4-12-year-old cattle in endemic areas of Turkey.[29] The areas of the bladder affected are the ventral and lateral walls of the fundus and the trigone, which are sites in constant contact with urine. Epithelial and mesenchymal

tumors may develop, and in more than 50 percent of affected cattle the neoplasms are mixed epithelial-mesenchymal tumors. A variety of carcinogens and mutagens such as quercetin, shikimic acid, prunasin, ptaquiloside, and aquilide are contained in bracken fern.[29-31] In addition to carcinogens and mutagens, the fern contains powerful immunosuppressants. Feeding bracken to cattle or sheep for prolonged times will induce bladder and intestinal neoplasms as well as the other components of this syndrome. However, the disease occurs in areas without bracken and other related ferns, and often does not occur where the fern is growing.[29,31]

In addition to environmental carcinogens, there is strong circumstantial evidence of a role for the bovine papillomavirus (BPV-2) in the pathogenesis of urinary bladder oncogenesis.[28,31] DNA of BPV-2 was found in 69 percent and 46 percent of experimental and naturally occurring bovine bladder cancers. BPV-2 can induce cutaneous papillomas, and extracts of these can induce bladder tumors when injected into the urinary bladder of cows.[31] Bovine papilloma virus is the etiological agent of papillomas in the upper alimentary tract, and these lesions can serve as a focus for transformation to squamous cell carcinoma in animals feeding on bracken fern. Animals with carcinoma of the upper alimentary canal may also have adenomas and adenocarcinoma of the lower bowel, and carcinoma and hemangiosarcoma of the urinary bladder.

REFERENCES

1. Norris, A.M., Laing, E.J., Valli, V.E.O., et al. (1992) Canine bladder and urethral tumors: A retrospective study of 115 cases (1980-1985). *J Vet Intern Med* 6:145-153.
2. Eble, J.N., and Young, R.H. (2000) Tumors of the urinary tract. In Christopher Fletcher, *Diagnostic Histopathology of Tumors,* 2nd ed. Churchill Livingstone, Inc., pp. 475-565.
3. Valli, V.E., Norris, A., Jacobs, R.M., et al. (1995) Pathology of canine bladder and urethral cancer and correlation with tumor progression and survival. *J Comp Pathol* 113:113-130.
4. Clemo, F.A.S., DeNicola, D.B., Carolton, W.W., et al. (1995) Immunoreactivity of canine transitional cell carcinoma of the urinary bladder with monoclonal antibodies to tumor-associated glycoprotein 72. *Vet Pathol* 32:155-161.
5. Stone, E.A., George, T.F., Gilson, S.D., et al. (1996) Partial cystectomy for urinary bladder neoplasia: Surgical technique and outcome in 11 dogs. *J Sm Anim Pract* 37:480-485.
6. Rocha, T.A., Nel Mauldin, G., et al. (2000) Prognostic factors in dogs with urinary bladder carcinoma. *J Vet Intern Med* 14:486-490.
7. Knapp, D.W., Glickman, N.W., et al. (2000) Naturally occurring canine transitional cell carcinoma of the urinary bladder. *Urologic Oncol* 5:47-59.
8. Stone, E.A., Withrow, S.J., Page, R.L., et al. (1988) Ureterocolonic anastomosis in ten dogs with transitional cell carcinoma. *Vet Surgery* 17:147-153.
9. Helfand, S.C., Hamilton, T.A., et al. (1994) Comparison of three treatments for transitional cell carcinoma of the bladder in the dog. *J Amer Anim Hosp Assoc* 30:270-275.
10. Chun, R., Knapp, D.W., et al. (1996) Cisplatin treatment of transitional cell carcinoma of the urinary bladder in dogs: 18 cases (1983-1993). *J Amer Vet Med Assoc* 209:1588-1591.
11. Walker, M., and Breider, M. (1987) Intraoperative radiotherapy of canine bladder cancer. *Vet Radiol* 28:200-204.
12. Knapp, D.W., Richardson, R.C., Chan, T.C.K., et al. (1994) Piroxicam therapy in 34 dogs with transitional cell carcinoma of the urinary bladder. *J Vet Intern Med* 8:273-278.
13. Rao, K.V., Detrisac, C.J., et al. (1996) Differential activity of aspirin, ketoprofen and sulindac as cancer chemopreventative agents in the mouse urinary bladder. *Carcinogenesis* 17:1435-1438.
14. Khan, K.N.M., Stanfield, K.M., et al. (2001) Expression of cyclooxygenase-2 in canine renal cell carcinoma. *Vet Pathol* 38:116-119.
15. Radomski, J.L., Glass, E.M., and Deichman, E.B. (1971) Transitional cell hyperplasia in the bladder of dogs fed DL-tryptophan. *Cancer Res* 31:1690-1694.
16. Broan, R.R., and Price. J.M. (1956) Quantitative studies on metabolites of tryptophan in the urine of the dog, cat, rat and man. *J Biol Chem* 219:985-997.
17. Leklem, J.E., Brown, R.R., et al. (1971) Tryptophan metabolism in the cat. *Amer J Vet Res* 32:335-344.
18. Macy, D.W., Withrow, S.J., and Hoopes, J. (1983) Transitional cell carcinoma of the bladder associated with cyclophosphamide therapy in a dog. *J Amer Anim Hosp Assoc* 19:965-969.
19. Glickman, L.T., Schofer, F.S., and McKee, L.J. (1989) Epidemiology study of insecticide exposures, obesity and risk of bladder cancer in household dogs. *J Toxicol Environ Health* 28:407-414.
20. Conzelman, G.M., Jr., and Moulton, J.E. (1972) Dose-response relationships of the bladder tumorigen 2-naphthylamine: A stude in beagle dogs. *J Natl Cancer Inst* 49:193-205.
21. Okajima, E., Hiramatsu, T., Hirao, K., et al. (1981) Urinary bladder tumors induced by nitrosamine in dogs. *Cancer Res* 41:1958-1966.
22. Wakui, S., Furusato, M., Sasaki, S., et al. (1999) Expression of vascular endothelial growth factor in nirosamine-induced rat bladder carcinogenesis. *Vet Pathol* 36:111-116.
23. Hayes, H.M., Hoover, R., and Tarone, R. (1981) Bladder cancer in pet dogs: A sentinel for environmental cancer? *J Epidemiol* 114:229-233.
24. Hayes, H.M. (1976) Canine bladder cancer: Epidemiological features. *Amer J Epidemiol* 104:673-677.
25. Warren, W., Biggs, P.J., et al. (1995) Mutations in the p53 gene in schistosomal bladder cancer. *Carcinogenesis* 16:1181-1189.
26. Gamblin, R.M., and Couto, C.G. (1997) Overexpression of p53 tumor suppressor protein in spontaneously arising neoplasms of dogs. *Amer J Vet Res* 58:857-863.
27. Baffa, R., Gomella, L.G., et al. (2000) Loss of FHIT expression in transitional cell carcinoma of the urinary bladder. *Amer J Pathol* 156:419-424.
28. Borzacchiello, G., Ambrosio, V., Galati, P., et al. (2001) The pagetoid variant of urothelial carcinoma in situ of urinary bladder in a cow. *Vet Pathol* 38:113-116.
29. Ozkul, I.A., and Aydin, Y. (1996) Tumours of the urinary bladder in cattle and water buffalo in the Black Sea region of Turkey. *Br Vet J* 152:473-475.
30. Pamukcu, A.M., Goksoy, S.K., and Price, J.M. (1967) Urinary bladder neoplasms induced by feeding bracken fern (*Pteris aqulinia*) to cows. *Cancer Res* 27:917-924.
31. Campo, M.S., Jarrett, W.F.H., et al. (1992) Association of bovine papillomavirus type 2 and bracken fern with bladder cancer in cattle. *Cancer Res* 52:6898-6904.
32. Nielsen, S.W., and Moulton, J.E. (1990) Tumors of the urinary system. *Tumors in Domestic Animals,* 3rd ed. University of California Press, Berkely, pp. 458-478.

Mesenchymal Tumors

Approximately 10 percent of canine urinary bladder neoplasms are mesenchymal. They are similar to the same tumors in other locations, and complete descriptions are best found in those sections of this book. The most frequent types are leiomyoma and leiomyosarcoma and hemangioma and hemangiosarcoma. The most interesting type is rhabodomyosarcoma because of this seemingly unusual location, its occurrence in young dogs, and the associated syndrome they produce, hypertrophic osteopathy. Mesenchymal tumors and mixtures of epithelial-mesenchymal tumors occur in cattle with enzootic hematuria.

Leiomyoma and Leiomyosarcoma

Clinical Characteristics

Similarly to other tumors of the urinary bladder, these occur primarily in dogs and are rare in all the other species. Earlier reports indicate they account for approximately 12 percent of all primary canine urinary bladder tumors,[1] but other surveys report only 4/137 (3 percent) (3 leiomyomas and 1 leiomyosarcoma), 2/115, or 1/213 canine bladder tumors;[2,3,4] table 10.4 shows 75/1547 for 5 percent. Dogs range in age from 2 to 14 years, with a mean of 12.5 for leiomyoma and 7 for leiomyosarcoma.[4] The chapter on muscle tumors in this book reports 29 leiomyomas and 15 leiomyosarcomas in the urinary bladder of dogs, from 20 years of archival material in the Cornell files (tables 6.1 and 6.2). These authors also observed them in cats (five benign and four malignant) and rarely in other species.

Gross Morphology and Histological Features

The gross and histological features are similar to those of smooth muscle tumors located in other organs. Leiomyomas produce discrete, bulging white-tan nodules that protrude into the lumen of the bladder or expand the muscular wall. They are more common in the lower urinary tract and genital system. They arise from smooth muscle in the wall of the bladder and are organized in long streams or pallisading waves of spindle shaped cells. Cell borders are usually indiscernible; nuclei are oval shaped, but if cut on cross section are circular. Histochemistry (Masson's and Van Gieson) can be used to differentiate them from fibromas or fibrosarcomas, and if necessary, they will be positive for desmin or smooth muscle actin. When the histological organization and/or the cellular features are anaplastic, or if there is invasion, giant cells, and a high mitotic index, the tumor is classified as a leiomyosarcoma. Despite the malignant classification, metastases are very rare, but local infiltration and recurrence is expected.[5] Mitotic indices and AgNORs have been used to distinguish benign and malignant smooth tumors in the intestinal, genital, and urinary tracts of dogs: mitotic index of 0.05 for leiomyoma and 1.65 for leiomyosarcoma, or 5 mitoses/100 400X fields vs. 1-2 mitoses/400X field.[6]

Rhabdomyosarcoma

Clinical Characteristics

These tumors are uncommon, occur most frequently in dogs[7-11] (23/1547, 1 percent; table 10.4), and are reported in the horse[13] and cat.[1,4] They originate from skeletal muscle located in the urethra and fundus or from undifferentiated mesenchyme that can differentiate into striated muscle. The skeletal muscle of the bladder is under the influence of the sympathetic nervous system and functions to cause constriction of the bladder and evacuation of urine. In the urinary bladder, rhabdomyosarcomas produce a grape-like bunch of tumors and hence are referred to as botryoid.[7-9] Subclassification schemes used for similar tumors in humans are described and illustrated in chapter 6 of this book.

Rhabdomyosacomas occur in young dogs (1-2 years of age), at a ratio of 2:1, females to males, and they may be overrepresented in basset hounds and large breeds such as the Saint Bernard.[8] Some urinary bladder rhabdomyosarcomas cause hypertrophic osteopathy.[8,9] Typically the patient is young, less than 2 years of age, and presents for problems referable to the skeletal system. The urinary tumor is found during workup of the bony problem and is associated with hematuria. The pathogenesis of hypertrophic osteopathy is unknown but is probably due to neurogenic or vasogenic stimuli from the space-occupying lesion in the bladder. After tumor removal, the bony lesions resolve.

Gross Morphology and Histological Features

The tumors arise in the trigone as botryoid or polypoid masses and protrude into the lumen of the bladder. They tend to be pleomorphic histologically and cytologically. In more differentiated regions they stream and interlace. There are long, well differentiated muscle fibers and cross striations that can be seen in about one-half of the cases (see fig. 6.19A, B). In undifferentiated regions they form unorganized sheets or lobules, appear sarcomatous, and have numerous mitotic figures. The presence in the more differentiated areas of some of the following features will help establish the diagnosis: elongated cells, multiple nuclei situated closely together, cross striations, and eosinophilic granular cytoplasm. Reducing the iris and/or field diaphragm, to enhance refractivity, can enhance both of these latter features, as will the use of PTAH or toluidene blue histochemical stains. The large multinucleated cells may be bizarre and help in the recognition of this tumor. Immunohistochemistry for desmin or myoglobin and other muscle markers will confirm the diagnosis if needed.[11]

Growth and Metastasis

Although there are multiple reports of this tumor in animals there are few long-term studies. Some references indicate the tumors metastasize, but most cases are euthanized at or near the time of initial diagnosis.[7-9,12] Surgical excision of urinary bladder rhabdomyosarcomas (and TCC) is difficult, and successes are limited due to the location of the tumors in the trigone and their infiltrative nature. These tumors are considered malignant and warrant a guarded to poor prognosis.

Fibroma and Fibrosarcoma

These tumors only account for 2 percent of the 1547 primary bladder tumors summarized in table 10.4. Histologically, fibromas and fibrosarcomas have the same features found in more "traditional" primary locations. There may be some overlap between the diagnoses of fibroma and fibrous polyps. Fibroma is in the wall of the bladder, between muscle and mucosa. Fibrosarcomas infiltrate the muscle layers. Neither tumor is encapsulated but both are well demarcated.

One report details the findings from a four year retrospective study of 51 dogs with fibromas of the urinary bladder.[14] A recent report describes the same lesion but classified their two cases as eosinophilic cystitis.[15] Histopathology slides from both studies were reviewed by several pathologists, but the interpretations were not unanimous. Some favored cystitis with fibroplasia and others diagnosed a mesenchymal tumor with inflammation. I felt the lesions were best interpreted as inflammatory, nonneoplastic masses with inflammation, ulceration of mucosa, granulation tissue, and marked fibroplasia with eosinohils. The osinophilopoiesis and fibrous tissue proliferation may be due to a synergistic relation between eosinophils, fibroblasts, and eotaxin production. In any event the lesions have diagnostic light microscopic features and a benign clinical course, and surgical excision is curative. A compromise on terminology may be to consider these lesions inflammatory fibrous polyps until further investigations clarify their origin. The fibrous mass is clearly not a smooth muscle tumor; for example, they stained negatively with desmin and muscle specific actin and stained strongly for collagen with Masson's trichrome. The lesions occurred in a variety of breeds of dogs ranging in age from 8 months to 15 years, with an average of 8 years.[14] As with tumors in the bladder, hematuria was the most common clinical problem and was present in 47 of 50 dogs; surgical excision corrected the hematuria and resulted in long periods without clinically detectable problems. Three dogs were euthanized because of continued or recurrent problems. Twelve of 18 dogs had bacterial growth in their urine and 16 dogs had bladder calculi. In 37 of 50 dogs, the lesions were singular, often pedunculated, and in the wall of the bladder at various locations but were predominantly in the lamina propria and submucosa and not in the deeper muscle layers. They ranged in size from 0.5 to 7.5 cm. The masses were covered by hyperplastic epithelium that was often ulcerated. Foci of cystitis glandularis were present in some cases and extended into the fibrous tissue component (see fig. 10.12 A,B). The masses consisted of fusiform cells, often with abundant stroma; they were nonencapsulated but demarcated from adjacent tissues. Inflammation was present subjacent to ulcers and disseminated throughout the mass. Neutrophils and eosinophils were common, and foci of lymphocytes and plasma cells were also present. Eosinophilopoiesis with mitoses and eosinophils in various stages of maturation are distinctive features (see fig. 10.12 D). Lesions were well vascularized. The authors cited literature on similar lesions in humans that are associated with bacterial cystitis and that are heavily infiltrated with eosinophils and produce a fibrous nodule subjacent to hyperplastic transitional epithelium.[15]

Smooth muscle tumors and fibromas look similar macroscopically and microscopically, and additional studies beyond H&E should be performed on spindle cell tumors in the bladder, although a benign biological behavior is likely for both tumors. The chapter on muscle cell tumors (chapter 6) in this book provides information that tumors of muscle cell origin were originally misclassified under a variety of diagnoses. Studies of spindle cell tumors in the gastrointestinal tract or the subcutis indicate that although these lesions look similar with H&E staining, it becomes apparent that they are a morphologically diverse group when additional studies are performed. Responses to treatment and long-term survival studies for dermal spindle cell tumors correlate better with the grade of the tumor than with the morphological classification. Perhaps the grade of the spindle cell tumor in the bladder may be more predictive of biological behavior than the morphological diagnosis.

Hemangioma and Hemangiosarcoma

These are uncommon primary or secondary tumors of the bladder.[1,4,16] They appear grossly and histologically as blood vessel tumors seen elsewhere, and can be benign or malignant. The gross appearance can be confused with polyps, trauma, or congested neoplasms of some other derivation. Less well differentiated tumors can be confirmed if they stain positively with antibodies to factor VIII related antigen.

In cattle these vascular tumors are part of the complex, enzootic hematuria. BPV-2 has been detected in experimentally induced hemangiosarcoma of the urinary bladder; however, the exact role of BPV in malignant transformation is obscure.

Metastatic Tumors

Other than lymphoma and direct extension by a prostate, rectal, or uterine tumor, secondary neoplasms of the urinary bladder are extremely rare. Although primary lymphomas of the bladder are reported,[17,18] the vast majority (99 percent) are part of generalized lymphoma. A chemodectoma has been reported in the bladder of a dog.[19] Differentiation of primary adenocarcinoma of the bladder and tumors of prostate or other epithelial origins was discussed previously.

REFERENCES

1. Osborne, C.A., Low, D.G., et al. (1968) Neoplasms of the canine and feline urinary bladder: Incidence, etiologic factors, occurrence and pathologic features. *Amer J Vet Res* 29:2041-2053.
2. Norris, A.M., Laing, E.J., Valli, V.E.O., et al. (1992) Canine bladder and urethral tumors: A retrospective study of 115 cases (1980-1985). *J Vet Intern Med* 6:145-153.
3. Strafuss, A.C., and Dean, M.J. (1975) Neoplasms of the canine urinary bladder. *J Amer Vet Med Assoc* 166:1161-1163.
4. Caywood, D.D., Osborne, C.A., and Johnston, G.R. (1980) Neoplasms of the canine and feline urinary tracts. *Current Veterinary Therapy VIII*, W.B. Saunders Co., Philadelphia, pp. 1203-1212.
5. Seely, J.C., Cosenza, S.F., and Montgomery, C.A. (1978) Leiomyosarcoma of the canine urinary bladder with metastases. *J Amer Vet Med Assoc* 172:1427-1429.
6. Johnson, G.C., Miller, M.A., and Ramos-Vara, J.A. (1995) Comparison of argyrophilic nucleolar organizer regions (AgNORs) and mitotic index in distinguishing benign from malignant canine smooth muscle tumors and in separating inflammatory hyperplasia from neoplastic lesions of the urinary bladder mucosa. *J Vet Diagn Invest* 7:127-136.
7. Kelly, D.F. (1973) Rhabdomyosarcoma of the urinary bladder in dogs. *Vet Pathol* 10:375-384.
8. Van Vechten, M., Goldschmidt, M.H., and Wortman, J.A. (1990) Embryonal rhabdomyosarcoma of the urinary bladder in dogs. *Comp Cont Ed* 12:783-793.
9. Halliwell, W.H., and Ackerman, N. (1971) Botryoid rhabdomyosarcoma of the urinary bladder and hypertrophic osteoarthropathy in a young dog. *J Amer Vet Med Assoc* 165:911-913.
10. Pletcher, J.M., and Dalton, L. (1981) Botryoid rhabdomyosarcoma of the urinary bladder of a dog. *Vet Pathol* 18:695-697.

11. Andreasen, C.B., White, M.R., et al. (1988) Desmin as a marker for canine botyroid rhabdomyosarcoma. *J Comp Pathol* 98:23-29.

12. Kuwamura, M., Yoshida, H., et al. (1998) Urinary bladder rhabdomyosarcoma (sarcoma botryoides) in a young newfoundland dog. *J Vet Med Sci* 60(5): 619-621.

13. Turnquist, S.E., Pace, L.W., et al. (1993) Botryoid rhabdomyosarcoma of the urinary bladder in a filly. *J Vet Diag* 5:451-453.

14. Esplin, D.G. (1987) Urinary bladder fibromas in dogs:51 cases (1981-1985). *J Amer Vet Med Assoc* 190:440-444.

15. Fuentealba, I.C., and Illanes, O.G. (2000) Eosinophilic cystitis in 3 dogs. *Can Vet J* 41:130-131.

16. Martinez, S.A., and Schulman, A.J. (1988) Hemangiosarcoma of the urinary bladder in a dog. *J Amer Vet Med Assoc* 192:655-656.

17. Sweeney, R.W., Hamir, A.N., et al. (1999) Lymphosarcoma with urinary bladder infiltration in a horse. *J Amer Vet Med Assoc* 199:1177-1178.

18. Maiolino, P., and DeVico, G. (2000) Primary epitheliotropic T-cell lymphoma of the urinary bladder in a dog. *Vet Pathol* 37:184-186.

19. Patnaik, A.K., Peter, F., and Liu, S.K. (1974) Chemodectoma of the urinary bladder in a dog. *J Amer Vet Med Assoc* 164:797-800.

Tumor-Like Lesions

Polypoid (Papillary) Cystitis

This lesion is observed in many species. Younger male dogs are the predominant patient group. The lesion may be mistaken for TCC in maloriented or small surgical specimens.[3] Grossly, the mucosal surface of the bladder is elevated by multiple nodular to polypoid lesions, 2-3 cm in diameter, that protrude into the lumen (fig. 10.11). The bladder wall may be thickened by edema and inflammation. Microscopically the polyp consists of transitional cell hyperplasia covering a core of proliferating connective tissue. There is usually edema, congestion, and a variable inflammatory cell infiltrate with areas of ulceration and hemorrhage. The polyps may undergo mucoid degeneration, and there may be metaplasia to mucus-secreting glands.

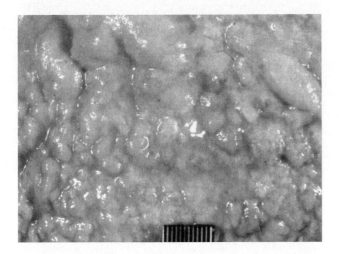

Fig. 10.11. Polypoid cystitis is characterized by multiple, bulging nodules, of various sizes, consisting of hyperplastic transitional epithelium, a fibromatous core and variable amounts and types of inflammation that can form lymphoid follicles. Rule = 1 cm.

Eosinophilic Cystitis

The characteristic features are hyperplastic transitional epithelium covering a nodule of fibrous tissue that contains fibrocytes, fibroblasts, lymphocytes, plasma cells, abundant blood vessels, and numerous eosinophils (fig. 10.12 A,B). Foci of granulopoiesis and eosinophilopoiesis are present in some lesions (fig. 10.12 C,D). The hyperplastic epithelium is typically ulcerated in one or more regions.[4,5] There often are foci of cystitis glandularis and Brunn's nests. Eosinophils are disseminated throughout the fibrous proliferation and tend to aggregate around blood vessels. They are an easily recognized feature of this lesion, and their presence may be due to the production of eotaxin by the proliferating fibroblasts.[6] A few lymphoid follicles may be present in the deeper portions. The fibrous proliferation can be marked and form a discrete lesion that has been interpreted as fibroma. The fibrous mass is located in the submucosa and not the muscle layers.[4,5] In developing lesions the fibroblast proliferation is perpendicular to blood vessels, and the stroma is loose and edematous. The most proliferative areas of connective tissue will contain a few mitoses. The lesions stain positively for collagen histochemically and negatively for muscle immunohistochemically (desmin and muscle specific actin). Eosinophilic cystitis may be a variant of polypoid cystitis, one in which eosinophils are a predominant component. Hematuria is the most common clinical problem, and some are culture positive for bacteria. The section on fibromas in this chapter discussed the duplication of names for this benign lesion of dogs[4,5] and suggested the alternative name of inflammatory fibrous polyps.

Metaplasia

These three forms of metaplasia often occur concurrently and are usually associated with hyperplasia of transitional epithelium and cystitis.[1,2]

Squamous Metaplasia

Foci of transitional epithelium that has converted to squamous epithelium with or without keratinization. There is usually concurrent transitional epithelial hyperplasia and evidence of inflammation.

Glandular Metaplasia (Cystitis Glandularis)

Foci of transitional epithelium that converted to columnar epithelial cells formed acini or tubules of varying sizes in the lamina propria or submucosa (fig. 10.13 C,D). The columnar cells may contain mucus (goblet epithelial cells). Cystitis glandularis is most often subjacent to hyperplastic transitional epithelium but can protrude above the mucosa. Occasionally the tubules are large and cystic. Concurrent cystitis, inflammation, edema,

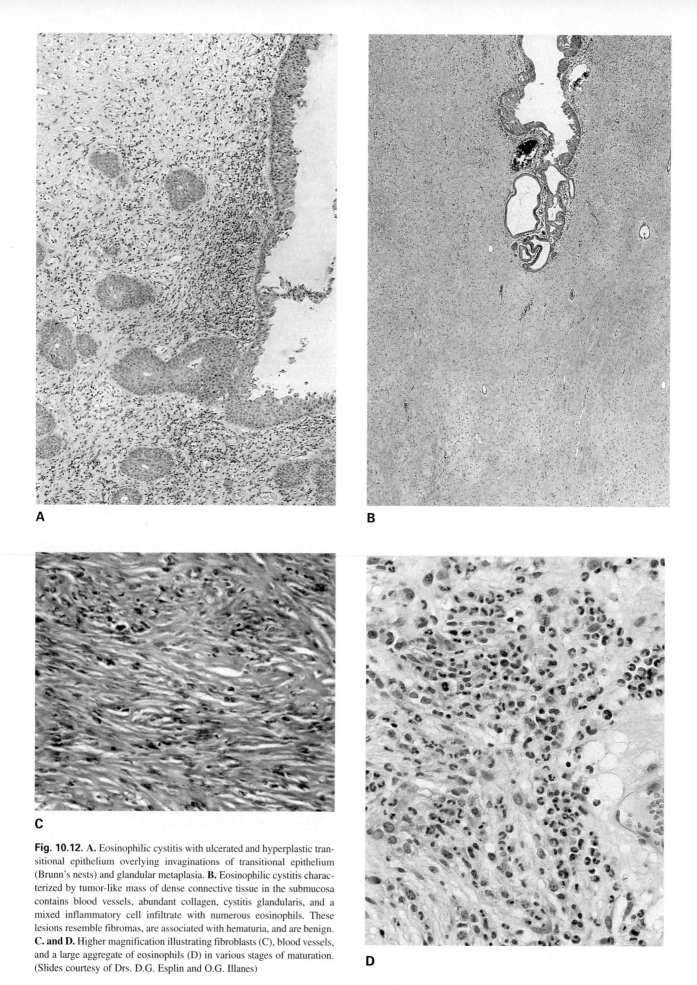

Fig. 10.12. A. Eosinophilic cystitis with ulcerated and hyperplastic transitional epithelium overlying invaginations of transitional epithelium (Brunn's nests) and glandular metaplasia. **B.** Eosinophilic cystitis characterized by tumor-like mass of dense connective tissue in the submucosa contains blood vessels, abundant collagen, cystitis glandularis, and a mixed inflammatory cell infiltrate with numerous eosinophils. These lesions resemble fibromas, are associated with hematuria, and are benign. **C. and D.** Higher magnification illustrating fibroblasts (C), blood vessels, and a large aggregate of eosinophils (D) in various stages of maturation. (Slides courtesy of Drs. D.G. Esplin and O.G. Illanes)

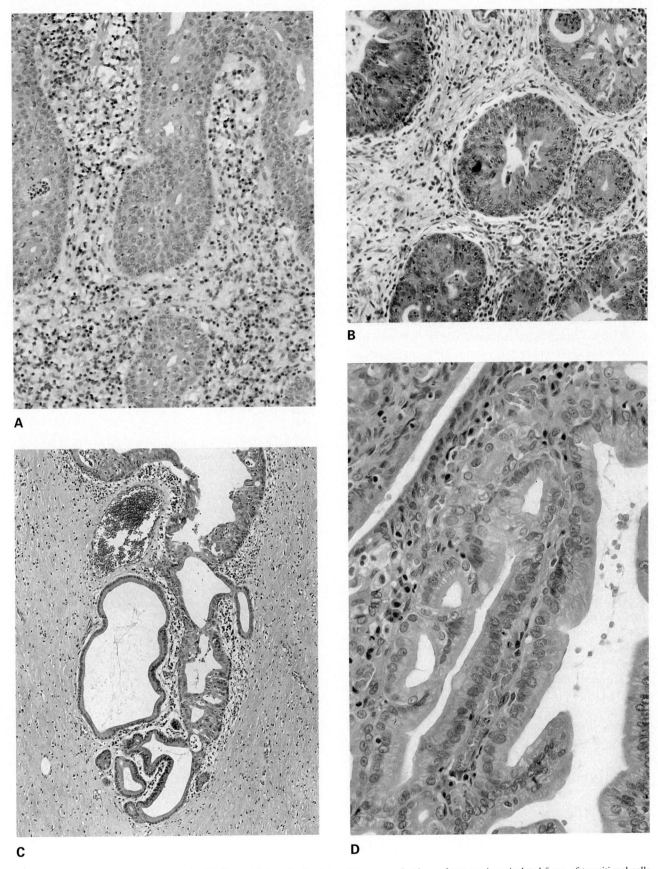

Fig. 10.13. **A.** Hyperplastic transitional epithelium with invagination into submucosa and at base of one peg is an isolated focus of transitional cells (Brunn's nest). Small spaces are present in the centers of these islands of hyperplastic urothelium. Inflammation is primarily lymphocytic. **B.** Brunn's nests in submucosa of bladder consist of varying sized foci of transitional epithelium. Some are solid nests and others have open centers resembling acini and tubules. Typically these are subjacent to hyperplastic transitional epithelium and are associated with edema, inflammation, and fibrosis. **C.** Marked glandular metaplasia (cystitis glandularis) in a dog with eosinophilic cystitis. **D.** Cystitis glandularis is characterized by acini and tubules lined by well-differentiated columnar epithelium, and a few goblet cells resembling intestinal epithelium. These lesions are often accompanied by hyperplasia of overlying urothelium and evidence of cystitis. (Slides courtesy of Drs. D.G. Esplin and O.G. Illanes)

and fibrosis are usually present. Intestinal metaplasia is a variant in humans in which the mucin-secreting epithelium on the mucosal surface of the bladder resembles intestine.[2]

Brunn's Nests

These are foci of transitional cells of various sizes within the lamina propria or submucosa that are near to or are continuous with the overlying urothelium, which is usually hyperplastic (fig. 10.13 A,B). They form solid nests or have central spaces resembling acini and tubules. The isolated nests probably form from invaginations of hyperplastic urothelium that are cut tangentially (fig. 10.13 A). The cells are uniform and well differentiated, polygonal, with oval to round nuclei, evenly dispersed chromatin, a single nucleolus, and a moderate amount of cytoplasm. Their location and appearance at low magnification are similar to those of cystitis glandularis, and often the two lesions are concurrent. Cystitis with associated edema, inflammation, and fibrosis is present in many cases. They are considered to be a preneoplastic lesion in humans, and they have been reported adjacent to neoplasms in animals.

Urethral Tumors

Primary urethral tumors are rare, and a retrospective study representing 966,000 hospital visits from 14 veterinary teaching hospitals identified only 40 dogs with urethral cancer.[7] They are seen primarily in the dog and cat and have morphological classifications similar to those in the urinary bladder.[7-10] In dogs there is a clear predominance for females; of 103 urethral tumors for which data was collected, 79 occurred in females and 19 in males.[7-10] The authors of one study speculated that the lower frequency of tumors in male dogs was due to resting prostatic secretions, approximately 2 ml/hour, which would dilute residual urine in the urethra and potential carcinogens in the urine.[7] The cause of the tumors is unknown, but an association with urethritis and urethral tumors has been shown in women.[2,7]

Urethral tumors occur in older (mean 10.4 years) dogs, and beagles are overrepresented.[7] Hematuria and stranguria are the most common clinical signs. Metastases are seen in approximately one-third of the cases, and regional lymph nodes are the most common site.[7] In a report of 115 tumors of the lower urinary tract, 14 were located in the urethra only, and all were diagnosed as malignant.[9] Approximately one-third of dogs are reported to have a concurrent malignancy in the bladder.[7]

In 103 canine urethral tumors, there were 51 TCCs, 27 SCCs, and 9 adenocarcinomas, a total of 84 percent.[7,9,10] Other tumors reported include adenoma, undifferentiated carcinoma, myxosarcoma, hemangiosarcoma, and embryonic rhabdomyosarcoma. The high prevalence of squamous cell carcinoma in the urethra is in contrast to the pattern seen in the urinary bladder and is likely attributable to the histology of the urethra. In the female dog the distal two-thirds of the urethra is lined by squamous epithelium, and the proximal one-third is lined by transitional epithelium. In the male dog the entire urethra is lined by transitional epithelium, and only the external opening of the urethra is lined by squamous epithelium.[8]

Dogs with tumors in the urethra or bladder have a better prognosis and longer survival than dogs with tumors located in both the urethra and the bladder.[7,9]

REFERENCES

1. Zachary, J.F. (1981) Cystitis cystica, cystitis glandularis, and Brunn's nests in a feline urinary bladder. *Vet Pathol* 18:113-116.
2. Eble, J.N., and Young, R.H. (2000) Tumors of the urinary tract. In Christopher Fletcher, *Diagnostic Histopathology of Tumors,* 2nd ed. Churchill Livingstone, Inc., pp. 475-565.
3. Johnston, S.D., Osborne, C.A., et al. (1975) Canine polypoid cystitis. *J Amer Vet Med Assoc* 166:1155-1160.
4. Fuentealba, I.C., and Illanes, O.G. (2000) Eosinophilic cystitis in 3 dogs. *Can Vet J* 41:130-131.
5. Esplin, D.G. (1987) Urinary bladder fibromas in dogs: 51 cases (1981-1985). *J Amer Vet Med Assoc* 190:440-444.
6. Miyamasu, M., Nakajima, T., et al. (1999) Dermal fibroblasts represent a potent major source of human eotaxin: In vitro production and cytokine regulation. *Cytokine* 11:751-758.
7. Wilson, G.P., Hayes, H.M., and Casey, H.W. (1979) Canine urethral cancer *J Amer Anim Hosp Assoc* 15:741-744.
8. Tarvin, G., Patnaik, A., and Greene, R. (1978) Primary urethral tumors in dogs. *J Amer Vet Med Assoc* 172:931–933.
9. Norris, A.M. Laing, E.J., Valli, V.E.O, et al. (1992) Canine bladder and urethral tumors: A retrospective study of 115 cases (1980-1985) *J Vet Intern Med* 6:145-153.
10. Caywood, D.D., Osborne, C.A., and Johnston, G.R. (1980) Neoplasms of the canine and feline urinary tracts. *Current Veterinary Therapy VIII,* W.B.Sauders Co., Philadelphia, pp. 1203-1212.

11 Tumors of the Genital Systems

N. J. MacLachlan and P. C. Kennedy

INTRODUCTION AND EMBRYOLOGY

An understanding of the embryology of the reproductive tract is relevant to classification of the various tumors that occur therein. The determination of genetic sex is fixed at the time of fertilization. The genetic sex is then imposed on the undifferentiated gonad. While the mechanism by which this occurs is not entirely clear, the Y chromosome clearly is male determining in all eutherian mammals, and a protein encoded by the Y chromosome (a DNA-binding protein called *testis-determining factor*) apparently dictates conversion of the undifferentiated gonad to a testis. Ovarian differentiation occurs in the absence of a Y chromosome. All other differences between the sexes are secondary effects due to hormones or factors produced by the gonads. To a considerable extent the determination of a sex is, therefore, equivalent to testis determination, although much remains to be determined regarding the mechanisms and regulation of gonadal differentiation.[1-3]

The urogenital system arises from mesoderm. Primordial germ cells originate in the fetal yolk sac and migrate into the gonadal ridge. The gonads then form within the gonadal ridge. The nongonadal portion of the genital tract of both sexes derives from either the mesonephric (Wolffian) or paramesonephric (Mullerian) ducts, and the bipotential sinusal and external genital primordia. The paramesonephric ducts arise as invaginations of the coelomic epithelium adjacent to the urogenital ridge, whereas the mesonephric ducts arise from the mesonephros. Female differentiation occurs in the absence of male gonadal hormones, which are secreted by the fetal testicle; thus, in the male fetus, Sertoli cells in the fetal testicle secrete anti-Mullerian hormone that brings about Mullerian duct regression, and interstitial (Leydig) cells secrete testosterone, which prevents mesonephric duct regression and so induces development of the male tubular tract. Dihydrotestosterone induces development of the male external genitalia. Female differentiation, and atro-phy of the mesonephric duct system, occurs in the absence of these male gonadal hormones.[1,4]

Classification of tumors of the reproductive system in this chapter will follow the system utilized in the most recent WHO fascicle.[5]

REFERENCES

1. Greenfield, A., Koopman, P. (1996) SRY and mammalian sex determination. *Curr Top Devel Biol* 34:1-23.
2. Koopman, P., Gubbay, J., Vivian, N., Goodfellow, P., and Lovell-Badge, R. (1991) Male development of chromosomally female mice transgenic for SRY. *Nature* 351:117-121.
3. McLaren, A. (1990) What makes a man a man? *Nature* 346:216-217.
4. McEntee, K. (1990) Embryology of the reproductive organs. In *Reproductive Pathology of Domestic Animals.* Academic Press Inc., San Diego, pp. 1-7.
5. Kennedy, P.C., Cullen, J.M., Edwards, J.F., Goldschmidt, M., Larsen, S., Munson, L., and Nielsen, S. (1998) World Health Organization. *Histological Classification of Tumors of the Genital System of Domestic Animals.* Armed Forces Institute of Pathology, Washington D.C.

TUMORS OF THE OVARY

Introduction

Current classification of tumors of the gonads in domestic animals is primarily based upon the histological appearance of the tumor, specifically upon the similarity of the appearance of the neoplastic cells to cellular constituents of the normal gonad.[1-4] Classification also is based on the purported embryological derivation of the predominant cellular constituent of each tumor; thus, tumors of the ovary (table 11.1) are considered to arise from three broad embryological origins: (1) the epithelium of the ovary, which includes the lining (surface) epithelium of modified mesothelium, the rete ovarii, and in the bitch, the subsurface epithelial structures (SES), (2) the germ cells, and (3) the ovarian stroma including the sex cords

Table 11.1. Distinguishing features of the principal ovarian tumors

Epithelial Tumors
    Adenoma/carcinoma of the ovarian epithelium
    Variety of origins including the lining epithelium of the ovary, subsurface epithelial structures (SES), and rete ovarii
    Most common in the bitch and derived from the SES
    Cystic multinodular enlargement of the ovary or proliferative growths that project from the ovarian surface
    Less commonly originate in the medulla of the ovary from the rete ovarii
    Consist of epithelial-lined arboriform papillae that project into the lumen of cystic cavities

Sex Cord–Stromal Tumors
    Solid or cystic, uni- or bilateral, nodular or symmetrical enlargement of the ovary
    The most common ovarian tumor of the mare, cow, and queen
    Variety of histological patterns and named according to their resemblance to the normal constituents of the ovarian endocrine
       apparatus: granulosa cell tumor, granulosa-theca cell tumor, thecoma, luteoma, Sertoli cell tumor of the ovary, lipid cell tumor, etc.
    Frequently produce reproductive hormones, progesterone, estrogen, and/or inhibin. Associated endocrine effects include
       anestrus, persistent estrus, nymphomania, masculinization, and hematologic aberrations (blood dyscrasias)

Germ Cell Tumors
    Dysgerminoma
       Often large tumors; gray/white, firm, and homogeneous
       Occur in all species but rare
       Cellular tumors with broad sheets of large cells with prominent nuclei and little cytoplasm
    Teratoma
       Composed of two or more germinal layers
       Most common in the bitch but occur in all species
       Solid or cystic enlargement of the ovary; may include bone, cartilage, teeth, hair. Dermoid cysts very common in cattle

(sex-cord stromal or gonadostromal elements), which together contribute the endocrine apparatus of the ovary.

Germ cells (ova) that migrate from the fetal yolk sac into the gonadal ridge become surrounded by cords of cells termed the *sex cords,* which are precursors of the follicular granulosa in the developing ovary.[5,6] Thus the association of germ cells and sex cords during development leads to the formation of primary follicles. The precise origin of the sex cords is conjectural, and it is unresolved if they are derived from the rete ovarii, primitive gonadal mesenchyme, or the mesothelial lining of the developing gonad.[7,8] All of these structures ultimately are derived early in development from nephrogenic tissue, and it may be that the precise origin of the somatic elements of the ovary is species dependent.[7] Sex-cord stromal elements of the differentiated ovary include the theca and granulosa cells, as well as their luteinized derivatives.

Epithelial Tumors

Tumors that arise from the ovarian epithelium occur in all domestic species.[1-3,9-16] Most epithelial tumors of the ovary arise from the surface epithelium, and the SES in the bitch, but they can arise less frequently in the hilus of the ovary from the rete ovarii. Epithelial tumors of the ovary are common only in the bitch because the SES are unique to the canine among the domestic species.[9]

Sites and Gross Morphology

Epithelial tumors of the ovary can be either uni- or bilateral, and characteristically appear as cystic, multinodular enlargements. The cut surface typically has multiple cysts that contain thin yellow to brown fluid, interspersed between solid regions. Carcinomas also may appear as proliferative cauliflower-like growths that project from the surface of the ovary to involve adjacent struc-

tures. Small tumors may be localized to their site of origin; specifically, those that arise from the surface epithelium or the SES initially are confined to the cortex of the ovary, whereas those that arise from the rete ovarii are initially confined to the medulla adjacent to the hilus of the ovary.

Histological Features

Both adenomas and carcinomas of the ovary usually consist of arboriform papillae that project into the lumen of cystic cavities. They sometimes are further subclassified as papillary (papillary adenoma or carcinoma) or cystic (cystadenoma or cystadenocarcinoma). The papillae that characterize these tumors consist of connective tissue stalks that are lined by single or multiple layers of cuboidal or columnar epithelial cells that may or may not be ciliated (fig. 11.1 C,D). The wall of each cyst usually is lined by single or multiple layers of epithelium, and the lumen of the cyst may contain proteinaceous material. Anaplastic carcinomas that lack the characteristic arboriform pattern occur occasionally and consist of broad, disorganized sheets of neoplastic cells.

In the absence of metastasis or obvious vascular invasion, malignant tumors (ovarian carcinomas) are identified as such on the basis of their larger size, the presence of foci of necrosis and hemorrhage, cellular atypia and a tendency for the neoplastic cells to pile up on one another, mitotic index, and in particular, stromal invasion. The cyst wall, the connective tissue papillae, or the stroma of the adjacent ovary may be invaded and these invasions are features of malignancy. Extension of the tumor into adjacent structures such as the ovarian bursa or peritoneum is unequivocal evidence of malignancy.

Epithelial tumors of the canine ovary usually arise from the SES.[3,9] The incidence of hyperplasia of the SES also increases with age; thus neoplasia and hyperplasia of

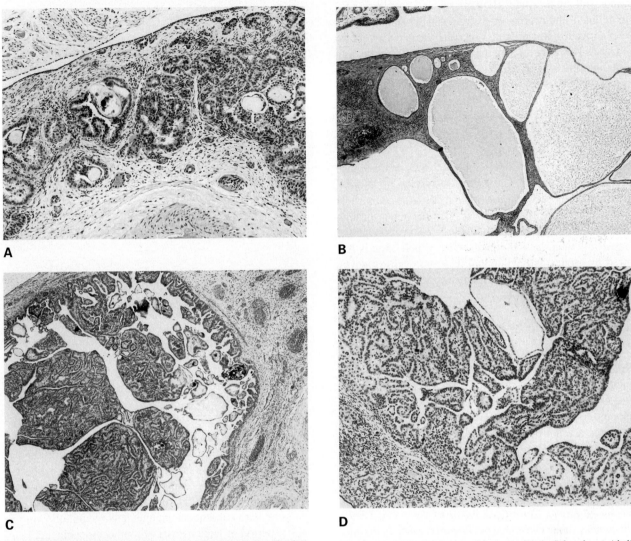

A

B

C

D

E

Fig. 11.1. Epithelial tumors of the ovary. Bitch. *Subsurface epithelial structures (SES):* **A.** Adenomatous hyperplasia of the SES. **B.** Cysts of the SES. **C.** Cystadenoma of the SES. **D.** Cystadenoma. *Rete:* **E.** Adenoma of the ovarian rete.

distinguished from hyperplasia because of the focal nature of the former as compared to the multicentric distribution of SES hyperplasia (fig. 11.1 A and C), although the two conditions may coexist in the ovaries of older bitches. Similarly, distinction of age-related hyperplasia of the rete ovarii from adenoma of this structure (rete adenoma, fig. 11.1 E) is difficult, and it usually is based arbitrarily on the size of the lesion. Tumors of the rete ovarii may be distinguished from those that arise from the surface epithelium or SES only on the basis of their location in the medulla of the ovary, as their histological appearances are similar.

Immunohistochemistry

Immunohistochemical staining is used increasingly to characterize ovarian tumors of animals, but definitive criteria available for use in identifying ovarian tumors of

the SES can occur together and may be difficult to differentiate. Whereas the SES do not normally extend into the ovary beyond the level of the primary follicles, tumors of the SES can invade and efface the gonad or protrude from its surface. Adenomas of the SES (SES adenoma) may be women still are lacking.[17] Hyperplastic and neoplastic proliferations of the ovarian epithelium usually stain strongly for cytokeratins; however, they also may stain positively for vimentin. This positive staining for vimentin is a reflection of the mesothelial derivation of the ovarian surface (lining) epithelium. In contrast, tumors derived from the sex-cord stromal elements of the ovary stain positively for vimentin and are negative or only weakly express cytokeratins.

Biological Behavior

Adenomas and carcinomas of the ovary cause enlargement of the affected gonad. Metastasis of carcinomas frequently occurs transcoelomically after rupture of cysts within the neoplasm or invasion of the tumor through the capsule of the ovary, leading to implantation of the neoplasm within the abdominal cavity, which often is followed by ascites and abdominal distention subsequent to lymphatic blockage. Metastasis also can occur after lymphatic or venous invasion.

Sex-Cord Stromal Tumors

These are tumors that are derived from, or which histologically resemble, the normal cellular constituents of the endocrine apparatus of the ovary. They are considered to arise from the theca, follicular granulosa, or their luteinized derivatives. The precise embryological origins of these structures are not determined and might be species specific.[6-8] Included in this group of tumors are neoplasms with a diverse array of histological appearances that have been given an equally diverse, and confusing, array of names including *granulosa cell tumor, granulosa-theca cell tumor, luteoma, thecoma, Sertoli cell tumor of the ovary, Leydig cell tumors, androblastoma, arrhenoblastoma, interstitial gland tumor,* and *lipid cell tumor of the ovary.* The term *sex-cord stromal* (gonadostromal) is preferred as it reflects the uncertainty of the embryological and histogenetic origin of cells in these tumors, which may include gonadal stroma, follicles, sex cords, interstitial glands of the ovary, and undifferentiated rest cells. In many of these tumors there is coexistence of multiple cell types in the same tumor.[1-4]

Tumors derived from sex-cord stromal tissues of the ovary share the potential to be hormonally active and to secrete steroid hormones.[1-3,9,11-16,18-27] They are the principal, but not exclusive, source of hormonally functional ovarian tumors (fig. 11.2). Ovarian sex-cord stromal tumors are capable of producing a diverse mixture of female and male sex hormones as, in the normal ovary, progesterone is converted in the theca interna to androgen by cytochrome $P450_{17\alpha}$, and in turn, androgens are converted to estrogen by P450 aromatase in the follicular granulosa in a process termed *aromatization.*[28] Sex-cord stromal tumors can produce varying amounts of progesterone, estrogen, testosterone, and inhibin, and these hormones can profoundly influence the reproductive behavior of the affected animal and induce changes in extraovarian

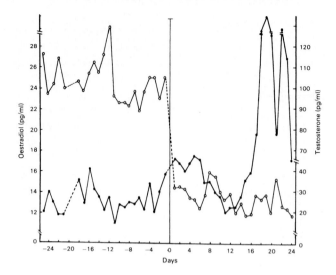

Fig. 11.2. Testosterone (○) and estradiol-17-beta (●) patterns in a mare (BMM) with an ovarian tumor before and after surgery (Day 0). The mare exhibited male-like behavior and no cyclical ovarian activity before surgery. [Stabenfeldt, G.H., Hughes, J.P., Kennedy, P.C., Meagher, D., and Neely, D.P. (1979) Clinical findings, pathological changes, and endocrinological secretory patterns in mares with ovarian tumors. *J Reprod Fert Suppl* 27: 277-285; with permission.]

tissues. Animals with hormonally productive sex-cord stromal tumors often exhibit abnormal reproductive behavior that may manifest as persistent anestrus, intermittent or continuous estrus, or masculinization. Bitches with sex-cord stromal tumors also may manifest signs of hyperestrinism including endocrine alopecia, bone marrow suppression with consequent anemia, leukopenia following an initial period of leukocytosis, thrombocytopenia and hemorrhagic diathesis, and cystic endometrial hyperplasia.[1,3,9,11,15,16,21] These changes are reversible by removal of the tumor. Hyperadrenocorticism also has been described in a bitch with an ovarian sex-cord stromal tumor.[29]

Tumors of the endocrine apparatus of the ovary are not readily classified on the basis of their endocrine products, as the types and amounts of the different hormones secreted by individual tumors varies considerably. The products of ovarian tumors other than steroid hormones also can influence reproductive behavior. For instance, mares with granulosa-theca cell tumors exhibit abnormal reproductive activity and atrophy of the contralateral gonad. It appears that inhibin, rather than elevated levels of plasma testosterone, is responsible for some of these effects. Inhibin is a normal glycoprotein secretory product of granulosa cells that decreases pituitary secretion of follicle stimulating hormone (FSH), and the high levels of inhibin in mares with granulosa cell tumors likely prevent normal FSH mediated stimulation of the unaffected ovary.[30] Rarely, however, mares with granulosa-theca cell tumors continue to cycle, and folliculogenesis occurs in the unaffected, contralateral ovary.[31]

Sites and Gross Morphology

With the possible exceptions of the sow and bitch, sex-cord stromal tumors are the most common ovarian neoplasms in domestic species. They clearly are the most common ovarian tumors in the cow and mare. Sex-cord stromal tumors are more common in older animals but occur in animals of all ages and even the very young. These frequently are large tumors that are either multinodular or symmetrical, uni- or bilateral, and they include both solid and cystic areas, with or without scattered areas of hemorrhagic necrosis. The cysts frequently contain yellow to red thin fluid. Some tumors contain a single large central cystic cavity.

Histological Types

Classification of sex-cord stromal tumors is based on the appearance of the predominant cell population and its resemblance to the normal constituents of the ovarian endocrine apparatus. It must be stressed, however, that more than one cell type often is present in a single neoplasm and that the histological appearance of an individual tumor may vary markedly in different areas.

Granulosa Cell Tumor

Granulosa cell tumor is the most common sex-cord stromal tumor. It consists of irregular accumulations of granulosa cells separated by a supporting stroma of spindle cells, imparting a distinct resemblance to disorganized attempts at follicle formation (Figs. 11.3 A, 11.3 B). In some, the stroma resembles thecal tissue, giving rise to the designation *granulosa-theca cell tumor*. Within the follicular structures are multiple layers of cells that resemble granulosa cells, with palisading at the periphery. The follicular pattern may be less prominent in some tumors, with the neoplastic granulosa cells being arranged in solid sheets, cords, trabeculae, or nests. A variety of patterns may occur in different areas within the same tumor. The appearance of some granulosa cell tumors, particulary in the bitch but also in the mare, closely resembles that of testicular Sertoli cell tumors, thus the designation of *Sertoli cell tumor of the ovary* for tumors with this appearance (fig. 11.3 C). Tumor cells in this variant are spindle shaped and are arranged in tubules that frequently are separated by a fibrous stroma. The term *Sertoli cell tumor of the ovary* may be inappropriate because cells with a similar histological appearance are present in the granulosa cell cords that are characteristic of the normal canine ovary.[9] Variably sized areas of apparent luteinization may occur in some granulosa-theca cell tumors, especially in the mare; these areas are characterized by accumulations of polyhedral cells, with abundant vacuolated eosinophilic cytoplasm, that usually are prominent adjacent to the margins of follicular structures (fig. 11.3 D). Call-Exner bodies are present in some granulosa cell tumors (fig. 11.3 A) and, when present, are a useful diagnostic feature. Call-Exner bodies consist of a radial aggregate of tumor cells about a central deposit of eosinophilic proteinaceous material.

Luteoma, Leydig Cell Tumor of the Ovary, and Lipid Cell Tumor

Luteoma, Leydig cell tumor of the ovary, and lipid cell tumors are, respectively, composed of cells that resemble those of the corpus luteum in all species, and those of the interstitial glands of the normal feline ovary.[3] These tumors consist of multiple lobules of neoplastic cells separated by a well-vascularized connective tissue stroma. The neoplastic cells are polygonal with abundant granular eosinophilic cytoplasm that contains lipid vacuoles.

Thecoma

Thecoma consists of irregular, loosely arranged unencapsulated aggregates of spindle shaped cells (fig. 11.3 F). Individual cells have elongated nuclei, and the cytoplasm may contain lipid vacuoles, which are indicative of steroid hormone production. The distinction between a thecoma and mesenchymal tumors such as leiomyoma and fibroma can be difficult. However, a thecoma has the capacity to produce steroid hormones, elevated levels of which often can be detected in blood. Cytoplasmic lipid vacuoles in the cells of thecoma can be stained with fat stains such as Sudan Black. If necessary, histochemical or immunohistochemical staining can be used to identify muscle or collagen to distinguish thecoma from mesenchymal tumors.

Miscellaneous

Other types of sex-cord stromal tumors have been described, usually based on comparison of their histological appearance to that of ovarian tumors that have been described in women. These include androblastoma (Sertoli-Leydig cell tumor or arrhenoblastoma) in the cow, mare, ewe, and queen.[3,32,33] These are tumors that include elements that resemble both granulosa cell tumor and luteoma; however, foci of apparent luteinization within granulosa-theca cell tumors can produce this same appearance.

Granulosa or granulosa-theca cell tumors are especially common in the mare and cow, although thecomas and luteomas also have been described in the latter. Granulosa cell tumors in cattle frequently have a solid pattern, whereas the thecal component and follicular pattern usually are more prominent in similar tumors in mares, hence the usual designation of granulosa-theca cell tumor in the latter species. Some sex-cord stromal tumors of the ovary of both the cow and the mare resemble Sertoli cell tumors. A variety of patterns of sex-cord stromal tumors have been described in the bitch, including granulosa cell tumors, Sertoli cell tumors of the ovary, luteomas, and nonspecific stromal tumors. The histological appearance of granulosa cell tumors of the bitch is variable, ranging from follicular to solid. Sex-cord stromal tumors with the Sertoli cell pattern are proposed to have a better prognosis than those with the typical granulosa cell pattern. In the queen, granulosa cell tumors, luteomas (including lipid cell tumor), and androblastomas have been described. Luteomas or lipid cell tumors of the queen are composed

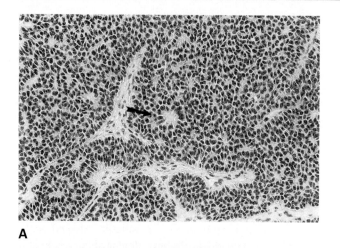

A

B

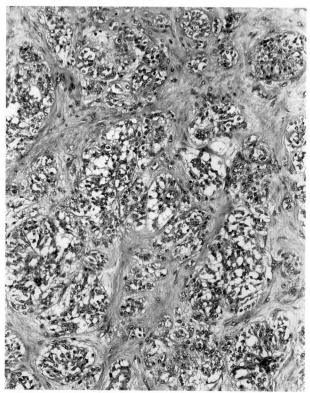

C

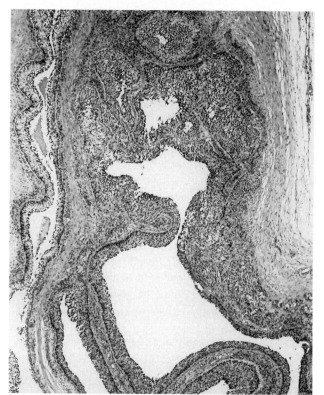

D

Fig. 11.3. Sex-cord stromal tumor. **A.** Granulosa cell tumor. Benign, well differentiated, with Call-Exner body (arrow). Cow. **B.** Granulosa cell tumor. Macrocystic pattern. Mare. **C.** Granulosa cell tumor. Cords of poorly differentiated tumor cells are embedded in a dense fibrous stroma, creating the Sertoli cell tumor-like pattern. Bitch. **D.** Granulosa cell tumor with patchy areas of luteinization of the theca (arrow). Mare. (continued)

of cells that closely resemble those found in the so-called interstitial glands that are a feature of the normal feline ovary.

Immunohistochemistry

Immunohistochemical staining of sex-cord stromal tumors has not been adequately described for domestic species, and preliminary findings are somewhat contradictory. Specifically, while tumors of this type generally stain for intermediate filaments, some also stain for cytokeratins, which perhaps reflects the different embryological derivation of the cells that actually constitute tumors derived from the sex-cord stromal elements of the

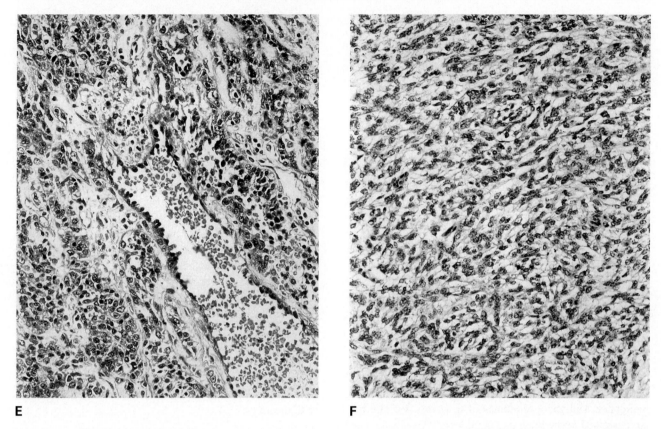

E   F

Fig. 11.3. (continued)   **E.** Malignant granulosa cell tumor. The poorly differentated tumor cells are invading blood vessels. Bitch. **F.** Thecoma. Tumor cells are spindle shaped with vacuolated cytoplasm that contains lipid. Cow. (Courtesy of Dr. J.F. Edwards.)

ovary.[4-8] Immunohistochemical staining for reproductive hormones is used to classify sex-cord stromal tumors in women, but this approach has yet to be adequately described in domestic animals.

Biological Behavior

All sex-cord stromal tumors share the propensity to be hormonally active, producing signs of hyperestrinism, masculinization, or persistent anestrus. The metastatic behavior of the various sex-cord stromal tumors also differs among the species. Granulosa cell tumors in mares almost invariably are benign, whereas metastasis is relatively common in the queen and, less so, the bitch. Reported malignancy of bovine sex-cord stromal tumors has varied considerably among studies, but metastasis, if it occurs, is late. Metastasis can occur to the regional lymph nodes, via the blood to a variety of organs or, rarely, by implantation into the peritoneal cavity. Malignant sex-cord stromal tumors are disorganized as compared to their benign counterparts, and may exhibit cellular anaplasia, with numerous mitotic figures, foci of necrosis and/or hemorrhage, and vascular invasion by the tumor cells (fig. 11.3 E).

Germ Cell Tumors

Germ cells initially are found in the yolk sac and, early in differentiation, migrate to the gonadal ridge. In the developing ovary, association of germ cells and sex cords precedes formation of primary follicles. Dysgerminomas and teratomas are tumors of domestic animals derived from germ cells. Other ovarian germ cell tumors that occur in women and laboratory animals, such as embryonal carcinoma, choriocarcinoma, and endodermal sinus tumor, have yet to be adequately described in domestic animals.

Dysgerminoma

Dysgerminoma is the female equivalent of testicular seminoma. This is an uncommon ovarian tumor in domestic animals, but it has been described in most species and appears to be most common in the bitch and queen.[1-3,9,11-15,23,34-36] There is an especially high incidence of dysgerminoma in the maned wolf.[37] Aged animals typically are affected and occasionally may manifest signs of hyperestrinism. Mares with disseminated germ cell tumors also may manifest hypertrophic osteopathy.[38] Dysgerminomas can be large tumors that produce spherical or ovoid enlargement of the affected ovary. On cut surface the tumor characteristically is white or gray, firm, and homogenous, although hemorrhage and/or necrosis can produce areas of discoloration and cysts of variable size. Dysgerminomas are highly cellular tumors, consisting of broad sheets, cords, and nests of cells separated by occasional thin connective tissue septa. Individual tumor cells resemble primitive germ cells; they are large and polyhedral, with vesicular nuclei, prominent nucleoli, and scant amphophilic or basophilic cytoplasm (fig. 11.4 A). Mitotic figures, which often are abnormal, may be very numerous (several per high power field). Multinucleate tumor cells and focal aggregations of lymphocytes are regularly present. Metastasis can occur, either to regional lymph nodes and adjacent organs or transcoelomically.

Teratoma

Teratoma is composed of abnormal tissue derived from at least two, and often all three, germinal layers. They presumably arise from pluripotential germ cells that have undergone differentiation.[39] Ovarian teratomas are uncommon in domestic animals, but they have been described in most species and are most common in the bitch.[1-3,9,12,15,16,23,35,36,40] They cause spherical or ovoid enlargement of the affected ovary, with solid and cystic areas on cut surface. The latter may contain sebaceous material and hair. A variety of other tissues may be present, including bone, cartilage, and teeth (fig. 11.4 B-G). Teratomas of the bovine ovary frequently are dermoid cysts, especially in zebu cattle. Most teratomas are benign and are composed of well-differentiated mature tissues, but any of the tissues that make up a teratoma may be malignant. Malignant teratomas of the ovary are rare but are described in the bitch and mare.[3,16,36,41,42]

Other Tumors

Mixed Tumors

Ovarian tumors that include elements of more than one of the three traditional lineages occur, but these must be distinguished from the presence of two different tumors in the same ovary or histological variation within a single tumor. Mixed tumors include both epithelial and sex-cord stromal elements or both germ cells and sex-cord stromal cells, although definitive descriptions currently are lacking. Gonadoblastoma is a specific mixed tumor of human ovary or testicle that includes germ cells and sex-cord stromal derivatives. It occurs in individuals with abnormal sexual development and dysgenic gonads. Ovarian gonadoblastoma has yet to be described in animals.

Mesenchymal Tumors

Tumors derived from the mesenchymal elements of the ovary also occur. These include fibromas, hemangiomas, leiomyomas, and their malignant counterparts. Hemangioma is the most common ovarian neoplasm of the sow, although it still is rare and usually occurs only in older animals.[14,43] These tumors consist of numerous endothelium-lined channels filled with blood that manifest grossly as discrete, rubbery, red-brown nodules within the affected ovary. Morphologically similar lesions have been described in the ovary of older cows, mares, and beagle bitches.[3,9] Ovarian fibroma and leiomyoma have the same appearance as tumors of these cell types in other tissues, as do their malignant counterparts.[1-3,15,23,24] They can be difficult to distinguish from thecomas. The presence of lipid droplets in the cytoplasm of tumor cells is consistent with thecoma.

Metastatic Nonovarian Cancer

Secondary tumors of the ovary do occur in domestic animals, but their frequency is uncertain because detailed examinations are rarely made. Lymphosarcomas can occur at this site, especially in the bitch, sow, queen, cow, and mare.[3,24,44] Other tumors are less common, but carcinomas and sarcomas of other sites clearly do metastasize to the ovary and, because of its rich vasculature, the corpus luteum may be especially prone.[3,15,23]

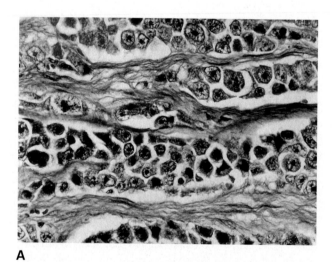

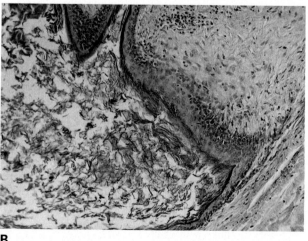

A   B

Fig. 11.4. Germ cell. **A.** Dysgerminoma in a bitch; clusters of tumor cells are separated by connective tissue septa similar to seminoma of the testis. (Courtesy of Armed Forces Institute of Pathology.) **B.–G.** Teratoma in the ovary of a bitch. The tumor consists of a variety of mature, but disorganized, tissues. **B.** Cyst lined by stratified squamous epithelium with keratosis. This suggests epidermis. (continued)

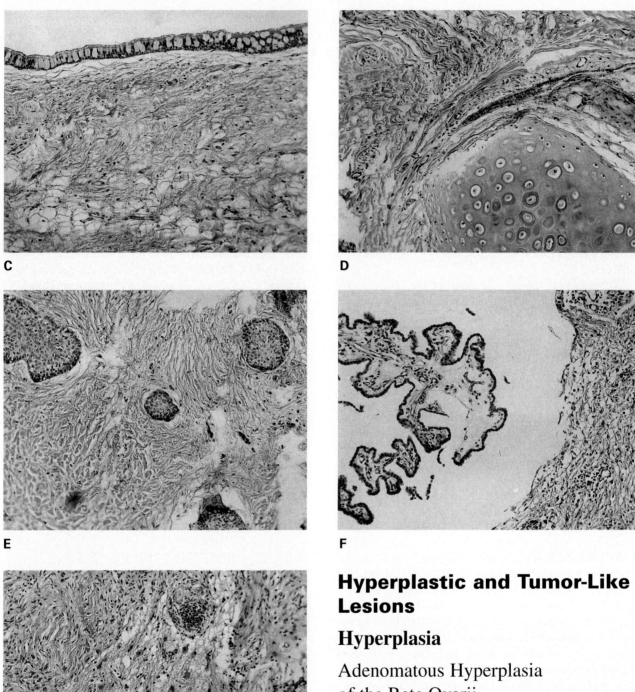

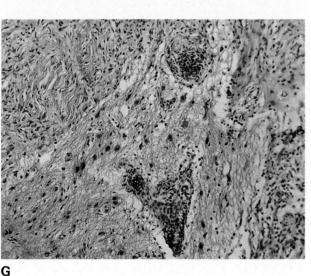

Fig. 11.4. (continued) **C.** Ciliated columnar epithelium showing mucin production. This resembles respiratory epithelium. **D.** Large plate of hyaline cartilage. **E.** Clumps of squamous epithelium. **F.** Cyst-containing papillary structure covered by cuboidal epithelium, suggestive of tela choroidea. **G.** Nerve fibers adjacent to central nervous gray matter.

Hyperplastic and Tumor-Like Lesions

Hyperplasia

Adenomatous Hyperplasia of the Rete Ovarii

The rete ovarii includes intra- and extraovarian portions. Cysts of the rete ovarii are relatively common in both the bitch and queen, and adenomatous hyperplasia of the ciliated lining epithelium sometimes accompanies cystic dilatation of the structure. The rete ovarii enlarges with age, and distinction between adenomatous hyperplasia and rete adenoma is arbitrary, with larger lesions being considered adenomas.[3,9]

Hyperplasia of the Subsurface Epithelial Structures

The ovary of the bitch is distinctive because of the presence of cords, tubules, and nests of cells beneath the surface epithelium, the so-called subsurface epithelial structures (SES), that arise from the surface epithelium lining the ovary. These structures are very prominent at certain stages of development in the fetal ovary and again increase in prominence and number with advancing age. Hyperplasia and cystic dilatation of the SES occur commonly in geriatric bitches (see fig. 11.1 A,B), often with papillary infolding of the lining epithelium. Cystic dilatation can become very extensive, such that the entire cortex of the affected ovary is involved. Cysts arising from the SES are rarely more than 5 mm in diameter, but these cysts can be difficult to distinguish from cystic epithelial neoplasms on occasion. Cysts tend to be multiple, bilateral, and lined by a single layer of epithelium, whereas tumors can be single or multiple, uni- or bilateral, and may have a complex arboriform pattern that is not consistent with SES cysts.[3,9,45]

The surface lining epithelium of the canine ovary also normally changes with age, progressing from simple cuboidal to pseudostratified columnar.

Hyperplasia of the Granulosa Cell Cords of the Canine Ovary

The granulosa cell cords are a characteristic feature of the canine ovary. They consist of elongate, spindle shaped cells arranged in tubules. Granulosa cell cords are most numerous near the corticomedullary junction, and enlarged, hyperplastic cords frequently are present adjacent to the medullary blood vessels of the ovary of older bitches.[3,9]

Cysts

Ovarian Cysts

A wide variety of cysts occur in and around the ovary.[1,2,9,45] Some may interfere with normal reproductive cyclicity, but most are innocuous. Cysts that occur within the ovarian parenchyma include cysts derived from anovulatory Graafian follicles (luteal and follicular cysts), cystic corpora lutea, cystic rete ovarii, inclusion cysts derived from the ovarian surface epithelium, and cysts of the SES.

Luteal and follicular cysts both are derived from anovulatory Graafian follicles and differ only in the degree of luteinization of the cyst wall. Cysts derived from anovulatory Graafian follicles are most common in the cow and sow, but also occur sporadically in the bitch and queen. They often cause altered reproductive activity through secretion of steroid hormones. Affected animals, especially bitches, may show marked manifestations of hyperestrinism such as altered reproductive behavior, anemia, and hemorrhagic diathesis. In the cow and sow they may be associated with anestrus, persistent estrus, or nymphomania. These signs can mimic those in animals with hormonally productive sex-cord stromal tumors. Anovulatory cysts persist longer than the normal mature follicle, and

they frequently are larger than normal follicles. These cysts are lined by multiple layers of granulosa cells (follicular cyst) or with luteal cells that result from luteinization of the theca (luteal cyst). The two types of cyst can coexist in the same ovary. In contrast, cystic corpora lutea are otherwise apparently normal corpora lutea with a central cavity, but because they are derived from postovulatory follicles, they typically have a discrete ovulation papilla. Cystic corpora lutea are clinically silent and consist of normal luteal cells, but contain a central cavity. Cysts of the surface epithelium are most common in the mare and the bitch. SES cysts of the bitch may be lined by an attenuated epithelium and are distinguished from atretic follicles and follicular cysts by the lack of theca interna and follicular granulosa.[9] Epithelial cysts of the mare's ovary are clustered adjacent to the ovulation fossa, hence the name *fossa cyst*. Fossa cysts are variably sized but can become large (several centimeters in diameter).[3] They are lined by cuboidal epithelium. Cystic rete ovarii is most common in the bitch and queen. Rete cysts appear as dilated epithelium-lined tubules that may become so large as to compress the cortex of the affected ovary.[45,46]

Parovarian Cysts

Cysts that occur adjacent to the ovary can derive from a variety of structures, including the mesonephric duct and tubule, paramesonephric duct, uterine tube, and mesosalpinx.[1-3] These are fluid filled cysts that are located adjacent to the ovary or uterine tube. They can become quite large, especially in the mare (up to 7 cm). Cysts derived from the paramesonephric duct (cystic epoophoron) usually are lined by a single layer of cuboidal epithelium that includes both ciliated and nonciliated secretory cells, and a thin layer of smooth muscle surrounds the cyst.

Vascular Hamartoma

Vascular hamartoma of the ovary has been described in cattle, swine and horses.[47,48] These manifest as cystic, blood filled spaces in the affected ovary and can be difficult to distinguish from vascular neoplasms, especially hemangioma and ovarian hematoma. Both hemangioma and vascular hamartoma include proliferations of vessels with prominent endothelial lining, thus differentiation is very difficult. The difference is that vascular hamartoma is a congenital lesion, whereas hemangioma is acquired. Thrombosis can occur in the tortuous vessels within vascular hamartomas.

Ovarian Hematoma

Ovarian hematoma is common in mares and is thought to arise from excessive hemorrhage into the follicular cavity following ovulation.[19,49] They can become large (up to 10 cm) but generally resolve spontaneously.

Ovarian Choristoma

Choristoma is normal tissue in an ectopic location. Ectopic adrenal gland may occur within the ovary, particularly in the mare.[50]

REFERENCES

1. Kennedy, P.C., and Miller, R.B. (1993) The female genital system. In Jubb, K.V.F., Kennedy, P.C., and Palmer, N. (eds.) *Pathology of Domestic Animals,* 4th ed. Academic Press, San Diego.
2. MacLachlan, N.J. (1987) Ovarian disorders in domestic animals. *Environ Health Pers* 73:27-33.
3. McEntee, K. (1990) Ovarian neoplasms. In *Reproductive Pathology of Domestic Animals.* Academic Press Inc., San Diego, pp. 69-93.
4. Scully, R.E. (1977) Ovarian tumors: A review. *Amer J Pathol* 87:686-720.
5. McEntee, K. (1990) Embryology of the reproductive organs. In *Reproductive Pathology of Domestic Animals.* Academic Press Inc., San Diego, pp. 1-7.
6. Byskov, A.G. (1986) Differentiation of the mammalian embryonic gonad. *Physiology Reviews* 66:71-117.
7. Ullman, S.L. (1996) Development of the ovary in the brushtail possum *Trichosurus vulpecula (Marsupiala). J Anat* 189:651-665.
8. Byskov, A.G., Skakkebaek, N.E., Stafanger, G., and Peters, H. (1977) Influence of the ovarian surface epithelium and rete ovarii on follicle formation. *J Anat* 123:77-86.
9. Andersen, A.C., and Simpson, M.E. (1973) *The Ovary and Reproductive Cycle of the Dog (Beagle).* Geron-X, Los Altos, CA.
10. Anderson, L.J., and Sandison, A.T. (1969) Tumors of the female genitalia in cattle, sheep, and pigs found in a British abbatoir survey. *J Comp Pathol* 79:53-63.
11. Cotchin, E. (1961) Canine ovarian neoplasms. *Res Vet Sci* 2:133-142.
12. Gelberg, H.B., and McEntee, K. (1985) Feline ovarian neoplasms. *Vet Pathol* 22:572-576.
13. Jergens, A.E., and Shaw, D.P. (1987) Tumors of the canine ovary. *Comp Cont Educ Pract Vet* 9:489-495.
14. Nelson, L.W., Todd, G.C., and Migaki, G. (1967) Ovarian neoplasms in swine. *J Amer Vet Med Assoc* 151:1331-1333.
15. Norris, H.J., Garner, F.M., and Taylor, H.B. (1970) Comparative pathology of ovarian neoplasms. IV. Gonadal stromal tumors of canine species. *J Comp Pathol* 80:399-405.
16. Patnaik, A.K., and Greenlee, P.G. (1987) Canine ovarian neoplasms: A clinicopathologic study of 71 cases, including histology of 12 granulosa cell tumors. *Vet Pathol* 24:509-514.
17. Park, S.H., and Kim, I. (1994) Histogenic consideration of ovarian sex cord-stromal tumors analyzed by expression pattern of cytokeratins, vimentin, and laminin. *Path Res Pract* 190:449-456.
18. Arthur, G.H. (1972) Granulosa cell tumor of the bovine ovary. *Vet Rec* 91:78.
19. Bosu, W.T.K., Van Camp, S.C., and Miller, R.B. (1982) Ovarian disorders: Clinical and morphological observations in 30 mares. *Can Vet J* 23:6-14.
20. Farin, P.W., and Estill, C.T. (1993) Infertility due to abnormalities of the ovaries in cattle. *Vet Clin N Amer Food Anim Pract* 9:291-308.
21. McCandlish, I.A., Munro, C.D., Breeze, R.G., and Nash, A.S. (1979) Hormone producing ovarian tumors in the dog. *Vet Rec,* pp. 9-11.
22. Meinecke, B., and Gips, H. (1987) Steroid hormone secretory patterns in mares with granulosa cell tumors. *J Vet Med* A34:545-560.
23. Norris, H.J., Garner, F.M., and Taylor, H.B. (1969) Pathology of feline ovarian neoplasms. *J Pathol* 97:138-143.
24. Norris, H.J., Taylor, H.B., and Garner, F.M. (1969) Comparative pathology of ovarian tumors II. Gonadal stromal tumors of bovine species. *Vet Pathol* 6:45-58.
25. Norris, H.J., Taylor, H.B., and Garner, F.M. (1968) Equine granulosa cell tumors. *Vet Rec* 82:419-420.
26. Stabenfeldt, G.H., Hughes, J.P., Kennedy, P.C., Meagher, D., and Neely, D.P. (1977) Clinical findings, pathological changes and endocrinological secretory patterns in mares with ovarian tumors. *J Reprod Fert, Suppl* 27:277-285.
27. Whitacre, M.D., Van Camp, S.D., MacLachlan, N.J., and Umstead, J.A. (1988) Premature lactation in a heifer with a sex cord-stromal tumor. *J Amer Vet Med Assoc* 193:946-948.
28. Sasano H. (1994) Functional pathology of human ovarian steroidogenesis: Normal cycling ovary and steroid producing neoplasms. *Endocrin Pathol* 5:81-94.
29. Yamini, B., VanDenBrink, P.L., and Refsal, K.R. (1997) Ovarian steroid cell tumor resembling luteoma associated with hyperadrenocorticism (Cushing's Disease) in a dog. *Vet Pathol* 34:57-60.
30. Piquette, G.N., Kenney, R.M., Sertich, P.L., Yamoto, M., and Hsueh, J.W. (1990) Equine granulosa–theca cell tumors express inhibin α- and β$_A$-subunit messenger ribonucleic acids and proteins. *Biol Reprod* 43:1050-1057.
31. Hinrichs, K., Watson, E.D., and Kenney, R.M. (1990) Granulosa cell tumor in a mare with a functional contralateral ovary. *J Amer Vet Med Assoc* 197: 1037-1038.
32. Hoffman, W., Arbiter, D., and Scheele, D. (1980) Sex cord stromal tumor of the cat: So-called androblastoma with Sertoli-Leydig cell pattern. *Vet Pathol* 17:508-513.
33. Mills, J.H.L., Fretz, P.B., Clark, E.G., and Ganjam, V.K. (1977) Arrhenoblastoma in a mare. *J Amer Vet Med Assoc* 171:754-757.
34. Andrews, E.J., Stookey, J.L., Helland, D.R., and Slaughtor, L.J. (1974) A histopathological study of canine and feline ovarian dysgerminomas. *Can J Comp Med* 38:85-89.
35. Dehner, L.P., Norris, H.J., Garner, F.M., and Taylor, H.B. (1970) Comparative pathology of ovarian neoplasms. III. Germ cell tumors of canine, bovine, feline, rodent, and human species. *J Comp Pathol* 80:299-306.
36. Greenlee, P.G., and Patnaik, A.K. (1985) Canine ovarian tumors of germ cell origin. *Vet Pathol* 22:117-122.
37. Munson, L., and Montali, R.J. (1991) High prevalence of ovarian tumors in maned wolves (*Chrysocyon brachyurus*) at the National Zoological Park. *J Zoo Wildlife Med* 22:125-129.
38. Meuten, D.J., and Rendano, V. (1978) Hypertrophic osteopathy in a mare with dysgerminoma. *J Equine Med Surg* 2:445-450.
39. Linder, D., McCaw, B.K., and Hecht, F. (1989) Parthenogenic origin of benign ovarian teratomas. *N Eng J Med* 292:790-793.
40. Basaraba, R.J., Kraft, S.L., Andrews, G.A., Leipold, H.W., and Small, D. (1998) An ovarian teratoma in a cat. *Vet Pathol* 35:141-144.
41. Frazer, G.S., Robertson, J.T., and Boyce, R.W. (1988) Teratocarcinoma of the ovary in a mare. *J Amer Vet Med Assoc* 193: 953-955.
42. Van Camp, S.D., Mahler, J., Roberts, M.C., Tate, L.P., and Whitacre, M.D. (1989) Primary ovarian adenocarcinoma associated with teratomatous elements in a mare. *J Amer Vet Med Assoc* 194:1728-1730.
43. Hsu, F. (1983) Ovarian hemangioma in swine. *Vet Pathol* 20:401-409.
44. Neufeld, J.L. (1973) Lymphosarcoma in the horse: A review. *Can Vet J* 14:129-135.
45. McEntee, K. (1990) Cysts in and around the ovary. In *Reproductive Pathology of Domestic Animals.* Academic Press Inc., San Diego, pp. 52-68.
46. Gelberg, H.B., McEntee, K., and Heath, E.H. (1984) Feline cystic rete ovarii. *Vet Pathol* 21:304-307.
47. Lee, C.G., and Ladds, P.W. (1976) Vascular hamartoma in the ovary of a cow. *Aust Vet J* 52:236.
48. Rhyan, J.C., D'Andrea, G.H., and Smith, L.S. (1981) Congenital ovarian vascular hamartoma in a horse. *Vet Pathol* 18:131.
49. Hughes, J.P., Stabenfeldt, G.H., and Evans, J.W. (1972) Estrous cycle and ovulation in the mare. *J Am Vet Med Assoc* 161:1367-1374.
50. McEntee, K. (1990) The ovary. In *Reproductive Pathology of Domestic Animals.* Academic Press Inc., San Diego, pp. 31-51.

TUMORS OF THE UTERINE TUBE (OVIDUCT) AND UTERUS

Epithelial Tumors

Tumors of the Uterine Epithelium

Epithelial tumors of both the uterus and oviduct are rare in domestic animals. Adenoma of the uterus is very rare. It consists of a proliferative mass of glandular elements, and must be distinguished from uterine carcinoma, uterine stromal polyp, and focal areas of adenomyosis, although distinction often is very difficult. Carcinoma of the uterus also is rare in domestic animals, in marked contrast to the prevalence of this tumor in women. Among the domestic species, it is most often reported in the cow, and it is fairly common in older cows at slaughter. There are a number of reports of similar tumors in the mare, ewe, bitch, and queen.[1-9] There is some controversy as to the validity of some published descriptions of canine uterine carcinomas because hyperplastic lesions of the canine endometrium and carcinomas metastatic to the uterus can be confused with primary endometrial carcinomas.[2,9]

Uterine carcinomas in cattle manifest as discrete, firm enlargements of the uterus that are composed of very firm, dense, white to yellow tissue. Widespread metastasis also can occur. These tumors tend to be solitary and develop in the uterine horn. The histological appearance of these tumors is characterized by nests and cords of anaplastic epithelium in a dense and abundant fibrous connective tissue stroma (fig. 11.5 A). The tumor develops deep in the endometrium and often extends into the myometrium early in the disease. Invasion of the tumor into veins and/or lymphatics frequently is present, and lymphatic spread initially is via the internal iliac and sublumbar nodes. Metastasis to other parenchymal organs such as lungs and liver also can occur, and the neoplasm can implant in the abdomen.

Tumors of the Chorionic Epithelium

Chorioepithelioma and hydatiform mole are tumors of women that arise from the placental chorionic epithelium. Initial descriptions of similar tumors in animals have not been substantiated; thus, it is not clear whether placental tumors occur in domestic animals. Tumors of placental origin must be distinguished from nonneoplastic infiltration of placental trophoblastic cells, as occurs in subinvolution of placental sites in the bitch.[1,2,9,13]

Mesenchymal Tumors

A variety of mesenchymal tumors occur in the uterus of domestic animals, including leiomyoma, fibroma, fibroleiomyoma and, far less commonly, their malignant counterparts. Unquestionably, different titles have been applied to similar tumors, and the specific designation frequently reflects the bias of individual pathologists. Leiomyomas of the myometrium are most common, especially in the bitch, queen, and cow, and they are more common in older animals.[1,2,8,9] Those in the bitch typically are accompanied by similar, concurrent tumors in the vagina.

Gross Morphology

Mesenchymal tumors manifest as a firm, nodular proliferation within the myometrium that may project into the uterine lumen. Mesenchymal tumors of the tubular tract tend to be multiple.

Histological Types

Leiomyoma of the myometrium has the expected appearance of a tumor of smooth muscle with interlacing bundles of muscle fibers admixed with variable amounts of collagenous stroma (fig. 11.5 B), hence the designation *fibroleiomyoma* that is preferred by some pathologists. Fibroma, on the other hand, is exclusively composed of fibrous connective tissue and is devoid of smooth muscle. Malignant mesenchymal tumors, especially leiomyosarcomas, also can occur. These usually are larger than their benign counterparts, and cells within the tumor exhibit cellular atypia and a relatively high mitotic index. Immunohistochemical staining for the presence of vimentin and desmin can be used to distinguish tumors derived from smooth muscle and fibrous tissue (see chapter 6).

A variety of other mesenchymal tumors can occur in the tubular tract, including lipoma within the broad ligament and ovarian bursa in the bitch and lymphosarcoma. Lymphosarcoma frequently involves the uterus of adult cattle with the disseminated form of enzootic leukosis, and it is the most common neoplasm of the uterus in cows. Lymphosarcomas involving the uterine wall can be very extensive; they have the homogeneous gray/yellow appearance that is characteristic of these tumors. The histological appearance is similar to those in other locations of the tumor, with frequent accumulation of neoplastic lymphocytes within the endometrium and effacement of normal tissue architecture. Disseminated lymphosarcoma also may involve the uterus in the mare.[2]

Hyperplastic and Tumor-Like Lesions of the Uterus

Adenomyosis

Adenomyosis is a nonneoplastic proliferation of uterine glands characterized by multicentric infiltration of these glands into the myometrium. It is most often seen in the dog, cat, and cow, but also can occur in other species.[2]

Cystic Endometrial Hyperplasia

Cystic endometrial hyperplasia (CEH) is a diffuse proliferation of the endometrial glands and stroma. In

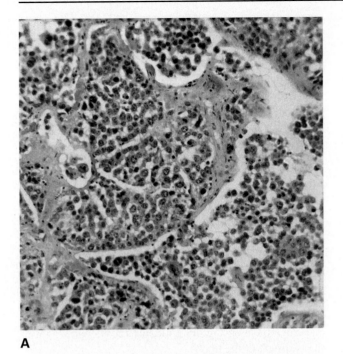

A

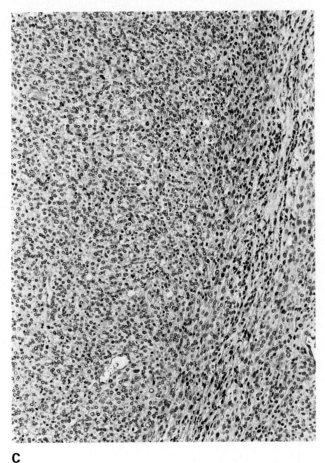

C

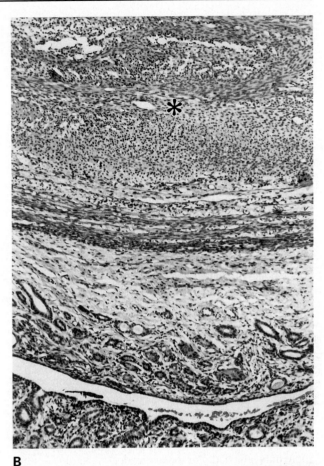

B

Fig. 11.5. Uterus/vagina. **A.** Uterine carcinoma. Adenocarcinoma in the uterus of a cow. Observe neoplastic glands formed by large hyperchromatic cells and adjacent noncancerous glands. The stroma shows fibrosis and infiltration of inflammatory cells. (Courtesy of Armed Forces Institute of Pathology.) **B.** Leiomyoma of the uterus. A well-differentiated leiomyoma (*) that compresses the subjacent endometrium. Bitch. **C.** Leiomyoma of the vagina. Bitch.

CEH in the bitch; however, spontaneous CEH in the bitch and queen most often is the result of a heightened sensitivity of the endometrium to stimulation by endogenous progesterone.[1,2,9,10] Both the bitch and the queen normally retain their corpora lutea for extended periods after ovulation regardless of whether or not they are pregnant. Irritation of the endometrium under the influence of progesterone leads to CEH; if the irritation is due to bacterial infection, it also can result in pyometra. The histological appearance of CEH induced by estrogen and progesterone is quite different. The epithelium of the endometrium is cuboidal to low columnar under estrogenic stimulation and tall columnar with extensively vacuolated cytoplasm under progestational influence.

Uterine Stromyl Polyp

Endometrial stromyl polyp of the bitch and queen consists of a focal proliferation of both glandular and stromal elements of the endometrium, and may be single or multiple. These polyps usually project into the lumen of

ruminants it is induced by excessive estrogenic stimulation of the endometrium from either exogenous sources such as estrogenic plants (such as specific varieties of clover) or from endogenous production of estrogens by sex-cord stromal tumors of the ovary or cystic follicles.[1,2] Iatrogenic administration of exogenous estrogen also can induce the affected uterus as sessile or pedunculated masses emanating from the endometrium. They can become large and may readily be confused with tumors of the uterus. Polyps consist of dilated uterine glands within a proliferative endometrial stroma.[2,9,11] Idiopathic nodular endometrial hyperplasia occurs sporadically in mares, and focal regions of apparent endometrial hyperplasia may develop at sites of adventitial placentation in ruminants.[2,12]

Subinvolution of Placental Sites

Subinvolution of placental sites occurs in young bitches. Failure of the endometrial sites of placental implantation to regress following whelping leads to a persistent discharge from the vulva. The histological appearance of these sites of placentation is characterized by inflammation with persistence of placental trophoblast cells within the endometrium.[1,2,13]

Miscellaneous Uterine Cysts

A variety of cysts that occur in the uterine wall have been described in domestic animals.[1,3,9] Lymphatic cysts, which may be transmural, are most common adjacent to the uterine bifurcation of multiparous mares. Remnants of the ducts and embryonic structures associated with sexual development also can give rise to cysts in all species, and remnants of the mesonephric duct are especially commonly affected. Mesonephric duct cysts are epithelium lined and have a muscular wall. Serosal inclusion cysts may be single or multiple, thin-walled cysts on the serosal surface of the uterus. Endometrial cysts derived from very dilated uterine glands occur in the endometrium of old bitches.

REFERENCES

1. Kennedy, P.C., and Miller, R.B. (1993) The female genital system. In Jubb, K.V.F., Kennedy, P.C., and Palmer, N. (eds.), *Pathology of Domestic Animals,* 4th ed. Academic Press, San Diego.
2. McEntee, K. (1990) The uterus: atrophic, metaplastic, and proliferative lesions. In *Reproductive Pathology of Domestic Animals.* Academic Press Inc., San Diego, pp. 167-190.
3. Baldwin, C.J. (1992) Uterine adenocarcinoma in dogs. *Comp Cont Educ* 14:731-737.
4. Chaffin, M.K., Fuentealba, I.C., Schmitz, D.G., and Read, W.K. (1990) Endometrial adenocarcinoma in a mare. *Cornell Vet* 80:65-73.
5. Cotchin, E. (1964) Spontaneous uterine cancer in animals. *Brit J Cancer* 18:209-227.
6. Migaki, G., Carey, A.M., Turnquest, R.U., and Garner, F.M. (1970) Pathology of bovine uterine adenocarcinoma. *J Amer Vet Med Assoc* 157:1577-1584.
7. Preiser, H. (1964) Endometrial adenocarcinoma in a cat. *Vet Pathol* 1:485-490.
8. Stein, B.S. (1981) Tumors of the feline genital tract. *J Amer Anim Hosp Assoc* 17:1022-1025.
9. Andersen, A.C., and Simpson, M.E. (1973) *The Ovary and Reproductive Cycle of the Dog (Beagle).* Geron-X, Los Altos, CA.
10. Nomura, K., Kawasoe, K., and Shimada, Y. (1990) Histological observations of canine cystic endometrial hyperplasia induced by uterine scratching. *Jpn J Vet Sci* 52:237-240.
11. Gelberg, H.B., and McEntee, K. (1983) Hyperplastic endometrial polyps in the dog and cat. *Vet Pathol* 21:570-573.
12. Hamir, A.N., Hunt, P.R., and Kenney, R.M. (1989) Hyperplastic endometrial polyp in a two-year-old filly. *Vet Pathol* 26:185-187.
13. Dickie, M.B., and Arbeiter, K. (1993) Diagnosis and therapy of the subinvolution of placental sites in the bitch. *J Reprod Fert, Suppl* 47:471-475.

TUMORS OF THE CERVIX, VAGINA, AND VULVA

Epithelial Tumors

Primary epithelial tumors of the cervix are extremely uncommon in domestic animals, in contrast to the frequency of these tumors in women. Carcinomas of the vagina and vulva, on the other hand, are relatively common, particularly squamous cell carcinomas in ruminants and carcinomas of urinary epithelial (urothelial) origin in the vestibule of the bitch.

Papilloma

Papilloma is a virus induced epithelial proliferation that may affect the skin over any part of the body, including the external genitalia (see chapter 2).[1-3] The appearance is that of a typical "wart" with papillary projections of epithelium with a scant fibrovascular stroma. The lesions usually undergo spontaneous regression. Transmissible genital papilloma is a specific, virus induced papilloma in swine which manifests as a raised epithelial proliferation that emanates from the vaginal mucosa of the sow and the prepuce in the boar. Virus induced fibropapilloma is a similar tumor that occurs in cattle and will will be described elsewhere in this chapter.

Squamous Cell Carcinoma

Squamous cell carcinoma of the vulva is well recognized in sheep, goats, and cattle in areas where they are exposed to high levels of solar irradiation.[1,2] Unpigmented regions of the body that are not protected by wool or hair are most commonly affected by squamous cell carcinoma.[4] These lesions in the vulva may be either ulcerative or proliferative, and histologically are typical squamous cell carcinomas. They are occasionally invasive but rarely metastatic. Progression from focal epidermal hyperplasia and dysplasia to squamous papilloma and eventually squamous cell carcinoma occurs with time and actinic exposure in cattle.

Carcinoma of the Vestibule

Carcinoma of the vestibule is a distinct entity in the bitch, with the majority likely being of urothelial origin.[2,5,6] The distal two-thirds of the bitch's urethra is lined with stratified squamous, rather than transitional, epithelium. The majority of urethral carcinomas in the bitch arise in the distal urethra, and thus the vagina and vestibule adjacent to the urethral papillae typically are affected. The histological appearance is that of a carcinoma with islands and nests of anaplastic epithelial cells within a fibrous stroma. Metastasis to regional lymph nodes is common. Adenocarcinoma of the vestibular gland (Bartholin's gland) is an extremely rare tumor of the vestibule that has been described in a cow.[7]

Mesenchymal Tumors

Mesenchymal tumors of the lower genital tract are relatively common, producing firm nodules within the wall of the tract, which may encroach on the lumen. The canine transmissible venereal tumor will be described elsewhere in this chapter.

Leiomyoma is a common tumor of the vagina of the bitch (see fig. 11.5 C) and, less commonly, other species, and resembles the same tumor in the uterus.[1,2,8,9] Leiomyomas may be solitary or multiple, extraluminal or intraluminal, and they can become large (up to 12 cm in diameter in the bitch). These tumors are hormonally dependent as they often regress after ovariectomy and do not occur in neutered bitches. Fibroma of the vagina is less common than leiomyoma, with which it may be confused. Lipoma sporadically may occur in the wall of the canine vagina.

Miscellaneous tumors that may involve the vulva and vagina include melanomas in gray mares, lymphosarcoma, embryonal sarcoma of the porcine vagina, and metastatic tumors such as metastatic mammary carcinoma.[2]

Tumor-Like Lesions of the Vagina and Vulva

Cysts of mesonephric duct remnants are most common in cattle. These are fluid filled structures on the serosal surface of the tubular genitalia.[2]

REFERENCES

1. Kennedy, P.C., and Miller, R.B. (1993) The female genital system. In Jubb, K.V.F., Kennedy, P.C., and Palmer, N. (eds.), *Pathology of Domestic Animals,* 4th ed. Academic Press, San Diego.
2. McEntee, K. (1990) Cervix, vagina, and vulva. In *Reproductive Pathology of Domestic Animals.* Academic Press Inc., San Diego.
3. Campo, M.S. (1997) Bovine papillomavirus and cancer. *Vet J* 154:175-188.
4. Mendez, A., Perez, J., Ruiz-Villamor, E., Garcia, R., Martin, M.P., and Mozos, E. (1997) Clinicopathological study of an outbreak of squamous cell carcinoma in sheep. *Vet Rec* 141:597-600.
5. Magne, M.L., Hoopes, P.J., Kainer, R.A., Olson, P.N., Husted, P.W., Allen, T.A., Wykes, P.M., and Withrow, S.J. (1985) Urinary tract carcinomas involving the canine vagina and vestibule. *J Amer Anim Hosp Assoc* 21:767-772.
6. Tarvin, G., Patnaik, A., and Greene, R. (1978) Primary urethral tumors in dogs. *J Amer Vet Med Assoc* 172:931-933.
7. Tanimoto, T., Fukunaga, K., and Ohtsuki, Y. (1994) Adenocarcinoma of the major vesticular gland in a cow. *Vet Pathol* 31:246-247.
8. Andersen, A.C., and Simpson, M.E. (1973) *The Ovary and Reproductive Cycle of the Dog (Beagle).* Geron-X, Los Altos, CA.
9. Manothaiudom, K., and Johnson, S.D. (1991) Clinical approaches to vaginal/vestibular masses in the bitch. *Vet Clin N Amer* 21:509-521.

TUMORS OF THE TESTICLE

Introduction

The histogenesis of tumors of the testicle is similar to that of the ovary; however, only two of the three potential embryological derivations are significant; specifically, testicular tumors of domestic animals generally arise from either the sex-cord stromal elements of the gonad or from germ cells (table 11.2). Seminoma is the testicular homolog of ovarian dysgerminoma, with both being derived from germ cells. Teratomas also are derived from germ cells. Sex-cord stromal tumors of the testicle include Leydig (interstitial) and Sertoli cell tumors, which closely resemble some forms of ovarian granulosa cell tumors and luteomas (and related lipid cell tumors and ovarian Leydig cell tumor). The Sertoli cell tumor, like many sex-cord stromal tumors of the ovary, frequently is hormonally productive. Whereas tumors of the ovarian surface epithelium (adenomas and carcinomas of the surface epithelium and SES) are common in the bitch, the rare mesothelioma is the only tumor of the testicle in domestic animals that is derived from the lining epithelium of modified mesothelium.[1,2]

Sex-Cord Stromal Tumors

Sertoli Cell Tumor

Sertoli cell tumor of the testicle arises from the supporting cells within the seminiferous tubules, hence its synonym, sustentacular cell tumor. Sertoli cell tumor is common in dogs, especially in cryptorchid testicles, but also has been reported in the stallion, ram, cat, and bull.[1,2] It most often occurs in older animals, but also has been described in newborn calves. An especially high incidence has been reported in miniature schnauzer dogs with persistent Mullerian duct syndrome. Sertoli cell tumors are usually unilateral, but there is a significant incidence of bilateral tumors. Perhaps one-half of all canine Sertoli cell tumors arise in cryptorchid testicles, and the incidence of Sertoli cell tumors is more than 20 times higher in cryptorchid than in scrotal testes.[3]

Approximately 20 to 30 percent of dogs with Sertoli cell tumor manifest signs of hyperestrinism, characterized by any combination of feminization, gynecomastia, atrophy of the contralateral testicle, squamous metaplasia within the prostate gland (often with accompanying suppurative prostatitis), alopecia, and bone marrow atrophy.[1,2,4,5] It is not proven that estrogen solely is responsible

TABLE 11.2.   Distinguishing features of the principal testicular tumors

Sertoli Cell Tumors
   Most common in the dog, especially in cryptorchid testicles
   Often hormonally active, producing manifestations of hyperestrinism
   Very firm to hard, multinodular, white to gray
   Typically consist of variable sized aggregates of Sertoli cells (tubular and diffuse forms) separated by an abundant fibrous tissue
      stroma

Seminomas
   Most common in the dog, but also common in the stallion, especially in cryptorchid testicles
   May produce enlargement of the affected testicle
   Generally soft with a homogeneous gray/white appearance on cut surface
   Consist of tubules or sheets of large polyhedral (germ) cells with large vesicular nuclei, prominent nucleoli, and scant basophilic
      cytoplasm with necrosis and mitotic figures
   Intratubular and diffuse types

Interstitial Cell Tumors
   Most common in the dog but also common in the bull
   Sharply delineated, rubbery, bulging yellow/tan nodules; hemorrhage, cysts
   Consist of polyhedral cells with small dark nuclei and abundant eosinophilic cytoplasm that may contain lipid droplets

Teratomas
   Uncommon but most often seen in young horses, especially in cryptorchid testicles
   Include more than one tissue type

for all of these manifestations; in fact, serum estrogen is not increased in some dogs with apparent hyperestrinism associated with testicular Sertoli cell tumor. Other secretory products of the tumor, such as inhibin, contribute to this syndrome and likely also are responsible for the development of the signs and lesions. Inhibin produced by the neoplastic Sertoli cells reduces testosterone production through inhibition of trophic pituitary hormone secretion.[4] Feminization of dogs with Sertoli cell tumors can manifest as attractiveness to other male dogs, lethargy, loss of libido, pendulous swelling of the penile sheath, and redistribution of body fat. The bone marrow suppressive effects accompanying Sertoli cell tumors can be so severe as to cause anemia, leukopenia, and thrombocytopenia. Thrombocytopenia may precipitate a hemorrhagic diathesis. Changes in the hair coat of dogs with hyperestrinism are those of bilaterally symmetrical alopecia and epidermal atrophy, similar to that which occurs in other endocrinopathies such as Cushing's disease and hypothyroidism. There is marked atrophy of adnexal structures, epidermal thinning, and atrophy of hair follicles in the affected skin. Marked squamous metaplasia of the columnar epithelium lining the ducts and glands of the prostate occurs in some dogs with Sertoli cell tumors. Keratinization of the squamous epithelium can become extensive, as can accumulation of neutrophils and other inflammatory cells. Gynecomastia, especially of the caudal two sets of glands, also occurs in some dogs with Sertoli cell tumors. This manifests as elongation of the mammary nipples, with or without enlargement of the glands themselves. These signs disappear after castration, if the tumor has not already metastasized.

Sites and Gross Morphology

Sertoli cell tumors are very firm, discrete nodular or multinodular tumors that are well demarcated within the affected testicle. They can become quite large and cause marked distortion of the affected testicle. Most Sertoli cell tumors are fully contained within the testicle, and only large malignant tumors extend into adjacent structures of the tunica albuginea, epididymis, or spermatic cord. On cut surface the tumor is white or gray, and it sometimes has tan or yellow areas of hemorrhage. A rim of compressed, atrophic normal testicular tissue typically is peripheral to the tumor. The Sertoli cell tumor is much firmer than either seminoma or interstitial cell tumor, the other common tumors of the canine testicle.

Histological Features

Sertoli cell tumors are subdivided on the basis of their histological appearance into intratubular and diffuse forms. Cells within the tumor variably resemble Sertoli cells that normally populate the seminiferous tubules, and are arranged into islands or tubular structures that are separated by an abundant stroma of dense, mature fibrous connective tissue (fig. 11.6 A,B). The tumor cells are elongate, with small, round to elongate nuclei and have either vacuolated or dense eosinophilic cytoplasm that frequently contains lipochrome pigment granules. In the intratubular form the tumor consists of well-formed tubules that are lined by multiple layers of neoplastic Sertoli cells. The tumor cells are arranged perpendicularly to the basement membrane. In contrast, the diffuse form lacks an orderly tubular architecture, and the neoplastic Sertoli cells are present in broad sheets or islands divided by dense fibrous stroma. The cells in such tumors are more irregular in their size and shape, and in malignant tumors may infiltrate tissues adjacent to the testicle or invade vessels.

Biological Behavior

The vast majority of Sertoli cell tumors are benign. Metastasis is more likely to occur in larger Sertoli cell tumors. The rate of metastasis reported from different studies has varied widely. The metastatic rate is very low for small tumors (less than 2 cm), especially when treated by castration. The diffuse histological pattern is more likely to be associated with malignant behavior, whereas the intratubular form usually is benign. Metastasis occurs to the adjacent lymph nodes of the sublumbar and pelvic regions and to internal organs. The metastatic nodules have a histological appearance similar to the primary tumor, and they also may be hormonally active.

Interstitial (Leydig) Cell Tumor

Testicular interstitial cell tumors arise from and histologically resemble the interstitial (Leydig) cells of the normal testicle. They are most common in the dog, but also occur in the bull, cat, and stallion.[1,2,6] Those that occur in the stallion most often occur in cryptorchid testicles. There is some uncertainty as to whether the majority of the focal interstitial cell proliferations that occur in the testicles of old animals, especially dogs and bulls, reflect hyperplastic nodules or adenomas, given the extremely low incidence of malignant behavior of these masses in either species. Criteria to distinguish interstitial cell hyperplasia from neoplasia are arbitrary and may be as simple as the size of the lesion. Macroscopic nodules are generally considered to be adenomas, whereas microscopic nodules are considered hyperplasias. More definitive criteria of neoplasia would include encroachment and compression of adjacent testicular tissue by the tumor.

Sites and Gross Morphology

Interstitial cell tumors usually develop in older animals and may be uni- or bilateral, single or multiple. Although interstitial cells normally secrete androgens, interstitial cell tumors produce no obvious manifestations of excessive androgen secretion. The gross appearance of interstitial cell tumors is distinctive. They normally are small, frequently producing little or only subtle distortion of the affected testicle. They are yellow/brown, soft, well circumscribed, and sharply delineated from the adjacent testicle. They tend to bulge on cut surface, and some contain areas of hemorrhage or cysts.

Histological Features

The tumor cells resemble normal interstitial cells, being round to polyhedral, with abundant eosinophilic cytoplasm that varies from finely granular to vacuolated, and containing prominent lipid accumulations (fig. 11.6 C). Nuclei typically are small, dark, and round, and mitotic figures are extremely unusual. The tumor cells can be arranged in solid sheets or an irregular acinar (glandular) pattern, and they have a supporting fine stroma of connective tissue and blood vessels. Cysts lined by tumor cells are present in some tumors (fig. 11.6 D).

Biological Behavior

The vast majority of interstitial cell tumors are benign, although malignant forms (interstitial cell carcinoma) have been described. Within an interstitial cell carcinoma, cells often are more irregular, mitotic figures more

numerous, and vascular invasion may be evident; however, distinction between benign and malignant forms on purely histological criteria, in the absence of metastasis, often is difficult.

Germ Cell Tumors

Seminoma, teratoma, embryonal carcinoma, and yolk sac carcinoma are all derived from germ cells.[1,2,7] Seminoma is the only one of these that occurs frequently in the testicles of domestic animals.

Seminoma

Seminoma is derived from the germ cells that constitute the spermatogenic epithelium within the seminiferous tubules. They are most common in the dog, in which they are relatively common, but seminoma also has been reported in the stallion, ram, bull, goat, and cat.[2] Cryptorchidism predisposes to development of seminoma, as it does to development of Sertoli cell tumor. Seminomas most often occur in older animals, with boxer dogs apparently being predisposed.

Sites and Gross Morphology

Seminomas may be uni- or bilateral, solitary or multiple, and they are more common in the right testicle than the left. Seminoma is of variable size, and larger tumors can cause enlargement of the affected testicle. The tumor is soft or somewhat firm, but markedly less so than Sertoli cell tumor, and has a homogeneous glistening gray/white appearance on cut surface. Some tumors include obvious areas of discoloration that reflect hemorrhage or necrosis.

Histological Features

Seminomas are subdivided into intratubular (fig. 11.7 A,C) and diffuse forms based upon their histological appearance. The former is the earlier form and consists of aggregates of germ cells that fill the lumen of affected seminiferous tubules, replacing the normal lining of spermatogenic and Sertoli cells (fig. 11.7 A). The appearance of the tumor cells is highly characteristic and is similar to those in ovarian dysgerminoma: very large, polyhedral, with sharp borders, vesicular nuclei and prominent nucleoli, and scant basophilic or amphophilic cytoplasm (fig. 11.7 A,B). Mitotic figures are numerous and frequently bizarre. Focal aggregates of lymphocytes are present in many tumors. In the diffuse form, tumor cells are not confined to the seminiferous tubules; instead they form broad sheets (fig. 11.7 B). Necrosis of individual cells produces a "starry sky" effect within the neoplasm.

Biological Behavior

The incidence of malignant seminoma is low, although malignant forms clearly occur. Metastasis is more likely in affected horses than dogs.[2,8,9] It usually is difficult to distinguish malignant and benign forms of seminoma

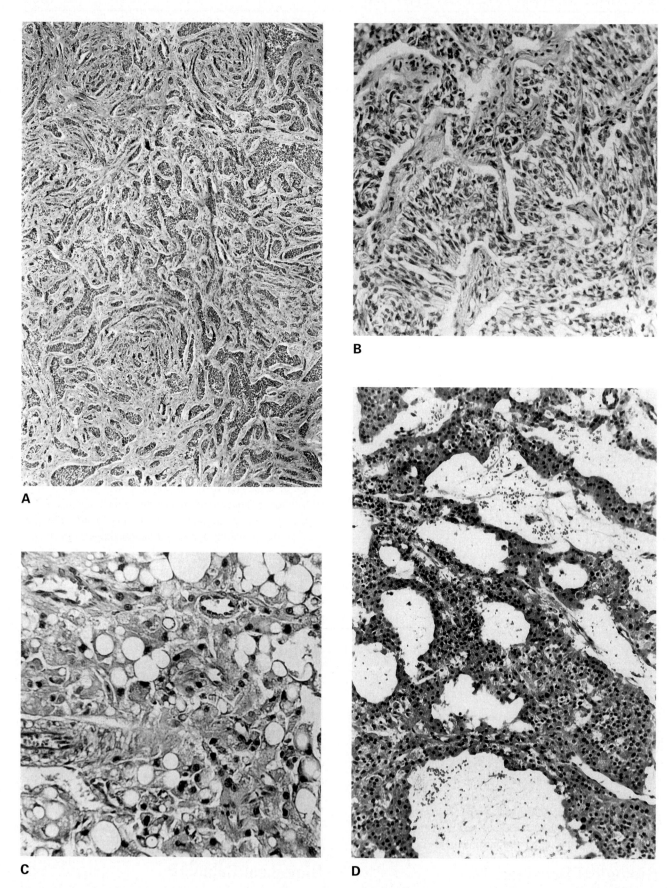

Fig. 11.6. Sex cord–stromal. **A.** Sertoli cell tumor. The tumor cells form cords in a dense fibrous stroma. Dog. **B.** Sertoli cell tumor in the testis of a dog. Note tubules of elongated, vacuolated tumor cells of the testis in parallel arrangement. **C.** Interstitial cell adenoma in the testis of a dog. Tumor cells with lipid vacuoles. **D.** Interstitial (Leydig) cell tumor. The tumor cells are arranged in a cystic-vascular pattern. Dog.

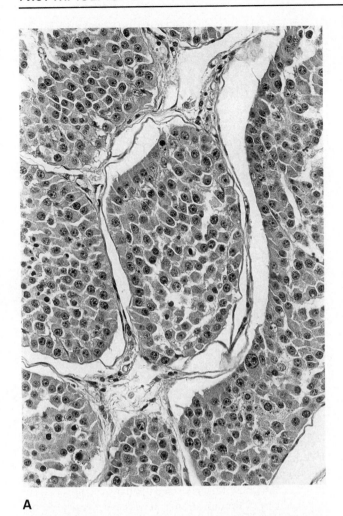

A

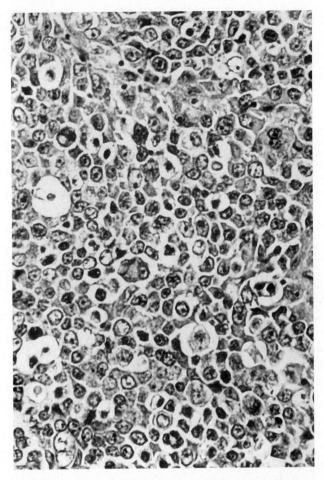

B

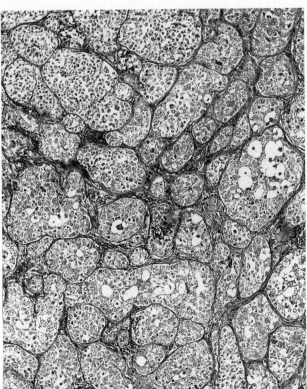

C

Fig. 11.7. Germ cell. Dog. **A.** Intratubular seminoma. The tumor cells are confined to preexisting tubules. **B.** Seminoma in the testis. Diffuse seminoma with starry sky pattern. **C.** Seminoma in the testis. Intratubular growth of tumor cells without stromal invasion.

based solely on histological evaluation of the primary neoplasm, as both have a malignant histological appearance. The infiltration of tumor cells into vessels or tissues adjacent to the testicle, such as the tunica albuginea, epididymis, or spermatic cord is evidence of malignancy. Metastasis often occurs to the regional lymph nodes, but widespread dissemination to internal organs also can occur.

Teratoma

A teratoma is a tumor consisting of tissues from more than one germinal layer; thus it presumably arises from a multipotential germ cell that has undergone partial differentiation. Teratomas of the testicle have been described in the stallion and, rarely, in the dog, cat, bull, and boar.[1,2] In the stallion they occur in cryptorchid testicles, and the fact that they can occur in young colts and are most commonly reported in stallions of between 1 and 5 years of age suggests that they may be a congenital neoplasm. Development of the tumor may prevent normal descent of the affected testicle.[10]

Sites and Gross Morphology

Teratomas can be uni- or bilateral, single or multiple, and produce obvious uniform or irregular enlargement of the affected gonad. They can include both solid and cystic areas and may contain foci of cartilage, bone, fat, or haired skin.

Histological Features

The histological appearance of teratomas is highly variable and ranges from tumors that resemble a dermoid cyst within the affected gonad to very complex tumors that can include multiple tissue types such as any combination of haired skin with adnexal structures, glandular tissue or epithelium, fibrous connective tissue, fat, muscle, lymphoid tissue, bone, cartilage, teeth, nervous tissue, and choroid plexus. Even parenchymal organs such as liver, kidney, and spleen rarely may be included in a teratoma. A teratocarcinoma is a teratoma in which one or more of the tissues are poorly differentiated and malignant.[2,11]

Biological Behavior

Teratomas may be either benign or malignant (teratocarcinoma), the latter being an undifferentiated teratoma with both mature and embryonal elements. Teratocarcinomas have been described in both stallions and dogs, but most teratomas are benign.

Embryonal Carcinoma

Embryonal carcinoma is a rare testicular neoplasm in animals.[2] It is derived from poorly differentiated embryonal epithelium of uncertain derivation. The histological appearance is that of a poorly differentiated carcinoma that may include solid, papillary, or tubular areas embedded in an abundant stroma of fibrous connective tissue. Ultrastructural features include closely packed cells with large nuclei and intercellular desmosomes. A single case of metastatic embryonal carcinoma has been reported in a stallion.[12] The tumor can be difficult to distinguish from anaplastic seminoma and carcinoma of the rete testis, and the diagnosis of testicular embryonal carcinoma is based on the histopathologic and ultrastructural appearance and positive immunohistochemical staining for alpha-fetoprotein.[12]

Yolk Sac Carcinoma

Yolk sac carcinoma or endodermal sinus tumor is a malignant tumor of apparent germ cell origin that occurs in the ovaries and testes of humans and rodents. A disseminated case of testicular yolk sac carcinoma recently was described in a calf.[13] This tumor exhibited a variety of patterns including solid nests and pseudopapillary structures with varying degrees of epithelial differentiation. The tumor cells contained cytoplasmic lipid and PAS-positive eosinophilic inclusions and were stained immunohistochemically with antibodies to alpha-fetoprotein and placental alkaline phosphatase. Yolk sac carcinoma is distinguished in calves from congenital mesothelioma by the abundant presence of types I and III collagen in the stroma of the latter tumor.

Mixed Tumors of the Testicle

Multiple tumors can occur in the testes of an individual animal, particularly in cryptorchid dogs. These can be any combination of Sertoli cell tumor, interstitial cell tumor, and/or seminoma. In contrast, true mixed tumors are single tumors that include a mixture of different neoplastic cells.

Mixed Germ Cell–Sex-Cord Stromal Tumors

Mixed germ cell–sex-cord stromal tumors include neoplastic elements derived from both the germ cell and sex-cord stromal elements of the testicle. A series of such tumors has been described in dogs, and a single case has been described in a stallion.[14,15] Mixed germ cell–sex-cord stromal tumors include features of both seminoma and Sertoli cell tumor within a single tumor. Seminomas occasionally abut on Sertoli cell tumors, thus creating tumors with features of both seminoma and Sertoli cell tumor. These have properly been designated as *collision tumors,* reflecting the interpretation that they represent the interface between two distinct tumors. In true mixed tumors, however, both Sertoli and germ cell elements are intimately admixed in variably sized tubular structures that are separated by a fibrous stroma of variable density. Either the germ cell or Sertoli cell component may predominate in individual tumors. Immunohistochemical staining with neuron specific enolase, desmin, and vimentin can be useful in establishing that the tumor includes two distinct cell populations. Sertoli cells are stained for both neuron specific enolase and desmin, whereas germ cells are not stained for either. Furthermore, Sertoli cells are stained diffusely for vimentin, whereas staining of germ cells is focal. Neither Sertoli cells nor germ cells are stained for cytokeratins. These tumors are more common in cryptorchid testicles and can be either uni- or bilateral. Their behavior is similar to that of seminoma and Sertoli cell tumor, although they apparently do not induce hyperestrinism syndromes and usually are benign.

Gonadoblastoma

A single putative case of gonadoblastoma, which also is a mixed gonadal tumor that includes germ cell and sex-cord elements, has been described in a dog.[16] In humans, additional features of gonadoblastoma are that they occur in genetic females with abnormal external genitalia and gonads, and the tumor cells have an abnormal karyotype. These neoplasms often are hormonally active in humans and frequently include foci of interstitial cells, along with tubular structures populated by a mixture of neoplastic Sertoli and germ cells.

Other Tumors of the Testicle

Mesothelioma

Other primary tumors of the testicle are sufficiently uncommon that they might best be regarded as oddities in domestic animals.[2] These include mesothelioma (derived from the mesothlelial lining of the vaginal tunics), fibroma/fibrosarcoma, hemangioma/hemangiosarcoma, and leiomyoma/leiomyosarcoma, which are not morphologically distinguished from similar tumors at other sites in the body. Mesothelioma of the testicle is described in dogs and bulls. Primary mesothelioma of the gonad must be distinguished from metastasis of peritoneal mesothelioma, especially in young cattle. The appearance is typical of mesothelioma, with irregular papillary proliferations over the testicular tunics. Mast cell tumors also rarely occur in the testicle.

Adenoma/Carcinoma of the Rete Testis

Carcinomas of the testicle that likely arose from the rete testis have been described in the stallion, dog, and ram.[2] They typically are cystic tumors that involve variable amounts of the affected testicle and consist of irregular cords and papillary projections of epithelium supported by connective tissue septae. Necrosis and hemorrhage can occur, especially in malignant tumors.

Metastatic Tumors

Metastatic tumors that involve the testicle have not been commonly reported, although metastatic lymphosarcoma and hemangiosarcoma occasionally involve the testicle, in the boar and dog in particular.[2]

Tumor-Like Lesions of the Tissues Adjacent to the Testicle

Cysts

Cysts derived from remnants of the ducts and embryonic structures associated with sexual development may occur adjacent to the testicle, epididymis, or spermatic cord. These cysts are lined by a single layer of epithelium, which distinguishes them from teratomas composed of multiple tissues. Furthermore, monophasic teratomas usually manifest as dermoid cysts that have a stratified squamous epithelial lining. Cysts derived from the epididymis also have a characteristic subepithelial

layer of smooth muscle. Cells lining cysts of the rete testis and efferent ductule, like the mesothelial lining of the testicle, are variably stained immunohistochemically for cytokeratins, vimentin, and desmin. Cells derived from the efferent ductules may be ciliated, whereas those from the rete testis or lining mesothelium are not, a fact that also can be useful in determining the origin of testicular cysts.[2,17,18]

Choristoma

Ectopic adrenal tissue occasionally may be present within or adjacent to the testicle, epididymis, or spermatic cord.[2]

REFERENCES

1. Ladd, P.W. (1993) The male genital system. In Jubb, K.V.F., Kennedy, P.C., and Palmer, N. (eds.) *Pathology of Domestic Animals.* 4th ed. Academic Press, Inc., San Diego.
2. McEntee, K. (1990) Scrotum, spermatic cord, and testis: Proliferative lesions. In *Reproductive Pathology of Domestic Animals.* Academic Press Inc., San Diego, pp. 279-306.
3. Hayes, H.M, and Pendergrass, T.W. (1976) Canine testicular tumors: Epidemiologic features of 410 dogs. *Intl J Cancer* 18:482-487.
4. Grootenhuis, A.J., van Sluijs, F.J., Klaij, I.A., Steenbergen, J., Tillerman, M.A., Bevers, M.M., Dieleman, S.J., and de Jong, F.H. (1990) Inhibin, gonadotrophins and sex steroids in dogs with Sertoli cell tumors. *J Endocrinol* 127: 235-242.
5. Morgan, R.V. (1982) Blood dyscrasias associated with testicular tumors in the dog. *J Amer Anim Hosp Assoc* 18:970-975.
6. Gelberg, H.B., and McEntee, K. (1987) Equine testicular interstitial cell tumors. *Vet Pathol* 24:231-234.
7. Bosl, G.J., and Motzer, R.J. (1997) Testicular germ-cell cancer. *N Eng J Med* 337:242-253.
8. Trigo, F.J., Miller, R.A., and Torbeck, R.L. (1984) Metastatic equine seminoma: Report of two cases. *Vet Pathol* 21:259-260.
9. Villancourt, D., Fretz, P., and Orr, J.P. (1979) Seminoma in the horse: Report of two cases. *J Equine Med Surg* 3:213-218.
10. Cotchin, E. (1977) A general survey of tumors in the horse. *Equine Vet J* 9:16-21.
11. Shaw, D.P., and Roth, J.E. (1986) Testicular teratocarcinoma in a horse. *Vet Pathol* 23:327-328.
12. Valentine, B.A., and Weinstock, D. (1986) Metastatic testicular embryonal carcinoma in a horse. *Vet Pathol* 23:92-96.
13. Kagawa, Y., Ohosaki, A., Ohosaki, R., Katsuta, O., Tsuchitani, M., and Taniyama, H. (1998) Testicular yolk sac carcinoma in a calf. *Vet Pathol* 35:220-222.
14. Cullen, J.M., Whiteside, J., Umstead, J.A., and Whitacre, M.D. (1987) A mixed germ cell-sex cord-stromal neoplasm of the testis in a stallion. *Vet Pathol* 24:575-577.
15. Patnaik, A.K., and Mostofi, F.K. (1993) A clinicopathologic, histologic, and immunohistochemical study of mixed germ cell-stromal tumors of the testis in 16 dogs. *Vet Pathol* 30:287-295.
16. Turk, J.R., Turk, M.A.M., and Gallina, A.M. (1981) A canine testicular tumor resembling gonadoblastoma. *Vet Pathol* 18:201-207.
17. Schumaker, J., Lenz, S.D., and Walker, W. (1994) Cystic rete testis associated with cryptorchidism in a horse. *Vet Pathol* 31:115-117.
18. Wakui, S., Fursato, M., Yokoo, K., and Ushigome, S. (1997) Testicular efferent ductule cysts of a dog. *Vet Pathol* 34:230-232.

TUMORS OF THE SPERMATIC CORD, EPIDIDYMIS, AND ACCESSORY SEX GLANDS

Tumors of the Spermatic Cord and Epididymis

Tumors of the spermatic cord and epididymis are extremely uncommon in domestic animals.[1,2] The most common tumors in the male tubular genitalia are testicular tumors that have invaded these adjacent structures. Papillary carcinoma of the epididymis has been described in the dog and bull, and mesenchymal tumors (fibroma/fibrosarcoma and leiomyoma/leiomyosarcoma) can develop at this site. Adenomyosis is a nonneoplastic proliferation of the epithelial lining of the epididymis into the muscle of the duct. It is usually caused by excessive exposure to estrogen. Causes include iatrogenic administration of estrogen or endogenous production of estrogen by hormonally productive testicular tumors such as Sertoli cell tumor. Histologically the lesion consists of proliferation of branching tubules and ducts from the lining epithelium into the adjacent smooth muscle of the epididymis.

Tumors of the accessory sex glands are very uncommon in domestic animals, and only those that affect the canine prostate are of significance. Tumors of the accessory glands other than the prostate, specifically the ampullae, seminal vesicles, and bulbourethral glands, clearly can occur, but they are not well documented. Similarly, hyperplastic and tumor-like lesions such as cysts can occur in these structures and must be distinguished from neoplasms.

Tumors and Tumor-Like Lesions of the Prostate

Squamous Metaplasia

Squamous metaplasia and enlargement of the prostate occurs after excessive estrogenic stimulation, as occurs in ruminants grazing certain estrogenic plants and in dogs with hormonally productive Sertoli cell tumors.[1,3]

Hyperplasia and Hypertrophy

Incidence and Age

This is a benign enlargement of the prostate that results from hyperplasia of the glandular epithelium and/or the fibromuscular stroma.[1,3-6] It is extremely common in intact male dogs. Almost all intact dogs develop the condition with aging. It may develop as early as 2 years of age, but in rare cases it may be delayed until 10 years. In most dogs hyperplasia is well developed by 6 years. The cause of the condi-tion is only partially understood; the incidence increases with age, but it is clearly hormonally controlled. It occurs only in intact animals and is reversible with castration.

Histological Features

There are two primary patterns of prostatic hyperplasia in the dog. In the benign diffuse glandular form, there is an increase in secretory epithelium with an increase in size of lobules and papillary projections of secretory epithelium into alveoli. These papillary projections are more elaborate than normal, and the size of the individual cells is increased. This pattern of hyperplasia is most often uniform throughout the gland, but nodules may develop. In the complex form of prostatic hyperplasia, areas of glandular hyperplasia are intermixed with cystic alveoli (fig. 11.8 A). The epithelium that lines these cystic alveoli may be thin and atrophic or plump columnar. The fibromuscular stroma of the gland is increased in amount. Chronic inflammation is often seen in the complex form of prostatic hyperplasia. It is thought that the complex form is a sequela to the diffuse glandular form.

Adenocarcinoma

Incidence, Age, and Sex

This malignant tumor arises from prostatic glandular epithelium. It is uncommon in the dog and extremely rare in other domestic animals.[1,3,7-9] Hyperplasia does not appear to be a precancerous change, but since hyperplasia occurs in essentially all aged intact male dogs and prostatic adenocarcinoma of the dog is a tumor affecting dogs 8 years and older, the two conditions may occur concurrently. A benign counterpart (adenoma) has not been described.

The incidence of this tumor in dogs is not clear because not all carcinomas of the prostate develop from glandular epithelium, and many of the reported cases of adenocarcinoma arose not from the secretory prostatic epithelium but from urothelium of the prostatic urethra or the periurethral ducts and were urothelial (transitional cell) carcinomas (fig. 11.8 B). The frequency of prostatic invasion by urothelial carcinoma in the dog is not yet accurately documented, but it clearly is very substantial. Urothelial carcinomas of the prostatic urethra can easily escape detection at their primary site and invade the prostate. The distinction between these two carcinomas can be very difficult and requires careful gross dissection, the examination of multiple sections, and the use of immunohistochemical staining. Polyclonal antibodies to prostatic acid phosphatase can be useful in identifying tumors of prostatic glandular epithelium.[10] Prostatic acid phosphatase is not present in urothelial (transitional cell) tumors, but these tumors express cytokeratin 7, which secretory cells of the prostate do not.

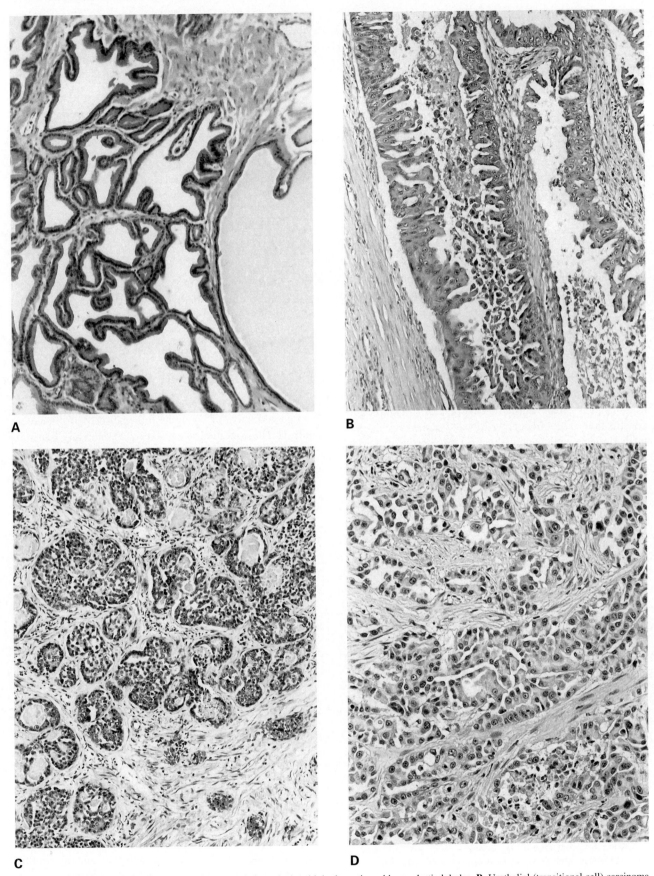

Fig. 11.8. Prostate. Dog. **A.** Benign complex prostatic hyerplasia with both cystic and hyperplastic lobules. **B.** Urothelial (transitional cell) carcinoma invading the prostate. **C.** Prostatic adenocarcinoma. Intra-alveolar pattern. **D.** Prostatic adenocarcinoma. Tumor cells in a dense fibrous stroma.

Histological Features

The establishment of a satisfactory histological characterization of prostatic adenocarcinomas of dogs is difficult at this time because relatively few tumors have been studied in detail and because urothelial carcinomas have been included in some reports. The most common pattern of growth of canine prostatic adenocarcinoma is intra-alveolar. Here, the cells form large alveoli filled with papillary projections of glandular epithelium (fig. 11.8 C). The tumor cells are round or cuboidal; some are vacuolated and produce mucus. The nuclei are moderately hyperchromatic, and mitotic figures are present. A second pattern of canine prostatic adenocarcinoma is acinar, in which the neoplastic cells, usually cuboidal, are arranged in acini. The neoplastic lining cells are most often one to two cells thick, but the acini may be filled with solid masses of neoplastic cells. Mucus may be present in the acini, and the neoplastic acini are often embedded in a fibrous stroma (fig. 11.8 D).

Biological Behavior

Carcinomas of the prostate, whether adenocarcinomas of the glandular epithelium or urothelial carcinomas extending into the prostate, produce nonsymmetrical enlargement of the gland. The tumors usually are firm and irregular. They may cause clinical signs of stranguria and constipation. They frequently are associated with hematuria. If they extend beyond the prostatic capsule, they may fix the prostate to adjacent structures. Carcinomas of the prostate are aggressive and often metastasize to the pelvic and sublumbar lymph nodes, but widespread metastasis to a variety of organs including bone and brain also occurs.

Other Tumors of the Prostate

Other mesenchymal tumors of the prostate gland occur uncommonly, including lymphosarcoma, fibroma/fibrosarcoma, leiomyoma/leimyosarcoma, and hemangioma/hemangiosarcoma.[3]

REFERENCES

1. Ladd, P.W. (1993) The male genital system. In Jubb, K.V.F., Kennedy, P.C., and Palmer, N. (eds.) *Pathology of Domestic Animals.* 4th ed. Academic Press Inc., San Diego.
2. McEntee K. (1990) Scrotum, spermatic cord, and testis: Proliferative lesions. In *Reproductive Pathology of Domestic Animals.* Academic Press Inc., San Diego, pp. 279-306.
3. McEntee K. (1990) Bulbourethral, vesicular, and prostate glands. In *Reproductive Pathology of Domestic Animals.* Academic Press Inc., San Diego, pp. 333-358.
4. Berry S.J., Coffey, D.S., and Ewing, L.L. (1986) Effects of aging on prostate growth in beagles. *Amer J Physiol* 250:R1039-R1046.
5. Berry, S.J., Strandberg, J.D., Saunders, W.J., and Coffey, D.S. (1986) Development of canine benign prostatic hyperplasia with age. *Prostate* 9:363-373.
6. Lowseth, L.A., Gerlach, R.F., Gillett, N.A., and Muggenburg, B.A. (1990) Age-related changes in the prostate and testes of the beagle dog. *Vet Pathol* 27:347-353.
7. Bell, F.W., Klausner, J.S., Hayden, D.W., Feeney, D.A., and Johnson, S.D. (1991) Clinical and pathologic features of prostatic adenocarcinoma in sexually intact and castrated dogs: 31 cases (1970-1978). *J Amer Vet Med Assoc* 199:1623-1630.
8. Caney, S.M., Holt, P.E., Day, M.J., Rudorf, H., and Gruffydd-Jones, T.J. (1998) Prostatic carcinoma in two cats. *J Small Anim Pract* 39:140-143.
9. Leav, I., and Ling, G.V. (1973) Adenocarcinoma of the canine prostate. *Cancer* 22:1329-1345.
10. McEntee, M., Isaacs, W., and Smith, C. (1987) Adenocarcinoma of the canine prostate: Immunohistochemical examination for secretory antigens. *Prostate* 11:163-170.

TUMORS OF THE EXTERNAL GENITALIA

These are tumors of the penis and prepuce, although it also is to be stressed that tumors of the skin obviously can affect the scrotum and skin adjacent to the external genitalia.

Epithelial Tumors

Fibropapilloma of Cattle

This is a virus induced, transmissible tumor of the vagina and vulva of young heifers and the penis of young bulls.[1-4] The condition is caused by a venereally transmitted papovavirus, and transmission frequently occurs as a consequence of homosexual activity among bulls. Fibropapillomas are elevated, fleshy, multinodular proliferations that emanate from the affected mucosa and may be ulcerated. The tumors predominantly consist of abundant proliferating fibrous tissue with an epithelial covering of variable thickness (fig. 11.9 A). Pegs of epithelium typically extend into the subjacent connective tissue. Although benign, potentially adverse consequences of these tumors include secondary infection and/or adhesions between the prepuce and penis.

Papilloma

Transmissible Genital Papilloma of the Pig

A pox virus has been suggested as the cause of this virus induced papilloma. It consists of extensive thickening of the affected epithelium with little proliferation of the underlying connective tissue.[4] Similar lesions occur on the mucosa of the vagina or vulva of affected sows. The papillomas regress with time in both sexes.

Squamous Papilloma

These are benign epithelial proliferations.[4] They are most common in the horse, and some contain papillomavirus antigen.[5] Squamous papillomas consist of keratinized epithelial proliferations with sparse fibrous stroma.

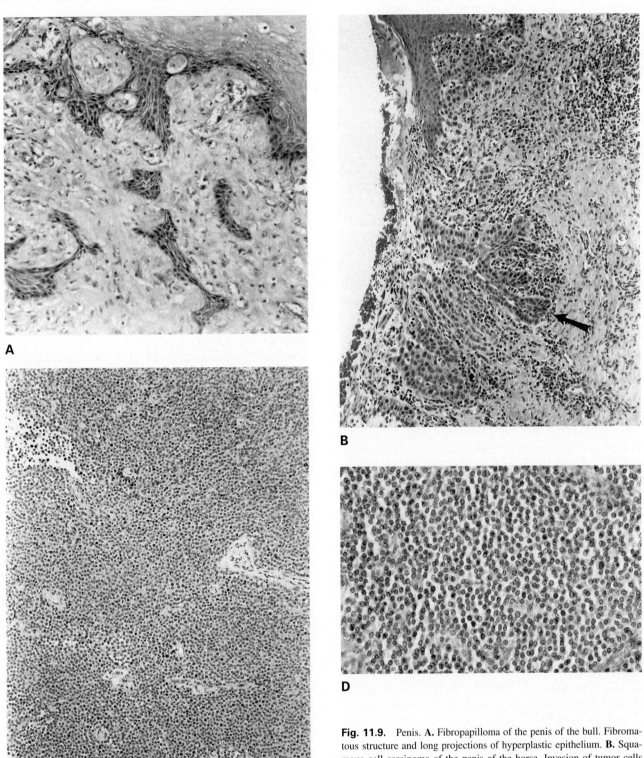

Fig. 11.9. Penis. **A.** Fibropapilloma of the penis of the bull. Fibromatous structure and long projections of hyperplastic epithelium. **B.** Squamous cell carcinoma of the penis of the horse. Invasion of tumor cells (arrow) beneath an area of ulceration. **C.** Transmissible venereal tumor. Homogeneous sheet of tumor cells. **D.** Transmissible venereal tumor. Microscopic features showing uniform size tumor cells that resemble immature lymphoid cells but are not of lymphocytic origin. (Courtesy of Dr. D.A. Higgins and *Vet. Rec.*)

571

Papilloma is distinguished from squamous cell carcinoma by the absence of stromal invasion.

Squamous Cell Carcinoma

Squamous cell carcinoma of the penis and prepuce is most common in the stallion but also is described in the dog.[3-6] Irritation from smegma is considered to be important in the promotion of these tumors, but ultraviolet irradiation from sunlight also may contribute, as it does to carcinomas of the vulva, because penile squamous cell carcinomas often are located on unpigmented or lightly pigmented areas. Lesions associated with the tumor may be primarily proliferative or ulcerative, and often are multicentric (fig. 11.9 B). Metastasis can occur, although this generally is late in the course of disease; lymphatic metastasis occurs first to the inguinal lymph nodes. Grossly, squamous cell carcinoma of the equine penis can resemble cutaneous habronemiasis, but the two conditions can occur together.

Mesenchymal Tumors

Transmissible Venereal Tumor of the Dog

The canine transmissible venereal tumor (TVT) is a transplantable tumor that is most often disseminated during coitus; thus TVT is a naturally occurring allogeneic tumor transmitted from dog to dog by living cells rather than by transformation of cells in the affected host. The histogenesis of the tumor cells is poorly defined. Previous studies have suggested a histiocytic origin for TVT based on positive immunohistochemistry for lysozyme;[11] however, lysozyme is not specific for histiocytes because it also stains neutrophils, serous glands, and other cell types.[12] Recent studies indicate that TVT is composed of immature leukocytes, likely myeloid in origin, that express CD45 and CD45RA but neither beta-2 nor CD1 (P.F. Moore, personal communication). Remarkably, there appears to be a common cellular origin to all TVT worldwide. Tumor cells collected from various parts of the world have a near constant karyotypic variation. The normal number of diploid chromosomes in the dog is 78, whereas there are only 58 or 59 chromosomes in cells of TVT. Further evidence of a common cellular origin of TVT is the demonstration of a common rearrangement of oncogenes in TVT from various geographical locations.[7,8] TVT cells consistently harbor a retrotransposon upstream from the c-myc oncogene that is a molecular fingerprint for the tumor.[13,14]

Sites and Gross Appearance

The tumor develops most often on the external genitalia, but it can be implanted on the oral, nasal, and conjunctival mucosa or, less commonly, the skin. The tumor can consist of a single mass or form multiple nodules. If the tumor has been implanted in a mucous membrane, it grows in the submucosa and stretches the covering epithelium, which may be ulcerated. A TVT can become large at the primary site of implantation (up to approximately 10 cm in diameter) and may invade adjacent tissues. Growth is rapid for 1 to 2 months, after which the tumor usually regresses spontaneously. Tumors rarely persist more than 6 months in animals that are not immunologically suppressed. Regression is followed by transplantation immunity.

Histological Features

The histological appearance of the tumor depends on the stage of growth or regression.[9] The tumor cells initially are uniformly round or oval and resemble lymphoblasts; they are arranged in sheets or clusters (fig. 11.9 C,D). They have centrally located, large, oval or round nuclei that contain a single prominent nucleolus and coarsely aggregated chromatin. The cytoplasm is scant, pale blue, and finely granular and may contain vacuoles. Mitotic figures are common. The fibrovascular stroma is scanty early in tumor development and becomes more abundant in older tumors. Lymphocytes and other inflammatory cells infiltrate tumors undergoing spontaneous regression, at which stage individual tumor cells degenerate.

Biological Behavior

TVT usually develops as a local tumor, but metastasis, at least transient, is frequent, most often involving the inguinal and iliac nodes. The precise incidence of regional metastasis is not known because local nodes are not often examined. Distant metastasis is rare and occurs in dogs that are immunologically suppressed. Large tumors induce polycythemia (erythrocytosis). In such tumors the level of erythropoietin is raised, and erythropoietin can be extracted from the tumor.

Other Tumors

A variety of tumors can occur on the prepuce and penis including papilloma, equine sarcoid, melanoma (especially in gray horses), lymphosarcoma, mast cell tumor, hemangioma, and hemangiosarcoma.[3,4,10]

REFERENCES

1. Campo, M.S. (1997) Bovine papillomavirus and cancer. *Vet J* 154:175-188.
2. Jarrett, W. (1985) The natural history of bovine papilloma virus infections. *Adv Virol Oncol* 5:83-102.
3. McEntee K. (1990) Penis and prepuce. In *Reproductive Pathology of Domestic Animals*. Academic Press Inc., San Diego.
4. Ladd, P.W. (1993) The male genital system. In Jubb, K.V.F., Kennedy, P.C., and Palmer, N. (eds), *Pathology of Domestic Animals*, 4th ed. Academic Press, San Diego.

5. Junge, R.E., Sundurg, J.P., and Lancaster, W.D. (1984) Papillomas and squamous cell carcinomas of horses. *J Amer Vet Med Assoc* 185:656-659.

6. Cotchin, E. (1977) A general survey of tumors in the horse. *Equine Vet J* 9:16-21.

7. Cohen, D. (1985) The canine transmissible venereal tumor: A unique result of tumor progression. *Adv Cancer Res* 43:75-112.

8. Katzir, N., Arman, E., Cohen, D., Givol, D., and Rechavi, G. (1987) Common origin of transmissible venereal tumors (TVT) in dogs. *Oncogene* 1:445-448.

9. Mozos, E., Mendez, A., Gomez-Villamandos, J.C., Martin de las Mula, J., and Perez, J. (1996) Immunohistochemical characterization of canine transmissible venereal tumor. *Vet Pathol* 33:257-263.

10. Roberts, S.J. (1986) Obstetrics and Genital Diseases. Edwards Bros., Ann Arbor.

11. Marchal, T., Chabanne, L., et al. (1997) Immunophenotype of the canine transmissible venereal tumor. *Vet Immunol Immunopathol* 57:1-11.

12. Moore, P.F. (1986) Utilization of cytoplasmic lysozyme in canine histiocytic disorders. *Vet Pathol* 23:757-762.

13. Choi, Y., Ishiguro, N. et al. (1999) Molecular structure of canine LINE-1 elements in canine transmissible venereal tumor. *Anim Genet* 30:51-53.

14. Chu, R.M., Sun, T.J., et al. (2001) Heat shock proteins in canine transmissible venereal tumor. *Vet Immunol Immunopathol* 82:9-21.

12 Tumors of the Mammary Gland

W. Misdorp

GENERAL CONSIDERATIONS

Incidence

Dog

Mammary cancer is the most common malignant neoplasm in the bitch.[1] The annual incidence rate has been estimated at 198/100,000.[2] When canine and human incidences were adjusted to the same population distribution, age-adjusted canine incidence rate was three times higher. Female age-specific rates increased at the same magnitude for both species; the canine rates (in contrast to the human rates) continued to increase as approximately the same exponential value as in the younger age group. [2]

The exact incidence of mammary tumors and the benign/malignant ratio are difficult to determine since particularly small benign tumors are either not brought to the veterinarian's attention or are not surgically removed. Based on histological and biological criteria (from follow-up studies), it can be estimated that approximately 30 percent of the surgically removed mammary tumors are malignant.

Dysplasias and benign and malignant mammary tumors increased in frequency from anterior to posterior glands. Dysplasias appeared before palpable tumors in a study of beagles.[3,4] Multiple tumors, mostly of different histological cell types, are frequent in the dog.

Cat

Mammary tumors are third in frequency after skin tumors and lymphoma, and among tumors in cats they account for 12 percent of all tumors and 17 percent of the tumors in queens.[1] The annual incidence was estimated at 12.8 per 100,000 cats and 25.4 per 100,000 female cats. [1] The average age at first detection is 10-11 years, with a range of 2.5-13 years.[5] The ratio of malignant to benign tumors was estimated at 9:1[6] and 4:1.[7] Multiple tumors, of either similar or different histological type, are relatively common.[8] In the former case the possibility of metastatic lymphogenous involvement from a neighboring primary tumor has to be considered.

REFERENCES

1. Dorn, C.R., Taylor, D.O.N., Frye, F.L., and Hibbard, H.H. (1968) Survey of animal neoplasms in Alameda and Contra Costa Counties, California I. Methodology and description of cases. *J Natl Cancer Inst* 40:295-305.
2. Schneider, R. (1970) Comparison of age, sex and incidence rates in human and canine breast cancer. *Cancer* 26:419-426.
3. Warner, M.R. (1976) Age incidence and site distribution of mammary dysplasia in young beagle bitches. *J Natl Cancer Inst* 57:57-61.
4. Else, R.W., and Hannant, D. (1979) Some epidemiological aspects of mammary neoplasia in the bitch. *Vet Rec* 194:296-304.
5. Hayes, H.M., Milne, K.L., and Mandell, C.P. (1981) Epidemiological studies of feline mammary carcinoma. *Vet Rec* 108:476-479.
6. Hayes, A.A., and Mooney, S. (1985) Feline mammary tumors. *Vet Clin N Amer* 15:513-520.
7. Misdorp, W., Romijn, A., and Hart, A.A.M. (1991) Feline mammary tumors: a case-control study of hormonal factors. *Anticancer Res* 11:1793-1798.
8. Weyer, K., Head, K.W., Misdorp, W., and Hampe, J.F. (1972) Feline malignant mammary tumors. I. Morphology and biology. Some comparisons with human and canine mammary carcinomas. *J Natl Cancer Inst* 49:1696-1704.

Etiology

Hormones and Growth Factors

Endogenous

Mammary tumors occur almost exclusively in female dogs and cats. Some mammary tumors in male dogs are associated with hormonal abnormalities such as estrogen secreting Sertoli cell tumor of the testis.

In bitches and queens, early ovariectomy offers a considerable protective effect against mammary carcinoma.[1,2] If carried out later in life ovariectomy may still reduce the risk of developing benign canine mammary tumors.[3] Based on morphological studies of the pituitary gland and on serum hormone levels, it was suggested that either growth hormone or prolactin imbalance might be associated with mammary carcinogenesis in the dog.[4-6] However, in other studies neither growth hormone nor prolactin concentrations at rest or during dynamic function tests were significantly different in dogs with benign or malignant mammary tumors than in control dogs (matched for endogenous or exogenous progesterone exposure).[7,8] Some tumor bearing dogs appeared to be overresponsive to stimulation of prolactin secretion with thyrotrophin releasing hormone. The concentrations of hormones in the plasma of tumor bearing animals, however, do not necessarily reflect conditions present during the process of tumorigenesis.[9] The possibility that having many litters offers some protection should be investigated further.[10] Data on the effect of pseudopregnancy related lactation are conflicting. No relation has been observed between irregularities in estrous cycles and mammary tumor risk in the bitch.[11]

Exogenous

Injectable progestins are used in some European countries to prevent estrus in the bitch and the queen. Such treatment was found to slightly enhance the risk of benign, but not malignant, mammary tumors in dogs.[3] In cats, regular administration of progestins was associated with a significantly increased risk for malignant and benign mammary tumors.[12] Irregular treatment did not increase the risk of mammary tumors, either benign or malignant, in cats. Benign mammary lesions in the cat, particularly fibroadenomatous change (feline mammary hypertrophy), are associated with either endogenous progestins (during pregnancy) or exogenous progestins.[13-15]

Much attention has been focused on the effects of administration of estrogen and progestins to dogs in toxicity studies. Prolonged administration of diethylstilbestrol or other synthetic estrogens alone did not increase the incidence of mammary tumors. Long-term treatment with progesterone or synthetic progestins induced mammary hyperplasia and benign mammary tumors.[16-20]

Malignant mammary tumors occurred in particular during treatment with progestin-estrogen combinations or with high doses of progesterone, whereas low doses seemed to offer some degree of protection.[12] Contraceptive steroids are, under certain conditions, associated with mammary tumor development in the dog, rodents, cats, and monkeys.[21,22] Prolonged oral contraceptive use by women at young ages is associated with increased risk of development of breast cancer at an early age.[23] Those findings contradict both the concept of "the uniqueness of the dog in its sensitivity to the induction of mammary neoplasia by progestins" and an earlier statement that "the beagle findings are irrelevant to the human situation."[24]

In the dog, endogenous progesterone and synthetic progestins can increase the production of growth hormone (GH), resulting in acromegaly and insulin resistance. Progestin induced GH excess was found to have characteristics of autonomous secretion.[25] Hypophysectomy in ovariohysterectomized bitches treated with progestins did not result in a significant decrease in plasma growth hormone levels. Subsequent analysis of the GH content of various tissues revealed that the highest GH immunoreactivity was found in the mammary gland, particularly in focal areas of hyperplastic ductular epithelium resembling end buds.[26,27] It can be speculated that GH stimulates the proliferation of mammary stem cells in the end buds as a first step in the process of mammary carcinogenesis. Ectopic production of GH in the mammary gland was confirmed by the lowering of plasma GH values into reference range within 2 hours after complete mammectomy and by arteriovenous GH gradients.[26] Expression of the gene encoding GH was demonstrated in mammary gland tumors of dogs and cats and subsequently also in normal and neoplastic human mammary glands.[28,29]

Receptors

Dog

The growth of normal and neoplastic mammary tissue may be stimulated by steroid and peptide hormones or by growth factors, binding to receptors (high affinity binding system) in target cells.

In most studies, receptors for estrogen (ER), progesterone (PR), prolactin (PRL-R), and epidermal growth factors (EGF-R) have been found in normal mammary glands from either nonaffected dogs[30-34] or tumor bearing dogs.[34] It was reported that benign and malignant mammary tumors were positive for ERs, PRs, and PRL-Rs, in a range of 40-60 percent,[34-40] as well as androgen receptors[39] and EGF-Rs.[33,34,41] In many tumors there was simultaneous occurrence of several receptors. It can be expected that receptor values from malignant mammary tumors can be falsely positive due to the admixture of normal epithelium (with high ER and PR content). Indeed, it was demonstrated that receptor positivity was more frequent and levels of receptors significantly higher in carcinomas admixed with normal tissue than in "pure" carcinomas.[31] Regional and distant metastases were frequently steroid receptor negative[31] and also EGF-R negative,[32] indicating that in advanced disease the expression of genes encoding ERs, PRs, and EGF-Rs is lost.

Undifferentiated mammary carcinomas had lower numbers of receptors than more differentiated mammary carcinomas.[34] A positive ER and PR status was significantly more common in *complex* carcinomas than in *simple* carcinomas[33]; complex carcinomas have a better prognosis.[42] Receptor-rich carcinomas were associated with longer postsurgical survival.[43-46] An inverse correlation was reported in canine mammary tumors between ER status and the activity of two enzymes (glucose-6-phosphatase and 6-phosphogluconate dehydrogenase) known for their association with malignancy.[47]

Cat

Normal mammary tissue and benign mammary tumors were mostly positive for ERs and PRs.[46,48,49] ER and PR positivity was found to be significantly higher for benign tumors than for carcinomas.[49] In other studies, feline mammary carcinomas were either ER negative[48,50] or positive in only a few cases.[43,46,51, 52] Interestingly, progesterone receptors were detected in seven ER negative feline mammary carcinomas.[50]

REFERENCES

1. Schneider, R., Dorn, C.R., and Taylor, D.O.N. (1969) Factors influencing canine mammary cancer development and post-surgical survival. *J Natl Cancer Inst* 43:1249-1261.

2. Misdorp, W., Romijn, A., and Hart, A.A.M. (1991) Feline mammary tumors: A case-control study of hormonal factors. *Anticancer Res* 11:1793-1798.

3. Misdorp, W. (1988) Canine mammary tumours: Protective effect of late ovariectomy and stimulating effect of progestins. *Vet Quarterly* 10:26-33.

4. El Etreby, M.F., Muller-Peddinghaus, R., Bhargava, A.C., Fath El Bar, M.R., Graf, K.J., and Trautwein, G. (1980) The role of the pituitary gland in spontaneous canine mammary carcinogenesis. *Vet Pathol* 17:2-16.

5. Attia, M.A. (1982) Cytological study of the anterior pituitary gland of senile untreated bitches with spontaneous mammary tumours. *Arch Toxicol* 50:34-45.

6. Saluja, P.G., Hamilton, J.M., Gronow, M., and Misdorp, W. (1974) Pituitary prolactin levels in canine mammary cancer. *Eur J Cancer* 10:63-66.

7. Rutteman, G.R., Misdorp, W., Van den Brom, W.E., and Rijnberk, A. (1989) Anterior pituitary function in female dogs with mammary tumors. I. Growth hormone. *Anticancer Res* 9:235-240.

8. Rutteman, G.R., Bevers, M.M., Misdorp, W., and Van den Brom, W.E. (1989) Anterior pituitary function in female dogs with mammary tumors. II. Prolactin. *Anticancer Res* 9:241-246.

9. Rutteman, G.R. (1990) Hormones and mammary tumor disease: an update. *In Vivo* 4:33-40.

10. Chrisp, C.E., and Spangler, W.L. (1980) The canine malignant tumor as a model for the study of human breast cancer. In Shifrine, M., and Wilson, P.D. (eds.), *The Canine as a Biomedical Research Model: Immunological, Hematological and Oncological Aspects.* U.S. Department of Energy, Washington, D.C.

11. Brodey, R.S., Fidler, I.J., and Howson, A.E. (1966) The relationship of estrous irregularity, pseudopregnancy and pregnancy to the development of canine mammary gland neoplasms. *J Amer Vet Med Assoc* 149:1047-1049.

12. Misdorp, W. (1991) Progestagens and mammary tumours in dogs and cats. *Acta Endocr (Copenhagen)* 125:27-31.

13. Allen, H.L. (1973) Feline mammary hypertrophy. *Vet Pathol* 10:501-508.

14. Hinton, M., and Gaskell, C.J. (1977) Non-neoplastic mammary hypertrophy in the cat associated either with pregnancy or with oral progestagen therapy. *Vet Rec* 100:277-280.

15. Hayden, D.W., Johnston, S.D., Kiang, D.T., Johnston, K.H., and Barnes, D.M. (1981) Feline mammary hypertrophy / Fibroadenoma complex. Clinical and hormonal aspects. *Amer J Vet Res* 42:1699-1703.

16. Giles, R.C., Kwapiem, R.P., Geil, R.G., and Casey, H.W. (1978) Mammary nodules in beagle dogs administered investigational contraceptive steroids. *J Natl Cancer Inst* 60:1351-1364.

17. Frank, D.W., Kirton, K.I., Murchison, T.E., Quinlan, W.J., Coleman, M.E., Gilbertson, T.J., Feenstra, E.S., and Kimball, F.A. (1979) Mammary tumors and serum-hormones in the bitch treated with medroxyprogesterone acetate for four years. *Fertil Steril* 31:340-346.

18. Casey, H.W., Giles, R.C., and Kwapiem, R.P. (1979) Mammary neoplasia in animals. Pathologic aspects and the effect of contraceptive steroids. *Recent Res Cancer Res* 66:129-160.

19. El Etreby, M.F., and Graf, K.J. (1979) Effect of contraceptive steroids on the mammary gland of female dogs and its relevance to human carcinogenicity. *Pharm Ther* 5:369-402.

20. Concannon, P.W., Spraker, T.R., Casey, H.W., and Hansel, W. (1981) Gross and histopathologic effects of medroxyprogesterone on the mammary gland of adult beagle bitches. *Fertil Steril* 36:373-387.

21. Rutteman, G.R. (1992) Contraceptive steroids and the mammary gland. Is there a hazard? *Breast Cancer Res Treat* 23:29-41.

22. Tavasolli, F.A., Casey, H.W., and Norns, H.J. (1988) The morphologic effects of progestins on the mammary gland of rhesus monkeys. *Amer J Pathol* 131:213-214.

23. Van Leeuwen, F. (1991) Epidemiologic aspects of exogenous progestagens in relation to their role in pathogenesis of human breast cancer. *Acta Endocrinol (Copenhagen)* 125:13-26.

24. Briggs, M. (1983) The beagle dog and contraceptive steroids. *Life Sci* 21:275-284.

25. Selman, P.J., Mol, J.A., Rutteman, G.R., and Rijnberk, A. (1991) Progestins and growth hormone excess in the dog. *Acta Endocrinol (Copenhagen)* 125:43-47.

26. Selman, P.J., Mol, J.A., Rutteman, G.R., Van Garderen, E., and Rijnberk, A. (1994) Progestin-induced growth hormone excess in the dog originates in the mammary gland. *Endocrinology* 134:287-292.

27. Van Garderen, E., De Wit, M., Voorhout, W.F., Rutteman, G.R., Mol, J.A., Nederbragt, H., and Misdorp, W. (1997) Expression of growth hormone in canine mammary tissue and mammary tumors. *Amer J Pathol* 150(3): 1037-1047.

28. Mol, J.A., Van Garderen, E., Selman, P.J., Wolfswinkel, J., Rijnberk, A., and Rutteman, G.R. (1995) Growth hormone mRNA in mammary gland tumors of dogs and cats. *Clin Invest* 95:2028-2034.

29. Mol, J.A., Henzen-Logmans, S.C., Hageman, P.H., Misdorp, W., Blankenstein, M.A., and Rijnberk, A. (1995) Expression of the gene encoding growth hormone in the human mammary gland. *J Clin Endocrinol Metab* 80(10): 3094-3096.

30. Rutteman, G.R., Willekes-Koolschijn, N., Bevers, M.M., Van der Gugten, A.A., and Misdorp, W. (1986) Prolactin binding in benign and malignant mammary tissue of female dogs. *Anticancer Res* 6:829-835.

31. Rutteman, G.R., Misdorp, W., Blankenstein, M.A., and Van den Brom, W.E. (1988) Oestrogen (ER) and progestin receptors (PR) in mammary tissue of the female dog: Different receptor profile in non-malignant and malignant states. *Brit J Cancer* 58:594-599.

32. Rutteman, G.R., Foekens, J.A., Blankenstein, M.A., Vos, J.H., and Misdorp, W. (1990) EGF-receptors in non-affected and tumorous dog mammary tissues. *Eur J Cancer* 26:182-186.

33. Rutteman, G.R., and Misdorp, W. (1993) Hormonal background of canine and feline mammary tumours. *J Reprod Fert, Suppl* 47:483-487.

34. Donnay, I., Rauis, J., Wouters-Ballman, P., Devleeschouwer, N., Leclerq, G., and Versteegen, J.P. (1993) Receptors for estrogen, progesterone and epidermal growth factors in normal and tumorous canine mammary tissues. *J Reprod Fert, Suppl* 47:501-512.

35. Hamilton, J.M., Else, R.W., and Forshaw, P. (1977) Oestrogen receptors in canine mammary tumours. *Vet Rec* 101:258-260.

36. Monson, K.R., Malbica, J.O., and Hubben, K. (1977) Determination of estrogen receptors in canine mammary tumors. *Amer J Vet Res* 38:1937-1939.

37. Raynaud, J.P., Cotard, M., et al. (1981) Spontaneous canine mammary tumors: A model for human endocrine therapy? *J Steroid Biochem* 15, 201-207.

38. McEwen, E.G., Patnaik, A.K., Harvey, H.J., and Panko, W.B. (1982) Estrogen receptors in canine mammary tumors. *Cancer Res* 42:2255-2259.

39. Elling, H., and Ungenach, F.R. (1983) Simultaneous occurrence of receptors for estradiol, progesterone and dihydrotestosterone in canine mammary tumors. *J Cancer Res Clin* 105:321-237.

40. Pierrepoint, C.G., Thomas, S.E., and Eaton, C.L. (1984) Studies with mammary tumours in the bitch. In Bresciani, F. (ed.), *Progress in Cancer Research and Therapy.* Raven Press, New York, p. 31.

41. Nerurkar, V.R., Seshadri, R., Mulherkar, R., Ishwad, C.S., Lalitha, V.S., and Naik, S.N. (1987) Receptors for epidermal growth factor and estradiol in canine mammary tumors. *Intl J Cancer* 40:230-232.

42. Misdorp, W., and Hart, A.A.M. (1976) Prognostic factors in canine mammary cancer. *J Natl Cancer Inst* 56:779-786.

43. Parodi, A.L., Mialot, J.P., Martin, P.M., Cotard, M., and Raynaud, J.P. (1984) Canine and feline mammary cancers as animal models for hormone-dependent human breast tumors: Relationship between steroid receptor profiles and survival rates. *Prog Cancer Ther* 31:357-365.

44. Mialot, J.P., Andre, F., Martin, P.H., Cotard, M.P., et Raynaud, J.P. (1982) Etude de recepteurs des hormones steroides dans les tumeurs mammaires de la chienne. Mise en evidence, caracterisation et relation avec le type histologique. *Rec Med Vet* 158:215-221.

45. Mialot, J.P., Andre, F., Martin, P.M., Cotard, M., et Raynaud, J.P. (1982) Etude des recepteurs steroides dans les tumeurs mammaires de la chienne. II. Correlation avec quelques caracteristiques cliniques. *Rec Med Vet* 158:513-521.

46. Martin, P.M., Cotard, M., Mialot, J.P., et al. (1984) Animal models for hormone dependent human breast cancer. Relationship between steroid acceptor profiles in canine and feline mammary tumors and survival rate. *Cancer Chemother Pharmacol* 12:13-17.

47. Nerurkar, V.R., Ishwed, C.S., Seshadri, R., Naik, S.N., and Lalitha, V.S. (1990) Glucose-6-phosphate dehydrogenase and 6-phosphogluconate dehydrogenase activities in normal canine mammary gland and in mammary tumours and their correlation with oestrogen receptors. *J Comp Pathol* 102:191-195.

48. Weyer, K. (1980) Feline mammary tumours and dysplasias. *Vet Quarterly* 2(2): 69-74.

49. Rutteman, G.R., Blankenstein, M.A., Minke, J.M.H.M., and Misdorp, W. (1991) Steroid receptors in mammary tumours of the cat. *Acta Endocrinol (Copenhagen)* 125:32-37.

50. Johnston, S.D., Hayden, D.W., Kiang, D.T., Handschein, B., and Johnson, K.H. (1984) Progesterone receptors in feline mammary adenocarcinoma. *Amer J Vet Res* 45:379-382.

51. Hamilton, J.M., and Else, R.W. (1976) Oestrogen receptors in feline mammary carcinoma. *Vet Rec* 99:477-479.

52. Martín de las Mulas, J., VanNiel, M., Millán, Y., Blankenstein, M.A., Van Mil, F., and Misdorp, W. (2000) Immunohistochemical analysis of estrogen receptors in feline mammary gland benign and malignant lesions: Comparison with biochemical assay. *Dom Anim Endocrinol* 18:111-125.

Food, Virus, and Irradiation

Animal experiments and human epidemiological studies have suggested that a high fat diet and obesity increase the risk of breast cancer. Recent epidemiological studies have produced conflicting evidence. In dogs neither a high fat diet nor obesity 1 year before diagnosis increased the risk of mammary cancer. However, in spayed dogs the risk was found to be significantly reduced in those that had been thin at 9-12 months of age.[1]

Nutritional factors operating early in life may be of etiologic importance in canine and feline mammary cancer, by modifying the concentration and availability of female sex hormones, for example. More detailed study in this relatively new field of veterinary oncology is required.

Several investigators have demonstrated the presence of virus particles in feline mammary carcinomas.[2,3] Moreover, FeLV and RD 114 antigens were demonstrated in 30.6 percent and 55.5 percent of the analyzed carcinomas but not in benign tumors or normal mammary tissue.[4] Since it was not possible to induce mammary carcinomas in fetal cats with cell-free filtrate, it seems likely that these viruses must be regarded as passenger viruses.[4]

The total incidence of mammary tumors was the same in x-ray irradiated dogs and in control beagle dogs, but in the former group mammary neoplasms occurred at an earlier age.[5-7]

REFERENCES

1. Sonnenschein, E.G., Glickman, L.T., Goldschmidt, M.H., and McKee, L.J. (1991) Body conformation, diet and risk of breast cancer in pet dogs: A case-control study. *Amer J Epidemiol* 133(7): 694-702.

2. Feldman, D.G., and Gross, L. (1971) Electron microscopic study of spontaneous mammary carcinomas in cats and dogs: Virus-like particles in cat mammary carcinomas. *Cancer Res* 31:1261-1267.

3. Weyer, K., Calafat, J., Daams, J.H., Hagemans, P.C., and Misdorp, W. (1974) Feline malignant mammary tumors. II. Immunologic and electronmicroscopic investigations into a possible viral etiology. *J Natl Cancer Inst* 52:673-679.

4. Calafa, J., Weyer, K., and Daams, J.H. (1977) Feline malignant mammary tumours. III. Presence of C particles and intracisternal A particles and their relationship with feline leukemia virus. *Intl J Cancer* 20:759-767.

5. Andersen, A.C., and Rosenblatt, L.S. (1969) The effect of whole body X radiation on the median life span of female dogs (beagles). *Rad Res* 39:177-200.

6. Moulton, J.E., Taylor, D.O.N., Dorn, C.R., and Andersen, A.C. (1970) Canine mammary tumors. *Pathol Vet* 7:289-320.

7. Moulton, J.E., Rosenblatt, L.S., and Goldman, M. (1986) Mammary tumors in a colony of beagle dogs. *Vet Pathol* 23:741-749.

Genetic Factors

Breed Disposition

Purebred dogs were found to be significantly overrepresented among cases of mammary cancer. The median inbreeding coefficients in the mammary cancer group and the comparison group (consisting of other cancers) were approximately twice that of the nonneoplastic group.[1] A significantly increased risk was calculated for the dachshund and the pointer,[2,3] and a low risk for the collie and the boxer.[2,4]

Two maternal families in a beagle life-span study were shown to have markedly different phenotypes, one susceptible and one resistant to mammary neoplasia. Neither $p53$ nor $p185^{erB2}$ was the basis for the familial predisposition.[5]

Siamese cats were found to have a significantly increased risk, and the age at first diagnosis tends to be younger.[6]

Chromosomes and DNA Ploidy

Cytogenetic studies may reveal chromosomal changes associated with amplification of oncogenes and/or deletion of repressor genes. Thus far, only a few cases of primary canine mammary tumors have been studied cytogenetically. The chromosomal changes reported were divergent and complex: translocation in a complex adenocarcinoma,[7] isochromosomes in two osteochondrosarcomas,[8] and a deleted chromosome in two benign mammary tumors.[9]

Two cell lines derived from a single spontaneous feline mammary carcinoma had several marker chromosomes in either one or both subpopulations. These data suggest that the two lines arose from a hypothetically single cell ancestor which diverged during tumor progression.[10] Cell lines derived from metastases of a mammary carcinoma in a dog had various chromosomal aberrations, including deletion and amplification.[11]

Aneuploidy is a rather frequent (62 percent) phenomenon in canine mammary cancer and significantly more frequent in malignant (62 percent) than in benign mammary tumors.[12-14] Analysis of primary mammary tumors and metastases failed to reveal significant differences in DNA ploidy.[12,15] DNA ploidy was not related to histological tumor type, nuclear grade, steroid receptor presence, tumor size, or nodal status.[12,13] Strikingly, the most malignant mammary cancers in the dog, the anaplastic carcinoma and the osteosarcoma, were either diploid or near diploid.[15]

The S phase fraction was significantly higher in malignant than in benign mammary tumors and also higher in aneuploid than in diploid tumors.[13] In a multivariate study of dogs dying from mammary cancer, DNA aneuploidy and elevated S phase fraction were found to be associated with unfavorable prognosis.[16]

Aneuploidy is also recognized in feline mammary carcinomas.[17] Among the aneuploid tumors, hypodiploidy was relatively frequent.[17,18] Aneuploidy was not found to be correlated with tumor type, vascular invasion, tumor size, or histological malignancy grade.[17]

Oncogenes and Suppressor Genes

The types of genetic alterations that have been found in human mammary tumors include oncogene amplification, inactivation of tumor suppressor genes, point mutations, and translocations. Some oncogenes code for growth factors and growth factor receptors and thus promote cell growth in normal cells and, by amplification or overexpression, contribute to uncontrolled growth.

One such oncogene (c-erB2 or neu) was found to be overexpressed in the majority of primary canine mammary cancers examined (not in benign tumors) but was not associated with vascular invasion or regional metastasis.[19] In two of seven canine mammary tumor cell lines, expression of c-erB2 was also found to be stable and thus not associated with progression during the culture period. In contrast, amplification of epidermal growth factor receptor gene (EGF-R) was found only at high passage numbers in a feline mammary carcinoma cell line.[10] In that study no rearrangements or amplifications of the c-myc and c-erB2 oncogenes were detected in a primary feline mammary carcinoma and the two cell lines derived from it. Expression of the c-myc gene by mammary tumors was found to be increased in 1 of 12 tumors, an undifferentiated carcinoma, but no amplification or other rearrangements in the gene locus were detected.[20]

Among the suppressor genes, p53 is currently the most prominent ("gene of the year"). After partial characterization of the canine p53 gene, loss of one allele and a mutation in the remaining allele were detected in three of nine mammary tumor cell lines, leading to complete loss of the normal ("wild") alleles. Identical point mutations were found in two of three corresponding tumors from which the lines were derived, but not in the corresponding normal tissue.[21]

REFERENCES

1. Dorn, C.R., and Schneider, R. (1976) Inbreeding and canine mammary cancer. A retrospective study. *J Natl Cancer Inst* 57(3): 545-548.

2. Frye, F.L., Dorn, C.R., Taylor, D.O.N., Hibbard, H.H., and Klauber, M.R. (1967) Characteristics of canine mammary gland tumor cases. *Anim Hosp* 3:1-12.

3. McVean, D.W., Monlux, A.W., Anderson, P.S., Silverberg, S.L., and Roszel, J.F. (1978) Frequency of canine and feline tumors in a defined population. *Vet Pathol* 15:700-715.

4. Howard, E.B., and Nielsen, S.W. (1965) Neoplasms of the boxer dog. *Amer J Vet Res* 26:1121-1131.

5. Schater, K.A., Kelly, G., Schrader, R., Griffith, C., Muggenburg, A., Tierney, A., Lechner, J.F., Janorvitz, E.B., and Hahn, F.F. (1998) A canine model of familial mammary gland neoplasia. *Vet Pathol* 35:168-177.

6. Hayes, H.M., Milne, K.L., and Mandell, C.P. (1981) Epidemiological studies of feline mammary carcinoma. *Vet Rec* 108:476-479.

7. Mayr, B., Swindersky, W., and Schleger, W. (1990) Translocation (+ .4:27) in a canine mammary complex adenocarcinoma. *Vet Rec* 126:42.

8. Mayr, B., Kramberger-Kaplan, E., Loupal, G., and Schleger, W. (1992) Analysis of complex cytogenetic alterations in three canine mammary sarcomas. *Res Vet Sci* 53:205-211.

9. Mayr, B., Plasser, J., Schleger, W., Loupal, G., and Burtscher, H. (1992) Deleted chromosome 32 in mammary neoplasms in two domestic dogs. *J Small Anim Pract* 33:277-278.

10. Minke, J.M.H.M., Schuuring, E., Van den Berghe, R., Stolwijk, J.A.M., Boonstra, J., Cornelisse, C., and Misdorp, W. (1991) Isolation of two distinct epithelial cell lines from a single feline mammary carcinoma with different tumorigenic potential in nude mice and expressing different levels of epidermal growth factor receptors. *Cancer Res* 51:4028-4037.

11. Mellink, C.H.M., Bosma, A.A., and Rutteman, G.R. (1989) Cytogenetic analysis of cell lines derived from metastases of a mammary carcinoma in a dog. *Anticancer Res* 9:1241-1244.

12. Rutteman, G.R., Cornelisse, C.J., Dijkshoorn, N.J., Poortman, J., and Misdorp, W. (1988) Flow cytophotometric analysis of DNA ploidy in canine mammary tumors. *Cancer Res* 48:3411-3417.

13. Perez Alenza, M.D., Rutteman, G.R., Kuipers-Dijkshoorn, N.J., Pena, L., Montoya, A., Misdorp, W., and Cornelisse, C.J. (1995) DNA flow cytometry of canine mammary tumours: The relationship of DNA ploidy and S-phase in relation to clinical and histological features. *Res Vet Sci* 58:238-243.

14. Hellmén, E., Lindgren, A., Linell, F., Mattson, P., and Nilsson, A. (1988) Comparison of histology and clinical variables to DNA ploidy in canine mammary tumors. *Vet Pathol* 25:219-226.

15. Hellmén, E., and Svensson, S. (1995) Progression of canine mammary tumours as reflected by DNA ploidy in primary tumors and their metastases. *J Comp Pathol* 113:327-342.

16. Hellmén, E., Bergstrom, R., Holmberg, L., Spangberg, I.B., Hannson, K., and Lindgren, A. (1993) Prognostic factors in canine mammary tumors: A multivariate study of 202 consecutive cases. *Vet Pathol* 30:20-27.

17. Minke, J.M.H.M., Cornelisse, C.J., Stolwijk, J.A.M., Kuipers-Dijkshoorn, N.J., Rutteman, G.R., and Misdorp, W. (1990) Flow

cytometric DNA ploidy analysis of feline mammary tumors. *Cancer Res* 50:4003-4007.

18. Prop, F.J.A., Weyer, K., Spies, J., Souw, L., Peters, K., Erich, T., Rijnhart, P. and Misdorp, W. (1986) Feline mammary carcinomas as a model for human breast cancer. I. Sensitivity of mammary tumor cells in culture to cytostatic drugs. A preliminary investigation of a predictive test. *Anticancer Res* 6:989-994.

19. Ahern, T.E., Bird, R.C., Allison, E., Bird, E.C., and Wolfe, L.G. (1996) Expression of the oncogene c-*erB2* in canine mammary cancers and tumor-derived cell lines. *Amer J Vet Res* 57(5): 693-696.

20. Engstrom, W.E., Barrios, C., Azawedo, E., Mollermark, G., Kangstrom, L.E., Eliason, I., and Larsson, O. (1987) Expression of c-*myc* in canine mammary tumours. *Anticancer Res J* 1:1235-1238.

21. Van Leeuwen, I.S., Hellmén, E., Cornelisse, C.J., Van der Burg, B., and Rutteman, G.R. (1996) *p53* mutations in mammary tumor cell lines and corresponding tumor tissues in the dog. *Anticancer Res* 16:3737-3743.

Pathogenesis

Some genes are known to increase cellular transformation (*TGF-alpha*) or growth by overexpression (*EGF*, c-*erB2*) or by mutation (*p53*). Gene amplifications and mutations have recently been reported in canine mammary carcinoma (see Oncogenes and Suppressor Genes section). Hypoploidy was found relatively frequently in canine and feline mammary carcinomas, perhaps reflecting loss of (protecting) suppressor genes. There is ample evidence that a protein, E cadherin, acts as an invasion suppressor molecule.[1] However, it appeared from an in vitro invasion study of canine mammary carcinoma cells that invasion may also depend on additional factors in the stromal microenvironment.[2] Not only invasion but also growth of tumor cells can be influenced by (growth) factors in the stroma.

Relatively little is known about the time of initiation or what agents cause mammary cancer. Experimental studies in the rat demonstrated that the types of mammary lesions that appeared after administration of DBMA-application were associated with mammary gland development and hence with hormonal status. Mammary carcinomas arose in the *terminal end buds* in the most primitive ductal structures in the very young animal. Adenomas, fibroadenomas, and cysts arose from more differentiated structures, such as *alveolar buds,* in slightly older animals.[3] From epidemiological and cell kinetic studies in women, it appears that differentiation induced during pregnancy and lactation constitutes a powerful protective element.[3]

High proliferative activity of epithelial cells, probably stem cells, was found in the terminal end buds of women and rats. Medroxy progesterone acetate, a progestin, was found to increase the DNA labeling index of terminal end buds of rats.[4] Growth hormone production was demonstrated in structures resembling terminal end buds in dogs under endogenous or exogenous progesterone stimulation, possibly indicating autocrine or paracrine induction of proliferation.[5] This finding is particularly interesting since expression of growth hormone was also demonstrated in the majority of mammary tumors examined.

From the sparing effect of ovariectomy and the stimulating effect of progestins, it seems likely that hormones play a (promotor) role in mammary carcinogenesis in the dog and the cat. Growth hormone and other growth factors produced either in the epithelium or in the stroma may play a joint role.

Is there progression from either a preneoplastic condition or a preneoplastic lesion to carcinoma or from a hormonally dependent carcinoma to an autonomous, hormonally independent tumor? Based on studies[3] in the rat and human and also from the recent study on growth hormone producing terminal end bud–like structures in the dog,[5] it is possible to speculate that hormonally induced proliferation of stem cells is a preneoplastic condition (or lesion?) associated with an increased risk of cancer.

Preneoplastic lesions, in the sense of an increased risk of cancer arising from such lesions, were detected by microanatomic studies of dog mammary gland. The most common lesion was the *hyperplastic alveolar nodule* (HAN), and the frequency of this lesion increased with age.[6] The strongest evidence for the preneoplastic nature of hyperplastic alveolar nodules was the morphological continuum of lesions toward very large, hyperplastic, lobular lesions containing neoplastic foci.[6] Aneuploidy is infrequently observed in canine mammary dysplasia and benign tumors, and it may indicate a precancerous state.[7] Although foci of atypical cells can occasionally be observed in some otherwise benign appearing lesions, evidence of true malignant transformation is infrequent.

Carcinoma in situ is the most frequent premalignant lesion, but it is not possible to predict what percentage of those lesions will progress to invasive carcinomas, remain in situ, or disappear.

Benign mammary lesions are often responsive to various hormones and also contain high numbers of hormone receptors.[8] Carcinomas containing estrogen and progesterone receptors were found to be particularly sensitive (in terms of proliferation) to estradiol and progesterone stimulation.[9] It can be expected that many primary and metastatic mammary carcinomas that lack hormone receptors are not, or are no longer, hormone dependent. Therefore, they may be good models for study of autocrine or paracrine growth, the mechanisms of which can be dissected by using cell cultures in media supplemented with serum treated to inactivate growth factors.[10]

REFERENCES

1. Mareel, M., Vleminckx, K., Bracke, M., and Van Roy, F. (1992) E-cadherin expression: A counterbalance for cancer cell invasion. *Bull Cancer* 79:347-355.

2. Spieker, N., Mareel, M., Bruyneel, E.A., and Nederbragt, H. (1995) E-cadherin expression and in vitro invasion of canine mammary tumour cells. *Eur J Cell Biol* 68:427-436.

3. Russo, J., and Russo, I.H. (1987) Biology of disease. Biological and molecular basis of mammary carcinogenesis. *Lab Invest* 75(2): 112-137.

4. Russo, I.H., and Russo, J. (1991) Progestagens and mammary development: Differentiation versus carcinogenesis. *Acta Endocrinol (Copenhagen)* 125:7-12.

5. Van Garderen, E., De Wit, M., Voorhout, W.F., Rutteman, G.R., Mol, J.A., Nederbragt, H., and Misdorp, W. (1997) Expression of growth hormone in canine mammary tissue and mammary tumours. *Amer J Pathol* 150(3): 1037-1047.

6. Cameron, A.M., and Faulkin, L.J. (1971) Hyperplastic and inflammatory nodules in the canine mammary gland. *J Natl Cancer Inst* 47:1277-1287.

7. Hellmén, E. (1996) The pathogenesis of canine mammary tumors. *Cancer J* 9(6): 282-286.

8. Warner, M.R. (1977) Response of beagle mammary dysplasia to various hormone supplements in vitro. *Cancer Res* 37:2062-2067.

9. Lespagnard, L., Kiss, R., Danguy, A., Legros, N., Lengler, G., Devleeschouwer, N., and Paridaens, R. (1987) In vitro studies of canine mammary tumors: Influence of 17-B-estradiol and progesterone on cell-kinetic parameters. *Oncology* 44:292-301.

10. Van den Burg, B., Van Selm-Miltenburg, A.J.P., Van Maurik, M., Rutteman, G.R., Misdorp, W., De Laat, S., and Van Zoelen, E.J.J. (1989) Isolation of autonomously growing dog mammary tumor cell lines cultured in medium supplemented with serum treated to inactivate growth factors. *J Natl Cancer Inst* 81(20): 1545-1551.

Histogenesis

Canine mammary tumors are known for their structural complexity and disputed histogenesis. Of veterinary and comparative interest (human pleomorphic adenoma of the salivary gland) is the intriguing question concerning the possible role of basal epithelial/myoepithelial cells in the histogenesis of complex and mixed tumors and mammary carcinomas. The application of immunohistochemical techniques, the establishment of cell lines, and transplantation experiments have provided useful information.

Immunohistochemical studies of intermediate filaments (keratins, vimentin, desmin, etc.) and microfilaments (actin) have demonstrated that the distribution of those filaments is tissue specific. Studies with monoclonal and polyclonal antibodies made it possible to recognize various subtypes of keratin in secretory luminal epithelium and in basal epithelium/myoepithelium (table 12.1). Keratins 14 and 17 and alpha-actin appeared to be exclusively present in the myoepithelium, but the presence of vimentin in these cells was controversial.[1,2] In two studies the myoepithelial cells stained distinctly positive for vimentin,[3,4] in another weakly positive,[5] and in another negative.[1] Myoepithelial cells were believed to be the source of the basal membrane components laminin, type IV collagen, and type VII collagen. Basal membranes were intact in normal mammary gland and benign mammary lesions, discontinuous in well-differentiated carcinomas, and missing in poorly differentiated carcinomas.[6]

Many studies have been performed on the characterization of the spindle/stellate cells in complex/mixed tumors and their eventual role in the production of cartilaginous and osseous ground substance. Spindle cells in those tumors were characterized as myoepithelial cells on the basis of electronmicroscopic and enzyme histochemical (alkaline phosphatase) studies.[7,8] In another study, the vast majority of spindle cells (alpha-actin negative, K14 negative, vimentin positive) appeared to be fibroblastic rather than myoepithelial.[9] Progressive transformation

TABLE 12.1.   Normal canine mammary gland. Reactivity of luminal epithelium, basal epithelium-myoepithelium, and stromal fibroblasts with monoclonal antibodies directed against keratins, vimentin, and alpha-actin

Specificity	Secretory Luminal Epithelium	Basal Epithelium Myoepithelium	Fibroblasts	References*
Keratin 4	±	–	–	1
Keratin 5+8	+	+	–	1
Keratin 7	+	–	–	1,2
Keratin 8	+	–	–	1
Keratin 8+18	+	–	–	2,4
Keratin 10	±	–	–	1
Keratin 13	+	–	–	5
Keratin 14	–	+	–	1,2
Keratin 14+17	–	+	–	1
Keratin 18	+	–	–	2,3
Keratin 19	+	+	–	1,4
Vimentin	– – –	+ + –	+ + +	1,3,4
α-Actin	–	+	–	1,4

Note: +, positive; ±, weakly positive; –, negative.
*1. Vos, J.H., et al. (1993) *Vet Quarterly* 15(3): 96-102. 2. Walter, J.H., and Kling, S. (1995) *Eur J Vet Pathol* 1(3): 105-111. 3. Hellmen, E., and Lindgren, A. (1989) *Vet Pathol* 26:420-428. 4. Destexhe, E., et al. (1993) *Vet Pathol* 30:146-154. 5. Griffey, S.M., et al. (1993) *Vet Pathol* 30:155-161.

from myoepithelial cells to cartilaginous cells was suggested by the production of type IX collagen in proliferative myoepithelial cells followed by the switch of cytokeratins to vimentin.[4, 10] The expression of several adhesion molecules (NCAM), tenascin, and fibronectin demonstrated in myoepithelial cells decreased in chondroblast-like cells and disappeared in chondrocytes.[11] Cells in early stages of chondroid metaplasia expressed type XI collagen, whereas mature cartilage was labeled for type II collagen.[12] A gradual change from mucopolysaccharide secreting myoepithelial cells to pseudocartilaginous ground substance to mature cartilage was demonstrated in an enzyme histochemical study.[7]

Several benign and malignant mammary tumors were found to simultaneously express different types of intermediate filaments (cytokeratin, vimentin, desmin, neurofilaments), indicating a possible stem cell origin in most canine mammary tumors.[3,19] Two cell lines derived from a mammary adenocarcinoma and a benign mixed tumor showed duct formation in collagen, one of the criteria for the recognition of stem cells. The former line also formed ducts when inoculated into nude mice.[13,14] Two cell lines from benign mixed tumors gave rise to different tumor phenotypes when inoculated into nude mice, indicating a multipotent stem cell origin.[13]

In conclusion, four lines of thinking have developed about the histogenesis of mixed tumors: (1) stem cell origin,[13,14] (2) metaplasia from myoepithelial cells,[4,7,8] (3) metaplasia from epithelial cells,[15] and (4) metaplasia from connective tissue.[9]

Canine mammary carcinomas have been subdivided into luminal and basal on the basis of the reactivity of their keratin subtypes.[5] Dual reactivity was indicative of noninvasive carcinomas.[5] These carcinomas probably represent *complex carcinomas,* which are associated with a relatively favorable prognosis (see Biological Behavior and Prognosis section). In another study a molecular marker of malignant transformation (type I 57 KD cytokeratin) was recognized.[16] Myoepithelium was found to be a major component in the majority of canine mammary carcinomas in one study.[4]

Chondroitin sulphate was often found around clusters of mammary carcinoma cells, and it also accumulated between tumor cells in canine complex and mixed hyperplasias and tumors. In the third pattern chondroitin sulphate was found in fibrillar structures, probably representing basement membranes.[17]

From in vitro invasion studies with two canine mammary carcinoma cell lines, it was concluded that TGF-β mediated chondroitin sulphate production stimulated invasion into collagen gel.[18]

REFERENCES

1. Vos, J.H., Van den Ingh, T.S.G.A.M., Misdorp, W., Molenbeek, R.F., Van Mil, F.N., Rutteman, G.R., Ivanyi, D., and Ramaeckers, F.C.S. (1993) Immunohistochemistry with keratin, vimentin, desmin and alpha smooth muscle actin monoclonal antibodies in canine mammary glands: Normal mammary tissue. *Vet Quarterly* 15(3): 96-102.

2. Walter, J.H., and Kling, S. (1995) Biochemical and immunohistochemical characterization of cytokeratins in normal and neoplastic canine mammary glands. *Eur J Vet Pathol* 1(3): 105-111.

3. Hellmén, E., and Lindgren, A. (1993) The expression of intermediate filaments in canine mammary glands and their tumours. *Vet Pathol* 26:420-428.

4. Destexhe, E., Lespagnard, L., Degeyter, M., Heymann, R., and Coignoul, E. (1993) Immunohistochemical identification of myoepithelial and connective tissue cells in canine mammary tumors. *Vet Pathol* 30:146-154.

5. Griffey, S.M., Madewell, B.R., Dairkee, S.H., Hunt, J.E., Maydan, D.K., and Higgins, R.J. (1993) Immunohistochemical reactivity of basal and luminal epithelium specific cytokeratin antibodies within normal and neoplastic canine mammary glands. *Vet Pathol* 30:155-161.

6. Pena, L., Castano, M., Sanchez, M.A., Rodriques, A., and Flores, J.M. (1995) Immunohistochemical study of type IV collagen and laminin in canine mammary tumours. *J Vet Med A.* 42:50-61.

7. Pulley, L.T. (1973) Ultrastructural and histochemical demonstration of myoepithelium in mixed tumors of the canine mammary gland. *Amer J Vet Res* 34:1513-1522.

8. Tateyma, S., and Cotchin, E. (1977) Alkaline phosphatase reaction of canine mammary mixed tumours: A light and electronmicroscopic study. *Res Vet Sci* 23(3): 356-364.

9. Vos, J.H., Van den Ingh, T.S.G.A.M., Misdorp, W., Molenbeek, F.R., Van Mil, F.N., Rutteman, G.R., Ivanyi, D., and Ramaeckers, F.C.S. (1993) Immunohistochemistry with keratin, vimentin, desmin and alpha smooth muscle actin monoclonal antibodies in canine mammary glands: Benign mammary tumours and duct ectasias. *Vet Quarterly* 15(3): 89-95.

10. Arai, K., Uehara, K., and Naoi, M. (1995) Simultaneous expression of type IX collagen and an inhibin-related antigen in proliferative myoepithelial cells with pleomorphic adenoma of canine mammary glands. *Jpn J Cancer Res* 86:577-584.

11. Arai, K., Uehara, K., and Naoi, M. (1994) Immunohistochemical examination of neural adhesion molecule (NCAM), tenascin and fibronectin on the development of cartilaginous tissue in canine mammary mixed tumors. *J Vet Med Sci* 56(4): 809-811.

12. Arai, K., Uehara, K., and Naoi, M. (1989) Expression of type II and type XI collagens in canine mammary mixed tumors and demonstration of collagen production by tumor cells in collagen gel culture. *Jpn J Cancer Res* 80:840-847.

13. Hellmén, E. (1992) Characterization of four in vitro established canine mammary carcinoma and one atypical benign mixed tumor cell line. *In Vitro Cell Devel Biol* 28A:309-319.

14. Hellmén, E. (1993) Canine mammary tumour cell lines established in vitro. *J Reprod Fert, Suppl* 47:489-499.

15. Monlux, A.W., Roszel, J.F., MacVean, D.W., and Palmer, T.W. (1977) Classification of epithelial mammary tumors in a defined population. *Vet Pathol* 14:194-217.

16. Arai, K., Kaneko, S., Naoi, M., Suzuki, K., Maruo, K., and Uehara, K. (1994) Expression of stratified squamous epithelia-type cytokeratin by canine mammary epithelial cells during tumorigenesis. Type I (acidic) 57 kilodalton cytokeratin could be a molecular marker for malignant transformation of mammary epithelial cells. *J Vet Med Sci* 56:51-58.

17. Hinrichs, U., Rutteman, G.R., and Nederbragt, H. (1999) Stromal accumulation of chondroitin sulphate in mammary tumors of dogs. *Brit J Cancer* 80(9):1359-1365.

18. Hanekamp, E.E., Van Garderen, E., van Schalke, N., and Nederbragt, H. (1998) TGF-beta mediated chondroitin sulphate production as a stimulator of collagen gel contraction and tumor cell invasion. Proceedings Dutch Society of Pathology.

19. Hellmén, E., Moller, M., Blankenstein, M.A., Andersson, L., and Westermark, R. (2000) Expression of different phenotypes in cell lines from canine mammary spindle-cell tumours and osteosarcomas indicating a pluripotent mammary stem cell origin. *Breast Cancer Res Treat* 61:197-210.

Immunological Factors

Immune responses and experimental immunotherapy of canine and feline mammary carcinoma has been reviewed.[1] Many authors have reported the occurrence of large amounts of circulating immune complexes in dogs with mammary neoplasia. Tumor antigen and immunoglobulins were found to be incorporated in the immune complexes.[2-4] Immune complexes favor the progression of neoplasms by their immunosuppressive and cytotoxicity blocking effects. Their partial removal leads to the redistribution of tumor associated antibodies.

Two types of cellular infiltrates were recognized adjacent to mammary tumors in dogs[5]: (1) Diffuse plasmacytic infiltration, especially around undifferentiated carcinomas, and (2) perivenous infiltrates of small lymphocytes near precancerous lesions.

Survival time in dogs with peritumorous lymphoid infiltrates tended to be longer than in dogs lacking such reactions, but in cats the reverse was true.[6,7] A more detailed morphologic and functional identification of these infiltrates may be helpful in elucidating these conflicting results.

In vitro, cytotoxicity of lymphocytes against autologous canine mammary carcinoma cells has been demonstrated.[8-10] Cytotoxicity could be blocked by autologous serum. In cats with mammary carcinoma no specific cell mediated cytotoxicity could be demonstrated.[11]

REFERENCES

1. Rutten, V.P.M.G., Misdorp, W., Gauthier, A., Estrada, M., Mialot, J.P., Parodi, A.L., Rutteman, G.R., and Weyer, K. (1990) Immunological aspects of mammary tumors in dogs and cats: A survey including own studies and pertinent literature. *Vet Immumol Immunopathol* 26:211-225.

2. Hannant, D., Else, R.W., and Crighton, G.W. (1978) Antigens associated with canine spontaneous mammary carcinoma. *Vet Rec* 1033:441-443.

3. Holohan, T.V., Philips, T.M., Bowles, C., and Deisseroth, A. (1982) Regression of canine mammary carcinoma after immuno-absorbtion therapy. *Cancer Res* 42:3663-3668.

4. Balint, J., Nagai, T., Ikeda, Y., Meek, K., and Terman, D.S. (1982) IgA containing immune complexes in dogs bearing a spontaneous mammary adenocarcinoma. *Clin Exp Immunol* 49:433-440.

5. Gilbertson, J.R., Kurzman, I.D., Zachrau, R.E., Hurvitz, A.E., and BLack, M.M. (1983) Canine mammary epithelial neoplasms: Biological implication of morphologic characteristics assessed in 232 dogs. *Vet Pathol* 20:127-142.

6. McEwen, E.G. (1986) Current concepts in cancer therapy: Biologic therapy and chemotherapy. *Sem Vet Med Surg* 1:5-16.

7. Weyer, K., and Hart, A.A.M. (1983) Prognostic factors in feline mammary carcinoma. *J Natl Cancer Inst* 70:709-716.

8. Fidler, I.J., Brodey, R.S., and Bech-Nielsen, S. (1974) In vitro immune stimulation of spontaneous canine mammary tumors of various histologic types. *J Immunol* 112:1051-1060.

9. Ulvund, M.J. (1975) Cellular immunity to canine mammary tumor cells by leucocyte migration technique. *Acta Vet Scand* 16:95-114.

10. Betton, G.R., and Gorman, N.T. (1978) Cell-mediated responses in dogs with spontaneous neoplasms. *J Natl Cancer Inst* 61:1085-1093.

11. Weyer, K. (1980) Feline mammary tumors and dysplasias. Conclusions based on personal studies and some suggestion for future research. *Vet Quarterly* 2:69-74.

Treatment

Surgery

Surgery remains the treatment of choice for dogs and cats with most types of mammary gland tumors; the exceptions are inoperable disease (e.g., *inflammatory carcinoma* of the dog) and distant (organ) metastases. For both the dog and the cat, clinical evaluation should include a thorough physical examination and routine hematologic and chemistry profiles prior to anesthesia.[1] Thoracic radiographs should be taken to evaluate for metastasis.

Clinical evaluation requires assessment of the following factors: (1) signalment, (2) general condition, (3) duration of signs, (4) rate of tumor growth, (5) recurrence, (6) size, (7) location, (8) consistency of tumors, (9) number of glands involved, (10) mode of growth, (11) ulceration, (12) fixation to skin or body walls, (13) lymph node enlargement, (14) lymphedema of extremity, (15) nipple deformity, and (16) presence of distant metastasis.[2] Factors 6, 11, 12, 13, and 16 contribute to the assessment of the clinical stage of the tumor disease according to the World Health Organization TNM (tumor, node, metastasis) system.[3] Multiple tumors occur in over 50 percent of the affected dogs[2] and in approximately 40 percent of the cats.[4]

Multiple tumors reflect simultaneous primary neoplasms and/or spread by direct extension or metastasis.

Early and complete resection and microscopic diagnostic examination are advocated. Delaying surgery may result in a larger tumor and more difficult removal. The extent of the resection is determined by the size, the degree of infiltration and the location of the tumor, the number of tumors, and the status of the regional lymph nodes. The age of the patient and the owner's expectations also influence the decision. Location is important because of the pattern of the lymphatic drainage.[5,6] Complete resection (wide margins) is followed by examination of the excisional biopsy. Lumpectomy or nodulectomy should be restricted to small (less than 5mm), firm, nonfixed nodules. It is contraindicated in dogs with multiple lesions or any clinical sign of malignancy. Simple mastectomy may be indicated if there is a single tumor in the first thoracic gland, since no lymphatic connection exists with other glands.[5] Nodulectomy and simple mastectomy have increased risks of local recurrence, as compared to block resection or chain resection if the tumor is malignant and invades lymph vessels.[7]

Block resection or regional mastectomy is considered in dogs with tumors that involve the abdominal and inguinal glands or the second thoracic glands. If there are multiple tumors or suspected malignancy (fixation, ulceration), single chain resection is advocated, particularly since connection of lymphatics between abdominal and thoracic glands has been demonstrated in 10 percent of the dogs.[5]

During resection of the caudal glands, by either regional or chain resection, the superficial inguinal lymph nodes are also removed. This is recommended because of the intimate anatomical association between the inguinal lymph nodes and the caudal glands, as well as the possibility that tumor cells are in draining lymphatics or are already present in the regional lymph nodes (approximately 50 percent)[8]. Axillary lymph nodes are removed only if there is clinical or cytologic suspicion of metastasis. Both mammary chains and inguinal lymph nodes should be removed in cases of bilateral, multiple, mammary tumors. Drainage to the regional lymph nodes is ipsilateral. Chain resection is the treatment of choice for feline mammary tumors because it significantly reduces local recurrence.[9]

It is expected that malignant mammary tumors *without detectable* metastasis at first presentation will develop (or already have) micrometastases in most dogs and cats (see Biological Behavior and Prognosis section).

Adjuvant Therapies

Radiation Therapy and Chemotherapy

Radiation therapy has been tried in a few dogs with inoperable tumors and in inflammatory carcinoma, but the short term mortality is high.[2] No single therapeutic or adjuvant chemotherapy protocol has been reported to be effective in the dog. Combination chemotherapy (doxorubicin and cyclophosphamide) has been shown to induce short-term partial and complete response in 50 percent of cats with metastatic or nonresectable local disease.[10] Doxorubicin did not influence growth of feline mammary carcinomas transplanted in nude mice.[11]

In short-term cultures feline mammary carcinomas proved to be most sensitive to doxorubicin and 5-fluorouracil.[12] In order to develop a reliable in vitro–predictive test, in vitro and in vivo response of feline mammary carcinoma to doxorubicin was tested. The best sensitivity (100 percent) was obtained using 2.00 μg doxorubicin in vitro and 5×30 mg/m^2 in vivo. Tumors recurring after treatment demonstrated resistance in vitro.[13]

Ovariectomy

Adjuvant ovariectomy has not produced impressive benefits in dogs with mammary cancer, which is not surprising since most metastases lack hormone receptors.[14] Tamoxifen, an antiestrogen, was reported to produce serious side effects in dogs.[15] A clonal canine mammary carcinoma cell line containing estrogen receptors appeared to be sensitive to tamoxifen or tamoxifen with estradiol.[16]

Nonspecific Immunotherapy

Nonspecific immunotherapy using biologic substances BCG and *Corynebacterium parvum* (Cp) vaccine did not influence survival of dogs with mammary carcinoma when injected into the tumor before mastectomy.[17] An encouraging study on the beneficial effect of repeated intravenous BCG[18] after mastectomy in dogs was not confirmed by a larger study that used intravenous BCG and Cp.[19] Although the intravenous treatment with liposomes containing muramyl-tripeptide-compound positively influenced postsurgical survival in dogs with osteosarcoma, this is not true for dogs or cats with mammary carcinoma.[20,21]

Immunization with neuraminidase-treated autologous tumor cells appeared to be successful in dogs with mammary tumor.[22] Extracorporeal perfusion over *Staphlococcus aureus* led to extensive necrosis of spontaneous canine mammary carcinomas.[23] With the advent of monoclonal antibodies that recognize canine and feline mammary carcinoma antigens, the detection and the eradication of micrometastases may become possible.[24,25] Intrafetal subcutaneous injection of two cell lines of feline mammary carcinoma resulted in metastasizing tumors that could be identified by the use of radiolabeled monoclonal antibodies.[26] This feline model is interesting for future studies on the diagnosis and eradication of micrometastases.

REFERENCES

1. McEwen, E.G., and Withrow, S.J. (1989) Tumors of the mammary gland. In Withrow, S.J., and McEwen, E.G. (eds.) *Clinical Veterinary Oncology.* Lippincott Co., pp. 292-304.

2. Madewell, B.B. and Theilen, G.H. (1987) Tumors of the mammary gland. In Theilen, G.H., and Madewell, B.R. (eds.), *Veterinary Cancer Medicine,* 2nd ed. Lea and Lebiger, pp. 327-343.

3. Owen, L.N. (1980) *TNM Classification of Tumours in Domestic Animals.* World Health Organization, Geneva, pp. 16-20.

4. Weyer, K., Head, K.W., Misdorp, W., and Hampe, J.F. (1972) Feline malignant mammary tumors I. Morphology and biology: Some comparisons with human and canine mammary carcinomas. *J Natl Cancer Inst* 49:1679-1704.

5. Sautet, J.Y., Ruberte, J., et al. (1992) Lymphatic system of the mammary glands in the dog: An approach to the surgical treatment of malignant mammary tumors. *Canine Pract* 17:30-33.

6. Norris, A.M., Harayz, G., Ege, G.N., Broxup, B., Valli, V.E.O., and Leger, L. (1982) Lymphoscintigraphy in canine mammary neoplasia. *Amer J Vet Res* 42(2):195-199.

7. Rutteman, G.R. (1997) Mammary tumors in the dog. In Kirk, R.W. (ed.), *Current Veterinary Therapy.* W.B. Saunders Co., pp. 518-523.

8. Misdorp, W., and Hart, A.A.M. (1979) Canine mammary cancer. II. Therapy and causes of death. *J Small Anim Pract* 20:395-404.

9. McEwen, E.G., Hayes, A.A., Harvey, J.H., Patnaik, A.K., Mooney, S., and Passe, S. (1984) Prognostic factors for feline mammary tumors. *J Amer Vet Med Assoc* 185(2):201-204.

10. Jeglum, K.A., and Young, K.M. (1985) Chemotherapy of advanced mammary adenocarcinoma in 14 cats. *J Amer Vet Med Assoc* 187:157-160.

11. Ladiges, W.C., and Van Hoosier, G.L. (1980) Heterotransplantation of feline malignant tumors in nude thymus less mice. *Amer J Vet Res* 41(5):840-842.

12. Prop, F.J.A., Weyer, K., Spies, J., Souw, L., Peters, K., Erich, T., Rijnhart, P., and Misdorp, W. (1986) Feline mammary carcinomas as a model for human breast cancer. I. Sensitivity of mammary tumor cells in culture to cytostatic drugs. A preliminary investigation of a predictive test. *Anticancer Res* 6:989-994.

13. Stolwijk, J.A.M., Minke, J.M., Rutteman, G.R., Hoekstra, J., Prop, F.J.A., and Misdorp, W. (1989) Feline mammary carcinomas as a model for human breast cancer. II. Comparison of in vivo and in vitro adriamycin sensitivity. *Anticancer Res* 91:1045-1048.

14. Rutteman, G.R. (1990) Hormones and mammary tumour disease in the female dog: An update. *In Vivo* 4:33-40.

15. Morris, J.S., Dobson, J.M., and Bostock, D.E. (1993) Use of tamoxifen in the control of canine mammary neoplasia. *Vet Rec* 133:539-542.

16. Sartin, E.A., Barnes, S., Toito-Kinnucan, M., Wright, J.C., and Wolfe, L.G. (1993) Heterogenic properties of clonal cell lines derived from canine mammary carcinomas and sensitivity to tamoxifen and doxorubicin. *Anticancer Res* 13:229-236.

17. Parodi, A.L., Misdorp, W., Mialot, J.P., Mialot, M., Hart, A.A.M., Hurtrel, M., and Salomon, J.C. (1983) Intratumoral BCG and *Corynebacterium parvum* therapy of canine mammary tumours before radical mastectomy. *Cancer Immunol Immunother* 15:172-177.

18. Bostock, D.E., and Gorman, N.T. (1978) Intravenous BCG therapy of mammary carcinoma in bitches after surgical excision of the primary tumor. *Eur J Cancer* 14:879-883.

19. Rutten, V.P.M.G., Misdorp, W., Gauthier, A., Estrada, M., Mialot, J.P., Parodi, A.L., Rutteman, G.R., and Weyer, K. (1990) Immunological aspects of mammary tumors in dogs and cats: A survey including studies and pertinent literature. *Vet Immunol Immunopathol* 26:211-225.

20. Teske, E., Rutteman, G.R., Van der Ingh, T.S.G.A.M., Vanhoort, R., and Misdorp, W. (1998) Liposome-encapsulated muramyl tripeptide phosphatidyl-ethanolamine (L-MTP-PE): A randomized clinical trial in dogs with mammary carcinoma. *Anticancer Res* 18:1015-1020.

21. Fox, L.E., McEwen, E.G., et al. (1994) L^1-MTPPE treatment of feline mammary adenocarcinoma. Proceeding 14th Annual Conference Veterinary Cancer Society, pp. 107-108.

22. Sedlacek, H.H., Weise, M., Lemmer, A., and Seiler, F.R. (1979) Immunotherapy of spontaneous mammary tumors in mongrel dogs

with autologous tumor cells and neuraminidase. *Cancer Immunol Immunother* 6:47-58.

23. Terman, D.S., Yamamoto, T., Mattioli, M., Cook, G., Tillquist, R., Henry, J., Poser, R., and Daskal, Y. (1980) Extensive necrosis of spontaneous canine mammary adenocarcinoma after extracorporeal perfusion over *Staphylococcus aureus. J Immunol* 124:795-805.

24. Mottolese, M., Morelli, L., Agrimi, U., Benevols, M., Sciaretta, F., Antonucci, G., and Natale, P.G. (1994) Spontaneous canine mammary tumors: A model for monoclonal antibody diagnostics and treatment of human breast cancer. *Lab Invest* 71(2):182-187.

25. Minke, J.M.H.M. (1990) Feline mammary carcinoma: Characterization and development of an allogenic host-tumor model for immunodiagnosis. Thesis Utrecht, pp. 135-155.

26. Minke, J.M.H.M., Weyer, K., and Misdorp. W. (1991) Allotransplantation of K248 feline mammary carcinoma cell line in cats. *Lab Invest* 65(4):421-432.

Comparative Model Aspects: Dogs, Cats, and Humans

Canine and feline mammary tumors share various characteristics with human mammary tumors. Mammary tumors are frequent in all three species, with the age-adjusted incidence ratios being three times higher in dogs than in women.[1] Among the benign tumors (incidence: woman, 40 percent; dog, 60-70 percent; cat, 20 percent), fibroadenomas are the most frequent in women and cats, while complex adenomas and benign mixed tumors are the most common in dogs. The latter tumors are extremely interesting because of their suspected histogenesis from either multipotent stem cells or from myoepithelial cells. There is some structural similarity to the pleomorphic adenoma of the salivary gland in the human.

The cells of origin of mammary carcinoma in all three species may be undifferentiated stem cells in the terminal ductulolobular unit.[2,3] It appears from studies on rat and human mammary tumors that the first steps of tumorigenesis occur early in life.[4] The type of mammary proliferations that develop seem to be associated with the development of anatomic structures (e.g., ductal end buds) that are under hormonal influences. In structures resembling ductal end buds, growth hormone secretion was demonstrated in canine mammary glands under progestational influence.[5] Growth hormone expression has also been demonstrated in mammary tumors of dogs, cats, and humans. The significance of growth hormone and of other growth factors and their possible association with oncogenes needs to be explored.

Hormonal factors, endogenous and exogenous, appear to play a promoting role in the development of mammary tumors. Metastases, at the end point of tumor progression in the dog and the cat, were found to contain few or no hormone receptors, indicating autonomous growth possibly associated with autocrine or paracrine secretion. Thus, at least this segment of canine and feline mammary cancers may serve as a pathogenetic and therapeutic model for those carcinomas in humans that are hormone independent.

Many dogs, cats, and humans with mammary carcinoma will be cured by early and complete resection. In

TABLE 12.2. Prognostic factors of women, dogs, and cats with mammary cancer

Prognostic Factor	Woman	Dog[a]	Cat[b]
Delay in operating	–	–	+
Localization	–	±	–
Clinical stage primary tumor	+	+	
Size, volume tumor	+	+	+
Histological type	+	+	–
Histological grade of malignancy	+	+	
Type of growth (mode of infiltration)	+	+	+
Type of treatment (mastectomy versus block-dissection)	–		+
Regional lymph node involvement	+	–	+

Note: – indicates "not a prognostic factor."
[a]Based on multivariate prognostic study: Misdorp, W. and Hart, A.A.M. (1976) *J Small Anim Prac* 56:395-404.
[b]Based on multivariate prognostic study: Weyer, K., and Hart, A.A.M. (1983) *J Natl Cancer Inst* 70:709-716.

40-60 percent of the cases however, micrometastases that are already present at first presentation of the patient will grow and kill the patient. Future efforts should be directed toward detection and elimination of micrometastases. Monoclonal antibodies that recognize canine and feline mammary cancer cells may be instrumental in achieving that goal. Several established cell lines of canine mammary carcinomas cause tumors when inoculated into nude mice.[6-9] Intermediate models to help study metastases are also available: metastasizing feline mammary carcinomas in juvenile cats after intrafetal injection with feline mammary carcinoma cell lines[10] and metastasizing canine mammary carcinoma in nude mice[11] and in puppies.[12] Prognostic factors for mammary carcinoma in the woman, dog, and cat have many similarities (table 12.2). The use of canine and feline mammary cancer as models has been reviewed.[13,14]

REFERENCES

1. Schneider, R. (1970) Comparison of age, sex and incidence rates in human and canine breast cancer. *Cancer* 26:419-426.

2. Hellmén, E. (1992) Characterization of four in vitro established canine mammary carcinoma and one atypical benign mixed tumor cell line. *In Vitro Cell Devel Biol* 28A:309-319.

3. Ivanyi, D., Groeneveld, E., Calafat, J., Minke, J.M.H.M., and Van Doornweerd, G. (1993) Modulation of mammary carcinoma cell phenotype and keratin expression patterns by retinoid acid. *Cancer Lett* 73:191-205.

4. Russo, A.J., and Russo, I.H. (1987) Biology of disease. Biological and molecular bases of mammary carcinogenesis. *Lab Invest* 57(2): 112-137.

5. Van Garderen, E., De Wit, M., Voorhout, W.F., Rutteman, G.R., Mol, J.A., Nederbragt, H., and Misdorp. W. (1997) Expression of growth hormone in canine mammary tissue and mammary tumors. *Amer J Pathol* 150(3): 1037-1047.

6. Thomas, S.E. (1983) Growth and histology of 4 canine mammary tumour lines established in nude mice. *Eur J Cancer Clin Oncol* 19:979-987.

7. Norval, M., Maingay, J., and Else, R.W. (1984) Studies of three canine mammary carcinoma cell lines II. In vitro profiles. *Eur J Clin Oncol* 20:1501-1508.

8. Wolfe, L.G., Smith, B.B., Toivo-Kinnucan, M.A., Sartin, E.A., Kwapiem, R.P., Henderson, R.A., and Barnes, S. (1986) Biologic properties of cell lines derived from canine mammary carcinoma. *J Natl Cancer Inst* 77:783-792.

9. Van den Burg, B., Van Selm-Miltenburg, A.J.P., Van Maurik, P., Rutteman, G.R., Misdorp, W., De Laet, S., and Van Zoelen, E.J. (1989) Isolation of autonomously growing dog mammary tumor cell lines, cultured in medium supplemented with serum treated to inactivate growth factors. *J Natl Cancer Inst* 81(20): 1545-1551.

10. Minke, J.M.H.M., Weyer, K., and Misdorp, W. (1991) Allotransplantation of K248 feline mammary carcinoma in cats. *Lab Invest* 65(4): 421-435.

11. Hellmén, E. (1996) The pathogenesis of canine mammary tumors. *Cancer J* 9(6): 282-286.

12. Owen, L.N., Morgan, D.R., Bostock, D.E., and Flemans, R.J. (1977) Tissue culture and transplantation studies on canine mammary carcinoma. *Eur J Cancer* 13:1445-1449.

13. Owen, L.N. (1979) A comparative study of canine and human breast cancer. *Invest Cell Pathol* 2: 257-275.

14. Stolwijk, J.A.M., Minke, J.M.H.M., and Misdorp, W. (1987) Feline mammary carcinoma. Breast tumor model 202. In *Handbook: Animal Models of Human Disease.* Fascicle 16.

Diagnosis: Benign or Malignant

Although some clinical signs (rapid growth, tumor size, ulceration, and fixation to skin and underlying tissues) may point to malignancy, it is often impossible to differentiate between benign and malignant mammary tumors clinically, particularly in the dog. Cytological differentiation between benign and malignant canine mammary tumors is difficult, however, an irregular chromatin pattern was reported to be a significant criterion for malignancy.[1] The accuracy of cytological differentiation was 19 percent, sensitivity was 65 percent, and specificity was 94 percent.[1] DNA ploidy in cytological specimens and in specimens obtained from defined tumor samples was highly correlated to malignancy.[2]

Preoperative incisional biopsy and postoperative excisional biopsy followed by histopathologic examination offer the best methods to determine diagnosis, including tumor type, and prognosis. In excisional biopsy specimens, the margins must be evaluated. Malignant mammary tumors often have some degree of infiltrative/destructive growth into adjacent tissues and/or invasion of vessels. Discontinuous or missing basement membranes are indicative of malignancy in canine and feline mammary tumors.[3] Immunohistochemical staining for Von Willebrand factor demonstrated a slightly higher degree of vascular invasion (36.5 percent versus 23 percent) by mammary tumors in dogs than did routine histological staining.[4] Benign mammary tumors lack destructive-invasive growth and are often encapsulated. Exceptions to this are the hyperplastic-lobular lesions and fibroadenomatous lesions of cats. Necrosis is more frequent in malignant than in benign mammary tumors. Significantly more mitotic figures are present in malignant than in benign tumors in the dog, but not in the cat. Mitotic index clearly correlated with nuclear grade in canine mammary cancer but less significantly so

in feline mammary cancer.[5] The proliferation markers AgNOR's[6,7] and PCNA[5] were significantly higher in malignant than in benign canine mammary tumors. The same is true for DNA-aneuploidy.[8, 9]

Anaplasia (loss of differentiation) occurs more often in malignant mammary tumors than in benign ones. Cellular and nuclear pleomorphism (variation in size and shape) is more frequent in malignant than in benign mammary tumors of the dog and cat. Polymorphism (the occurrence of various types of cells often organized in an unorderly way) can be observed in benign and malignant, complex and mixed canine mammary tumors. Some monoclonal antibodies recognizing human breast cancer-associated antigens appear to discriminate benign from malignant canine mammary tumors.[10]

REFERENCES

1. Allen, S.W., Prasse, K.W., and Mahaffey, E. 1986. Cytologic differentiation of benign from malignant canine mammary tumors. *Vet Pathol* 23:649-655.

2. Hellmén, E., and Lindgren, A. (1989) The accuracy of cytology in diagnosis and DNA analysis of canine mammary tumours. *J Comp Pathol* 101:443-450.

3. Benazzi, C., Sarzi, G., Galeotti, N., and Marcato, P.S. (1993) Basement membrane components in mammary tumours of the dog and the cat. *J Comp Pathol* 109:241-252.

4. Gutberlet, K., and Rudolph, R. (1994) Immunohistochemical identification of vessels in cancer cell invasion in canine mammary tumours. *Eur J Vet Pathol* 1(1): 11-14.

5. Preziosi, R., Sarli, G., Benazzi, C., and Marcato, P.S. (1995) Detection of proliferating cell nuclear antigen (PCNA) in canine and feline mammary tumours. *J Comp Pathol* 113:301-313.

6. Bostock, D.E., Moriarty, J., and Crocker, J. (1993) Correlation between histologic diagnosis, mean nuclear organizer region count and prognosis in canine mammary tumors. *Vet Pathol* 29:381-385.

7. Destexhe, E., Vanmanshoven, P., and Coignoult, F. (1995) Comparison of argyrophilic nuclear organizer regions by counting and image analysis in canine mammary tumors. *Amer J Vet Res* 56(2):185-187.

8. Hellmén, E., Lindgren, A., Linell, F., Mattson, P., and Nilsson, A. (1988) Comparison of histology and clinical variables to DNA ploidy in canine mammary tumors. *Vet Pathol* 25:219-226.

9. Rutteman, G.R., Cornelisse, C.J., Dijkshoorn, N.J., Poortman, J., and Misdorp, W. (1988) Flow cytometric analysis of DNA ploidy in canine mammary tumors. *Cancer Res* 48:3411-3417.

10. Mottolese, M., Morelli, L., Agrimi, U., Benevolo, M., Sciaretta, F., Antonucci, G., and Natale, P.G. (1994) Spontaneous canine mammary tumors: A model for monoclonal antibody diagnosis and treatment of human breast cancer. *Lab Invest* 71(2):182-187.

Biological Behavior and Prognosis

Dogs

There are no published data relevant to the clinical course of bitches with untreated mammary gland tumors.

Prospective, follow-up studies compared prognosis of dogs with benign mammary tumors, noninfiltrating carcinomas, and infiltrating mammary cancer.[1-5] The latter cat-

TABLE 12.3. Canine mammary cancer; the prognostic significance of tumor and host characteristics

Characteristics	U²	U³	U⁵	M⁵	U⁶	M⁶	U⁷	M⁷	U⁸	U¹³
Age			+	+	−					
Delay	−	−		−	−	−				
Tumor site		−	−	−	−				+	
Size, volume	+	−	−	−	+	+		+	+	
Tumor type	+	±	+	+	+	+	+	+	+	±
Infiltration soft tissue, skin	+	+	+	−	+	+	+	−	+	+
Vascular invasion				−	−	−			+	
Histological grade of malignancy					+	±	+	+	+	
Positive lymph nodes			+	−	−	−			+	+
Completeness of excision							+		+	
Local recurrence							+	−		
Distant metastasis										+

Note: +, correlated with a poor prognosis; −, no correlation with prognosis; blank, not examined; U, univariate; M, multivariate; superscript numbers refer to references at the end of section on Biological Behavior and Prognosis.

egory was, as expected, associated with a significantly shorter postsurgical survival. In addition, follow-up studies were performed on dogs diagnosed with histologically malignant mammary tumors. Multiple statistical studies are presented in table 12.3. Three of these studies included both univariate and multivariate analyses, the latter being a superior method because it selects independent prognostic factors.[5-7] Another study examined the development of de novo or recurrent invasive mammary cancer less than 2 years after mastectomy.[4] Among the prognostic variables (table 12.3), tumor type was found to be an important independent factor in nearly all studies. In three studies[3,6,8] a range of increasing malignancy from complex carcinoma to simple carcinoma to sarcoma was observed. In another study, sarcomas were considered the most malignant tumor type.[5]

Within the group of simple carcinomas, the increasing order of malignancy was found to be noninfiltrating carcinoma to tubulopapillary carcinoma to solid carcinoma to anaplastic carcinoma.[2]

A histological grading system that quantifies anaplasia, tubule formation, mitotic activity, and nuclear pleomorphism has been used for canine and feline mammary carcinoma (table 12.4). The sum of individual scores determines the histological grade of malignancy. The histological grade of malignancy is of prognostic significance, but the individual grades for anaplasia, mitotic activity, and pleomorphism are not. Infiltration into skin and soft tissues, and invasion of tumor cells into vessels were the best criteria (95 percent and 70 percent) of malignant behavior of mammary tumors in a study of beagles.[9] Microscopic infiltration was a prognostic factor in most univariate analyses but not so in two multivariate analyses.[5,7] Metastatic involvement of regional (superficial inguinal) lymph nodes found in 50 percent of dogs treated by block-resection[10,11] was found of prognostic importance in three univariate analyses[5,8,13] but not in two multivariate analyses.[5,6]

The extent of mammary cancer (and other neoplastic diseases) can be determined by using the TNM system based on clinical investigations.[12] The tumor category

TABLE 12.4. Histologic grading system of canine and feline mammary carcinoma

Characteristic	Score		
1. *Tubule formation.* One point if the section has well-marked tubule formation; three points if there are very few or no tubules	1	2	3
2. *Hyperchromatism and mitoses.* One point if only an occasional hyperchromatic or mitotic figure per high power field is seen; two points if there are two or three such figures; three points if the number is higher	1	2	3
3. *Irregular size and shape of nuclei.* One point if the nuclei are fairly uniform in size, shape, and staining; three points if pleomorphism is marked	1	2	3

Evaluate each characteristic and add the scores together to determine histological grade of malignancy:

Total Score	Grade of Malignancy
3–5	I
6–7	II
8–9	III

Note: There is no grading system for mammary sarcomas.

includes the size of the primary tumor and the degree of infiltration into surrounding tissues. Dogs with mammary cancer were clinically staged, and in one study the clinical stage of complex carcinomas had significant prognostic importance.[6] Tumor size was a prognostic factor in most prospective studies (see table 12.3). Only one study concerned the significant prognostic impact of complete TNM staging and determined that size of the primary tumor (T), lymph node involvement (N), and distant metastasis (M) were associated with prognosis.[13] Ductular carcinomas were overrepresented among the total carcinomas in a beagle life-time study.[14]

Other unfavorable variables are elevated S phase fraction,[5] high percentage of protein and fat in the diet,[7] absence of hormone receptors,[15] and increased nucleolar organizer region (NOR) count.[16]

Most prognostic studies have been based on groups of dogs and their tumors. Therefore, the prognostic significance of some variables will not necessarily apply for each individual case. It is advocated that the pathologist's report to the clinician include the diagnosis (tumor type) and other factors of possible prognostic significance, such as histological grade of malignancy (I, II, III), degree of infiltration, and vascular invasion.

The prognosis is often expressed as the percentage of animals surviving 1 or 2 years after initial mastectomy. In dogs, the 2-year survival in several studies ranged from 25 to 40 percent. Survival, however, is a problematic end point influenced by factors unrelated to mammary neoplasms.[4] Therefore, postoperative cancer free interval was chosen as a more useful and reasonable end point in two studies.[4,8] The 2-year, cancer-free survival rates in dogs were 27 percent and 55 percent, respectively.[4,8]

The main cause of death in dogs after mastectomy for mammary cancer was metastasis (75 of 178 cases), and dyspnea (n = 45) was the most important clinical sign of metastasis. Involvement of distant organs (liver, bones) and pleura without involvement of the lungs (*bypassing*) occurred but was very unusual.[11] Bypassing of regional lymph nodes was also unusual, indicating that regional lymph nodes and lungs function at least initially as filters in the process of metastasis. Local recurrence (39 of 178) and other concurrent diseases (63 of 178) were also major causes of death.

Cats

Mammary carcinomas in cats are highly infiltrating tumors (infiltration into soft tissues, 88 percent; vascular invasion, 53 percent). Regional lymph nodes were found to be involved in 27 percent of surgical block resection specimens.[17]

Old age, large diameter of primary tumor, high number of mitoses, large amount of necrosis, metastasis to regional lymph nodes, and incompleteness of surgical excision as judged by the pathologist were found to be independent unfavorable prognostic factors in a multivariate study.[17]

In a univariate study the volume of the mammary tumor was found to be the single most important prognostic factor: cats with tumors of less than 8 cm³ had a significantly longer disease free interval and overall survival time than cats with tumors of greater than 8 cm.[3,18] Cats that had undergone radical surgery had a significantly longer disease free interval than cats treated conservatively, but the survival time was not improved.[18] The cause of death in most cats (61 percent) was associated with metastasis, recurrent tumor, or both. Metastasis to lungs (76 percent) and pleura (40 percent) was observed frequently at postmortem examination.[17]

REFERENCES

1. Fowler, E.H., Wilson, G.R., and Koestner, A. (1974) Biologic behavior of canine mammary neoplasms based on a histogenetic classification. *Vet Pathol* 30:20-27.

2. Bostock, D.E. (1975) The prognosis following the surgical excision of canine mammary neoplasms. *Eur J Cancer* 11:389-396.

3. Else, R.W., and Hannant, D. (1979) Some epidemiological aspects of mammary neoplasia in the bitch. *Vet Rec* 194:296-304.

4. Gilbertson, S.R., Kurzman, I.D., Zachrau, R.E., Hurvitz, A.I., and Black, M.M. (1983) Canine mammary epithelial neoplasms: Biologic implications of morphologic characteristics assessed in 232 dogs. *Vet Pathol* 20:127-142.

5. Hellmén, E., Bergstrom, R., Holmberg, L., Spangberg, I.B., Hansson, K., and Lindgren, A. (1993) Prognostic factors in canine mammary tumors: A multivariate study of 202 consecutive cases. *Vet Pathol* 11:212-229.

6. Misdorp, W., and Hart, A.A.M. (1976) Prognostic factors in canine mammary cancer. *J Natl Cancer Inst* 56:779-786.

7. Shofer, F.C., Sonnenschein, E.G., Goldschmidt, M.H., Laster, L.L., and Glickman, L.T. (1989) Histopathologic and dietary prognostic factors for canine mammary carcinoma. *Breast Cancer Res Treat* 13:49-60.

8. Parodi, A.L., Misdorp, W., Mialot, J.P., Mialot, M., Hart, A.A.M., Hurtrel, M., and Salomon, J.C. (1983) Intratumoral BCG and *Corynebacterium parvum* therapy of canine mammary tumours before radical mastectomy. *Cancer Immunol Immunother* 15:172-177.

9. Chrisp, C.E., and Spangler, W.L. (1980) The malignant mammary tumor as a model for the study of human breast cancer. In Shifrine, M., and Wilson, F.D. (eds.), *The Canine as a Biomedical Research Model: Immunological, Hematological and Oncological Aspects*, 17. U.S. Department of Energy, Washington, D.C., pp. 331-349.

10. Fidler, I.J., Abt, D.A., and Brodey, R.S. (1967) The biological behavior of canine mammary gland neoplasms. *J Amer Vet Med Assoc* 151:1311-1318.

11. Misdorp, W., and Hart, A.A.M. (1979) Canine mammary cancer. II. Therapy and causes of death. *J Small Anim Pract* 20:395-404.

12. Owen, L.N. (1980) TNM classification of tumours in domestic animals. World Health Organization, Geneva, pp. 16-20.

13. Yamagami T., Kobayashi, T., Takahaski, K., and Sugiyama, M. (1996) Prognosis for canine malignant mammary tumors based on TNM and histologic classification. *J Vet Med Sci* 58(11): 1079-1083.

14. Benjamin, S.A., Lee, A.C., and Saunders, W.J. (1998) Classification and behavior of canine epithelial neoplasms based on life-span observations in beagles. *Vet Pathol* 36(5): 423-430.

15. Martin, P.M., Cotard, M., Mialot, J.P., Andre, F., and Raynaud, J.P. (1984) Animal models for hormone dependent human breast cancer. Relationship between steroid receptor profiles in canine and feline mammary tumors and survival rate. *Cancer Chemother Pharmacol* 12:13-17.

16. Bostock, D.E., Moriarty, J., and Crocker, J. (1993) Correlation between histologic diagnosis, mean nuclear organizer region count and prognosis in canine mammary tumors. *Vet Pathol* 29:381-385.

17. Weyer, K., and Hart, A.A.M. (1983) Prognostic factors in feline mammary carcinoma. *J Natl Cancer Inst* 70:709-716.

18. McEwen, E.G., Hayes, A.A., Harvey, H.J., Patnaik, A.K., Mooney, S., and Passe, S. (1984) Prognostic factors for feline mammary tumors. *J Amer Vet Med Assoc* 185: 201-204.

Methods of Classification

Three primary methods are used to classify mammary tumors: (1) histogenetic, (2) histological descriptive, and (3) prognostic.

Histogenetic classification is hampered by the uncertainty of the specific cell of origin of many mammary tumors.[1,2] We therefore agree with Moulton[3] that the term *duct carcinomas* should not be used. Similarly, we don't use the term *lobular carcinoma*. It is likely that many dysplastic and tumorous lesions originate from stem cells situated in the *terminal ductulolobular units*.

A previous classification was based on descriptive morphology.[4] This classification has been employed in several clinical (prognostic) and investigational (progestin) studies in Europe and the United States. The classification was judged "unnecessarily complex" by Moulton, who added that "its use, however, may be justified in the future, particularly if additional behavioral differences in neoplasms can be related to histological types."[3] It seems now justified, based on the results of statistical follow-up studies (see table 12.3) to reclassify canine mammary carcinomas, in order of increasing malignancy, as follows: noninfiltrating carcinoma, complex carcinoma (two cell types), simple carcinoma (one cell type), simple carcinoma (tubulopapillary type), simple carcinoma (solid type), and simple anaplastic carcinoma. The classification presented here is the same as the recently prepared WHO-AFIP classification of canine mammary tumors, which is partly based on prognosis. Inflammatory carcinoma is not a separate type of mammary tumor. It is a generic name given to a mammary carcinoma that has considerable inflammation within the tumor. Mammary carcinomas that have a marked inflammatory component tend to be aggressive and are associated with decreased survival and short, tumor-free intervals.

In the dog and the cat, many carcinomas have a heterogeneous histomorphology. We classify such carcinomas by using combined diagnoses with the predominant pattern indicated first. The present knowledge acquired from two prognostic studies does not permit reclassification of the feline carcinomas according to their prognostic histological features.[5,6]

DESCRIPTIONS OF MAMMARY TUMORS

Malignant Mammary Tumors in the Dog and Cat

Carcinomas

Noninfiltrating (in Situ) Carcinomas

These lesions are often multicentric and are usually not visible grossly. They may be part of fibrocystic disease or are found incidentally near infiltrating carcinomas or other mammary tumors. Noninfiltrating carcinomas of simple type (one cell type) are frequently found in the dog and the cat. Noninfiltrating complex carcinoma has not been reported.

Tumor cells not invading the basement membrane can be arranged in several patterns: cribriform (sievelike pattern) (fig. 12.1); solid, eventually with central necrosis (*comedo*); and clincing (scattered cells covering the basement membrane). Only those lesions that display histological and cytological characteristics similar to their invasive counterparts should be classified as in situ cancers (fig. 12.1; see also fig. 12.15). The difference between in situ carcinoma and atypical or even typical, regular epithelial hyperplasia can be difficult. This holds especially true for the small-cell types. It can also be very difficult to exclude the possibility of incipient invasion of the ductal wall or of intraductal propagation from a neighboring invasive carcinoma In the latter case the myoepithelial layers of the duct may be at least partially intact.

Complex Carcinoma

This type of tumor is relatively common in the dog and rare in the cat. Grossly, these tumors are usually lobulated. This type of carcinoma has both epithelial and myoepithelial components (fig. 12.1). The luminal epithelium-like cells can be arranged in either a tubulopapillary or a solid fashion (fig. 12.2). Squamous metaplasia of a portion may occur. The spindle cell type of myoepithelium-like cells are frequently arranged in a more or less stellate, reticulated pattern (fig. 12.3). The intercellular mucoid substance (fig. 12.4) occasionally found in these tumors must be differentiated from young cartilage as found in carcinosarcomas, which is characterized by the presence of cells embedded in lacunae of cartilaginous matrix. Expansive growth is quite common, and growth within lymphatics is rare (about 10 percent). Differentiation between highly differentiated complex carcinomas and complex adenomas can be difficult. Absence of a capsule, infiltrative growth, high cellularity, necrosis, and high mitotic index are indicative of malignancy; median survival time is 10 months.

Simple Carcinomas

These tumors are the most common malignant mammary tumor in the dog and the cat. Carcinomas of this type are composed of one type of cell. These tumors have a strong tendency to infiltrate into surrounding tissues and vessels (up to 50 percent). Lymphogenous and hematogenous spread are common; median survival is 10-12 months.[8] The amount of stroma can vary considerably. Peritumoral lymphocytes are common, either in association with necrosis or not. Based on their differentiation and their biologic behavior, simple carcinomas can be graded in terms of increasing malignancy as tubulopapillary, solid, or anaplastic (fig. 12.2).

Tubulopapillary Carcinoma

These tumors are characterized by the formation of tubules with or without papillary projections (fig. 12.5). In the dog, tubular carcinomas can be accompanied by marked proliferation of stromal fibroblasts in the primary and/or metastatic tumor. The stromal component is usually scanty in the papillary type, which occurs frequently in the dog and the cat. In the cat, it should be differentiated from the common cribriform type. A special variant is the cystic papillary type, which is usually well demarcated and can be difficult to differentiate from benign lesions such as papil-

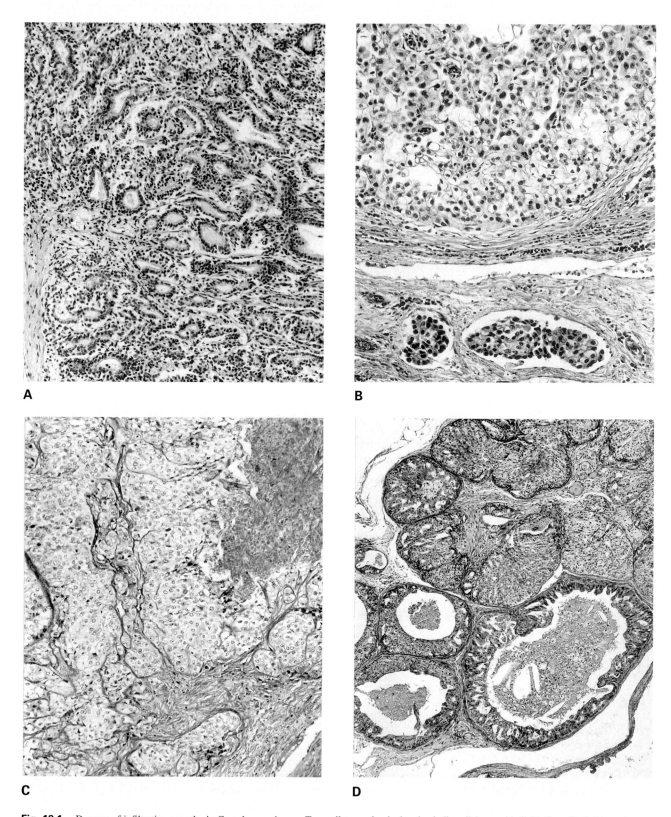

Fig. 12.1. Degrees of infiltrative growth. **A.** Complex carcinoma. Two cell types, luminal and spindle cell (myoepithelial). Dog. **B.** Solid carcinoma. Appears to be well defined but has metastasized along lymphatics. **C.** Solid carcinoma, moderately infiltrating. Cat. **D.** Cribriform carcinoma. Partly intraductal (DCIS) partly intralobular (LCIS), some infiltrative growth, cat.

590

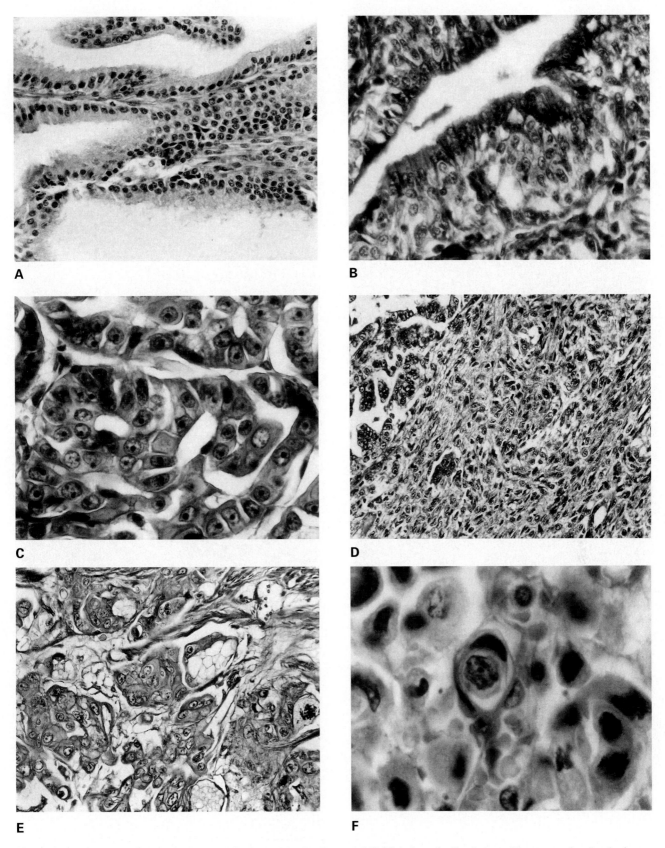

Fig. 12.2. Histologic grades of malignancy. The histologic grade of malignancy (I, II, III) is determined by the sum of the scores assigned to the degrees of nuclear pleomorphism, tubule formation and the mitotic index (see table 12.4). **A.** Simple carcinoma: papillary cystic type. Grade I, Dog. **B.** Complex carcinoma. Grade I, Dog. **C.** Simple carcinoma: tubular type. Grade II, Dog. **D.** Complex carcinoma. Grade II, Cat. **E.** Simple carcinoma: solid type. Grade III, Cat. **F.** Anaplastic carcinoma. Grade III, Dog.

591

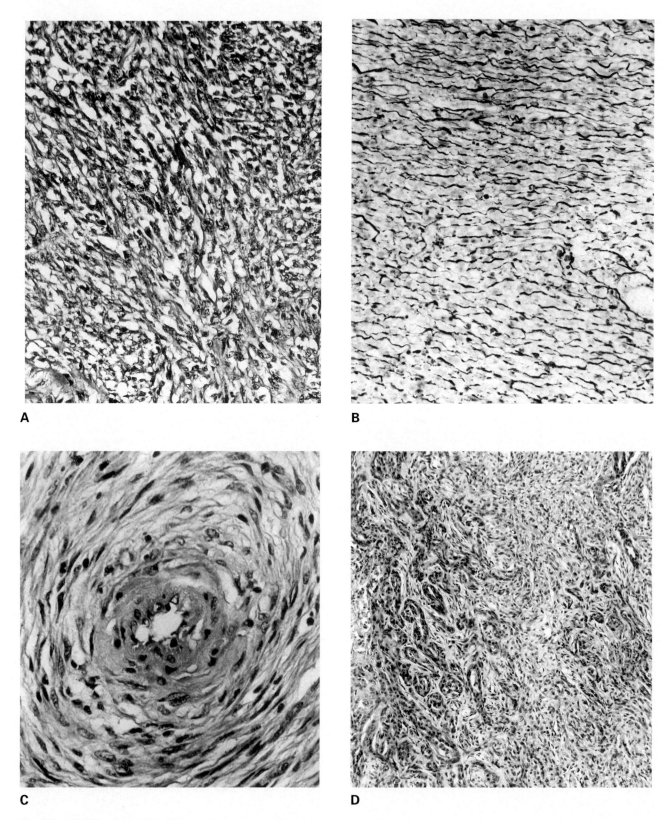

Fig. 12.3. Spindle cells. Spindle cells in mammary tumors can be neoplastic or nonneoplastic (stromal). Neoplastic spindle cells can be of epithelial, myoepithelial, or myofibroblastic origin. Fibrosarcoma can be differentiated from spindle cell carcinoma by use of reticulum fiber stain. **A.** Spindle cell carcinoma, cat. **B.** Fibrosarcoma, fine reticulin fiber network around individual tumor cells, dog. **C.** Concentric arrangement of spindle cells around prominent blood vessels, hemangiopericytoma-like pattern of fibrosarcoma, dog. **D.** Complex carcinoma, neoplastic spindle cells possibly of myoepithelial origin, dog.

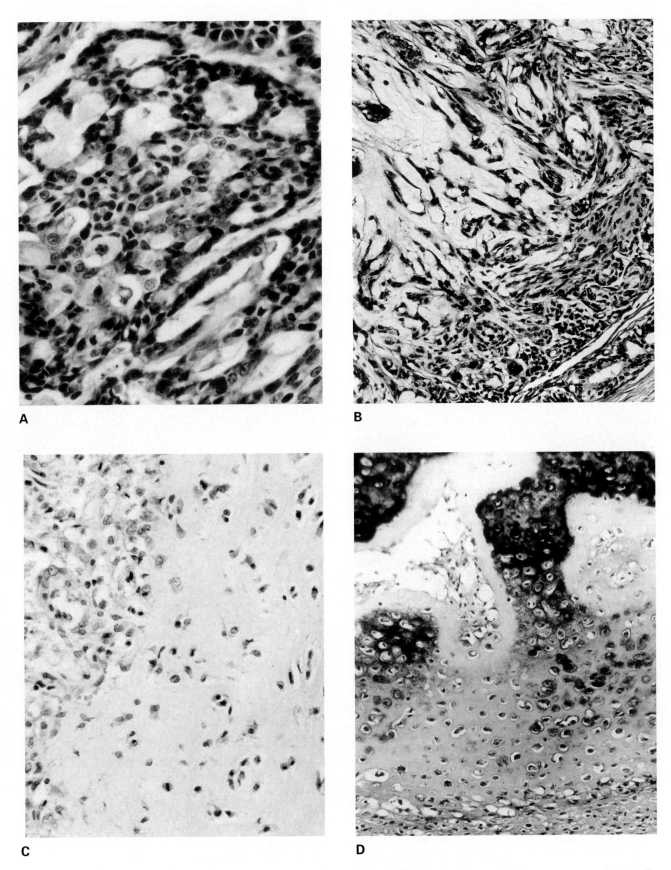

Fig. 12.4. Mucin and cartilage. Mucinous and mucoid material is found in many mammary tumors. Mucin appears to be formed by epithelial cells, mucoid material probably by myoepithelial or stromal cells. Mucoid material must be differentiated from young cartilage (chrondrocytes embedded in lacunae = cartilage). Calcifying cartilage should be differentiated from "true bone" formation (osteoid, woven bone). **A.** Mucinous carcinoma, mucin formation by epithelial cells, cat. **B.** Complex carcinoma, mucoid material apparently produced by myoepithelial cells, low grade, dog. **C.** Carcinosarcoma, cartilage formation, dog. **D.** Mammary sarcoma, calcifying and ossifying cartilage, dog.

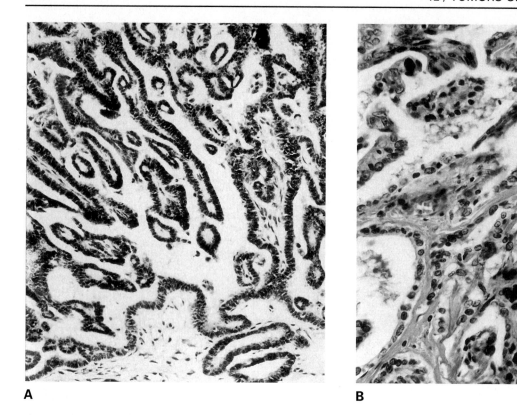

A

B

Fig. 12.5. **A.** Papillary carcinoma infiltrating into a vessel. Uniform cylindrical cells on stromal papillae, low grade of malignancy, cat. **B.** Papillary cystic carcinoma, highly differentiated with intraepithelial calcification, dog.

lomatous ductal hyperplasia. Unexpected metastasis from a highly differentiated cystic papillary lesion to regional lymph nodes (see fig. 12.8) has been reported in the dog.[7]

Solid Carcinoma

This carcinoma type is rather frequent in the dog and the cat. Solid carcinomas are usually ill defined, but some are rather well defined. Tumor cells are arranged in solid sheets, cords, or nests (see fig. 12.1). Some solid carcinomas are composed of cells with vacuolated cytoplasm (clear cell type), possibly of myoepithelial origin. The amount of stroma ranges from small to moderate.

Cribriform Carcinoma

This carcinoma type is common in the cat. It is usually highly invasive. Cribriform carcinomas are basically solid carcinomas with small apertures like a sieve (see 12.1). It should be differentiated from papillary carcinoma and from solid carcinoma with foci of necrosis.

Anaplastic Carcinoma

This type of tumor occurs in dogs but has not been reported in the cat.[8] These tumors are ill defined grossly. Occasionally small foci of anaplastic carcinomas are found in mastectomy specimens removed for another mammary tumor or dysplasia. These tumors infiltrate diffusely and are composed of large, pleomorphic cells, often with bizarre nuclei that are rich in chromatin. Some cells may

be multinucleated. Neutrophils and eosinophils are present in the tumor and in the stroma. Collagenous stroma is abundant. Differentiation between extremely anaplastic carcinoma and anaplastic (rhabdomyo-) sarcoma can be difficult. Anaplastic carcinoma cells are often positive for keratin and vimentin by immunohistochemistry; rhabdomyosarcoma cells are positive for muscle cell markers. Anaplastic carcinomas may be differentiated from inflammatory lesions with highly reactive macrophages by the use of immunohistochemical markers (keratin vs. histiocyte markers). This type of carcinoma has a poor prognosis because it frequently recurs and metastasizes. Surgery alone is of questionable value.

Special Types of Carcinomas
Spindle Cell Carcinoma

This tumor is relatively rare in the dog and very rare in the cat.[7] It is composed of spindle cells that are usually arranged in an epithelial fashion (see fig. 12.3): groups of cells are wrapped by reticulin fibers, in contrast to fibrosarcomas in which individual tumor cells are wrapped by reticulin fibers (see fig. 12.3). Moreover, immunohistochemical markers (cytokeratin, vimentin) may be useful in differentiation between the two spindle cell cancers. It seems likely that some spindle cell carcinomas are of myoepithelial origin.

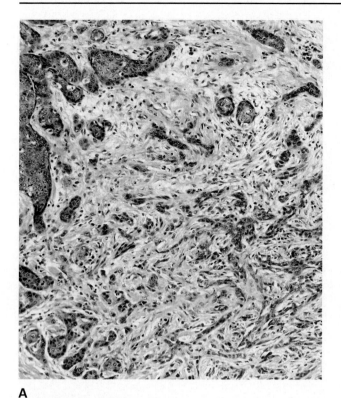

A

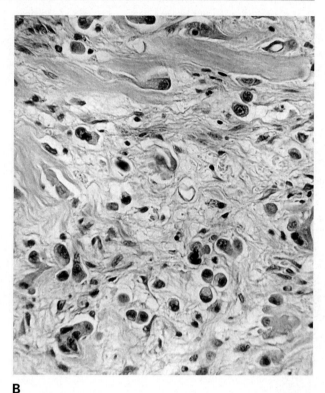

B

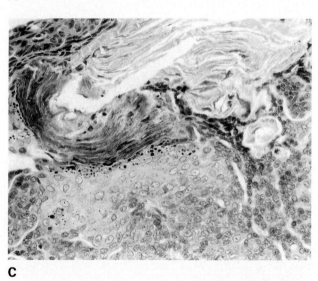

C

Fig. 12.6. **A.** Squamous cell carcinoma with marked desmoplasia, severely infiltrating, dog. **B.** Anaplastic carcinoma, marked infiltration, dog. **C.** Malignant basaloid tumor, dog. This tumor has the same characteristics as the basaloid adenoma (palisading, cornification) but is more cellular, has local invasion, and metastasized to the lymph node.

trative type (fig. 12.6), and invasion of lymphatics is common. Squamous cell carcinomas originating in the mammary gland or in the teat canal should be distinguished not only from squamous cell carcinomas derived from the skin and adnexa, but also from squamous metaplasia of larger ducts due to inflammation. In the carcinomas, the cells often have atypia and have invaded adjacent tissue. In addition, a rare type of carcinoma that to some extent resembles *basaloid adenoma,* but with invasive and metastasizing properties, is also included under this heading (fig. 12.6).

Mucinous Carcinoma

This type of tumor is rare in the dog and the cat (see fig. 12.4). A predominant feature is the presence of large amounts of mucinous material that stains positively with PAS, with and without diastase and alcian blue stains. Transition of mucinous to chondroid-like intercellular material is sometimes recognized. It is not certain whether the mucin has been produced by secretory epithelial cells or by myoepithelial cells. The tumor cells are polyhedral with vacuolated cytoplasm.

Lipid-Rich Carcinoma

This tumor is extremely rare in dogs (and in women) and is characterized by cells that have an abundant foamy cytoplasm which contains a large amount of neutral lipid.

Carcinomas with Squamous Differentiation

This type of carcinoma is uncommon in the dog and is not reported to occur in the cat (fig. 12.6). Classical squamous cell carcinomas and adenosquamous carcinomas should be classified under this heading. Classical squamous cell carcinomas consist of solid sheets and cords with areas of cornification. Basal cells are predominant in the peripheral parts of the sheets. The central parts consist of lamellated keratin in which necrotic tumor cells (shadow cells) can be recognized. The adenosquamous carcinoma contains adenomatous tissue and areas of squamous differentiation.

Most squamous cell carcinomas are of a highly infil-

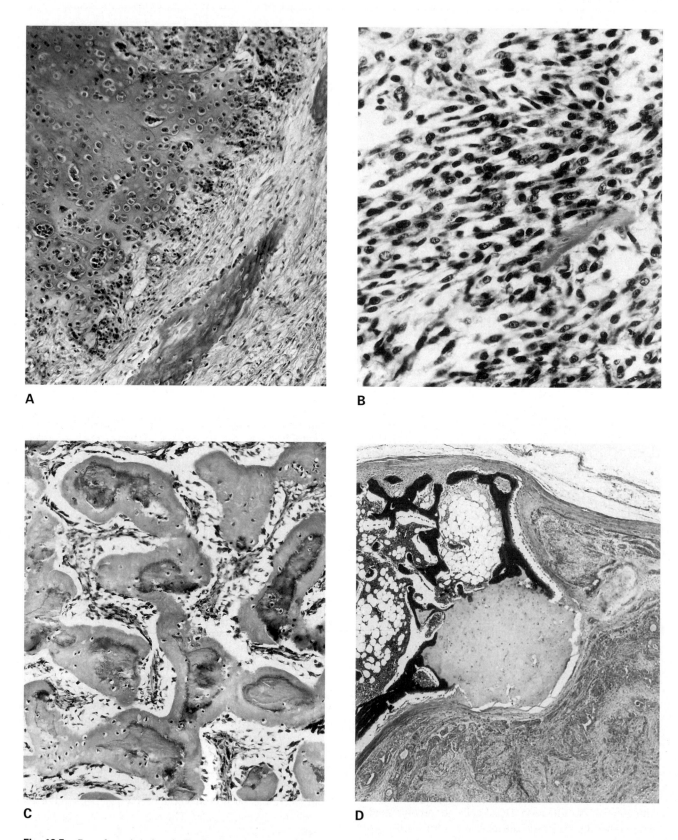

Fig. 12.7. Bone formation, dog. **A.** Carcinosarcoma with osteoid formation in connective tissue. **B.** Osteosarcoma, poorly differentiated, few spicules of osteoid. **C.** Mammary osteosarcoma with extensive bone formation. **D.** Benign mixed tumor, formation of well-differentiated bone and bone marrow, from a cartilaginous intermediate stage (osteochondroma-like pattern).

Sarcomas

Mammary sarcomas comprise approximately 10-15 percent of mammary neoplasia in the dog and are rare in the cat. In older cats fibrosarcomas are common in soft tissues, and some may occur in the mammary gland.[9]

Sarcomas are usually large, often seemingly well demarcated, and firm to bony (fig. 12.7). Fibrosarcomas and osteosarcomas are the most frequent mammary sarcomas in the dog. Chondrosarcomas are rare. Mammary sarcomas are associated with an unfavorable prognosis due to a high tendency for local recurrence and metastases to regional lymph nodes and/or lungs; median survival is 10 months.[8]

Fibrosarcoma

Tumors of this type are composed of spindle cells that have formed reticulin and collagenous fibers (see fig. 12.3). The fibers can be arranged in parallel fashion (bundles) or haphazardly. In some sarcomas there is concentric arrangement of fibers around proliferating blood vessels as in hemangiopericytoma (see fig. 12.3C). Necrotic and hemorrhagic fibrosarcomas may be difficult to distinguish from encapsulated abscesses or hemorrhages, but the peripheral areas of the lesions usually indicate the correct diagnosis. Differentiation from spindle cell carcinomas is usually possible by the use of reticulin fiber staining (wrapping of individual cells by fibers = fibrosarcoma). In cats, as in women with cystosarcoma, fibroadenomas can contain very cellular areas resembling fibrosarcoma. It is not known whether these areas represent true progression toward mammary sarcoma (and subsequent metastasis) or are merely areas of enhanced kinetic activity.

Osteosarcoma

These tumors are characterized by osteoid production by neoplastic cells (fig. 12.7). This type of direct bone formation should be differentiated from indirect bone formation that goes through a cartilaginous intermediate stage, as in chondrosarcomas. Osteosarcomas are either pure osteosarcomas or combinations of bone, fibrous, and cartilaginous components (combined sarcomas). The latter tumors are composed of malignant osseous and cartilaginous cells and possibly malignant fibrous and/or adipose cells. Generally the matrix is most dense in the center, and the more cellular areas are usually situated at the periphery. Pleomorphism and mitotic activity are usually prominent; however, the combined sarcomas and their metastases can look highly differentiated.[9]

Carcinosarcoma

This type of tumor (fig. 12.8; see also fig. 12.4) is uncommon in the dog and rare in the cat. Grossly, these tumors are usually well circumscribed, and the cut surface is firm to bony. These tumors are composed of cells morphologically resembling malignant epithelial cells (luminal epithelial and/or myoepithelial) and cells resembling malignant connective tissue (fig. 12.7). Mixtures of all types of carcinomatous components can be recognized. Some carcinosarcomas have a benign histological pattern. Merging between carcinomatous and chondrosarcomatous parts is suggestive of transformation (fig. 12.9). Postsurgical survival is relatively long: mean 18 months.[8] The metastases are of mixed, sarcomatous, or carcinomatous type.

Carcinomas or Sarcomas Arising in Benign Tumors

Foci, or even nodules, of atypical cells can be recognized occasionally in complex adenomas and benign mixed tumors in the dog. Osteosarcomas may arise in benign mixed tumors. The malignant component may have largely replaced the benign tumor, at the time of histological examination. Insufficient information is available about the prognosis of these tumors.

Benign Mammary Tumors in the Dog and Cat

Benign mammary tumors are far more frequent in the dog than in the cat (ratio benign/malignant in the dog 70/30 and in the cat 20/80). Most benign tumors are well demarcated. Their internal structure, particularly in the dog, can be disorderly, with participation of several types of cells: epithelial, myoepithelial, and/or stromal.

Simple Adenoma

This lesion is rare in the dog and the cat, and it is usually well demarcated. Simple adenomas may be of tubular type, consisting of well-differentiated luminal epithelial cells (fig. 12. 10). Some of these tubular adenomas have a secretory product. In the dog, the solid type, consisting of benign spindle cells, has been labeled as *myoepithelioma* by pathologists in the United States.

Basaloid Adenoma

These tumors were first reported to occur in beagle dogs that had received investigational progestins.[10] The tumors were usually small and well circumscribed and had not metastasized. Some of these lesions appear to grow as adenosis rather than as discrete adenomas. The tumors are composed of uniform cords and clusters of monomorphic epithelial cells that may have cornified. The peripheral cells palisade along a thin basal membrane, and it is this characteristic that differentiates these from a simple adenoma (see fig. 12.6). A rare metastasizing type has been recognized and categorized as a carcinoma with squamous differentiation. Further studies are required for proper categorization of basaloid lesions.

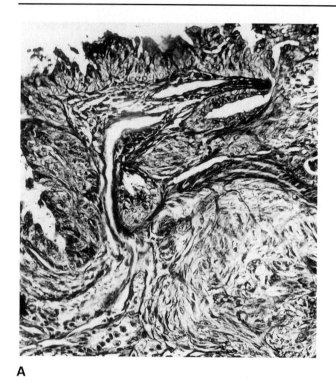

A

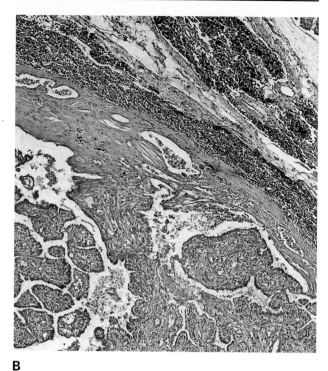

B

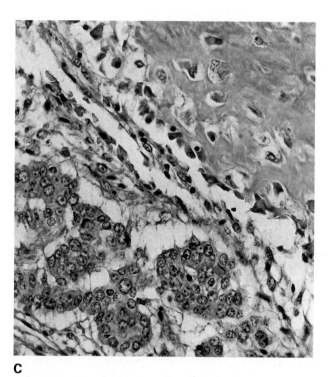

C

Fig. 12.8. Malignant versus benign? Complex and mixed tumors in the dog are too often considered malignant, probably because of their structural complexity and unorderly arrangement. In contrast, there are tumors that appear "benign" but metastasize. This is also true for some papillary "carcinomas" in which the papillae don't consist exclusively of tumor cells, as in regular papillary carcinomas, but of stalks of stroma covered by uniform cylindrical cells. **A.** Complex adenoma, dog. Contains unorderly arranged ductules and spindle cell formation and has low mitotic index, low grade of anaplasia, and no metastasis. **B.** Unexpected metastasis of low grade complex cystic papillary carcinoma to a regional lymph node, dog. **C.** Carcinosarcoma, well differentiated but metastatic to lungs, dog.

Complex Adenoma

These tumors are common in the bitch and less common in the queen. Complex adenomas are composed of luminal epithelial cells together with spindle shaped or stellate cells resembling myoepithelial cells (fig. 12. 10). The latter cells appear to produce a mucin-like substance that can be mistaken for chondroid material characteristic of benign mixed tumors. Differentiation of complex adenoma from benign mixed tumors,

fibroadenomas, and lobular hyperplasia may be difficult. Encapsulation, low mitotic index, absence of necrosis, and low atypia are characteristics of complex adenomas (see fig. 12.8).

Benign Mixed Tumor

These tumors are frequent in the dog and very rare in the cat. They are composed of benign cells resembling luminal epithelium and myoepithelium mixed with mesenchymal cells that have produced fibrous tissue *in combination* with cartilage, bone, and/or fat (fig. 12.10; see also fig. 12.7). Differentiation from fibroadenoma (basically also a mixed tumor) is based on the presence (mixed tumors) or absence (fibroadenoma) of distinct cartilage, bone, and/or fat.

Fibroadenoma

Fibroadenoma (fig. 12.11) is relatively common in the dog and the cat. It consists of a mixture of luminal epithelial cells and fibroblastic stromal cells, sometimes

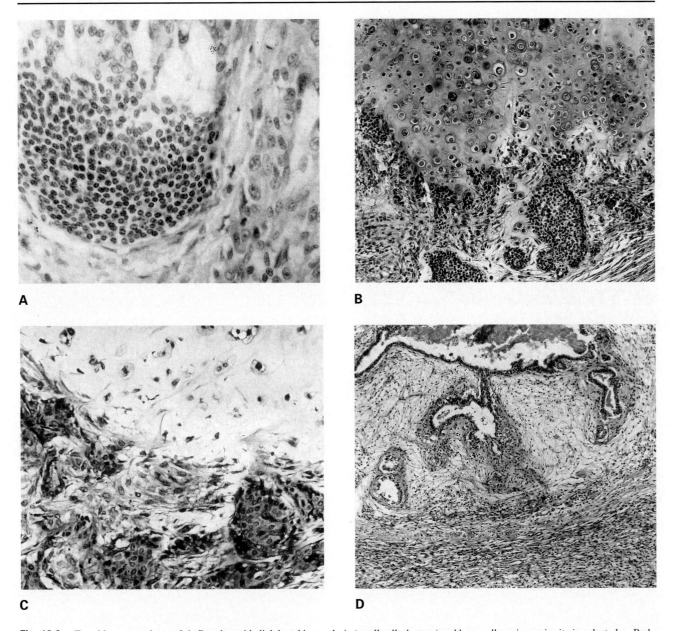

Fig. 12.9. Transition or coexistence? **A.** Regular epithelial ductal hyperplasia (small cells, bottom) and large cell carcinoma in situ in a duct, dog. Probably coexistence rather than transition. **B.** Carcinosarcoma , dog. Transition of solid carcinoma to chondrosarcoma. **C.** Atypical, borderline tumor of mixed type. Transition? **D.** Fibrosarcoma arising in a fibroadenoma or cellular fibroadenoma, dog.

admixed with myoepithelial cells. The latter fact can cause difficulties in the differentiation from complex adenomas. Periductal and intraductal subtypes can be recognized. The stroma can be extremely cellular and rich in mitotic figures, as in *cystosarcoma phyllodes* in women.

Fibroadenomatous Change

Lesions of fibroadenomatous change (synonyms: feline mammary hypertrophy, fibroepithelial hypertrophy) occur in progestin treated, pregnant, and very young cats and are induced by exogenous and endogenous proges-

terone (fig. 12.12). Progesterone receptors are usually present in high concentrations. The lesion(s) is(are) usually nonencapsulated. Lesions may occupy one or several mammary glands. They grow rapidly and cause clinical problems. They regress after ovariohysterectomy or termination of pregnancy or progestin treatment.

Duct Papilloma

This is a rare lesion in the dog and the cat, often found by chance in a duct distended by fibrocystic disease. Structurally it is branching or lobulated and composed of epithelial and/or myoepithelial cells.

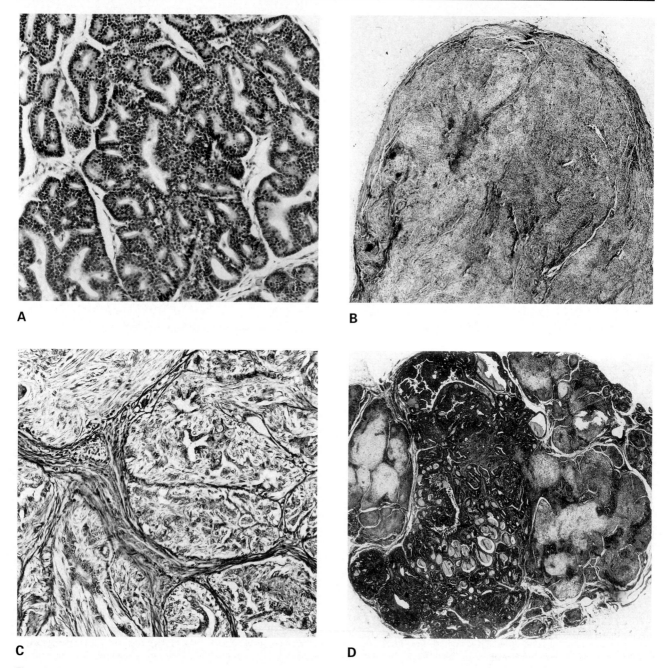

Fig. 12.10. **A.** Simple adenoma, tubular type, dog. Tubules formed by uniform epithelial cells. **B.** Simple adenoma, solid type (*myoepithelioma*), dog. **C.** Complex adenoma, dog. Two cell types: (1) epithelial cells forming tubules and (2) spindle cells or myoepithelial cells forming solid sheets. **D.** Benign mixed tumor, dog. Mixture of epithelial, myoepithelial, and chondromatous tissue. Multilobular growth of coalescent lesions.

Multiple duct papillomas, originating from ductal epithelium/myoepithelium must be differentiated from ductal papillomatosis, which is basically an adenosis with an intraductal component.

Unclassified Tumors in the Dog and Cat

The following are benign or malignant tumors that cannot be placed in any of the above categories.

Mammary Dysplasia: Fibrocystic Disease

This is a benign condition in the dog and the cat (and women) characterized by a spectrum of proliferative and regressive alterations of mammary tissue with an abnormal interplay of epithelial, myoepithelial, and connective tissue elements.[11] These alterations combine variously and may produce a palpable lump. Most of these epithelial proliferations probably begin in the terminal duct and manifest

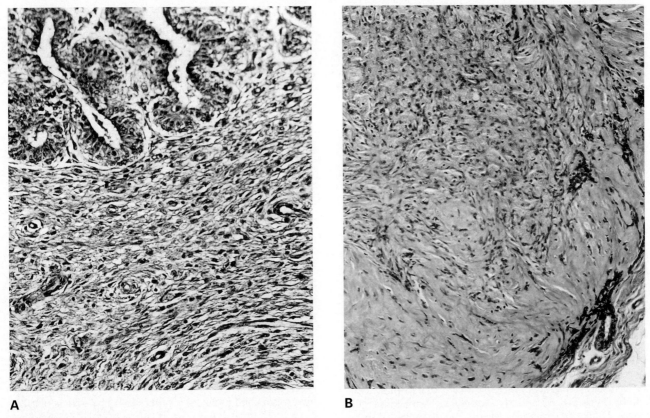

Fig. 12.11. **A.** Cellular fibroadenoma, concentric arrangement of spindle cells (fibroblasts) around tubules and vessels, dog. **B.** Fibrosclerosis, nodule consisting of spindle cells (myo-fibroblasts) and abundant collagen, dog.

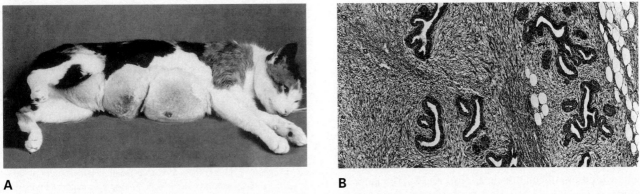

Fig. 12.12. **A.** Cat with diffuse fibroadenomatous change (*fibroepithelial hyperplasia*) after treatment with progestins. The lesion was characterized by rapid growth and ulceration. **B.** Fibroadenomatous change, cellular fibroadenomatous tissue, infiltrating into surrounding fat, cat.

themselves as hyperplastic changes of extralobular (ducts/ductal hyperplasia) and/or intralobular ductules (lobular hyperplasia). In some cases, distinction between these two is difficult, if not impossible.

Ductal Hyperplasia

This condition is characterized by a hyperplasia of epithelial cells in either normal or abnormal (e.g., distended) ducts (figs. 12.13, 12.14). It may eventually lead to partial or total obliteration of the duct. The hyperplasia may be diffuse or multifocal and has been referred to as papillomatosis or epitheliosis. Small size and uniformity of cells and nuclei, lack of mitoses, and the presence of readily recognizable myoepithelial layers indicate the lesion is benign; this is regular ductal hyperplasia (fig. 12.14). When atypia is pronounced, the term *atypical ductal hyperplasia* (fig. 12.14) is used. Differentiation from intraductal carcinoma (fig. 12.15) is based on degree of cellular and nuclear atypia. Epithelial cells that slough into the lumen of ducts may resemble macrophages or even anaplastic carcinoma cells. Ductal hyperplasia with moderate and marked atypia was considered precancerous and

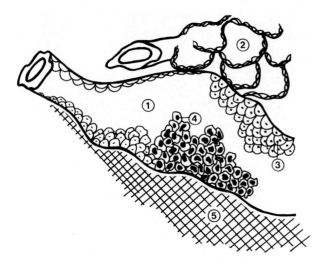

Fig. 12.13. Intraductal and intraductular lesions. The following proliferations of mammary epithelium can be difficult to distinguish: regular epithelial hyperplasia, atypical hyperplasia, and carcinoma in situ. They all carry a "good" prognosis, and it is not known if they represent a continuum. Carcinoma in situ is characterized by cytologic characteristics of malignancy such as pleomorphism, high mitotic index, and anaplasia, but the focus of epithelial proliferation is well confined. Regular epithelial hyperplasia is characterized by proliferation of uniform, mostly cylindrical shaped cells with darkly stained nuclei. Differentiation between atypical epithelial hyperplasia and carcinoma in situ can be extremely difficult and may not be possible. Another diagnostic problem in intraductular lesions is the differentiation among sloughed epithelial cells, macrophages, and anaplastic carcinoma cells. *Ductal epithelial hyperplasia and ductectasia:* 1. Ectasia of larger duct. 2. Ectasia of ductules (*spongy breast*). 3. Regular epithelial hyperplasia. 4. Ductal carcinoma in situ. 5. Adjacent stroma.

was associated with a greater chance of developing into invasive carcinomas than was ductal hyperplasia with normotypic cells.[12]

Lobular Hyperplasia

There are two types of lobular hyperplasia (see figs. 12.16, 12.17): (1) adenosis, an increase in the number of ductules, and (2) epitheliosis, a proliferation of epithelial cells within intralobular ductules (fig. 12.17). The latter is similar to that seen in extralobular ducts: papillomatosis or epitheliosis. Proliferation of ductules leading to an increase in the number of tubules is known as adenosis. Adenosis consists of the following components in varying proportions: ductules, secretory epithelium, myoepithelium, and specific and/or nonspecific connective tissue (fig. 12.16). When proliferation of fibrous tissues is prominent, the term sclerosing adenosis is used (see fig. 12.18). This lesion is far less frequent in dogs and cats than in women. It may simulate infiltrating carcinoma. The retention of a lobular pattern and lack of infiltration favor a benign process. The most frequent growth pattern in dogs and cats is intramural, exophytic in the lumen, or periductal. Lobular hyperplasia of the adenosis type is often present in dogs and cats as unilobular hyperplasia and as coa-

lescence of multilobular hyperplasia (fig. 12.17) or adenomatoid hyperplasia (an intermediate phase between lobular hyperplasia and adenoma or benign mixed tumor). Inflammatory cells can be prominent in the stroma. Partial or total fibroadenomatous change in the cat can be regarded as a type of adenosis with excessive proliferation of connective tissue.

Cysts and Ductectasia

Cysts are often multiple and may form part of fibrocystic disease. The epithelium may be atrophic or show some degree of hyperplasia and papillary growth. Cyst formation can be prominent (*spongy breast*) in the cat (see fig. 12.19).

Ductectasia is a progressive dilatation of the mammary duct system. When the continuity of the epithelial lining is broken, lipid material enters the stroma and provokes a foreign body reaction. Ductectasia can be difficult to differentiate from cysts, but spaces in the former are generally smaller and of recognizable ductal origin.

Focal Fibrosis (Fibrosclerosis)

Most of the dysplasias listed above will show some degree of fibrosis. Focal fibrosis can occur in lobular hyperplasia and in ductal proliferation. The term is usually used as a qualifier and is rarely used as a final diagnosis.

Gynecomastia

Enlarged mammary glands in male dogs due to hyperplasia of ducts and stroma is referred to as gynecomastia. Acini of mammary glands may be present. This condition is often part of the feminizing syndrome in dogs with Sertoli cell tumors.

REFERENCES

1. Destexhe, E., Lespagnard, L., Degeyter, M., Heymann, R., and Coignoul, E. (1993) Immunohistochemical identification of myoepithelial and connective tissue cells in canine mammary tumors. *Vet Pathol* 30:146-154.
2. Fowler, E.H., Wilson, G.R., and Koestner, A. (1974) Biologic behavior of canine mammary neoplasms based on a histogenetic classification. *Vet Pathol* 30:20-27.
3. Moulton, J.E. (1990) Tumors of the mammary gland. In *Tumors in Domestic Animals,* 3rd ed. University of California Press, Berkeley, pp. 518-552.
4. Hampe, J.E., and Misdorp, W. (1974) Tumours and dysplasias of the mammary gland. *Bull WHO* 50:111-133.
5. Weyer, K., and Hart, A.A.M. (1983) Prognostic factors in feline mammary carcinoma. *J Natl Cancer Inst* 70:709-716.
6. McEwen, E.G., Hayes, A.A., Harvey, H.J., Patnaik, A.K., Mooney, S., and Passe, S. (1984) Prognostic factors for feline mammary tumors. *J Amer Vet Med Assoc* 1852):201-204.
7. Misdorp, W., Cotchin, E., Hampe, J.F., Jabara, A.G., and Von Sandersleben, J. (1972) Canine malignant mammary tumours. II. Adenocarcinomas, solid carcinomas and spindle cell carcinomas. *Vet Pathol* 9:447-470.

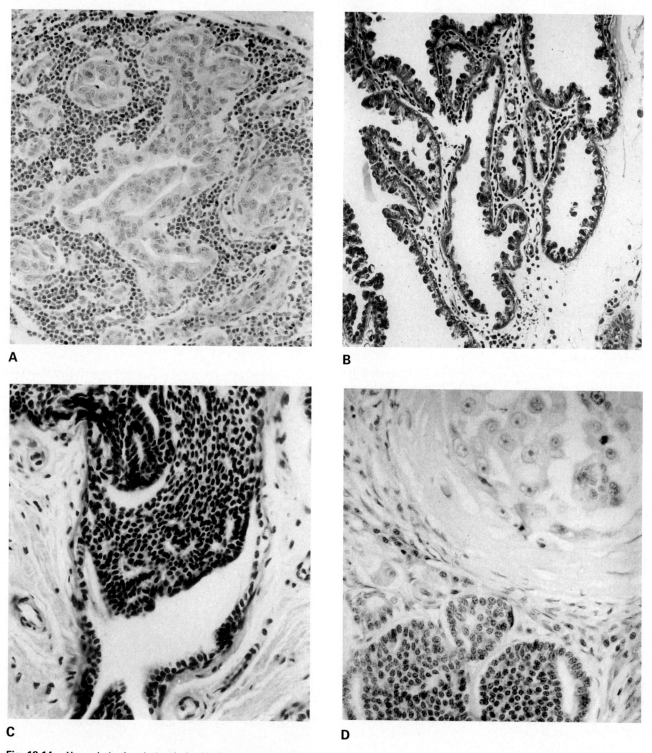

Fig. 12.14. Hyperplasia, dog. **A.** Atypical epithelial ductular hyperplasia. Marked lymphoid reaction. **B.** Regular hyperplasia of apocrine epithelial cells in distended duct. **C.** Regular hyperplasia of small cell type. **D.** Regular epithelial ductular hyperplasia (bottom) and growth of carcinoma (top) in lymphatic vessel.

8. Misdorp, W., Cotchin, E., Hampe, J.F., Jabara, A.G., and Von Sandersleben, J. (1973) Canine malignant mammary tumours. III. Special types of carcinomas, malignant mixed tumors. *Vet Pathol* 10:241-256.

9. Misdorp, W., Cotchin, E., Hampe, J.F., Jabara, A.G., and Von Sandersleben, J. (1971) Canine malignant mammary tumours. I. Sarcomas. *Vet Pathol* 8:99-117.

10. Kwapiem, R.P., Giles, R.C., Geil, R.G., and Casey, H.W. (1977) Basaloid adenomas of the mammary gland in beagle dogs administered investigational steroids. *J Natl Cancer Inst* 59(3):933-939.

11. World Health Organization. (1981) *Histological Typing of Breast Tumours,* 2nd ed. Geneva.

12. Gilbertson, S.R., Kurzma I.D., Zachrau, R.E., Hurvitz, A.I., and Black, M.M. (1983) Canine mammary epithelial neoplasms: Biologic implications of morphologic characteristics assessed in 232 dogs. *Vet Pathol* 20:127-142.

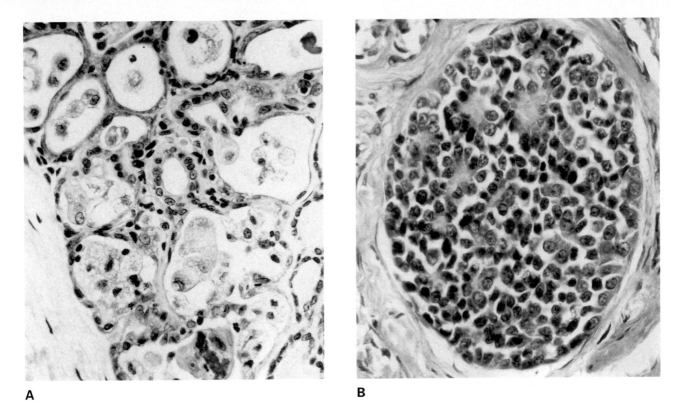

A

B

Fig. 12.15. Carcinoma in situ, dog. **A.** Intraductular accumulation of pleomorphic vacuolated cells. The diagnosis of *carcinoma in situ* rather than that of *reactive macrophages* was made because of cellular and nuclear pleomorphism. **B.** Noninfiltrating, in situ, ductal carcinoma (DCIS). Duct completely filled with moderately pleomorphic cells.

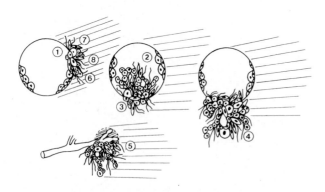

Fig. 12.16. Lobular lesions. *Patterns of lobular hyperplasia, adenosis.* 1. Intramural. 2. Exophytic in the lumen. 3. Intramural and/or periductal. 4. Infiltrating into periductule connective tissue. 5. Lobular localization. *All types of consist of the following components in varying proportions:* 6. Secretory epithelium. 7. Myoepithelium. 8. Connective tissue. (Drawings prepared by the late Professor J.F. Hampe, my teacher and friend. Reproduced with permission of Dr. K. Weyer from his doctoral thesis: Feline mammary tumors and hyperplasia. 1979.)

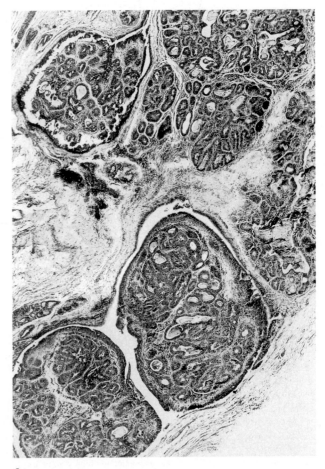

A

Fig. 12.17. **A.** Lobular hyperplasia, adenosis. Intramural-exophytic growth (right) and periductal growth (left top), cat. (continued)

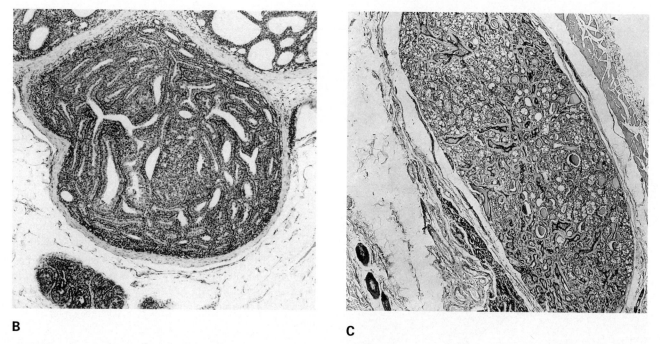

B

C

Fig. 12.17. (continued) **B.** Adenosis of intraductal type (*duct papillomatosis*), dog. **C.** Multilobular adenosis, well demarcated, cat.

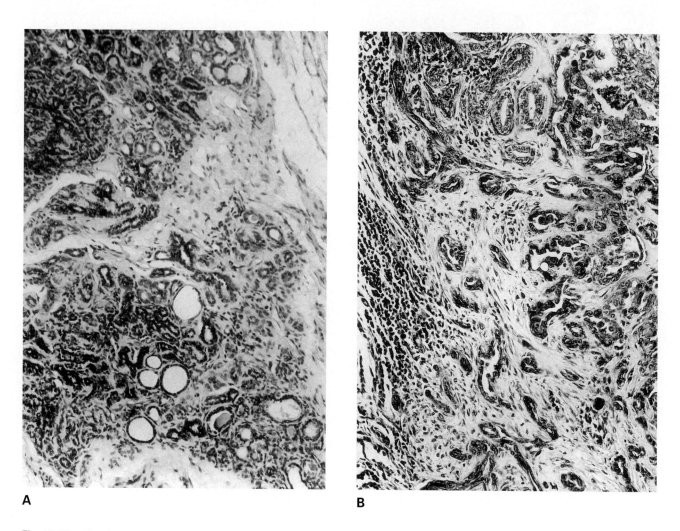

A

B

Fig. 12.18. Fibrosing adenosis, cat. **A.** Poorly demarcated. **B.** Sample showing some similarity to tubular adenocarcinoma. The presence of the myoepithelial layer points to adenosis.

605

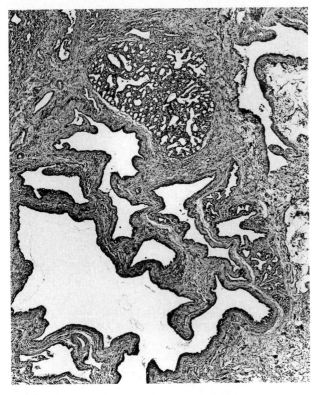

Fig. 12.19.   Extensive ectasia of ducts (*spongy breast*), cat.

Spontaneous Mammary Tumors of Other Species

This subject has been reviewed previously.[1,2] Mammary gland neoplasms are extremely rare in herbivorous animals, particularly the cow. The rare occurrence in cows is interesting because dairy cows lactate for many years and are generally allowed to survive to "cancer age." Among the 22 reported cases of mammary neoplasms in cows, eight were carcinomas and two sarcomas.[3] Papillomas of the teat have the highest incidence and are the most common tumor in the mammary gland of dairy cattle.[3]

Mammary tumors in goats, sheep, and horse are extremely rare. Ten of 4000 examined goats had fibrocystic disease, a well-recognized precancerous condition in women, and two had intraductal carcinomas.[4] Most mammary tumors reported to occur in horses were carcinomas.[1]

Mammary gland neoplasms are fairly common in female nonhuman primates and are histologically and biologically (metastasis) similar to mammary carcinomas in women.[5] Spontaneous mammary tumors constitute the most common tumor in laboratory mice and are common in rats, less common in guinea pigs, and rare in rabbits and hamsters.

REFERENCES

1. Kaiser, H.E. (1989) Comparative aspects of mammary cancer in other species. In *Cancer Growth and Progression,* 5. Kluwer Academic Publishers, Dordrecht, The Netherlands, pp. 142-151.
2. Madewell, B.R., and Theilen, G.H. (1987) Tumors of the mammary gland. In *Veterinary Cancer Medicine.* 2nd ed. Lea and Fibiger, Philadelphia, pp. 327-344.
3. Povey, R.C., and Osborne, A.D. (1969) Mammary gland neoplasia in the cow. A review of the literature and report of a fibrosarcoma. *Vet Pathol* 9:441-443.
4. Singh, B., and Her, P.K.P. (1972) Mammary intraductal carcinoma in goats. *Vet Pathol* 9:441-443.
5. Appleby, E.C., Keymer, L.F., and Hime, J.M. (1974) Three cases of suspected mammary neoplasia in non human primates. *J Comp Pathol* 84:351-357.

13 Tumors of the Endocrine Glands

C. C. Capen

INTRODUCTION

Endocrine glands are collections of specialized cells that synthesize, store, and release their secretions directly into the bloodstream. Because they lack a duct system, they are often referred to as ductless glands of internal secretion. Secretory products of specialized endocrine cells are hormones that are released into the extracellular fluids and transported via the blood. They affect the rates of specific chemical reactions in target cells and other body tissues. Endocrine glands in concert with the nervous system are involved in integrating and coordinating a wide variety of activities concerned with the maintenance of internal homeostasis of the body.

Endocrine glands are small in relation to many other body organs, widely distributed in the body, and connected with one another only by the bloodstream. They are richly supplied with blood, and there is a close anatomical relationship between endocrine cells and the capillary network. Peripheral cytoplasmic extensions of capillary endothelial cells have numerous fenestrae covered by a single membrane that facilitate rapid transport of raw materials and secretory products between the bloodstream and endocrine cells.

Hormones secreted by mammals are divided chemically into three major groups: polypeptides (about 80 percent), steroids (about 15 percent), and tyrosine derivatives (about 5 percent). By knowing the chemical nature of a hormone, it is possible to predict much about its mechanism of action, receptors, solubility, half-life in blood, and its plasma protein-binding characteristics (table 13.1).

Polypeptide hormones produced by organs such as the adenohypophysis, pancreatic islets, parathyroid glands,

thyroid C cells, and gastrointestinal tract share the following characteristics: (1) their primary site of action is the plasma membrane of target cells, (2) specific receptors for the hormone are proteins that are an integral part of the plasma membrane, often with transmembrane domains, (3) they are water soluble, (4) they have a short half-life in blood (usually measured in minutes), and (5) they lack specific plasma-binding proteins (table 13.1). There appears to be a single common intracellular pathway for many different polypeptide hormones. It begins with the activation of the enzyme adenylate cyclase in the plasma membrane of target cells, followed by the intracellular formation of cyclic adenosine monophosphate (cAMP) from adenosine triphosphate (ATP), and subsequent activation of cAMP-dependent protein kinases.

Steroid hormones produced by organs such as the adrenal cortex and gonads account for approximately 15 percent of mammalian hormones and share the following characteristics: (1) primary site of action is the nucleus of target cells, (2) high affinity "functional" receptors are proteins in the nucleus of target cells, (3) they are lipid soluble, which facilitates their easy entry and transport through the cell membrane, (4) they have a long half-life in blood (typically measured in hours or days), and (5) they reversibly bind to high affinity, specific-binding proteins in plasma for transport to target cells. After steroid hormones are within target cells they may bind initially to cytoplasmic receptors; the hormone-receptor complex subsequently is translocated into the nucleus, where it binds to the high affinity receptors and increases genomic expression. The interaction of steroid hormones with the genetic information in the nucleus results in increased transcription of messenger ribonucleic acid (mRNA), which directs

TABLE 13.1. Comparison of major classes of hormones

Hormone Class	Primary Site of Action	Receptors	Solubility	Half-Life in Blood	Plasma-Binding Protein
Polypeptides (catecholamines)	Plasma membrane	Proteins in plasma membrane	Aqueous	Minutes	None
Steroids (iodothyronines)	Nucleus	High affinity functional receptors in nucleus	Lipophilic	Hours > days	Specific binding proteins

new protein synthesis (e.g., enzymes, binding or structural proteins) by specific target cells (table 13.1).

The third chemical group of hormones are the tyrosine derivatives. They account for approximately 5 percent of mammalian hormones and include the catecholamines (epinephrine and norepinephrine) secreted by the adrenal medulla and the iodothyronines [thyroxine (T_4) and triiodothyronine (T_3)] produced by follicular cells of the thyroid gland. Catecholamines share a similar mechanism of action with polypeptide hormones, whereas iodothyronines more closely resemble steroid hormones (table 13.1).

There are certain morphological differences among endocrine cells that secrete polypeptide and steroid hormones. These structural differences that normally exist are also found in neoplastic cells derived from the different endocrine glands. Normal and neoplastic cells concerned with the synthesis of polypeptide hormone have a well-developed endoplasmic reticulum with many attached ribosomes for assembly of hormone. They also have a prominent Golgi apparatus for packaging hormone into small granules for intracellular storage and transport.

Secretory granules are unique for cells that secrete polypeptide hormones (and catecholamines) and provide a mechanism for intracellular storage of preformed hormone. These membrane-limited granules represent macromolecular aggregations of active hormone, often in association with a specific-binding protein and chromogranin A. Upon receipt of an appropriate signal for hormone secretion, the contraction of microfilaments and microtubules moves secretory granules to the periphery of the endocrine cell, where the limiting membrane of the granule fuses with the plasma membrane of the cell. The hormone-containing granule core is extruded into the extracellular perivascular space either by emiocytosis or exocytosis from the endocrine cell. Neoplasms derived from endocrine cells that secrete polypeptide hormone or catecholamine may release recently synthesized hormone on a continuous or episodic basis and often have only a few characteristic secretory granules in their cytoplasm.

Neoplasms derived from polypeptide hormone secreting endocrine cells usually consist of one predominant cell type and are associated with the secretion of one major polypeptide hormone. However, there is evidence from immunocytochemical and electron microscopic investigations that some endocrine tumors may be composed of more than one type of neoplastic cell and be capable of synthesizing multiple hormones (e.g., pancreatic islet cell tumors may stain positive for insulin, glucagon, somatostatin, and pancreatic polypeptide); however, an overproduction of one hormone (e.g., insulin) usually predominates and is responsible for the clinical disease syndrome.

Neoplasms derived from steroid hormone secreting endocrine cells are characterized by having large lipid bodies in their cytoplasm that contain cholesterol, cholesterol esters, and other precursor molecules for hormone synthesis. The lipid bodies are in close proximity to an extensive

tubular network of smooth endoplasmic reticulum and large mitochondria that contains the hydroxylase and dehydrogenase enzyme systems necessary for the attachment of various side chains and radicals to the basic steroid nucleus. Steroid hormone producing cells lack secretory granules and are unable to store significant amounts of preformed hormone. They are dependent on continued synthesis to maintain the normal secretory rate for a particular steroid hormone.

The histopathological separation between nodular hyperplasia, adenoma, and carcinoma often is more difficult in endocrine glands than in most other organs of the body. However, criteria for the separation should be established and applied in a uniform manner in the evaluation of proliferative lesions in endocrine glands. For many endocrine glands (especially thyroid C cells, secretory cells of the adrenal medulla, thyroid follicular cells, parathyroid chief cells, endocrine cells of the pancreas, and specific trophic hormone secreting cells of the adenohypophysis) there appears to be a continuous spectrum of proliferative lesions between focal (nodular) hyperplasia and adenomas derived from a specific population of secretory cells.[1]

It appears to be a common feature of endocrine glands that prolonged stimulation of a population of secretory cells predisposes to the subsequent development of a higher incidence of tumors than expected in a control population. Long-continued stimulation may lead to the development of clones of cells within the hyperplastic endocrine glands that grow more rapidly than the rest and are more susceptible to genetic alterations that lead to neoplastic transformation when exposed to the right combination of promoting agents.

Focal (nodular) hyperplasia usually appears as multiple small areas in one or both (for paired) endocrine gland(s) that are well-demarcated but not encapsulated from normal cells. There usually is only minimal compression of adjacent cells in the normal endocrine tissue. Cells making up an area of focal hyperplasia closely resemble the cells of origin; however, the cytoplasmic area may be slightly enlarged and the nucleus more hyperchromatic than in the normal endocrine cell.

Excessive focal growth of endocrine cells is the consequence of aberrant secretion of growth stimulating and/or function stimulating hormone(s) and has been referred to as *nonneoplastic endocrine hyperplasia*.[2] Lesions in endocrine organs of this type are considered to be largely reversible upon cessation of the inciting stimulus. Nodules arising in hyperplastic endocrine glands may be of polyclonal as well as of clonal origin.[2] Hyperfunction and cellular hypertrophy associated with nonneoplastic endocrine hyperplasia are completely reversible when the overstimulation ceases; however, chronic and severe hyperplasia of endocrine tissues may not be fully reversible.[2] Examples of pathogenic mechanisms that can result in nonneoplastic endocrine hyperplasia include (1) pathologic overproduction of trophic hormones (e.g.,

ACTH by a corticotroph adenoma) or hormone-like factor(s) [e.g., long-acting thyroid stimulator (LATS) in Grave's disease] of human patients, (2) disruption of negative feedback control system as in iodine-deficient goiter or parathyroid chief cell hyperplasia associated with chronic renal disease or nutritional imbalances, and (3) exogenous administration of trophic hormones (e.g., estrogen stimulation of prolactin secreting cells in the pituitary of rats).

There are several characteristics of nonneoplastic endocrine hyperplasia that can not be explained solely on the basis of simple systemic overstimulation and that emphasize the overlap between nonneoplastic and neoplastic growth in endocrine glands. These unique characteristics of nonneoplastic endocrine hyperplasia include the following: (1) hyperplasia is not a fully reversible process, (2) hyperplasia often is focal or nodular and not uniformly diffuse, (3) hyperplastic nodules may grow autonomously, (4) hyperplastic nodules may secondarily acquire the features of autonomous growth, (5) hyperplastic endocrine nodules may be clonal as well as polyclonal or be of both types within the same gland, (6) clonal nodules may become heterogeneous, polymorphic, and indistinguishable from polyclonal lesions, and (7) both hypo- and hyperfunction may develop in hyperplastic nodules of endocrine organs.[2]

Adenomas are solitary nodules in one endocrine gland (or occasionally in both for paired endocrine glands) that usually are larger than the multiple areas of focal hyperplasia. They are sharply demarcated from the adjacent normal glandular parenchyma by a thin, partial to complete, fibrous capsule. The adjacent parenchyma is compressed to varying degrees depending on the size of the adenoma. Cells composing an adenoma are phenotypically uniform and may closely resemble the cells of origin morphologically and in their architectural pattern of arrangement. However, adenomas often have histological differences from normal glands such as multiple layers of cells lining follicles and vascular trabeculae or solid clusters of secretory cells subdivided into packets by a fine fibrovascular stroma. The term *adenoma* should be used to designate *true neoplasms* arising in an endocrine organ that appear as nodular lesions that grow autonomously in the absence of known systemic or locally acting growth stimulating agents. It should be emphasized that the separation of adenoma from focal hyperplasia in endocrine organs solely on the basis of histological criteria is unreliable and arbitrary using existing morphological methods.

Carcinomas often are larger than adenomas and result in a macroscopically detectable enlargement in one (or occasionally both, for paired) endocrine gland(s). The accurate separation between adenoma and carcinoma of an endocrine gland also can be difficult using only morphological criteria. Histopathologic features that are suggestive of malignancy in an endocrine tumor include intraglandular invasion, invasion into and through the capsule of the gland with establishment of secondary foci

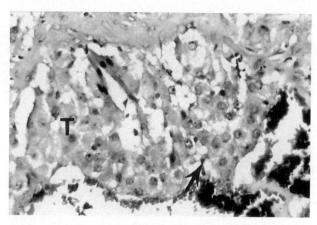

Fig. 13.1.   Subendothelial growth of tumor (T) cells in a pheochromocytoma of a rat. The blood filled space is lined by endothelial cells.

of growth in the periglandular fibrous and adipose connective tissues, formation of tumor cell thrombi within vessels (especially muscular walled), and the establishment of metastases at distant sites. The spread of neoplastic endocrine cells subendothelially in highly vascular benign tumors should not be mistaken for vascular invasion (fig. 13.1). Malignant endocrine cells may be more pleomorphic (including oval or spindle shaped) than normal, but nuclear pleomorphism and other cytological characteristics are not consistent criteria to distinguish an adenoma from a carcinoma in endocrine organs. Mitotic figures may be frequent in malignant endocrine cells, but the significance of this criterion can vary considerably with the degree of background stimulation of the endocrine gland. Therefore, predicting biological behavior (benign vs. malignant) of endocrine tumors is difficult based only upon histopathologic evaluation and clinically should be correlated with careful retrospective analysis of a substantial number of similar cases in a particular animal species.

Many neoplasms derived from endocrine glands are functionally (endocrinologically) active, secrete an excessive amount of hormone either continuously or episodically, and result in dramatic clinical syndromes of hormone excess. Examples in animals that are described in this chapter include, among others, the hypoglycemia of beta-cell neoplasms of the pancreatic islets in dogs; hyperthyroidism associated with adenomas and carcinomas derived from thyroid follicular cells in cats and dogs; hypercalcemia produced by parathyroid hormone producing parathyroid tumors in dogs and cats; growth hormone secreting pituitary tumors in cats and dogs; hypercalcitoninism in bulls and other animal species with thyroid C cell tumors; hyperadrenocorticism associated either with adrenocorticotropin (ACTH) secreting pituitary corticotroph adenomas or neoplasms derived from the adrenal cortex (zona fasciculata) in dogs; hypertension resulting from overproduction of catecholamines by tumors of the adrenal medulla; and gastric ulceration associated with gastrin producing tumors of the endocrine pancreas.[3]

Quantitation of hormone levels in serum or plasma in the basal, stimulated, or suppressed state and/or the measurement of hormonal metabolites in the urine over a 24 hour period of excretion often is essential to confirm that an endocrine tumor is functional and is releasing hormone at an abnormally elevated rate. Morphologically, an endocrine tumor often can be interpreted as endocrinologically active if the rim of normal tissue around the tumor, the opposite of paired endocrine glands, or the nontumorous endocrine glands undergo trophic atrophy due to negative feedback inhibition by the elevated hormone levels or by an altered blood constituent (e.g., elevated blood calcium). In response to the autonomous secretion of hormone by the tumor, the nonneoplastic secretory cells (especially in the cytoplasmic area) become smaller than normal, and eventually the number of cells is decreased. Functional pituitary neoplasms secreting an excess of a particular trophic hormone (e.g., ACTH) will be associated with striking hypertrophy and hyperplasia of target cells in the adrenal cortex (e.g., zonae fasciculata and reticularis) or follicular cells in the thyroid glands in response to thyroid stimulating hormone (TSH).

REFERENCES

1. Capen, C.C. (2001) Toxic responses of the endocrine system. In: C.D. Klaassen (ed.), *Casarett and Doull's Toxicology: The Basic Science of Poisons*, 6th ed. McGraw Hill, New York, pp. 711-759.
2. Studer, H., and Derwahl, M. (1995) Mechanisms of nonneoplastic endocrine hyperplasia—a changing concept: A review focused on the thyroid gland. *Endocrine Rev* 16:411-425.
3. Capen, C.C.. and Martin, S.L. (1989) Mechanisms that lead to disease of the endocrine system in animals. *Toxicol Pathol* 17:234-249.

TUMORS AND NONNEOPLASTIC CYSTS OF THE PITUITARY GLAND

Functional Corticotroph (Chromophobe) Adenoma in Pars Distalis

Incidence

Functional tumors arising in the pituitary gland in domestic animals are most commonly derived from corticotroph (ACTH secreting) cells in the pars distalis or pars intermedia (in dogs) and associated with a clinical syndrome of cortisol excess (Cushing's-like disease) (see fig. 13.2 A).[1] These neoplasms are encountered most frequently in dogs, occasionally in cats,[2] and infrequently in other animal species. They develop in adult to aged dogs and have been reported in a number of breeds.[3-6] Boxers and Boston terriers appear to be breeds having a higher incidence of functional (ACTH producing) pituitary

tumors. The spectrum of dramatic clinical manifestations and lesions that develop are primarily the result of a long-term overproduction of cortisol by hyperplastic adrenal cortices. These changes are the result of the combined gluconeogenic, lipolytic, protein catabolic, and antiinflammatory actions of glucocorticoid hormones on many organ systems of the body. There are other causes of cortisol excess in dogs, including functional (zona fasciculata) adrenal cortical neoplasms and suspected biochemical derangements in the hypothalamus that result in corticotroph hyperplasia that results in a similar clinical syndrome (refer to section on Tumors of the Adrenal Cortex and fig. 13.13 D).

Clinical Characteristics

A number of distinctive clinical and functional alterations develop in dogs with corticotroph (ACTH secreting) adenomas, resulting in the syndrome of hyperadrenocorticism.[5] Eighty-four percent of dogs with pituitary-dependent hyperadrenocorticism have been reported to have adenomas derived from cells either of the pars distalis or the pars intermedia.[7] Immunocytochemical staining of the tumor cells gave a positive reaction for ACTH, beta-lipotrophin, and beta-endorphin. Nearly all of the clinical and clinicopathologic abnormalities are due directly to the high circulating concentrations of cortisol (not ACTH). If blood cortisol levels are decreased by specific chemotherapy (o,p′-DDD or mitotane) of the hyperplastic adrenal cortices, the physical and laboratory abnormalities will return to normal even though the pituitary tumor continues to produce an excess of ACTH.

Centripetal redistribution of adipose tissue leads to prominent fat pads on the dorsal midline of the neck, giving the neck and shoulders a thick appearance. Appetite and intake of food may be increased or ravenous, either as a direct result of the hypercortisolism on the CNS or destruction of hypothalamic appetite control (satiety) centers in the ventromedial nucleus by a large pituitary tumor. The muscles of the extremities and abdomen are weakened and atrophied. The loss of tone of abdominal muscles and muscles of the abaxial skeleton results in gradual abdominal enlargement (pot belly), lordosis, muscle trembling, and a straight legged skeletal-braced posture to support the body's weight. Profound atrophy of the temporal muscles may result in obvious concave indentations and readily palpable prominences of underlying skull bones. A cortisol associated myopathy contributes to the pendulous abdomen and muscle weakness in dogs. Hepatomegaly due to increased glycogen deposition, fat accumulation, and vacuolation of smooth endoplasmic reticulum in liver cells due to enzyme induction by cortisol contributes to the development of the distended, often pendulous, abdomen.

Skin lesions occur in more than 90 percent of dogs with hyperadrenocorticism. The initial changes in the skin are over points of wear. The hair coat becomes thin, rough, and dry. Hair shafts can be easily broken and dislodged from their follicles. As the disease progresses these initial skin changes spread in a bilaterally symmetrical pattern to involve a significant portion of the body surface. The skin is of a fine and dry texture, coarsely wrinkled, and often "paper thin." The basic lesion in the skin, caused by the excessive secretion of cortisol, is a loss of collagen and elastin fibers in the dermis and subcutis, often with severe atrophy of the epidermis and pilosebaceous apparatus. The majority of hair follicles are inactive and are in the telogen phase of the growth cycle. The prominent comedones observed in the skin, particularly on the ventral abdomen, represent hair follicles distended with keratin and debris. The outer stratum corneum is thickened considerably, giving the skin surface a dry, roughened, scaly appearance.

Other distinctive skin changes in dogs with functional pituitary tumors include hyperpigmentation and mineralization. The accumulations of melanin pigment may be either focal or diffuse and consist of increased numbers of melanocytes in the basal epidermis, the stratum corneum, and the dermis and upper subcutis. Cutaneous mineralization is a characteristic lesion (detected clinically or in a skin biopsy) in up to 30 percent of dogs with hyperadrenocorticism. Numerous mineral crystals deposited along collagen and elastin fibers in the dermis may protrude through the atrophic and thinned epidermis. In less severe cases the epidermis remains intact and appears irregularly elevated by the opaque white deposits of mineral. A mild to moderate granulomatous inflammatory reaction often accompanies the deposition of mineral in soft tissues. Another common site for mineralization is the interalveolar septa of the lung. The pathogenesis of the mineralization is related to the increased gluconeogenesis stimulated by the cortisol excess that leads to increased protein catabolism and formation of an organic matrix that attracts and binds calcium and phosphorus. Dermal vessels often are prominent and readily visible through the thin skin. In an occasional dog with marked abdominal distension and loss of supporting dermal collagen and elastin fibers, the superficial vessels become severely stretched and dilated, forming striae similar to those described in human beings with Cushing's syndrome.

The syndrome of long-term cortisol excess often is complicated by an increased susceptibility to infection with the development of bacterial or fungal infections in the skin, urinary tract, conjunctiva, and lung. Multifocal areas of suppurative folliculitis and dermatitis develop near the lip folds and footpads and elsewhere in the skin.[8] A frequent serious complication in dogs with hyperadrenocorticism is a suppurative bronchopneumonia that can be fatal if not detected early and treated appropriately.

Clinical laboratory abnormalities due to cortisol excess in dogs are characteristic and include in the complete blood count leukocytosis (> 25,000/dl), mature neutrophilia (due to decreased migration and bone marrow stimulation), lymphopenia (due to lysis and lymphocyte redistribution), eosinopenia (due to lysis and sequestration in certain tissues), monocytosis, and erythrocytosis with nucleated red blood cells. Serum chemistry abnormalities include a marked increase in alkaline phosphatase (steroid and hepatic isoenzymes), a mild increase in alanine transaminase (associated with the steroid induced hepatopathy), and moderate hyperglycemia. Alkaline phosphatase concentrations greater than 1000 IU/l are highly suggestive of cortisol excess in dogs. Although electrolyte disturbances are common in human patients with Cushing's syndrome, it is uncommon for dogs to develop disturbances in circulating levels of sodium, chloride, or potassium.

Laboratory evaluation of adrenal cortical function became considerably more accurate with the development of satisfactory methods for measuring the concentration of corticosteroids in plasma. These methods permit adrenal cortical disease to be evaluated directly by measuring cortisol in the basal state or in response to suppression by exogenous dexamethasone (low or high dose) or stimulation by exogenous ACTH. The plasma levels of cortisol in unstressed caged dogs range from 1.0 to 2.5 µg/dl in our laboratory. Normal dogs not adapted to a veterinary medical hospital have higher plasma concentrations of cortisol, varying from 2.0 to 8.5 µg/dl.

The clinical diagnosis of hyperadrenocorticism usually can be confirmed by using one or more screening tests such as urine cortisol:creatinine (> 20), ACTH stimulation test (> 15 µg/dl), and low dose dexamethasone suppression (serum cortisol > 1.5 µg/dl at 8 hr). These tests are subsequently followed with confirming tests that attempt to differentiate whether the hyperadrenocorticism is pituitary or adrenal dependent, either by measuring the plasma ACTH concentration or by evaluating the response of serum cortisol to high dose dexamethasone suppression.

The basal concentration of cortisol in the plasma of dogs with hyperadrenocorticism ranges from 3 to 10 µg/dl or higher. Most dogs with bilateral adrenal cortical hyperplasia (either idiopathic or caused by an ACTH secreting pituitary tumor) respond to ACTH by an exaggerated increase in the plasma concentration of cortisol, ranging from 20 to 60 µg/dl at 2 hours postinjection. Some dogs respond with a lower but more prolonged elevation in cortisol concentration. The ACTH stimulation test also has proven useful in monitoring the response to o,p′-DDD therapy. Although a more expensive and time consuming test, the ACTH stimulation provides a more accurate assessment of adrenocortical destruction by chemotherapy than the urine cortisol:creatinine ratio.[9]

The plasma cortisol level in dogs with hyperadrenocorticism usually will fall after the injection of dexamethasone only if the adrenal gland remains under the trophic control of ACTH (as with idiopathic cortical hyperplasia or small adenomas of the adenohypophysis). If a dog has a larger corticotroph (ACTH secreting) adenoma of the adenohypophysis or if the adrenal cortex is functioning independently of endogenous ACTH (e.g., adenoma or carcinoma), the dexamethasone suppression test usually results in minimal or no significant decrease in plasma cortisol concentration. Low doses of dexamethasone (0.1 mg/kg) suppress ACTH production and subsequently plasma cortisol levels in normal dogs, but usually do not suppress cortisol levels in dogs with pituitary dependent hyperadrenocorticism or adrenal cortical neoplasms. High doses of dexamethasone (1.0 mg/kg) usually suppress plasma cortisol levels in dogs with pituitary dependent hyperadrenocorticism (< 1.5 μg/dl) but do not significantly suppress levels in dogs with adrenal cortical neoplasms (> 1.5 μg/dl).

Measurement of circulating levels of ACTH is another way to differentiate between pituitary dependent and adrenal dependent hyperadrenocorticism. Radioimmunoassays for plasma ACTH in the dog have reported a mean concentration of 46 pg/ml (range 17–98 pg/ml).[10] Dogs with functional adrenal cortical neoplasms have plasma ACTH concentrations two standard deviations or more below (< 20 pg/ml) the mean value for normal dogs, whereas dogs with pituitary dependent hyperadrenocorticism have plasma ACTH values of more than 40 pg/ml.[11] Pituitary and adrenal dependent hyperadrenocorticism usually can be differentiated by the laboratory methods described above.[12]

Macroscopic Pathology

The pituitary gland usually is enlarged in dogs with corticotroph adenomas and ranges in size from 0.7 × 0.6 × 0.5 cm to 4.0 × 2.5 × 2.5 cm. However, the occurrence or severity of functional disturbance has no consistent relationship to the size of the neoplasm. Small chromophobe adenomas (*microadenomas*) are as likely to be endocrinologically active as larger neoplasms. The magnitude of expansion of corticotroph adenomas was dependent upon the degree of insensitivity to negative feedback by glucocorticoids.[13] The larger adenomas are often firmly attached to the base of the sella turcica, but without evidence of erosion of the sphenoid bone. In the animal species most likely to develop pituitary neoplasms (dog and horse), the diaphragma sella is incomplete. Therefore, the line of least resistance in the dog and horse favors dorsal expansion of the gradually enlarging mass with resulting invagination into the infundibular cavity, dilatation of the infundibular recess and third ventricle, and eventual compression and replacement of the hypothalamus and thalamus. This differs from the situation in humans where the complete diaphragma sella, which is a tough reflection of dura mater separating the hypophysis from the cranial cavity, favors ventrolateral growth of the neoplasm and erosion of the sphenoid bones that form the walls and base of the sella turcica. Dorsal expansion of the larger pituitary neoplasms results in either a broad based indentation and compression of the overlying hypothalamus or extension into and replacement of the parenchyma of the hypothalamus and occasionally the thalamus; however, the dorsal extension of the tumor is not interpreted to be a criterion of malignancy for pituitary tumors (fig. 13.2 A). Focal areas of hemorrhage, necrosis, mineralization, and liquefaction are frequently encountered in the larger pituitary neoplasms. Pituitary macrotumors in dogs can be readily identified by magnetic resonance imaging and frequently are associated with neurological signs of disorientation and ataxia.[14,15]

Dogs with functional corticotroph adenomas have bilateral enlargement of the adrenal glands (fig. 13.2 A) due to chronic excessive stimulation by ACTH. The hypertrophy and hyperplasia often is striking and is due entirely to an increased amount of cortical parenchyma, primarily in the zona fasciculata and to a lesser extent in the zona reticularis. Nodules of yellow-orange cortical tissue often are identified outside the capsule in the periadrenal fat and extending into the medulla. The corticomedullary junction is irregular, and the medulla frequently is compressed.

Histopathology

Pituitary adenomas are composed of well-differentiated secretory cells supported by fine connective tissue septa. Chromophobe adenomas are subclassified into sinusoidal and diffuse types on the basis of the predominant pattern of arrangement of neoplastic cells. The tumor cells in the sinusoidal type are separated into compartments of varied sizes and shapes by delicate, often incomplete, connective tissue septa containing capillaries or small venules (fig. 13.2 B). The sinusoidal type of pituitary tumor is more vascular than the diffuse type, and in some areas the blood sinusoids attain considerable size and appear to be lined by neoplastic cells. When the tumor cells palisade along the connective tissue septa or blood sinusoids, they are more elongated and have oval or spindle shaped nuclei. The tumor cells in the diffuse type of adenoma lack a characteristic architectural arrangement and appear as sheets or masses of large chromophobic cells (fig. 13.2 C). Blood vessels are small and few in number. The connective tissue stroma is sparse.

Corticotroph adenomas are composed of either large or small chromophobic cells. Large-cell chromophobes make up the majority of adenomas of this type. They are polyhedral and have large vesicular nuclei with one or two prominent nucleoli and an abundant eosinophilic cytoplasm with distinct cell boundaries. The cytoplasm is devoid of secretory granules detectable by the conventional histochemical procedures employed for pituitary cytology. Small-cell chromophobes constitute the remaining pituitary adenomas of this type. They are roughly half the size of large-cell chromophobes and have small dark nuclei with indistinct nucleoli and a small amount of cytoplasm. Mitotic figures are infrequent in both types of chromophobic cells.

Remnants of the pars distalis may be identified near the periphery of the pituitary adenomas. Demarcation between the neoplasm and the pars distalis is not distinct. The separation is effected by an incomplete layer of condensed reticulum, and there usually is not a complete capsule. Acidophils and occasionally basophils are incorporated within the neoplasm near the margin. The pars

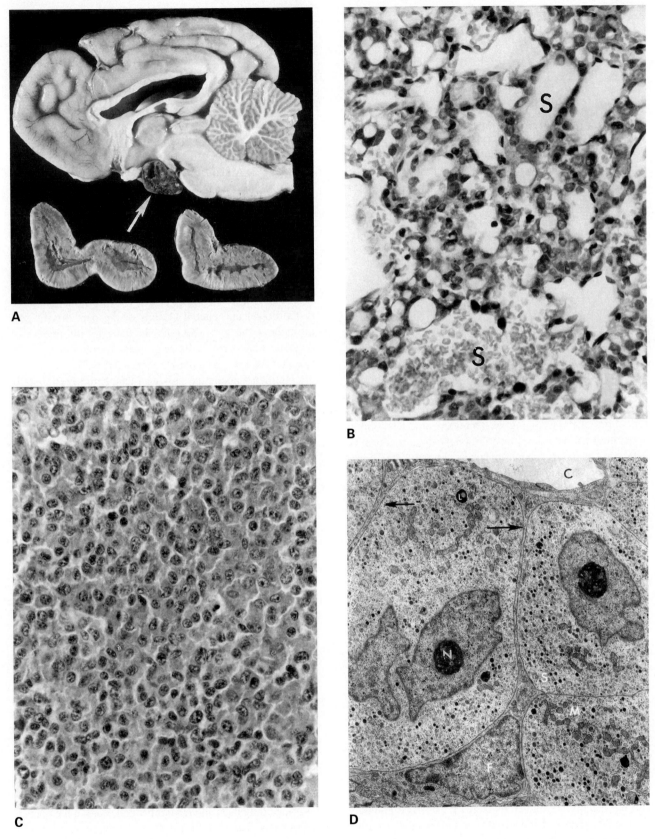

Fig. 13.2. Functional chromophobe adenoma. **A.** Corticotroph adenoma (arrow) in the hypophysis with bilateral adrenal cortical hyperplasia in a dog. The hypothalamus is compressed by the dorsally expanding pituitary adenoma. **B.** Corticotroph adenoma, sinusoidal type. The neoplastic cells are separated into compartments by the numerous endothelial-lined ascular sinusoids *(S)*. **C.** Corticotroph adenoma, diffuse type. The sheets of large chromophobic tumor cells lack a characteristic pattern of arrangement. Capillaries are small, indistinct, and few in number. **D.** Neoplastic corticotrophs. The tumor cells have irregularly shaped nuclei and prominent nucleoli *(N)* and are supported by a reticular framework of follicular cells *(F)* that extend long cytoplasmic processes (arrows) to the perivascular spaces *(C* is capillary). The cytoplasm of the neoplastic cells contains numerous small secretory granules *(S)* of varying electron density, occasional dense lipid bodies *(L),* and scattered mitochondria (M).

613

distalis is either partly replaced by the neoplasm or severely compressed and composed principally of heavily granulated acidophils. The posterior lobe and infundibular stalk are either infiltrated and disrupted by tumor cells or completely incorporated within the larger neoplasms. The hypothalamus is severely compressed or replaced by the large, dorsally expanding, corticotroph adenomas (fig. 13.2 A). There are increased numbers of fibrous astrocytes and hemosiderin laden macrophages, perivascular hemorrhages, a loss of neurons, and myelin degradation within the hypothalamus and occasionally in the thalamus around the dorsally expanding mass of neoplastic cells. Focal areas of hemorrhage, coagulation and liquefactive necrosis, mineralization, and cholesterol clefts often occur within the larger corticotroph adenomas.

Ultrastructural and Immunocytochemical Characteristics

Cells constituting functional corticotroph adenomas in dogs have definite evidence of secretory activity.[16] Organelles concerned with protein synthesis (endoplasmic reticulum) and packaging of secretory products (Golgi apparatus) are well developed in neoplastic corticotrophs. The predominating neoplastic cells are large, relatively electron dense, and roughly polyhedral or cuboidal (fig. 13.2 D). The outline of the neoplastic cells is irregular, and cytoplasmic projections extend between neighboring cells or encompass them completely. The nucleus usually is centrally located and irregular in shape with deep indentations and contains one or two dense nucleoli (fig. 13.2 D).

The neoplastic cells are supported by a reticular framework of follicular cells.[16,17] These cells are stellate and have long cytoplasmic processes that extend between the neoplastic cells and terminate on the extracellular accumulations of colloid or on perivascular spaces (fig. 13.2 D). The cytoplasmic matrix of the follicular cells is finely granular and comparatively electron dense because of the presence of numerous organelles.

Cells making up functional corticotroph adenomas contain mature secretory granules at the level of ultrastructure. This is in contrast to the absence of demonstrable secretory granules within the neoplastic cells as observed through light microscopy following the application of conventional histochemical procedures for pituitary cytology. Secretory granules vary in number from cell to cell but usually are numerous (fig. 13.2 D). The granules are roughly spherical and are surrounded by a delicate limiting membrane. The space between the secretory granule and its covering membrane is relatively wide compared with the granules in other cells of the adenohypophysis of the dog. The secretory granules, particularly those in the vicinity of the Golgi apparatus, are small (mean diameter 170 nm) and extremely electron dense, and they have a prominent submembranous space. Larger secretory granules may be admixed with the small secretory granules, particularly near the periphery of the neoplastic cells. They are uniformly less electron dense, finely granular, and limited by a definite membrane. Within the membranes of the Golgi apparatus are small prosecretory granules of variable size, presumably in the process of formation. Secretory granules are observed occasionally in the process of becoming detached from the Golgi membranes.

In the normal dog pituitary gland immunocytochemical staining has demonstrated cells that stain for ACTH and melanocyte stimulating hormone (MSH) [antisera to porcine ACTH, synthetic ACTH-beta (1-24), and ACTH-beta (17-39)] and bovine beta-MSH are polyhedral to round, sparsely granulated, and most numerous in the ventrocentral and cranial portions of the pars distalis in dogs, where they occur in large groups. They are less numerous in the dorsal and caudal regions of the pars distalis and throughout the pars tuberalis. In the pars intermedia of dogs most endocrine cells demonstrated immunoreactivity to either ACTH, alpha-MSH, or beta-MSH.[18]

Pituitary adenomas arising in both the pars distalis and the pars intermedia, associated with the syndrome of cortisol excess in dogs, are composed of polyhedral cells that immunocytochemically stain selectively for ACTH and MSH.[19,20] Focal areas of hyperplasia and microadenomas, composed of similar ACTH/MSH cells, also are present in both lobes of the adenohypophysis. Pituitary adenomas arising in both the pars distalis and pars intermedia have positive immunocytochemical staining for ACTH, beta-lipotrophin, and beta-endorphin.[7] In spite of hypercortisolemia and neoplastic transformation of corticotrophs in dogs with pituitary dependent hyperadrenocorticism, corticotrophs usually remain responsive to hypophysiotropic stimulation by corticotrophin releasing hormone and other factors.[21]

Cells constituting functional corticotroph adenomas in dogs share many histological and ultrastructural features with the *adrenalectomy cell* reported in the hypophysis of rats.[22] They can be differentiated from acidophils and basophils of the canine hypophysis by the smaller size and lesser density of their secretory granules. The ACTH producing cell in the hypophysis is a large chromophobic cell. Following adrenalectomy this chromophobic cell had the highest content of tritium and the fastest rate of both incorporation (hormone synthesis) and loss (hormone secretion) of tritium of all the hypophyseal cell types. The adrenalectomy cell is morphologically distinct from gonadectomy or thyroidectomy cells and from other cell types in the normal hypophysis. The cytoplasm often is compressed between or indented by the neighboring pituitary cells. Chromophobe adenomas that possess secretory activity have been reported in humans and are associated with an increased secretion of ACTH. Cushing's disease was described initially in association with basophil adenomas of the hypophysis in human patients.

Nonfunctional Chromophobe Adenoma in Pars Distalis

Incidence

Nonfunctional (endocrinologically inactive) pituitary tumors are most common in dogs, cats, and parakeets and are rare in other species.[5,23] In contrast to the functional adenomas, there is no indication of any breed or sex predisposition. Although these chromophobe adenomas appear to be endocrinologically inactive, they may result in significant functional disturbances by virtue of compression atrophy of the pars nervosa and pars distalis or extension into the overlying brain.

Clinical Characteristics

Animals with nonfunctional pituitary adenomas usually are presented with clinical disturbances related to dysfunction of the central nervous and neurohypophyseal systems or lack of secretion of pituitary trophic hormones with diminished end-organ function (e.g., thyroid follicular cells, adrenal cortex, and gonads). The clinical history often includes depression, incoordination and other disturbances of balance, weakness, collapse with exercise, and a marked change in personality. Animals may become unresponsive to people and develop a tendency to hide at the slightest provocation. In long-standing cases there may be evidence of blindness with dilated and fixed pupils.[24] The body condition varies from a progressive loss of weight to obvious obesity. The animals often appear to be dehydrated, as evidenced by a lusterless dry hair coat, and the owner may have noticed increased water consumption and frequent urination. Parakeets with chromophobe adenomas often develop exophthalmos due to extension of neoplastic cells along the optic nerve, disturbances of balance and falling down from a perch, and diarrhea (associated with disturbances in water balance).

A consistent finding with both functional and nonfunctional pituitary tumors is the excretion of large volumes of dilute urine with a low specific gravity (approximately 1.007).[5] Water intake is increased correspondingly, and the owner often complains that the animal, previously housebroken, urinates frequently in the house. Disturbances of water balance (diabetes insipidus) are the result of either a direct diuretic effect exerted on the kidney by the elevated cortisol level or an interference with the synthesis and release of antidiuretic hormone (ADH).[25] The posterior lobe, infundibular stalk, and hypothalamus often are compressed or disrupted by the infiltration of neoplastic cells in dogs with pituitary tumors. This interrupts the nonmyelinated axons that transport ADH from the site of production in the hypothalamus (primarily in the supraoptic nucleus) to the site of release in the capillary plexus of the posterior lobe. Compression of neurosecretory neurons in the hypothalamus by the tumor may result in decreased ADH synthesis.

Clinical signs in animals with nonfunctional pituitary adenomas and hypopituitarism are not highly specific and could be confused with other disorders of the central nervous system, such as brain tumors and encephalitis (e.g., toxoplasmosis) or chronic renal disease. Hypopituitarism caused by pituitary tumors should be included in the differential diagnosis of adult to older animals with signs of incoordination, depression, polyuria, blindness, and a sudden change in personality. Since the blindness is central in origin, ophthalmoscopic evaluation of the eye usually fails to reveal significant lesions.

The daily administration of calcitonin to Sprague-Dawley and to a lesser degree Fischer 344 rats for 1 year has been reported to increase the incidence of nonfunctional pituitary adenomas.[26] Immunohistochemical analysis revealed that the tumor cells were negative for all of the major pituitary hormones, and serum levels of growth hormone, prolactin, ACTH, luteinizing hormone (LH), and follicle stiumlating hormone (FSH) were unchanged in calcitonin treated rats.[27] Immunohistochemistry and in situ hybridization analysis demonstrated that the nonfunctional pituitary tumors expressed the glycoprotein hormone alpha-subunit, and serum levels of alpha-subunit were markedly increased (approximately 20-fold).

Macroscopic Pathology

Nonfunctional pituitary adenomas usually reach considerable size before they cause obvious clinical signs and kill the animal (fig. 13.3 A). The proliferating tumor cells incorporate the remaining structures of the adenohypophysis and infundibular stalk. The neoplasms are firmly attached to the base of the sella turcica, but there usually is no evidence of erosion of the sphenoid bone. In dogs and cats the diaphragma sella is incomplete, so the line of least resistance favors dorsal expansion of the progressively enlarging adenoma, resulting either in a broad based indentation or extension into the overlying brain (fig. 13.3 B). The entire hypothalamus may be compressed and replaced by the tumor, which extends through the thalamus and protrudes into the lateral ventricles. The optic nerves are compressed and incorporated within the large neoplastic mass on the ventral aspect of the brain, accounting for the blindness observed clinically (fig. 13.3 A).

The adrenal glands of animals with large nonfunctional pituitary adenomas are small and often difficult to find at necropsy. The adrenals consist primarily of medullary tissue surrounded by a narrow zone of atrophic cortex (fig. 13.3 B). The adrenal cortex appears as a thin yellow-brown rim composed of a moderately thickened capsule and secretory cells of the outer layer, zona multiformis (glomerulosa). The zonae fasciculata and reticularis are severely atrophied compared with those in normal adrenal glands and secrete subnormal amounts of glucocorticoid hormones. Thyroid glands in animals with large pituitary adenomas may be either near normal or reduced in size, although to a much lesser degree than is the adrenal cortex (fig. 13.3 B). The

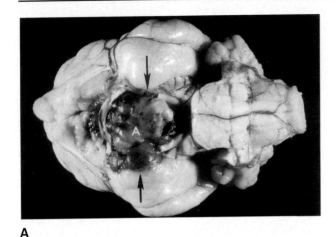

A

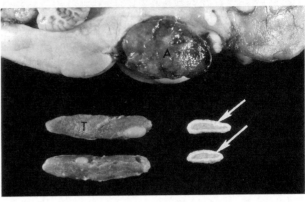

B

Fig. 13.3. Nonfunctional chromophobe adenoma of the pituitary gland. **A.** Ventral view of the brain of a 4-year-old male Siamese cat illustrating a large chromophobe adenoma *(A)*. The neoplasm has completely incorporated the pituitary, extended into the brain, and destroyed the optic nerves. Arrows mark the junction between the neoplastic tissue and brain parenchyma. **B.** Nonfunctional chromophobe adenoma *(A)* in a dog with expansion into the hypothalamus. There is severe trophic atrophy of the adrenal cortex (arrows), but the thyroid glands *(T)* are nearly normal size due to distention of follicles with colloid in the absence of thyrotropin.

majority of follicles are large, lined by flattened (atrophic) cuboidal follicular cells, and distended with a densely stained colloid showing little evidence of endocytotic activity because of a lack of thyroid stimulating hormone (TSH, thyrotrophin). Seminiferous tubules in the testis are small and have little evidence of active spermatogenesis.

Histopathology

The tumor cells are cuboidal to polyhedral and either are arranged in diffuse sheets or subdivided into small packets by fine connective tissue septa. Numerous small capillaries are present throughout the neoplasm. Special histochemical techniques for pituitary cytology fail to demonstrate specific secretory granules within the cytoplasm of tumor cells. The histogenesis of these tumors is uncertain, but they appear to be derived from pituitary cells that have not differentiated sufficiently to synthesize and secrete a specific trophic hormone.

Adenoma of the Pars Intermedia

Incidence

Adenoma derived from cells of the pars intermedia is the most common type of pituitary tumor in horses, the second most common type in dogs, infrequent in certain strains of laboratory rats and nonhuman primates,[28] and rare in other species. It develops in older horses, with females being affected more frequently than males. Nonbrachycephalic breeds of dogs develop adenomas in the pars intermedia more often than brachycephalic breeds.[5]

Clinical Characteristics

Adenomas of the pars intermedia in dogs either are endocrinologically inactive and associated with varying degrees of hypopituitarism and diabetes insipidus or are endocrinologically active and secrete excessive adrenocorticotropin (ACTH), leading to bilateral adrenal cortical hyperplasia and the syndrome of cortisol excess. The clinical signs in these dogs are similar to those described previously for corticotroph adenomas of the pituitary gland.

A sparsely granulated adenoma reportedly arising in the pars intermedia of a male *Macaca mulatta* was associated with gynecomastia, galactorrhea, and testicular atrophy.[28] The polygonal tumor cells were negative for prolactin, somatotropin, ACTH, LH, and thyrotropin by the peroxidase-antiperoxidase method, but occasional large (600 to 700 nm) secretory granules were demonstrated by electron microscopy.

Two cell populations have been identified in the pars intermedia of normal dogs by immunocytochemistry.[29] The predominant cell type (A cell) stains strongly for alpha-MSH as in the pars intermedia of other species. A second cell type (B cell) in the canine pars intermedia stains intensely for ACTH but not for alpha-MSH. This second cell population accounts for the high bioactive ACTH concentration found in the pars intermedia of dogs[29] and most likely gives rise to corticotroph adenomas of the pars intermedia in dogs with the syndrome of cortisol excess.[5]

The clinical syndrome associated with tumors of the pars intermedia in horses is characterized by polyuria, polydipsia, ravenous appetite, muscle weakness, somnolence, intermittent hyperpyrexia, and generalized hyperhidrosis.[30] The affected horses often develop a striking hypertrichosis (hirsutism) because of failure of the cyclic seasonal shedding of hair.[31-33] The hair over most of the trunk and extremities is long (as much as 4 or 5 inches), abnormally thick, wavy, and often matted together (fig. 13.4 A). Horses with larger tumors may have hyperglycemia (insulin resistant) and glycosuria,[32,34] probably the result of a down regulation of insulin receptors on tar-

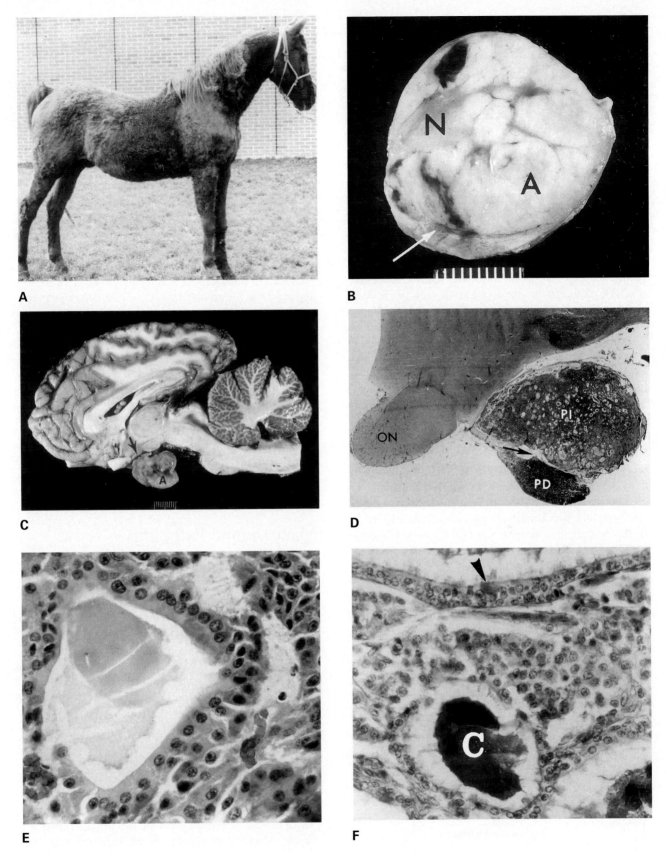

Fig. 13.4. Adenoma of the pars intermedia. **A.** Hirsutism resulting from a failure of cyclic shedding in a horse. **B.** Longitudinal section of adenoma *(A)* of same horse, incorporating the pars nervosa *(N)* and compressing the pars distalis (arrow). Scale = 1 cm. **C.** Large pars intermedia adenoma *(A)* in a horse with dorsal extension out of the sella turcica along lines of least resistance into the overlying hypothalamus. Many of the dramatic clinical signs with this tumor in horses are the result of disruption in hypothalamic and neurohypophyseal function. Scale = 1 cm. **D.** The tumor *(PI)* in a dog is sharply demarcated from the compressed pars distalis *(PD)*. The arrow indicates the residual hypophyseal lumen. Numerous colloid-containing follicles are present within the adenoma. *ON* refers to optic nerve. **E.** Tumor cells are large, cylindrical, or polyhedral, with oval nuclei, and are arranged around a colloid filled follicle. **F.** Adenoma from a dog illustrating nests of chromophobic cells interspersed between colloid-containing follicles *(C)* lined by cuboidal to low columnar, partially ciliated epithelium (arrowhead).

get cells induced by the chronic excessive intake of food and hyperinsulinemia.

The disturbances in carbohydrate metabolism and ravenous appetite, hirsutism, and hyperhidrosis are considered to be primarily a reflection of deranged hypothalamic function caused by the large pituitary tumors. Adenomas of the pars intermedia in horses often extend out of the sella turcica, expand dorsally because of the incomplete diaphragma sella, and severely compress the overlying hypothalamus (fig. 13.4 C). The hypothalamus is known to be the primary center for homeostatic regulation of body temperature, appetite, and cyclic shedding of hair.

In addition to the space-occupying effects, adenomas of the pars intermedia may be endocrinologically active. Plasma cortisol and immunoreactive adrenocorticotropin (iACTH, molecular weight 4500) levels may be modestly elevated in horses with pars intermedia adenomas.[35] The cortisol levels often lack the normal diurnal rhythm and are not suppressed by either high or low doses of dexamethasone.

Tumor tissue and plasma from horses with the adenoma contain high concentrations of immunoreactive peptides, such as corticotropin-like intermediate lobe peptide (CLIP), alpha and beta melanocyte stimulating hormones (alpha- and beta-MSH), and beta-endorphin (beta-END), which are derived from pro-opiolipomelanocortin (pro-OLMC) and processed in the pars intermedia.[36] This biosynthetic precursor of ACTH and other pituitary peptides is a high molecular weight (31,000 to 37,000 daltons) glycoprotein that undergoes different posttranslational processing in the pars distalis and pars intermedia (fig. 13.5). In the normal pars distalis, pro-OLMC is processed to ACTH (4500 daltons), beta-lipoprotein (beta-LPH), and gamma-LPH, whereas in the normal pars intermedia the same precursor molecule is cleaved into alpha-MSH, CLIP that contains amino acids 18-39 of the ACTH molecule, beta-MSH, and beta-END. Plasma cortisol strongly inhibits ACTH secretion by the pars distalis, but has a much smaller effect on peptides secreted by the pars inter-

media, which are under tonic dopaminergic inhibitory control.

The modest elevations of plasma immunoreactive ACTH (4500 daltons) appear to be due to the different processing of pro-OLMC in tumors derived from cells of the pars intermedia. This may explain the normal or slightly elevated blood cortisol levels and normal or mildly hyperplastic adrenal cortices observed in some horses with adenomas of the pars intermedia. The tumor concentration of ACTH has been reported to be six times that of the normal pars intermedia and only approached the levels found in the pars distalis of normal horses.[36] The plasma and tumor levels of pars intermedia–derived peptides (CLIP, alpha-MSH, beta-MSH, and beta-END) are disproportionately elevated (40 times or more) compared to those of ACTH, apparently as the result of selective posttranslational processing of pro-OLMC in a manner similar to the normal pars intermedia.

Three immunoreactive peptides have been found in pars intermedia tumor extracts that have a larger molecular weight than those present in normal pituitary tissue.[36] All three peptides had both ACTH (11-24) and beta-END/beta-LPH immunoreactivity. The smallest (38,500 daltons) of these peptides could represent pre–pro-OLMC with an attached signal or leader sequence of approximately 26 amino acid residues. The larger peptides (47,000 and 63,000 daltons) may be derived from improper intranuclear processing of pro-OLMC mRNA with retention of additional coding nucleotide sequences.

Macroscopic Pathology

Adenomas of the pars intermedia in dogs produce only a moderate enlargement of the pituitary gland. The pars distalis is readily identifiable and sharply demarcated from the anterior margin of the neoplasm. The tumor may extend across the residual hypophyseal lumen and result in compression atrophy, but usually does not invade the parenchyma of the pars distalis. The posterior lobe is incorporated within the tumor, but the infundibular stalk is intact. Degenerative changes within the neoplasm are minimal. Adenomas of the pars intermedia in horses result in symmetrical enlargement of the hypophysis. These large tumors extend out of the sella turcica and may severely compress the overlying hypothalamus (see fig. 13.4 C). The optic nerves often are displaced and compressed by the tumor; however, visual deficits infrequently are noted clinically. The adenomas are yellow to white, multinodular, and incorporate the pars nervosa. On sectioning of the pituitary mass, multiple areas of hemorrhage often are present, and the pars distalis can be identified as a compressed subcapsular rim of tissue on the anterior margin (see fig. 13.4 B). A sharp line of demarcation remains between the neoplasm and the atrophic pars distalis.

Histopathology

Adenomas of the pars intermedia in horses are partly encapsulated and sharply delineated from the compressed

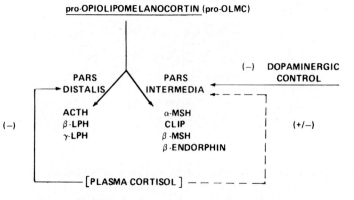

Fig. 13.5. The precursor of ACTH and related peptides proopiolipomelanocortin (pro-OLMC) is processed differently in the pars distalis and pars intermedia. Plasma cortisol exerts primary negative feedback control on the pars distalis, whereas the pars intermedia is predominantly under dopaminergic control.

parenchyma of the pars distalis. The tumors are subdivided into nodules or compartments by fine septa of connective tissue that contain numerous capillaries. Areas of hemorrhage and necrosis are infrequent even in large neoplasms, although hemosiderin laden macrophages may be present within the connective tissue septa. The tumor cells are arranged in cords and nests along the capillaries and connective tissue septa. Tumor cells are large, cylindrical, spindle shaped or polyhedral, and have an oval hyperchromatic nucleus. The histological pattern often is reminiscent of the prominent pars intermedia of normal horses. Cuboidal tumor cells often form follicular structures that contain dense eosinophilic colloid. In other areas the spindle shaped cells form a sarcomatous pattern and palisade around vessels. The cytoplasm is lightly eosinophilic and distinctly granular. Mitotic figures are uncommon. The compressed remnant of pars distalis is atrophic but contains granulated acidophils and basophils. The neurohypophysis often is infiltrated at the periphery by an extension of neoplastic cells, compressed, and replaced by fibrous astrocytes and hemosiderin laden macrophages. The hypothalamus also is compressed to varying degrees, depending upon the size of the adenoma, and has increased glial cells and a loss of nerve cell bodies.

Adenomas of the pars intermedia in dogs appear to arise from the lining epithelium of the residual hypophyseal lumen covering the infundibular process. They are relatively small and more strictly localized than corticotroph (chromophobe) adenomas in dogs arising in the pars distalis. Adenomas of the pars intermedia extend across the residual hypophyseal lumen to compress the pars distalis (see fig. 13.4 D) and are sharply demarcated from the pars distalis (usually by an incomplete layer of condensed reticulum and focal accumulations of lymphocytes), but they are not encapsulated. The histological appearance is strikingly different from adenomas arising in the pars distalis in that there are numerous large colloid filled follicles interspersed between nests of chromophobic cells of varying size (see figs. 13.4 E,F). The follicles are lined by simple columnar epithelium, which is partly ciliated and contains interspersed mucin secreting goblet cells. The follicular colloid is densely eosinophilic and periodic acid-Schiff (PAS) positive. The nests of cells between the follicles are primarily chromophobic, but an occasional cell is observed that contains secretory granules of simple protein (acidophilic) or mucoprotein (basophilic).

Endocrinologically active (ACTH secreting) adenomas of the pars intermedia in dogs have prominent groups of large corticotrophs with abundant eosinophilic cytoplasm and more widely scattered follicles. Dense bands of fibrous connective tissue are occasionally interspersed between the follicles and nests of chromophobic cells, particularly in the endocrinologically inactive adenomas of the pars intermedia. Mitotic figures are observed infrequently. The neoplastic cells compress and frequently invade the pars nervosa and infundibular stalk.[5]

Ultrastructural and Immunohistochemical Characteristics

Electron microscopy of adenomas of the pars intermedia in horses reveals numerous membrane-limited secretory granules in the cytoplasm of tumor cells (fig. 13.6 A). Their mean diameter is approximately 300 nm, and they are surrounded by a closely applied limiting membrane. The rough endoplasmic reticulum and Golgi apparatus are particularly well developed in cells consti-

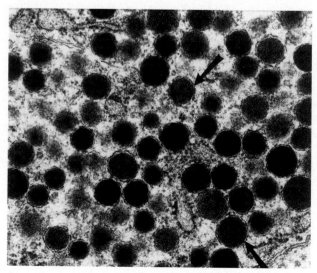

A

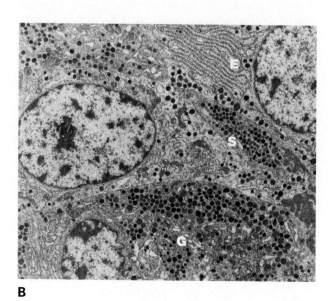

B

Fig. 13.6.   Adenoma in the pars intermedia of the horse. **A.** Secretory granules are approximately 300 nm in diameter. The limiting membrane (arrows) is closely applied, and the granule core is electron dense. **B.** Neoplastic cells with large lamellar arrays of rough endoplasmic reticulum *(E)*, prominent Golgi apparatuses *(G)*, and numerous electron-dense secretory granules *(S)*.

tuting adenomas of the pars intermedia in horses, suggesting they are synthesizing and packaging considerable amounts of protein (e.g., pro-OLMC) for secretion (fig. 13.6 B).

Immunocytochemical staining of adenomas of the pars intermedia has been reported to be similar to that of the nonneoplastic equine pars intermedia.[37,38] There was a strong diffuse cytoplasmic reaction for proopiomelanocortin (POMC), a moderate strong reaction for alpha-MSH and beta-END, a weak reaction for ACTH, and negative immunostaining for prolactin, glial fibrillary acidic protein, and neuron specific enolase. Two antisera directed against different parts of the N-terminal fragment of human POMC differed in their immunoreactivity. Anti-h[1]-[48]N-POMC had stronger immunostaining of the tumor cells than antisera h[1]-[76]N-POMC. The significance of the differences in immunostaining of POMC derived peptides and the specificity of the two antibodies generated against different portions of the N-terminal fragment of human POMC in the horse has not been determined.

These immunocytochemical findings support the biochemical studies that suggest horses with pituitary adenomas derived from the pars intermedia develop a unique clinical syndrome that is the result of hypothalamic and neurohypophyseal derangement as well as an autonomous production of excess amounts of POMC derived peptides. Although many of the functional disturbances in horses with pituitary adenomas (e.g., diabetes insipidus, polyphagia, hyperpyrexia, hyperhidrosis, and hirsutism) appear to be the result of hypothalamic or neurohypophyseal dysfunction (see fig. 13.4 C), other behavioral signs (e.g., docility and diminished responsiveness to painful stimuli) may be related to elevated plasma and cerebrospinal fluid (CSF) levels of beta-END.[39] The clinical syndrome in horses with pituitary tumors is distinctly different than Cushing's disease that occurs in dogs, cats, and human patients.[32,37,38] Although ACTH was demonstrated in adenomas of the pars intermedia, the staining intensity was patchy and considerably weaker than that of POMC, alpha-MSH, and beta-END. The immunocytochemical findings are in agreement with biochemical studies that reported markedly elevated concentrations of circulating immunoreactive POMC and POMC derived peptides (including alpha- and beta-MSH, CLIP, and beta-END) in adenomas and plasma of affected horses relative to ACTH.[35,36,39] The overall processing of peptides in adenomas of the pars intermedia appears to be similar to that in the normal equine pars intermedia.[36,39,40] Diurnal variations in plasma cortisol concentrations were not statistically different between horses with pars intermedia adenomas and control horses.[41] Neither an ACTH stimulation test nor a combined dexamethasone suppression/ACTH stimulation test was able to distinguish between horses with adenomas of the pars intermedia and control horses.

Corticotrophs in the pars distalis of normal horses have strong immunostaining for ACTH, whereas only a few cells stain for alpha-MSH. These immunocytochemi-

cal findings illustrate the differences between adenomas of the pars intermedia in horses and corticotroph adenomas of the pars distalis (also pars intermedia in dogs) that result in classical Cushing's disease in the dog[42] and human beings.[43] Corticotroph adenomas in dogs and human beings associated with Cushing's disease are characterized by strong immunostaining for ACTH and weak to moderate immunostaining for alpha-MSH.

Acidophil Adenoma of Pars Distalis

Incidence

Neoplasms derived from granulated acidophils are uncommon in all domestic animal species, but are common in many strains of adult rats. Acidophil adenomas and an adenocarcinoma have been reported in dogs,[44-46] sheep,[47] and cat.[48,49]

Clinical Characteristics

A spectrum of clinical problems have been associated with acidophil adenomas including metahypophyseal diabetes, diabetes insipidus, cranial nerve deficits, and muscular atrophy.[44,45,50,51] Clinical laboratory evaluation often reveals acidosis, hyperglycemia and glycosuria, and resistance to insulin therapy.

Acidophil adenomas in cats have been associated with clinical signs of diabetes mellitus with degranulation of the pancreatic islets and vacuolar changes in beta cells,[48] suggesting that the tumors were secreting excess growth hormone, which resulted in a down regulation of insulin receptors and resistance to the action of insulin at the target cell level. Several reports have described feline acidophil adenomas that were associated with insulin resistant diabetes mellitus and acromegalic features[49,52] and with immunocytochemical localization of growth hormone in the cytoplasm of tumor cells.[53] The circulating growth hormone levels were approximately 100 times normal and were not suppressible by an exogenous glucose load.[54] Clinical evidence of acromegaly included an enlarged abdomen and prognathia inferior. Cats with growth hormone secreting pituitary adenomas also develop degenerative arthritis with joint cartilage proliferation and chronic renal disease associated with periglomerular fibrosis and mesangial proliferation in the glomerulus.

Acidophil adenomas in sheep (that have a complete diaphragma sella separating the pituitary region from the brain) may attain considerable size and remain confined to the sella turcica (fig. 13.7 A). The remaining adenohypophysis and neurohypophysis are compressed severely, and the sella turcica is enlarged and deepened due to pressure induced osteolysis (figs. 13.7 B,C). Increased development of mammary tissue and galactorrhea has been observed in sheep with acidophil adenomas, suggesting an overproduction of prolactin by the tumor cells.

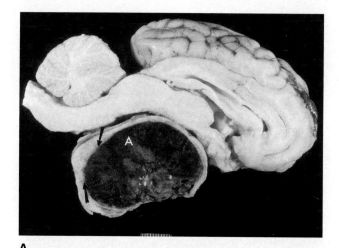

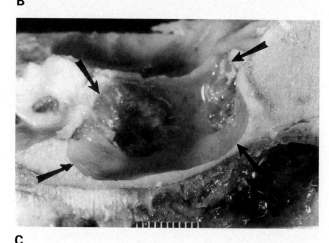

Fig. 13.7. Acidophil adenoma *(A)* of a ewe. **A.** Severe compression of the pars distalis (arrows) and overlying brain. **B.** Erosion of sella turcica (arrows). The adenoma remained confined to the sella turcica due to the complete diaphragma sellae. **C.** Enlargement and deepening of sella turcica (arrows).

Histopathology

Acidophil adenomas enlarge the pituitary gland and indent the overlying hypothalamus to varying degrees. The enlarged hypophysis is composed of irregular columns of acidophils interspersed between numerous large, blood filled sinusoids (fig. 13.8 A). The fibrous stroma is sparse. Although the degree of cytoplasmic granulation of acidophils varies from cell to cell, the predominating type of neoplastic acidophil usually contains many secretory granules. The nuclei of the densely granulated acidophils are small, oval, and hyperchromatic. Sparsely granulated (chromophobic) cells often are interspersed between the densely granulated acidophils. Their cytoplasm is more abundant, lightly acidophilic, and contains only an occasional secretory granule. The nucleus is large, round, and vesicular; mitotic figures are observed infrequently. Secretory granules of the acidophils are evident on hematoxylin and eosin stained sections but are more readily visualized as bright red granules when stained either with acid fuchsin-aniline blue or Crossman's modification of Mallory's trichrome. Orange-G stains the granules an intense yellow-orange, but they are PAS negative.

Colloid-containing follicles lined by follicular cells are found occasionally within acidophil adenomas in dogs (fig. 13.8 A). The colloid is intensely PAS positive. Numerous sinusoids are distended with erythrocytes, detached neoplastic cells, and large masses of fibrin. The pars nervosa and infundibular stalk are compressed to varying degrees, partly replaced by fibrous astrocytes, and infiltrated at the periphery by neoplastic cells; however, this limited extension of neoplastic cells into adjacent parts of the pituitary gland is not interpreted as a criterion of malignancy.

Ultrastructural and Immunocytochemical Characteristics

Two types of acidophils have been found within pituitary acidophil tumors (fig. 13.8 B).[46] The predominating type of acidophil is smaller and contains many secretory granules. The plasma membranes of adjacent cells are relatively straight with uncomplicated interdigitations and are connected by an occasional desmosome. The Golgi apparatus is comparatively small and associated with few prosecretory granules. The rough endoplasmic reticulum is composed of small, flattened membranous sacs with attached ribosomes. A few mitochondria are distributed randomly throughout the cytoplasm. Acidophils of this type are interpreted to be in the *storage phase* of the secretory cycle.

The less common type of neoplastic acidophil has a greater cytoplasmic and nuclear area, and the cytoplasm contains numerous organelles but few mature secretory granules. The rough endoplasmic reticulum is extensive and consists of aggregates of lamellar arrays of granular membranes. The Golgi apparatuses are prominent and are composed of agranular membranes associated with numerous small prosecretory granules. Mitochondria are observed more frequently in the cytoplasm of this type of acidophil. These hypertrophied acidophils are considered

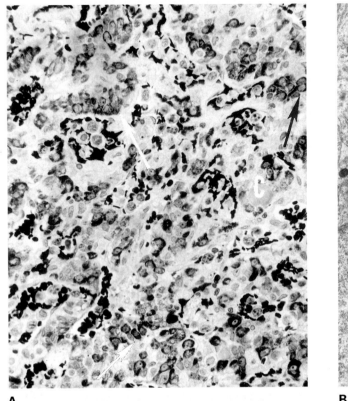

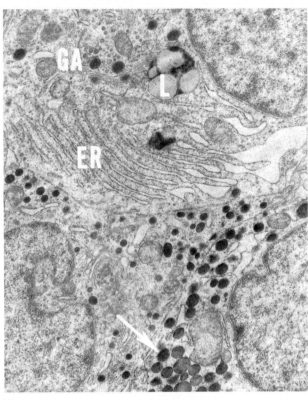

A   **B**

Fig. 13.8.   Acidophil adenoma of a dog. **A.** Densely granulated acidophils (arrows) and chromophobic cells arranged in cords along capillaries. Accumulations of colloid *(C)* surrounded by follicular cells also are present. Acid fuchsin-aniline blue. **B.** Acidophils in the storage phase that have many large secretion granules (arrow). Actively synthesizing acidophils have well-developed rough endoplasmic reticulum *(ER)* and Golgi apparatus *(GA)* but few secretory granules, and they appear chromophobic by light microscopy. Lipofuscin granule *(L)* in tumor cell.

to be actively synthesizing and secreting cells. Cells with varying intergrades of organellar development and a number of mature secretory granules are observed between the extremes of acidophils in the storage phase and those that are actively synthesizing.

The neoplastic acidophils often contain numerous large mature secretory granules at the level of ultrastructure (fig. 13.8 B). The granules are spherical to oval, uniformly electron dense, finely granular, and surrounded by a delicate limiting membrane. The submembranous space of the granule is narrow. Secretory granules are occasionally observed in the process of becoming detached from membranes of the Golgi apparatus. The mean diameter of mature secretory granules in the neoplastic acidophils was 420 nm (range 320–600 nm).[46]

Immunoreactive prolactin cells occur in small groups of large polygonal cells with prominent granules in the ventrocentral and cranial parts of the normal canine pars distalis. A diffuse increase in this population of cells occurs in female dogs near parturition[20] and in pregnant sheep near parturition. Growth hormone secreting cells are present singly along capillaries in the dorsal region of the pars distalis near the pars intermedia. They are small, round to oval, and have fine cytoplasmic granules. Somatotrophs frequently undergo diffuse hyperplasia and hyper-

trophy in old dogs, especially females with mammary dysplasia or neoplasia.[20]

Pituitary Chromophobe Carcinoma

Incidence

Pituitary carcinomas are uncommon compared with pituitary adenomas, but they have been seen in older dogs and cows.[55] These carcinomas are usually endocrinologically inactive, but may cause significant functional disturbances by destruction of the pars distalis and neurohypophyseal system, leading to panhypopituitarism and diabetes insipidus. A corticotroph carcinoma has been reported in a dog with intracerebral metastases that stained positive by immunohistochemistry for ACTH and alpha-, beta-, and gamma-MSH.

Macroscopic Pathology and Histopathology

Pituitary carcinomas are large, extensively invade the overlying brain, and aggressively infiltrate into the sphenoid bone of the sella turcica (fig. 13.9 A). Metastasis infrequently occurs in regional lymph nodes or to distant sites, such as the spleen or liver (fig. 13.9 B).

Malignant tumors of pituitary chromophobes are highly cellular and often have large areas of hemorrhage and necrosis. Giant cells, nuclear pleomorphism, and mitotic figures are encountered more frequently than in chromophobe adenomas; however, pituitary cytology is not a dependable criterion of malignancy, especially in tumors developing in the commonly utilized strains of laboratory rats. Invasion of neoplastic cells into the adjacent sphenoid bone, vascular invasion with formation of tumor cell thrombi, extensive aggressive invasion (not just extension along lines of least resistance) into the overlying brain, and establishment of metastases at distant sites are criteria for the diagnosis of pituitary carcinoma. Limited extension of neoplastic cells into the adjacent pars nervosa and infundibular stalk are observed frequently with larger pituitary adenomas. This finding is not considered evidence for malignancy of a pituitary neoplasm.

Craniopharyngioma (Intracranial Germ Cell Tumor)

Incidence

Craniopharyngioma is a benign tumor that is derived from epithelial remnants of the oropharyngeal ectoderm of

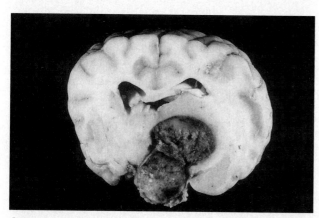

A

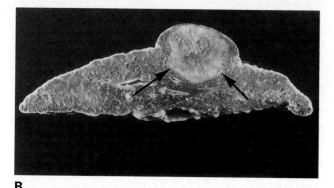

B

Fig. 13.9. Pituitary chromophobe carcinoma. **A.** Extensive dorsal invasion into the brain. **B.** Metastasis to the spleen (arrows).

dorsal extensions of the craniopharyngeal duct (Rathke's pouch). They occur in animals younger than those with other types of pituitary neoplasms and are present either in a suprasellar or infrasellar location. Craniopharyngiomas are one cause of panhypopituitarism and dwarfism in young dogs resulting from a subnormal secretion of somatotropin and other trophic hormones beginning at an early age, prior to closure of the growth plates[54]; however, most pituitary neoplasms of this type develop in young adult (2- to 4-year-old) dogs.

It has been proposed recently that pleomorphic neoplasms in the suprasellar region of younger dogs be classified as germ cell tumors rather than craniopharyngiomas.[56,57] The diagnosis of germ cell tumors was based upon three criteria: (1) midline suprasellar location, (2) presence within the tumor of several distinct cell types (one population resembling a seminoma or dysgerminoma and others suggesting teratomatous differentiation into secretory glandular and squamous elements), and (3) positive staining for alpha-fetoprotein.[56]

Clinical Features

The clinical signs are due to the large size of this type of pituitary tumor and are usually a combination of several factors, including (1) lack of secretion of pituitary trophic hormones resulting in trophic atrophy and subnormal function of the adrenal cortex and thyroid gland (fig. 13.10 A),[58] gonadal atrophy and, occasionally, a failure to attain somatic maturation due to a lack of growth hormone secretion, (2) disturbances in water metabolism (diabetes insipidus with polyuria, polydipsia, low urine specific gravity and osmolality) from interference in the release and synthesis of ADH by the large tumor,[59] (3) deficits in cranial nerve function, and (4) central nervous system dysfunction due to extension into the overlying brain.

Macroscopic Pathology

Craniopharyngiomas often are large and grow along the ventral aspect of the brain where they can incorporate several cranial nerves and destroy much of the pars distalis and pars nervosa. In addition, they may extend dorsally into the hypothalamus and thalamus (fig. 13.10 A); however, dorsal growth of the tumor is not considered to be evidence of malignancy but rather extension along lines of least resistance.

Histological Characteristics

Craniopharyngiomas have alternating solid and cystic areas.[3] The histological characteristics of craniopharyngiomas are distinctive and unique for any intracranial tumor occurring on the ventral aspect of the brain. The solid areas are composed of nests of epithelial cells (cuboidal, columnar, or squamous cells) with prominent focal areas of keratinization (fig. 13.10 B) and occasional mineralization that compress the overlying hypothalamus (fig. 13.10 C). The areas of keratinization are densely eosinophilic and frequently are associated with fragments

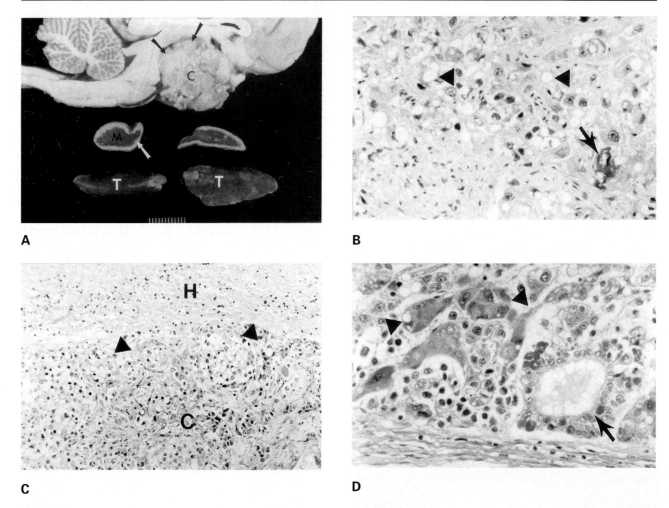

Fig. 13.10. Craniopharyngioma in the dog. **A.** Dorsal extension and compression of the hypothalamus and thalamus (black arrows). The large neoplasm *(C)* has incorporated the adenohypophysis and neurohypophysis, resulting in severe trophic atrophy of the adrenal cortex (white arrow). The adrenal glands consist predominantly of medulla *(M)* surrounded by a thin rim of cortex (capsule plus zona glomerulosa). Although the thyroid follicular cells were flattened and atrophic, the overall gland *(T)* size was within normal limits due to distension of the follicles with colloid. Scale = 1 cm. **B.** Keratinization (arrow) and numerous characteristic cytoplasmic vacuoles (arrowheads) in tumor cells. H&E. **C.** Dorsal extension of tumor cells *(C)* into the overlying hypothalamus *(H)* along lines of least resistance. The tumor is sharply demarcated from the compressed hypothalamus (arrowheads). H&E. **D.** Colloid-containing follicles lined by single or multiple layers of cuboidal cells (arrow) and large pleomorphic neoplastic cells (arrowheads). H&E.

of nuclear chromatin (fig. 13.10 B). The neoplastic epithelial cells are large and pleomorphic with vesicular nuclei and prominent nucleoli (fig. 13.10 D), and they frequently have discrete vacuoles in their cytoplasm (fig. 13.10 B). There frequently is an admixture with smaller cuboidal to polyhedral cells that have acidophilic secretory granules that stain positive for either prolactin or growth hormone by immunocytochemistry. The cystic spaces are lined by either columnar or squamous cells and contain keratin debris and colloid. Colloid-containing follicles may be formed that are lined either by cuboidal or by columnar cells and contain variable amounts of eosinophilic colloid.

An alternative interpretation is that these suprasellar pleomorphic neoplasms in dogs are of germ cell origin and that the secretory (glandular) and squamous elements represent teratomatous differentiation.[56] Additional cases need to be studied utilizing a spectrum of immunocytochemical stains for the protein and glycoprotein pituitary hormones,

alpha subunit, chorionic gonadotropin, alpha-fetoprotein, and placental alkaline phosphatase to determine which of the pleomorphic neoplasms in the suprasellar region are derived from remnants of the oropharyngeal epithelium of the craniopharyngeal duct and which have their origin from multipotential germ cells.

Basophil Adenoma of Pars Distalis

Tumors composed of granulated basophils are one of the most rare pituitary tumors in all animal species. Cushing's disease in humans was initially attributed to a hypersecretion of adrenocorticotropin by small basophilic adenomas in the pars distalis. Current evidence suggests they are a possible cause for a small percentage of patients with Cushing's disease. Several of the early reports on corticotropin secreting pituitary tumors in dogs with hyperadrenocorticism reflected this concept and considered them to be basophil adenomas.[60] Corticotroph (chromophobe) adenomas of the pars distalis and pars intermedia are responsible for the great majority of cases of Cushing's-like disease in dogs.

Basophil adenomas in humans may secrete thyrotropin (TSH), resulting in bilateral enlargement of both thyroid lobes (*goiter*).[61] Serum thyroxine, triiodothyronine, and TSH are elevated and responsive to thyrotropin releasing hormone. The neoplastic cells contain small secretory granules (diameter < 150 nm) with prominent rough endoplasmic reticulum and Golgi apparatuses, characteristic of pituitary thyrotrophs.

A well-circumscribed chromophobe adenoma reported in a male monkey (*Macaca mulatta*) was composed of round or polyhedral cells arranged either into follicles or diffuse sheets.[62] Although the neoplastic cells lacked basophilic or acidophilic granules, the small secretory granules (mean diameter 151 nm) and positive immunohistochemical staining for TSH suggested that the tumor was derived from thyrotrophic basophils in the pars distalis. However, the thyroid gland did not show evidence of stimulation, but rather was composed of involuted follicles lined by atrophic follicular cells and filled with colloid, suggesting that the tumor was not endocrinologically active.

Metastatic Tumors to the Pituitary Gland

The pituitary gland occasionally is either partially or completely destroyed by metastatic tumors from distant sites. Examples include lymphoma of cattle and dogs, malignant melanoma of horses and dogs, transmissible venereal tumor, and adenocarcinoma in the mammary gland of dogs. In addition, the pituitary gland may be destroyed by local infiltration or compression from an osteosarcoma of the sphenoid bone, ependymoma arising in the infundibular recess of the third ventricle, meningioma (fig. 13.11), and a glioma (*infundibuloma*) of the infundibular stalk.[63]

Nonneoplastic Cysts of the Pituitary Gland

Cysts of the Distal (Sellar) End of the Craniopharyngeal Duct

Cysts may develop from remnants of the distal (sellar) end of the craniopharyngeal duct, which normally disappears by birth in most animal species. The cysts are lined by ciliated, cuboidal to columnar epithelial lining and contain mucin.[64] In dogs, especially of the brachycephalic breeds, cysts from these remnants frequently are found at the periphery of the pars tuberalis and pars distalis. In one survey cystic remnants of the craniopharyngeal duct were

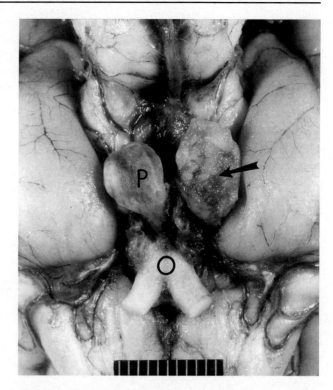

Fig. 13.11. Meningioma (arrow) arising on ventral aspect of brain in a dog that exerted pressure on the hypothalamic-hypophyseal portal system and infundibular stalk. *O,* optic nerve; *P,* pituitary.

found histologically in 53 percent of dogs of several breeds.

Craniopharyngeal duct cysts occasionally become large enough to exert pressure on the infundibular stalk and hypophyseal-hypothalamic portal system, median eminence, or pars distalis. Structures adjacent to the cysts undergo atrophy to varying degrees owing to compression and interference with the blood supply. Disruption of a large cyst with escape of the proteinic contents into adjacent tissues may incite an intense, local inflammatory reaction with subsequent fibrosis that interferes with normal pituitary function. Clinical signs may include visual difficulties due to pressure on the optic chiasma, diabetes insipidus, obesity, and hypofunction of the adenohypophysis (gonadal atrophy, decreased basal metabolic rate, and hypoglycemia).

Cysts Derived from the Proximal End of the Craniopharyngeal Duct (Pharyngeal Hypophysis)

The proximal portion of the adenohypophyseal anlage (i.e., craniopharyngeal duct) may persist in the dorsal aspect of the oral cavity in adults as undifferentiated remnants of cells along the craniopharyngeal canal or as differentiated cells similar to those of the definitive adenohypophysis. These remnants, called the *pharyngeal hypophysis,* have been described in dogs, cats, other animal species, and humans.[65] The pharyngeal hypophysis is physically separated from the sellar adenohypophysis in dogs, but in cats these structures may be continuous because of persistence of the craniopharyngeal canal.

The pharyngeal hypophysis is seen most frequently in brachycephalic breeds of dogs. It is a tubular structure lined by ciliated columnar epithelium and located on the midline of the nasopharynx, and it is frequently continuous with a multilocular cyst that is lined by squamous, ciliated, cuboidal or columnar epithelium. The cyst contains colloid material and cellular debris. A mass of differentiated acidophilic, basophilic, and chromophobic cells similar to those of the adenohypophysis in the sella turcica usually extends from the cyst wall.

A cyst (as much as several centimeters in diameter) may be derived from the oropharyngeal end of the craniopharyngeal duct and project as a space-occupying mass into the nasopharynx in dogs. The predominant clinical sign is related to respiratory distress due to ventral displacement of the soft palate and occlusion of the posterior nares.[66] The cyst wall is hard on palpation because of the presence of partially mineralized woven bone. The contents of the cyst are often yellow-gray and caseous due to the accumulation of keratin and desquamated epithelial cells from the cyst lining. The squamous epithelial lining of the cyst appears to be derived from metaplasia of the remnants of the primitive oropharyngeal epithelium.

Cysts Associated with Pituitary Dwarfism

Pituitary dwarfism in German shepherd dogs usually is associated with a failure of the oropharyngeal ectoderm of Rathke's pouch to differentiate into trophic hormone secreting cells of the pars distalis. This results in a progressively enlarging, multiloculated cyst in the sella turcica and a partial to complete absence of the adenohypophysis.[67] The cyst is lined by pseudostratified, often ciliated, columnar epithelium with interspersed, mucin secreting, goblet cells. The mucin filled cysts eventually occupy the entire pituitary area in the sella turcica and severely compress the pars nervosa and infundibular stalk (fig. 13.12 A). A few differentiated trophic homone secreting chromophils may be present in the pituitary cyst; these stain immunocytochemically for one or more of the specific trophic hormones. An occasional small nest or rosette of poorly differentiated epithelial cells is interspersed between multiloculated cysts, but the cell cytoplasm is usually devoid of hormone-containing secretory granules.

Cysts associated with pituitary dwarfism morphologically are distinct from the cysts that develop following the abnormal accumulation of colloid in the residual lumen of Rathke's pouch (fig. 13.12 B). In the latter, the normally developed pars distalis and pars nervosa are compressed to varying degrees by the abnormal accumulation of colloid in a preformed normal cavity of the pituitary gland.

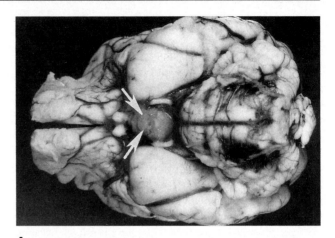

A

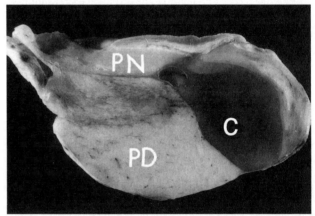

B

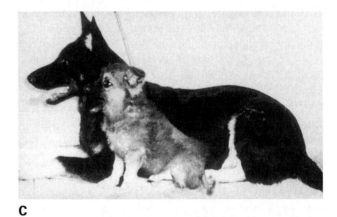

C

Fig. 13.12. Pituitary cysts. **A.** Pituitary cysts resulting from a failure of the primitive oropharyngeal ectoderm of Rathke's pouch to differentiate into secretory cells of the adenohypophysis. The pituitary region is occupied by a large multiloculated cyst (arrows) that compressed adjacent structures. The dog developed panhypopituitary dwarfism due to a failure of secretion of growth hormone and other trophic hormones by the cystic pituitary gland. **B.** Cystic distention of residual hypophyseal lumen with colloid *(C)* compressing the pars distalis *(PD)* and pars nervosa *(PN)*. Bovine hypophysis. **C.** Panhypopituitarism (pituitary dwarfism) in a 5-month-old German shepherd dog. An unaffected littermate weighed 60 pounds and the dwarf pup 8.8 pounds. Note the retention of the puppy hair coat on the dwarf. [From Alexander, J.E. (1962) *Can Vet J* 3:83.]

Pituitary dwarf pups appear normal or are indistinguishable from littermates at birth and until about 24 months of age. Subsequently, a slower growth rate than littermates, retention of puppy hair coat, and lack of primary guard hairs gradually become evident in dwarf pups (fig. 13.12 C). German shepherd dogs with pituitary dwarfism appear coyote-like or fox-like due to their diminutive size and soft woolly coat.[68] A bilaterally symmetrical alopecia develops gradually and often progresses to complete alopecia except for the head and tufts of hair on the legs. There is progressive hyperpigmentation of the skin until it is uniformly brown-black over most of the body. Adult German shepherd dogs with panhypopituitarism vary in size from as tiny as 4 pounds up to nearly half normal size, apparently depending on the degree of penetrance of the inherited defect and whether the failure of formation of the adenohypophysis is nearly complete or only partial.

Panhypopituitarism in German shepherd dogs often occurs in littermates and related litters, suggesting a simple autosomal recessive mode of inheritance.[69-73] The activity of somatomedin (a cartilage growth promoting peptide whose production in the liver and plasma activity are controlled by somatotrophin) is low in dwarf dogs.[72] Intermediate somatomedin activity is present in the phenotypically normal ancestors suspected to be heterozygous carriers. Assays for somatomedin (a non–species-specific, somatotropin dependent peptide) provide an indirect measurement of circulating growth hormone activity in dogs with suspected pituitary dwarfism.[70,74]

REFERENCES

1. Capen, C.C. (1996) Functional and pathologic interrelationships of the pituitary gland and hypothalamus in animals. In Jones, T.C., Capen, C.C., and Mohr, U. (eds.), *Endocrine System. Series II. Monographs on the Pathology of Laboratory Animals,* 2nd ed. International Life Sciences Institute Series. Springer-Verlag, Inc., Berlin, Heidelberg, New York, pp. 3-32.

2. Schwedes, C.S. (1997) Mitotane (*o,p'*-DDD) treatment in a cat with hyperadrenocorticism. *J Small Anim Pract* 38:520-524.

3. White, E.G. (1938) A suprasellar tumor in a dog. *J Pathol Bacteriol* 47:323-326.

4. Lesbouyries, G., Drieux, H., Charton, A., and Macharka, K. (1942) Adénome chromophobe de l'hypophyse et syndrome pluriglandulaire chez un chien. *Bull Acad Vet Fr* 15:298-316.

5. Capen, C.C., Martin, S.L., and Koestner, A. (1967) Neoplasms in the adenohypophysis of dogs: A clinical and pathologic study. *Pathol Vet* 4:301-325.

6. Rijnberk, A., der Kinderen, P.J., and Thijssen, J.H.H. (1968) "Cushing's syndrome" (spontaneous hyperadrenocorticism) in the dog. *J Endocrinol* 41:397-406.

7. Peterson, M.E., Kreiger, D.T., Drucker, W.D., and Halmi, N.S. (1982) Immunocytochemical study of the hypophysis in 25 dogs with pituitary-dependent hyperadrenocorticism. *Acta Endocrinol* 101:15-24.

8. Hall, E.J., Miller, W.H., Jr., and Medleau, L. (1984) Ketoconazole treatment of generalized dermatophytosis in a dog with hyperadrenocorticism. *J Amer Anim Hosp Assoc* 20:597-602.

9. Angles, J.M., Feldman, E.C., Nelson, R.W., and Feldman, M.S. (1997) Use of urine cortisol:creatinine ratio versus adrenocorticotropic hormone stimulation testing for monitoring mitotane treatment of pituitary-dependent hyperadrenocorticism in dogs. *J Amer Vet Med Assoc* 211:1002-1004.

10. Feldman, E.C., Bohannon, N.V., and Tyrrell, J.B. (1977) Plasma adenocorticotropin levels in normal dogs. *Amer J Vet Res* 38:1643-1645.

11. Feldman, E.C. (1983) Distinguishing dogs with functioning adrenocortical tumors from dogs with pituitary dependent hyperadrenocorticism. *J Amer Vet Med Assoc* 183:195-200.

12. Peterson, M.E. (1984) Hyperadrenocorticism. *Vet Clin N Amer* 14:731-749.

13. Kooistra, H.S., Voorhout, G., Mol, J.A., and Rijnberk, A. (1997) Correlation between impairment of glucocorticoid feedback and the size of the pituitary gland in dogs with pituitary-dependent hyperadrenocorticism. *J Endocrinol* 152:387-394.

14. Bertoy, E.H., Feldman, E.C., Nelson, R.W., Duesberg, C.A., Kass, P.H., Reid, M.H., and Dublin, A.B. (1995) Magnetic resonance imaging of the brain in dogs with recently diagnosed but untreated pituitary-dependent hyperadrenocorticism. *J Amer Vet Med Assoc* 206:651.

15. Duesberg, C.A., Feldman, E.C., Nelson, R.W., Bertoy, E.H., Dublin, A.B., and Reid, M.H. (1995) Magnetic resonance imaging for diagnosis of pituitary macrotumors in dogs. *J Amer Vet Med Assoc* 206:657.

16. Capen, C.C., and Koestner, A. (1967) Functional chromophobe adenomas of the canine adenohypophysis: An ultrastructural evaluation of a neoplasm of pituitary corticotrophs. *Pathol Vet* 4:326-347.

17. Kagayama, M. (1965) The follicular cell in the pars distalis of the dog pituitary gland: An electron microscope study. *Endocrinology* 77:1053-1060.

18. El Etreby, M.F., and Dubois, M.P. (1980) The utility of antisera to different synthetic adenocorticotrophins (ACTH) and melanotrophins (MSH) for immunocytochemical staining of the dog pituitary gland. *Histochemistry* 66:245-260.

19. Attia, M.A. (1980) Cytological study on pituitary adenomas in senile untreated beagle bitches. *Arch Toxicol* 46:287-293.

20. El Etreby, M.F., Muller-Peddinghaus, R., Bhargava, A.S., and Trautwein, G. (1980) The Role of the pituitary gland in spontaneous canine mammary tumorigenesis. *Vet Pathol* 17:109-122.

21. Meij, B.P., Mol, J.A., Bevers, M.M., and Rijnberk, A. (1997) Alterations in anterior pituitary function of dogs with pituitary-dependent hyperadrenocorticism. *J Endocrinol* 154:505-512.

22. Siperstein, E.R., and Allison, V.F. (1965) Fine structure of the cells responsible for secretion of adrenocorticotrophin in the adrenalectomized rat. *Endocrinology* 76:70-79.

23. Zaki, F.A., and Liu, S.K. (1973) Pituitary chromophobe adenoma in a cat. *Vet Pathol* 10:232-237.

24. Heavner, J.E., and Dice, P.F. (1977) Pituitary tumor as a cause of blindness in a dog. *Vet Med Small Anim Clin* 72:873-876.

25. Koestner, A., and Capen, C.C. (1967) Ultrastructural evaluation of the canine hypothalamic-neurohypophyseal system in diabetes insipidus associated with pituitary neoplasms. *Pathol Vet* 4:513-536.

26. Brown, W.R., Fetter, A.D., Van Ryzin, R.J., and Langloss, J.M. (1993) Proliferative pituitary lesions in rats treated with salmon or porcine calcitonin. *Toxicol Pathol* 21:81.

27. Jameson, J.L., Weiss, J., Polak, J.M., Childs, G.V., Bloom, S.R., Steel, J.H., Capen, C.C., Prentice, D.E., Fetter, A.W., and Langloss, J.H. (1992) Glycoprotein hormone alpha-subunit-producing pituitary adenomas in rats treated for one year with calcitonin. *Amer J Pathol* 140:75-84.

28. Chalifoux, L.V., MacKey J.J., and King, N.W. (1983) A sparsely granulated, nonsecreting adenoma of the pars intermedia associated with galactorrhea in a male rhesus monkey (*Macaca mulatta*). *Vet Pathol* 20:541-547.

29. Halmi, N.S., Peterson, M.E., Colurso, G.J., Liotta, A.S., and Kreiger, D.T. (1981) Pituitary intermediate lobe in dogs: Two cell types and high bioactive adrenocorticotrophin content. *Science* 211:72-74.

30. Urman, H.K., Ozean, H.C., and Tekeli, S. (1963) Pituitary neoplasms in two horses. *Zbl Vet Med* 10:257-262.

31. Eriksson, K., Dyrendahl, S., and Grimfelt, D. (1956) A case of hirsutism in connection with hypophyseal tumor in a horse. *Nord Vet Med* 8:807-814.

32. Loeb, W.F., Capen, C.C., and Johnson, L.E. (1966) Adenomas of the pars intermedia associated with hyperglycemia and glycosuria in two horses. *Cornell Vet* 56:623-639.

33. Holscher, M.A., Linnabarry, R.L., Netsky, M.G., and Owen, H.D. (1978) Adenoma of the pars intermedia and hirsutism in a pony. *Vet Med Small Anim Clin* 73:1197-2000.

34. King, J.M., Kavanaugh, J.R., and Bentinck-Smith, J. (1962) Diabetes mellitus with pituitary neoplasms in a horse and a dog. *Cornell Vet* 52:133-145.

35. Orth, D.N., Holscher, M.A., Wilson, M.G., Nicholson, W.E., Plue, R.E., and Mount, C.D. (1982) Equine Cushing's disease: Plasma immunoreactive proopiolipomelanocortin peptide and cortisol levels basally and in response to diagnostic tests. *Endocrinology* 110:1430-1442.

36. Wilson, M.G., Nicholson, W.E., Holscher, M.A., Sherrell, B.J., Mount, C.D., and Orth, D.N. (1982) Proopiomelanocortin peptides in normal pituitary, pituitary tumor and plasma of normal and Cushing's horses. *Endocrinology* 110:941-954.

37. Heinrichs, M., Baumgärtner, W., and Capen, C.C. (1990) Immunocytochemical demonstration of proopiomelanocortin-derived peptides in pituitary adenomas of the pars intermedia in horses. *Vet Pathol* 27:419-425.

38. Boujon, C.E., Bestetti, G.E., Meier, H.P., Straub, R., Junker, U., and Rossi, G.L. (1993) Equine pituitary adenoma: A functional and morphological study. *J Comp Pathol* 109:163-178.

39. Millington, W.R., Dybdal, N.O., Dawson, R., Jr., Manzini, C., and Mueller, G.P. (1988) Equine Cushing's disease: differential regulation of beta-endorphin processing in tumors of the intermediate pituitary. *Endocrinology* 123:1598-1604.

40. Orth, D.N., and Nicholson, W.E. (1982) Bioactive and immunoreactive adrenocorticotropin in normal equine pituitary and in pituitary tumors of horses with Cushing's disease. *Endocrinology* 111:559-563.

41. Dybdal, N., Hargreaves, K.M., Madigan, J.E., Gribble, D.H., Kennedy, P.C., and Stabenfeldt, G.H. (1994) Diagnostic testing for pituitary pars intermedia dysfunction in horses. *J Amer Vet Med Assoc* 204:627-632.

42. Peterson, M.E., Orth, D.N., Halmi, N.S., Zielinksi, A.C., Davis, D.R., Chavez, F.T., and Drucker, W.D. (1986) Plasma immunoreactive proopiomelanocortin peptides and cortisol in normal dogs and dogs with Addison's disease and Cushing's syndrome: basal concentrations. *Endocrinology* 119:720-730.

43. Lloyd, R.V., Chandler, W.F., McKeever, P.E., and Schteingart, D.E. (1986) The spectrum of ACTH-producing pituitary lesions. *Amer J Surg Pathol* 10:618-626.

44. King, J.M., Kavanaugh, J.R., and Bentinck-Smith, J. (1962) Diabetes mellitus with pituitary neoplasms in a horse and a dog. *Cornell Vet* 52:133-145.

45. Hottendorf, G.H., Nielsen, S.W., and Lieberman, L.L. (1966) Acidophil adenoma of the pituitary gland and other neoplasms in a boxer. *J Amer Vet Med Assoc* 148:1046-1050.

46. Capen, C.C., Martin, S.L., and Koestner, A. (1967) The ultrastructure and histopathology of an acidophil adenoma of the canine adenohypophysis. *Pathol Vet* 4:348-365.

47. Olson, D.P., Ohlson, D.L., Davis, S.L., and Laurence, K.A. (1981) Acidophil adenoma in the pituitary gland of a sheep. *Vet Pathol* 18:132-135.

48. Gembardt, C., and Lopponow, H. (1976) Zur Pathogenese des spontanen Diabetes Mellitus der Katze. II. Mitteilung: Azidophile Adenome des Hypophysenvorderlappens und Diabetes Mellitus in zwei Fallen. *Berl Muench Tierärztl Wochenschr* 89:336-340.

49. Eigenmann, J.E., Wortman, J.A., and Haskins, M.E. (1984) Elevated growth hormone levels and diabetes mellitus in a cat with acromegalic features. *J Amer Anim Hosp Assoc* 20:747-752.

50. Jubb, K.F., and Kennedy, P.C. (1957) Tumors of the Nonchromaffin Paraganglia in Dogs. *Cancer* 10:89-99.

51. van Keulen, L.J.M., Wesdorp, J.L., and Kooistra, H.S. (1996) Diabetes mellitus in a dog with a growth hormone-producing acidophilic adenoma of the adenohypophysis. *Vet Pathol* 33:451-453.

52. Lichtensteiger, C.A., Wortman, J.A., Eigenmann, J.E. (1986) Functional pituitary acidophilic adenoma in a cat with diabetes mellitus and acromegalic features. *Vet Pathol* 23:518-521.

53. Heinrichs, M., Baumgärtner, W., and Krug-Manntz, S. (1989) Immunohistochemical demonstration of growth hormone in a acidophilic adenoma of the adenohypophysis in a cat. *Vet Pathol* 26:179-180.

54. Eigenmann, J.F., Lubberink, A.A.M.E., and Koemann, J.P. (1983) Panhypopituitarism caused by a suprasellar tumor in a dog. *J Amer Anim Hosp Assoc* 19:377-382.

55. Powers, R.D., and Winkler, J.K. (1977) Pituitary carcinoma with extracranial metastasis in a cow. *Vet Pathol* 14:524-526.

56. Valentine, B.A., Summers, B.A., de Lahunta, A., White, C.L., III, and Kuhajda, F.F. (1988) Suprasellar germ cell tumors in the dog: A report of five cases and review of the literature. *Acta Neuropathol* 76:94-100.

57. Hare, W.R. (1993) primary suprasellar germ cell tumor in a dog. *J Amer Vet Med Assoc* 203:1432-1433.

58. Neer, T.M., and Reavis, D.U. (1983) Craniopharyngioma and associated central diabetes insipidus and hypothyroidism in a dog. *J Amer Vet Med Assoc* 182:519-520.

59. Saunders, L.Z., and Rickard, C.G. (1952) Craniopharyngioma in a dog with apparent adiposogenital syndrome and diabetes insipidus. *Cornell Vet* 42:490-494.

60. Dämmrich, K. (1959) Ein Polymorphzelliges basophiles Adenom der Hypophyse beim Hund. *Berl Muench Tierärztl Wochenschr* 24:109-113.

61. Yovos, J.G., Falko, J.M., O'Dorisio, T.M., Malarkey, W.B., Cataland, S., and Capen, C.C. (1981) Thyrotoxicosis and a thyrotropin-secreting pituitary tumor causing unilateral exophthalmos. *J Clin Endocrinol Metab* 52:338-343.

62. Tsuchitani, M., and Narama, I. (1984) Pituitary thyrotroph cell adenoma in a cynomolgus monkey (*Macaca fascicularis*). *Vet Pathol* 21:444-447.

63. Saunders, L.Z., Stephenson, H.C., and McEntee, K. (1951) Diabetes insipidus and adiposogenital syndrome in a dog due to an infundibuloma. *Cornell Vet* 41:445-458.

64. Rao, R.R., and Bhat, N.G. (1971) Incidence of cysts in pars distalis of mongrel dogs. *Indian Vet J* 48:128-133.

65. McGrath, P. (1974) The pharyngeal hypophysis in some laboratory animals. *J Anat* 117:95-115.

66. Slatter, D.H., Schirmer, R.G., and Krehbiel, J.D. (1976) Surgical correction of cystic Rathke's cleft in a dog. *J Amer Anim Hosp Assoc* 12:641.

67. Alexander, J.E. (1962) Anomaly of craniopharyngeal duct and hypophysis. *Can Vet J* 3:83.

68. Muller, G.H., and Jones, S.R. (1973) Pituitary dwarfism and alopecia in a German shepherd with cystic Rathke's cleft. *J Amer Anim Hosp Assoc* 9:567-572.

69. Andresen, E., Willeberg, P., and Rasmussen, P.G. (1974) Pituitary dwarfism in German shepherd dogs. *Nord Vet Med* 26:692-701.

70. Willeberg, P., Kastrup, K.W., and Andresen, E. (1975) Pituitary dwarfism in German shepherd dogs: Studies on somatomedin activity. *Nord Vet Med* 27:448-454.

71. Andresen, E., and Willeberg, P. (1976) Pituitary dwarfism in German shepherd dogs: Additional evidence of simple, autosomal recessive inheritance. *Nord Vet Med* 28:481-486.

72. Lund-Larsen, T.R., and Grondalen, J. (1976) Ateliotic dwarfism in the German shepherd dog: Low somatomedin activity associated with apparently normal pituitary function (2 cases) and with panadenopituitary dysfunction (1 case). *Acta Vet Scand* 17:293-306.

73. Nicholas, F. (1978) Pituitary dwarfism in German shepherd dogs: A genetic analysis of some Australian data. *J Small Anim Pract* 19:167-174.

74. Van Wyk, J.J., Underwood, L.E., Hintz, R.L., Clemmons, D.R., Voina, S.J., and Weaver, R.P. (1974) The somatomedins: A family of insulin-like hormones under growth hormone control. *Recent Prog Horm Res* 30:259-318.

TUMORS OF THE ADRENAL GLAND

Tumors of the Adrenal Cortex: Adenoma, Carcinoma, Myelolipoma

Incidence

Adenomas of the adrenal cortex are seen most frequently in old dogs (8 years and older) and sporadically in cats, horses, cattle, goats, and sheep.[1-5] Castrated male goats are reported to have a much higher incidence of cortical adenomas than intact mates.[6]

Adrenal cortical carcinomas occur less frequently than adenomas. They have been reported most often in cattle,[7] sporadically in old dogs,[5,8,9] and rarely in other species. Carcinomas develop in adult to older animals, and there is no particular breed or sex prevalence.

Clinical Characteristics

Adenomas and carcinomas of the adrenal cortex in dogs may be functional (endocrinologically active) and secrete excessive amounts of cortisol. There are multiple pathogenic mechanisms that can result in the syndrome of cortisol excess (see fig. 13.13 D). The clinical signs of functional adrenal cortical tumors in dogs usually are the result of cortisol excess and are essentially similar to those described previously for corticotroph (ACTH secreting) adenomas of the pituitary. The clinical picture of adrenal cortical carcinoma may be complicated by compression of adjacent organs by the large tumor; invasion into the aorta or posterior vena cava, leading to intra-abdominal hemorrhage or blockage of venous blood flow to the heart; and metastasis to distant sites. Ultrasonography and/or radiographic detection of adrenal enlargement with or without calcification has proven to aid in the diagnosis of adrenal neoplasms in dogs.[10] In horses, adrenal tumors have been reported to be associated with endocrine disturbances. The clinical signs of cortisol excess caused by a functional cortical adenoma or carcinoma usually can not be reversed by *o,p'*-DDD, an adrenal cytotoxic drug,[5] unless the tumors are small and remain responsive to ACTH.

The mean basal plasma cortisol has been reported to be high (6.3 µg/dl) in dogs with functional adrenal cortical neoplasms compared to clinically normal control dogs (1.6 ± 1.0 µg/dl).[11] In 59 percent of dogs with cortical adeno-

mas and carcinomas, there was an exaggerated increase in plasma cortisol following administration of exogenous ACTH (20 units ACTH gel intramuscularly). The mean concentration of plasma cortisol was 37.9 µg/dl at 2 hours post-ACTH in dogs with adrenal cortical tumors. The plasma cortisol levels were approximately fourfold higher at 2 hours post-ACTH in dogs with functional carcinomas than in those with cortical adenomas. Although the low dose dexamethasone (0.01 mg/kg IV) suppression test is used frequently as a screening procedure to distinguish between dogs with cortisol excess and normal ("stressed") dogs, recent reports indicate the test also is useful in distinguishing between dogs with pituitary dependent hyperadrenocorticism and those associated with cortisol producing adrenal tumors.[12] The high dose dexamethasone test (0.1 mg/kg IV) was useful in dogs with hyperadrenocorticism that did not suppress with the low dose of dexamethasone. In addition to adrenalectomy, high doses of mitotane (*o,p'*-DDD) have been reported to be an alternative to surgical adrenalectomy in some dogs with cortisol secreting adrenal cortical neoplasms.[13]

Adrenal tumors are being recognized with greater frequency in ferrets as they are being kept as household pets and living to a more advanced age. The adrenal enlargements are either bilateral (approximately 45 percent) due to diffuse (most frequent) or nodular hyperplasia, or unilateral (approximately 55 percent) due to adrenal cortical carcinoma (more common) or cortical adenoma.[14] Clinical signs in ferrets with adrenal cortical tumors include vulvar enlargement; bilaterally symmetrical alopecia, especially on the ventral abdomen and medial aspects of the rear legs; polyuria; polydipsia; and the presence of a palpable mass at the cranial pole of the kidney (left side greater frequency than right).[15] Adrenal tumors develop in adult ferrets (mean age 5 years), with females more frequently affected than males (sex ratio of 2:1 or greater). The history frequently indicates the ferrets were gonadectomized at an early age (5 or 6 weeks). Other functional disturbances including anemia, thrombocytopenia, pyometra, and endometrial hyperplasia are consistent with an overproduction of estrogenic steroids by the adrenal tumors. Some of the functional disturbances resemble intact females with persistent or prolonged estrus, ferrets being seasonally polyestrous and induced ovulators. About one-third of ferrets with adrenal cortical tumors also have neoplasms derived from the insulin producing beta cells of the pancreatic islets, which can be associated with hypoglycemia and elevated levels of serum insulin, resulting in seizures, episodic lethargy, ptyalism, ataxia, and hind leg weakness.[16-19]

The most consistent endocrinologic change in ferrets with adrenal tumors is an elevation in plasma levels of estradiol-17-beta. It is presumed that the estradiol-17-beta is produced by the tumor directly, but an alternative possibility would be that the adrenal tumors secrete androgenic steroids that are aromatized in the skin and possibly elsewhere to estrogenic steroids. There is no increase in circulating estradiol-17-beta levels in response to exogenous ACTH, but plasma levels decrease following adrenalectomy. Plasma cortisol and corticosterone levels in ferrets with adrenal tumors are in the range of normal or below and do not show an exaggerated increase in response to exogenous ACTH.[20] There is not a decrease in plasma cortisol following unilateral adrenalectomy, and the contralateral adrenal cortex is not atrophic, as would be expected if the adrenal tumor was secreting excess cortisol. However, the urinary cortisol:creatinine ratio has been found to be elevated in ferrets with adrenal cortical tumors (5.98 × 10^{-6}) compared to controls (0.34 × 10^{-6}).[21] The clinical signs in ferrets with adrenal cortical tumors can be effectively reversed by adrenalectomy[22] (especially of the left side if there is no macroscopic enlargement), but not by chemotherapy with o,p'-DDD. Complete regrowth of hair usually occurs by 2-3 months postadrenalectomy.

Macroscopic Pathology

Cortical adenomas usually are well-demarcated single nodules in one adrenal gland, but they may be bilateral. Larger cortical adenomas are yellow to red, distort the external contour of the affected gland, and are partially or completely encapsulated. Adjacent cortical parenchyma is compressed, and the tumor may extend into the medulla.

Smaller cortical adenomas are more yellow or similar in color to the normal adrenal cortex because of the high lipid content. They are surrounded on all sides by mildly compressed cortex with early attempts at fibrous encapsulation and may be difficult to distinguish from areas of nodular cortical hyperplasia observed frequently in old dogs. Nodular hyperplasia usually consists of multiple foci of various sizes in both adrenals with no evidence of encapsulation and often is associated with extracapsular nodules of hyperplastic cortical tissue extending into the periadrenal connective tissues and into the adrenal medulla (fig. 13.13 E).

Adrenal cortical carcinomas are larger than adenomas and may be more likely to develop in both glands. In dogs they are composed of a variegated, yellow to brownish red, friable tissue that incorporates most or all of the affected adrenal gland. They often are fixed in location because of extensive invasion of surrounding tissues and the posterior vena cava, forming a large tumor cell thrombus. Carcinomas may attain considerable size in cattle (as much as 10 cm or more in diameter) and have multiple areas of mineralization or ossification.

Functional (cortisol secreting) adrenal cortical adenomas and carcinomas are associated with profound cortical atrophy of the contralateral gland because of negative feedback inhibition of the pituitary ACTH secretion by the elevated blood cortisol levels (fig. 13.13 A,D). The atrophic cortex consists primarily of the adrenal capsule and zona multiformis (glomerulosa), with only few secretory cells remaining in the zonae fasciculata and reticularis. A similar parenchymal atrophy is present in the uncompressed cortex around functional adenomas. The adrenal medulla appears expanded and relatively more conspicuous because of the lack of surrounding cortical parenchyma.

Histopathology

Cortical adenomas are composed of well-differentiated steroid hormone producing cells that resemble secretory cells of the normal zona fasciculata or reticularis (fig. 13.13 B). Tumor cells are arranged in broad trabeculae or nests separated by small vascular spaces. The abundant cytoplasmic area of tumor cells is lightly eosinophilic, often vacuolated, and filled with many lipid droplets. Adenomas are partially or completely surrounded by a thin fibrous connective tissue capsule of varying thickness and a rim of compressed cortical parenchyma. Focal areas of mineralization, extramedullary hematopoiesis, and accumulations of fat cells may be found in cortical adenomas. Extramedullary hematopoiesis with megakaryocytes and erythroid and granulocytic colonies is a characteristic lesion of canine adrenal cortical adenomas. Larger adenomas have areas of necrosis and hemorrhage near the center.

Adrenal cortical carcinomas are composed of more highly pleomorphic cells than adenomas, which are subdivided into groups by a fibrovascular stroma of varying thickness. The architecture of the affected adrenal is completely obliterated by the carcinoma. The pattern of growth varies between individual tumors and within the same carcinoma, resulting in the formation of trabeculae, lobules, or nests of tumor cells (fig. 13.13 C). Tumor cells usually are large and polyhedral with a vesicular nucleus, prominent nucleoli, and densely eosinophilic or vacuolated cytoplasm. Anaplastic carcinomas may have spindle shaped cells with a smaller and more lightly eosinophilic cytoplasm.[23] Areas of hemorrhage within the tumors are common because of rupture of thin-walled vessels. Invasion of tumor cells through the adrenal capsule into adjacent tissues and into vessels and lymphatics, forming emboli, is frequently detected in carcinomas of the adrenal cortex.[24]

Nodular cortical hyperplasia and myelolipoma are two discrete cortical lesions that must be differentiated histologically from adrenal cortical adenomas. The presence of a partial or complete fibrous capsule surrounding one or two progressively expanding areas of proliferating cortical cells suggests an adenoma rather than nodular hyperplasia.

Myelolipoma is a benign lesion commonly encountered in the adrenal glands of cattle and nonhuman primates and infrequently in other animals. It is composed of accumulations of well-differentiated adipose cells and hematopoietic tissue, including both myeloid and lymphoid elements. Focal areas of mineralization or bone formation may occur in myelolipomas. Although the origin of these nodular aggregations of fat, bone, and myeloid cells is uncertain, they appear to develop by metaplastic transformation of cells in the adrenal cortex or cells lining adrenal sinusoids.

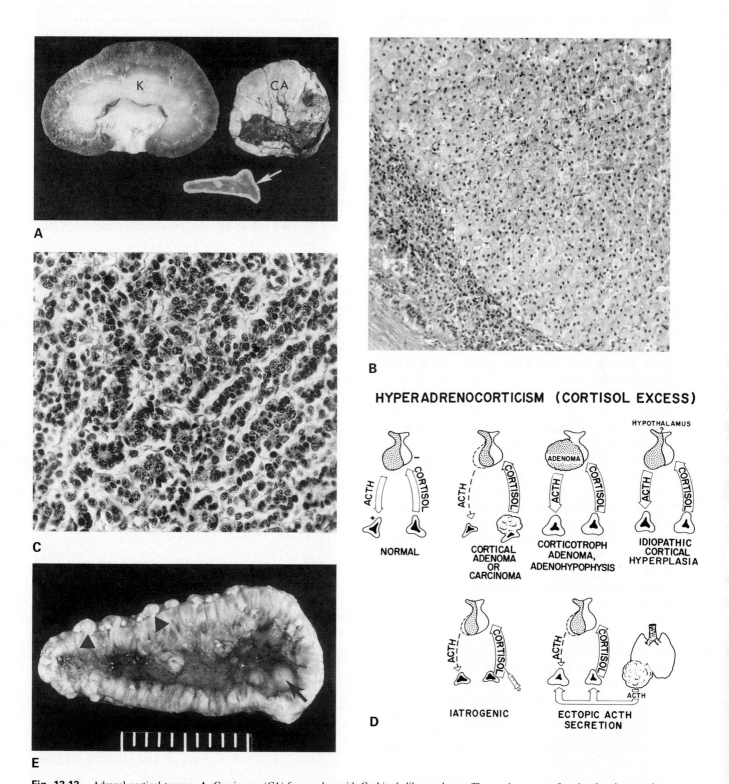

Fig. 13.13. Adrenal cortical tumors. **A.** Carcinoma *(CA)* from a dog with Cushing's-like syndrome. The carcinoma was functional and secreted an excess of cortisol that resulted in prominent cortical atrophy (white arrow) of the contralateral adrenal gland. A longitudinal section of kidney *(K)* is at the left. **B.** Adenoma from a dog is composed of large, lipid laden cells with a vacuolated cytoplasm and small hyperchromatic nucleus. A rim of compressed adrenal cortex and adrenal capsule is at the upper left. **C.** Carcinoma in a cow. Cords of tumor cells with prominent hyperchromatic nuclei are separated by small vascular sinusoids. **D.** Multiple pathogenic mechanisms of cortisol excess in dogs. **E.** Nodular cortical hyperplasia in a dog with multiple extra-capsular (arrowheads) and intramedullary (arrow) extensions. Scale = 1 cm.

Growth and Metastasis

Adrenal cortical adenomas usually are slow growing, relatively small tumors that may be associated with a hypersecretion of cortisol or infrequently other adrenal steroid hormones (e.g., aldosterone, androgens, or estrogens). Carcinomas of the adrenal cortex are larger, locally invasive, and metastasize to distant sites.[24] They often invade through the thin wall of the posterior vena cava, forming a large tumor cell thrombus, and into the adventitial layer of the abdominal aorta in dogs and cattle. Metastases are found primarily in the liver, kidney, and mesenteric lymph nodes.

REFERENCES

1. Sikora, A. (1953) Beitrag zur Nebennierenkarzinomatose des Pferdes. *Mh Vet Med* 8:241-243.
2. Richter, W.R. (1957) Tubular adenomata of the adrenal of the goat. *Cornell Vet* 47:558-577.
3. Richter, W.R. (1958) Adrenal cortical adenomata in the goat. *Amer J Vet Res* 19:895-901.
4. Sandison, A.T., and Anderson, L.J. (1968) Tumours of the endocrine glands in cattle, sheep and pigs found in a British abattoir survey. *J Comp Pathol* 78:435-444.
5. Vince, M.E., and Watson, A.D.J. (1982) Functioning adrenocortical tumour in a dog. *Aust Vet J* 58:156-158.
6. Altman, N.H., Streett, C.S., and Terner, J.Y. (1969) Castration and its relationship to tumors of the adrenal gland in the goat. *Amer J Vet Res* 30:583-589.
7. Wright, B.J., and Conner, G.H. (1968) Adrenal neoplasms in slaughtered cattle. *Cancer Res* 28:251-263.
8. Chaistain, C.B., Mitten, R.W., and Kluge, J.P. (1978) An ACTH-hyperresponsive adrenal carcinoma in a dog. *J Amer Vet Med Assoc* 172:586-588.
9. van Sluijs, F.J., Sjollema, B.E., Voorhout, G., van den Ingh, T.S.G.A.M., and Rijnberk, A. (1995) Results of adrenalectomy in 36 dogs with hyperadrenocorticism caused by adrenocortical tumour. *Vet Quarterly* 17:113-116.
10. Penninck, D.G., Feldman, E.C., and Nyland, T.G. (1988) Radiographic features of canine hyperadrenocorticism caused by autonomously functioning adrenocortical tumors: 23 cases (1978-1986). *J Amer Vet Med Assoc* 192:1604.
11. Peterson, M.E., Gilbertson, S.R., and Drucker, W.D. (1982) Plasma cortisol response to exogenous ACTH in 22 dogs with hyperadrenocorticism caused by adrenocortical neoplasia. *J Amer Vet Med Assoc* 180:542-544.
12. Feldman, E.C., Nelson, R.W., and Feldman, M.S. (1996) Use of low- and high-dose dexamethasone tests for distinguishing pituitary-dependent from adrenal tumor hyperadrenocorticism in dogs. *J Amer Vet Med Assoc* 209:772-775.
13. Kintzer, P.P., and Peterson, M.E. (1994) Mitotane treatment of 32 dogs with cortisol-secreting adrenocortical neoplasms. *J Amer Vet Med Assoc* 205:54.
14. Williams, B., and Heffess, C. (1994) Proliferative lesions of the ferret adrenal cortex. *Vet Pathol* 31:5.
15. Weiss, C.A., and Scott, M.V. (1997) Clinical aspects and surgical treatment of hyperadrenocorticism in the domestic ferret: 94 cases (1994-1996). *J Amer Anim Hosp Assoc* 33:487-493.
16. Luttgen, P.J., Storts, R.W., Rogers, K.S., and Morton, L.D. (1986) Insulinoma in a ferret. *J Amer Vet Med Assoc* 189:920-921.
17. Jergens, A.E., and Shaw, D.P. (1989) Hyperinsulinism and hypoglycemia associated with pancreatic islet cell tumor in a ferret. *J Amer Vet Med Assoc* 194:269-271.
18. Marini, R.P., Ryden, E.V., Rosenblad, W.D., Murphy, J.C., and Fox, J.G. (1993) Functional islet cell tumor in six ferrets. *J Amer Vet Med Assoc* 202:430-433.
19. Ehrhart, N., Withrow, S.J., Ehrhart, EJ., and Wimsatt, J.H. (1996): Pancreatic beta cell tumor in ferrets: 20 cases (1986-1994). *J Amer Vet Med Assoc* 209:1737-1740.
20. Rosenthal, K.L., Peterson, M.E., Quesenberry, K.E., Hillyer, E.V., Beeber, N.L., Moroff, S.D., and Lothrop, C.D., Jr. (1993) Hyperadrenocorticism associated with adrenocortical tumor or nodular hyperplasia of the adrenal gland in ferrets: 50 cases (1987-1991). *J Amer Vet Med Assoc* 203:271-275.
21. Gould, W.J., Reimers, T.J., Bell, J.A., Lawrence, H.J., Randolph, J.F., Rowland, P.H., and Scarlett, J.M. (1995) Evaluation of urinary cortisol: Creatinine ratios for the diagnosis of hyperadrenocorticism associated with adrenal gland tumors in ferrets. *J Amer Vet Med Assoc* 206:42-46.
22. Lawrence, H.J., Gould, W.J., Flanders, J.A., Rowland, P.H., and Yeager, A.E. (1993) Unilateral adrenalectomy as a treatment for adrenocortical tumors in ferrets: Five cases (1990-1992). *J Amer Vet Med Assoc* 203:267-270.
23. Monlux, A.W., Anderson, W.A., and Davis, C.L. (1956) A survey of tumors occurring in cattle, sheep, and swine. *Amer J Vet Res* 17:646-677.
24. Kelly, D.F., Siegel, E.T, and Berg, P. (1971) The adrenal glands in dogs with hyperadrenocorticalism. *Vet Pathol* 8:385-400.

Tumors of the Adrenal Medulla: Pheochromocytoma, Neuroblastoma, Ganglioneuroma

Incidence and Classification

Pheochromocytomas are the most common tumors in the adrenal medulla of animals, although other tumors may develop from the neuroectodermal cells, which differentiate into either secretory cells or sympathetic ganglion cells (fig. 13.14). Neuroblastomas arise from primitive neuroectodermal cells, often in younger animals, and form a large intra-abdominal neoplasm that may metastasize to peritoneal surfaces. Ganglioneuromas usually are well-differentiated small tumors that have sympathetic ganglion cells and neurofibrils.

Pheochromocytomas develop most often in cattle and dogs and infrequently in other domestic animals[1-4]; however, they also occur frequently in certain strains of commonly used laboratory rats.[5,6] A recent study of 61 cases of pheochromocytomas in dogs found they usually developed in middle-aged to older dogs with no apparent gender or breed predisposition.[7] In bulls and humans pheochromocytomas may develop concurrently with calcitonin secreting C cell (ultimobranchial) tumors of the thyroid gland.[8-12] This appears to represent a multicentric neoplastic transformation of multiple types of endocrine cells of neuroectodermal origin in the same individual and resembles the syndrome of multiple endocrine neoplasia reported in human patients.[13] Most affected animals are 6 years of age or more. Boxers appear to be the breed of dogs that are most predisposed to develop pheochromocytomas.[14] A

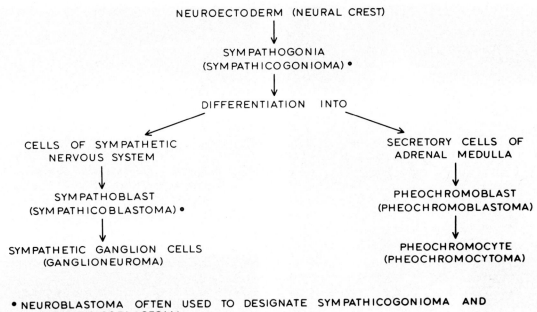

NEUROECTODERM (NEURAL CREST)

↓

SYMPATHOGONIA
(SYMPATHICOGONIOMA) •

↓

DIFFERENTIATION INTO

CELLS OF SYMPATHETIC   SECRETORY CELLS OF
NERVOUS SYSTEM   ADRENAL MEDULLA

↓   ↓

SYMPATHOBLAST   PHEOCHROMOBLAST
(SYMPATHICOBLASTOMA) •   (PHEOCHROMOBLASTOMA)

↓   ↓

SYMPATHETIC GANGLION CELLS   PHEOCHROMOCYTE
(GANGLIONEUROMA)   (PHEOCHROMOCYTOMA)

• NEUROBLASTOMA OFTEN USED TO DESIGNATE SYMPATHICOGONIOMA AND
  SYMPATHICOBLASTOMA.

Fig. 13.14.   Histogenesis of tumors of the adrenal medulla.

comprehensive review has been published recently on the selected etiologic factors involved in the frequent occurrence of proliferative lesions in the adrenal medulla in laboratory rats.[15]

Clinical Characteristics

Functional pheochromocytomas have been reported infrequently in animals. Tachycardia, edema, and cardiac hypertrophy observed in several dogs and horses with pheochromocytomas were attributed to excessive catecholamine secretion.[14] Arteriolar sclerosis and widespread medial hyperplasia of arterioles has been reported in dogs with pheochromocytomas that were associated with clinical signs suggestive of paroxysmal hypertension. Hypertension was detected in 43 percent of dogs with pheochromocytomas tested; all hypertensive dogs had concurrent diseases that may have contributed to the elevation in blood pressure.[7] Infrequently, hyperadrenocorticism may occur concurrently in dogs with pheochromocytoma and may contribute to the development of hypertension, particularly during digital manipulation of the affected adrenal gland during surgery.[16]

Norepinephrine is the principal catecholamine extracted from pheochromocytomas in dogs. This is similar to normal pups, where norepinephrine is the predominant catecholamine, but in adult dogs epinephrine predominates. The catecholamine content in pheochromocytomas from bulls with concurrent C cell tumors of the thyroid gland has been found to be higher than in the normal adrenal medulla.[17] Urinary excretion of vanillylmandelic acid and free unconjugated catecholamines was elevated in bulls with pheochromocytomas.

Many adrenal medullary tumors in animals are found as incidental findings at necropsy surgery.[18] However, pheochromocytomas often are large and invade into the posterior vena cava, forming an extensive tumor cell thrombus (fig. 13.15 A) that may be detected on abdominal radiographs. The vena cava is distended greatly and partially occluded by the thrombus, leading to impaired venous return from the posterior extremities (fig. 13.15 B). In a study of 50 pheochromocytomas, local tumor invasion was present in 52 percent, regional lymph node metastasis in 12 percent, and distant metastases in 24 percent.[18] Large vascular pheochromocytomas with invasion of the posterior vena cava may undergo extensive hemorrhage and form a blood filled cyst near the kidney in horses.[19]

Macroscopic Pathology

Pheochromocytomas are tumors of chromaffin cells and are almost always located in the adrenal gland, although a few extra-adrenal tumors have been found along the posterior aorta and vena cava in sites analogous with the organ of Zuckerkandl in humans.[14] They usually are unilateral and infrequently bilateral. Although size varies considerably, pheochromocytomas can be large (10 cm or more in diameter) and incorporate the majority of the affected adrenal. A small remnant of the adrenal gland usually can be found at one pole. Smaller tumors are completely surrounded by a thin compressed rim of adrenal cortex (fig. 13.15 C).

Large pheochromocytomas are multilobular and are variegated light brown to yellowish red or pink due to areas of hemorrhage and necrosis. A valuable aid in macroscopic diagnosis of pheochromocytoma is the Henle chromoreaction with either potassium dichromate or

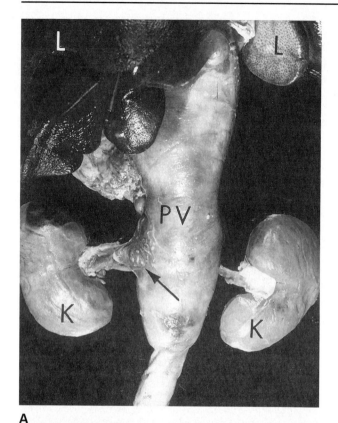

A

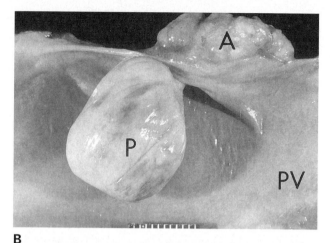

B

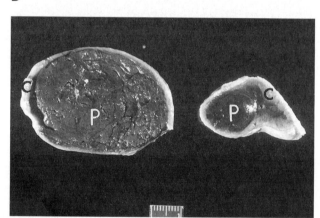

D

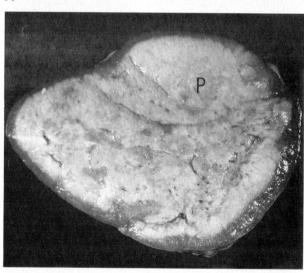

C

Fig. 13.15. Pheochromocytoma. **A.** Neoplasm in adrenal medulla (arrow) of a dog. The posterior vena cava *(PV)* is greatly distended due to invasion through the vessel wall and formation of a large tumor cell thrombus. Chronic passive congestion is evident in the liver *(L)* (*K* is kidney). Scale = 1 cm. **B.** Pheochromocytoma *(P)* extending from the region of the adrenal gland *(A)* to the wall of the posterior vena cava *(PV)* and forming a tumor cell thrombus in the lumen. Scale = 1 cm. **C.** Pheochromocytoma *(P)* in adrenal medulla from a bull that also had a C cell tumor of the thyroid. The surrounding adrenal cortex is thin and is compressed by the expanding tumor in the medulla. **D.** Chromaffin positive reaction in bilateral pheochromocytomas (P) in the bovine adrenal gland. The surrounding cortex *(C)* is compressed to varying degrees. Scale = 1 cm.

iodate (fig. 13.15 D). Application of Zenker's solution to the flat cut surface of a freshly sectioned tumor results in oxidation of catecholamines, forming a dark brown pigment within 5 to 20 minutes.

Malignant pheochromocytomas have a thin fibrous capsule that is invaded at several points. They exert pressure on the posterior vena cava or infiltrate the vessel, forming a tumor cell thrombus.

Histopathology

Tumor cells in pheochromocytomas vary from small cuboidal or polyhedral cells, similar to those in the normal

adrenal medulla, to large pleomorphic cells with multiple hyperchromatic nuclei. The cytoplasmic area is lightly eosinophilic, finely granular, and often indistinct because of early onset of autolysis in adrenal medullary tissue. Tumor cells characteristically are subdivided into small lobules by a fine connective tissue septa and capillaries (fig. 13.16 A). Vascular sinusoids may be lined directly by polyhedral to spindle shaped tumor cells. Primary fixation with potassium dichromate (e.g., Zenker's solution) gives a positive chromaffin reaction and a brown granular appearance to the cytoplasm of tumor cells. The chromaffin reaction is helpful in distinguishing anaplastic pheochromocytomas from poorly differentiated adrenal cortical carcinomas.

The term *pheochromoblastoma* has been used to designate poorly differentiated anaplastic tumors derived from of catecholamine secreting cells in the adrenal medulla. *Malignant pheochromocytoma* often is used to designate adrenal medullary tumors that invade through the adrenal capsule and into adjacent structures (e.g., posterior vena cava and periadrenal fat) and/or metastasize to distant sites (e.g., liver, regional lymph nodes, or lungs). Multiple areas of coagulation necrosis and hemorrhage often are present in larger malignant pheochromocytomas. The neoplastic cells completely incorporate the medulla of the affected adrenal, invade most or all of the surrounding cortex, and often penetrate the adrenal capsule and grow in the periadrenal connective tissues. There is frequent evidence for invasion into adrenal sinusoids and lymphatics and the formation of distinct tumor cell emboli; however, vascular invasion in adrenal medullary proliferative lesions should be evaluated carefully due to the frequent growth of tumor cells in a subendothelial location. The pattern of arrangement of neoplastic cells varies between different areas of the malignant pheochromocytoma, but includes small lobules, solid sheets, and palisading along blood sinusoids. Neoplastic cells tend to be larger and more pleomorphic (polyhedral and spindle shaped) and tend to have more frequent mitotic figures than those of more benign pheochromocytomas.

Diffuse or nodular adrenal medullary hyperplasia appears to precede the development of pheochromocytoma in bulls, laboratory rats, and humans with C cell tumors of the thyroid gland (fig. 13.16 B).[17,20] Adrenal medullary hyperplasia is detected by an increased total adrenal weight, a decreased corticomedullary ratio (fig. 13.16 C) due to an increase in the size and number of medullary cells, and the presence of frequent mitotic figures in the adrenal medulla.

Neuroblastomas are differentiated from pheochromo-

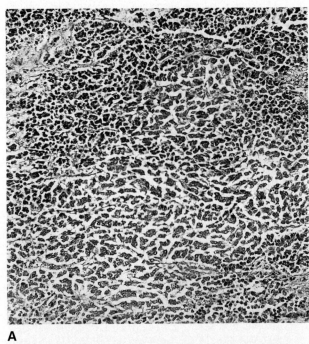

A

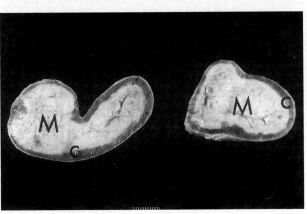

C

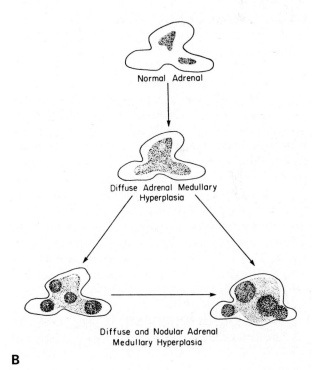

B

Fig. 13.16. Adrenal medullary hyperplasia. **A.** Pheochromocytoma of a dog. Groups of small and large tumor cells are arranged along vascular sinusoids. The adrenal cortex (top) is compressed. [From DeLellis, R.A., et al. (1976) *Amer J Pathol* 83:177-196.] **B.** Histogenesis of pheochromocytoma from diffuse and/or nodular adrenal medullary hyperplasia in humans with thyroid C cell neoplasms. [From Yarrington, J.T., and Capen, C.C. (1981) *Vet Pathol* 18:316-325.] **C.** Bilateral diffuse hyperplasia of adrenal medulla in a bull with a concomitant C cell carcinoma of the thyroid gland. The expanded adrenal medulla *(M)* compresses the surrounding adrenal cortex *(C)*. Scale = 1 cm.

cytomas by being composed of small tumor cells with a hyperchromatic nucleus and a scant amount of cytoplasm. They develop as a centrally located expansive mass that compresses the surrounding cortex (fig. 13.17 A). Cells comprising neuroblastomas resemble lymphocytes and tend to form pseudorosettes (fig. 13.17 B). Neurofibrils or unmyelinated nerve fibers usually can be demonstrated in neuroblastomas.

Ganglioneuromas usually are small benign tumors arising in the medulla and compressing the surrounding cortex (fig. 13.17 C). They are composed of multipolar sympathetic ganglion cells and neurofibrils with a prominent fibrous connective tissue stroma. Neoplastic cells in medullary tumors occasionally differentiate along two lines, resulting in adjacent pheochromocytomas and ganglioneuromas in the same adrenal gland (fig. 13.17 D). The two adjacent masses in the same adrenal gland have typical microscopic characteristics of a ganglioneuroma (fig. 13.17 E) and pheochromocytoma (fig. 13.17 F).

Ultrastructural Characteristics

Pheochromocytomas are composed of epinephrine secreting cells, norepinephrine secreting cells, or both.[17,21] The principal distinguishing ultrastructural feature between these two populations of medullary cells is in the fine structure of their secretory granules. Pheochromocytomas from which norepinephrine is the principal catecholamine extracted are composed of cells of the type illustrated in figure 13.18 A. The secretory granules have an eccentrically situated, small, electron dense core that is surrounded by a wide submembranous space. When epinephrine is the principal catecholamine secreted by the pheochromocytoma, the secretion granules in tumor cells have a coarsely granular internal core of lower density and a narrow submembranous space (fig. 13.18 B). Golgi apparatuses are prominent, and there are lamellar arrays of endoplasmic reticulum in many tumor cells.[17]

Growth and Metastasis

Small pheochromocytomas are well encapsulated and remain confined to the affected adrenal gland. Malignant pheochromocytomas often are larger and exert pressure on and invade adjacent tissues, particularly the vena cava and aorta. Tumor cells often invade the capsule and wall of the posterior vena cava, forming either a large thrombus that partially occludes the venous return from the posterior extremities or a blood filled cyst. Metastases have been reported in approximately 50 percent of pheochromocytomas in dogs to the liver, regional lymph nodes, spleen, and lungs[14]; however, recent studies of 50 and 61 cases found metastases to distant sites in 24 and 13 percent, respectively.[7,18] Malignant pheochromocytomas have been reported to metastasize to a lumbar vertebral body (L_2), resulting in localized osteolysis and progressive paraparesis,[22] as well as to the femur in a dog, predisposing to the development of a pathological fracture.

REFERENCES

1. Wright, B.J., and Conner, G.H. (1968) Adrenal neoplasms in slaughtered cattle. *Cancer Res* 28:251-263.
2. Buckingham, J.D.E. (1970) Case report: Pheochromocytoma in a mare. *Can Vet J* 11:205-208.
3. West, J.L. (1975) Bovine pheochromocytoma: Case report and review of literature. *Amer J Vet Res* 36:1371-1373.
4. Froscher, B.G., and Power, H.T. (1982) Malignant pheochromocytoma in a foal. *J Amer Vet Med Assoc* 181:494-496.
5. DeLellis, R.A., Nunnemacher, G., and Wolfe, H.J. (1977) C cell hyperplasia, an ultrastructural analysis. *Lab Invest* 36:237–248.
6. Capen, C.C., DeLellis, R.A., and Yarrington, J.T. (1991) Endocrine system. In Haschek, W.M. and Rousseaux C.G.(Eds.), *Handbook of Toxicologic Pathology*. Ch. 21. Academic Press Inc., New York, pp. 675-760.
7. Barthez, P.Y., Marks, S.L., Woo, J., Feldman, E.C., and Matteucci, M. (1997) Pheochromocytoma in dogs: 61 cases (1984-1995). *J Vet Intern Med* 11:272-278.
8. Sipple, J.H. (1961) The association of pheochromocytoma with carcinoma of the thyroid gland. *Amer J Med* 31:163-166.
9. Voelkel, E.F., Tashjian, A.H., Jr., Davidoff, F.F., Cohen, R.B., Perlia, C.P., and Wurtman, R.J. (1973) Concentrations of calcitonin and catecholamines in pheochromocytomas, a mucosal neuroma and medullary thyroid carcinoma. *J Clin Endocrinol Metab* 37:297-307.
10. Black, H.E., Capen, C.C., and Young, D.M. (1973) Ultimobranchial thyroid neoplasms in bulls: A syndrome resembling medullary thyroid carcinoma in man. *Cancer* 32:865-878.
11. Khairi, M.R.A., Dexter, R.N., Burzynski, N.J., and Johnston, C.C., Jr. (1975) Mucosal neuroma, pheochromocytoma and medullary thyroid carcinoma: Multiple endocrine neoplasia, type 3. *Medicine* 54:89-112.
12. Spoonenberg, D.P., and McEntee, K. (1983) Pheochromocytomas and ultimobranchial (C-cell) neoplasms in the bull: Evidence of autosomal dominant inheritance in the guernsey breed. *Vet Pathol* 20:396-400.
13. Sizemore, G.W., Carney, J.A., Gharib, H., and Capen, C.C. (1992) Multiple endocrine neoplasia type 2B: 18-year follow-up of a four generation family. *Henry Ford Hosp Med J* 40:236-244.
14. Howard, E.B., and Nielsen, S.W. (1965) Pheochromocytomas associated with hypertensive lesions in dogs. *J Amer Vet Med Assoc* 147:245-252.
15. Lynch, B.S., Tischler, A.S., Capen, C.C., Monroe, I.C., McGirr, L.M., and McClain, R.M. (1996) Low digestible carbohydrates (polyols and lactose): Significance of adrenal medullary proliferative lesions in the rat. *Regul Toxicol Pharmacol* 23:256-297.
16. von Dehn, B.J., Nelson, R.W., Feldman, E.C., and Griffey, S.M. (1995) Pheochromocytoma and hyperadrenocorticism in dogs: Six cases (1982-1992). *J Amer Vet Med Assoc* 207:322.
17. Yarrington, J.T., and Capen, C.C. (1981) Ultrastructural and biochemical evaluation of adrenal medullary hyperplasia and pheochromocytoma in aged bulls. *Vet Pathol* 18:316-325.
18. Gilson, S.D., Withrow, S.J., Wheeler, S.L., and Twedt, D.C. (1994) Pheochromocytoma in 50 dogs. *J Vet Int Med* 8:228-232.
19. Yovich, J.V., and Ducharme, N.G. (1983) Ruptured pheochromocytoma in a mare with colic. *J Amer Vet Med Assoc* 183:452-464.
20. DeLellis, R.A., Wolfe, H.J., Gagel, R.F., Feldman, Z.T., Miller, H.H., Gang, D.L., and Reichlin, S. (1976) Adrenal medullary hyperplasia. A morphometric analysis in patients with familial medullary thyroid carcinoma. *Amer J Pathol* 83:177-196.
21. Lauper, N.T., Tyce, G.M., Sheps, S.G., and Carney, J.A. (1972) Pheochromocytoma: Fine structural, biochemical and clinical observations. *Amer J Cardiol* 30:197-204.
22. Berzon, J.L. (1981) A metastatic pheochromocytoma causing progressive paraparesis in a dog. *Vet Med Small Anim Clin* 76:675-679.

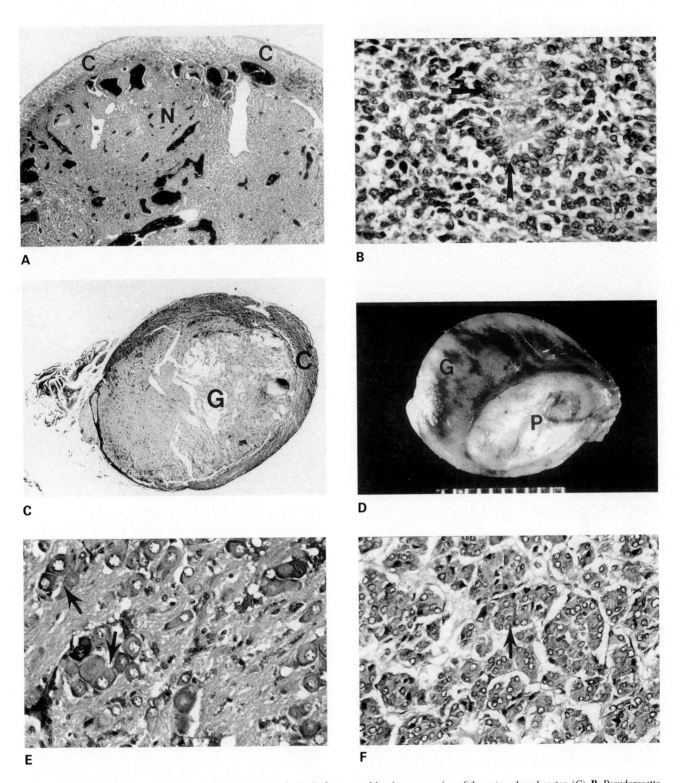

Fig. 13.17. **A.** Neuroblastoma *(N)* developing in the adrenal gland of a rat resulting in compression of the outer adrenal cortex *(C)*. **B.** Pseudorosette (arrows) formation in a neuroblastoma. The tumor cells have a small hyperchromatic nucleus and a small amount of poorly defined cytoplasm. **C.** Ganglioneuroma *(G)* arising in adrenal medulla of a rat resulting in compression of the adrenal cortex *(C)*. **D.** Adrenal medullary tumor in a rat with dual differentiation to form an adjacent ganglioneuroma *(G)* and pheochromocytoma *(P)*. **E.** Ganglioneuroma *(G)* portion of tumor in figure 13.17 C composed of numerous ganglion cells (arrows) and neurofibrils. **F.** Pheochromocytoma *(P)* portion of tumor in figure 13.17 D composed of typical neuroendocrine packets of chromaffin cells (arrow).

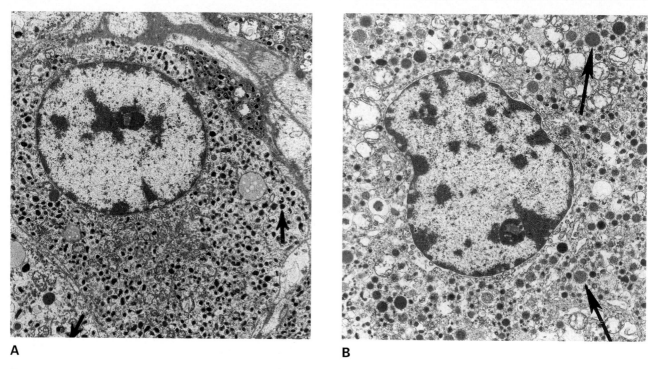

Fig. 13.18. Ultrastructure of pheochromocytoma. **A.** Norepinephrine secreting cell in pheochromocytoma from a bull in storage phase. Secretory granules have a wide space (arrows) between the core and limiting membrane. **B.** Epinephrine secreting cell in storage phase from a pheochromocytoma of a bull. Secretion granules (arrows) are less dense and have a narrow submembranous space. Cytoplasmic organelles are poorly developed.

TUMORS, HYPERPLASIA, AND CYSTS OF THYROID FOLLICULAR CELLS

Tumors of Thyroid Follicular Cells: Adenoma, Carcinoma

Incidence

Tumors of thyroid follicular cells are encountered most often in dogs, cats, and horses, with other species affected only infrequently.[1-3] They are classified either as adenomas or carcinomas, with various subtypes based on histopathological or behavioral characteristics. Earlier reports suggested that the incidence of thyroid tumors may be higher in iodine deficient areas where many animals have long-standing diffuse hyperplastic goiter; however, an increased incidence of thyroid tumors has not been documented conclusively in either animals or humans living in iodine deficient areas. Most animals with thyroid tumors are adult or aged. The mean ages of dogs and cats with thyroid adenoma have been reported as 10.7 years and 12.4 years, respectively, and those with thyroid carcinoma as 9 years and 15.8 years, respectively.[4] Thyroid carcinomas occur more frequently than adenomas in dogs, whereas adenomas are diagnosed more frequently in cats.[4,5] Unlike the situation in humans where females are more often affected with thyroid carcinomas, no sex

prevalence has been observed in dogs. Boxers are reported to develop thyroid carcinomas more frequently than any other breed of dog.[6] Three breeds of dogs (beagle, boxer, and golden retriever) appear to have a significantly greater risk for thyroid carcinoma than all other breeds of dogs combined.[1]

In cats, there has been a dramatic increase in the incidence of thyroid neoplasms and other focal proliferative lesions that result in hyperthyroidism since the late 1970s, and at present hyperthyroidism is one of the two most common endocrine diseases in adult cats (diabetes mellitus being the other common endocrinopathy in this species). Prior to 1980 clinical hyperthyroidism was diagnosed infrequently in cats. The reasons for the apparent increased incidence are uncertain, but appear to be related, in part, to (1) a larger population of old cats seeking veterinary medical care since 1980, (2) improved assays for thyroid hormones, and (3) detailed characterization of the clinical syndrome and increased awareness of its common occurrence in adult to aged cats by veterinary clinicians. In addition, there does appear to be a "real" increase in the incidence of feline hyperthyroidism over the last 30 years. Potential risk factors have been reported to include a predominantly indoor environment, regular treatment with flea powders, exposures to herbicides and fertilizers, a diet primarily of canned food, and non-Siamese breeds (10 times greater occurrence).[7] It has been suggested that wide variations (excessive to inadequate) in dietary iodine intake over prolonged periods may play a role in the pathogenesis of thyroid disorders in cats.[8]

The disease in cats is mechanically different from Grave's disease in human patients as hyperthyroid cats do not have elevated circulating levels of thyroid stimulating immunoglobulins comparable to long acting thyroid stimulator (LATS) (an autoantibody that binds to the TSH receptor and activates follicular cells).[9] Purified immunoglobulin G (IgG) preparations from hyperthyroid cats significantly increased ^{3}H-thymidine in DNA and stimulated cell proliferation 15-fold but did not stimulate intracellular cAMP.[10] Thymidine uptake could be inhibited completely by a specific TSH receptor blocking antibody. These data suggest that elevated titers of thyroid growth IgGs are present in cats with hyperthyroidism and most likely act by the TSH receptor. This important thyroid disease in cats most closely resembles toxic nodular goiter in human patients.[11,12] Hyperplastic and neoplastic thyroid tissue from cats is transplantable into athymic (nude) mice and continues to overproduce T_4 and T_3 in a subcuticular location.

Studies utilizing primary cultures of enzymatically dissociated follicles from thyroid proliferative lesions from cats with hyperthyroidism have reported that organification and ^{3}H-thymidine labeling continues in the absence of TSH, in contrast to follicles from normal cat thyroids.[13] These findings suggest that an intrinsic alteration in follicular cell function occurs in thyroids of cats with multinodular goiter, leading to autonomy of cell growth and persistent overproduction of thyroid hormones. A recent study reported an overexpression of the c-ras oncogene in areas of nodular hyperplasia and adenomas derived from follicular cells in cats with hyperthyroidism, suggesting that mutations in this oncogene may play a role in the pathogenesis of these proliferative lesions.[14]

Point mutations in the thyrotropin receptor (TSHR) gene cause two forms of thyrotoxicosis in humans, namely, autonomously functioning toxic follicular adenomas and hereditary (autosomal dominant) toxic thyroid hyperplasia. The normal feline TSHR sequence between codons 480 and 640 is highly homologous to that of other mammalian TSHRs, with 95 percent, 92 percent, and 90 percent amino acid identity between the feline, canine, human, and bovine TSHRs, respectively.[15] Analysis of single stranded conformational polymorphisms in thyroid DNA from 11 sporadic cases of feline thyrotoxicosis and leukocyte DNA from two cases of familial hyperthyroidism in cats failed to identify mutations between codons 480 and 640 of the TSHR gene. These interesting findings suggest that TSHR gene mutations are not a common cause of the focal proliferative lesions of thyroid follicular cells that result in feline thyrotoxicosis.[15]

Clinical Characteristics

Disturbances of growth involving the thyroid gland are common in cats. The literature and our experience suggest that adenomas and multinodular hyperplasia of follicular cells are encountered more commonly than thyroid carcinomas (approximately 5 percent) in hyperthyroid

cats.[4,5,16-19] Adenomas and carcinomas are most likely encountered in aged cats, whereas multinodular hyperplasia can occur at any age. The mean age of cats with benign tumors was reported as 12.4 years and those with thyroid carcinomas as 15.8 years.[4]

Until recently most proliferative lesions encountered in the feline thyroid gland were found incidentally at necropsy and were not recognized as being associated with obvious clinical disturbances. Recent reports have described a syndrome of hyperthyroidism in aged cats associated with multinodular goiter, adenomas, and occasionally adenocarcinomas derived from follicular cells of the thyroid.[16,20-22] Large adenomas and carcinomas may be detected by palpation of swellings in the cranioventral cervical region; however, thyroid tumors in cats occasionally are displaced caudally to the level of the first rib and anterior mediastinum. Arterial thrombosis has been reported in a cat with a bilateral thyroid carcinoma. The cat was unable to use the left front leg, which was cool to the touch as a result of a tumor cell embolus occluding the left brachial artery. Dyspnea and dysphagia were reported in a cat with a rapidly growing anaplastic giant cell adenocarcinoma of the left thyroid.[23] The mass had partially enclosed the trachea and esophagus.

In a report of 26 cases of hyperthyroidism in aged cats, all affected cats were short- or longhaired crossbreeds ranging in age from 9 to 22 years.[16] Both sexes were equally represented. The most common clinical sign was weight loss in spite of a normal or increased appetite (fig. 13.19 A). Polydipsia and polyuria occurred in some cats. Increased frequency of defecation and increased volume of stools were observed in about half of affected cats. Restlessness and increased activity occurred in some previously quiet cats.

A common clinical finding in hyperthyroidism is tachycardia accompanied by premature heartbeats, a systolic murmur, or both. Electrocardiographic changes are common in cats with hyperthyroidism and include sinus tachycardia, often with heart rates exceeding 240 beats/minute, and increased R wave voltages, indicative of left ventricular enlargement. Cardiomegaly may be evident on radiographs; however, congestive heart failure develops infrequently (10-12 percent) in cats with hyperthyroidism. The changes usually regress after treatment of the hyperthyroidism.

One or both thyroid lobes are enlarged in hyperthyroid cats. Solitary adenomas derived from thyroid follicular cells are the most common lesions associated with hyperthyroidism in cats (fig. 13.19 B,C). The affected thyroid lobe is partially or completely incorporated by the adenoma. The adenomas often develop in thyroid glands with areas of multinodular hyperplasia of follicular cells.

Cats with hyperthyroidism usually have markedly elevated serum thyroxine (T_4) and triiodothyronine (T_3) concentrations (fig. 13.19 D).[19] The serum T_4 levels in cats with hyperthyroidism range from 3.4 to 30 µg/dl (normal range 1.5-5.0 µg/dl),[16] and serum T_3 levels range from 179 to 470 ng/dl (normal 60-200 ng/dl). Moderately increased serum enzyme levels, including ALT (alanine transaminase), AST (aspartate transaminase), and especially alkaline phosphatase, occur in hyperthyroid cats.

A small percentage of hyperthyroid cats have T_4 concentrations within the upper limits of the reference range when first evaluated. This most likely is due to early detection of the disease attributable to clinician awareness and readily available screening tests. Hyperthyroidism usually can be confirmed in these cats by repeating the thyroid hormone assays or performing a T_3 suppression test.[24] In addition, a wide variety of nonthyroidal illnesses in hyperthyroid cats also may suppress the serum T_4 concentration into the normal range.[25] Hyperthyroid cats with increased circulating T_4 and T_3 levels do not respond to exogenous TSH stimulation by increasing hormone levels two- or threefold as in normal cats. The neoplastic follicular cells are unable to recognize and respond to the exogenous TSH, and follicular cells in the adjacent normal rim of thyroid have undergone trophic atrophy and colloid involution of follicles and are unable to increase blood T_4 and T_3 levels after only short-term stimulation by TSH.

Hyperthyroid cats often have disturbances of calcium homeostasis and diffuse chief cell hyperplasia in the parathyroid glands.[26] Blood ionized (not total) calcium and plasma creatinine concentrations were significantly decreased and plasma phosphate and intact parathyroid hormone levels were increased compared to reference ranges. Hyperparathyroidism occurred in 77 percent of hyperthyroid cats with parathyroid hormone levels elevated up to 19 times the upper limit of the reference range. Hyperphosphatemia was present in approximately 40 percent of hyperthyroid cats.[26] The mechanisms for the development of hyperphosphatemia in feline hyperthyroidism are uncertain but may be related, in part, to polyphagia with increased intestinal phosphate absorption, increased catabolism of muscle proteins and release of phosphate due to the gluconeogenic effects of the elevated thyroid hormone levels, and increased bone resorption with release of phosphate into the blood. The hyperparathyroidism and chief cell hyperplasia appear to be related to the reciprocal decline in circulating levels of ionized calcium in response to the hyperphosphatemia. An elevated blood phosphate also could inhibit the renal 1-alpha-hydroxylase and decrease the production of the active form of vitamin D, thereby reducing intestinal calcium absorption; however, circulating levels of 1,25-dihydroxycholecalciferol were not decreased in the limited number of hyperthyroid cats evaluated.[26]

Serum levels of alkaline phosphatase (bone isoenzyme) are elevated consistently in cats with hyperthyroidism; however, there is no correlation between the magnitude of increase of alkaline phosphatase, osteocalcin, and serum T_4 concentrations. Although the total calcium usually is in the reference range, the serum ionized calcium often (approximately 50 percent of cases) is reduced.[27] These findings suggest that hyperthyroid cats have altered bone metabolism; however, bone disease usually is not clinically significant in adult to aged cats with hyperthyroidism.

Surgical excision of affected thyroid lobe(s) and medical management by thyroid blocking drugs (e.g., methimazole, propylthiouracil) and radioactive iodine are the treatments available for cats with hyperthyroidism. Bilateral thyroidectomy is performed if both glands are abnormal in appearance at surgery. At least one parathyroid gland should be left with an intact blood supply if bilateral thyroidectomy is performed. A thyroid blocking agent, such as methimazole or propylthiouracil, can be used before surgery to alleviate some of the severe clinical effects of hyperthyroidism.[16]

When bilateral thyroidectomy has been performed, careful monitoring of the serum calcium level is indicated immediately postoperation to detect hypocalcemia secondary to hypoparathyroidism. If the serum calcium level drops below 8 mg/dl, dietary supplementation with cal-

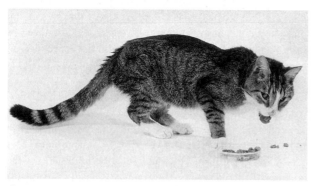

A

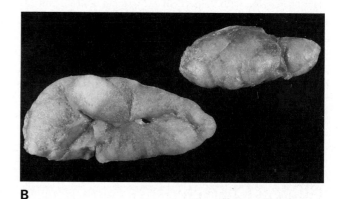

B

Fig. 13.19. Functional thyroid neoplasms in the cat. **A.** Hyperthyroid cat with a functional adenoma derived from thyroid follicular cells. The cat had lost a considerable amount of body weight in spite of its ravenous appetite. **B.** Functional thyroid adenoma excised from a hyperthyroid cat, illustrating cut (left) and external (right) surfaces. The adenoma was coarsely nodular and firm in consistency. (continued)

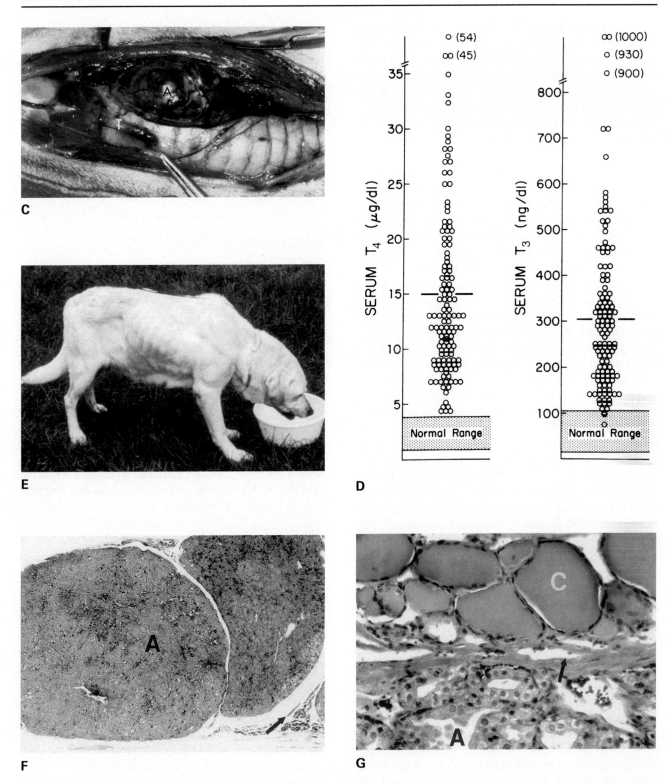

Fig. 13.19. (continued)   **C.** Surgical dissection of the ventral cervical region reveals a large unilateral thyroid adenoma (A) and a small thyroid (T) gland on the opposite side. **D.** Serum thyroid hormone levels in cats with hyperthyroidism. There is a marked elevation of serum thyroxine (mean 15 μg/dl) and triiodothyronine (mean 300 μg/dl) in cats with hyperthyroidism. [From Peterson, M.E., et al. (1983) *J Amer Vet Med Assoc* 183:103-110.] **E.** Hyperthyroidism associated with a follicular cell carcinoma (arising from ectopic thyroid tissue at the base of the tongue) in a dog with severe weight loss, muscle atrophy, and polydipsia. **F.** Multilobular follicular cell adenoma *(A)* in a cat with hyperthyroidism. The tumor is sharply demarcated from a rim of normal thyroid (arrow). **G.** Endocrinologically active follicular cell adenoma *(A)* in a cat illustrating colloid *(C)* involution of follicles in adjacent rim of normal thyroid. The follicular cells have undergone marked trophic atrophy due to suppression of TSH production by the elevated T_4 and T_3 levels, resulting in the intrafollicular accumulation of colloid. In the tumor the cuboidal to columnar cells line partially collapsed follicles containing minimal colloid. A thin fibrous connective tissue capsule (arrow) separates the adenoma from the adjacent thyroid.

cium and vitamin D should be given until the calcium level is stabilized. These cats eventually (1 to 3 months) stabilize their calcium metabolism and no longer require calcium or vitamin D supplementation. After bilateral thyroidectomy, replacement therapy with thyroxine also is required to maintain a euthyroid state. Sodium levothyroxine at 0.05 to 0.1 mg given starting 5 to 7 days after surgery is adequate to maintain normal serum T_4 and T_3 levels in most cats.

Thyroid follicular cell adenomas in horses may grow large enough to result in a multinodular enlargement in the anterioventral cervical region. Many well-demarcated thyroid adenomas are of C cell origin in horses and are amenable to complete surgical excision. Thyroid adenocarcinomas are much less common in horses and may metastasize to the retropharyngeal lymph nodes.[28]

In dogs only about 15 percent of thyroid adenomas, compared with at least 60 percent of carcinomas, are detected clinically by palpation of a firm mass in the neck or by evidence of respiratory distress.[4] However, approximately 90 percent of clinically apparent thyroid tumors in the dog are carcinomas. Carcinomas often are fixed in position by extensive local invasion of adjacent structures, whereas adenomas are freely movable under the skin.

Although the majority of dogs with thyroid follicular cell tumors are euthyroid, some thyroid tumors secrete sufficient thyroid hormone (T_4 and/or T_3) to produce mild clinical signs of hyperthyroidism.[29,30] It is surprising that hyperthyroidism occurs in dogs even with functional tumors since experimental induction of hyperthyroidism in the dog requires daily administration of about 25 times the normal replacement dose of desiccated thyroid or L-thyroxine to overload the very efficient enterohepatic excretory mechanism in this species. Polyuria is the most consistent clinical finding in hyperthyroid dogs with functional thyroid tumors, but other frequent clinical signs include weight loss despite increased appetite, polydipsia, muscle weakness and fatigue, intolerance to heat, and nervousness (fig. 13.19 E).[31] An occasional dog with a functional thyroid adenocarcinoma has been described with a mitral valve insufficiency that improved markedly following surgical excision of the tumor.[32] Rarely, dogs with bilateral thyroid carcinoma have destruction of both thyroid lobes, leading to clinical evidence of hypothyroidism with hypercholesterolemia and corneal lipidosis.[33]

Serum T_4 and T_3 levels in dogs with clinical hyperthyroidism only are mildly elevated (5-7 µg/dl and 300-400 ng/dl, respectively) compared with hyperthyroid cats, where thyroid hormone levels are markedly increased (fig. 13.19 D). In general, the likelihood of developing clinical hyperthyroidism associated with thyroid neoplasms in animals depends upon (1) the capability of tumor cells to synthesize T_4 and T_3 (e.g., well-differentiated thyroid tumors that form follicles and produce colloid are more likely to synthesize thyroid hormones than poorly differentiated

solid neoplasms) and (2) the degree of elevation of circulating levels of T_4 and T_3, which depends upon a balance between the rate of secretion of thyroid hormones by the tumor and the rate of degradation of thyroid hormones. Dogs have a much more efficient enterohepatic excretory mechanism for thyroid hormones than cats. Cats are very sensitive to phenol and phenol derivatives[34] and have a poor ability to conjugate phenolic compounds (such as T_4) with glucuronic acid and excrete the T_4-glucuronide into the bile. The capacity for conjugation of T_3 with sulfate is also limited and is easily overloaded.

Macroscopic Pathology

Thyroid Adenoma

Adenomas are usually white to tan, relatively small, usually solid nodules that are well demarcated from the adjacent thyroid parenchyma. The affected thyroid lobe is only moderately enlarged and distorted in contour. A distinct, white, fibrous connective capsule of variable thickness separates the adenoma from the compressed parenchyma (fig. 13.20 A). Only a single adenoma usually is present in a thyroid lobe.

Other thyroid adenomas are composed of thin-walled cysts filled with a yellow to red fluid (fig. 13.20 B). The external surface is smooth and covered by an extensive network of blood vessels. Small masses of neoplastic tissue remain in the wall and form rugose projections into the cyst lumen. The thyroid parenchyma of the affected lobe may be completely obliterated.

Thyroid Carcinoma

Carcinomas are larger than adenomas, are coarsely multinodular, and often have large areas of hemorrhage and necrosis near the centers. Unilateral involvement by thyroid carcinoma is about twice as frequent in dogs as involvement of both thyroid lobes[4] (fig. 13.20 C). Carcinomas are poorly encapsulated and invade locally into the wall of the trachea, cervical muscles, esophagus, larynx, nerves, and vessels. Early invasion into branches of the cranial and caudal thyroid veins, with the formation of tumor cell thrombi (fig. 13.21), leads to multiple pulmonary metastases, often before involvement of the retropharyngeal and caudal cervical lymph nodes. White, gritty, focal areas of mineralization or bone formation are scattered throughout some thyroid carcinomas.

Although adenomas and carcinomas derived from follicular cells usually arise in the neck from the thyroid lobes, they may develop from ectopic thyroid parenchyma in the anterior mediastinum and must be included in the differential diagnosis of *heart base tumors* in dogs.[35,36] Invasive ectopic thyroid carcinomas that arose at the base of the heart and metastasized to the lung, pancreas, and kidney have been reported in dogs.[37] The neoplastic cells

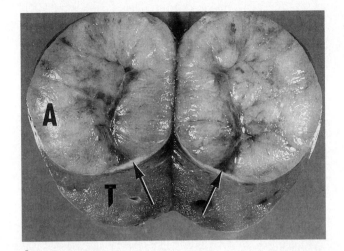

A

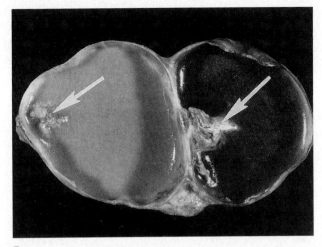

B

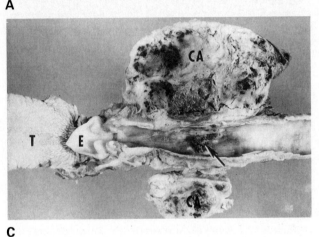

C

Fig. 13.20. Macroscopic gross features of thyroid neoplasms. **A.** Follicular adenoma from the thyroid gland of a horse. The adenoma (A) is solid and is separated from the adjacent compressed thyroid (T) by a prominent fibrous capsule (arrows). **B.** Cystic adenoma from the thyroid gland of a dog. The cyst wall is primarily fibrous tissue, but a few masses of neoplastic cells (arrows) project into the lumen. **C.** Bilateral thyroid carcinoma (CA) in a dog with local invasion through the wall of the trachea (arrow) (E = epiglottis, T = tongue).

Cystic adenomas consist of one or two large cavities filled with proteinic fluid, necrotic debris, and erythrocytes. Focal accumulations of tumor cells, forming either follicles or solid nests, are present in the capsule of dense fibrous connective tissue. These adenomas may develop by progressive cystic degeneration of one of the several types of follicular adenomas. Oxyphilic adenomas are composed predominantly or entirely of large cells with a densely eosinophilic granular cytoplasm arranged in indistinct follicles with little or no colloid formation. *Oxyphil (Hürthle) cells* appear to be metabolically altered follicular cells that accumulate abnormally

ultrastructurally formed intra- or intercellular lumens with microvillar projections and contained large lysosomes and arrays of rough endoplasmic reticulum.

Histopathology

Thyroid Adenoma

The adenomas are classified into *follicular* and *papillary* types. They are sharply demarcated and partially to completely encapsulated from the adjacent compressed thyroid parenchyma by a fibrous capsule of varying thickness. Adenomas that retain the ability to form follicles are by far more common than papillary adenomas in animals (fig. 13.22 A). Each follicular adenoma tends to have a consistent growth pattern throughout the tumor.

There are several different patterns of growth similar to those of the normal thyroid for the species involved. *Microfollicular adenomas* consist of tumor cells arranged in miniature follicles with small amounts of colloid or an absence of colloid. Macrofollicular adenomas are formed by large, irregularly shaped follicles that are greatly distended with colloid and lined by flattened follicular cells. There may be extensive hemorrhage and desquamation of follicular cells into the lumens of the distended follicles.

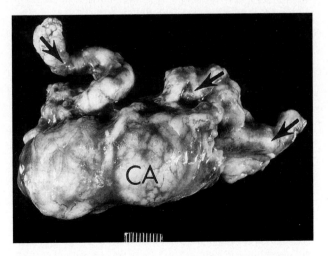

Fig. 13.21. Prominent tumor cell thrombi distending thyroid veins (arrows) of a dog with an adenocarcinoma (CA) derived from thyroid follicular cells. Scale is 1 cm.

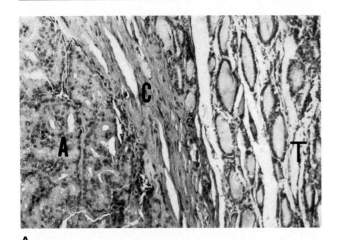

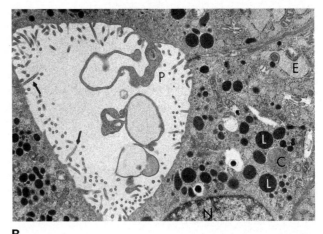

A   **B**

Fig. 13.22. Thyroid adenoma. **A.** Follicular adenoma *(A)* from a horse with a prominent fibrous capsule *(C)* separating it from the adjacent compressed thyroid parenchyma *(T)*. **B.** Functional adenoma of the cat. The neoplastic cells are arranged into a follicle with numerous, long, cytoplasmic processes *(P)* extending from the luminal surface to engulf colloid by endocytosis. There are many large lysosomal *(L)* bodies in follicular cells associated with colloid droplets *(C)* and long microvilli (arrows) on the surface bordering the colloid. Profiles of rough endoplasmic reticulum *(E)* often are dilated by a finely granular material (*N* is nucleus of follicular cell).

large numbers of mitochondria in their cytoplasm. Trabecular adenomas are the most poorly differentiated of the follicular type. The tumor cells are small and are arranged in narrow columns separated by an edematous fibrous stroma, and there is little evidence of follicle formation.

Papillary adenomas are recognized infrequently in most animal species in comparison to human beings, where this is the most common pattern of arrangement of follicular cells in thyroid neoplasms. Columnar or cuboidal follicular cells are arranged in a single layer around a thin vascular connective tissue stalk. These papillary projections extend into the lumens of cystic spaces of various sizes. The cysts contain desquamated tumor cells, colloid, erythrocytes, and occasionally laminated foci of mineralization resembling psammoma bodies.

Follicular adenomas are the most common thyroid lesion in cats with hyperthyroidism. They appear as solitary, soft, lobulated nodules that enlarge and distort the contour of the affected lobe (see fig. 13.19 F). A thin, fibrous connective tissue capsule separates the adenoma from the adjacent, often compressed, thyroid parenchyma (see fig. 13.19 G). The neoplastic cells form irregularly shaped follicles with occasional papillary infoldings of epithelium and variable amounts of colloid. Focal areas of necrosis, mineralization, and cystic degeneration are present in larger adenomas. Multiple sections of adenomas fail to reveal histological evidence of either vascular or capsular invasion by tumor cells.

Thyroid adenomas also must be differentiated from multinodular (*adenomatous*) hyperplasia (*goiter*) that occurs frequently in certain species such as old cats. These multiple areas of thyroid hyperplasia usually are microscopic and do not enlarge the affected lobe of thyroid unless they are numerous. In contrast to adenomas, the

areas of nodular hyperplasia are not encapsulated, and the adjacent thyroid parenchyma is not compressed. Histopathologically, the hyperplastic nodules are composed of irregularly shaped follicles lined by cuboidal follicular cells and contain variable amounts of colloid. Follicles between the nodules of hyperplasia often have undergone colloid involution, suggesting that these focal proliferative lesions of follicular cells are producing thyroid hormones at an autonomous rate resulting in decreased TSH production.

Functional thyroid adenomas in cats associated with a clinical syndrome of hyperthyroidism are composed of cuboidal to columnar follicular cells that form follicles of varying sizes and shapes. The follicles usually are partially collapsed and contain little colloid because of the intense endocytotic activity of neoplastic follicular cells. Long cytoplasmic projections often extend from the follicular cells into the lumen to phagocytize colloid (fig. 13.22 B). As a result of the marked endocytotic activity, numerous colloid droplets are present in the apical cytoplasm of follicular cells in close proximity to the many electron dense lysosomal bodies. The neoplastic follicular cells are considerably larger (two to four times) the size of the atrophic cells lining the follicles in the rim of normal thyroid.

Functional thyroid adenomas are partially or completely separated from remnants of the adjacent normal thyroid by a fine connective tissue capsule. Follicles in the rim of normal thyroid around a functional adenoma are enlarged and distended by an accumulation of colloid (i.e., colloid involution). The follicular cells are low cuboidal and atrophied, with little evidence of endocytotic activity in response to the elevated levels of thyroid hormones and decreased circulating levels of TSH.

The opposite thyroid lobe should be carefully evaluated in cats with solitary adenomas for evidence of focal (adenomatous) hyperplasia or microadenomas. The opposite thyroid lobe in cats with unilateral functional adenoma often has discrete, small areas of multinodular hyperplasia of follicular cells that may cause recurrence of hyperthyroidism several months to a year or more after surgical removal of the tumor. The multifocal areas of follicular cell hyperplasia appear to be precursor lesions for the development of follicular adenomas in the thyroid glands of old cats.

Thyroid Carcinoma

Malignant tumors of thyroid follicular cells are generally more highly cellular and have a greater degree of cellular pleomorphism than adenomas. There appears to be a good correlation between fine needle aspiration cytology and histopathologic evaluation of thyroid biopsies in the diagnosis of thyroid carcinomas in dogs.[38] On the basis of the predominant histological pattern of growth, *differentiated thyroid carcinomas* are subdivided into *follicular, papillary,* and *compact cellular (solid)* types.[4] In dogs, where thyroid carcinomas are encountered most frequently, they often have both a follicular and compact cellular growth pattern, whereas papillary carcinomas are rare. Papillary carcinoma is the most common type of thyroid carcinoma in humans.

Follicular adenocarcinomas are diagnosed when the majority of tumor cells are arranged in a recognizable follicular pattern. It is possible to subdivide follicular carcinomas further on the basis of degree of follicle formation, as described for follicular adenomas, but that often is difficult because of the admixture of growth patterns present in any one tumor. Such a subdivision of thyroid carcinomas appears to be of little prognostic value in animals. The tumor cells are tall cuboidal to columnar and form follicles of varying size, shape, and colloid content. Mitotic activity in the tumor cells usually is minimal. The colloid in follicular lumens occasionally is clumped and extensively mineralized (fig. 13.23 A).

In *compact cellular thyroid carcinomas,* tumor cells form compact aggregations or solid sheets of cells, often separated by a fibrous stroma with little or no attempt at follicle formation and colloid secretion. The polyhedral cells are closely arranged and have an eosinophilic cytoplasm that is finely granulated or vacuolated. Immunocytochemical and ultrastructural studies have demonstrated that compact cellular (solid) carcinomas of the canine thyroid are derived from follicular cells[4] and not from C cells, as previously suggested.[39] Thyroglobulin immunoreactivity has been demonstrated in compact cellular thyroid tumors of dogs by the peroxidase-antiperoxidase technique, but there is a lack of calcitonin positive cells.[40] The major patterns of thyroglobulin immunoreactivity included diffuse cytoplasmic staining, apical staining on the border of follicular lumens and intracytoplasmic droplets, and staining of colloid in the follicular lumens. The stroma has bands of fibrous connective tissue of varying thickness, but

does not contain amyloid as was reported in C cell (medullary) carcinomas of the thyroid.

Compact cellular carcinomas in the thyroid of dogs have been reported to respond to TSH by increased phosphatide turnover, especially phosphatidic acid and phosphatidylinositol. The malignant tumor cells appeared to retain at least one complete control system from TSH receptors to the final metabolic product.

Follicular–compact cellular carcinoma, which has approximately equal follicular and compact cellular (solid) growth patterns, is the most common histological type of malignant thyroid tumor in dogs (fig. 13.23 B). The follicles formed often are smaller and contain less colloid than in pure follicular carcinoma. The tumor cells arranged in compact nests appear to be morphologically and functionally less differentiated than those that form follicles and secrete colloid.

Papillary carcinomas, in which tumor cells predominantly form papillae extending into cystic spaces, are rare in animals in contrast to their frequent occurrence in humans. Single or multiple layers of cuboidal cells are arranged around fibrovascular stalks that project into cystic spaces. The nuclei of tumor cells are vesicular and pleomorphic with prominent nucleoli. The nuclear vacuoles or inclusions observed by light microscopy have been shown by electron microscopy to represent cytoplasmic evaginations into the nucleus.[41] Other areas of papillary thyroid tumors may form small follicles or solid sheets.

Infiltration of tumor cells through the fibrous connective tissue capsule (fig. 13.23 C) and into adjacent tissues is observed frequently in thyroid carcinomas of dogs. The early formation of tumor cell emboli by invasion of thin-walled veins results in pulmonary metastasis in dogs prior to the development of secondary foci of growth in regional lymph nodes draining the affected thyroid lobe.

Undifferentiated thyroid carcinomas lack a characteristic architectural pattern of arrangement of tumor cells. They are an uncommon form of thyroid carcinoma in animals and are composed of sheets of spindle cells forming interlacing bands and whorls. The spindle cells have a large oval nucleus with a prominent nucleus and abundant eosinophilic cytoplasm. The mitotic index often is high, up to 10-15 mitoses/high power field. The abundant cytoplasmic area stains diffusely or focally for thyroglobulin.[42] The neoplastic cells ultrastructurally have abundant rough endoplasmic reticulum, numerous free ribosomes, distinct intercellular junctional complexes, and large membrane-bound granules in the cytoplasm.

Small cell carcinoma is one type of undifferentiated thyroid carcinoma. It is composed of highly malignant follicular cells, with either a diffuse or compact pattern of growth, that rarely form follicles. The small tumor cells are uniform in appearance and are closely packed together in clusters separated by a fibrous stroma (fig. 13.23 D). The scant cytoplasm is eosinophilic, and the oval nucleus is densely hyperchromatic. Mitotic figures are frequent.

Giant cell carcinoma is the second type of undifferentiated thyroid carcinoma. It is a highly malignant tumor composed of poorly differentiated thyroid follicular cells. The anaplastic tumor cells are large, pleomorphic, and often spindle shaped, making a differentiation from fibrosarcoma difficult (fig. 13.23 E).[23] A metastasizing fibrosarcoma in the thyroid gland has been reported in a sheep that had received 5 microcuries of radioactive iodine (^{131}I) for 53 months beginning at weaning.[43,44] The demonstration of identifiable epithelial structures may require multiple sections from several areas of the tumor. Ultrastructural studies of giant cell carcinomas from humans have demonstrated microvilli, numerous dense bodies, and other nuclear and cytoplasmic characteristics similar to those of follicular cells.[45] Follicular remnants and transi-

tional forms suggest that giant cell carcinomas are derived from thyroid follicular cells.[46]

Malignant mixed thyroid tumors contain both malignant follicular cells and mesenchymal (usually osteogenic or cartilaginous) elements.[47-49] An interesting case of bilateral thyroid neoplasms in a dog (follicular–compact cellular on the left and malignant mixed tumor on the right) was accompanied by severe multifocal myxedema with a low normal serum thyroxine level.[48] There was a marked accumulation of glycosaminoglycans, particularly hyaluronic acid, leading to increased water-binding capacity in the dermis and subcutis over the head, footpads, elbows, and elsewhere.

Thyroid carcinomas occur less frequently in cats than either adenoma or multinodular hyperplasia of follicular cells. They often result in considerable enlargement of one

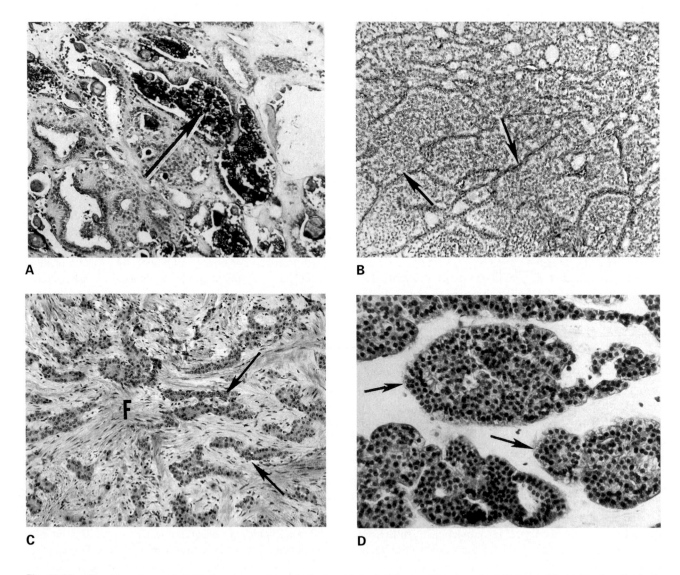

Fig. 13.23. Thyroid carcinoma. **A.** Follicular adenocarcinoma in the thyroid gland of the dog. Many irregular follicles are filled with mineralized colloid (arrow). **B.** Follicular compact cellular carcinoma of the thyroid gland from a dog. Small colloid-containing follicles are interspersed between compact aggregations of tumor cells. Fine connective tissue septa with capillaries (arrows) subdivide the carcinoma into small lobules. **C.** Invasion of thyroid carcinoma (arrows) through the fibrous capsule (F) into adjacent tissues in a dog. **D.** Small cell carcinoma in the thyroid gland of a dog. Clusters of small tumor cells (arrows) are separated by an edematous fibrous stroma with capillaries. (continued)

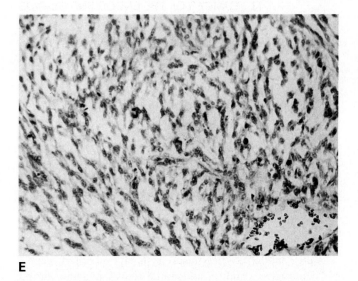

E

Fig. 13.23. (continued) **E.** Giant cell carcinoma in the thyroid gland of a dog. The tumor cells are spindle shaped, and there is a lack of follicle formation. (continued)

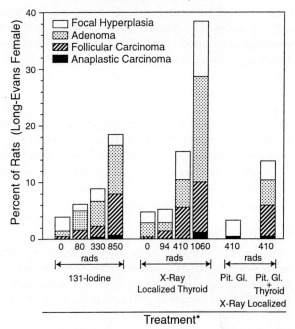

F

Disruption of Hypothalamic, Pituitary, Thyroid Triad by Xenobiotic Chemicals

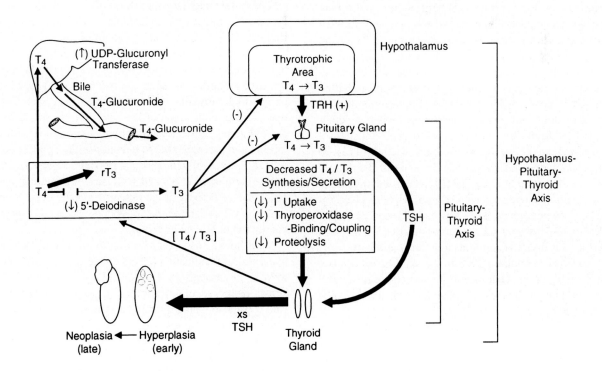

G

Fig. 13.23. (continued) **F.** Thyroid follicular cell lesions vs radiation exposure. [From Capen, C.C. et al. (1999) In: *Radiation and Thyroid Cancer,* World Scientific Publishing.] **G.** Disruption of hypothalamic-pituitary-thyroid triad by xenobiotic chemicals. [From Capen, C.C. (1997) *Toxicol Pathol* 25:39–48.]

or both thyroid lobes and may invade adjacent structures. Carcinomas are characterized by the invasion of vessels and the connective tissue capsule by neoplastic cells. Metastases to regional lymph nodes (retropharyngeal, mandibular, and deep cervical) and distant sites have been reported in less than 50 percent of thyroid carcinomas in cats.[4] The well-differentiated thyroid carcinomas are relatively solid and composed of a uniform pattern of small follicles containing little colloid and occasional compact cellular areas; however, many thyroid carcinomas in cats can not be distinguished microscopically from thyroid adenomas. Strands of dense connective tissue with an abundant capillary network and foci of lymphocytes subdivide the neoplastic cells into small lobules.

Growth and Metastasis

Thyroid adenomas grow slowly and occasionally result in a palpable enlargement that is detected clinically in the anterior cervical region. Thyroid carcinomas are larger and more frequently produce a palpable enlargement and respiratory distress that is apparent clinically. The probability of metastasis increases in proportion to the size and duration of the thyroid carcinoma in dogs.[4] For example, metastases were found in only 14 percent of dogs with carcinoma when the tumor volume was less than 21 ml, but they were found in 78 percent when the tumor was larger than 21 ml. Therefore, it appears that early surgical removal of thyroid carcinomas before they attain a large size is critical for long-term survival in dogs. Follicular carcinomas in dogs appear to enlarge more rapidly than those with a compact cellular (solid) component. Radioisotope imaging has proven useful in determining the extent of local tissue involvement by a thyroid carcinoma.[50]

Carcinomas often grow rapidly, invade adjacent structures such as the trachea, esophagus, and larynx, and often are fixed in position. Metastasis has been reported in 38 percent of dogs with thyroid carcinomas,[4] whereas other studies have found an even higher incidence.[6] The earliest and most frequent site of metastasis is the lung because thyroid carcinomas tend to invade branches of the thyroid vein. Tumor cell emboli may be palpated in the thyroid or jugular veins in some dogs with thyroid carcinoma (see fig. 13.21).[6] The retropharyngeal and caudal cervical lymph nodes are less frequent sites of tumor metastasis. Although metastasis of thyroid carcinoma to bone is rare in the dog, an occasional case may spread to the skull bones or elsewhere, resulting in focal osteolysis and persistent hypercalcemia that is suggestive clinically of a functional parathyroid tumor.[51]

Thyroid carcinomas are less frequent in cats than in dogs.[4,49,52] Functional thyroid carcinomas are well differentiated histologically and often difficult to distinguish from an adenoma. The tumor cells form follicles in lymph node metastases that contain variable amounts of colloid, take up radioiodine, and synthesize thyroid hormones at an uncontrolled rate. Canine thyroid carcinoma has been successfully transplanted to puppies treated with total body irradiation and nitrogen mustard. A thyroid carcinoma cell line of canine origin has been established that had a regular growth pattern after 50 passages.[53]

Transgenic Animal Models of Thyroid Carcinogenesis

Transgenic mice with thyroid targeted expression of the *ret/PTC1* oncogene develop thyroid carcinomas similar to papillary carcinomas in human patients.[54] The *ret/PTC1* oncogene is a rearranged form of the *ret* protooncogene which encodes for a receptor of tyrosine kinase. Germ line mutations of the *ret/PTC1* oncogene have been reported to predispose to the development of three variants of the multiple endocrine neoplasia Type II inherited cancer syndromes[55] and a congenital developmental defect (Hirschsprung's disease) of the intestine.[56] The tissues affected in these syndromes are derived from cells of neural crest origin where the *ret/PTC1* oncogene is constitutively or transiently expressed.[57] All *ret/PTC1* oncogenes have been found to be restricted to papillary thyroid cancer in humans,[58,59] although follicular thyroid carcinoma shares a common histogenesis from follicular cells.

To target the expression of *ret/PTC1* to the thyroid gland, a hybrid gene (*Tg-PTC1*) was cloned into the plasmid *pRc/CMV*. The *Tg-PTC1* was comprised of the bovine thyroglobulin gene promoter and the coding region for the *ret/PTC1* oncogene.[54] The thyroid carcinomas had a mixture of solid, cribriform, and follicular architecture with relatively few papillary infoldings. Colloid formation was infrequent, and tumor cell nuclei were variable in size, irregular in shape, and had frequent nuclear grooves and occasional cytoplasmic inclusions. Despite a lack of microscopic evidence of local or distant metastasis in mice up to 5 months of age, extensive intrathyroidal and periglandular invasion was present in all mice. The finding that targeted expression of the *ret/PTC1* oncogene in the thyroid gland causes bilateral thyroid carcinoma with cellular features comparable to human papillary cancer is significant because it indicates that *ret/PTC1* oncogene is not only a biomarker associated with papillary thyroid cancer, but it also is the only proven specific genetic event leading to the development of the most common type of thyroid carcinoma in human patients.[54]

Although transgenic mice with thyroid-targeted expression of the *ret/PTC1* oncogene developed bilateral thyroid carcinomas by 1 month of age, the tumors were slowly progressive, with limited invasion beyond the thyroid capsule and an absence of distant metastasis. The thyroid carcinomas were studied further for responsiveness to increased endogenous TSH by feeding a low iodide diet for 3 to 6 months to evaluate the effect of TSH on thyroid tumor progression.[60] The low iodine diet resulted in a progressive increase in thyroid weight and tumor cellularity with the development of a prominent spindle cell component in the carcinomas after 6 months; however, there was no evidence of extensive local invasion or distant metastasis. Despite the lack of histological differentiation, the spindle cell population retained focal immunoreactivity for thyroglobulin. Although *ret/PTC1* induced thyroid carcinomas retained TSH responsiveness, they maintain a benign biological behavior despite histological evidence of anaplasia.[61] Exogenous thyroxine administration with corresponding decreased circulating levels of TSH retarded the development and progression of the thyroid carcinoma in this transgenic animal model; however, prior TSH stimulation induced tumor nodules that failed to regress following suppression of TSH by the elevated thyroxine levels.[61]

Immunohistochemical analysis of thyroid tumors in transgenic mice did not reveal p53 protein overexpression. Mutations in the *p53* tumor suppressor gene have been associated with progression of differentiated thyroid carcinomas to anaplastic types in humans.[62-64] The lack of p53 alterations, retention of thyroglobulin expression, and failure of metastatic progression suggests that the TSH induced spindle cell areas in thyroid papillary carcinomas in transgenic mice with targeted expression of the *ret/PTC1* oncogene are different from the areas of anaplastic transformation of differentiated thyroid carcinomas in human patients.[60]

Thyroid Carcinogenesis and Radiation

Epidemiological studies in humans and animals have suggested that the risk of developing thyroid cancer following exposure to external (localized) X rays is greater than exposure to internal ^{131}I irradiation.[65,66] However, results of a large study in female Long-Evans rats (3000 animals divided into 10 equal treatment groups administered a single dose of irradiation at 6 weeks of age) revealed that the proportion of rats with thyroid carcinomas was similar for ^{131}I and X-ray irradiation within the dose range of 0-1000 rads.[67]

There was a significant dose dependent increase in follicular cell carcinomas in rats administered ^{131}I or exposed to external X-ray irradiation (fig. 13.23 F). Of rats given the high dose (HD) of ^{131}I, 7.3 percent developed follicular cell carcinomas compared to 0.4 percent of controls. By comparison, 8.9 percent of rats administered the HD of X rays developed follicular cell carcinomas compared to 0.4 percent of control rats. A small number of anaplastic carcinomas were observed in the HD irradiation group for both ^{131}I and X rays. If these rats were included, the respective figures increased to 8.1 percent for the HD ^{131}I group and 10.1 percent for the HD X-ray group.[68] There also was a significant dose dependent increase in follicular cell adenomas in rats administered ^{131}I or exposed to external X-ray irradiation (fig. 13.23 F). Of the rats receiving the HD ^{131}I, 8.5 percent developed adenomas compared to 1.1 percent in controls. External X rays resulted in an 18.6 percent incidence of adenomas in rats administered the HD compared to 2.6 percent in controls.

When the total thyroid follicular cell tumor incidence (adenoma and carcinoma) was evaluated, there was a significant increase to 16.6 percent in the HD ^{131}I group compared to 1.4 percent in controls and a 28.7 percent incidence in the HD X-ray group compared to 3.0 percent in controls.

Thyroid Carcinogenesis and Xenobiotic Chemicals

Xenobiotic chemicals in large doses may disrupt thyroid function in rodents either by a direct effect on the thyroid, influencing synthesis or secretion of thyroxine (T_4) and triiodothyronine (T_3), or by adversely influencing the peripheral metabolism of thyroid hormones.[69,70] Review of the *U.S. Physician's Desk Reference* (1994) reveals a number of marketed drugs that result in a thyroid tumorigenic response when tested at high doses in rodents, particularly in rats. A broad spectrum of product classes is represented including antibiotics, calcium channel blockers, antidepressants, and hypolipidemic agents, among others. Amiodarone (an antiarrhythmic drug) and iodinated glycerol (an expectorant) are highly iodinated molecules that disrupt thyroid hormone economy by mechanisms similar to the food color FD&C Red No. 3.[71]

The major mechanisms by which nongenotoxic chemicals disrupt the hypothalamic-pituitary-thyroid axis can be summarized (fig. 13.23 G) as follows: (1) a direct thyroid effect by blocking the uptake of iodine, inhibiting the important thyroperoxidase enzyme that disrupts iodine binding and the coupling reaction, or interfering with the proteolysis of colloid and the release of thyroid hormones, all of which result in low blood levels of T_4 and T_3; (2) inhibition of 5'-deiodinase in peripheral tissues (such as liver and kidney) that normally convert T_4 (the major secretory product of the thyroid) to T_3 (the principal thyroid hormone that interacts with nuclear receptors in target cells). When the 5'-deiodinase is inhibited by highly iodinated compounds such as Amiodarone and FD&C Red No. 3, T_4 is preferentially converted to reverse T_3 (rT_3), which is biologically inactive and does not exert negative feedback control on the pituitary gland and hypothalamus; (3) induction of hepatic microsomal enzymes such as thyroxine-UDP glucuronyl transferase, which increases the conjugation of thyroid hormones with glucuronic acid and excretion of conjugated T_4 and T_3 in the bile, resulting in lower blood levels of thyroid hormones. A number of xenobiotic chemicals have been reported to act by this mechanism, including drugs acting on the CNS, calcium channel blockers, steroids, retinoids, chlorinated hydrocarbons, and polyhalogenated biphenyls.[70,72]

With each of these seemingly different pathogenic mechanisms, the hypothalamus-pituitary axis senses the lower circulating thyroid hormone levels and increases the production of TSH. The rodent thyroid is very sensitive to TSH, and follicular cells respond by undergoing hypertrophy and hyperplasia initially and, if sustained, by the development of thyroid tumors (usually adenomas, occasionally carcinomas). The thyroid glands of most domestic animal species and human beings respond in a much different manner to chronic increased blood levels of TSH, frequently by undergoing hyperplasia (resulting in goiter or clinical enlargement of the thyroid) but rarely developing thyroid tumors as a response to long-term stimulation by TSH.

The proliferative lesions that develop from rodent thyroid follicular cells in response to a chronic increase in TSH represent a morphological continuum from hyperplasia, to benign tumors (adenomas), and occasionally to malignant tumors (carcinomas). It is difficult with the techniques currently available to accurately determine when a focal proliferative lesion becomes autonomous and continues to proliferate in the absence of the inciting stimulus. Reversibility studies with compounds that produce a high incidence of focal proliferative lesions early, such as methimazole, have been useful and suggest that many of the small focal lesions classified as adenomas in the thyroid of rodents are reversible when the hormonal imbalances return to normal.[73]

A number of chemicals disrupt thyroid function in rodents by inhibiting thyroperoxidase. These include thiourea, propylthiouracil sulfonamides, methimazole, aminotriazole, and acetoacetamide, among others. Chemicals that inhibit thyroperoxidase result in decreased iodination of tyrosine due to a failure of oxidation of iodide ion (I^-) to iodine (I_2) and the inhibition of the coupling of iodotyrosines to active iodothyronines such as T_4 and T_3. A contemporary example of a chemical acting as a thyroperoxidase inhibitor is sulfamethazine. This is a widely used antibacterial compound in food-producing animals and has a current permissible tissue residue level of 100 ppb. Carcinogenicity studies completed at the National Center for Toxicologic Research reported a significant increase in thyroid tumors in male Fischer 344 rats administered the HD (2400 ppm) of sulfamethazine. The incidence of thyroid tumors also was increased in both male and female $B_6C_3F_1$ mice after 2 years in the HD (4800 ppm) group but not in the lower dose groups.[74]

Hyperplasia of Thyroid Follicular Cells: Hyperplastic, Colloid, Nodular, and Congenital Goiter

Incidence

Nonneoplastic and noninflammatory enlargement of the thyroid (goiter) can develop in all domestic mammals, birds, and submammalian vertebrates from one of several pathogenic mechanisms. Iodine deficiency causing diffuse thyroid hyperplasia was common in certain enzootic goitrogenic areas throughout the world before the widespread addition of iodized salt to animal diets. Although iodine deficient goiter still occurs worldwide in domestic animals, the outbreaks are sporadic, and fewer animals are affected than prior to the widespread use of iodized salt. Animals born to dams on iodine deficient diets are more likely to develop severe thyroid hyperplasia and have clinical evidence of hypothyroidism. Offspring of iodine deficient mothers may be stillborn or aborted late in pregnancy. Of the animals born alive, some are weak and partly hairless with subcutaneous edema of the head and neck. Foals with hyperplastic goiter have been reported to have rupture of the common digital extensor tendons, forelimb, contracture, and mandibular prognathism.[75]

Certain goitrogenic substances that interfere with thyroid hormone synthesis may precipitate the development of hyperplastic goiter in animals on a diet that is marginally iodine deficient (fig. 13.24 A). These substances include thiouracil, propylthiouracil (PTU), sulfonamides, complex anions [perchlorate (ClO_4^-), pertechnetate (TcO_4^-), perrhenate (ReO_4^-), and tetrafluoroborate (BF_4^-)], and a number of plants from the genus *Brassica* that contain thioglycosides, which after digestion release thiocynate and isothiocyanate (fig. 13.24 A). A particularly potent thioglycoside, goitrin (L-5-vinyl-2 thiooxazolidone), from plants is excreted in milk. Both lateral lobes of the thyroid are uniformly enlarged in diffuse hyperplastic goiter (fig. 13.24 B). The enlargements may be extensive and result in palpable swelling in the cranial cervical area. The affected lobes are firm and dark red because an extensive interfollicular capillary network develops under the influence of long-term TSH stimulation. The thyroid enlargements are the result of intense hypertrophy and hyperplasia of follicular cells lining thyroid follicles, with the formation of papillary projections into the lumens of collapsed follicles that contain little colloid (fig. 13.24 C). Endocytosis of colloid often proceeds at a rate greater than synthesis, resulting in progressive depletion of colloid and partial collapse of follicles.

Isolated outbreaks of hyperplastic goiter develop in calves, lambs, kids, and pups as a consequence of an inability to synthesize thyroglobulin or due to an enzyme defect in the biosynthesis of the thyroid hormones by follicular cells.[76,77] The more prevalent forms of inherited goiter in human patients include defects in the iodination of tyrosine, deiodination of iodotyrosines, synthesis and proteolysis of thyroglobulin, coupling of iodotyrosines to form iodothyronines, and a disruption in iodide transport.

Congenital dyshormonogenetic goiter is inherited by an autosomal recessive gene in sheep (Corriedale, Dorset horn, merino, and Romney breeds),[77] Afrikander cattle,[78] and Saanen dwarf goats (fig. 13.24 D).[79] The subnormal growth rate, absence of normal wool development or presence of a rough sparse hair coat, myxedematous swellings of the subcutis, weakness, and sluggish behavior suggest that the affected kids are clinically hypothyroid. Most lambs with congenital goiter either die shortly after birth or are highly sensitive to the effects of adverse environmental conditions. Thyroid glands are symmetrically enlarged at birth due to an intense diffuse hyperplasia of follicular cells.[80] Thyroid follicles are lined by tall columnar cells, but follicles often have collapsed because of lack of colloid resulting from the marked endocytotic activity. The tall columnar follicular cells lining thyroid follicles have extensively dilated profiles of rough endoplasmic reticulum and large mitochondria, but there are relatively

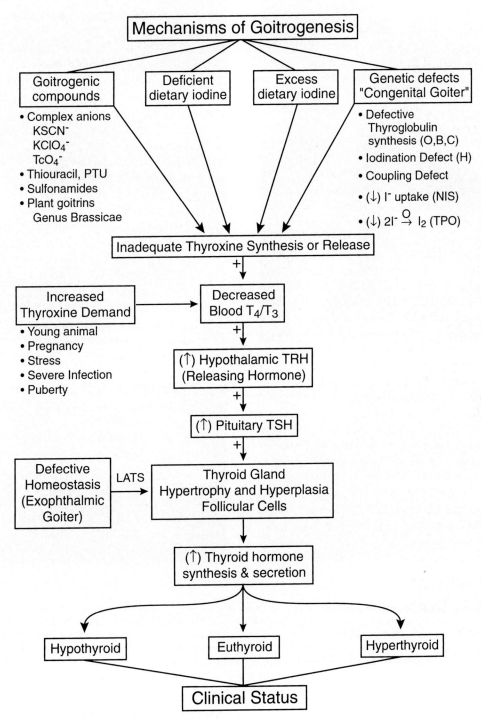

Fig. 13.24. A. Mechanisms of goitrogenesis. Multiple pathogenic factors (goitrogenic compounds, deficient and excess dietary iodine intake, and genetic defects) result in inadequate thyroxine/triiodothyronine synthesis and leads to long-term stimulation of thyroid follicular cells (hypertrophy and hyperplasia) by an increased secretion of pituitary thyroid stimulating hormone (TSH). LATS = long acting thyroid substance, an autoantibody that binds to the TSH receptor to stimulate the synthetic and secretory activity of follicular cells. TPO = thyroperoxidase. PTU = propylthiouracil. NIS = sodium iodine symporter. H = Human. O = Ovine. B = Bovine. C = Caprine. $KClO_4^-$ = potassium perchlorate. TcO_4^- = Pertechnetate. $KSCN^-$ = potassium thiocynate. TRH = thyrotropin releasing hormone. (continued)

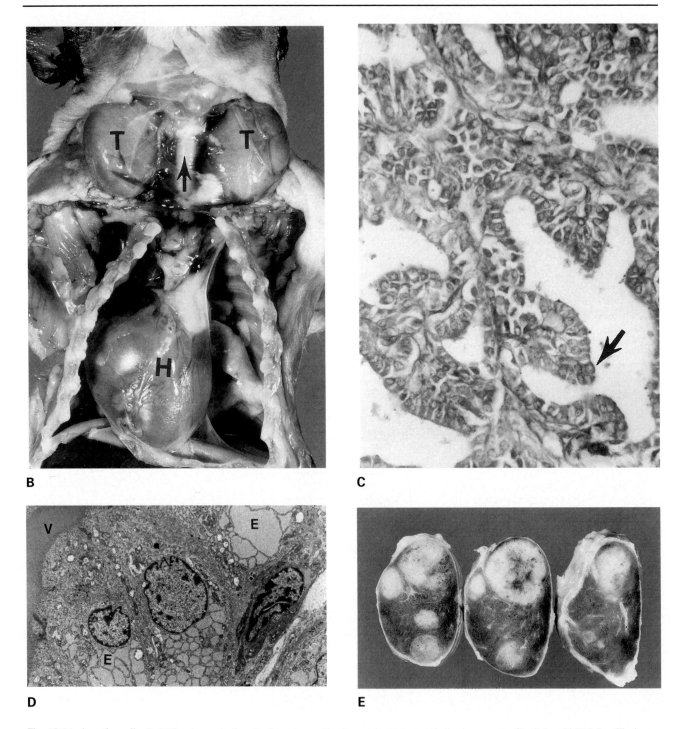

Fig. 13.24. (continued)   **B.** Diffuse hyperplastic goiter in a pup resulting in prominent symmetrical enlargements of both thyroid *(T)* lobes. The hyperplastic thyroids were freely movable from the trachea (arrow) in the cervical region. (*H* = heart.) **C.** Diffuse hyperplastic goiter illustrating papillary projections (arrow) into follicular lumens and partial collapse of follicles due to increased endocytosis of colloid in a pup. **D.** Dyshormonogenetic goiter in a lamb illustrating hypertrophied thyroid follicular cells. Profiles of rough endoplasmic reticulum *(E)* are dilated by finely granular material and long microvilli *(V)* extend into the colloid. Few thyroglobulin-containing apical vesicles are present in the luminal aspect of the cell. **E.** Multifocal hyperplasia of thyroid follicular cells (Anodular goiter) in an old horse. The light tan nodules of hyperplasia are not encapsulated, and there is minimal compression of the adjacent thyroid parenchyma.

few dense granules associated with the Golgi apparatus and few thyroglobulin-containing apical vesicles near the luminal plasma membrane (fig. 13.24 D). Numerous long microvilli extend from apical surfaces of follicular cells into the follicular lumen.

A closely related or similar defect appears to be responsible for congenital goiter in sheep, cattle, and goats. Although thyroidal uptake and turnover of ^{131}I are greatly increased compared with euthyroid controls, circulating T_4 and T_3 levels are consistently low. The protein-bound iodine levels in animals with inherited congenital goiter are markedly elevated; however, this appears to be the result of iodination of albumin and other plasma proteins by the thyroid gland under long-term TSH stimulation. There is no defect in the iodide transport mechanism, organification, or dehalogenation, but normal 19S thyroglobulin in goitrous thyroids is absent, and only minute amounts of thyroglobulin related antigens (0.01 percent of normal) are present, suggesting an impairment in thyroglobulin biosynthesis in animals with congenital goiter. Although thyroglobulin mRNA sequences are present in the goitrous tissue, their concentration is markedly reduced (1/10 to 1/40 that of normal thyroid), and the intracellular distribution is abnormal (nuclear, 42 percent of normal; cytoplasmic, 7 percent; membrane fraction, 1 to 2 percent). The lack of thyroglobulin in these examples of congenital goiter in animals appears to be due to a defect in thyroglobulin mRNA, leading to aberrant processing of primary transcripts and/or transport of the thyroglobulin mRNA from the nucleus to the ribosomes on the endoplasmic reticulum in the cytoplasm of follicular cells.

Hypothyroid goats with congenital goiter can be returned to a state of euthyroidism by the addition of iodide (1.0 mg/day) to the diet. Although the goats remain unable to synthesize thyroglobulin, supplementation with additional iodide results in sufficient formation of T_4 and T_3 in the abnormal iodoproteins to make the animals euthyroid.

Although seemingly paradoxical, an excess of iodide in the diet can also result in thyroid hyperplasia in animals and humans (fig. 13.24 A). Foals of mares fed dry seaweed containing excessive iodide may develop thyroid hyperplasia and clinically evident goiter.[81] The thyroid glands of the foal are exposed to higher blood iodide levels than the mare because of concentration of iodide first by the placenta and subsequently by the mammary gland. High blood iodide interferes with one or more steps of thyroid hormone synthesis and secretion (especially proteolytic cleavage of thyroid hormones from thyroglobulin), leading to lowered blood T_4 and T_3 levels and a compensatory increase in pituitary TSH secretion.

Goiter in adult animals usually is of little clinical significance, and the general health of the animal is not impaired, except for occasional local pressure influences. It is of significance as a disease of the newborn, although the previous drastic losses in endemic areas are now controlled by the prophylactic use of iodized salt. Congenital hypothyroidism in domestic animals may be associated with iodine deficient hyperplastic goiter, even though the dam shows no evidence of thyroid dysfunction. Gestation may be prolonged, and the larger goiters may cause dystocia (difficult birth), with retention of the fetal placenta. Affected foals with iodine deficient goiter are weak and die within a few days after birth with moderately enlarged thyroids. Calves with goiter are born partially or completely hairless and either are born dead or die soon after birth. Newborn goitrous pigs, goats, and lambs frequently have myxedema and hair loss. The mortality rate is high, with the majority born dead or dying within a few hours of birth. Enlarged thyroid glands are readily palpable or visible in kids and lambs, but are not apparent in piglets because of the combination of short neck and myxedema. Asphyxiation also may result from pressure by the enlarged thyroid gland. Young goitrous animals that are treated and survive usually do not show permanent harmful effects.

Multinodular goiter in most animals (except cats) is endocrinologically inactive and is encountered only as an incidental lesion at necropsy. However, there is evidence that functional thyroid adenomas in old cats with hyperthyroidism often develop in a gland with multinodular hyperplasia and that certain cats with thyroid hormone excess only have multinodular hyperplasia in their thyroids. In contrast to thyroid adenomas (see fig. 13.20 A), the areas of nodular hyperplasia are *not* encapsulated and result in minimal compression of adjacent parenchyma.

Macroscopic Pathology

Nodular hyperplasia (goiter) in thyroid glands of old horses appears as multiple white to tan nodules of varying size (fig. 13.24 E). The affected lobes are moderately enlarged and irregular in contour. In contrast to thyroid adenomas, the areas of nodular hyperplasia are not encapsulated and result in minimal compression of adjacent thyroid parenchyma.

Both lateral lobes and the isthmus of the thyroid in ruminants are uniformly enlarged in young animals with diffuse hyperplastic goiter associated with iodine deficiency. The enlargements may be extensive in severe cases and result in palpable swellings in the anterior cervical area. The affected lobes are firm and dark red because an extensive interfollicular capillary network develops under the influence of long-term TSH stimulation.

In colloid goiter both thyroid lobes are diffusely enlarged but are more translucent and are not dark red in color as with diffuse hyperplastic goiter. The differences in macroscopic appearance are the result of a lower degree of vascularity in colloid goiter and the development of macrofollicles due to involution and distention of follicles by colloid.

Histopathology

Nodular goiter consists of multiple foci of hyperplastic follicular cells that are sharply demarcated but not encapsulated from the adjacent thyroid. The microscopic appearance within a nodule is variable. Some hyperplastic cells form small follicles with little or no colloid. Other nodules are formed by larger irregularly shaped follicles lined by one or more layers of columnar cells that may form papillary projections into the lumen. Some of these follicles are involuted and filled with densely eosinophilic colloid. These changes appear to be the result of alternating periods of hyperplasia and colloid involution in the thyroid glands of old animals. The areas of nodular hyperplasia may be microscopic (as in old cats) or grossly visible and causing asymmetrical enlargement of the thyroid (as in old horses).

The histological changes in diffuse hyperplastic and colloid goiters are more consistent throughout the diffusely enlarged thyroid lobes and are essentially similar in all animal species. The follicles are irregular in size and shape in hyperplastic goiter because of varying amounts of lightly eosinophilic and vacuolated colloid. Some larger follicles are collapsed due to a lack of colloid. The lining epithelial cells are columnar with a deeply eosinophilic cytoplasm and small hyperchromatic nuclei that are often situated in the basilar part of the cell. The follicles are lined by single or multiple layers of hyperplastic follicular cells that in some follicles may form papillary projections into the lumen. Similar proliferative changes are present in ectopic thyroid parenchyma in the neck or anterior mediastinum of certain species (especially dogs).

Colloid goiter represents the involutionary phase of diffuse thyroid hyperplasia, which may develop in young adult to adult animals either after sufficient amounts of iodide have been added to the diet or after the requirements for thyroid hormones have diminished in an older animal. Blood thyroid hormone levels return to normal, and the secretion of TSH by the pituitary gland is correspondingly decreased. Follicles are progressively distended with densely eosinophilic colloid because of diminished TSH induced endocytosis of colloid. The follicular cells lining the macrofollicles are flattened and atrophic. The interface between the colloid and luminal surface of follicular cells is smooth and lacks the characteristic endocytotic vacuoles of actively secreting follicular cells. Interfollicular capillaries are less well developed than with diffuse hyperplastic goiter.

Tumors of Thyroglossal Duct Remnants

Incidence

Tumors arising in remnants of the thyroglossal duct are rare in animals, but have been encountered in the dog.[82]

The canine thyroid originates as a thickened plate of epithelium in the floor of the pharynx. It is intimately related to the aortic sac in its development, and this association leads to the frequent occurrence of accessory thyroid parenchyma, which may undergo neoplastic transformation, in the mediastinum of the adult dog.[35,83,84] Branched cell cords develop from the pharyngeal plate and migrate dorsolaterally, but remain attached to the pharyngeal area by the narrow thyroglossal duct. A portion of the thyroglossal duct may persist postnatally and form a cyst because of the accumulation of proteinic material secreted by the lining epithelium. Thyroglossal duct cysts are present in the ventral aspect of the anterior cervical region in dogs and are lined by thyroidogenic epithelium with vari-

able numbers of colloid-containing follicles. Their lining epithelium may undergo neoplastic transformation and give rise to well-differentiated papillary thyroid carcinomas.

Macroscopic Pathology

Tumors of thyroglossal duct remnants appear as well-circumscribed, fluctuant, movable enlargements (approximately 2 to 4 cm in diameter) on the ventral midline in the anterior cervical region. The clinical history usually indicates a slowly progressive expansion of the cervical mass. On cross section they have multilocular cystic areas containing a translucent proteinic fluid alternating with white solid areas (fig. 13.25 A).

The cervical thyroid glands appear to be normal in the few cases studied in the dog. These tumors develop de novo from the epithelium of the thyroglossal duct and are not a cystic metastasis from a primary carcinoma in the thyroid gland.

Histopathology

The tumors appear as well-differentiated papillary carcinomas. Multiple papillary outgrowths, covered by several layers of tall cuboidal to columnar epithelial cells, extend from the cyst wall into the lumen (fig. 13.25 B). The lining of the cyst may undergo squamous metaplasia to form a keratinizing epithelium.[82] The cyst wall is composed of dense fibrous connective tissue with focal areas of hemorrhage and cholesterol clefts. Aggregations of thyrogenic epithelium in the form of small follicles and cell cords often are present within the fibrous capsule and in the surrounding connective tissue. These follicles are lined by a low cuboidal epithelium and contain variable amounts of eosinophilic colloid.

Growth and Metastasis

Carcinomas of thyroglossal duct remnants are well differentiated and slow growing. They infrequently recur following complete surgical resection of the multilocular cyst and adjacent tissue.

REFERENCES

1. Hayes, H.H., Jr. (1975) canine thyroid neoplasms: Epidemiologic features. *J Natl Cancer Inst* 55:931-934.
2. Vitovec, J. (1976) Epithelial thyroid tumors in cows. *Vet Pathol* 13:401-408.
3. Hillidge, C.J., Sanecki, R.K., and Theodorakis, M.C. (1982) Thyroid carcinoma in a horse. *J Amer Vet Med Assoc* 181:711-714.
4. Leav, I., Schiller, A.L., Rijnberk, A., Kegg, M.A., and der Kinderen, P.J. (1976) Adenomas and carcinomas of the canine and feline thyroid. *Amer J Pathol* 83:61-64.
5. Brodey, R.S. (1970) Canine and feline neoplasia. *Adv Vet Sci* 14:309-354.
6. Brodey, R.S., and Kelly, D.F. (1968) Thyroid neoplasms in the dog: A clinicopathologic study of fifty-seven cases. *Cancer* 22:406-416.
7. Scarlett, J.M. (1994) Epidemiology of thyroid diseases of dogs and cats. *Vet Clin N Amer Small Anim Pract* 24:477-486.

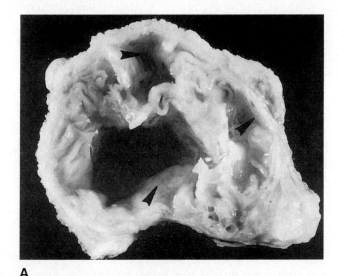

A

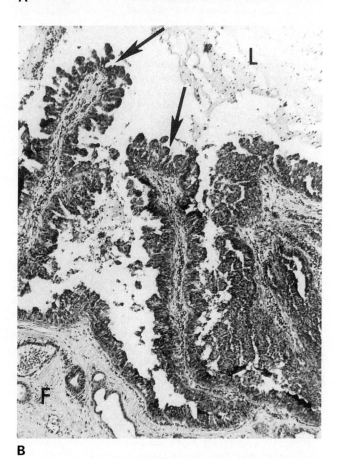

B

Fig. 13.25. Tumors of thyroglossal duct remnants. **A.** Carcinoma in the thyroglossal duct remnants of a dog. The multicystic tumor (arrowheads) was removed from the ventral midline of the anterior cervical region. **B.** Papillary carcinoma of thyroglossal duct remnants from a dog. Papillary outgrowths covered with multiple layers of tall cuboidal to columnar cells (arrows) project from the fibrous capsule *(F)* into the cyst lumen *(L)*.

8. Johnson, L.A., Ford, H.C., Tarttelin, M.F., et al. (1992) Iodine content of commercially prepared cat foods. *N Z Vet J* 40:18-20.

9. Peterson, M.E., Livingston, P., and Brown, R.S. (1987) Lack of circulating thyroid stimulating immunoglobulins in cats with hyperthyroidism. *Vet Immunol Immunopathol* 16:277-282.

10. Brown, R.S., Keating, P., Livingston, P.G., and Bullock, L. (1992) Thyroid growth immunoglobulins in feline hyperthyroidism. *Thyroid* 2:125.

11. Peter, H.J., Gerber, H., Studer, H., and Smeds, S. (1985) Pathogenesis of heterogeneity in human multinodular goiter: A study on growth and function of thyroid tissue transplanted onto nude mice. *J Clin Invest* 76:1992-2002.

12. Gerber, H., Peter, H., Ferguson, D.C., and Peterson, M.E. (1994) Etiopathology of feline toxic nodular goiter. *Vet Clin N Amer Small Anim Pract* 24, 541-565.

13. Peter, H.J., Gerber, H., Studer, H., Peterson, M.E., Becker, D.V., and Groscurth, P. (1991) Autonomous growth and function of cultured thyroid follicles from cats with spontaneous hyperthyroidism. *Thyroid* 1:331.

14. Merryman, J.I., Buckles, E.L., Bowers, G., and Neilsen, N.R. (1999) Overexpression of c-*ras* in hyperplasia and adenomas of the feline thyroid gland: An immunohistochemical analysis of 34 cases. *Vet Pathol* 36(2):117-124.

15. Pearce, S.H.S., Foster, D.J., Imrie, H., Myerscough, N., Beckett, G.J., Thoday, K.L., and Kendall-Taylor, P. (1997) Mutational analysis of the thyrotropin receptor gene in sporadic and familial feline thyrotoxicosis. *Thyroid* 7:923-927.

16. Holzworth, J., Theran, P., Carpenter, J.L., Harpster, N.K., and Todoroff, R.J. (1980) Hyperthyroidism in the cat: Ten cases. *J Amer Vet Med Assoc* 176:345-353.

17. Clark, S.T., and Meier, H. (1958) A clinicopathological study of thyroid disease in the dog and cat. Part 1. Thyroid pathology. *Zbl Vet Med* 5, 17-32.

18. Hoenig, M., Goldschmidt, M.H., Ferguson, D.C., Koch, K., and Eymontt, M.J. (1982) Toxic nodular goitre in the cat. *J Small Anim Pract* 23:1-12.

19. Peterson, M.E., Kintzer, P.P., Cavanagh, P.G., Fox, P.R., Ferguson, D.C., Johnson, G.F., and Becker, D.V. (1983) Feline hyperthyroidism: Pretreatment clinical and laboratory evaluation of 131 cases. *J Amer Vet Med Assoc* 183:103-110.

20. O'Brien, S.E., Riley, J.H., and Hagemoser, W.A. (1980) Unilateral thyroid neoplasm in a cat. *Vet Rec* 107:199-200.

21. Martin, S.L., and Capen, C.C. (1983) The endocrine system. In Pratt, P.W. (ed.), *Feline Medicine and Surgery,* 3rd ed. American Veterinary Publications, Santa Barbara, pp. 321-362.

22. Peterson, M.E. (1984) Feline hyperthyroidism. *Vet Clin North Amer* 14:809-826.

23. Patnaik, A.K., and Lieberman, P.H. (1979) Feline anaplastic giant cell adenocarcinoma of the thyroid. *Vet Pathol* 16:687-692.

24. Peterson, M.E., Graves, T.K., and Gamble, D.A. (1990) Triiodothyronine (T3) suppression test: An aid in the diagnosis of mild hyperthyroidism in cats. *J Vet Int Med* 4:233-238.

25. Peterson, M.E., and Gamble, D.A. (1990) Effect of nonthyroidal illness on serum thyroxine concentration in cats: 494 cases (1988). *J Amer Vet Med Assoc* 197:1203-1208.

26. Barber, P.J., and Elliott, J. (1996) Study of calcium homeostasis in feline hyperthyroidism. *J Small Anim Pract* 37:575-582.

27. Archer, F.J., and Taylor, S.M. (1996) Alkaline phosphatase bone isoenzyme and osteocalcin in the serum of hyperthyroid cats. *Can Vet J* 37:735-739.

28. Joyce, J.R., Thompson, R.G., Kyzar, J.R., and Hightower, D. (1976) Thyroid carcinoma in a horse. *J Amer Vet Med Assoc* 168:610-612.

29. Chaistain, C.B., Hill, B.L., and Nichols, C.E. (1980) Excess triiodothyronine production by a thyroid adenocarcinoma in a dog. *J Amer Vet Med Assoc* 177:172-173.

30. Ackerman, L.J., Silver, J.N., and Ginsberg, E.B. (1984) Thyroid adenocarcinoma in a dog. *Mod Vet Pract* 64:303-304.

31. Rijnberk, A., and der Kinderen, P.J. (1969) Toxic thyroid carcinoma in the dog. *Acta Endocrinol* 138:177.

32. Reid, C.F., Pensinger, R.R., Ferrigan, L.W., and Parkes, L. (1963) Functioning adenocarcinoma of the thyroid gland in a dog with mitral insufficiency. *Amer Vet Radiol Soc* 4:36-40.

33. Harrington, G.A., and Kelly, D.V. (1980) Corneal lipoidosis in a dog with bilateral thyroid carcinoma. *Vet Pathol* 17:490-517.

34. Jernigan, A.D. (1989) Idiosyncrasies of feline drug metabolism. In *Proceedings 12th Annual Kal Kan Symposium for Treatment of Small Animal Diseases*. Veterinary Learning Systems, Trenton, NJ.

35. Cheville, N.F. (1972) Ultrastructure of canine carotid body and aortic body tumors: Comparison with tissues of thyroid and parathyroid origin. *Vet Pathol* 9:166-189.

36. Walsh, K.M., and Diters, R.W. (1984) Carcinoma of ectopic thyroid in a dog. *J Amer Anim Hosp Assoc* 20:665-668.

37. Stephens, L.C., Saunders, W.J., and Jaenke, R.S. (1982) Ectopic thyroid carcinoma with metastases in a beagle dog. *Vet Pathol* 19:669-675.

38. Thompson, E.J., Stirtzinger, T., Lumsden, J.H., and Little, P.B. (1980) Fine needle aspiration cytology in the diagnosis of canine thyroid carcinoma. *Can Vet J* 21:186-188.

39. Williams, E.D., Brown, C.L., and Doniach, I. (1966) Pathological and clinical findings in a series of 67 cases of medullary carcinoma of the thyroid. *J Clin Pathol* 19:103-113.

40. Moore, F.M., Kledzik, G.S., Wolfe, H.J., and DeLellis, R.A. (1984) Thyroglobulin and calcitonin immunoreactivity in canine thyroid carcinomas. *Vet Pathol* 21:168-173.

41. Gould, V.E., Gould, N.S., and Benditt, E.P. (1972) Ultrastructural aspects of papillary and sclerosing carcinomas of the thyroid. *Cancer* 29:1613-1625.

42. Anderson, P.C., and Capen, C.C. (1986) Undifferentiated spindle cell carcinoma of the thyroid gland in a dog. *Vet Pathol* 23:203-204.

43. Bustad, L.K., George, L.A., Jr., Marks, S., Warner, D.E., Barnes, C.M., Herde, K.E., and Kornberg, H.A. (1957) Biological effects of I[131] continuously administered to sheep. *Rad Res* 6:380-413.

44. Marks, S., George, L.A., Jr., and Bustad, L.K. (1957) Fibrosarcoma involving the thyroid gland of a sheep given I[131] daily. *Cancer* 10:587-591.

45. Graham, H., and Daniel, C. (1974) Ultrastructure of an anaplastic carcinoma of the thyroid. *Amer J Clin Pathol* 61:690-696.

46. Gaal, J.M., Horvath, E., and Kovacs, K. (1975) Ultrastructure of two cases of anaplastic giant cell tumor of the human thyroid gland. *Cancer* 35:1273-1279.

47. Buergelt, C.D. (1968) Mixed thyroid tumors in two dogs. *J Amer Vet Med Assoc* 152:1658-1663.

48. Johnson, J.A., and Patterson, J.M. (1981) Multifocal myxedema and mixed thyroid neoplasm in a dog. *Vet Pathol* 18:13-20.

49. Clark, S.T., and Meier, H. (1958) A clinicopathological study of thyroid disease in the dog and cat. Part 1. Thyroid pathology. *Zbl Vet Med* 5:17-32.

50. Branam, J.E., Leighton, R.L., and Hornof, W.J. (1982) Radioisotope imaging for the evaluation of thyroid neoplasia and hypothyroidism in a dog. *J Amer Vet Med Assoc* 80:1077-1079.

51. Krook, L., Olsson, S., and Rooney, J.R. (1960) Thyroid carcinoma in the dog: A case of bone-metastasizing thyroid carcinoma simulating hyperparathyroidism. *Cornell Vet* 50:106-114.

52. Johnson, K.H., and Osborne, C.A. (1970) Adenocarcinoma of the thyroid gland in a cat. *J Amer Vet Med Assoc* 156:906-912.

53. Kasza, L. (1964) Establishment and characterization of a canine thyroid adenocarcinoma and canine melanoma cell lines. *Amer J Vet Res* 25:1178-1185.

54. Jhiang, S.M., Sagartz, J.E., Tong, Q., Parker-Thornburg, J., Capen, C.C., Cho, J.-Y., Xing, S., and Ledent, C. (1996) Targeted expression of the *ret*/PTC[1] oncogene induces papillary thyroid carcinomas. *Endocrinology* 137:375-377.

55. Mulligan, L.M., and Ponder, B.A.J. (1995) Genetic basis of endocrine disease: Multiple endocrine neoplasia type 2. *J Clin Endocrinol Metab* 80:1989-1995.

56. Romeo, G., Ronchetto, P., Luo, Y., Barone, V., Seri, M., Ceccherini, I., Pasini, B., Bocciardi, R., Lerone, M., Kaariainen, H., and Martucciello, G. (1994) Point mutation affecting the tyrosine kinase domain of the ret proto-oncogene in Hirschsprung's disease. *Nature* 367:377-378.

57. Nakamura T., Ishizaka, Y., Nagao, M., Hara, M., and Ishikawa, T. (1994) Expression of the ret proto-oncogene product in human normal and neoplastic tissues of neural crest origin. *J Pathol* 172:225-260.

58. Jhiang, S.M., Caruso, D.R., Gilmore, E., Ishizaka, Y., Tahira, T., Nagao, M., Chiu, I.M., Mazzaferri, E.L. (1992) Detection of the *ret*PTC[1] oncogene in human thyroid carcinomas. *Oncogene* 7:1331-1337.

59. Santoro, M., Carlomagno, F., Hay, I.D., Herrmann, M.A., Grieco, M., Melillo, R., Pierotti, M.A., Bongarzone, I., Della Porta, G., Berger, N., Peix, J.L., Paulin, C., Fabien, N., Vecchio, G., Jenkins, R.B., and Fusco, A. (1992) *Ret* oncogene activation in human thyroid neoplasms is restricted to papillary cancer subtype. *J Clin Invest* 89:1517-1522.

60. Sagartz, J.E., Jhiang, S.M., Tong, Q., and Capen, C.C. (1997) Thyroid-stimulating hormone promotes growth of thyroid carcinomas in transgenic mice with targeted expression of the *ret*/PTC[1] oncogene. *Lab Invest* 76:307-318.

61. Sagartz, J.E., Jhiang, S.M., Tong, Q., and Capen, C.C. (2001) Thyroxine suppresses the development and progression of papillary thyroid carcinoma in transgenic mice with targeted expression of *ret*/PTC[1] oncogene. *Toxicol Pathol* 27, in press.

62. Ito, T., Seyama, T., Mizuno, T., Tsuyama, N., Hayashi, T., Dohi, K., Nakamura, N., and Akiyama, M. (1993) Genetic alterations in thyroid tumor progression: Association with p53 gene mutations. *Jpn J Cancer Res* 84:526-531.

63. Holm, R., and Nesland, J.M. (1994) Retinoblastoma and p53 tumors suppressor gene protein expression in carcinomas of the thyroid gland. *J Pathol* 172:267-272.

64. Matias-Guiu, X., Cuatrecasas, M., Musulen, E., and Prat, J. (1994) p53 expression in anaplastic carcinomas arising from thyroid papillary carcinomas. *J Clin Pathol* 47:337-339.

65. Doniach, I. (1963) Effects including carcinogenesis of ^{131}I and X ray on the thyroid of experimental animals: A review. *Health Phys* 9:1357-1362.

66. Maxon, H.R., Thomas, S.R., Saenger, E.L., Buncher, C.R., Kereiakes, J.C. (1977) Ionizing radiation and the induction of clinically significant disease in the human thyroid gland. *Amer J Med* 63:967-978.

67. Lee, W., Chiacchierini, R.P., Shleien, B., Telles, N.C. (1982) Thyroid tumors following ^{131}I or localized X irradiation to the thyroid and pituitary glands in rats. *Radiat Res* 92:307-319.

68. Capen, C.C., DeLellis, R.A., and Williams, E.D. (1999) Experimental thyroid carcinogenesis in rodents: Role of radiation and xenobiotic chemicals. In Thomas, G., Karaoglou, A., and Williams, E.D. (eds.), *Radiation and Thyroid Cancer*. World Scientific Publishing, Singapore, New Jersey, London, Hong Kong, pp. 167-176.

69. Capen, C.C. (1997) Toxic responses of the thyroid gland. In Sipes, I.G., McQueen, C.A., and Gandolfi, A.J. (eds.-in-chief), *Comprehensive Toxicology*. Vol. 10, Boekelheide, K., et al. (eds.), *Reproductive and Endocrine Toxicology*. Ch. 52. Elsevier Science/Pergamon, Oxford, New York, Tokyo, pp. 691-708.

70. Capen, C.C. (1997) Mechanistic data and risk assessment of selected toxic end points of the thyroid gland. *Toxicol Pathol* 25:39-48.

71. Capen, C.C. (1996) Hormonal imbalances and mechanisms of chemical injury of thyroid gland. In Jones, T.C., Capen, C.C., and Mohr, U. (eds.), *Endocrine System. Series II. Monographs on the Pathology of Laboratory Animals*, 2nd ed. International Life Sciences Institute Series. Springer-Verlag, Inc., Berlin, Heidelberg, New York, pp. 217-238.

72. Hotz, K.J., Wilson, A.G.E., Thake, D.C., Roloff, M.V., Capen, C.C., Kronenberg, J., and Brewster, D.W. (1997) Mechanism of thiazopyr-induced effects on thyroid hormone homeostasis in male Sprague-Dawley rats. *Toxicol Appl Pharmacol* 142:133-142.

73. Todd, G.C. (1986) Induction and reversibility of thyroid proliferative changes in rats given an antithyroid compound. *Vet Pathol* 23:110-117.

74. McClain, R.M. (1995) The use of mechanistic data in cancer risk assessment: Case example-sulfanamides. In *Low Dose Extrapolation of Cancer Risk: Issues and Perspectives*. International Life Sciences Institute Series (ILSI), Washington, D.C., pp. 163-173.

75. McLaughlin, B.G. and Doige, C.E. (1981) Congenital musculoskeletal lesions and hyperplastic goiter in foals. *Can Vet J* 22:130-133.

76. Falconer, I.R. (1966) Studies of the congenitally goitrous sheep: The iodinated compounds of serum, and circulating thyroid-stimulating hormone. *Biochem J* 100:190-196.

77. Rac, R., Hill, G.N., Pain, R.W., and Mulhearn, C.J. (1968) Congenital goiter in merino sheep due to an inherited defect in the biosynthesis of thyroid hormone. *Res Vet Sci* 9:209-223.

78. Pammenter, M., Albrecht, C., Liebenberg, W., and van Jaarsveld, P. (1978) Afrikander cattle congenital goiter: Characteristics of its morphology and iodoprotein pattern. *Endocrinology* 102:954-965.

79. Rijnberk, A., de Fijlder J.J.M., van Dijk, J.E., Jorna, T.J., and Tegelaers, W.H. (1977) Clinical aspects of iodine metabolism in goats with congenital goitre and hypothyroidism. *Brit Vet J* 133:495-503.

80. Capen, C.C. (1980) Criteria for the development of animal models of diseases of the endocrine system. *Amer J Pathol* 101:S141.

81. Baker, H.J., and Lindsey, J.R. (1968) Equine goiter due to excess dietary iodide. *J Amer Vet Med Assoc* 153:1618-1630.

82. Harkema, J.R., King, R.R., and Hahn, F.F. (1984) Carcinoma of thyroglossal duct cysts: A case report and review of the literature. *J Amer Anim Hosp Assoc* 20:319-324.

83. Thake, D.C., Cheville, N.F., and Sharp, R.K. (1971) Ectopic thyroid adenomas at the base of the heart of the dog: Ultrastructural identification of dense tubular structures in endoplasmic reticulum. *Vet Pathol* 8:421-432.

84. Kameda, Y. (1972) The accessory thyroid glands of the dog around the intrapericardial aorta. *Arch Histol Jpn* 34:375-391.

TUMORS OF THYROID C (PARAFOLLICULAR) CELLS (ULTIMOBRANCHIAL DERIVATIVES): ADENOMA, CARCINOMA

Incidence

Tumors derived from C cells (parafollicular cells) of the thyroid gland are encountered most frequently in adult to aged bulls,[1,2] certain strains of laboratory rats,[3] and adult to aged horses,[4,5] but infrequently in other domestic species.[6,7] Approximately 30 percent of aged bulls have been reported to develop C cell neoplasms, and an additional 15 to 20 percent have hyperplasia of C cells and ultimobranchial derivatives.[8] These frequently occurring hyperplastic and neoplastic changes in C cells have been observed often in bulls fed high calcium diets but rarely in cows. A progressive increase in the incidence of thyroid C cell tumors has been reported in bulls with advancing age.[9] This coincided with an increase in the development of vertebral osteophytes (table 13.2).

The high incidence of C cell tumors in bulls differs from the situation in humans in which medullary carcinoma accounts for only 6 to 10 percent of all thyroid tumors. The development of C cell tumors in both humans and bulls is preceded by a multifocal C cell hyperplasia.

TABLE 13.2.   Vertebral osteophytosis and C cell tumors related to age

Age (Years)	No. of Bulls	C cell Tumors	Osteophytosis	Vertebral Fractures
5 to 8	469	52 (11.1%)*	100 (21.3%)*	2 (0.4%)
8 to 11	162	48 (29.6%)	79 (48.8%)	11 (6.7%)
11 to 14	119	52 (43.7%)	62 (52.1%)	6 (5.0%)
14 to 18	32	21 (65.6%)	22 (68.8%)	4 (12.5%)
Total	782	173 (22.1%)	263 (33.6%)	23 (2.9%)

Source: From McEntee, K., et al. (1980) Proceedings of the Eighth Technical Conference on Artificial Insemination Reproduction, pp. 45-47.
*Percentages of total number of bulls in each age group with that particular lesion.

Medullary (C cell) carcinoma in humans is the only type of thyroid tumor known to have a genetic basis, and it appears to be transmitted as an autosomal dominant trait in certain families. Thyroid C cell tumors in humans frequently develop in patients with neoplasms in multiple endocrine organs.[10]

The syndrome of C cell tumors in bulls shares many similarities with medullary thyroid carcinoma in humans.[2] Multiple endocrine tumors, especially bilateral pheochromocytomas and occasionally pituitary adenomas, are coincidentally detected in bulls with C cell tumors.[11,12] This may represent a simultaneous neoplastic transformation of multiple endocrine cell populations of neural crest origin in the same individual.[13] A high frequency of thyroid C cell tumors and pheochromocytomas has been reported in a family of guernsey bulls, suggesting an autosomal dominant pattern of inheritance.[14] A diffuse or focal (nodular) hyperplasia of secretory cells in the adrenal medulla appears to precede the development of pheochromocytoma.

An occasional thyroid C cell carcinoma has been reported in dogs that also had a pheochromocytoma and parathyroid chief cell hyperplasia.[15] Immunoreactive calcitonin levels were elevated approximately 10-fold, but the dog was hypercalcemic (12.9 mg/dl) because of primary parathyroid hyperplasia and moderate elevations in circulating levels of immunoreactive parathyroid hormone. In a recent report of 33 thyroid carcinomas in dogs, 36 percent were demonstrated by immunohistochemical methods to be of C cell origin, whereas 64 percent were derived from follicular cells.[16]

Clinical Characteristics

Thyroid C cell adenomas in bulls may result in a slight palpable enlargement of the anterioventral cervical region. C cell carcinomas often attain considerable size and cause extensive multinodular enlargements along the ventral aspect of the neck because of the primary tumor in the thyroid and metastasis in anterior cervical lymph nodes (fig. 13.26 A).

Severe vertebral osteosclerosis with ankylosing spondylosis deformans, osteophytes, vertebral fractures, and degenerative osteoarthrosis resulting in clinical lameness often is detected in bulls with thyroid C cell neo-

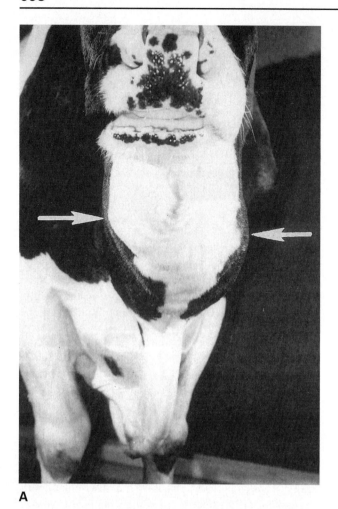

A

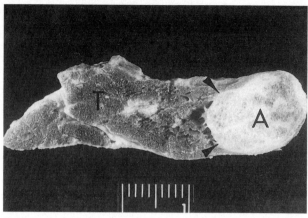

B

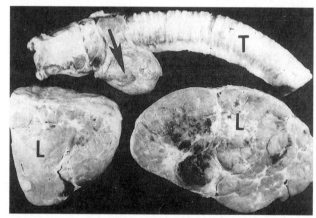

C

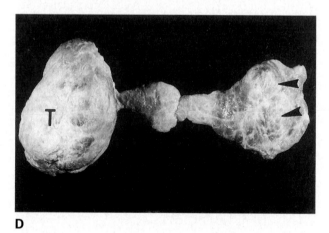

D

Fig. 13.26. Macroscopic features of thyroid C cell tumors. **A.** C cell carcinoma in a Holstein bull causing massive enlargement of ventral cervical region (arrows). **B.** Discrete C cell adenoma *(A)* in thyroid lobe *(T)* of a bull. Scale = 1 cm. **C.** C cell carcinoma illustrating multiple nodules in the thyroid (arrow) on the trachea (T). Two anterior cervical lymph nodes *(L)* are extensively enlarged due to metastases of the C cell carcinoma. **D.** Multiple nodules (arrowheads) in both thyroid lobes *(T)* of bull with C cell carcinoma.

plasms (table 13.3). Skeletal lesions of this type have been reported to occur frequently in adult bulls, but are rare in cows of the same age and breed.[17] The relationship of excess calcitonin secretion by C cell hyperplasia or neoplasia to the pathogenesis of skeletal lesions in bulls is uncertain and requires additional investigation. Prominent bone lesions have not been reported in human patients with medullary thyroid carcinoma despite the secretion of excessive calcitonin by the tumor.[18,19]

The blood calcium level is usually in the normal or low normal range in animals with C cell tumors. A bilateral medullary (C cell) carcinoma in the thyroid of a dog was reported to be associated with hypocalcemia (5 to 6 mg/dl) that returned to slightly above normal (12.8 mg/dl) following surgical excision of the tumor.[20] The hypocalcemia recurred with regrowth of the C cell carcinoma in regional lymph nodes.

Macroscopic Pathology

C cell adenomas appear as discrete, single or multiple, gray to tan nodules in one or both thyroid lobes (fig. 13.26 B). Adenomas are smaller (approximately 1 to 3 cm in diameter) than carcinomas and are separated from the thyroid parenchyma by a thin fibrous connective tissue capsule. The adjacent thyroid is compressed, but not invaded, by neoplastic C cells.

TABLE 13.3.   Vertebral osteophytosis and C cell tumors with different dietary calcium intake

| | | | | Vetebral Lesions | | | |
Time Periods	No. of Bulls	Mean Age (Years)	Vetebrae Normal	Osteophytes	Fusion of Vertebrae	Vetebral Fractures	C cell Tumors
High calcium intake (1959 to 1969)	275	7.7	172 (62.5%)	103 (37.5%)	38 (36.9%)	6 (2.2%)	62 (22.6%)[a] 52 (30.2%)[b] 10 (9.7%)[c]
Transition period (1969 to 1976)	248	—	180 (72.6%)	68 (27.4%)	40 (58.8%)	4 (1.6%)	40 (16.1%)[a] 27 (15.0%)[b] 13 (19.1%)[c]
Reduced calcium intake	143	6.9	96 (67.1%)	47 (32.9%)	24 (51.1%)	0.00	22 (15.4%)[a] 15 (15.5%)[b] 7 (14.9%)[c]
Total	666	——	448	218	102	10	124 (18.6%)[a] 94 (21.0%)[b] 30 (13.8%)[c]

Source: From McEntee, K., et al. (1980) Proceedings of the Eighth Technical Conferene on Artifical Insemination Reproduction, pp. 45-47.
[a]Tumors in total sample.
[b]Tumors in bulls with normal vertebrae.
[c]Tumors in bulls with vertebral osteophytosis.

Thyroid C cell carcinomas result in extensive multinodular enlargements of one or both thyroid lobes (fig. 13.26 C,D). The entire thyroid gland may be incorporated by the proliferating neoplastic tissue. Multiple metastases in anterior cervical lymph nodes (fig. 13.26 C) usually are large, have areas of necrosis and hemorrhage, and result in palpable enlargements in the ventral cervical region (fig. 13.26 A). Pulmonary metastases are present less frequently and appear as discrete tan nodules throughout all lobes of the lung.

Histopathology

Focal and/or diffuse hyperplasia of C cells often precedes the development of C cell neoplasms in animals and humans (fig. 13.27 A).[21] C cells appear normal, with an abundant, lightly eosinophilic, granular cytoplasm. Nodular hyperplasia of C cells consists of focal accumulations less than the size of a colloid filled follicle. Calcitonin immunoreactivity has been localized to the cytoplasm of the hyperplastic C cells.[22]

The calcitonin producing C cells were described initially in dogs as light or gray cells and are particularly prominent in this species.[23-30] Nodular aggregations of C cells are especially prominent in dogs either near the thyroid hilus in the perithyroidal connective tissues (fig. 13.27 B) or within the thyroid lobes along the course of the major branches of the thyroid artery (fig. 13.27 C). The ultimobranchial body (last, usually fifth, pharyngeal pouch) that delivers the neural crest–derived C cells to the postnatal thyroid gland fuses with each thyroid lobe at the hilus and distributes C cells throughout each lobe to varying degrees in different species. In the dog nodular aggregations of C cells frequently persist along the course of the major vessels to the thyroid; therefore, C cell hyperplasia in dogs should be diagnosed only when there is a definite increase in C cell numbers throughout each thyroid lobe compared to age-matched controls. Both thyroid lobes should be sectioned longitudinally in a consistent manner for micro-

scopic evaluation. This will minimize the prominent regional differences of C cells in the thyroid glands of normal dogs that can result in the overinterpretation of these focal aggregations of C cells as a significant lesion. The C cells in the focal aggregations have an abundant, lightly eosinophilic to amphophilic, finely granular cytoplasm and a spherical to oval nucleus. There are occasional ultimobranchial derived, colloid-containing follicles within the focal accumulations of C cells along the course of vessels within the thyroid lobe or in the connective tissues of the thyroid hilus in dogs (fig. 13.27 D).

C cell adenomas present as a discrete, expansive mass of cells greater in size than a colloid distended follicle. They are well circumscribed or partially encapsulated from adjacent follicles that are compressed to varying degrees. C cell adenomas may be subdivided into packets of cells by fine connective tissue septa and capillaries. The coarse fibrous connective tissue septa that divide neoplastic cells in C cell adenomas into small groups or nests originate from the capsule. Other cells are columnar or tall cuboidal and form small acinar or ductal structures that contain a colloid-like material. The formation of follicles and secretion of thyroglobulin have also been reported in medullary thyroid carcinoma in humans. The neoplastic C cells are well differentiated and have an abundant cytoplasmic area that is lightly eosinophilic or clear on sections stained with hematoxylin and eosin (fig. 13.28 A). The nucleus has one or more nucleoli and evenly distributed chromatin.

C cell carcinomas are more highly cellular than C cell adenomas, and the tumor cells are more pleomorphic. They often show evidence of intrathyroidal and/or extracapsular invasion, occasionally with metastases to distant sites. The neoplastic cells are polyhedral to spindle shaped, with a lightly eosinophilic, finely granular, indistinct, cytoplasmic area. The vesicular nuclei are oval or elongate and have more frequent mitotic figures than in adenomas. C cells are often subdivided into small groups

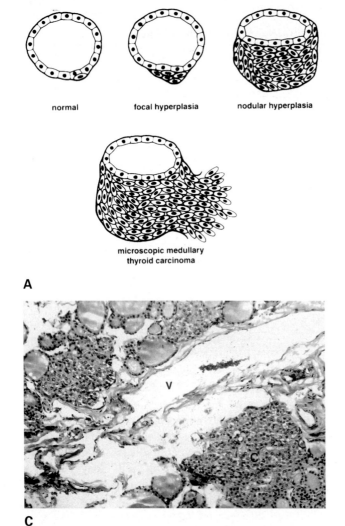

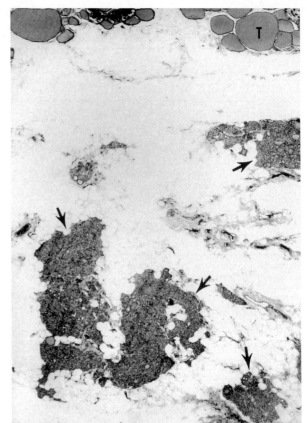

Fig. 13.27. **A.** Focal and/or nodular hyperplasia of C cells preceding the development of C cell neoplasms. **B.** Ectopic C cells (arrows) near thyroid hilus in a normal dog. T = colloid filled follicle. H&E. **C.** Nodular aggregations of C cells *(C)* along the course of major vessels *(V)* in normal canine thyroid gland. C cells often occur in prominent nodules in the thyroids of dogs and should not be over interpreted as multifocal C cell hyperplasia. H&E. **D.** Prominent nodular aggregations of C cells *(C)* in normal canine thyroid with an occasional colloid-containing follicle. H&E. **A** from Burek, CRC Press, 1978.

by fine connective tissue septa that contain small capillaries (fig. 13.28 B). Only occasional ducts and acini are present in C cell carcinomas. A similar histological pattern also is present in the metastatic lesions in cervical lymph nodes and lung.

Ultimobranchial tumors in the thyroid glands of bulls often have a more complex histological structure than the typical C cell (medullary) carcinoma in humans, dogs, horses, and many strains of laboratory rats. Areas in the tumor composed of differentiated C cells consist of focal accumulations of neoplastic cells with an abundant lightly eosinophilic cytoplasm in the wall of thyroid and ultimobranchial follicles, or they may be present as larger nod-

ules with a solid histological structure. Ultimobranchial thyroid tumors often are accompanied by a multifocal hyperplasia of C cells in other parts of the thyroid lobes and hilus. The neoplastic C cells often are embedded in an increased amount of hyalinized stroma that may contain amyloid. In bulls, parts of this thyroid neoplasm that appear to be derived from less differentiated ultimobranchial remnants consist of follicle-like structures, cysts, and tubules composed of immature, small, basophilic cells. These tumors in bulls and other species closely resemble undifferentiated or stem cells of the normal ultimobranchial body that can differentiate into both C cells and follicular cells. Thyroid follicles and cribriform structures with colloid-like material formed by cells that resemble differentiated follicular cells often are present in the neoplasms in close association with these more primitive ultimobranchial derived structures. The heterogeneous histological structure of ultimobranchial neoplasms in bulls resembles a variant of thyroid carcinoma in humans. This tumor, designated as an intermediate type of differentiated carcinoma, has structural and immunocytochemical characteristics of both medullary (C cell) and follicular carcinomas.[31,32]

Ultrastructural Characteristics

C cell neoplasms of bulls are composed of several types of cells with different ultrastructural features.[12] The most characteristic cell type has large perinuclear aggregations of concentric or interwoven microfilaments, often situated near the Golgi apparatus (fig. 13.28 C). In some neoplastic C cells the nucleus is partially indented by the extensive clusters of microfilaments. The formation of fine protein microfilaments appears to be one of the distinctive characteristics of C cells and other polypeptide hormone secreting cells of the amine precursor uptake decarboxylase (APUD) series.

Secretion granules are scattered between the networks of microfilaments and elsewhere in the cytoplasm. The secretory granules are membrane limited, composed of fine dense particles, and appear to be similar to those in normal C cells of control bulls. There are numerous aggregations of free ribosomes and dispersed profiles of rough endoplasmic reticulum in the cytoplasm.

The predominant type of neoplastic cell in C cell carcinomas is polyhedral or spindle shaped and appears to be poorly differentiated. The relatively small cytoplasmic area contains clusters of free ribosomes, prominent Golgi apparatuses associated with small vesicles, and scattered mitochondria, but few mature secretion granules (fig. 13.28 D). Other neoplastic cells are more columnar and assume a ductal or acinar pattern. Single or multiple layers of cells are arranged around a lumen containing finely granular material of moderate electron density. The plasma membranes of adjacent cells often are intricately interdigitated, and the apical cytoplasm contains numerous lipofuscin granules. Long microvilli and cytoplasmic projections extend into ductal lumens. Groups of mitochondria, clusters of ribosomes, and numerous vacuoles are present in the cytoplasm.

C cell tumors in both bulls and humans are firm, and in some areas the stroma consists of dense bands of fibrous connective tissue.[33,34] In both adenomas and carcinomas there often are deposits of a homogenous eosinophilic material that stains positively for amyloid. Large aggregations of fine amyloid fibrils are observed ultrastructurally between the bundles of collagen fibers, particularly in C cell adenomas (fig. 13.28 E).

The etiology of the localized amyloid deposits in the thyroid C cell neoplasms is uncertain, but it appears to be produced by the tumor cells and is not associated with amyloid deposition in other organs. Amyloid production is consistently associated with medullary thyroid carcinoma in humans and also has been reported in certain other endocrine tumors.[35-37] Amyloid in C cell tumors is present between tumor cells, around vessels, and in the interstitium of bulls, horses, dogs, and laboratory rats, but in amounts that vary (minimal to substantial) from case to case. Chemical differences exist between amyloid fibrils of immunoglobulin origin and those produced by endocrine tumors.[38]

The predominate cells that form ultimobranchial thyroid neoplasms in bulls resemble differentiated C (parafollicular) cells more closely than follicular cells in the thyroid gland. Differentiated C cells in normal bulls are found wedged between follicular cells lining thyroid follicles. They have a prominent Golgi apparatus, lamellar arrays of rough endoplasmic reticulum, and large aggregations of membrane-limited secretion granules in those portions of the cytoplasm bordering interfollicular capillaries. The granules are of a size and shape similar to those observed in cells of thyroid C cell tumors, but are more numerous than in the less differentiated neoplastic cells.

The ultimobranchial derived neoplastic cells lining the colloid filled follicles in bulls often have prominent microvilli that extend into the lumen. An occasional cytoplasmic pseudopodium may be observed to partially surround a portion of the colloid. Large dense bodies and colloid droplets are present in the cytoplasm, but no small, membrane-limited secretion granules are observed as in C cells. The endoplasmic reticulum appears as an extensive tubular network containing material of moderate density and usually is not aggregated into prominent lamellar arrays as in C cells. Other colloid filled follicles in ultimobranchial tumors developing in the thyroid glands of bulls represent normal follicles surrounded by the invading neoplastic cells.

Parathyroid glands from bulls with C cell neoplasms usually have ultrastructural evidence of secretory inactivity and atrophy of chief cells, probably as a result of the high calcium intake. Cytoplasmic organelles in chief cells are poorly developed, and secretion granules are infrequent. The large cytoplasmic area contains numerous lipofuscin granules and cytosegresomes. Parathyroid hyperplasia and adenoma, reported in humans with familial medullary thyroid carcinoma, have not been observed in bulls with C cell tumors. Prominent aggregations of amyloid fibrils are observed occasionally around the inactive chief cells in the parathyroid glands.

Bioassay for Calcitonin Activity

Bioassay of C cell adenoma and carcinoma from bulls demonstrates the presence of calcitonin activity [466 ± 93 MRC (Medical Research Council) milliunits/g] in these neoplasms,[12,39] and calcitonin has been detected at higher than normal levels in plasma of bulls by immunoassay.[40] Calcium infusion to raise serum calcium to 12.6 ± 0.6 mg/100 ml increases plasma calcitonin-like activity

(210 percent ± 31 percent above preinfusion levels) after 1 hour (fig. 13.29).[12] Mean serum calcium levels in bulls with calcitonin secreting thyroid tumors (9.51 mg/100 ml) are only slightly lower than in adult control bulls (9.92 ± 0.2 mg/100 ml). The near normal serum electrolyte values

in bulls with chronic hypersecretion of calcitonin most likely are a result of the low turnover rate of bone in old bulls and the compensatory mechanisms of other endocrine organs.

By comparison, cells constituting medullary thyroid

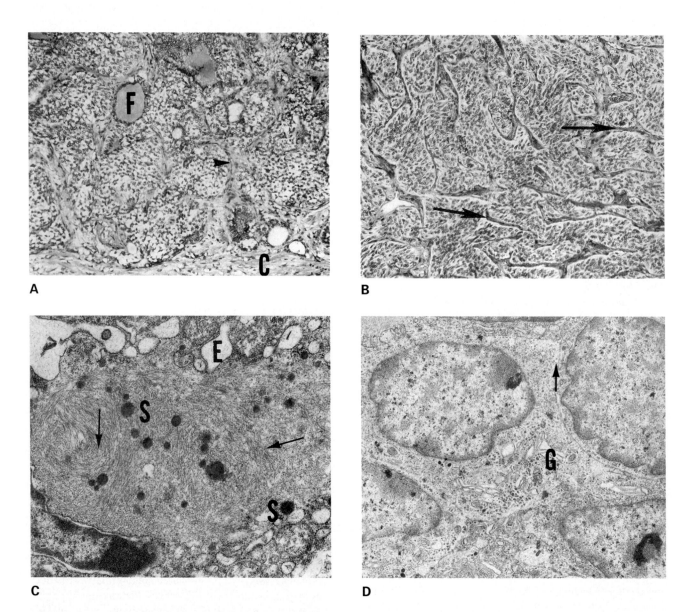

Fig. 13.28. Microscopic features of thyroid C cell tumors. **A.** C cell adenoma of a bull. Neoplastic cells are subdivided into small groups by prominent connective tissue septa (arrowhead) arising from the capsule *(C)*. There are scattered colloid-containing follicles *(F)* in the adenoma. **B.** C cell carcinoma of a bull. The neoplastic C cells are spindle shaped or polyhedral and are subdivided into discrete groups by fine connective tissue septa with capillaries (arrows). **C.** Extensive network of microfilaments (arrows) in a C cell carcinoma of a bull. Membrane-limited secretory granules *(S)* are scattered in the network of microfilaments. The nucleus is indented by the microfilaments, and profiles of rough endoplasmic reticulum *(E)* are distended. **D.** Poorly differentiated C cells in an ultimobranchial carcinoma from a bull. There are numerous clusters of free ribosomes (arrow) and a prominent Golgi apparatus *(G)* with small vesicles but few secretory granules in the cytoplasm. **E.** C cell tumor from a bull illustrating large aggregations of fine amyloid fibrils *(A)* interspersed in the stroma between bundles of collagen fibers *(C)*.

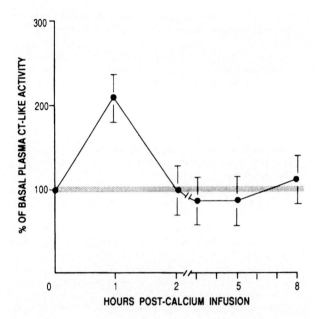

Fig. 13.29. Increased plasma calcitonin-like activity in bulls with thyroid C cell tumors following intravenous infusion of calcium. Note the brisk increase at 1 hour after the calcium infusion and rapid return to baseline by 2 hours. [From Black, H.E., et al. (1973) *Cancer* 32:865-878.]

carcinomas in humans have been reported to be more differentiated C cells than in bulls and have well-developed cytoplasmic organelles with more numerous membrane-limited secretion granules. An increased concentration of calcitonin in neoplastic tissue and peripheral plasma also appears to be a consistent finding in humans with medullary thyroid carcinoma.[19,41] The higher level of calcitonin activity reported in medullary carcinomas in humans than was observed in C cell tumors of bulls is interpreted to be a reflection of the degree of differentiation of neoplastic thyroid C cells.

Etiology

Although the etiology of C cell neoplasms is unknown, a possible relationship has been suggested between the long-term dietary intake of excessive calcium and the high incidence of these tumors in bulls. Adult bulls frequently ingest from 3.5 to approximately 6 times the amount of calcium normally recommended for maintenance of the blood calcium concentration.[42] The chronic stimulation of C cells and ultimobranchial derivatives by high levels of calcium absorbed from the digestive tract may be related to the pathogenesis of the thyroid C cell neoplasms in bulls.

There has been significant decline in the incidence of C cell tumors in bulls (with normal vertebrae) switched from a high calcium intake to a reduced calcium intake period (30.2 percent vs. 15.6 percent incidence, respectively) (see table 13.3).[9] There was no significant difference in the incidence of C cell tumors in bulls with verte-

bral lesions switched from a high calcium intake to a period of reduced calcium intake (9.7 percent vs. 14.9 percent incidence, respectively). The decline in incidence of C cell tumors in the total sample from 22.6 percent during the high calcium intake period to 15.4 percent in the reduced calcium period was not significant (see table 13.3).

Cows do not develop proliferative lesions of C cells under similar dietary conditions, possibly because of the high physiological requirements for calcium imposed by pregnancy and lactation. The demonstration that prolonged feeding of high calcium diets during pregnancy did produce C cell hyperplasia in nonlactating cows suggests that lactation, not pregnancy, is the mechanism that protects the cow from diet induced proliferative lesions in thyroid C cells. C cell proliferation in humans has been reported as a response to chronic hypercalcemia and has been suggested as being one etiological factor in the pathogenesis of thyroid medullary (C cell) carcinoma.[43] The fine structural changes suggesting secretory inactivity of parathyroid chief cells in bulls with C cell tumors also are interpreted to be an effect of the long-term feeding of high calcium diets.

Growth and Metastasis

C cell adenomas in bulls grow slowly, often near the thyroid hilus, and compress the adjacent parenchyma. Thyroid C cell carcinomas are larger and cause observable enlargements in the anterior cervical region of bulls. Carcinomas often metastasize to anterior cervical lymph nodes, invade adjacent tissues, and occasionally metastasize to the lungs. Medullary thyroid carcinomas in humans infrequently may be anaplastic and associated with widespread metastasis to lumbar vertebrae, heart, kidney, scapula, and cerebral dura mater[44]; however, C cell carcinomas in animals usually are well circumscribed and resectable in contrast to thyroid follicular cell adenocarcinomas.[45] The diagnosis of C cell carcinoma can be confirmed by demonstrating large amounts of immunoreactive calcitonin in tumor extracts and by immunocytochemical staining (species specific) for calcitonin. C cell tumors also may produce increased amounts of prostaglandins, serotonin, and 5-hydroxytryptophan. C cell tumors in horses usually are slow growing and well-encapsulated adenomas that are amenable to complete surgical excision.[5]

REFERENCES

1. Krook, L., Lutwak, L., and McEntee, K. (1969) Dietary calcium, ultimobranchial tumors and osteopetrosis in the bull: Syndrome of calcitonin excess? *Amer J Clin Nutr* 22:115-118.

2. Capen, C.C., and Black, H.E. (1974) Calcitonin-secreting ultimobranchial neoplasms of the thyroid gland in bulls: An animal model

for medullary thyroid carcinoma in man. *Amer J Pathol* 74:377-380.

3. Lindsay, S., Nichols, C.W., Jr., and Chaikoff, I.L. (1968) Naturally occurring thyroid carcinoma in the rat. *Arch Pathol* 86:353-364.

4. Hillidge, C.J., Sanecki, R.K., and Theodorakis, M.C. (1982) Thyroid carcinoma in a horse. *J Amer Vet Med Assoc* 181:711-714.

5. Turk, J.R., Nakata, Y.J., Leathers, C.W., and Gallina, A.M. (1983) Ultimobranchial adenoma of the thyroid gland in a horse. *Vet Pathol* 20:114-117.

6. Leav, I., Schiller, A.L., Rijnberk, A., Kegg, M.A., and der Kinderen, P.J. (1976) Adenomas and carcinomas of the canine and feline thyroid. *Amer J Pathol* 83:61-64.

7. Wadsworth, P.F., Lewis, D.J., and Jones, D.M. (1981) Medullary carcinoma of the thyroid in a mouflon (*Ovis musimon*). *J Comp Pathol* 91:313-316.

8. Jubb, K.V., and McEntee, K. (1959) The relationship of ultimobranchial remnants and derivatives to tumors of the thyroid gland in cattle. *Cornell Vet* 49:41-69.

9. McEntee, K., Hall, C.E., and Dunn, H.O. (1980) The relationship of calcium intake to the development of vertebral osteophytosis and ultimobranchial tumors in bulls. In Proceedings of the Eighth Technical Conference on Artificial Insemination Reproduction, pp. 45-47.

10. Sizemore, G.W., Carney, J.A., Gharib, H., and Capen, C.C. (1992) Multiple endocrine neoplasia type 2B: 18-year follow-up of a four generation family. *Henry Ford Hosp Med J* 40:236-244.

11. Wilkie, B.N., and Krook, L. (1970) Ultimobranchial tumor of the thyroid and pheochromocytoma in the bull. *Pathol Vet* 7:126-134.

12. Black, H.E., Capen, C.C., and Young, D.M. (1973) Ultimobranchial thyroid neoplasms in bulls: A syndrome resembling medullary thyroid carcinoma in man. *Cancer* 32:865-878.

13. Weichert, R.F., III. (1970) The neural ectodermal origin of the peptide-secreting endocrine gland: A unifying concept for the etiology of multiple endocrine adenomatosis and the inappropriate secretion of peptide hormones by nonendocrine tumors. *Amer J Med* 49:232-241.

14. Spoonenberg, D.P., and McEntee, K. (1983) Pheochromocytomas and ultimobranchial (C-cell) neoplasms in the bull: Evidence of autosomal dominant inheritance in the guernsey breed. *Vet Pathol* 20:396-400.

15. Peterson, M.E., Randolph, J.F., Zaki, F.A., and Heath, H., III. (1982) Multiple endocrine neoplasia in a dog. *J Amer Vet Med Assoc* 180:1476-1478.

16. Carver, J.R., Kapatkin, A., and Patnaik, A.K. (1995) A comparison of medullary thyroid carcinoma and thyroid adenocarcinoma in dogs: A retrospective study of 38 cases. *Vet Surg* 24:315-319.

17. Thomson, R.G. (1969) Vertebral body osteophytes in bulls. *Pathol Vet* 6:1-46.

18. Fletcher, J.R. (1970) Medullary (solid) carcinoma of the thyroid gland. *Arch Surg* 100:257-262.

19. Melvin, K.W., Miller, H.H., and Tashjian, A.H., Jr. (1971) Early diagnosis of medullary carcinoma of the thyroid gland by means of calcitonin assay. *N Engl J Med* 285:1115-1120.

20. Patnaik, A.K., Lieberman, P.H., Erlandson, R.A., Acevedo, W.M., and Liu, S.-K. (1978) Canine medullary carcinoma of the thyroid. *Vet Pathol* 15:590-599.

21. DeLellis, R.A., Nunnemacher, G., and Wolfe, H.J. (1977) C cell hyperplasia, an ultrastructural analysis. *Lab Invest* 36:237-248.

22. Deftos, L.J., Bone, H.G., III, and Parthemore, J.G. (1980) immunohistological studies of medullary thyroid carcinoma and C cell hyperplasia. *J Clin Endocrinol Metab* 51:857-862.

23. Nonidez, José F. (1931-32) The origin of the 'parafollicular' cell, a second epithelial component of the thyroid gland of the dog. *Amer J Anat* 49:479-505.

24. Tashiro, M. (1964) Electron microscopic studies of the parafollicular cells in the thyroid gland of a dog. *Okajimas Folia Anat Jpn* 39:191-211.

25. Pearse, A.G.E. (1966) The cytochemistry of the thyroid C cells and their relationship to calcitonin. *Proc Roy Soc B (Biol Ser)* 164:478-487.

26. Pearse, A.G.E. (1968) Common cytochemical and ultrastructural characteristics of cells producing polypeptide hormones (the *APUD* series) and their relevance to thyroid and ultimobranchial C cells and calcitonin. *Proc Roy Soc B* 170:71-80.

27. Bussolati, G., and Pearse, A.G.E. (1967) Immunofluorescent localization of calcitonin in the 'C' cells of pig and dog thyroid. *J Endocrinol* 37:205-209.

28. Teitelbaum, S.L., Moore, K.E., and Shieber, W. (1970) C cell follicles in the dog thyroid: Demonstration by in vivo perfusion. *Anat Rec* 168:69-78.

29. Kalina, M., and Pearse, A.G.E. (1971) Ultrastructural localization of calcitonin in C-cells of dog thyroid: An immunocytochemical study. *Histochemie* 26:1-8.

30. Kameda, Y. (1973) Electron microscopic studies on the parafollicular cells and parafollicular cell complexes in the dog. *Arch Histol Jpn* 36:89-105.

31. Ljungberg, O., Ericsson, U.-B., Bondeson, L., and Thorell, J. (1983) A compound follicular-parafollicular cell carcinoma of the thyroid: A new tumor entity? *Cancer* 52:1053-1061.

32. Ljungberg, O., Bondeson, L., and Bondeson, A.-G. (1984) Differentiated thyroid carcinoma, intermediate type: A new tumor entity with features of follicular and parafollicular cell carcinoma. *Human Pathol* 15:218-228.

33. Hazard, J.B., Hawk, W.A., and Crile, G., Jr. (1959) Medullary (solid) carcinoma of the thyroid: A clinicopathologic entity. *J Clin Endocrinol* 19:152-161.

34. Williams, E.D., Brown, C.L., and Doniach, I. (1966) Pathological and clinical findings in a series of 67 cases of medullary carcinoma of the thyroid. *J Clin Pathol* 19:103-113.

35. Manning, P.C., Jr., Molnar, G.D., Black, B.M., Priestly, J.T., and Woolner, L.B. (1963) Pheochromocytoma, hyperparathyroidism and thyroid carcinoma occurring coincidentally. *N Eng J Med* 268:68-72.

36. McDermott, F.T., and Hart, J.A.L. (1970) Medullary carcinoma of the thyroid with hypocalcaemia: Clinical and ultrastructural observations. *Brit J Surg* 57:657-661.

37. Bordi, C., Anversa, P., and Vitali-Mazza, L. (1972) Ultrastructural study of a calcitonin-secreting tumor: Cytology of the tumor cells and origin of amyloid. *Virchows Arch* 357:145-161.

38. Pearse, A.G.E., Ewen, S.W.B., and Polak, J.M. (1972) The genesis of APUD amyloid in endocrine polypeptide tumours: Histochemical distinction from immunamyloid. *Virchows Arch B* 10:93-107.

39. Young, D.M., Capen, C.C., and Black, H.E. (1971) Calcitonin activity in ultimobranchial neoplasms from bulls. *Vet Pathol* 8:19-27.

40. Deftos, L.J., Habener, J.R., Mayer, G.P., Bury, A.E., and Potts, J.T., Jr. (1972) Radioimmunoassay for bovine calcitonin. *J Lab Clin Med* 79:480-490.

41. Voelkel, E.F., Tashjian, A.H., Jr., Davidoff, F.F., Cohen, R.B., Perlia, C.P., and Wurtman, R.J. (1973) Concentrations of calcitonin and catecholamines in pheochromocytomas, a mucosal neuroma and medullary thyroid carcinoma. *J Clin Endocrinol Metab* 37, 297-307.

42. Krook, L., Lutwak, L., McEntee, K., Henrickson, P., Braun, K., and Roberts, S. (1971) Nutritional hypercalcitoninism in bulls. *Cornell Vet* 61:625-639.

43. Ljungberg, O., and Dymling, J.R. (1972) Pathogenesis of C-cell neoplasia in thyroid gland: C-cell proliferation in a case of chronic hypercalcaemia. *Acta Pathol Microbiol Scand* 80:577-588.

44. Long, G.G., Clemmons, R.M., and Heath, H., III (1980) Metastatic canine medullary thyroid carcinoma. A case report. *Vet Pathol* 17:323-330.

45. Carver, J.R., Kapatkin, A., and Patnaik, A.K. (1995) A comparison of medullary thyroid carcinoma and thyroid adenocarcinoma in dogs: A retrospective study of 38 cases. *Vet Surg* 24:315-319.

TUMORS AND NONNEOPLASTIC CYSTS OF THE PARATHYROID GLAND

Chief Cell Adenoma and Carcinoma

Introduction

Functional adenomas and carcinomas of parathyroid glands secrete parathyroid hormone (PTH) in excess of normal, resulting in a syndrome of primary hyperparathyroidism.[1] The normal control mechanism by the concentration of blood calcium ion is lost in functional parathyroid tumors. Parathyroid hormone secretion by functional tumors is excessive in spite of an increased level of blood calcium. Cells of the renal tubules are very sensitive to alterations in the amount of circulating parathyroid hormone. The hormone acts on these cells initially to promote the excretion of phosphorus and retention of calcium. A prolonged increased secretion of parathyroid hormone accelerates osteocytic and osteoclastic bone resorption. Mineral is removed from the skeleton and replaced by immature fibrous connective tissue. The bone lesion of fibrous osteodystrophy is generalized throughout the skeleton but is accentuated in local areas such as the maxillae, mandibles, and a subperiosteal location of long bones.[2]

Incidence

Adenomas or adenocarcinomas of parathyroid glands are encountered infrequently in older dogs,[3-6] cats,[7-9] laboratory rats, and mice. Inadequate numbers of cases have been studied to determine any breed or sex predisposition. Tumors of parathyroid chief cells do not appear to be a sequela of long-standing secondary hyperparathyroidism of renal or nutritional origin. Parathyroid carcinoma is rare in animals, but has been diagnosed in older dogs and cats. It is the parathyroid lesion responsible for approximately 4 percent of the cases of primary hyperparathyroidism in humans.[10] The incidence of parathyroid adenomas is increased in a dose dependent manner by both internal (^{131}I) and external (localized X ray) irradiation in rats (fig. 13.30 F).[11,12]

Clinical Characteristics

The clinical disturbances observed with functional parathyroid tumors are the result of the persistent hypercalcemia, increased urinary calcium and phosphorus excretion with the formation of calculi, and weakening of bones by excessive resorption. Lameness due to fractures of long bones may occur after relatively minor physical trauma. In long-standing cases compression fractures of vertebral bodies may exert pressure on the spinal cord and nerves, resulting in motor or sensory dysfunction or both. Facial hyperostosis with partial obliteration of the nasal cavity, and loosening or loss of teeth from alveolar sockets have been observed in dogs with primary hyperparathyroidism, due in part to the anabolic effect of PTH on stimulation of osteoblasts to form poorly mineralized osteoid. These lesions, however, are more common and severe with secondary (renal, nutritional) hyperparathyroidism. Hypercalcemia results in anorexia, vomiting, constipation, depression, polyuria, polydipsia, and generalized muscular weakness due to decreased neuromuscular excitability.

Primary hyperparathyroidism should be considered in older dogs and cats if they have a history of multiple fractures associated with generalized skeletal demineralization and the formation of urinary calculi but with otherwise normal renal function. Radiographic evaluation reveals areas of subperiosteal cortical bone resorption, loss of lamina dura dentes around the teeth, soft tissue mineralization, bone cysts, and a generalized decrease in bone density, with multiple fractures in advanced cases.

The most practical laboratory tests to aid in establishing the diagnosis of primary hyperparathyroidism are quantitation of total blood calcium and phosphorus, and circulating levels of parathyroid hormone [N-terminal or immunoradiometric assay (IRMA)]. Although other laboratory findings may be variable, hypercalcemia (> 12 mg/dl) is a consistent finding and is the result of accelerated release of calcium from bone. Dogs evaluated with primary hyperparathyroidism often have had a greatly elevated (13 to 20 mg/dl or higher) blood calcium level. Repeated palpation of a functional parathyroid adenoma may result in thrombosis of the parathyroid artery, leading to diffuse ischemic necrosis of the gland (fig. 13.30 G). This may result in the development of a rapidly progressive hypocalcemic tetany, similar to that which develops following the surgical removal of a functional parathyroid neoplasm.

The blood phosphorus level is low (4 mg/dl) or in the low to normal range because of inhibition of renal tubular resorption of phosphorus by excess parathyroid hormone. Serum alkaline phosphatase activity may be increased due to increased osteoblastic activity as a response to mechanical stress on bones weakened by excessive resorption or due to direct (receptor mediated) stimulation of osteoblasts by the elevated PTH level. The urinary excretion of calcium and phosphorus is increased and may predispose to the development of nephrocalcinosis and urolithiasis. Primary hyperparathyroidism may be a contributing factor in the development of calcium oxalate urolithiasis in cats.[8] Accelerated bone matrix catabolism is reflected by an increased excretion of hydroxyproline in the urine. The detection of elevated circulating levels of parathyroid hormone by radioimmunoassay in humans and animals has greatly facilitated early diagnosis of hyperparathyroidism.[13,14] Double-phase scintigraphy of the parathyroid glands using technetium (Tc) 99m can be helpful in localizing parathyroid adenomas in dogs with primary hyperparathyroidism.[15]

Macroscopic Pathology

Chief cell adenomas usually result in considerable enlargement of a single parathyroid gland. They are light brown to red and are located either in the cervical region near the thyroids or, rarely, within the thoracic cavity near the base of the heart.[3,16] Parathyroid neoplasms in the precardial mediastinum are derived from ectopic parathyroid tissue displaced into the thorax along with the expanding thymus during embryonic development. The adenomas are sharply demarcated and encapsulated from the adjacent thyroid gland (fig. 13.30 A). Multiple white foci may be seen in the thyroids of dogs with functional parathyroid tumors. These represent areas of C cell hyperplasia in response to the long-term hypercalcemia (fig. 13.30 A,C). All parathyroid glands should be evaluated at surgery for evidence of primary multinodular chief cell hyperplasia that can result in macroscopic enlargement of multiple glands and persistent hypercalcemia. All visibly enlarged parathyroid glands should be surgically removed.[6]

Hyperparathyroidism due to chief cell hyperplasia is common in animals as part of the compensatory reaction to chronic renal disease and nutritional imbalances. Chief cells undergo organellar hypertrophy initially and cellular hyperplasia later to increase parathyroid hormone synthesis and secretion in response to a hypocalcemic stimulus. In secondary (compensatory) chief cell hyperplasia, all four parathyroids are enlarged two to five times their normal size (fig. 13.30 B). A parathyroid adenoma enlarges a single gland to a much greater degree (fig. 13.30 C), while the remaining parathyroids will be atrophic and smaller than normal. Histopathological demonstration of a compressed rim of parathyroid parenchyma and a fibrous capsule in an enlarged gland points to the diagnosis of adenoma rather than chief cell hyperplasia.

Primary parathyroid hyperplasia has been described in German shepherd pups associated with hypercalcemia, hypophosphatemia, increased immunoreactive parathyroid hormone, and increased fractional clearance of inorganic phosphate in the urine.[17] Clinical signs include stunted growth, muscular weakness, polyuria, polydipsia, and a diffuse reduction in bone density. Intravenous infusion of calcium fails to suppress the autonomous secretion of parathyroid hormone by the diffuse hyperplasia of chief cells in all parathyroids. Lesions include nodular hyperplasia of thyroid C cells and widespread mineralization of the lungs, kidney, and gastric mucosa. The disease is inherited as an autosomal recessive.

Hypercalcemia and *hypophosphatemia* develop in certain dogs affected with several different types of malignant neoplasms (e.g., carcinomas of the kidney, lung, or ovary) in the absence of bone metastasis and functional lesions in the parathyroid glands. A syndrome of pseudo-

hyperparathyroidism (cancer-associated hypercalcemia) has been reported in dogs and cats with disseminated malignant lymphoma.[15,16] Antemortem differentiation between primary hyperparathyroidism and pseudohyperparathyroidism can be difficult, especially if there are no overt clinical signs of lymphoma, since both have hypercalcemia, hypophosphatemia, and often increased alkaline phosphatase. The degree of skeletal demineralization is usually less severe with pseudohyperparathyroidism.

Histopathology

Parathyroid adenomas are composed of closely packed chief cells subdivided into small groups by fine connective tissue septa with many capillaries (fig. 13.30 D). The chief cells are cuboidal or polyhedral, and the cytoplasm stains lightly eosinophilic. Neoplastic chief cells can form follicle-like structures with a lumen containing minimal proteinic material that could (at low power) be confused with a thyroid follicular cell tumor. Occasional oxyphil cells, water-clear cells, and transitional forms may be distributed throughout the adenoma or, infrequently, oxyphil cells or water-clear cells may be the predominant cell in the parathyroid adenoma. Fat cells and mast cells are often present in the stroma of the tumor. Adenomas are surrounded by a fine, partial to complete connective tissue capsule and may compress the adjacent thyroid gland (fig. 13.30 A). A rim of compressed parathyroid parenchyma usually is present outside the capsule of small adenomas. These atrophic chief cells are small and irregular in shape and have a densely eosinophilic cytoplasm and a pyknotic nucleus.[18]

(Focal/multifocal) chief cell hyperplasia may affect the parathyroid in a distinctly focal or multifocal distribution. In focal parathyroid hyperplasia, there are single or multiple nodules in one or multiple glands in which there are an increased number of closely packed chief cells, often with an expanded cytoplasmic area. The focal areas of chief cell hyperplasia are poorly demarcated and not encapsulated from adjacent parenchyma. Chief cells within the nodules have a relatively uniform composition with a high ratio of cytoplasm to nucleus and a slightly more hyperchromatic nucleus than adjacent normal chief cells. There may be slight compression of adjacent chief cells around the larger focal areas of hyperplasia. Focal chief cell hyperplasia often is difficult to separate from a chief cell adenoma using only morphological criteria. The presence of multiple nodules of varying sizes and uniform cellularity in one or multiple parathyroids with minimal compression and no encapsulation is more compatible with an interpretation of focal hyperplasia than with one of chief cell adenoma.

Parathyroid carcinomas are rare and occur less frequently than chief cell adenomas; they occur primarily in dogs and cats.[7] They usually are larger than adenomas, incorporate completely the parathyroid gland of origin, are more fixed in position, and have clear microscopic evidence of invasion (i.e., parathyroid capsule, adjacent thyroid gland, perathyroidal connective tissues, adjacent cervical muscles, occasionally veins or lymphatics). Some of the parathyroid enlargement is due to hemorrhage and necrosis within the carcinoma. Most carcinomas are composed of well-differentiated chief cells that are similar to those in parathyroid adenomas. However, the mitotic index may be increased moderately in some carcinomas, and the chief cells often are more pleomorphic. The malignant chief cells may be arranged in solid sheets, be subdivided into lobules by a fibrovascular stroma, palisade along blood sinusoids, or form infrequent acinar structures. The cytoplasmic area stains lightly eosinophilic, and boundaries of adjacent cells are indistinct. Metastases to distant sites (e.g., regional lymph nodes and lungs) are uncommon in parathyroid carcinomas in animals.

Ultrastructural Characteristics

Chief cells comprising *functional parathyroid adenomas* usually are in the actively synthesizing stage of the secretory cycle (fig. 13.30 E). Multiple large lamellar arrays of rough endoplasmic reticulum and clusters of free ribosomes are present in the cytoplasm. However, few mature secretory (storage) granules are present in the cytoplasm, suggesting that parathyroid hormone is secreted at a faster rate than synthesis and storage in autonomous chief cells (fig. 13.30 E). Large mitochondria and prominent Golgi apparatuses are present in neoplastic chief cells. The annulate lamellae that occur frequently in parathyroid adenomas from human patients have not been reported in either normal or neoplastic chief cells of animals.[19]

Parathyroid adenomas may contain secretory granules in chief cells as well as mature oxyphil cells and transitional forms with well-developed organelles concerned with hormonal synthesis and packaging. This is in marked contrast to the oxyphil cell of normal parathyroid glands, which has a cytoplasm filled with tightly packed mitochondria but a poorly developed endoplasmic reticulum and Golgi apparatus.[19] Occasional parathyroid adenomas in both dogs and human beings may be composed predominately of large eosinophilic oxyphil cells.

Parathyroid carcinomas are composed of chief cells with a highly variable development of cytoplasmic organelles. Alterations of the nuclear morphology have been described in malignant chief cells.[19] There usually is a greater degree of cellular pleomorphism than in chief cell adenomas, with more frequest mitotic figures and microscopic evidence of invasion into the adjacent parathyroid, thyroid, or periglandular connective tissues.

Chromogranin A

In addition to parathyroid hormone, secretory granules in chief cells also contain chromogranin A (CGA) (parathyroid secretory protein). Chromogranin A was first isolated from secretory granules of the bovine adrenal medulla.[20] Chromogranin A, a 49 kD peptide, is a major constituent of secretory granules of the adrenal medulla, pituitary, parathyroid, thyroid C cells, pancreatic islets, endocrine cells of the gastrointestinal tract, and sympathetic nerves, and it comprises up to 50 percent of the total protein secreted by the parathyroid. Chromogranin A shares considerable homology between species. Immunologic cross reactivity to mammalian proteins has been observed in reptiles, amphibians, fish, and *Drosophila* tissues. Chromogranin A is synthesized as a preprotein and is directed to the internal cavity of the rough endoplasmic reticulum (RER) by the N-terminal preregion of the peptide. Once inside the RER, the preregion is cleaved by a signal peptidase.

Although the functions of CGA are still under investigation, several roles have been postulated. Chromogranin A is suspected to play an important role in the maturation of secretory granules. Inside the Golgi apparatus, CGA is involved in the packaging of contents into newly formed vesicles. Chromogranin A precipitates as it diffuses into the trans-Golgi network. Other secretory products such as parathyroid hormone become entrapped in the growing CGA conglomerate and subsequently are packaged into a

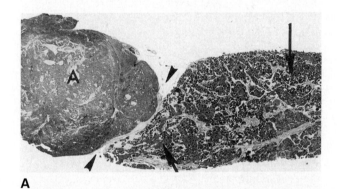

A

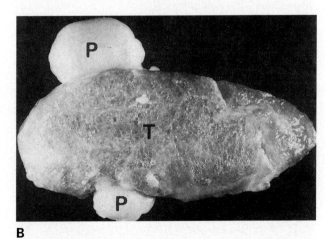

B

Fig. 13.30. Tumors of the parathyroid gland. **A.** Chief cell adenoma *(A)* in the external parathyroid gland of a dog with primary hyperparathyroidism. The adenoma is sharply demarcated and encapsulated (arrowheads) from the adjacent thyroid gland. The cranial pole of the thyroid is compressed and there are multifocal areas of C cell hyperplasia (arrows). **B.** Moderate enlargement of the internal and external parathyroids *(P)* in a dog with secondary chief cell hyperplasia associated with chronic renal failure (T is thyroid gland). Scale is 1 cm. (continued)

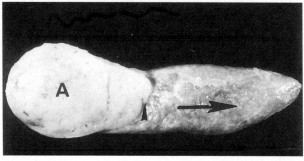

C

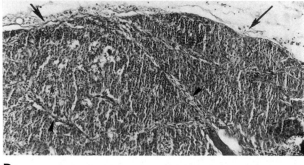

D

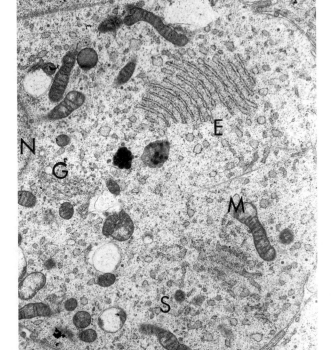

E

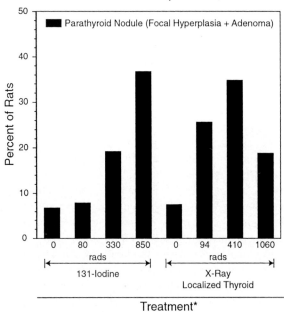

Parathyroid Nodular Proliferative Lesions vs Radiation Exposure*

F

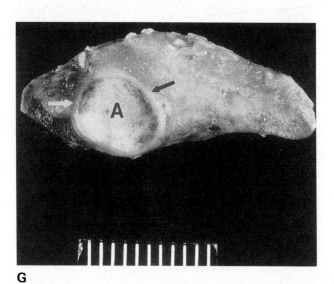

G

Fig. 13.30. (continued)   C. Parathyroid adenoma *(A)* causing extensive enlargement of one parathyroid gland. The tumor is encapsulated (arrowhead), and there are multicentric areas of C cell hyperplasia in the thyroid (arrow) as a response to the long-term hypercalcemia. D. Parathyroid adenoma illustrating closely packed chief cells subdivided into small groups by fine fibrous septa and capillaries (arrowheads). A thin capsule of fibrous connective tissue (arrows) surrounds the tumor. E. Active chief cell in a functional parathyroid adenoma from a dog with primary hyperparathyroidism. There are large lamellar arrays of rough endoplasmic reticulum *(E)*, a prominent Golgi apparatus *(G)*, large mitochondria *(M)*, but few secretory granules *(S)* in the abundant cytoplasmic area *(N* is nucleus). F. Parathyroid nodular proliferative lesions vs radiation exposure. [From Capen, C.C., et al. (1999) In: *Radiation and Thyroid Cancer,* World Scientific Publishing.] G. Functional chief cell adenoma *(A)* with a well-developed fibrous capsule (arrows) that sharply delineates the tumor from the adjacent thyroid. The dog was presented initially with persistent hypercalcemia; however, repeated palpations of the mass resulted in diffuse ischemic necrosis and the development of hypocalcemic tetany. Scale = 1 cm.

secretory granule.[21] Chromogranin A has a large calcium binding capacity which may enhance vesicle stability. As granules mature, they accumulate large amounts of calcium (up to 40 mM), which also may serve as a route of Ca^{++} secretion. However, free (ionized) calcium concentrations remain in the micromolar range since most Ca^{++} is bound to CGA. Chromogranin A–calcium complexes are important in maintaining the integrity of the secretory granule, since the absence of calcium will cause dissociation of protein complexes and result in osmotic lysis of the vesicle. Therefore, the intragranular functions of CGA include hormone packaging, stabilization of the granule against osmotic gradients, and excretion of intracellular calcium.

During the process of secretion, the contents of secretory granules are extruded into the pericapillary spaces. The pH and calcium concentration of the extracellular fluid promote dissociation of CGA complexes and solubilization of its bound calcium and other contents of the granule. Once solubilized, extracellular peptidases cleave CGA into biologically active peptides that act as paracrine or autocrine regulators of secretion.[22] Most of the CGA derived peptides have been reported to decrease hormone secretion.

Growth and Metastasis

Parathyroid adenomas usually are slow growing and compress the adjacent thyroid. They are well encapsulated and can be surgically excised without difficulty, considerably prolonging the life of the patient. Cervical ultrasonography has been reported to be more successful in localizing a parathyroid mass than multiple venous samplings (left and right jugular vein and one cephalic vein) for circulating levels of PTH.[23] Successful removal of a functional parathyroid adenoma results in a rapid decrease in circulating parathyroid hormone levels because the half-life of the hormone in plasma is less than 10 minutes. It should be kept in mind that plasma calcium levels in patients with functional chief cell adenomas and overt bone disease may decrease rapidly and be subnormal within 12 to 24 hours, resulting in life threatening hypocalcemic tetany. Postoperative hypocalcemia is the result of depressed secretory activity in the remaining atrophic parathyroid tissue, resulting from long-term suppression by the chronic hypercalcemia and decreased bone resorption combined with accelerated mineralization of organic matrix formed by the hyperplastic osteoblasts along bone surfaces. Infusion of calcium gluconate, high calcium diets, and supplemental vitamin D therapy in pharmacological doses will correct this postoperative complication. Repeated palpation of a functional parathyroid adenoma has led to thrombosis of the major arterial branches supplying blood to the tumor, resulting in diffuse ischemic necrosis of the tumor (fig. 13.30 G).[24] A hypocalcemic tetany similar to that following surgical removal of a functional parathyroid tumor may develop in these patients.

Parathyroid carcinomas are larger than adenomas, invade the capsule and adjacent structures (e.g., thyroid and parathyroid glands and cervical muscles), and may metastasize to regional lymph nodes and, infrequently, to the lung.

Nonneoplastic Parathyroid Cysts

Small cysts occur within the parenchyma of the parathyroid or in the immediate vicinity of the gland and are observed frequently in dogs and occasionally in other animal species (fig. 13.31 A). Parathyroid cysts are usually mutiloculated, are lined by a cuboidal to columnar (often ciliated) epithelium, and contain a densely eosinophilic proteinic material. The lining epithelial cells have an electron dense cytoplasm and numerous microvilli projecting into the lumen of the cyst, but the cells have poorly developed synthetic and secretory organelles (fig. 13.31 B). Chief cells adjacent to larger cysts may be moderately compressed. They are found microscopically in or adjacent to the parathyroid glands in the majority of dogs and occasionally are large enough to be seen macroscopically (fig. 13.31 A).

Parathyroid cysts (Kürsteiner's cyst) appear to develop from a persistence and dilatation of remnants of the duct that connects the parathyroid and thymic primordia (pharyngeal pouches III and IV) during embryonic development. Similar cysts may be present in the anterior mediastinum when remnants of the embryonic duct are displaced with the caudal migration of the thymus (fig. 13.31 C). They are lined by pseudostratified columnar epithelium, contain a proteinic material, and occasionally are large enough to act as a space occupying mass in the anterior mediastinum that exerts clinically significant pressure on the trachea, esophagus, or major vessels.

Parathyroid cysts are distinct from midline cysts derived from remnants of the thyroglossal duct. The latter are lined by multilayered thyrogenic epithelium that often has colloid-containing follicles and may be located near the midline from the base of the tongue caudally into the mediastinum.

Other cystic structures in the thyroid and parathyroid area include ultimobranchial cysts and branchial cysts. *Ultimobranchial duct cysts* are frequently present in the parenchyma of the thyroid of laboratory rats and near the hilus in ruminants; they have a squamous keratinizing epithelial lining. They are derived from remnants of the ultimobranchial body (last, usually fifth, pharyngeal pouch) that fuse with the lateral thyroid lobes during embryonic development and distribute calcitonin secreting C cells (derived from neural crest) into each thyroid lobe.

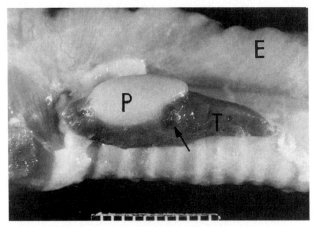

A

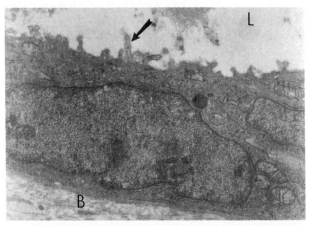

B

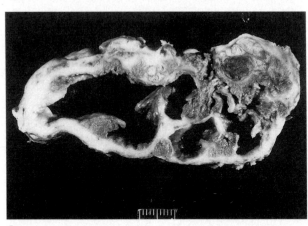

C

Fig. 13.31. Parathyroid cyst. **A.** Parathyroid cyst (arrow) derived from the persistence and distension of the embryonic duct that connects parathyroid-thymic primordia in pharyngeal pouches III and IV (Kürsteiner's cyst) (*T* = thyroid gland; and *E* = esophagus). Hyperplastic parathyroids *(P)* from a dog with chronic renal failure. Scale = 1 cm. **B.** Epithelial cell lining of Kürsteiner's cyst. The cuboidal cells have microvilli (arrow) projecting into the lumen *(L)* and contain proteinic material. The small cytoplasmic area has poorly developed secretory organelles (*B* = basement membrane of cyst wall). **C.** Multicompartmented cysts in the region of the thymus in the anterior mediastinum of a dog derived from persistence and dilatation of the embryonic duct that connects the parathyroid and thymic primordia in pharyngeal pouches (III and IV). Scale = 1 cm.

Branchial (lateral neck) cysts are located lateral to the thyroid and parathyroid area, often near the base of the ear near the angle of the mandible, attached deeply to cervical structures. They also are found in the anterior mediastinum in the thymus.[25] Branchial cysts are multicompartmented and lined by a pseudostratified columnar, partially ciliated epithelium that is derived from remnants of the second pharyngeal pouch.

Salivary mucoceles may also be present in the cervical region near the thyroid and parathyroid glands. These cysts are lined only by granulation tissue that develops in response to the escape of saliva into the interstitium following disruption of a salivary duct. The cyst wall also has evidence of lymphoplasmacytic or pyogranulomatous inflammation in response to the salivary secretions released into the interstitial tissues following disruption of a duct of one of the major glands (submaxillary, zygomatic, parotid).

REFERENCES

1. Capen, C.C. (1996) Pathobiology of parathyroid gland structure and function in animals. In Jones, T.C., Capen, C.C., and Mohr, U. (eds.), *Endocrine System.* Series II. *Monographs on the Pathology of Laboratory Animals,* 2nd ed. International Life Sciences Institute Series. Springer-Verlag, Inc., Berlin, Heidelberg, New York, pp. 293-327.

2. Capen, C.C. (1997) Chemically induced injury of the parathyroid glands: Pathophysiology and mechanistic considerations. In Thomas, J.A., and Colby, H. (eds.), *Endocrine Toxicology,* 2nd ed. Taylor and Francis, Washington, D.C., pp. 1-42.

3. Krook, L. (1957) Spontaneous hyperparathyroidism in the dog: A Pathological-anatomical study. *Acta Pathol Microbiol Scand Suppl.* 122(41): 1-88.

4. Stavrou, D. (1968) Beitrag zum Hyperparathyreoidismus des Hundes. *Dtsch Tierärztl Wochenschr* 75:117-121.

5. Berger, B., and Feldman, E.C. (1987) Primary hyperparathyroidism in dogs: 21 cases (1976-1986). *J Amer Vet Med Assoc* 191:350-356.

6. DeVries, S.E., Feldman, E.C., Nelson, R.W., and Kennedy, P.C. (1993) Primary parathyroid gland hyperplasia in dogs: Six cases (1982-1991). *J Amer Vet Med Assoc* 202:1132-1136.

7. Kallet, A.J., Richter, K.P., Feldman, E.C., and Brum, D.E. (1991) Primary hyperparathyroidism in cats: Seven cases (1984-1989). *J Amer Vet Med Assoc* 199:1767-1771.

8. Marquez, G.A., Klausner, J.S., and Osborne, C.A. (1995) Calcium oxalate urolithiasis in a cat with a functional parathyroid adenocarcinoma. *J Amer Vet Med Assoc* 206:817.

9. den Hertog, E., Goossens, M.M.C., van der Linde-Sipman, J.S., and Kooistra, H.S. (1997) Primary hyperparathyroidism in two cats. *Vet Quarterly* 19:81-84.

10. Roth, S.I., and Capen, C.C. (1974) Ultrastructural and functional correlations of the parathyroid gland. In Richter, G.W., and Epstein, M.A. (eds.), *International Review of Experimental Pathology.* Vol. 13. Academic Press, New York, pp. 161-221.

11. Lee, W., Chiacchierini, R.P., Shleien, B., Telles, N.C. (1982) Thyroid tumors following ^{131}I or localized X irradiation to the thyroid and pituitary glands in rats. *Radiat Res* 92:307-319.

12. Capen, C.C., DeLellis, R.A., and Williams, E.D. (1999) Experimental thyroid carcinogenesis in rodents: Role of radiation and xenobiotic chemicals. In Thomas, G., Karaoglou, A., and Williams, E.D. (eds.), *Radiation and Thyroid Cancer.* World Scientific Publishing, Singapore, New Jersey, London, Hong Kong, pp. 167-176.

13. Meuten, D.J., Segre, G.V., Capen, C.C., Kociba, G.J., Voelkel, E.F., Levine, L., Tashjian, A.H., Jr., Chew, D.J., and Nagode, L.A. (1983) Hypercalcemia in dogs with adenocarcinoma derived from apocrine glands of anal sac: Biochemical and histomorphometric investigations. *Lab Invest* 48:428-435.

14. Rosol T.J., Nagode, L.A., Couto, C.G., Hammer, A.S., Chew, D.J., Peterson, J.L., Ayl, R.D., Steinmeyer, C.L., and Capen, C.C. (1992) Parathyroid hormone (PTH)-related protein, PTH, and 1,25-dihydroxyvitamin D in dogs with cancer-associated hypercalcemia. *Endocrinology* 131:1157-1164.

15. Matwichuk, C.L., Taylor, S.M., Wilkinson, A.A., Dudzic, E.M., Matte, G.G., Outerbridge, C.A., Schmon, C.L., and Ihle, S.L. (1996) Use of technetium Tc 99m sestamibi for detection of a parathyroid adenoma in a dog with primary hyperparathyroidism. *J Amer Vet Med Assoc* 209:1733-1736.

16. Cheville, N.F. (1972) Ultrastructure of canine carotid body and aortic body tumors: Comparison with tissues of thyroid and parathyroid origin. *Vet Pathol* 9:166-189.

17. Thompson, K.G., Jones, L.P., Smylie, W.A., Quick, C.B., Segre, G.V., Meuten, D.J., and Petrites-Murphy, M.B. (1984) Primary hyperparathyroidism in German shepherd dogs: A disorder of probable genetic origin. *Vet Pathol* 21:370-376.

18. Rosol, T.J., and Capen, C.C. (1989) Tumors of the parathyroid gland and circulating parathyroid hormone-related protein associated with persistent hypercalcemia. *Toxicol Pathol* 17:346-356.

19. Roth, S.I., and Capen, C.C. (1974) Ultrastructural and functional correlations of the parathyroid gland. In Richter, G.W., and Epstein, M.A. (eds.), *International Review of Experimental Pathology*. Vol. 13. Academic Press, New York, pp. 161-221.

20. Winkler, H., and Fischer-Colbrie, R. (1992) Chromogranins A and B: The first 25 years and future perspectives. *Neuroscience* 49:497-528.

21. Cohn, D.V., Fasciotto, B.H., Zhang, J.-X., et al. (1994) Chemistry and biology of chromogranin A (secretory protein I) of the parathyroid and other endocrine glands. In Bilezikian, J.P. Levine, M.A., Marcus, R. (eds.), *The Parathyroids*. Raven Press, New York, pp. 107.

22. Deftos, L. (1991) Chromogranin A: Its role in endocrine function and as an endocrine and neuroendocrine tumor marker. *Endocrinol Rev* 12:181-187.

23. Feldman, E.C., Wisner, E.R., Nelson, R.W., Feldman, M.S., and Kennedy, P.C. (1997) Comparison of results of hormonal analysis of samples obtained from selected venous sites versus cervical ultrasonography for localizing parathyroid masses in dogs. *J Amer Vet Med Assoc* 211:54-56.

24. Rosol, T.J., Chew, D.J., Capen, C.C., and Sherding, R.G. (1988) Acute hypocalcemia associated with infarction of parathyroid gland adenomas in two dogs. *J Amer Vet Med Assoc* 192:212-214.

25. Liu, S.K., Patnaik, A.K., and Burk, R.L. (1983) Thymic branchial cysts in the dog and cat. *J Amer Vet Med Assoc* 182:1095-1098.

CANCER-ASSOCIATED HYPERCALCEMIA

Introduction

Hypercalcemia is a common disorder that affects animals and has many causes. The most common cause of hypercalcemia in animals and human beings is cancer associated hypercalcemia.[1,2] There are three mechanisms of increased serum calcium induced by neoplasms: (1) humoral hypercalcemia of malignancy, (2) hypercalcemia induced by metastases of solid tumors to bone, and (3) hematologic malignancies (see fig. 13.32 D). Hypercalcemia results from an imbalance of calcium released from bones, calcium excretion by the kidney, and/or calcium absorption from the intestinal tract.[1]

The clinical signs of hypercalcemia are similar regardless of underlying cause and depend on the rapidity of onset of increased serum ionized calcium levels.[3] Animals with serum calcium values in excess of 16.0 mg/dl (4.0 mmol/l) generally have the most severe clinical signs. Exceptions to this rule occur, and occasionally animals with severe hypercalcemia have mild clinical signs. Horses and rabbits have normal total serum calcium concentrations greater than other domestic animals, which should be considered before hypercalcemia is diagnosed in these species. Metabolic acidosis will enhance the severity of clinical signs since it will result in an increase in the ionized fraction of serum calcium.

Increased serum ionized calcium will induce clinical signs relating to the gastrointestinal, neuromuscular, cardiovascular, and renal systems.[3] Decreased contractility of the gastrointestinal smooth muscle may be associated with anorexia, vomiting, or constipation. There may be generalized locomotive weakness due to decreased neuromuscular excitability. Behavioral changes, depression, stupor, coma, seizures, and muscle twitching have been observed in dogs with hypercalcemia. Lameness and bone pain from demineralization of bone or pathological fractures may be clinical signs with long-standing hypercalcemia. Hypercalcemia results in increased myocardial excitability and diminished ventricular systole, which may result in weakness and syncope associated with cardiac dysrhythmia. There is shortening of the Q-T interval and prolongation of the P-R interval (first degree heart block). Ventricular fibrillation may develop in severe hypercalcemia. Hypercalcemia can predispose some animals to develop pancreatitis. The pathogenesis of pancreatitis associated with hypercalcemia is unknown, but may be related to degeneration of pancreatic acinar cells and leakage of cytoplasmic enzymes.[4]

Polyuria and polydipsia are commonly encountered and may be the reason for an animal owner to seek medical attention. Initially, polyuria and polydipsia are due to impaired renal concentrating ability. The mechanism of this defect is not completely understood, but it appears that hypercalcemia inhibits the antidiuretic hormone dependent resorption of NaCl in the diluting segment of the nephron by decreasing adenylate cyclase activity. Urine specific gravity often is low (< 1.020) and may be hyposthenuric (1.001-1.007). Sodium excretion usually remains unchanged due to the vasoconstrictor effect of hypercalcemia, which results in a reduction of the glomerular filtration rate.

Hypercalcemia also has a toxic effect on renal tubules either directly or from ischemia induced by vasoconstriction. Renal failure is an important consequence of severe or long-standing hypercalcemia.[5] Tubular epithelial cells undergo degeneration with the collecting system most severely affected. There is mineralization of epithelial cells and basement membranes of tubules. Glycosuria may occur due to failure of tubular reabsorption and granular cast formation from degenerate tubular epithelial cells. Azotemia will occur when renal injury is severe, and the polyuria and polydipsia are secondary to renal failure. The magnitude of mineralization and tubular damage can be reduced by phosphate restriction.

Humoral Hypercalcemia of Malignancy (Pseudohyperparathyroidism)

Humoral hypercalcemia of malignancy (HHM) is a syndrome associated with diverse malignant neoplasms in animal and human patients.[1,6] Characteristic clinical findings in patients with HHM include hypercalcemia, hypophosphatemia, hypercalciuria (often with decreased fractional calcium excretion), increased fractional excretion of phosphorus, increased nephrogenous cAMP, and increased osteoclastic bone resorption. Hypercalcemia is induced by humoral effects on bone, kidney, and possibly the intestine (fig. 13.32 E). Increased osteoclastic bone resorption is a consistent finding in HHM with increased calcium release from bone. The kidney plays a critical role in the pathogenesis of hypercalcemia and hypophosphatemia: renal calcium reabsorption is stimulated by parathyroid hormone related protein (PTHrP), and phosphorus reabsorption is inhibited due to binding to and activation of the renal PTH/PTHrP receptors. In some forms of HHM, there are increased serum 1,25-dihydroxy vitamin D levels, which may increase calcium absorption from the intestine.[7]

Malignant neoplasms that are commonly associated with HHM in animals include the adenocarcinoma derived from apocrine glands of the anal sac in dogs, some T cell lymphomas of dogs, myelomas, and miscellaneous carcinomas that sporadically induce HHM in various species, such as cats and horses (gastric squamous cell carcinoma).[1,8] Excessive secretion of biologically active PTHrP plays a central role in the pathogenesis of hypercalcemia in most forms of HHM; however, cytokines such as interleukin-1 (IL-1), tumor necrosis factor-alpha, or transforming growth factors alpha and beta, or 1,25-dihydroxy vitamin D may have synergistic or cooperative actions with PTHrP (fig. 13.32 E).[9-11] Before PTHrP was identified, it was well understood that nonparathyroid tumors associated with humoral hypercalcemia of malignancy induced a syndrome that mimicked primary hyperparathyroidism due to secretion of a PTH-like factor that was antigenically unrelated to PTH. Purification of the PTH-like activity from the adenocarcinoma derived from apocrine glands of the anal sac in dogs and multiple human tumors associated with HHM resulted in the discovery of PTHrP.[12,13] Parathyroid hormone related protein also can be demonstrated in a number of normal tissues, by immunohistochemical and biochemical analysis, where it appears to function primarily as a paracrine factor.[14]

PTHrP binds to the N-terminal PTH/PTHrP receptor in bone and kidney, but does not cross-react immunologically with native PTH (fig. 13.32 F). PTHrP stimulates adenylate cyclase and increases intracellular calcium ion in bone and kidney cells by binding to and activating the cell membrane PTH/PTHrP receptors. This results in a stimulation of osteoclastic bone resorption, increased renal tubular calcium reabsorption, and decreased renal tubular phosphate reabsorption. Interleukin-1 also stimulates bone resorption in vivo and in vitro and is synergistic with PTHrP.[1] Transforming growth factors alpha and beta can stimulate bone resorption in vitro and have been identified in tumors associated with HHM, including adenocarcinomas derived from apocrine glands of the anal sac in dogs.[9,10,15,16]

Clinical Characteristics

The clinical syndrome of pseudohyperparathyroidism has been well characterized in elderly female dogs associated with a perirectal adenocarcinoma.[17] The dogs had persistent hypercalcemia and hypophosphatemia that returned to normal following surgical excision of the neoplasm in the perirectal area. The hypercalcemia persisted following removal of the parathyroid glands. Immunoreactive parathyroid hormone (iPTH) levels were within range of normal for the dog, but were inappropriately high for the degree of hypercalcemia.

Detailed clinical, macroscopic, and histopathologic features of the adenocarcinomas arising from the apocrine gland of the anal sac have been reported in dogs.[18] This unique syndrome occurred in aged (mean 10 years), predominantly female dogs (92 percent), and was characterized by persistent hypercalcemia (91 percent) and hypophosphatemia (71 percent). Serum calcium values ranged from 11.4 to 24.0 mg/dl with a mean of 16.2 mg/dl. Tumor ablation resulted in a prompt return to normocalcemia, but the hypercalcemia recurred with tumor regrowth, suggesting that the neoplastic cells were producing a humoral substance that increased calcium mobilization. All tumors had histopathologic features of malignancy, and 96 percent had metastasized to iliac and sublumbar lymph nodes.

Macroscopic Pathology

Apocrine adenocarcinomas develop as a firm mass (81 percent unilateral) in the perirectal area, ventrolateral to the anus, in close association with the anal sac but usually are not attached to the overlying skin (fig. 13.32 A). The tumor arises in the wall of the anal sac and projects as a mass of variable size into its lumen (fig. 13.32 B).

Skeletal demineralization in dogs with pseudohyperparathyroidism is mild in comparison with primary hyperparathyroidism and usually undetectable by conventional roentgenographic methods. Neoplastic cells from the perirectal adenocarcinomas rarely metastasize to bone and cause osteolysis.[18] Variable numbers of osteoclasts have been detected on bone surfaces in dogs with marked hypercalcemia, possibly reflecting different states in the course of the disease and different phases of bone remodeling activity (fig. 13.32 C). Osteocytic osteolysis is not detected microscopically, and the cement lines are smooth and linear.[18,19]

Histomorphometric analyses indicate that dogs with apocrine adenocarcinomas and hypercalcemia have significantly decreased trabecular bone volume as compared to age matched control dogs. Total resorptive surface (Howship's lacunae with and without osteoclasts) is increased significantly, as are the number of osteoclasts per millimeter of trabecular bone. By comparison, dogs with primary hyperparathyroidism also have a significantly increased total resorptive surface and number of osteoclasts.[19]

Histopathology

This unique neoplasm that develops from apocrine glands of the anal sac (fig. 13.33 A) forms distinctive glandular acini with projections of apical cytoplasm extending into a lumen (fig. 13.33 B) and is histologically distinct from the more common perianal (circumanal) gland tumor in this region of dogs. The majority of neoplasms are histologically bimorphic, with glandular and solid areas (fig. 13.33 C). The solid pattern of arrangement of neoplastic cells is characterized by sheets, microlobules, and packets separated by a thin fibrovascular stroma. Pseudorosettes are common in solid areas adjacent to small blood vessels. Apocrine gland carcinomas with a predominately solid pattern must be differentiated from malignant circumanal (perianal) gland tumors in this region.

Renal mineralization is detected histologically in approximately 90 percent of dogs with pseudohyperparathyroidism associated with apocrine adenocarcinomas of the anal sac, particularly when the calcium times phosphorus product is 50 mg/dl or greater.[18] Tubular mineralization is most pronounced near the corticomedullary junction but also is present in cortical and deep medullary tubules, Bowman's capsule, and the glomerular tuft. Mineralization is present less frequently in the fundic mucosa of the stomach and endocardium.

Ultrastructural Characteristics

The tumor cells in adenocarcinomas derived from apocrine glands of the anal sac contain a well-developed rough endoplasmic reticulum, clusters of free ribosomes, large mitochondria, and prominent Golgi apparatuses.[20] Prominent blebs of apical cytoplasm project into the lumens of glandular acini (fig. 13.33 D). Small membrane-limited secretory granules often are present in the apical cytoplasm of neoplastic cells. These granules are similar in size and electron density to PTH-containing storage granules in the chief cells of normal parathyroid glands (fig. 13.33 E); however, additional studies are required to determine if they contain a hormone(s). It appears that these neoplastic cells secrete PTHrP in a constitutive rather than a regulated manner since most tumor cells have few secretory granules in their cytoplasm.

The parathyroid glands are small and difficult to locate or not visible macroscopically in approximately 70 percent of dogs with apocrine adenocarcinoma and hypercalcemia.[18] Atrophic parathyroid glands in dogs with apocrine adenocarcinoma are characterized by narrow cords of inactive chief cells with an abundant fibrous connective tissue stroma and widened perivascular spaces. The inactive chief cells have a markedly reduced cytoplasmic area, prominent hyperchromatic nuclei, and relatively straight cell membranes with uncomplicated interdigitations, and they are closely packed together. These findings indicate that the apocrine adenocarcinomas are not producing a substance that stimulates parathyroid hormone secretion by chief cells, but rather that the parathyroid glands are responding to persistent hypercalcemia by undergoing trophic atrophy. Thyroid parafollicular cells (C cells) often respond to the persistent elevation in blood calcium by undergoing diffuse or nodular hyperplasia.[18]

Laboratory Data

Early studies reported that the mean concentration of iPTH in the plasma of dogs with hypercalcemia and apocrine adenocarcinomas was 168 ± 40 pg/ml (fig. 13.34).[19] The concentration of iPTH in dogs with apocrine adeno-

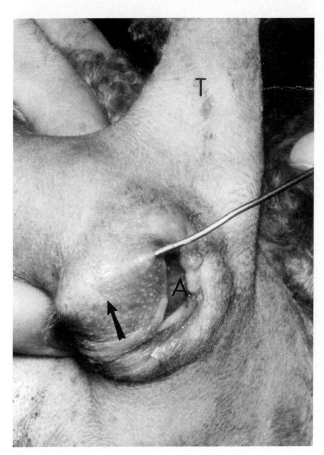

A

Fig. 13.32. Adenocarcinoma derived from apocrine glands of the anal sac. **A.** Perirectal region from a dog with hypercalcemia and a small adenocarcinoma (arrow) (A = anus; T = tail). (continued)

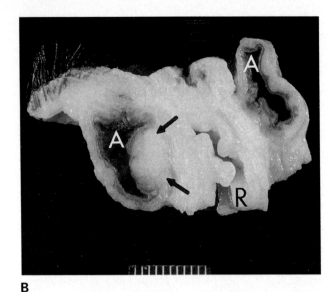

B

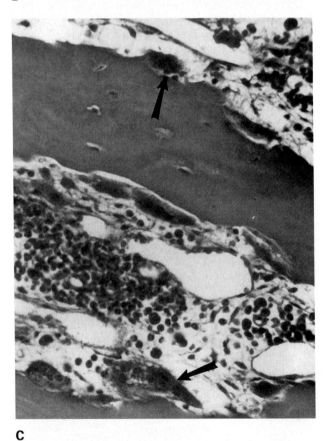

C

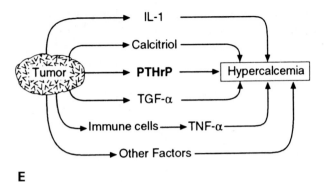

E

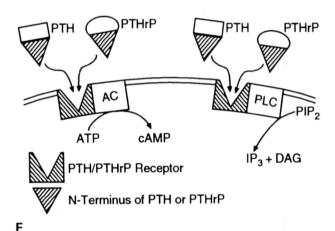

F

Fig. 13.32. (continued) **B.** Transverse section of perineum from a female dog with hypercalcemia and an adenocarcinoma. Anal sacs *(A)* are present on both sides of the rectum *(R)*. A 1 cm diameter tumor nodule (arrows) arising in the wall of the left anal sac protrudes into its lumen. Scale = 1 cm. [From Meuten, D.J., et al. (1981) *Vet Pathol* 18:454-471.] **C.** Osteoclastic osteolysis in the ilium of a dog with adenocarcinoma derived from apocrine glands of the anal sac. There are numerous osteoclasts (arrows) aligned along trabecular bone surfaces with excavations. [From Meuten, D.J., et al. (1981) *Vet Pathol* 18:454-471.] **D.** Pathogenesis of cancer associated hypercalcemia. Humoral and local forms of cancer associated hypercalcemia increase circulating concentrations of calcium by stimulating osteoclastic bone resorption and/or increased tubular reabsorption of calcium. [From Rosol, T.J., and Capen, C.C. (1992) *Lab Invest* 67:680-702.] **E.** Humoral factors, such as PTHrP, interleukin-1 (IL-1), tumor necrosis factors (TNF), or transforming growth factors (TGF), produced by tumors induce humoral hypercalcemia of malignancy (HHM) by acting as systemic hormones and stimulating osteoclastic bone resorption or increasing tubular reabsorption of calcium. [From Rosol, T.J., and Capen, C.C. (1992) *Lab Invest* 67:680-702.] **F.** A high degree of homology of the primary or tertiary structures of the N-terminal regions of parathyroid hormone (PTH) and PTHrP permits binding and activation of the PTH receptor. This results in stimulation of adenylate cyclase (AC) and phospholipase C (PLC) in target cells in bone and kidney with the formation of cyclic adenosine monophosphate (cAMP) and conversion of phosphotidylinositol diphosphate (PIP$_2$) to inositol triphosphate (IP$_3$) and diacylglycerol (DAG). [From Rosol, T.J., and Capen, C.C. (1992) *Lab Invest* 67:680-702.]

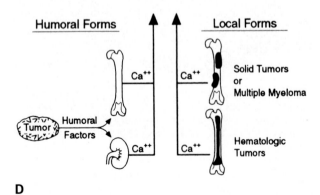

D

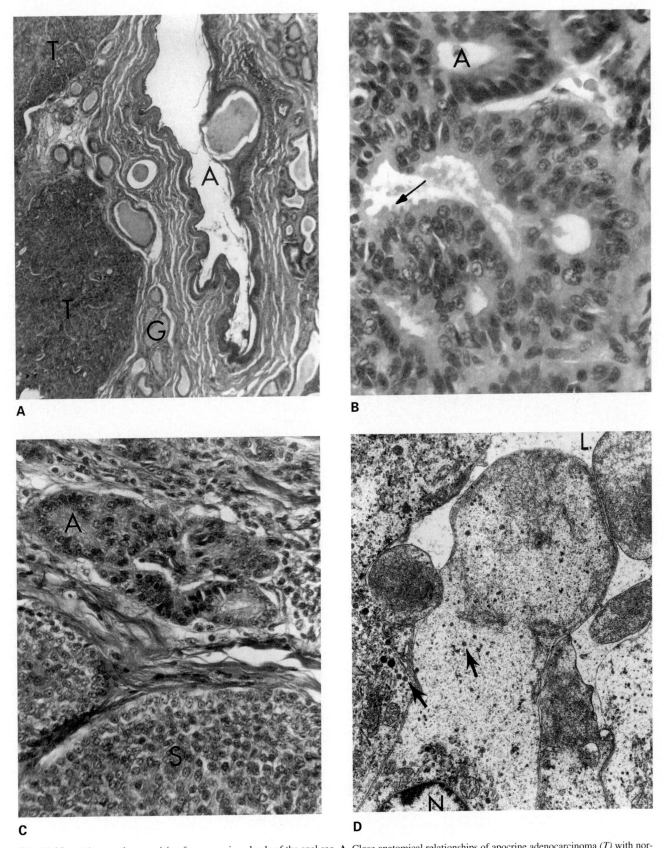

A

B

C

D

Fig. 13.33. Adenocarcinoma arising from apocrine glands of the anal sac. **A.** Close anatomical relationships of apocrine adenocarcinoma *(T)* with normal apocrine gland *(G)* in the wall of the anal sac. The anal sac *(A)* is lined by stratified squamous epithelium. [From Meuten, D.J., et al. (1981) *Vet Pathol* 18:454-471.] **B.** Adenocarcinoma arising from apocrine glands in wall of anal sac, illustrating glandular acini that are lined by single or multiple layers of columnar neoplastic cells with characteristic apical projections of cytoplasm into the lumen (arrow). The acini *(A)* contain varying amounts of colloid-like material and occasional inflammatory cells. [From Meuten, D.J., et al. (1981) *Vet Pathol* 18:454-471.] **C.** Bimorphic patterns of growth with adjacent solid (S) areas and acini *(A)* formed by neoplastic cells. [From Meuten, D.J., et al. (1981) *Vet Pathol* 18:454-471.] **D.** Characteristic projections of apical cytoplasm into lumen *(L)* of acinus. Small membrane-limited secretory granules (arrows) are present in the cytoplasm *(N* is nucleus of tumor cell). [From Meuten, D.J., et al. (1982) *Amer J Pathol* 107:167-175.] (continued)

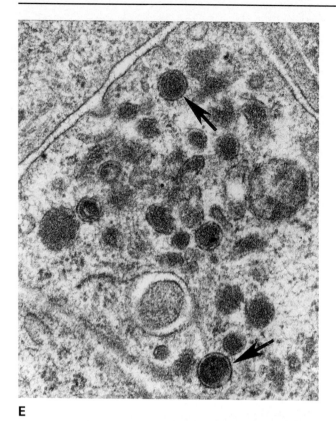

E

Fig. 13.33.   (continued) **E.** Small (200 to 400 nm diameter) electron-dense secretory-like granules (arrows) in neoplastic cells with an electron-dense core, closely applied limiting membrane, and narrow submembranous space. [From Meuten, D.J., et al. (1982) *Amer J Pathol* 107:167-175.]

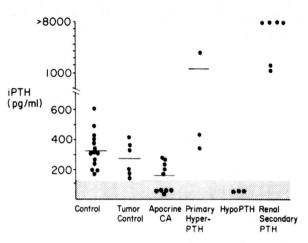

Fig. 13.34.   Plasma immunoreactive parathyroid hormone (iPTH) concentrations in dogs with hypercalcemia associated with adenocarcinoma derived from apocrine glands of the anal sac. Plasma iPTH was decreased in dogs with apocrine carcinomas compared to control dogs. Dogs with hypoparathyroidism (hypoPTH) had undetectable concentrations of iPTH, whereas dogs with primary (hyper-PTH) and secondary (renal hyper-PTH) hyperparathyroidism had increased concentrations of iPTH compared with control dogs. The limit of detectability for the iPTH assay (112 pg/ml) is indicated by the shaded area. Horizontal lines indicate the means for the various groups. [From Meuten, D.J., et al. (1983) *Lab Invest* 48:428-435.]

carcinomas was not significantly different from the concentration in control dogs (322 ± 33 pg/ml) or normocalcemic tumor controls (266 ± 46 pg/ml), but was significantly decreased compared to dogs with primary hyperparathyroidism. By comparison, the concentration of iPTH in dogs with chronic renal failure was markedly increased compared to control dogs. Plasma iPTH levels were undetectable in dogs with primary hypoparathyroidism, but were higher in dogs with primary hyperparathyroidism (mean 1540 pg/ml) (fig. 13.34).

Urea hydrochloric acid extracts of tumor tissue from apocrine adenocarcinomas, tumors from normocalcemic

control dogs, and lymph nodes from control dogs without tumors have been assayed for iPTH before and after precipitation with trichloroacetic acid. Immunoreactive PTH is not detected in tissue extracts from any tumor or lymph node. The iPTH concentrations in extracts of parathyroid glands from adult dogs have been reported to be greater than 200 μg/g.[19]

The mean serum concentration of 1,25-dihydroxy vitamin D [1,25-$(OH)_2$D] in dogs with apocrine adenocarcinomas and hypercalcemia was reported to be 23 pg/ml (table 13.4).[19] Although these dogs had hypercalcemia and normophosphatemia, the mean serum 1,25-$(OH)_2$D was not significantly different from either group of normocalcemic control dogs. Dogs with carcinomas derived from apocrine glands of the anal sac have a significantly greater urine calcium excretion [0.35 ± 0.11 mg/dl glomerular filtrate (GF)] than either control dogs (0.02 ± 0.01 mg/dl GF)

TABLE 13.4.   Serum and urine data from dogs with apocrine gland adenocarcinomas and control dogs

	Control Dogs (*n* = 15)	Normocalcemic Tumor Control Dogs (*n* = 6)	Apocrine Gland Carcinoma and Hypercalcemia (*n* = 10)
Serum calcium (mg/dl)	9.7 ± 013	9.4 ± 0.14	15.7 ± 0.56[a]
Serum phosphorus (mg/dl)	4.1 ± 0.13	4.2 ± 0.31	3.0 ± 0.42
Serum albumin (g/dl)	3.1 ± 0.12	2.8 ± 0.08	3.1 ± 0.13
Serum creatinine (mg/dl)	0.9 ± 0.05	1.0 ± 0.07	1.6 ± 0.25
Serum ALP (IU/l)	40 ± 4	54 ± 9	116 ± 34
Urine P (mg/dl glomerular filtrate)	0.76 ± 0.07	0.54 ± 0.12	2.00 ± 0.72
Serum 1,25-dihydroxy vitamin D (pg/ml)	26 ± 5 (6)[b]	16 ± 4	23 ± 5 (9)[b]

Source: From Meuten et al. (1983). *Lab Invest* 48:428-435.
Note: Values are expressed as mean ± SE.
[a]Significant differences (*p* < 0.05) as compared to control dogs and normocalcemic control dogs.
[b]Numbers in parentheses indicate a different number of dogs.

or normocalcemic tumor control dogs (0.04 ± 0.01 mg/dl GF), and have increased urine calcium compared to dogs with primary hyperparathyroidism (0.12 ± 0.06 mg/dl GF) (fig. 13.35 A).[19] In addition, the results for fractional excretion of calcium indicate that the urinary excretion of calcium in dogs with apocrine carcinoma is significantly increased compared to that of clinically normal dogs. Urinary cAMP concentrations are significantly higher in dogs with carcinomas derived from apocrine glands of the anal sac (mean 3.37 ± 0.44 nmol) compared to clinically normal dogs (mean 1.94 ± 0.16 nmol), but not compared to tumor control dogs (mean 2.70 ± 0.57 nmol) (fig. 13.35 A).[19]

More recent studies have reported that most dogs with HHM have increased circulating concentrations of PTHrP (fig. 13.35 B). Plasma concentrations of PTHrP are greatest (10-100 pmol) in dogs with adenocarcinomas derived from apocrine glands of the anal sac and sporadic carcinomas associated with HHM.[7,21] The serum calcium concentrations in these dogs correlate well with circulating PTHrP concentrations and are consistent with the concept that PTHrP plays a primary role in the pathogenesis of HHM in these dogs (fig. 13.35 C).

Some dogs with apocrine adenocarcinomas have inappropriate levels of 1,25-dihydroxy vitamin D (maintenance of normal range or increased) for the degree of hypercalcemia (fig. 13.35 D).[7] This suggests that the humoral factors produced by the neoplastic cells from some neoplasms are capable of stimulating renal 1-alpha-hydroxylase and increasing the formation of 1,25-dihydroxy vitamin D even in the presence of increased blood calcium. Plasma iPTH was not increased in hypercalcemic dogs and was significantly less than in dogs with primary hyperparathyroidism (fig. 13.35 E). Surgical removal or radiation therapy of the adenocarcinoma results in a rapid return to normal of serum calcium and phosphorus, increased serum PTH, and decreased 1,25-dihydroxy vitamin D.[7] Postsurgical survival in dogs with adenocarcinoma and hypercalcemia ranged from 2 to 21 months with a mean of 8.8 months.

An animal model of HHM utilizing the canine apocrine adenocarcinoma (CAC-8) has been developed and is characterized by severe hypercalcemia, hypophosphatemia, increased serum 1,25-$(OH)_2$-cholecalciferol levels, depressed serum PTH levels, and evidence of increased bone formation and resorption.[22,23] The tumor originated from a hypercalcemic dog, produced PTHrP in vivo, and resulted in clinical signs of HHM when transplanted into nude mice. The transplanted tumor maintained the histological pattern of the original adenocarcinoma for up to 31 passages. A spontaneous variant of the tumor, with altered morphology and function, has been developed that fails to induce HHM in tumor bearing mice.[24]

Mice bearing the CAC-8 (HiCa) tumor developed hypercalcemia (13.3 ± 0.5 mg/dl) compared with non–tumor bearing control mice (9.1 ± 0.2 mg/dl) and mice bearing CAC-8 (LoCa) tumor (10.0 ± 0.2 mg/dl)

(fig. 13.36 C). The mice bearing CAC-8 (LoCa) had mildly elevated serum calcium compared with controls. Serum PTHrP concentrations differed among the three experimental groups, with the highest serum PTHrP present in CAC-8 (HiCa) tumor bearing mice (30.4 ± 3.4 pmol), followed, in order of decreasing levels, by CAC-8 (LoCa) mice (5.9 ± 0.7 pmol), and non–tumor bearing controls (1.0 ± 0.1 pmol) (fig. 13.36 D). The neoplastic cells in CAC-8 (HiCa) were arranged predominately in acini; they showed strong positive staining for cytokeratin, but were negative for vimentin. The CAC-8 (LoCa) was a more solid tumor consisting of spindle shaped cells arranged in cords supported by a connective tissue stroma with a weak positive staining for cytokeratin and negative staining for vimentin.

Northern blot and phosphor image analysis revealed a 2.9-fold greater level of PTHrP mRNA in the CAC-8 (HiCa) tumor than in the CAC-8 (LoCa) tumor (fig. 13.36 E). CAC-8 (HiCa) had intense dark cytoplasmic staining for PTHrP mRNA by in situ hybridization; CAC-8 (LoCa) had much less intense staining; and connective tissue cells were negative (fig. 13.36 F). Both tumor lines expressed similar levels of steady state mRNA for transforming growth factor beta, tumor necrosis factor alpha, interleukin-1, and interleukin-6 (fig. 13.36 G). These findings support the central role of PTHrP in the pathogenesis of HHM. The HiCa line had a greater PTHrP mRNA and protein expression by neoplastic cells than the LoCa line, but the hypercalcemia was not the result of changes in mRNA expression of other cytokines or growth factors.

The effects of persistent hypercalcemia on parathyroid chief cells have included changes in the frequency and form of cytoplasmic organelles, including secretory granules and rough endoplasmic reticulum, and changes in the contour of the plasma membranes.[25] CAC-8 bearing mice and PTHrP infused mice had hypercalcemia and a significantly larger mean area of chief cells when compared with control mice and mice fed a LoCa diet. Chief cells in CAC-8 bearing mice had decreased tortuosity of plasma membranes and had only a few membranous interdigitations between adjacent cells. Severely hypercalcemic (15-25 mg/dl) CAC-8 bearing mice had the highest incidence of cytoplasmic membranous whorls (mean = 24 whorls/500 chief cells, range = 1-45).[25] The whorls consisted of membranes, presumably derived from the rough endoplasmic reticulum (RER), plus entrapped cytoplasmic organelles with lipid droplets near the center of the whorl. Formation of whorls in chief cells appears to be an indicator of suppressed secretory activity and results from the accumulation of membranous material derived from the RER.[25] Mice infused with PTH-rP had less severe hypercalcemia (12-16.5 mg/dl) but ultrastructural changes comparable to those in CAC-8 bearing mice. Control mice and mice fed a low calcium diet had chief cells with ultrastructural changes consistent with a resting or storage state: less cytoplasm and more electron-dense granules.

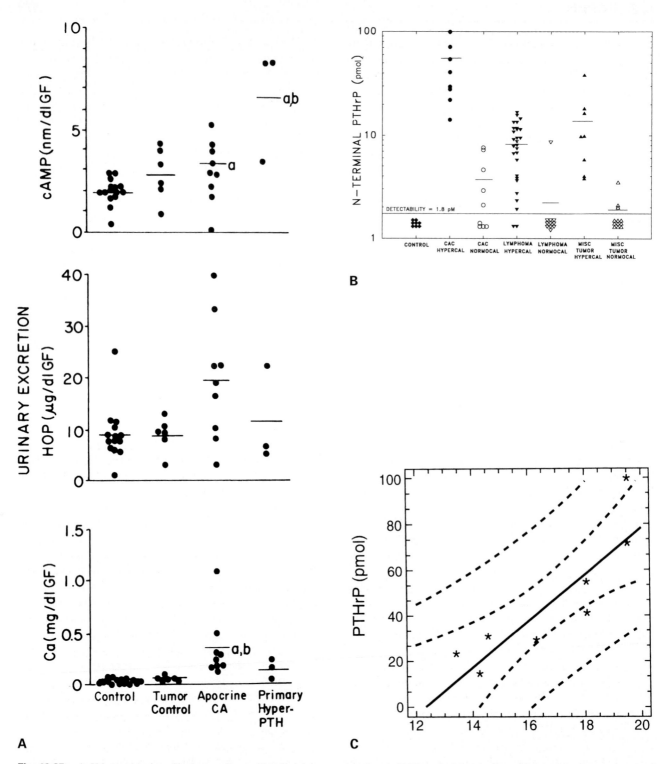

Fig. 13.35. **A.** Urinary excretion of hydroxyproline, cyclic adenosine monophosphate (cAMP), and calcium in dogs with apocrine adenocarcinoma of the anal sac compared to normocalcemic control dogs with and without other tumors and to dogs with primary hyperparathyroidism. Calcium and cAMP excretion were increased significantly in dogs with apocrine carcinomas compared to control dogs without tumors, but not when compared to control dogs with tumors. cAMP excretion was significantly greater (p < 0.05) in hyperparathyroid dogs than in any other group. Hydroxyproline in dogs with apocrine carcinomas [19.6 ± 3.9 µg/dl glomerular filtrate (GF)] was greater than in controls (9.5 ± 1.5 µg/dl GF), but this difference was not significant. Horizontal lines indicate the means for the various groups. Significant differences (p < 0.05) from control dogs are indicated by *a* and from tumor controls by *b*. [From Meuten, D.J., et al. (1983) *Lab Invest* 48:428-435.] **B.** Circulating N-terminal parathyroid hormone related protein (PTHrP) concentrations in normal dogs (control); dogs with hypercalcemia (> 12 mg/dl) and anal sac adenocarcinomas (CAC), lymphoma, or miscellaneous tumors (MISC TUMOR); and dogs with normocalcemia (< 12 mg/dl) and anal sac adenocarcinomas, lymphoma, or miscellaneous tumors. [From Rosol, T.J., et al. (1992) *Endocrinology* 131:1157-1164.] **C.** Regression of PTHrP and total calcium in dogs with anal sac carcinoma. There was a significant linear correlation (0.87, p < 0.01) between serum calcium and N-terminal PTHrP concentrations in dogs with humoral hypercalcemia of malignancy and adenocarcinomas derived from apocrine glands of the anal sac. [From Rosol, T.J., and Capen, C.C. (1997) Chapter 23 in *Clinical Biochemistry of Domestic Animals,* 5th ed., Academic Press, New York] (continued)

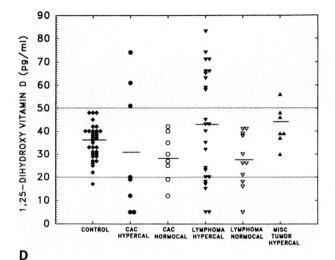

D

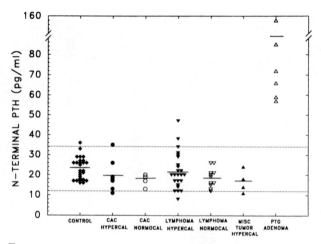

E

Fig. 13.35. (continued) **D.** Serum 1,25-dihydroxyvitamin D concentrations in normal dogs (control); dogs with hypercalcemia (> 12 mg/dl) and anal sac adenocarcinomas (CAC), lymphoma, or miscellaneous tumors (misc tumor); and dogs with normocalcemia (< 12 mg/dl) and anal sac adenocarcinomas, or lymphoma. The normal range was 20-50 pg/ml (dashed lines). Bar = mean. [From Rosol, T.J., et al. (1992) *Endocrinology* 131:1157-1164.]. **E.** Serum N-terminal PTH concentrations in normal dogs (control); dogs with hypercalcemia (> 12 mg/dl) and anal sac adenocarcinomas (CAC), lymphoma, miscellaneous tumors (misc tumor), or parathyroid adenomas (PTG adenoma); and dogs with normocalcemia (< 12 mg/dl) and anal sac adenocarcinomas or lymphoma. The normal range was 12-34 pg/ml (dashed lines). Bar = mean. [From Rosol, T.J., et al. (1992) *Endocrinology* 131:1157-1164.]

Growth and Metastasis

Biopsy specimens from adenocarcinomas derived from apocrine glands of the anal sac usually reveal histological evidence of malignancy, and approximately 95 percent metastasize to iliac and/or lumbar lymph nodes. Invasion of tumor cells into adjacent tissues in the perineal region (fig. 13.36 A) and endothelial-lined vessels forming emboli usually is present and often is extensive. Tumor cell emboli appear to be more common in lymphatic vessels than in blood vessels (fig. 13.36 B).

Differential Diagnosis of Humoral Hypercalcemia of Malignancy

Lymphoma is the most common neoplasm associated with hypercalcemia in dogs and cats.[26,27] Peripheral lymph node enlargement may or may not be detected, but evidence usually exists for anterior mediastinal or visceral involvement. Serum immunoreactive PTH levels have been found to be subnormal in hypercalcemic dogs with lymphoma, and plasma immunoreactive prostaglandin E_2 levels did not differ from levels in control dogs.[28] Culture media from normal lymphoid tissue and control media had no effect on release of ^{45}Ca from prelabeled fetal mouse forelimb bones; however, media from tumor tissue increased ^{45}Ca release. These early findings suggested that the local production of bone resorbing factors (e.g., osteoclast activating factor) was important in stimulating calcium release from bone in certain dogs with lymphoma and hypercalcemia.

Lymphoma

Malignant lymphoma is associated with hypercalcemia in 20-40 percent of the cases in dogs. Some dogs with lymphoma and hypercalcemia have HHM. Hypercalcemic lymphomas associated with HHM usually were of the T cell subset.[29] The affected dogs have increased fasting and 24-hour calcium excretion, increased fractional P excretion, and increased nephrogenous cAMP. Increased osteoclastic resorption was present in bones without evidence of tumor metastasis. Dogs with HHM and lymphoma may have a pathogenesis of hypercalcemia similar to that which occurs in humans with HTLV-1 induced lymphoma or leukemia. Neoplastic cells from humans with HTLV-1 induced lymphoma have increased PTHrP production due to stimulation of PTHrP transcription by the virally encoded tax transcription factor.[30]

Most dogs with lymphoma and HHM have significantly increased circulating PTHrP concentrations, but levels are lower (2-15 pmol) than dogs with carcinomas and HHM (see fig. 13.35 B), but there is no correlation with serum calcium concentration (fig. 13.37).[7] This indicates that although PTHrP is an important marker of dogs with HHM and lymphoma, it is not the sole humoral factor responsible for the stimulation of osteoclasts and the development of hypercalcemia. It is likely that cytokines such as interleukin-1 or tumor necrosis factor may function synergistically with PTHrP to induce HHM in dogs with lymphoma (see fig. 13.32 F).[1] Some dogs and human patients with lymphoma and hypercalcemia have increased serum 1,25-dihydroxy vitamin D levels, which may be responsible for or contribute to the induction of hypercalcemia (see fig. 13.35 D).[7,31] Parathyroid hormone (N-terminal) levels in dogs with lymphoma and hypercalcemia usually are in the normal range, although an occasional dog may have levels elevated slightly out of the normal range (see fig. 13.35 E).

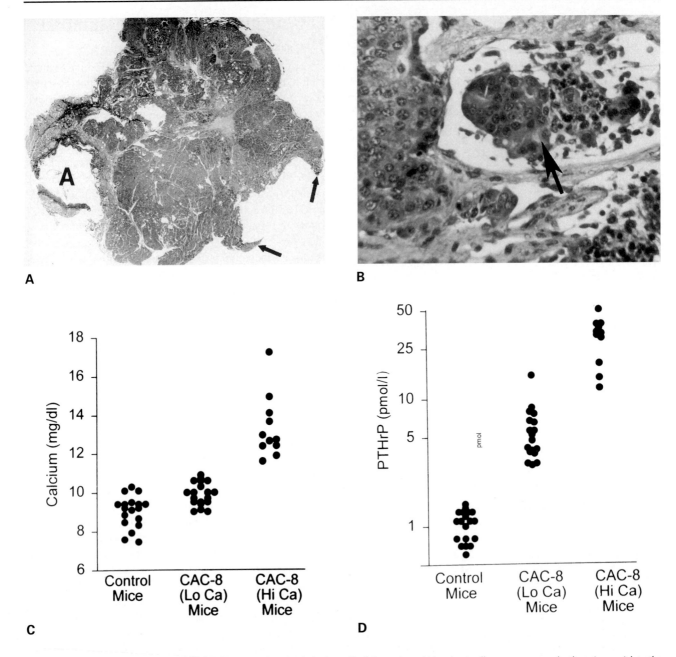

Fig. 13.36. **A.** Infiltrative carcinoma arising from apocrine glands in the wall of the anal sac *(A)* and extending numerous projections (arrows) into the surrounding perineal connective tissues and into the lymphatics in this region. [From Meuten, D.J., et al. (1981) *Vet Pathol* 18:454-471.] **B.** Tumor cell emboli (arrow) in lymphatic of a dog with an adenocarcinoma arising from apocrine glands of the anal sac. **C.** Canine adenocarcinoma model (CAC-8) of humoral hypercalcemia of malignancy. Serum calcium in non–tumor bearing controls and tumor bearing, low calcium, high calcium mice. [From Gröne, A., et al. (1998) *Vet Pathol* 35:344-351.] **D.** Serum PTHrP (pM) in non–tumor bearing controls and tumor bearing, low calcium, high calcium mice. [From Gröne, A., et al. (1998) *Vet Pathol* 35:344-351.] (continued)

Hematologic Malignant Neoplasms

Some forms of hematologic malignancies present in the bone marrow induce hypercalcemia by the local induction of bone resorption.[1] This occurs most commonly with multiple myeloma and lymphoma. There are a number of paracrine factors or cytokines that may be responsible for the stimulation of bone resorption. The cytokines most often implicated in the pathogenesis of local bone resorption include interleukin-1, tumor necrosis factor alpha, and tumor necrosis factor beta (lymphotoxin).[32] Other cytokines or factors that may play a role include interleukin-6, transforming growth factors alpha and beta, and PTHrP.[33] Production of low levels of PTHrP by a tumor in bone may stimulate local bone resorption without inducing a systemic response due to increased circulating concentrations of PTHrP. Prostaglandins (especially prostaglandin E$_2$) also may be

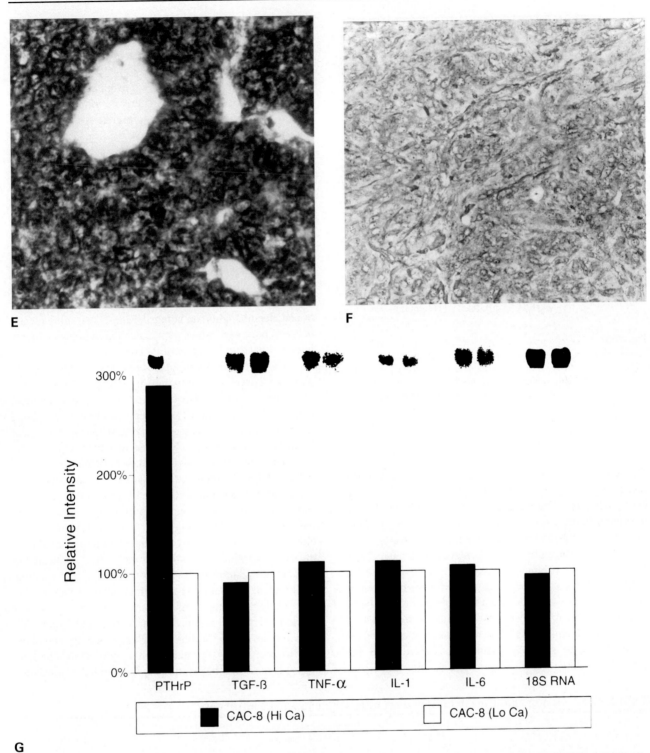

Fig. 13.36. (continued)   E. PTHrP mRNA expression in CAC-8 (HiCa) tumor analyzed by in situ hybridization. [From Gröne, A., et al. (1998) *Vet Pathol* 35:344-351.] **F.** PTHrP mRNA expression in CAC-8 (LoCa) tumor analyzed by in situ hybridization. [From Gröne, A., et al. (1998) *Vet Pathol* 35:344-351.] **G.** PTHrP mRNA expression in CAC-8 (HiCa) and CAC-8 (LoCa) tumors analyzed by Northern Blot analysis. PTHrP mRNA (after correction for background) was 2.9 fold greater in CAC-8 (HiCa) tumors than in CAC-8 (LoCa) tumors. There was similar mRNA expression by both tumors for TGF-beta, TNF-alpha, IL-1, and IL-6, with < 10 percent variation between tumor types. [From Gröne, A., et al. (1998) *Vet Pathol* 35:344-351.]

responsible for the local stimulation of bone resorption.

Some dogs with lymphoma and hypercalcemia have localized bone resorption associated with metastases to medullary cavities without evidence of increased bone resorption at sites distant from the tumor metastases.[34]

Hypercalcemic dogs with lymphoma and bone metastases had decreased serum PTH and 1,25-dihydroxy vitamin D levels, increased excretion of calcium, phosphorus, and hydroxyproline, and increased serum levels of the prostaglandin E$_2$ metabolite (13,14-dihydro-15-keto-

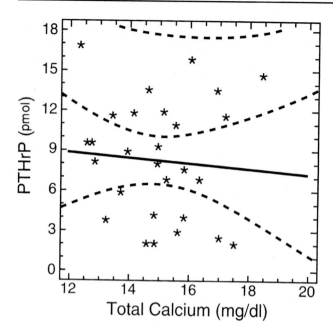

Fig. 13.37. Regression of PTHrP and total calcium in dogs with lymphoma. There was no correlation between serum calcium and N-terminal PTHrP concentrations in dogs with humoral hypercalcemia of malignancy and lymphoma, which suggests that PTHrP probably functions cooperatively with other cytokines to induce hypercalcemia. [From Rosol, T.J., and Capen, C.C. (1997) In *Clinical Biochemistry of Domestic Animals,* 5th ed., Academic Press, New York.]

prostaglandin E_2) (table 13.5). The mediator of local bone resorption has not been identified, but prostaglandin E_2 may be an important primary or secondary local mediator of bone resorption in these dogs. Other potential mediators include the cytokines, interleukin-1, and tumor necrosis factor.

Dogs with lymphoma and hypercalcemia have lower trabecular bone volume with more frequent osteoclastic osteolysis than control dogs and dogs with normocalcemia and lymphoma.[34] Only dogs with neoplastic cells in bone marrow have increased osteoclastic bone resorption. Dogs with hypercalcemic lymphoma often have osteoclasts on trabecular bone surfaces opposite a surface lined by osteoid and large columnar osteoblasts (fig. 13.38 A).

Bone surfaces in normocalcemic control dogs are smooth and lined by flattened osteoblasts and rare osteoclasts (fig. 13.38 B). Dogs with lymphoma that are normocalcemic do not have increased bone resorption.

Urine excretion of calcium, phosphorus, and hydroxyproline is higher in hypercalcemic dogs with lymphoma.[34] Light and electron microscopic examination of parathyroid glands reveals inactive or atrophic chief cells and evidence of secretory inactivity in dogs with lymphoma and hypercalcemia. Ultrastructurally lymphomas are composed of tumor cells with large nuclei and a paucity of cytoplasmic organelles.[34]

Tumors Metastatic to Bone

Solid tumors that metastasize widely to bone can produce hypercalcemia by the induction of local bone resorption associated with tumor growth. This is not common in animals, but it is an important cause of cancer associated hypercalcemia in human beings.[1] Tumors that often metastasize to bone and induce hypercalcemia in human patients include breast and lung carcinomas.

The pathogenesis of enhanced bone resorption is not well understood, but the two primary mechanisms include (1) secretion of cytokines or factors which stimulate local bone resorption and (2) indirect stimulation of bone resorption by tumor induced cytokine secretion from local immune or bone cells.[35] Cytokines or factors that may be secreted by tumor cells and stimulate local bone resorption include PTHrP,[36] transforming growth factors alpha and beta, and prostaglandins (especially prostaglandin E_2). In some cases, bone resorbing activity can be inhibited by indomethacin, which suggests that prostaglandins are either directly or indirectly associated with the stimulation of bone resorption. The cytokines most often implicated in indirect stimulation of bone resorption by local immune cells include interleukin-1 and tumor necrosis factor.

Malignant neoplasms with osseous metastases may cause moderate to severe hypercalcemia and hypercalciuria, but the serum alkaline phosphatase activity and phosphorus are usually normal or only moderately elevated. These changes are believed to be due to release of calcium

TABLE 13.5.   Serum and urine data from dogs with lymphoma and control dogs

	Control Dogs (n = 15)	Normocalcemic Tumor Control Dogs (n = 6)	Hypercalcemic Lymphoma (n = 10)	Normocalcemic Lymphoma (n = 9)
Serum calcium (mg/dl)	9.7 ± 0.1	9.4 ± 0.14	13.9 ± 0.3	8.7 ± 0.4
Serum phosphorus (mg/dl)	4.1 ± 0.1	4.2 ± 0.31	4.6 ± 0.3	5.1 ± 0.3
Serum albumin (g/dl)	3.1 ± 1.0	2.8 ± 0.08	3.0 ± 0.1	2.6 ± 0.2
Serum alkaline phosphatase (IU/l)	40 ± 4	54 ± 9	150 ± 38	260 ± 86
Serum creatinine (mg/dl)	0.9 ± 0.1	1.0 ± 0.07	2.7 ± 0.4	0.9 ± 0.1
Urine phosphorus (mg/dl glomerular filtrate)	0.76 ± 0.07	0.54 ± 0.12	3.10 ± 0.53 (14)[b]	1.12 ± 0.19 (6)[b]
Plasma PGE₂M[a] (pg/ml)	19 ± 4.2 (10)[b]	22 ± 9.9 (4)[b]	39 ± 5.7 (13)[b]	21 ± 5.6 (8)[b]

Source: From Meuten et al. (1983). *Lab Invest* 49:553-562.
Note: Values are expressed as mean ± SE.
[a]PGE₂M = 13,14-dihydro-15-keto-prostaglandin E_2.
[b]Numbers in parentheses indicate a different number of dogs.

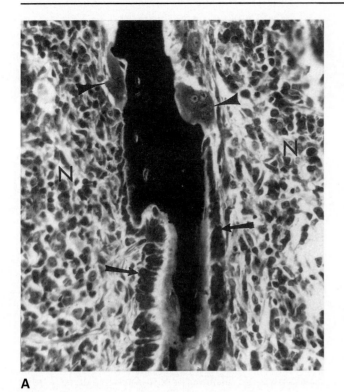

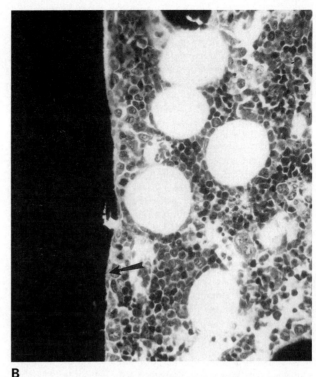

Fig. 13.38. Lymphoma with hypercalcemia of a dog. [von Kossa-tetrachromes from Meuten, D.J., et al. (1983) *Lab Invest* 48:428-435.]
A. Lumbar vertebrae with several large osteoclasts (arrowheads) present in lacunae along a thin bone trabecula. Hyperplastic osteoblasts (arrows) and prominent osteoid seams are present adjacent to the resorptive surfaces. The marrow contains neoplastic lymphoid cells *(N)*. **B.** Lumbar vertebrae from a normocalcemic control dog with smooth bone surfaces, no osteoclasts, and flattened osteoblasts (arrow) lining a large bone trabecula.

and phosphorus into the blood from areas of bone destruction at rates greater than can be cleared by the kidney and intestine. Bone involvement can be multifocal but usually is sharply demarcated and localized to the area of metastasis.

REFERENCES

1. Rosol, T.J., and Capen, C.C. (1992) Biology of disease: Mechanisms of cancer-induced hypercalcemia. *Lab Invest* 67:680-702.
2. Capen, C.C., and Rosol, T.J. (1993) Pathobiology of parathyroid hormone and parathyroid hormone-related protein: introduction and evolving concepts. Ch. 1. In LiVolsi, V.A., and DeLellis, R.A. (eds.), *Pathology of the Thyroid and Parathyroid Gland: An Update.* Williams and Wilkins Co., Philadelphia, pp. 1-33.
3. Rosol, T.J., Chew, D.J., Nagode, L.A., and Capen, C.C. (1995) Pathophysiology of calcium metabolism. *Vet Clin Pathol* 24:49-63.
4. Frick, T.W., Mithöfer, K., Fernandez-del Castillo, C., Rattner, D.W., and Warshaw, A.L. (1995) Hypercalcemia causes acute pancreatitis by pancreatic secretory block, intracellular zymogen accumulation, and acinar cell injury. *Amer J Surg* 169:167-172.
5. Kruger, J.M., Osborne, C.A., Nachreiner, R.F., and Refsal, K.R. (1996) Hypercalcemia and renal failure: Etiology, pathophysiology, diagnosis, and treatment. *Vet Clin N Amer Small Anim Pract* 26:1417-1445.
6. Rosol, T.J., and Capen, C.C. (1997) Calcium-regulating hormones and diseases of abnormal mineral (calcium, phosphorus, magnesium) metabolism. Ch. 23. In Kaneko, J.J., Harvey, J.W., and Bruss, M.L. (eds.), *Clinical Biochemistry of Domestic Animals,* 5th ed. Academic Press, New York, pp. 619-702.
7. Rosol T.J., Nagode, L.A., Couto, C.G., Hammer, A.S., Chew, D.J.,

   Peterson, J.L., Ayl, R.D., Steinmeyer, C.L., and Capen, C.C. (1992) Parathyroid hormone (PTH)-related protein, PTH, and 1,25-dihydroxy vitamin D in dogs with cancer-associated hypercalcemia. *Endocrinology* 131:1157-1164.
8. Rosol, T.J., Nagode, L.A., Robertson, J.T., Leeth, B.D., Steinmeyer, C.L., and Allen, C.M. (1994) Humoral hypercalcemia of malignancy associated with ameloblastoma in a horse. *J Amer Vet Med Assoc* 204:1930-1933.
9. Merryman, J.I., Capen, C.C., McCauley, L.K., Werkmeister, J.R., Suter, M.M., and Rosol, T.J. (1993) Regulation of parathyroid hormone-related protein production by a squamous carcinoma cell line in vitro. *Lab Invest* 69:347-354.
10. Merryman, J.I., DeWille, J., Werkmeister, J.R., Capen, C.C., and Rosol, T.J. (1994) Effects of transforming growth factor-beta on PTRrP production and RNA expression by a squamous carcinoma cell line in vitro. *Endocrinology* 134:2424-2430.
11. Gröne, A., Weckmann, M.T., Steinmeyer, C.L., Capen, C.C., and Rosol, T.J. (1996) Altered parathyroid hormone-related protein secretion and mRNA expression in squamous cell carcinoma cells in vitro. *Eur J Endocrinol* 135:498-505.
12. Weir, E.C., Burtis, W.J., Morris, C.A., Brady, T.G., and Insogna, K.L. (1988) Isolation of 16,000-dalton parathyroid hormone-like proteins from two animal tumors causing humoral hypercalcemia of malignancy. *Endocrinology* 123:2744-2751.
13. Moseley, J.M., and Gillespie, M.T. (1995) Parathyroid hormone-related protein. *Crit Rev Clin Lab Sci* 32:299-343.
14. Gröne, A., Werkmeister, J.R., Steinmeyer, C.L., Capen, C.C., and Rosol, T.J. (1994) Parathyroid hormone-related protein in normal and neoplastic canine tissues: Immunohistochemical localization and biochemical extraction. *Vet Pathol* 31:308-315.
15. Merryman, J.I., Rosol, T.J., Brooks, C.L., and Capen, C.C. (1989) Separation of parathyroid hormone-like activity from transforming growth factor-alpha and -beta in the canine adenocarcinoma (CAC-

8) model of humoral hypercalcemia of malignancy. *Endocrinology* 124:2456-2463.

16. Rosol, T.J., Merryman, J.I., Nohutcu, R.M., McCauley, L.K., and Capen, C.C. (1991) Effects of transforming growth factor-alpha on parathyroid hormone- and parathyroid hormone-related protein-mediated bone resorption and adenylate cyclase stimulation in vitro. *Domest Anim Endocrinol* 8:499-507.

17. Rijnberk, A., Elsinhorst, Th.A.M., Kolman, J.P., Hacking, W.H.L., and Lequin, R.M. (1978) Pseudohyperparathyroidism associated with perirectal adenocarcinomas in elderly female dogs. *T Diergeneesk* 103:1069-1075.

18. Meuten, D.J., Cooper, B.J., Capen, C.C., Chew, D.J., and Kociba, G.J. (1981) Hypercalcemia associated with an adenocarcinoma derived from the apocrine glands of the anal sac. *Vet Pathol* 18:454-471.

19. Meuten, D.J., Segre, G.V., Capen, C.C., Kociba, G.J., Voelkel, E.F., Levine, L., Tashjian, A.H., Jr., Chew, D.J., and Nagode, L.A. (1983) Hypercalcemia in dogs with adenocarcinoma derived from apocrine glands of anal sac: Biochemical and histomorphometric investigations. *Lab Invest* 48:428-435.

20. Meuten, D.J., Capen, C.C., Kociba, G.J., Chew, D.J., and Cooper, B.J. (1982) Ultrastructural evaluation of adenocarcinomas derived from apocrine glands of the anal sac associated with hypercalcemia in dogs. *Amer J Pathol* 107:167-175.

21. Rosol, T.J., Capen, C.C., Danks, J.A., Suva, L.J., Steinmeyer, C.L., Hayman, J., Ebeling, P.R., and Martin, T.J. (1990) Identification of parathyroid hormone-related protein in canine apocrine adenocarcinoma of the anal sac. *Vet Pathol* 27:89-95.

22. Rosol, T.J., Capen, C.C., Weisbrode, S.E., and Horst, R.L. (1986) Humoral hypercalcemia of malignancy in nude mouse model of a canine adenocarcinoma derived from apocrine glands of the anal sac. Biochemical, histomorphometric, and ultrastructural studies. *Lab Invest* 54:679-688.

23. Gröne, A., McCauley, L.K., Capen, C.C., and Rosol, T.J. (1997) Parathyroid hormone/parathyroid hormone-related protein receptor expression in nude mice with a transplantable canine apocrine adenocarcinoma (CAC-8) and humoral hypercalcemia of malignancy. *J Endocrinol* 153:123-129.

24. Gröne, A., Weckmann, M.T., Blomme, E.A., Capen, C.C., and Rosol, T.J. (1998) Dependence of humoral hypercalcemia of malignancy on parathyroid hormone-related protein expression in the canine anal sac apocrine gland adenocarcinoma (CAC-8) nude mouse model. *Vet Pathol* 35:344-351.

25. Gröne, A., Rosol, T.J., and Capen, C.C. (1992) Effects of humoral hypercalcemia of malignancy on the parathyroid gland in nude mice. *Vet Pathol* 29:343-350.

26. Osborne, C.A., and Stevens, J.B. (1973) Pseudohyperparathyroidism in the dog. *J Amer Vet Med Assoc* 16:125-135.

27. Zenoble, R.D., and Rowland, G.N. (1979) Hypercalcemia and proliferative, myelosclerotic bone reaction associated with feline leukovirus infection in a cat. *J Amer Vet Med Assoc* 175:591-595.

28. Heath, H., Weller, R.E., and Mundy, G.R. (1980) Canine lymphosarcoma: A model for study of the hypercalcemia of cancer. *Calcif Tissue Intl* 30:127-133.

29. Weir, E.C., Norrdin, R.W., Matus, R.E., Brooks, M.B., Broadus, A.E., Mitnick, M., Johnston, S.D., and Insogna, K.L. (1988) Humoral hypercalcemia of malignancy in canine lymphosarcoma. *Endocrinology* 122:602-608.

30. Prager, D., Rosenblatt, J.D., Ejima, E. (1994) Hypercalcemia, parathyroid hormone-related protein expression and human T-cell leukemia virus infection. *Leuk Lymphoma* 14:395-400.

31. Seymour, J.F., and Gagel, R.F. (1993) Calcitriol: The Major humoral mediator of hypercalcemia in Hodgkin's and non-Hodgkin's lymphomas. *Blood* 82:1383-1394.

32. Martin, T.J., and Grill, V. (1992) Hypercalcemia and cancer. *J Steroid Biochem Mol Biol* 43:123-129.

33. Black, K.S., and Mundy, G.R. (1994) Other causes of hypercalcemia: Local and ectopic secretion syndromes. In Bilezikian, J.P. Levine, M.A., Marcus, R. (eds.), *The Parathyroids*. Raven Press, New York, p. 341.

34. Meuten, D.J., Kociba, G.J., Capen, C.C. Chew, D.J., Segre, G.V., Levine, L., Tashjian, A.H., Jr., Voelkel, E.F., and Nagode, L.A. (1983) Hypercalcemia in dogs with lymphosarcoma: Biochemical, ultrastructural and histomorphometric investigations. Lab Invest 49:553-562.

35. Garrett, I. R. (1993) Bone destruction in cancer. *Sem Oncol* 20:4-9.

36. Powell, G. J., Southby, J., Danks, J. A., Stillwell, R. G., Hayman, J. A., Henderson, M.A., Bennett, R. C., and Martin, T. J. (1991) Localization of parathyroid hormone-related protein in breast cancer metastases: Increased incidence in bone compared to other sites. *Cancer Res* 51:3059-3061.

TUMORS OF THE PANCREATIC ISLET CELLS

Beta Cell (Insulin Secreting) Tumors: Adenoma, Carcinoma

Introduction

The most frequently ccurring tumors arising in pancreatic islets are adenomas and carcinomas derived from insulin secreting beta cells.[1,2] These neoplasms frequently are endocrinologically active and are associated with striking functional disturbances relating to the marked hypoglycemia.[3-6] Other pancreatic tumors appear to be derived from multipotential ductal epithelial cells with differentiation into one of the several other cell types of pancreatic islets that do not secrete insulin. In humans both insulin secreting and non–beta cell tumors have been reported to occur in pancreatic islets.[7] The non–beta cell islet neoplasms may be associated with a hypersecretion of gastrin, secretin, glucagon, somatostatin, vasoactive intestinal peptide, and other gastrointestinal hormones.[8]

Incidence

Beta cell neoplasms of pancreatic islets are seen most frequently in dogs from 5 to 12 years of age, with a mean of approximately 9 years. Although many different breeds of dogs are affected, boxers, fox terriers, standard poodles, and German shepherds appear to be overrepresented.[2,9-11] Both sexes appear to be affected equally.

Tumors of pancreatic islets are also reported to occur in older cattle,[12] in ferrets associated with adrenal cortical tumors,[13] and infrequently in cats.[14] They are derived from beta cells and may be functional and associated with periodic convulsive seizures and other signs associated with hypoglycemia. Insulin secreting beta cell tumors also are commonly encountered in ferrets with estrogen secreting tumors of the adrenal cortex.[15-19]

Clinical Characteristics

The clinical alterations observed with functional beta cell tumors are the result of excessive insulin secretion, leading to an increased rate of transfer of glucose from the blood into certain target cells of the body, and hence to the development of severe hypoglycemia. The clinical signs are a reflection of the hypoglycemia and are not specific for hyperinsulinism associated with beta cell neoplasms.[20] Initial signs include posterior weakness, fatigue after vigorous exercise, generalized muscular twitching and weakness, ataxia, mental confusion, and changes of temperament.[3,4,6,9,11] The dogs are easily agitated, and there are intermittent periods of excitability and restlessness. Periodic convulsive seizures of the tonic-clonic type occur later in the disease and increase progressively in frequency and intensity.

The clinical disturbances of functional beta cell neoplasms are characteristically episodic; they occur initially at widely spaced intervals, but become more frequent and prolonged as the disease progresses. In the initial stages the hypoglycemic attacks are precipitated by physical exercise or fasting (increased glucose utilization) as well as by the ingestion of food (stimulation of insulin release). The administration of glucose rapidly alleviates the clinical signs. Between hypoglycemic episodes affected dogs usually do not have abnormalities on physical examination, in contrast to other causes of hypoglycemia. Later in the disease there is no consistent pattern relating to the initiation of convulsive seizures and the dogs may become unresponsive to supplemental glucose therapy. Terminal comas of varying length often precede death.

The predominance of clinical signs relating to the central nervous system demonstrates the primary dependence of the brain on the metabolism of glucose for energy. When the brain is not supplied with glucose, there is a decrease in cerebral oxidation and manifestations of anoxia appear. The order in which different areas of the brain are affected by hypoglycemia is usually the reverse of the order in which the areas appear phylogenetically. If hypoglycemia is severe and prolonged it will induce laminar cortical necrosis in the cerebral hemispheres.

The failure to recognize that dogs with functional islet cell tumors may be presented with clinical signs that suggest primary diseases of the nervous system has frequently led to misdiagnoses, for periods of months or years, of idiopathic epilepsy, brain tumors, or other organic neurological diseases. Repeated episodes of prolonged and severe hypoglycemia will result in irreversible neuronal degeneration (laminal cortical necrosis) throughout the brain.[21] Permanent neurological disease probably accounts for the terminal coma, unresponsiveness to glucose, and eventual death in this disease. Affected dogs seem to recognize the temporary relief obtained from eating; therefore, the appetite often is good to excessive, and some dogs are obese.

The most important and practical laboratory test to confirm the diagnosis of hyperinsulinism is quantitation of blood glucose after an overnight fast. The finding of a fasting concentration of blood glucose of 40 mg/dl or less is strongly suggestive of hyperinsulinism in dogs, although fluctuations are not unusual and repeated assays may be necessary. A blood glucose determination should be part of the routine laboratory workup on all older dogs with a history of periodic convulsive seizures. The response of the fasting concentration of blood glucose to the administration of a glucose load (0.5 g/kg orally) may contribute to establishing the diagnosis in certain cases of hyperinsulinism.[20] Blood is collected after 0.5, 1, 2, and 3 hours. The resulting curve in dogs with hyperinsulinism is usually low and relatively flat compared with that in normal dogs, indicating an increased tolerance to exogenous glucose. The maximal blood glucose concentration attained is greater in normal dogs, and the return to fasting concentration is more prolonged, than in dogs with hyperinsulinism.

The amended insulin to glucose ratio (AIGR)

$$AIGR = \frac{\text{immunoreactive insulin } (\mu U/ml) \times 100}{\text{plasma glucose } (mg/dl) - 30}$$

in dogs with functional beta cell neoplasms has been reported to be markedly elevated to 1104 ± 1831 compared to 13.9 ± 4.6 in clinically normal dogs.[11] Mean basal immunoreactive insulin levels were 36.4 ± 27.2 μU/ml (range 5 to 96 μU/ml) in dogs with islet cell tumors and 11.7 ± 4.8 μU/ml in control dogs. A glucagon tolerance test was useful diagnostically only if repeated AIGR values were equivocal.

Other causes of hypoglycemia that must be considered in differential diagnosis are hepatic dysfunction, adenohypophyseal and/or adrenal cortical insufficiency, renal glycosuria, extrapancreatic mesodermal neoplasms, functional hypoglycemia, and surreptitious administration of insulin.

Macroscopic Pathology

Adenomas of the pancreatic islets (*insulinomas*) appear as single yellow to dark red, spherical, small (1 to 3 cm in diameter) nodules, usually visible from the serosal surface of the pancreas. They are of similar consistency or slightly firmer than the surrounding pancreatic parenchyma. Functional adenomas occur singly or occasionally as multiple nodules in the same or different lobes of the pancreas. A thin layer of fibrous connective tissue completely encapsulates adenomas from the adjacent parenchyma (fig. 13.39 A).

A review of our cases and those reported in the literature revealed that carcinomas of the pancreatic islets are more common (approximately 60 percent) in dogs than adenomas (approximately 40 percent).[1,2] This differs from the situation in humans, where adenomas are encountered much more often (as much as 90 percent of all pancreatic islet tumors) than islet cell carcinomas. Clinicopathological evidence suggesting hyperinsulinism has been reported more frequently with beta cell carcinoma than with adenoma in dogs. The duodenal (right) lobe of the pancreas appears to be a site of more frequent involvement with islet cell tumors in dogs than the splenic (left) part of the pancreas, although the numbers of islets per given area are greater in the splenic lobe.

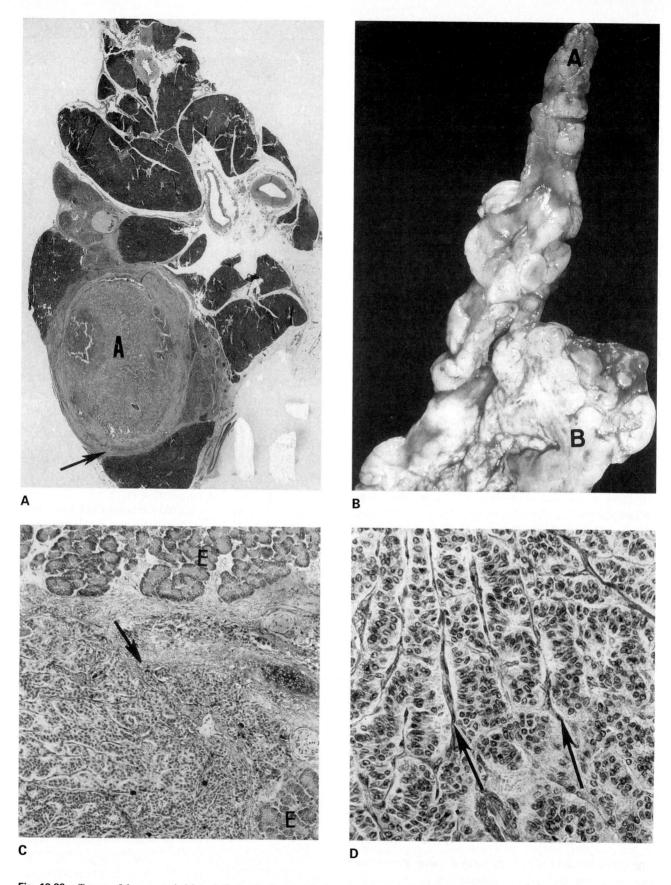

Fig. 13.39. Tumors of the pancreatic islets. **A.** Beta cell adenoma *(A)* of pancreatic islets in a dog. The neoplasm is well delineated from the exocrine pancreas by a fibrous capsule (arrow). **B.** Functional beta cell carcinoma of pancreatic islets *(B)* with invasion into the adjacent pancreas. The distal portion *(A)* of the pancreatic lobe is atrophic. **C.** Functional beta cell carcinoma of pancreatic islets invading through the fibrous connective tissue capsule (arrow) into adjacent exocrine pancreas *(E).* **D.** Beta cell carcinoma illustrating characteristic pattern of arrangement of cells that resembles the structure of normal pancreatic islets. The closely packed neoplastic beta cells are subdivided into small groups by fine connective tissue septa with capillaries (arrows).

Carcinomas of the pancreatic islets can be differentiated from adenomas by their larger size, multilobular appearance, extensive invasion into adjacent parenchyma (fig. 13.39 B) and lymphatics, and establishment of metastases in extrapancreatic sites. Important anatomical sites that must be examined for metastasis are the regional lymph nodes, liver, mesentery, and omentum. Larger neoplasms frequently have focal areas of necrosis, hemorrhage, and liquefaction. Carcinomas in the pancreatic angle may result in parenchymal atrophy of distal portions of the duodenal and splenic branches of the pancreas (fig. 13.39 B).

Histopathology

Islet cell adenomas are sharply delineated from the adjacent parenchyma and surrounded by a partial to complete, thin capsule of fibrous connective tissue. Small nests of acinar epithelial cells may be present throughout the neoplasm, but particularly near the periphery. Numerous connective tissue septa containing small capillaries radiate from the capsule into the neoplasm and subdivide the cells into small lobules or packets. The neoplastic cells are well differentiated, varying from cuboidal to columnar, and have a lightly eosinophilic and finely granular cytoplasm with indistinct cell membranes. The cellular structure and tinctorial properties of both adenoma and carcinoma are retained best in tissues fixed immediately in Bouin's fluid. Autolysis of neoplastic cells progresses rapidly if the interval between death and fixation is prolonged. The cytoplasm of the neoplastic cells is blue on sections stained with chromium hematoxylin phloxine after fixing or mordanting in Bouin's fluid. Scattered dark blue granules are observed in some neoplastic cells,, but they are not numerous. Islets in the surrounding pancreatic tissue appear normal or slightly reduced in size.

Irregularly shaped ducts and small nests of acinar cells are observed frequently within islet cell adenomas. The cuboidal to columnar lining epithelium has basal nuclei and eosinophilic cytoplasm. The ducts are intimately associated with the neoplastic cells, occur in greater numbers than would be expected for preexisting pancreatic ducts, and are considered to be part of the neoplasm. The findings of pancreatic ductal and acinar cells in a predominately islet cell tumor most likely reflect their common embryological origin from alimentary entoderm.

Islet cell carcinomas are consistently larger than adenomas, are multilobular, and invade the adjacent pancreatic parenchyma. Although there is a peripheral condensation of connective tissue in some areas, neoplastic cells invade into and through the fibrous capsule (fig. 13.39 C). The dense bands of fibrous tissue that course through the neoplasm give rise to fine connective tissue septa (with capillaries) that subdivide the cells into small cords or lobules (fig. 13.39 D). The well-differentiated neoplastic cells in islet cell carcinomas are closely packed and may be less uniform in size and shape than the cells composing adenomas. They are either cuboidal or polyhedral and have a granular eosinophilic cytoplasm. Mitotic figures are seen infrequently. Ductules are present within beta cell carcinomas, and there may be evidence of a transition of ductal epithelium into neoplastic beta cells.

Pathologists evaluating biopsies of islet cell tumors in dogs should be aware that even small neoplasms composed of well-differentiated beta cells may have already invaded lymphatics and vessels and metastasized to the liver and/or regional lymph nodes. Multiple sections often are necessary to demonstrate clear-cut evidence of lymphatic and vascular invasion and the formation of tumor cell emboli. Cytological features of the neoplastic cells often are not helpful in differentiating between islet cell adenomas and carcinomas; histological evidence of invasion by the tumor cells through the capsule and into adjacent pancreatic parenchyma is the most important criterion of malignancy.

Ultrastructural and Immunocytochemical Characteristics

The neoplastic beta cells are irregularly cuboidal or polyhedral, closely packed, and contain numerous electron dense cytoplasmic organelles (fig. 13.40 A).[1] The cytoplasmic area usually is abundant compared with the area of the nucleus. Insulin immunoreactivity can be demonstrated over the cytoplasmic area of neoplastic beta cells by peroxidase-antiperoxidase immunocytochemical techniques.[22] Although several pancreatic islet hormones may be demonstrated in islet cell tumors (e.g., somatostatin, pancreatic polypeptide, glucagon) by immunocytochemical evaluation, one hormone usually predominates (e.g., insulin) and is responsible for the clinical disturbances. Nuclei of neoplastic cells are irregularly indented and have peripheral condensations of nuclear chromatin. The plasma membranes of adjacent cells have uncomplicated interdigitations, and desmosomal attachments join adjacent cells.

Beta cells in different stages of secretory activity are observed in functional islet cell neoplasms. Sparsely granulated beta cells are considered to be in the *actively synthesizing phase* of their secretory cycle because of the extensive network of rough endoplasmic reticulum, large cytoplasmic area, numerous free ribosomes, and large mitochondria. Densely granulated beta cells are interpreted to be in the *storage phase* of the secretory cycle since they have less endoplasmic reticulum and fewer ribosomes. Cells with fine structural characteristics intermediate between these two extremes of organellar development and granulation are observed.

Secretory granules are present throughout the cytoplasm of neoplastic beta cells at the level of ultrastructure. The granules vary in shape, size, and electron density. The smallest granules are spherical in outline, are uniformly electron dense, and have a narrow electron-lucent space subjacent to the continuous limiting membrane. The mean diameter of this type of granule is approximately 200 mμ.

The larger oval or spherical granules with a wide sub-membranous space and bar shaped internal cores are considered to represent mature secretory granules since they are the most common type reported in beta cells of normal dogs.[23-26] They are encountered less frequently in neoplastic beta cells and are surrounded by a continuous agranular limiting membrane (fig. 13.40 B). The mature granules appear to develop from the uniformly electron dense, small, secretory granules in the Golgi apparatus by a central condensation of their contents. The finely granular internal core of the mature secretory granule is circular, bar, or V shaped, and is frequently situated eccentrically within the granule. A wide electron-lucent space (halo) separates the internal core from the outer limiting membrane. The margins of the internal cores are indistinct, and fine fibrils extend into the wide submembranous space. Limiting membranes of adjacent granules are sometimes fused together so that two internal cores are surrounded by a continuous membrane (fig. 13.40 B). The membranes of other adjacent granules are deeply interdigitated. Mature secretory granules of beta cells have a mean diameter of 340 mμ and internal cores measuring about 210 mμ. Bar shaped or rectangular internal cores measure 280 mμ in greatest length by 82 mμ in width and have a fibrillar or crystalline substructure. The granular cytoplasm of neoplastic beta cells stains positive for chromogranin A (fig. 13.40 C).[27,28]

There is no consistent polarity of secretory granules within the neoplastic beta cells, although large numbers of granules often are present in the portion of the cytoplasm bordering the perivascular space. Secretory granules frequently are aligned immediately subjacent to the plasma membrane of the cell. A portion of the limiting membrane of the secretory granule often fuses with the plasma membrane, and a hiatus is formed for extrusion of the granule contents into the extracellular space. This process of secretion of insulin from beta cells is termed *emiocytosis*.

The neoplastic beta cells can be differentiated readily from beta cells of the pancreatic islets in dogs by the unique rectangular or crystalloid internal cores and wide submembranous space of the mature secretory granules. Beta cells have round, extremely electron dense secretory granules with a closely applied limiting membrane in normal dogs.[25] The neoplastic beta cells also can be differentiated from the other cell types (F and D cells) normally found in the pancreatic islets by the ultrastructure of their secretory granules.[23,26,29]

Growth and Metastasis

Adenomas of beta cells usually grow slowly and compress the adjacent pancreatic parenchyma. Their sharp delineation and complete encapsulation permit successful surgical excision. Although beta cell adenomas are usually single in the dog, the entire pancreas should be examined by palpation for the presence of multiple tumors. Complete surgical removal of islet cell adenomas dramatically ame-liorates the hypoglycemia and associated neurological signs unless there have been irreversible changes in the central nervous system.[30]

Occasional small, insulin secreting, beta cell neoplasms may appear as well-delineated single nodules closely resembling an adenoma. However, tumor cells will have already invaded through the fibrous capsule into lymphatics and vessels and will have established multiple metastases in the liver. Islet cell carcinomas usually are considerably larger than adenomas and invade adjacent pancreatic parenchyma. Multiple metastases develop early in the liver and draining lymph nodes (duodenal, hepatic, splenic, and mesenteric). In a study of 73 dogs with insulin secreting pancreatic neoplasms (of which 52 underwent surgical techniques for tumor excision), it was reported that (1) dogs with higher preoperative serum insulin levels had shorter survival times, (2) dogs with tumors confined to the pancreas had longer disease-free intervals than dogs with regional lymph node or distant metastasis, and (3) younger dogs had a significantly shorter survival time than older dogs.[31] Chemotherapy with beta cell cytotoxins (e.g., streptozotocin) has not proven useful in the long-term management of carcinoma because of the development of nephrotoxicity.[32]

Non–Beta Cell (Gastrin Secreting) Tumors

Incidence

Gastrin secreting, non–beta islet cell tumors of the pancreas have been reported in humans, dogs,[33,34] and a cat.[35] The hypersecretion of gastrin in humans results in the well-documented Zollinger-Ellison syndrome, which consists of hypersecretion of gastric acid and recurrent peptic ulceration in the gastrointestinal tract. The non–beta islet cell tumors are derived from ectopic amine precursor uptake decarboxylase (APUD) cells in the pancreas that produce an excess of the hormone gastrin, which normally is secreted by gastrin secreting cells of the antral and duodenal mucosa. The incidence of gastrin secreting pancreatic tumors in dogs, cats, and other species is uncertain, but it appears to be rare compared to insulin secreting beta cell neoplasms.

Clinical Characteristics

The few cases studied in the dog and cat have been presented with clinical signs of anorexia, vomiting of blood tinged material, intermittent diarrhea, progressive weight loss, and dehydration. The most prominent functional disturbances appear to be the result of the multiple ulcerations of the gastrointestinal mucosa that develop from the gastrin hypersecretion.

Macroscopic Pathology

Animals with Zollinger-Ellison-like syndrome have single or multiple tumors of varying size in the pancreas.[33-35] They often are firm on palpation because of an increase of fibrous connective tissue in the stroma. There may be attempts at encapsulation, but the tumor usually extends into the surrounding pancreatic parenchyma.

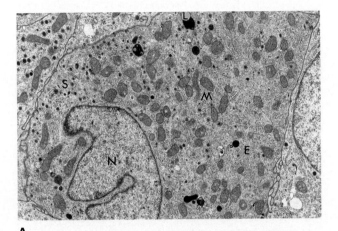

A

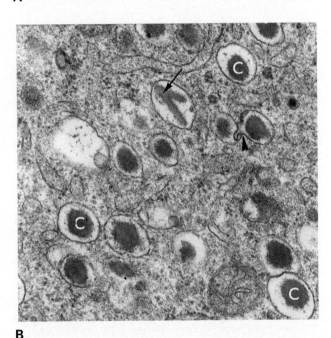

B

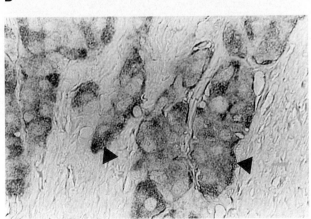

C

Histopathology

The basic histological pattern of pancreatic islet cell tumors in animals is similar whether they are secreting insulin or gastrin. Three histological patterns have been described in non–beta islet cell tumors in dogs: (1) a ribbon or trabecular arrangement of neoplastic cells with occasional pseudorosettes and an intimate relationship to capillaries, (2) solid nests of cells with a delicate, highly vascularized stroma, and (3) an acinar pattern with arrangement of cuboidal neoplastic cells around a central lumen.[34] The stroma may be prominent and hyalinized in some dogs with gastrin secreting tumors.

Ultrastructural and Immunocytochemical Characteristics

The abundant cytoplasmic area of gastrin secreting neoplastic cells contains scattered small secretory granules (100 to 150 nm in diameter).[34] They are surrounded by a closely applied limiting membrane and have a round internal core. The internal core of the secretory granule in gastrin secreting cells is different than that in the insulin secreting beta cell in the dog, which often is bar or V shaped, with a wide submembranous space. Localization of gastrin immunoreactivity to the cytoplasm of the neoplastic cells is the only reliable method for distinguishing gastrin producing from insulin secreting islet cell tumors of the pancreas.

The cat with a non–beta islet cell carcinoma had elevated serum gastrin levels (1000 pg/ml) compared to clinically normal cats (mean 87.6 pg/ml). Neoplastic cells stained by the unlabeled immunoperoxidase method were positive for gastrin and glucagon.[3]

Laboratory Data

Extracts of the pancreatic tumor have been reported to contain 1.72 and 0.03 µg gastrin equivalents per gram of wet tissue in dogs.[34] Gastrin component III was the prominent molecular form in the tumor in one dog, whereas in a second case gastrin components II and III were present in equimolar amounts.

Fig. 13.40. Beta cell carcinomas of pancreatic islets. **A.** Functional beta cell carcinoma. The neoplastic cells are polyhedral and have indented nuclei *(N)*. The plasma membranes of adjacent cells are straight, with uncomplicated interdigitations. The cytoplasm contains flat profiles of rough endoplasmic reticulum *(E)*, scattered secretory granules *(S)*, numerous mitochondria *(M)*, and lipofuscin *(L)*. **B.** Mature secretory granules in functional beta cell carcinoma. The internal cores *(C)* are circular or V shaped (arrow), surrounded by a wide halo, and often situated eccentrically within the granule. Fine fibrils extend outward from the indistinct margins of internal cores. The limiting membranes of adjacent granules appear fused or interdigitated (arrowhead). **C.** Pancreatic islet cell carcinoma from a dog. The neoplastic cells stained intensely positive for chromogranin A within a granular cytoplasm (arrowheads). Avidin-biotin-peroxidase immunohistochemistry.[From Doss, J.C., et al. (1998) *Vet Pathol* 35:312-315.]

Circulating levels of gastrin in a dog with a Zollinger-Ellison-like syndrome varied from 155 to 2780 pg/ml, whereas the mean serum gastrin in clinically normal control dogs (n = 17) was 70.9 ± 5.1 pg/ml.[34] Another well-documented non–beta islet cell tumor in a dog had a plasma immunoreactive gastrin level of 360 pg/ml.[33] Serum gastrin concentrations varied from 72 to 717 pg/ml in four dogs with well-documented pancreatic gastrinomas.

Growth and Metastasis

The gastrin secreting tumors (carcinomas) of the pancreas that have been studied in dogs appear to invade locally into the adjacent parenchyma and often metastasize to regional lymph nodes and liver. Dogs often have either single or multiple ulcerations in the gastric and/or duodenal mucosa associated with free blood in the lumen. Gastric and duodenal ulceration can be visualized by gastroduodenoscopy, and biopsies of the region of the ulcer revealed a severe localized inflammatory reaction. Additional cases of gastrinomas studied in dogs have confirmed that the tumors are highly malignant and that the long-term prognosis is poor due to frequent lymphatic metastasis.[36]

Localization of the tumors prior to surgery has been difficult due to their small size and frequent embedment within the pancreas. In addition to decreasing the tumor burden by surgery, proton pump inhibitors (H+, K+, ATPase) such as omeprazole (20 mg orally once/day) have proven helpful in diminishing gastric acid secretion.[37] The somatostatin analogues, pentetreotide and octreotide, have been evaluated to localize gastrinomas in dogs.[38] [111]Indium pentetreotide scintigraphy revealed multiple areas of activity in the abdomen that were similar to masses in the pancreas and liver. Immunohistochemistry, electron microscopy, and binding of ^{125}I-Tyr^3-octreotide in vitro confirmed the diagnosis of gastrinoma in a dog, which expressed somatostatin receptors.[38] The administration of octreotide (2, 4, and 8 μg/kg) resulted in a transient decrease in circulating gastrin levels.

REFERENCES

1. Capen, C.C., and Martin, S.L. (1969) Hyperinsulinism in dogs with neoplasia of the pancreatic islets: A clinical, pathologic, and ultrastructural study. *Pathol Vet* 6:309-341.
2. Njoku, C.O., Strafuss, A.C., and Dennis, S.M. (1972) Canine islet cell neoplasia: A review. *J Amer Anim Hosp Assoc* 8:284-290.
3. Grant, C.A. (1960) Pancreatic insuloma with clinical manifestations in a dog. *J Comp Pathol* 70:450-456.
4. Bullock, L. (1965) Two cases of a functioning islet cell tumor in the canine. *Calif Vet* 19:14-17.
5. Beck, A.M., and Krook, L. (1965) Canine insuloma: Two surgical cases with relapses. *Cornell Vet* 55:330-339.
6. Prescott, C.W., and Thompson, H.L. (1980) Insulinoma in the dog. *Aust Vet J* 50:502-505.
7. Bencosme, S.A., Allen, R.A., and Latta, H. (1963) Functioning pancreatic islet cell tumors studied electron microscopically. *Amer J Pathol* 42:1-22.

8. Greider, M.H., Rosai, J., and McGuigan, J.E. (1974) The human pancreatic islet cells and their tumors. II. Ulcerogenic and diarrheogenic tumors. *Cancer* 33:1423-1443.
9. Strafuss, A.C., Njoku, C.O., Blauch, B., and Anderson, N.V. (1971) Islet cell neoplasm in four dogs. *J Amer Vet Med Assoc* 159:1008-1011.
10. Mattheeuws, D., Rottiers, R., DeRijcke, J., DeRick, A., and DeSchepper, J. (1976) Hyperinsulinism in the dog due to pancreatic islet-cell tumour: A report on three cases. *J Small Anim Pract* 7:313-318.
11. Kruth, S.A., Feldman, E.D., and Kennedy, P.C. (1982) Islet cell tumors in the dog: A review of 25 cases. *J Amer Vet Med Assoc* 181:54- 58.
12. Tokarnia, C.H. (1961) Islet cell tumor of the bovine pancreas. *J Amer Vet Med Assoc* 138:541-547.
13. Caplan, E.R., Peterson, M.E., Mullen, H.S., Quesenberry, K.E., Rosenthal, K.L., Hoefer, H.L., and Moroff, S.D. (1996) Diagnosis and treatment of insulin-secreting pancreatic islet cell tumors in ferrets: 57 cases (1986-1994). *J Amer Vet Med Assoc* 209:1741-1745.
14. Hawks, D., Peterson, M.E., Hawkins, K.L., and Rosebury, W.S. (1992) Insulin-secreting pancreatic (islet cell) carcinoma in a cat. *J Vet Int Med* 6:193-196.
15. Luttgen, P.J., Storts, R.W., Rogers, K.S., and Morton, L.D. (1986) Insulinoma in a ferret. *J Amer Vet Med Assoc* 189:920-921.
16. Jergens, A.E., and Shaw, D.P. (1989) Hyperinsulinism and hypoglycemia associated with pancreatic islet cell tumor in a ferret. *J Amer Vet Med Assoc* 194:269-271.
17. Fix, A.S., and Harms, C.A. (1990) Immunocytochemistry of pancreatic endocrine tumors in three domestic ferrets. *Vet Pathol* 27:199-201.
18. Marini, R.P., Ryden, E.V., Rosenblad, W.D., Murphy, J.C., and Fox, J.G. (1993) Functional islet cell tumor in six ferrets. *J Amer Vet Med Assoc* 202:430-433.
19. Ehrhart, N., Withrow, S.J., Ehrhart, E.J., and Wimsatt, J.H. (1996) Pancreatic beta cell tumor in ferrets: 20 cases (1986-1994). *J Amer Vet Med Assoc* 209:1737-1740.
20. Rouse, B.T., and Wilson, M.R. (1966) A case of hypoglycaemia in a dog associated with neoplasia of the pancreas. *Vet Rec* 79:454-456.
21. Krook, L., and Kenney, R.M. (1962) Central nervous system lesions in dogs with metastasizing islet cell carcinoma. *Cornell Vet* 52:385-415.
22. Stromberg, P.C., Wilson, F., and Capen, C.C. (1983) Immunocytochemical demonstration of insulin in spontaneous pancreatic islet cell tumors in fischer rats. *Vet Pathol* 20:291-297.
23. Lacy, P.E. (1957) Electron microscopic identification of different cell types in the islets of Langerhans of the guinea pig, rat, rabbit and dog. *Anat Rec* 128:255-267.
24. Lacy, P.E. (1967) The pancreatic beta cell. structure and function. *N Eng J Med* 276:187-195.
25. Munger, B.L., Caramai, F., and Lacy, P.E. (1965) The ultrastructural basis for the identification of cell types in the pancreatic islets. II. Rabbits, dog and opossum. *Z Zellforsch* 67:776-798.
26. Sato, T., Herman, L., and Fitzgerald, P.J. (1966) The comparative ultrastructure of the pancreatic islets of Langerhans. *Gen Comp Endocrinol* 7:132-157.
27. Myers, N.C., III, Andrews, G.A., and Chard-Bergstrom, C. (1997) Chromogranin A plasma concentration and expression in pancreatic islet cell tumors of dogs and cats. *Amer J Vet Res* 58:615-620.
28. Doss, J.C., Gröne, A., Capen, C.C., and Rosol, T.J. (1998) Immunohistochemical localization of chromogranin A in endocrine tissues and endocrine tumors of dogs. *Vet Pathol* 35:312-315.
29. Legg, P.G. (1967) The fine structure of the beta and delta cells in the islets of Langerhans of the cat. *Z Zellforsch* 80:307-321.
30. Wilson, J.W., and Hulse, D.A. (1974) Surgical correction of islet cell adenocarcinoma in a dog. *J Amer Vet Med Assoc* 164:603-606.
31. Caywood, D.D., Klausner, J.S., O'Leary, T.P., Withrow, S.J., Richardson, R.C., Harvey, H.J., Norris, A.M., Henderson, R.A., and Johnston, S.D. (1988) pancreatic insulin-secreting neoplasms: Clin-

ical, diagnostic, and prognostic features in 73 dogs. *J Amer Anim Hosp Assoc* 24:577-584.

32. Meyer, D.J. (1976) Pancreatic islet cell carcinoma in a dog treated with streptozotocin. *J Amer Vet Med Assoc* 168:1221-1223.

33. Jones, B.R., Nicholls, M.R., and Badman, R. (1976) Peptic ulceration in a dog associated with an islet cell carcinoma of the pancreas and an elevated plasma gastrin level. *J Small Anim Pract* 17:593-598.

34. Happé, R.P., van der Gaag, I., Lamers, C.B.H.W., van Toorenburg, J., Renfeld, J.F., and Larsson, L.I. (1980) Zollinger-Ellison syndrome in three dogs. *Vet Pathol* 17:177-186.

35. Middleton, D.J., Watson, A.D.J., Vasak, E., and Culvenor, J.E. (1983) Duodenal ulceration associated with gastrin-secreting pancreatic tumor. *J Amer Vet Med Assoc* 183:461-462.

36. Green, R.A., and Gartrell, C.L. (1997) Gastrinoma: A retrospective study of four cases (1985-1995). *J Amer Anim Hosp Assoc* 33:524-527.

37. Brooks, D., and Watson, G.L. (1997) Omeprazole in a dog with gastrinoma. *J Vet Intern Med* 11:379-381.

38. Altschul, M., Simpson, K.W., Dykes, N.L., Mauldin, E.A., Reubi, J.C., and Cummings, J.F. (1997) Evaluation of somatostatin analogues for the detection and treatment of gastrinoma in a dog. *J Small Anim Pract* 38:286-291.

TUMORS OF THE CHEMORECEPTOR ORGANS

Aortic and Carotid Body: Adenoma, Carcinoma

Introduction

The chemoreceptor organs are sensitive barometers of changes in the blood carbon dioxide content, pH, and oxygen tension and aid in the regulation of respiration and circulation. Carotid and aortic bodies can initiate an increase in the depth, minute volume, and rate of respiration by way of parasympathetic nerves, which results in an increased heart rate and elevated arterial blood pressure by way of the sympathetic nervous system. They are normally composed of parenchymal (chemoreceptor and glomus) cells and stellate shaped sustentacular cells.[1,2] Nerve endings with synaptic vesicles and nerve fibers are seen in close association with the chemoreceptor cells. Although the embryological origin of chemoreceptor organs is not precisely known, there is considerable evidence to suggest that they arise from perivascular mesodermal cells that are invaded by cells of neuroectodermal origin.[3]

Chemoreceptor tissue is present at several sites in the body including the carotid body, aortic bodies, nodose ganglion of the vagus nerve, ciliary ganglion in the orbit, pancreas, bodies on the internal jugular vein below the middle ear, and glomus jugulare along the recurrent branch of the glossopharyngeal nerve. Normal aortic bodies of dogs consist of clusters of cells embedded in adventitia of major vessels at multiple sites including the innominate artery immediately below the origin of the right subclavian artery, on the anterior surface of the aortic arch, beneath the arch between the aorta and pul-

monary artery, between the ascending aorta and pulmonary artery near the left coronary artery, and scattered in the wall of the pulmonary artery.

Incidence

Although chemoreceptor tissue is widely distributed in the body, tumors develop principally in the aortic and carotid bodies in domestic animals. Aortic body tumors are encountered more frequently than neoplasms of the carotid body in animals,[4] but the reverse is true for humans.[5]

Chemodectoma and *nonchromaffin paraganglioma* are synonyms that are frequently used to designate neoplasms arising in chemoreceptor organs.[6] These tumors develop primarily in dogs[7,8] and infrequently in cats[9] and cattle.[10] Brachycephalic breeds of dogs such as the boxer and Boston terrier are highly predisposed to develop tumors of the aortic and carotid bodies (S.P. Bishop, personal communication).[6,11,12] The majority of dogs with chemodectomas are 8 years of age or older. Male dogs appear to have a greater frequency of chemodectomas than females.[4,8,12,13]

Clinical Characteristics

Tumors of the aortic and carotid bodies in animals are not functional (i.e., they do not secrete excess hormone into the circulation), but as space occupying lesions they may result in a variety of clinical signs. Clinical signs associated with larger aortic body adenomas and carcinomas usually are manifestations of cardiac decompensation due to pressure on the atria, vena cava, or both.[8] There may be evidence of dyspnea; coughing; vomiting; cyanosis; hydrothorax; hydropericardium; ascites; edema of the subcutaneous tissue of the head, neck, and forelimbs; and passive congestion of the liver. The accumulation of serous, often blood tinged, fluid in the pericardial sac results from the invasion of tumor cells into lymphatics at the base of the heart or the compression of small pericardial veins.

Dogs with carotid body tumors usually are presented with a palpable, slowly enlarging mass in the anterolateral cervical region near the angle of the mandible. Larger neoplasms interfere with swallowing because of pressure on the esophagus and result in circulatory disturbances from compression of the larger veins in the neck. Other clinical signs may be related to the presence of an aortic body tumor in the same animal. Dyspnea and coughing have been observed in dogs with malignant carotid body tumors that have multiple pulmonary metastases.[14]

Etiology

Although the etiology of chemodectomas is unknown, it has been suggested that a genetic predisposition aggravated by chronic hypoxia may account for the higher risk of certain brachycephalic breeds such as the boxer and Boston terrier to develop aortic and carotid body tumors.[13] Carotid bodies of several mammalian species, including dogs, have been shown to undergo hyperplasia when subjected to chronic hypoxia by living in a high altitude environment.[15] Humans living at high altitudes have been reported to have 10 times the frequency of chemodectomas seen in those living at sea level.[16]

Macroscopic Pathology

Aortic body tumors appear most frequently as single masses or occasionally as multiple nodules within the pericardial sac near the base of the heart.[8] They vary considerably in size from 0.5 to 12.5 cm, and carcinomas are generally larger than adenomas. Solitary small adenomas either are attached to the adventitia of the pulmonary artery and ascending aorta or are embedded in the adipose connective tissue between these major vascular trunks. They have a smooth external surface and on cross section are white and mottled with red to brown areas. Larger adenomas may indent the atria or displace the trachea. Their surface is more coarsely nodular, and large areas of hemorrhage or necrosis are present in the tumor. The larger aortic body adenomas are multilobular and partially surround the major arterial trunks at the base of the heart. Although the vessels may be completely surrounded by neoplastic tissue, there usually is little evidence of vascular constriction.

Malignant aortic body tumors occur less frequently in dogs than adenomas. Carcinomas may infiltrate the wall of the pulmonary artery to form papillary projections into the lumen or invade through the wall into the lumens of the atria (fig. 13.41 A). A large mural thrombus is attached occasionally to the neoplastic tissue extending into the atrium. Although tumor cells often invade blood vessels, metastasis to the lung and liver occurs infrequently in dogs with aortic body tumors.[8,17] However, local invasion of the pericardium, epicardium, myocardium, and walls of great vessels at the base of the heart by aortic body tumors occurs frequently.

Carotid body tumors arise near the bifurcation of the common carotid artery in the cranial cervical area. They usually appear as a unilateral, slow growing mass[4] and only rarely develop on both sides in the same animal.[6] Adenomas vary from approximately 1 to 4 cm in diameter, are well encapsulated, and have a smooth external surface. The bifurcation of the carotid artery is incorporated in the mass, and tumor cells firmly adhere to the tunica adventitia. A branch of the glossopharyngeal nerve may be traced into the capsule of the tumor by careful dissection. Adenomas are firm and white with scattered areas of hemorrhage and are extremely vascular. Biopsy and complete surgical excision often are difficult because of the high degree of vascularity and intimate relationship of the tumor with major arterial trunks in the neck.

Malignant carotid body tumors are larger (as much as 12 cm in diameter) and more coarsely multinodular than adenomas. Multiple areas of hemorrhage and cystic degeneration are present within the tumor. Although carcinomas appear to be encapsulated, tumor cells invade the capsule and the walls of adjacent vessels and lymphatics. The

external jugular vein and several cranial nerves, in addition to the carotid bifurcation, may be incorporated by the neoplasm. Larger tumors may result in extensive dorsolateral deviation of the trachea. In a review of 22 carotid body tumors in the dog, it was reported that approximately 30 percent of those with adequate descriptions of lesions had evidence of metastasis.[4] Metastasis of carotid body tumors has been found in the lung, bronchial and mediastinal lymph nodes, liver, pancreas, and kidney.[4,6,14] Occasionally the metastases to parenchymal organs, such as the kidney, may be extensive and nearly obliterate the affected organ.

Multicentric neoplastic transformation of chemoreceptor tissue occurs frequently in brachycephalic breeds of dogs. Approximately 65 percent of the reported carotid body tumors (i.e., those cases with adequate descriptions of lesions) also have aortic body tumors.[4,18]

Histopathology

The histological characteristics of chemoreceptor tumors are similar whether they are derived from the carotid or the aortic body. The neoplastic chemoreceptor cells are subdivided into lobules by prominent branching trabeculae of connective tissue that originate from the fibrous capsule.[6] They are further subdivided into small compartments by fine septa that contain collagen and reticulum fibers plus small capillaries (fig. 13.41 B). Tumor cells frequently are aligned along and around the small capillaries in chemodectomas. Focal accumulations of lymphocytes and hemosiderin laden macrophages often are present in the capsule and major connective tissue trabeculae.

The tumor cells of chemodectomas are discrete, cuboidal to polyhedral, and arranged in distinct packets (fig. 13.41 B). The cytoplasm is lightly eosinophilic, finely granular, and often vacuolated. Cells forming chemodectomas rapidly undergo autolysis. Cell boundaries become indistinct and the cytoplasm appears clear if the postmortem interval is prolonged. The nuclei are round to oval and usually are placed centrally in the cell. There is a finely granular chromatin pattern, and mitotic figures are infrequent.[11]

In larger aortic body adenomas or in carcinomas, there are scattered areas where the tumor cells are larger and more pleomorphic. Mononuclear tumor giant cells with bizarre shaped, multilobed, densely basophilic nuclei are intermingled with the cuboidal tumor cells. Although tumor giant cells are detected more consistently in carcinomas, they are by no means an unequivocal criterion of malignancy. Small, well-differentiated chemodectomas occasionally have a considerable number of tumor giant cells.

Aortic and carotid body tumors are very vascular and have numerous muscular arterioles, large thin-walled veins, and an abundant network of capillaries in the connective tissue septa.[8] Focal areas of hemorrhage from disruption of thin-walled vessels and areas of coagulation necrosis are a consistent finding in chemodectomas.[11] Cholesterol clefts and foci of mineralization often are present in the areas of necrosis. Several layers of tumor cells may radiate along fine connective tissue septa from the thin-walled vessels. Tumor cells frequently invade blood vessels and lymphatics and form emboli. Carcinomas show evidence of tumor cell invasion through the capsule and into the walls of large muscular arteries and adjacent structures (e.g., wall of the atrium, bifurcation of the trachea, and the pericardium). The invading tumor cells are pleomorphic, hyperchromatic with frequent mitotic figures, and arranged in broad sheets with little tendency to form distinctive packets of cells.

Adenomas and carcinomas derived from ectopic thyroid tissue account for approximately 5 to 10 percent of *heart base tumors* in dogs. They often compress or invade structures in the anterior mediastinum near the base of the heart.

Areas of ectopic thyroid tumors with a compact cellular (solid) pattern of arrangement are difficult to distinguish histologically from aortic body tumors. In general, cells of ectopic thyroid tumors are smaller than in aortic body tumors and have more hyperchromatic nuclei and eosinophilic cytoplasm. The neoplastic follicular cells are not consistently subdivided into small packets by fine strands of connective tissue. Tumor giant cells are infrequent in ectopic thyroid tumors, and the stroma is less prominent. Multiple sections usually reveal the formation of primitive follicular structures or colloid-containing follicles formed by neoplastic follicular cells in ectopic thyroid tumors, but not in aortic body tumors. Immunocytochemical localization of thyroglobulin or ultrastructural evaluation may be needed to differentiate thyroid tumors in the anterior mediastinum from aortic body tumors.

Ultrastructural and Immunocytochemical Characteristics

Cells of aortic and carotid body tumors in the dog[19] resemble those in normal chemoreceptor tissue,[1,20,21] but they lack the normal relationship to sustentacular, neural, and vascular elements. The large polyhedral chemoreceptor or parenchymal cells are arranged in small clusters. The cytoplasmic density of the neoplastic cell varies from light to dark depending on the development of secretory organelles and numbers of storage granules. Small spherical mitochondria, parallel arrays of rough endoplasmic reticulum, and Golgi apparatuses with prosecretory granules are scattered in the cytoplasm. Varying numbers of small, electron dense, membrane-limited secretory granules are present in the tumor cells and are important in establishing the diagnosis of an aortic or carotid body tumor (fig. 13.41 C). The electron density of secretory granules in chemoreceptor cells varies considerably with the fixative used, but the granules are well preserved with glutaraldehyde.[22] In general, secretory granules are more numerous in cells of adenomas than in those of carcinomas of the aortic and carotid bodies.[19]

Stellate cells often extend long cytoplasmic processes around and between the tumor cells in carotid body adenomas from dogs (fig. 13.41 C).[19] These processes appear to terminate near perivascular spaces. Cytoplasmic organelles are poorly developed, and secretory granules are few in number compared to the chemoreceptor cells. Similar sustentacular cells have been described in the carotid body of normal animals and are considered to have a supportive rather than a secretory function.[23,24]

Ultrastructural studies are helpful in differentiating between heart base tumors derived from chemoreceptor cells of the aortic body and ectopic thyroid follicular cells in the dog.[25] The neoplastic follicular cells are arranged predominantly in a compact cellular (solid) pattern with only an occasional colloid-containing follicle, and they may closely resemble an aortic body tumor. Although thyroid follicular cells contain large lysosomal (dense) bodies, they lack the small, membrane-limited secretory granules characteristic of chemoreceptor cells in the aortic and carotid bodies (fig. 13.41 D).[1,24] In addition, numerous microvilli project from the luminal surfaces of more differentiated follicular cells in ectopic thyroid adenomas. The neoplastic follicular cells consistently had long, electron dense, tubular structures within cisternae of the rough endoplasmic reticulum (fig. 13.41 D).[25] The cisternae are dilated by the tubules and the accumulation of a finely granular, electron dense material. These characteristic tubules are not observed in normal canine thyroid follicular cells, in nonadenomatous ectopic thyroid cells, or in aortic body tumors.[19,25-27]

Chromaffin granules can not be demonstrated in the cytoplasm of cells forming chemodectomas as they can in pheochromocytomas of the adrenal medulla, but the tumor cells do stain for chromogranin A (fig. 13.41 E).

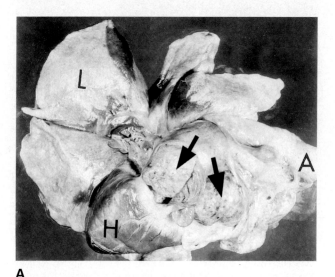

A

Fig. 13.41. Tumors of the chemoreceptors. **A.** Aortic body carcinoma of a dog with multiple nodules (arrow) at the base of the heart *(H)* and extension into the adjacent atrium (arrowhead) (*L* is diaphragmatic lobe of lung, *A* is aorta). (continued)

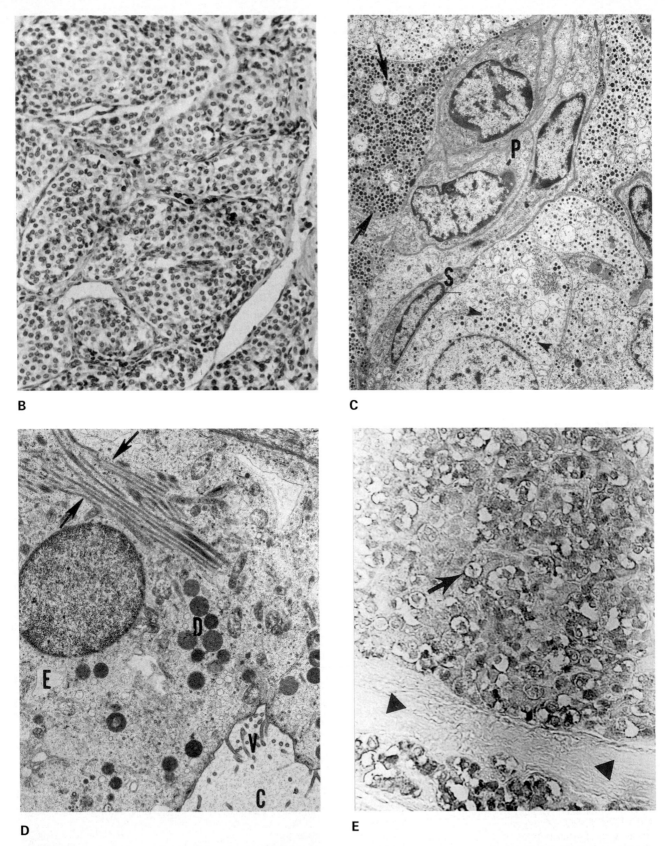

B

C

D

E

Fig. 13.41. (continued)   **B.** Characteristic histological pattern in a carotid body tumor from a dog. Tumor cells are subdivided into groups or lobules by fine connective tissue septa with many capillaries. [From Jubb, K.F., and Kennedy, P.C. (1957) *Cancer* 10:89-99.] **C.** Carotid body adenoma from a dog illustrating lightly (arrowheads) and densely (arrows) granulated tumor cells. The small secretory granules have a closely applied limiting membrane. A sustentacular cell *(S)* extends processes toward several perivascular cells (P). [From Cheville, N.F., (1972) *Vet Pathol* 9:166-189.] **D.** A follicular adenoma derived from ectopic thyroid tissue located at the base of the heart. The thyroid follicular cells contain dense bodies *(D)*, endoplasmic reticulum *(E)*, and numerous microvilli *(V)* projecting into the colloid *(C)* of the follicular lumen, but lack the small secretory granules found in aortic and carotid body tumors. Long dense tubules are present within the cisternae of endoplasmic reticulum in the tumor cells (arrows) [From Cheville, N.F., (1972) *Vet Pathol* 9:166-189.] **E.** Chemodectoma from a dog. The tumor cells stained intensely positive for chromogranin A (arrow) whereas the connective tissue capsule (arrowheads) was negative. Avidin-biotin-peroxidase immunohistochemistry. [From Doss, J.C., et al. (1998) *Vet Pathol* 35:312-315.]

Growth and Metastasis

Aortic body tumors in animals tend to be more benign than tumors of the carotid body. They grow slowly by expansion and exert pressure on the vena cava and atria. Aortic body carcinomas often invade locally into the atria, pericardium, and adjacent large, thin-walled vessels (see fig. 13.42). When they metastasize, secondary foci of growth are found most frequently in the lung and liver.[8,11]

Carotid body tumors tend to be more malignant, and metastases are present in approximately 30 percent of reported cases.[4,14] Metastases have been found in the lung, bronchial and mediastinal lymph nodes, liver, pancreas, and kidney. The presence of vascular or lymphatic emboli in a biopsy of the primary chemodectoma does not consistently indicate that metastases are present in distant organs.[5,6]

Ectopic thyroid carcinomas arising at the base of the heart in dogs may remain localized in the anterior mediastinum, where they enlarge and exert pressure on the heart and major vessels or occasionally metastasize to extrathoracic sites.[27]

A unique extra-adrenal paraganglioma has been reported in horses resulting primarily in clinical signs relating to exophthalmos.[28,29] The lesion appears to be derived from cells of neural crest origin, most likely nonchromaffin paraganglia near the ciliary ganglion. The neoplastic cells usually invade locally into the retrobulbar space but may infiltrate more aggressively through the optic canal into the cranial vault resulting in lysis of bone and extention into the nasal cavity.

The tumors are densely cellular with nests or packets of neoplastic cells subdivided by a fine fibrovascular (reticulin-positive) stroma characteristic of neuroectodermally derived tumors. The cytoplasmic area is abundant, lightly eosinophilic, and finely granular, often with indistinct individual cell boundaries. The neoplastic cells have a positive argyrophilic reaction (either by Pascual's silver impregnation method or the Grimelius technique), stain positive by immunohistochemical methods for chromogranin A and neuron-specific enolase but are negative for S-100 protein and glial fibrillary acidic protein.[28,29] Ultrastructurally, neoplastic cells of orbital paragangliomas in horses are similar to those in canine aortic and carotid body tumors with typical membrane-bound secretory granules and prominent arrays of rough endoplasmic reticulum.

Surgical removal of the tumors by transpalpebral orbital exenteration has been performed with variable success depending upon the degree of local tissue invasion of the tumor beyond the orbit.[29] Manipulation of the tumors during surgery may result in hypotension.

REFERENCES

1. Höglund, R. (1967) An ultrastructural study of the carotid body of horse and dog. *Z Zellforsch* 76:568-576.
2. Kobayashi, S. (1968) Fine structure of the carotid body of the dog. *Arch Histol Jpn* 30:95- 120.
3. Pryse-Davies, J., Dawson, I.M.P., and Westbury, G. (1964) Some morphologic, histochemical and chemical observations on chemodectomas and the normal carotid body, including a study of the chromaffin reaction and possible ganglion cell elements. *Cancer* 17:185-202.
4. Dean, M.J., and Strafuss, A.C. (1975) Carotid body tumors in the dog: A review and report of four cases. *J Amer Vet Med Assoc* 166:1003-1006.
5. Scotti, T.M. (1958) The carotid body tumor in dogs. *J Amer Vet Med Assoc* 132:413-419.
6. Jubb, K.F., and Kennedy, P.C. (1957) Tumors of the nonchromaffin paraganglia in dogs. *Cancer* 10:89-99.
7. Bloom, F. (1943) Structure and histogenesis of tumors of the aortic bodies in dogs: With a consideration of the morphology of the aortic and carotid bodies. *Arch Pathol* 36:1-12.
8. Johnson, K.H. (1968) Aortic body tumors in the dog. *J Amer Vet Med Assoc* 152:154-160.
9. Buergelt, C.D., and Das, K.M. (1968) Aortic body tumor in a cat: A case report. *Pathol Vet* 5:84-90.
10. Nordstoga, K. (1966) Carotid body tumor in a cow. *Pathol Vet* 3:412-420.
11. Nilsson, T. (1955) Heart-base tumours in the dog. *Acta Path Microbiol Scand* 37:385-397.
12. Howard, E.B., and Nielsen, S.W. (1965) Pheochromocytomas associated with hypertensive lesions in dogs. *J Amer Vet Med Assoc* 147:245-252.
13. Hayes, H.H., Jr. (1975) An hypothesis for the aetiology of canine chemoreceptor system neoplasms, based upon an epidemiological study of 73 cases among hospital patients. *J Small Anim Pract* 16:337-343.
14. Sander, C.H., and Whitenack, D.I. (1970) Canine malignant carotid body tumor. *J Amer Vet Med Assoc* 156:606-610.
15. Edwards, C., Heath, D., Harris, P., Castillo, Y., Krüger, H., and Arias-Stella, J. (1971) The carotid body in animals at high altitude. *J Pathol* 104:231-238.
16. Saldana, M.J., Salem, L.E., and Travezan, R. (1973) High altitude hypoxia and chemodectomas. *Human Pathol* 4:251-263.
17. Nillson, A. (1956) A case of metastasising tumour of the glomus aorticus in a dog. *Nord Vet Med* 8:875-881.
18. Hubben, K., Patterson, D.F., and Detweiler, D.K. (1960) Carotid body tumor in the dog. *J Amer Vet Med Assoc* 137:411-416.

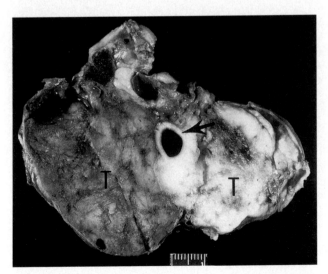

Fig. 13.42. Adenocarcinoma *(T)* arising from ectopic thyroid tissue surrounding the trachea (arrows) and other structures in the anterior mediastinum of a dog (scale = 1 cm).

19. Cheville, N.F. (1972) Ultrastructure of canine carotid body and aortic body tumors: Comparison with tissues of thyroid and parathyroid origin. *Vet Pathol* 9:166-189.

20. Ross, L.L. (1959) Electron microscopic observations of the carotid body of the cat. *J Biophys Biochem Cytol* 6:253-262.

21. deKock, L.L., and Dunn, A.E.G. (1966) An electron microscope study of the carotid body. *Acta Anat* 64:163-178.

22. Duncan, D., and Yates, R. (1967) Ultrastructure of the carotid body of the cat as revealed by various fixatives and the use of reserpine. *Anat Rec* 157:667-682.

23. Biscoe, T.J., and Stehbens, W.E. (1966) Ultrastrucrure of the carotid body. *J Cell Biol* 30:563-578.

24. Morita, E., Chiocchio, S.R., and Tramezzani, J.H. (1969) Four main types of cells in the carotid body of the cat. *J Ultrastruct Res* 28:399-410.

25. Thake, D.C., Cheville, N.F., and Sharp, R.K. (1971) Ectopic thyroid adenomas at the base of the heart of the dog: Ultrastructural identification of dense tubular structures in endoplasmic reticulum. *Vet Pathol* 8:421-432.

26. Pospischil, A., Hänichen, T., and von Bomhard, D. (1980) Ultrastrukturelle Untersuchungen an Schilddrüsentumoren beim Hund. *Schweiz Arch Tierheilk* 122:233-246.

27. Stephens, L.C., Saunders, W.J., and Jaenke, R.S. (1982) Ectopic thyroid carcinoma with metastases in a beagle dog. *Vet Pathol* 19:669-675.

28. Basher, A.W.P., et al. (1997) Orbital neuroendocrine tumors in three horses. *J Amer Vet Med Assoc* 210: 668-671.

29. Goodhead, A.D., Venter, I.J., and Nesbit, J.W. (1997) Retrobulbar extra-adrenal paraganglioma in a horse and its surgical removal by orbitotomy. *Vet Comp Ophthalmol* 7:96-100.

14 Tumors of the Nervous System

A. Koestner and R. J. Higgins

INTRODUCTION

General Considerations

Primary neoplasms of the nervous system (NS) are relatively rare in most domestic animal species with the exception of the dog and, to a lesser extent, the cat. Dogs and cats live mostly in close proximity to the families of their owners and are generally permitted to live their whole life span, reaching an age when both central nervous system (CNS) and peripheral nervous system (PNS) tumors become most prevalent. Based on the few published collections and our own experience, 60-80 percent of all NS neoplasms have been recognized in dogs and 10-20 percent in cats, leaving only 10-20 percent to all other animal species combined.[1,2] The variation in percentages among the various collections reflects the diversity of animal species represented within the institutions from which the statistics were calculated.

Neoplasia of the NS in domestic animals is primarily a problem of aged animals; over 70 percent of primary tumors of the CNS in dogs occur in dogs over 6 years of age. The incidence of CNS tumors in aged dogs is similar to that in the adult human population, amounting to 1-3 percent of all deaths where an autopsy was performed. In comparison to this relatively low tumor incidence in adult human beings, CNS tumors in children (up to 15 years of age) occupy a prominent position in cancer statistics. These tumors account for 25 percent of all childhood tumors, being surpassed only by leukemia. In contrast, CNS tumors in young dogs are of much less importance. Only 10 percent of all primary canine CNS tumors occurred in dogs 3 years of age or younger in our collections. Almost half of those tumors are of embryonal or neuronal origin; these include medulloblastomas, medulloepitheliomas, and craniopharyngiomas.

There are some differences in the prevalence of various tumor types both between and within species, and also among breeds. For instance, there is a relatively high incidence of meningiomas in cats and of nerve sheath cell tumors in cattle. While gliomas are more prevalent in dogs, this species best represents the spectrum of CNS tumors that occur in human beings. Within the canine species, over 50 percent of all gliomas occur in brachycephalic breeds such as boxers and Boston terriers. A genetic basis for this concurrence has not been established.

Classification

A classification of the various neoplasms recognized in the NS of animals is an essential means of communication between pathologists and clinicians as well as between veterinary medical and human medical specialists in the various branches of clinical and investigative neuroscience. The classification is generally based on histological and cytological criteria capable of determining the cell type of tumor origin, the growth characteristics, and the degree of differentiation. These determinations provide a valuable basis for prognosis and tumor therapy. Attempts to establish classification schemes of NS neoplasms go back to the early part of the twentieth century.[3] Diverse opinions by a number of leading neuropathologists from different schools and countries led to many controversies and created a need to establish a common language of understanding for tumor classification. In response to this need, the World Health Organization (WHO) initiated the formation of international committees of pathologists to create an internationally acceptable classification of tumors based on the most current methods available. The first international classification of NS tumors in domestic animals was published in 1974[4] and that of human NS tumors in 1979.

Since that time a remarkable development in cytogenetic analysis from electron microscopy, immunohistochemistry, and molecular pathology has provided a better understanding of some problems inherent in the first classification. The latest international classification of human brain tumors incorporating these findings was published in 1993.[5] An international committee of veterinary neuropathologists has updated the classification of tumors of the nervous system in domestic animals following the human classification. This updated classification will be followed in this text.

In general, we distinguish between tumors of the CNS and tumors of the PNS. We further separate primary tumors from secondary tumors. Primary tumors are those that originate from within the nervous system, while secondary tumors originate from extraneural organs and reach the brain by either extension or metastasis. Examples of secondary tumors reaching the brain by local extension (e.g., invasion, impingement) are nasal carcinomas invading the brain through the cribriform plate or osteosarcomas of the skull impinging on the brain by invasive growth. Metastatic tumors, such as carcinomas of the mammary gland, lungs, or kidneys reach the brain by intravascular immobilization.

Primary NS tumors are more frequently encountered than secondary tumors, with an approximate ratio of 3:1 in favor of primary neoplasms.

Clinical Characteristics

CNS neoplasms are space occupying lesions that affect the surrounding brain parenchyma by compression. Aggressive neoplasms may, in addition, lead to infiltration and parenchymal destruction, with resultant edema, hemorrhage, necrosis, and reactive inflammation. The consequences of CNS neoplasia depend upon location and size of the tumor as well as peritumoral changes. The severity of neurological deficits progresses with tumor growth, and localizing signs may become more diverse if the tumor infiltrates the nervous system more widely. Hydrocephalus may be a secondary effect if the flow of cerebrospinal fluid is partially or completely obstructed by the tumor. A clinical neurological examination is often inadequate to determine the location of confined mass lesions. Their location and size is best visualized by computerized tomography (CT) or by magnetic resonance imaging (MRI), which has become accessible to larger veterinary clinical centers and especially university veterinary hospitals. Follow-up CT-guided stereotactic biopsy techniques can lead to a precise neuropathological diagnosis of lesions.

A sizeable number of intracranial neoplasms is associated with epileptiform seizures. It has been reported that 46 percent of 79 dogs with intracranial neoplasms had epileptic seizures.[6] This incidence parallels that in human patients, where almost 50 percent of patients with brain tumors develop epileptic seizures.[7] In the McGrath collection, 80 percent of the tumors linked to epileptic seizures were located in the frontal and temporal lobes.[6,8] In such cases, seizures often appeared before any other neurological signs were observed. Seizures may also appear intermittently or at the terminal stage. In tumors located in the temporal or piriform area, epilepsy may be the only clinical neurological sign.

In addition to progressive localized signs and epilepsy, behavioral changes are frequently encountered in association with brain tumors.[9]

Clinical Pathology

The results from conventional examination (total and differential nucleated cell counts and total protein levels) of cerebrospinal fluid (CSF) from dogs with subsequently confirmed CNS tumors have not been demonstrated to be of much diagnostic specificity or usefulness.[10,11] Cytological assessment in these studies, however, was done only on cases with an elevated CSF cell count, using a cytospin technique. However there have been reports, using a membrane filter technique or a Kolmel sedimentation apparatus, where tumor cells were found in the CSF in 3 of 9 cases and in 9 of 17 cases of dogs with brain tumors.[12-14] In the latter report, two of five cytologically positive cases had nucleated cell counts within the normal reference range. The advent of new diagnostic neuroimaging techniques will further decrease the need for such routine analyses, and newer methods of cell identification (e.g., immunophenotyping) may prove to be diagnostically valuable.[15,16]

Brain Tumor Therapy in Animals

Since brain tumors form space-occupying masses within the cranial cavity, where expansion is limited by the cranial vault, the major objective of therapy is the elimination of the tumor mass. If this is only partially accomplished there will be only short-term clinical improvement. Long-term survival may depend on significant tumor reduction by surgical debulking, radiation, or chemotherapy or some combination of these. Glucocorticoids can temporarily diminish the mass effect by reducing the peritumoral edema that results from changes in blood-brain barrier permeability.

Surgical intervention has become more effective with the availability of neurodiagnostic imaging procedures of CT and MRI, since both provide an accurate location and size of mass lesions. With such information, superficially located neoplasms (e.g., meningiomas) can be removed more accurately and neurological deficits can be minimized. The possibility for the complete removal of deep-seated tumors and a successful outcome is much more guarded since neurological impairments are expected consequences of such surgical resection. Radiation therapy with or without tumor resection is a possible alternative, although there is no scientifically based information on the radiosensitivity of primary CNS tumors in animals. Newer techniques for brain tumor therapy presently being investigated (e.g., various types of gene therapy) may result in more effective brain tumor treatment in humans and animals.

New Techniques in Diagnostic Neuro-Oncology

The recent application in dogs and cats of modified procedures and equipment used in human neurosurgery for CT guided stereobiopsy has enhanced the capability for diagnosis and treatment of mass lesions detected by neuroimaging techniques. Small core tissue samples from such lesions can be taken with remarkable precision. Cytological evaluation of smear preparations from part of the core, fixed in 95 percent alcohol and rapidly stained with H&E, can be done within minutes. Diagnostically accurate information from this rapid technique is generally possible with both primary and metastatic nervous system tumors.[17] This cytological information can be subsequently confirmed with either frozen or paraffin-embedded sections. Degenerative or inflammatory lesions pose more of a challenge due to the heterogeneous nature of the histological changes. Immunohistochemistry has become an indispensable technique for the confirmation, diagnosis, and reclassification of nervous system tumors. The efficacy of proliferation indices (e.g., BrdU, AgNOR, Ki-67, MIB-1, PCNA) for prognostic use in animal nervous system tumors has not been evaluated. The recent development of a wide range of functional, cell specific, canine antibodies will probably lead to a better understanding of the immunobiology of nervous system tumors.[18] Molecular biology techniques in neuro-oncology in humans and small laboratory animals are demonstrating their usefulness, particularly in identifying amplification of genes for growth factors and cytokines and their receptors. They are also providing a better understanding of how molecular genetics and the expression of oncogenes and suppressor genes are involved in stages of tumor evolution.[19-21] This is as yet an unexplored area in tumors of the nervous system in domestic animals.

REFERENCES

1. Luginbühl H., Fankhauser R., and McGrath J.T. (1968) Spontaneous neoplasms of the nervous system in animals. *Prog Neurol Surg* 2:85-164.
2. Hayes H.M., Priester, W.A., and Prendergrass, T.W. (1975) Occurrence of nervous-tissue tumors in cattle, horses, cats and dogs. *Intl J Cancer* 15:39-47.
3. Bailey, P., and Cushing, H.A. (1926) *A Classification of the Glioma Group on a Histogenetic Basis with a Correlated Study of Prognosis.* J.B. Lippincott, Philadelphia, pp. 53-103.
4. Fankhauser R., Luginbühl H., McGrath, J.T. (1974) Tumors of the nervous system. *Bull WHO* 50(1-2):53-70.
5. Kleihues, P., Burger, P.C., and Scheithauer, B.W. (1993) Histological typing of tumors of the central nervous system. *WHO International Histological Classification of Tumors,* 2nd ed. Springer-Verlag, Berlin.
6. McGrath, J.T. (1960) Intracranial neoplasms. In *Neurologic Examination of the Dog,* 2nd ed. Lea and Febiger, Philadelphia, pp. 148-195.
7. Ketz, E. (1974) Brain tumors and epilepsy. In Vinken, P., and Bruyn, G.W. (eds.), *Handbook of Clinical Neurology.* North-Holland, Amsterdam, pp. 254-269.
8. Koestner, A.(1989) Neuropathology of canine epilepsy. In Indrieri, R.J. (ed.), *Problems in Veterinary Medicine. Epilepsy.* Lippincott, Philadelphia, pp. 516-534.
9. Bagly R.S., Gavin, P.R., Moore, M.P., Silver G.M., Harrington, M.L., Connors, R.L. (1999) Clinical signs associated with brain tumors in dogs: 97 cases (1992-1997). *J Amer Vet Med Assoc* 215:818-819.
10. Bailey, C.S., Higgins, R.J. (1986) Characteristics of cisternal cerebrospinal fluid associated with primary brain tumors in the dog: A retrospective study. *J Amer Vet Med Assoc* 188:414-417.
11. Bailey, C.S., and Vernau, W. (1997) Cerebrospinal fluid. In Kaneko, J.J., Harvey, J.W., and Bruss, M.L. (eds.) *Clinical Biochemistry of Domestic Animals.* 5th Ed. Academic Press, San Diego, pp. 785-827.
12. Bischel, P., Vandevelde, M., Vandevelde, E., Affolter, U., and Pfister, H. (1984) Immunoelectrophoretic determination of albumin and IgG in serum and cerebrospinal fluid in dogs with neurological diseases. *Res Vet Sci* 37:101-107.
13. Grevel, V., and Machus, B. (1990) Diagnosing brain tumors with a CSF sedimentation technique. *Vet Med Report* 2:403-408.
14. Grevel, V., Machus, B., and Steeb, C. (1992) Zytologie des Liquor cerebrospinalis bei Hirntumoren und Ruckenmarkskompressionen des hundes. Teil 4. *Tierarztl Prax* 20:419-428.
15. Xiao, S., Renshaw, A., Cibas, E.S., Hudson, T.J., and Fletcher, J.A. (1995) Novel fluorescence in situ hybridisation in solid tumors. *Amer J Pathol* 147:896-904.
16. Tipold, A., Moore, P.F., Jungi, T.W., Sager, H., Vandevelde, M. (1988) Lymphocyte subsets and CD45RA positive T-cells in normal canine cerebrospinal fluid. *J Neuroimmunol* 82:90-95.
17. Vernau, K.M., Higgins. R.J., Bollen, A.W., Jimenez, D.F., Anderson, J.V., Koblik, P.D., and LeCouteur, R.A. (2001) Primary canine and feline nervous system tumors: intraoperative diagnosis using the smear technique. *Vet Pathol* 38:47-57.
18. Moore, P.F., Affolter, V.K., Olivry, T., Schrenzel, M.D. (1988) The use of immunological reagents in defining the pathogenesis of canine skin diseases involving proliferation of leukocytes. In Kwocha, K.W., Willemse, T., and von Tscharner, C. (eds.), *Advances in Veterinary Dermatology,* vol. 3. Butterworth Heinemann, Oxford, pp. 77-94.
19. Kleihues, P., and Ohgaki, H. (1997) Genetics of glioma progression and the definition of primary and secondary glioblastoma. *Brain Pathol* 7:1131-1136.
20. Von Deimling, A. (1997) Molecular genetic classification of astrocytic and oligodendroglial tumors. *Brain Pathol* 7:1311-1313.
21. Cavenee, W.K., Furnari, F.B., Nagane M., et al. (2000) Diffusely infiltrating astrocytomas. In Kliehues, P., and Cavanee, W.K. (eds.), *Pathology and Genetics of Tumours of the Nervous System, WHO Classification of Tumours,* IARC Press, Lyon, pp. 10-21.

PRIMARY TUMORS OF THE CENTRAL NERVOUS SYSTEM

Glial Tumors

Astrocytoma

Classification

The new WHO international classification distinguishes three grades of human astrocytomas based on their degree of differentiation defined by grading criteria as follows[1]: diffuse astrocytoma (WHO grade II) (variants: fibrillary, protoplasmic, gemistocytic); anaplastic astrocytoma (WHO grade III); and glioblastoma multiforme (WHO grade IV).

Incidence and Sites

Glial tumors are among the common primary tumors of the CNS in dogs and cats but are rare in other domestic animal species.[2,3] Their prevalence is only exceeded by meningiomas in dogs and cats.[3] Canine astrocytomas and oligodendrogliomas each have about the same occurrence of about 10 percent of all primary tumors. Astrocytomas occur most frequently in the cerebral hemispheres, predominantly in the temporal-piriform region, but they may be located in most any area of the CNS including the brain stem, cerebellum, and spinal cord. They may arise from within either gray or white matter.

Gross Morphology

The gross appearance of astrocytomas depends upon their rate of growth and degree of differentiation. Slow growing, well-differentiated tumors are usually poorly defined and often barely distinguishable from normal brain by their often pinkish or, after fixation, white discoloration. Their growth may extend from the ependyma to the subpial cortex with blurring of anatomical gray and white matter boundaries (fig. 14.1 A). Exceptions are the canine gemistocytic and pilocytic variants which can be demarcated tumors (fig. 14.1 B). We have included both in this diffuse group, although more strictly the pilocytic astrocytoma belongs in a separate category.[1] Rapidly growing forms are more mottled and soft because of frequent associated intratumoral cysts, necrosis, hemorrhage, and edema.

Histological Features

Diffuse Astrocytoma

This tumor is usually composed of a fairly uniform population of loosely arranged cells, which infiltrate imperceptibly into adjacent normal tissue. The shape and size of the cells differ according to the histological subtype of astrocytoma. The most common fibrillary astrocytoma is composed of diffusely infiltrating elongate, spindloid, and occasionally polygonal cells that lead to a mild increase in overall cellularity (fig. 14.2 A). A reliable hallmark of neoplastic astrocytes is their nuclear atypia with enlarged or irregular hyperchromatic nuclei. There can be also marked variation in shape and size of cells and of their cytoplasmic processes. There may be cytological differences within the tumor, depending on regional anatomical involvement. Trapped neurons are often identified. Another histological variant is the less common gemistocytic astrocytoma, which consists of mostly large, irregular, globoid cells with eccentric nuclei and abundant, well-delineated, homogeneous eosinophilic cytoplasm with

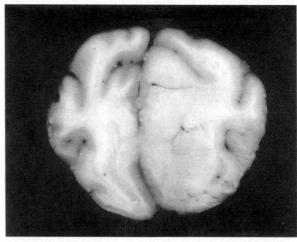

A

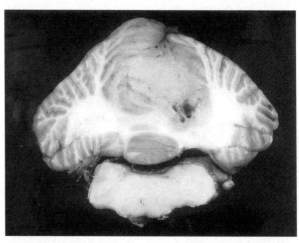

B

Fig. 14.1. Astrocytoma. **A.** Transverse section of a brain from a 9-year-old dog with a diffuse, low grade, fibrillary astrocytoma in the right frontal cortex. Note the enlargement and blurring of normal anatomical boundaries by the astrocytoma with the associated left midline shift. **B.** Transverse section of the brain of a dog with a well-demarcated gemistocytic astrocytoma in the cerebellum.

short, thick, intertwining processes (fig. 14.2 B). Their abundant cytoplasm is strongly positive for glial fibrillary acidic protein (GFAP) (fig. 14.2 C). The canine pilocytic variant is composed of fusiform cells within a dense fibrillary network. There can be other areas with a looser microcystic background. Compared with the human tumors, Rosenthal fibers are rare. In the rare protoplasmic type, cells are of small to medium size with poorly defined cytoplasmic borders and round, open faced nuclei, with a dispersed chromatic pattern and a prominent nucleolus. Numerous neuroglial fibrils and cytoplasmic processes are prominent in a microcystic background.[5] There is a low mitotic index (< 1/HP field) in all three variants of diffuse well-differentiated astrocytomas. Their proliferative index by MIB-1 staining is less than 3 percent.

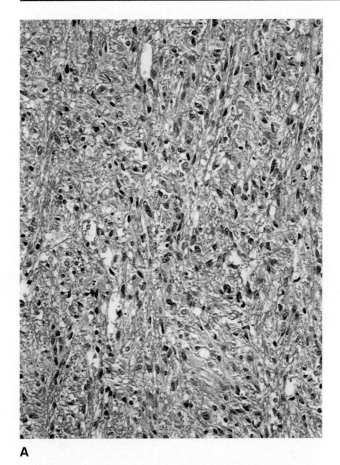

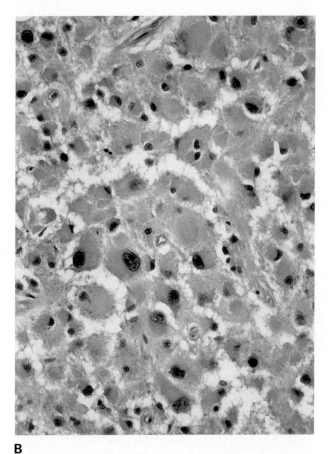

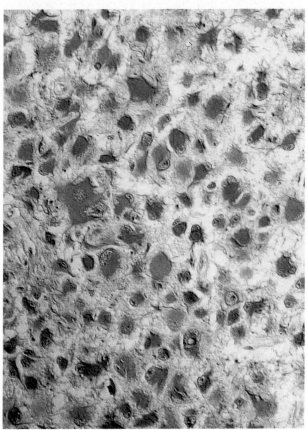

Fig. 14.2. Astrocytoma. **A.** Canine fibrillary astrocytoma with diffuse infiltration and low cellularity. **B.** Canine gemistocytic astrocytoma whose cells have abundant eosinophilic cytoplasm and eccentric nuclei. **C.** GFAP positive cell bodies in a gemistocytic astrocytoma.

Anaplastic Astrocytoma

These astrocytomas contain a pleomorphic more dense cell population consisting of fusiform, polygonal, or round shaped cells of variable sizes, often with distinct nuclear atypia; single and multinucleate giant cells may also be present (fig. 14.3). Nuclei are mostly larger than in differentiated astrocytomas and more hyperchromatic. There are also frequent mitoses (> 3/HP field). Anaplastic astrocytomas are highly cellular, fast growing, and infiltrative.

Glioblastoma multiforme

This rare tumor is also characterized by marked cellular pleomorphism, nuclear atypia, giant cell formation, a high mitotic index, and infiltrative growth similar to the anaplastic astrocytoma (fig. 14.4 A). Additionally, in human glioblastoma multiforme histological hallmarks are the serpentine foci of necrosis, with pseudopalisading when surrounded by radiating glial cells (fig. 14.4 B). Another distinguishing feature is the microvascular proliferations that occur mostly in the vicinity of necrotic foci or along the tumor margins (fig. 14.4 B).[1,14] Secondary structures of Scherer reflecting the migratory ability of high grade

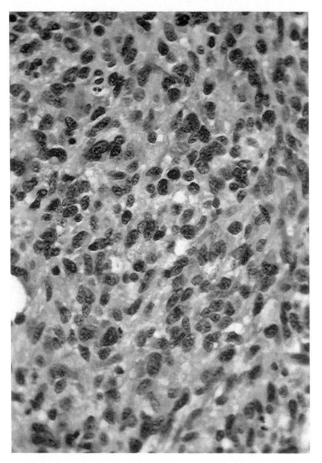

Fig. 14.3. Astrocytoma. Anaplastic astrocytoma with increased cellularity, hyperchromatic pleomorphic cells with nuclear atypia.

astrocytomas include neuronal satellitosis (fig. 14.4 C) and perivascular (fig. 14.4 C), subpial, and subependymal tumor cell infiltration.[4]

The term *glioblastoma multiforme* is actually a misnomer since it is not a tumor of glioblasts but of poorly differentiated astrocytes. The name *glioblastoma* is, however, so deeply ingrained within the vocabulary of neurologists, neurosurgeons, and neuropathologists that the WHO International Classification Committee decided to retain

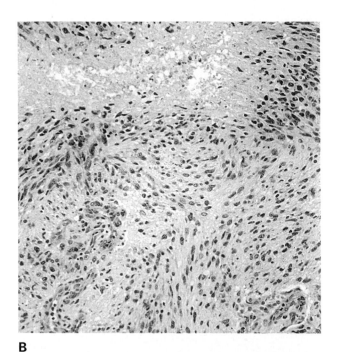

B

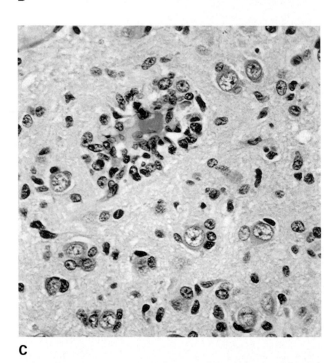

A   **C**

Fig. 14.4. Astrocytoma. **A.** Highly anaplastic astrocytoma (glioblastoma multiforme) with marked nuclear atypia and cellular pleomorphism. **B.** Characteristic serpentine necrosis with peripheral palisading and microvascular proliferation in a glioblastoma multiforme. **C.** Glioblastoma with neuronal satellitosis and perivascular infiltration by migratory neoplastic cells.

"glioblastoma multiforme" as another term for "high grade astrocytoma."[1] This recommendation has been followed in a recent classification of primary CNS tumors in animals.[5]

Cytology

The morphological appearance of smear preparations varies with the histological subtype; distinguishing features are the hypercellularity, nuclear atypia, and cytoplasmic processes with prominent fibrillarity (fig. 14.5). There is often a dense intertwining network formed by these processes, which often abut blood vessels. The nuclei tend to be larger, more irregular, more basophilic, and more pleomorphic than those of normal or reactive astrocytes. Reactive astrocytosis is usually a mixture of fibrillary and gemistocytic types with radiating processes, and it is less cellular than an astrocytoma.

Immunohistochemistry

A reliable marker for the identification of astrocytes is glial fibrillary acidic protein (GFAP), which is the main component of astrocytic intermediate filaments. Immuno-

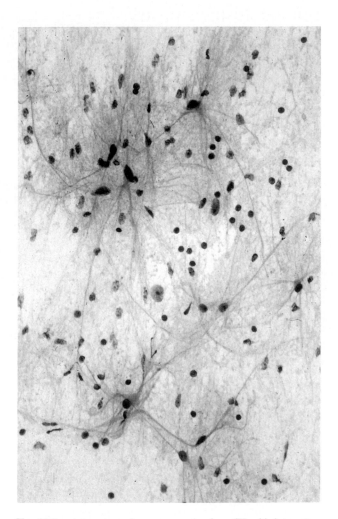

Fig. 14.5. Astrocytoma. Smear preparation from CT-guided stereotactic biopsy of an astrocytoma with increased cellularity, cellular pleomorphism, and prominent fibrillary processes.

cytochemical detection of GFAP is commonly used for the identification of normal, reactive, and neoplastic human and animal astrocytes. A large number of cells express GFAP in well-differentiated astrocytomas (e.g., fibrillary or gemistocytic astrocytomas) (see fig. 14.2 C), with less expression found in more anaplastic subtypes. Proliferative indices (e.g., MIB-1 staining) vary between 4 and 20 percent in low and high grade astrocytomas, respectively. Vimentin staining of astrocytomas is usually positive.

Differential Diagnosis

Confusion may occur between diffuse low grade and anaplastic astrocytomas and the so-called canine microgliomatosis.[3] The former tumors can be confirmed with positive staining for either GFAP or glutamine synthetase. The latter designation awaits confirmation as an entity.

Oligodendroglioma

Incidence and Sites

These tumors are derived from oligodendrocytes. Their overall incidence in dogs ranges from 5 to 12 percent, although they are reported to be the most common primary canine CNS tumor in one large European collection.[2] This difference may simply reflect a higher proportion of brachycephalic breeds in that series since oligodendrogliomas and other glial tumors have a relatively much higher frequency [at least 23 times greater] in brachycephalic breeds (e.g., boxers, Boston terriers, bull dogs, etc.) than in other breeds.[3,6] Oligodendrogliomas are generally located in the white or gray matter of the cerebral hemispheres, with decreasing frequency caudally from the olfactory bulbs and frontal, temporal, and piriform lobes to the parietal and occipital areas. Oligodendrogliomas rarely occur in the brain stem or spinal cord.[6] They are very rare in cats, horses, and cattle.[2,3,7-11]

Gross Morphology

Oligodendrogliomas are often large, generally with a grayish-blue, often gelatinous or mucoid, translucent matrix (fig. 14.6 A). On section, they are usually well demarcated, soft, and gray to pink, and they may break through the cortical surface. Intraventricular growth from local extension is common. In the cat there also can be extensive invasion of the meninges. Oligodendrogliomas can have multifocal areas of hemorrhage, yellowish to white areas of necrosis, and gelatinous cystic foci (fig. 14.6 B).

Histological Features

Oligodendrogliomas usually form dense sheets of uniform cells (fig. 14.7 A) but can be arranged in long straight or curving cords or in clusters (fig. 14.7 B). With a short interval before fixation, the cells have an irregular hyperchromatic nuclei set in a lightly staining cytoplasm with prominent cytoplasmic borders (fig. 14.7 C). A perinuclear halo effect is common with delayed fixation

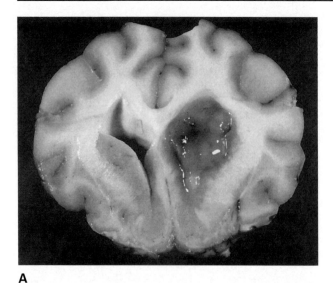

A

B

Fig. 14.6. Oligodendroglioma. **A.** Canine oligodendroglioma with the characteristic shiny gelatinous, mucoid transparent matrix. Note the sharp border of demarcation and intraventricular growth. **B.** An anaplastic canine oligodendroglioma with intratumoral necrosis and hemorrhage.

and results in the essentially artifactual but classically described "honeycomb" cell pattern (fig. 14.7 D). There is commonly a prominent microvascular proliferation, with the formation of vascular loops or glomerular-like tufts, often arranged in long lines or clusters, at the margins of or throughout the tumor (fig. 14.7 A,B). In more anaplastic tumors, there are also dilated thin-walled vessels near areas of hemorrhage. Variably sized foci of mineralization sometimes occur in tumors in both dogs and cats. Histologically the edges of the tumor are generally very sharp and discrete. There is minimal parenchymal reaction at the tumor margins, but neuronal satellitosis and perivascular accumulation of tumor cells can be prominent. Multifocal microcystic areas containing blue-staining, mucinous-like material and foci of recent hemorrhage may be found

(fig. 14.8). The tumors may also grow by extension along or through the leptomeninges and ependymal surfaces. Associated with intraventricular growth there can be widespread intraventricular metastases, with tumor foci impinging upon the ependymal surface or invading the underlying neuropil.

More anaplastic oligodendrogliomas are characterized by larger, more irregular, and less basophilic nuclei, a denser cytoplasm with scant vacuolization and increased mitoses (1-2/HP field). Microvascular proliferations tend to be more prominent. There are often areas of necrosis with peripheral glial cell palisading very similar to those seen in the more anaplastic astrocytomas.

Cytology

The most distinctive feature at low magnification is the formation of glomeruloid-like microvascular loops of varying size proliferating segmentally along blood vessels (fig. 14.9). Neoplastic oligodendrocytes are generally dispersed throughout the smear and have uniformly round nuclei with minimal eosinophilic cytoplasm with sharp borders.

Immunohistochemistry

There are no antibodies for specific markers for oligodendrogliomas that have been formalin fixed and paraffin embedded. The microvascular proliferations are partially composed of layers of factor VIII–related antigen positive cells. Most of the remaining cells have positive cytoplasmic staining for smooth muscle actin. In human glioblastomas, this smooth muscle cell hyperplasia has been correlated with platelet derived growth factors produced from tumor cells.[12] Canine oligodendrogliomas do not express myelin basic protein or myelin associated glycoprotein by immunostaining, although fresh-frozen tissue will stain positively with antibodies to galactocerebroside.[13] Intratumoral reactive gemistocytic astrocytes, presumably present as a result of entrapment, can be demonstrated in small numbers immunocytochemically.[13] Minigemistocytes may be part of the tumor cell phenotype.[8] The proliferation index, as determined by MIB-1 staining, varies between 2 and 15 percent in well-differentiated and anaplastic subtypes, respectively.

Ultrastructure

Ultrastructurally, oligodendrogliomas have no distinguishing features. Their cytoplasm contains sparse microtubules with few organelles. Structural myelin formation has not been found. Desmosomal junctions are common between cells.

Differential Diagnosis

The main differential diagnosis that needs to be considered, particularly in a tumor with intraventricular growth, is the central neurocytoma, but this rare tumor has so far only been identified in people.[14] Neurocytomas are

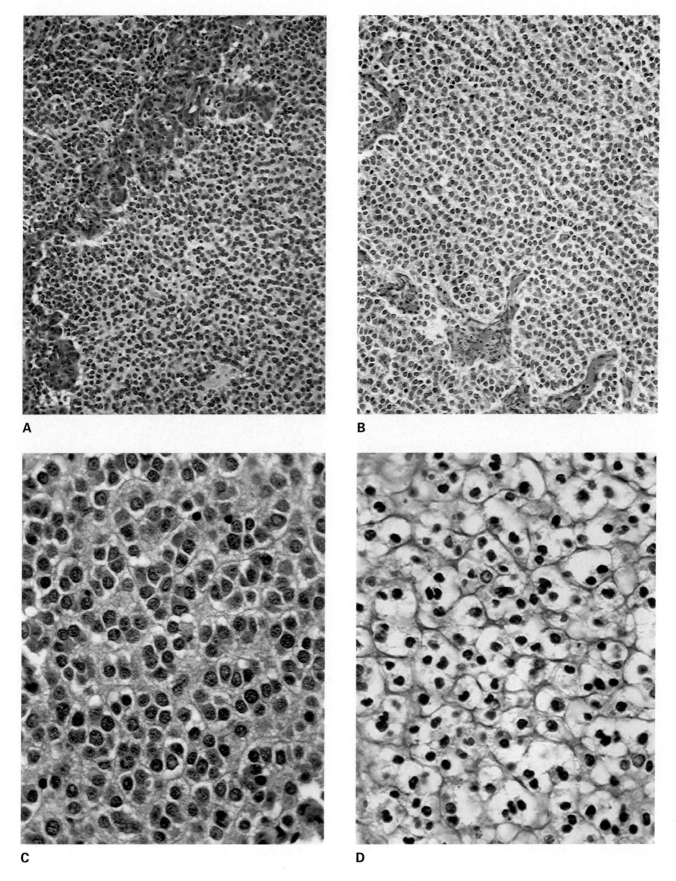

Fig. 14.7. **A.** A canine oligodendroglioma with sheets of round uniform cells and a line of microvascular proliferation. **B.** Oligodendrogliomas often have cells arranged in long lines, chords, or clusters. Note the characteristic microvascular proliferation. **C.** An oligodendroglioma with round uniform nuclei, eosinophilic cytoplasm and sharp cytoplasmic borders fixed after a very short (5 minute) postmortem interval. **D.** The classical honeycomb pattern described for oligodendrogliomas is an artifact of prolonged autolysis.

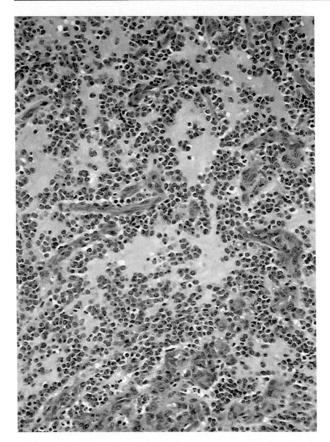

Fig. 14.8. Interstitial mucin-like microcystic lakes of varying size are often found in well-differentiated oligodendrogliomas.

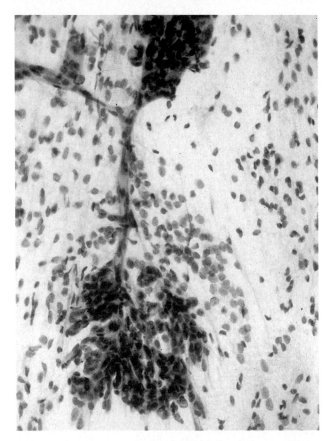

Fig. 14.9. A smear preparation from an oligodendroglioma with characteristic focal microvascular proliferations and evenly dispersed tumor cells.

strongly positive for synaptophysin and other neuronal markers and thus can be reliably differentiated from oligodendrogliomas. In the dog oligoastrocytomas have prominent areas of oligodendroglial differentiation.

Mixed Gliomas: Oligoastrocytoma

Several rare tumor types of glial origin are listed in classification tables of CNS tumors, but only one type occurs frequently enough to be worth including here with domestic animal neoplasms. Oligoastrocytoma is classified as a mixed glioma and is the most common subtype of this class. Grossly mixed gliomas may present either as a diffuse astrocytoma (see fig. 14.1 A) or as a more demarcated mass (fig. 14.10 A). It is a composite glial tumor consisting of both astrocytic and oligodendrocytic cell elements. These two cell types may be about equally admixed or they may appear juxtaposed in separate clusters (fig. 14.10 B). In canine oligoastrocytomas, oligodendroglioma cells are mostly in the majority. The astrocytic component can be strongly GFAP positive (fig. 14.10 C). It can be difficult to determine whether the astrocytic element consists of neoplastic astrocytes or whether they are just reactive, proliferating, regional astrocytes in an oligodendroglioma. In the latter case the number of astrocytes within the tumor is generally less than 30 percent of the total cell population of the neoplasm.

REFERENCES

1. Kliehues P., and Cavenee, W.K. (2000) *Tumors of the Nervous System: Pathology and Genetics. WHO Classification of Tumours.* 2nd ed. IARC Press, Lyon, pp. 9-52.
 2. Luginbühl, H., Fankhauser, R., McGrath, J.T. (1968) Spontaneous neoplasms of the nervous system in animals. *Prog Neurol Surg* 2:85-164.
 3. Summers, B.A., Cummings, J.F., and de Lahunta, A. (1995) *Veterinary Neuropathology.* Mosby, St. Louis, MO, pp. 362-373.
 4. Scherer, H.J. (1940) The forms of growth in gliomas and their significance. *Brain* 63:1-35.
 5. Koestner, A., Bilzer, T., Fatzer, R., Schulmer, F.Y.S., Summers, B.A., and Van Winkle, T.J. (1999) Histological classification of the tumors of the nervous system of domestic animals. In *International Histological Classification of Tumors of Domestic Animals.* 2nd series, vol. V. AFIP, Washington, D.C., pp. 1-71.
 6. Hayes, K.C., and Schiefer, B. (1969) Primary tumors in the CNS of carnivores. *Vet Pathol* 6:94-116.
 7. Wilson, R.B., and Beckman, S.L. (1995) Mucinous oligodendroglioma of the spinal cord in a dog. *J Amer Anim Hosp Assoc* 31:26-28.
 8. Dickinson, P.J., Keel, M.K., Higgins, R.J., Koblik, P.D., LeCouteur, R.A., Naydan, D.K., Bollen, A.W., Vernau, W. (2000) Clinical and pathological features of oligodendrogliomas in two cats. *Vet Pathol* 37:160-167.
 9. Reppas, G.P., and Harper, C.G. (1996) Sudden unexpected death in a horse due to a cerebral oligodendroglioma. *Equine Vet J* 28:163-165.
10. Baker, J.R., and Kippax, I.S. (1980) An oligodendroglioma in a bull. *Vet Rec* 107:42

11. Innes, J.R.M., and Saunders, L.Z. (1962) *Comparative Neuropathology*. Academic Press,London, pp. 85-98.

12. Haddad, S.F., Moore, S.A., Schelper, R.L., and Goeken, J.A. (1992) Vascular smooth muscle hyperplasia underlies the formation of glomeruloid vascular structures of glioblastoma multiforme. *J Neuropathol Exp Neurol* 51:488-492.

13. Vandevelde, M., Fankhauser, R., and Luginbuhl, H. (1985) Immunocytochemical studies in canine neuroectodermal brain tumors. *Acta Neuropathol* 66:111-116.

14. Burger, P.C., and Scheithauer, B.W. (1993) Tumors of the central nervous system. In *Atlas of Tumor Pathology*. 3rd series, Fasc 10. Armed Forces Institute of Pathology, Washington, D.C., pp. 178-184.

Tumors of the Ependyma and Choroid Plexus

Ependymoma

Incidence and Sites

Ependymomas are derived from cells lining the ventricular system of the central nervous system. Ependymomas have been reported in dogs, cats, cattle, and horses but are rare tumors.[1-10] Possible atypical ependymomas have been described in cattle.[9] Ependymomas occur mainly within the lateral ventricles, less often in the third and fourth ventricles, and rarely within the central canal of the spinal cord.[1]

Gross Morphology

Ependymomas are generally large intraventricular masses, mostly well demarcated, gray to red, with a smooth texture in the dog (fig. 14.11 A) but much more granular in the cat (fig. 14.11 B). There can be intratumoral cystic areas, necrosis, and focal hemorrhage. Although growth is usually intraventricular, ependymomas may infiltrate the adjacent neuropil. A secondary obstructive hydrocephalus may develop.

Histological Features

Cellular and papillary forms comprise the two major subtypes of ependymomas. The cellular ependymomas are moderately to densely cellular and well vascularized, with characteristic nuclear-free perivascular zones formed by tumor cell processes (fig. 14.12 A). These perivascular zones appear fibrillated and lead to the formation of pseudorosettes. The tumor cells are clustered without any orientation between the blood vessels. In contrast, feline cellular ependymomas are densely cellular, have minimal cytoplasm with darkly staining basophilic nuclei, and have more obvious perivascular pseudorosettes and ependymal rosettes than in the canine tumor (fig. 14.12 B). Ependymal rosette formation, most common in feline ependymomas, results from a radially arranged pattern of tumor cells centered around a miniature ependymal lumen (fig. 14.12 B,C). These lumens sometimes contain cilia whose anchoring blepharoblasts stain as dark blue dots with the phosphotungstic acid hematoxylin stain (fig. 14.12 C). Between the ependymal rosettes and the pseudorosette formations there are solid

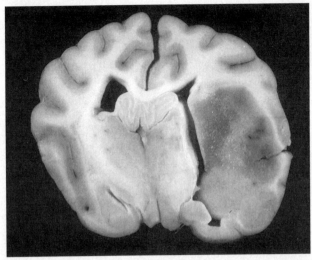

A

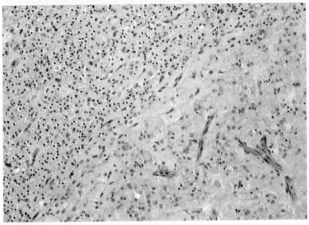

B

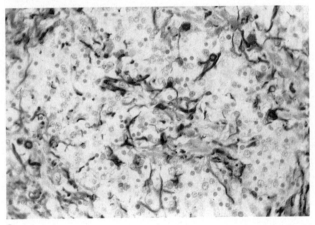

C

Fig. 14.10. **A.** A canine mixed glial tumor (oligoastrocytoma) with demarcated borders. **B.** Note the distinct areas of juxtaposed astroctytic and oligodendroglial differentiation. **C.** Note the positive GFAP staining of the astrocytic component.

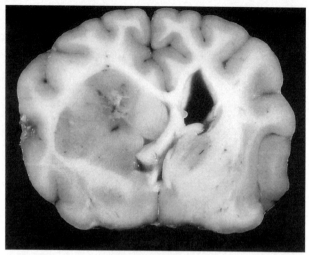

A

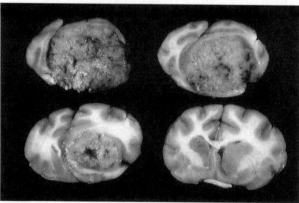

B

Fig. 14.11. Ependymoma. **A.** An intraventricular canine ependymoma with a solid appearance, grayish white color, a central area of necrosis and a well-demarcated border. **B.** A feline ependymoma, which usually has a more granular appearance than its canine counterpart.

sheets or clusters of cells without any pattern. Tumor cells contain round to ovoid nuclei and have an eosinophilic fibrillar cytoplasm with poorly defined borders. Nuclei are moderately hyperchromatic with a prominent nucleolus and punctate heterochromatin.

The papillary subtype of ependymoma in the dog, cat, and horse has a vascular core forming papillae whose surfaces are covered by single or multiple layers of columnar cells arranged in a pseudorosette pattern (fig. 14.12 D). Fibrillated or globular GFAP positive processes stream toward the central core. Ependymal rosettes are rare. A tanycytic subtype has been reported in a cat.[10] Malignant ependymomas are characterized by anaplasia, frequent mitoses (4/HP field), necrosis, and local neuropil invasion. In a calf an ependymoblastoma, interpreted as a poorly differentiated ependymoma, was diagnosed on the basis of age, the small round cells, and numerous mitotic figures.[6]

Cytology

Both cellular and papillary ependymomas have a distinctive appearance due to the formation of a highly branching vasculature with layers of perivascular palisading tumor cells. These cells have a polar nuclear location and elongated cytoplasmic attachments radially arranged around blood vessels. Individual cells have long tapered to oblong unipolar cytoplasm with distinctive processes.[11]

Immunohistochemistry

Well-differentiated ependymomas have a uniform and consistent cytoplasmic GFAP immunoreactivity.[7,13] Vimentin is also expressed uniformly but less intensely, while cytokeratin staining is negative.

Ultrastructure

Ependymomas contain large numbers of intermediate filaments, sometimes arranged in a whorling pattern.[7] Adjacent cells are connected by prominent desmosomal junctions of varying lengths (fig. 14.13). These junctions are most dense near the lumens of true rosettes. Microvilli and normally configured cilia protrude into the lumen of true rosettes, particularly in cats (fig. 14.13). Cilia extend from blepharoblasts. The basal poles of the cells rest on a basal lamina of vascular origin and are anchored there by hemidesmosomes.[7]

Differential Diagnosis

The differentiation between the papillary subtype of ependymoma and an anaplastic choroid plexus tumor may be difficult on H&E stained sections. True rosettes are present only in ependymomas. Together, the positive GFAP and negative cytokeratin immunostaining in ependymomas are the most reliable criteria for diagnosis.[7,12] Choroid plexus tumors stain positively for cytokeratins and possibly for transthyretin.[12,13] The choroid plexus tumor also has a fibrovascular stroma, while GFAP positive glial processes abut the vasculature in ependymomas. The spinal thoracolumbar tumor of young dogs has been commonly misdiagnosed as an ependymoma. Ependymomas can also be confused with neuroblastomas, but the latter have neuroblastic (Homer-Wright) rosettes and neuroblastomas may also stain positively with neuronal-specific cell markers.[13]

REFERENCES

1. Luginbühl, H., Fankhauser, R., and Mc Grath, J.T. (1968) Spontaneous neoplasms of the nervous system in animals. *Prog Neurol Surg* 2:85-164.
2. Fankhauser, R., Luginbühl, H., and McGrath, J.T. (1974) Tumors of the nervous system. *Bull WHO* 50:(1-2): pp. 53-70.
3. Ingwersen, W., Groom, S., and Parent, J. (1989) Vestibular syndrome associated with an ependymoma in a cat. *J Amer Vet Med Assoc* 195:98-100.
4. Fox, J.G., Snyder, S.B., Reed, C., and Campbell, L.H. (1973) Malignant ependymoma in a cat. *J Small Anim Pract* 14:23-26.

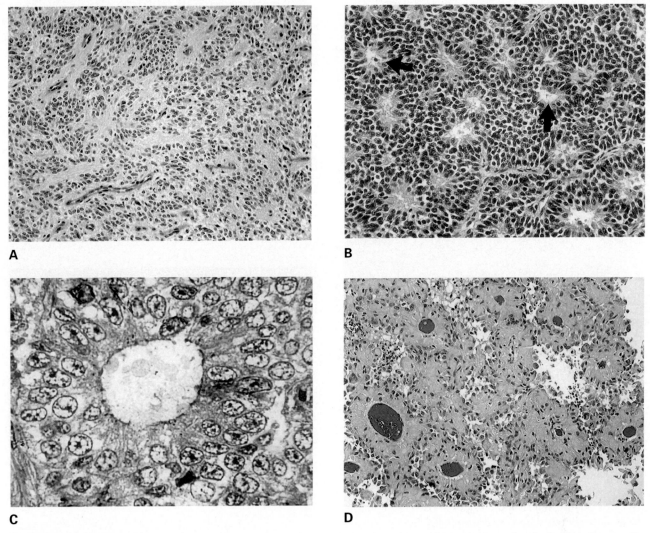

Fig. 14.12. **A.** A canine cellular ependymoma with prominent anuclear fibrillated perivascular zones between clusters of randomly oriented tumor cells. **B.** A feline ependymoma with perivascular palisading of tumor cells in both longitudinal and transverse orientation. Note also the prominent ependymal rosettes (arrows). **C.** An ependymal rosette of radially arranged tumor cells forming a central lumen. Blepharoblasts are prominent. **D.** An equine papillary ependymoma with cells radiating from a fibrillated anuclear vascular core. Nuclei are located peripherally.

5. Zaki, F.A., and Hurvitz, A.I. (1976) Spontaneous neoplasms of the cat. *J Small Anim Pract* 17:773-782.

6. Saunders, G.K. (1984) Ependymoblastoma in a dairy calf. *Vet Pathol* 21:528-529.

7. Carrigan, M.J., Higgins, R.J., Carlson, G.P., and Naydan, D.K. (1996) Equine papillary ependymoma. *Vet Pathol* 33:77-80.

8. Heath, S.E., Peter, A.T., Janovitz, E.B., Selvakumar, R., and Sandusky, G.E. (1995) Ependymoma of the neurohypophysis and hypernatremia in a horse. *J Amer Vet Med Assoc* 207:738-741.

9. McGill, I.S., and Wells, G.A.H. (1993) Neuropathological findings in cattle with clinically suspect but histologically unconfirmed bovine spongiform encephalopathy (BSE). *J Comp Pathol* 108:241-260.

10. Mckay, J.S., Targett, M.P., and Jeffrey, N.D. (1999) Histological characterisation of an ependymoma in the fourth ventricle of a cat. *J Comp Pathol* 120:105-113.

11. Vernau, K.M., Higgins, R.J., Bollen, A.W., Jimenez, D.F., Anderson, J.V., Koblik, P.D., and LeCouteur, R.A. (2001) Primary canine and feline nervous system tumors: Intraoperative diagnosis using the smear technique. *Vet Pathol* 38:47-57.

12. Vandevelde, M., Fankhauser, R., and Luginbuhl, H. (1985) Immunocytochemical studies in canine neuroectodermal brain tumors. *Acta Neuropathol* 66:111-116.

13. Burger, P.C., and Scheithauer, B.W. (1993) Tumors of the nervous system. In *Atlas of Tumor Pathology.* 3rd series, fasc. 10. Armed Forces Institute of Pathology, Washington, D.C., pp. 121-136.

Choroid Plexus Papilloma and Carcinoma

Incidence and Sites

These intraventricular tumors are derived from choroid plexus epithelium. The incidence of choroid plexus tumors is about 9 percent of all primary CNS tumors. They occur primarily in the dog but have been recognized rarely in the cat, horse, and cow.[1-5] Choroid plexus tumors can affect dogs 18 months and older, but generally affect those over 4 years of age. In one small series, they occurred almost three times more often in male than in female dogs.[1] There is no breed predilection. They may arise from the choroid plexi of the lateral,

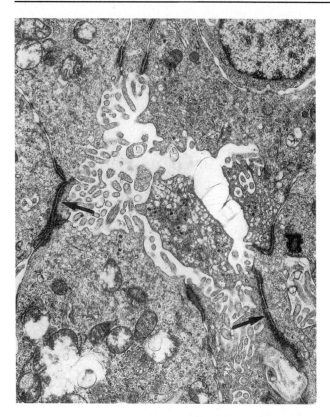

Fig. 14.13. An electronmicrograph of an ependymal rosette with microvilli and cilia protruding into the lumen. There are prominent, long, desmosomal-like attachments between the apical poles of the tumor cells (arrows).

third, or fourth ventricles. Besides local compression, these tumors may cause hydrocephalus by ventricular obstruction or possibly by excessive production of cerebrospinal fluid.

Gross Morphology

Choroid plexus papillomas are well-defined, nonencapsulated, grayish, white to red, granular or cauliflower-like masses either within a ventricle (fig. 14.14 A) or growing out into the cerebellopontine angle when arising from the plexus of the fourth ventricle (fig. 14.14 B). Plexus carcinomas may infiltrate locally from primary or metastatic foci into the adjacent neuropil through the ependymal lining. In the dog, widespread metastases may disseminate within cerebrospinal fluid pathways, especially in the spinal cord from a primary site in the brain (fig. 14.15).

Histological Features

Most of the choroid plexus tumors are papillomas. Their projection alone into the cerebellopontine angle does not define them as carcinomas. The typical architecture of the choroid plexus papilloma is the branching arboriform pattern, with a single layer of cuboidal or columnar cells covering a modest fibrovascular vascular stroma of lep-

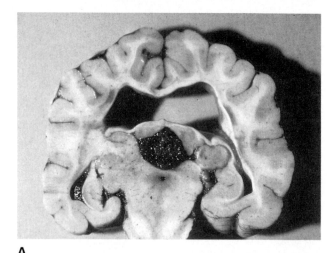

A

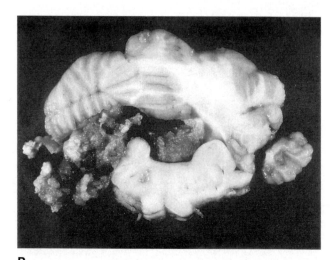

B

Fig. 14.14. Choroid plexus tumor. **A.** Choroid plexus papilloma in the third ventricle of a dog. Note the associated obstructive hydrocephalus proximally and the loss of the septum pellucidum. **B.** Choroid plexus papilloma in the fourth ventricle of a dog with local extension into the cerebellopontine angle.

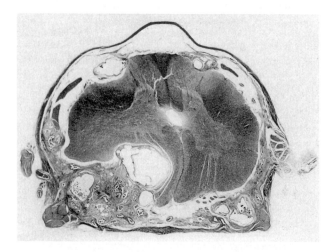

Fig. 14.15. Spinal cord of a dog with a primary choroid plexus carcinoma of the fourth ventricle with multiple metastatic foci resulting from spread within CSF pathways.

tomeningeal derivation (fig. 14.16 A). Edema, hemor-rhage, some necrosis, and mineralization can occur. Mitoses in these tumors are uncommon. Choroid plexus carcinomas are rare. They are distinguished from papillomas by cellular pleomorphism, nuclear atypia (fig. 14.17 A), frequent mitoses, and/or local invasion (fig. 14.16 B) and metastatic behavior within cerebrospinal fluid pathways. Metastases may occur within the ventricular system distant from the primary site (fig. 14.15).

Cytology

On smear preparations, papillomas form rafts of cells between which are evenly dispersed individual cells. The cells have abundant cytoplasm with round nuclei and may also line up in columns or form papillary fronds around a vascular core.

Immunohistochemistry

The most definitive immunocytochemical markers for the epithelial component of choroid plexus tumors are cytokeratins (fig. 14.17 B).[1] Any GFAP reactivity is extremely rare.

Differential Diagnosis

For most papillomas a histological diagnosis can be easily made. However, there may be some confusion between anaplastic choroid plexus carcinomas and papil-lary ependymomas. Choroid plexus tumors have a GFAP negative collagenous stroma, in contrast to the uniformly GFAP positive glial stroma of ependymomas. Thus cytokeratins and GFAP are reliable markers for differentiating choroid plexus tumors from ependymomas. Cilia have been reported ultrastructurally in both human choroid plexus tumors and ependymomas and therefore cannot be reliably used to differentiate between these tumors. Detailed ultrastructural studies have not been reported in animal choroid plexus tumors. Transthyretin (TTR) is described as an epithelial marker for some human choroid plexus tumors, but it is also present in some metastatic carcinomas of extraneural origin.[6] The application of TTR to animal choroid plexus tumors has not been reported.

REFERENCES

1. Luginbühl, H., Fankhauser, R., and McGrath, J.T. (1968) Spontaneous neoplasms of the nervous system in animals. In *Progress in Neurological Surgery.* Vol. 2. Karger, Basel, Chicago, pp. 85-164.
2. Ribas, J.L., Mena, H., Braund, K.G., Sesterhenn, I.A., and Toivio-Kinnucan, M. (1989) A histologic and immunocytochemical study of choroid plexus tumors in the dog. *Vet Pathol* 26:55-64.
3. Zaki, F.A., and Nafe, L.A. (1980) Choroid plexus tumors in the dog. *J Amer Vet Med Assoc* 176:328-330.
4. Summers, B.A., Cummings, J.F., and de Lahunta, A. (1995) *Veterinary Neuropathology.* Mosby, St. Louis, MO, pp. 373-375.

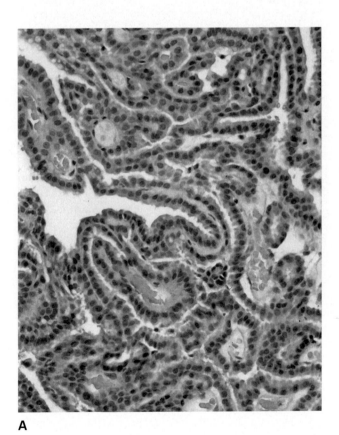

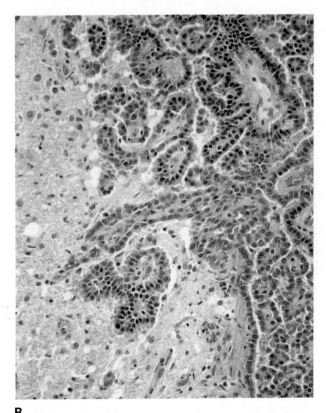

A   B

Fig. 14.16. **A.** Choroid plexus papilloma with arboriform pattern mimicking normal choroid plexus. **B.** Choroid plexus carcinoma with aggressive infiltration of adjacent neuropil.

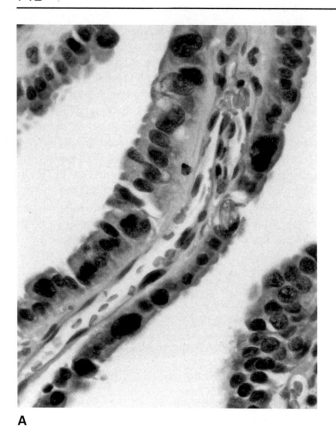

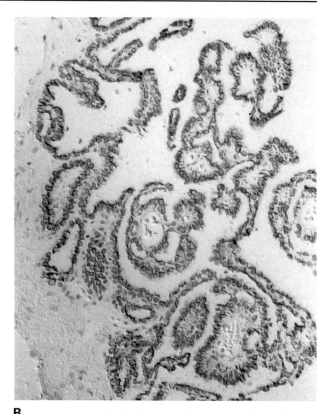

A

B

Fig. 14.17. **A.** Nuclear atypia in a choroid plexus carcinoma. **B.** Positive immunocytochemical staining for cytokeratins expressed in the cytoplasm of epithelial cells of a choroid plexus carcinoma.

5. Pirie, R.S., Mayhew, I.G., Clarke, C.J., and Tremaine, W.H. (1998) Ultrasonigraphic confirmation of a space occupying lesion in the brain of a horse: Choroid plexus papilloma. *Equine Vet J* 30:445-448.
6. Albrecht, S., Rouah, E., Becker, L.E., and Bruner, J. (1991) Transthyretin immunoreactivity in choroid plexus neoplasms and brain metastases. *Mod Pathol* 4:610-614.

Neuronal and Mixed Neuronal-Glial Tumors

Only neuronal tumors of adult animals are included in this section, following the WHO human classification scheme. The more frequent tumors of neuronal origin in young animals are discussed under embryonal neoplasms.

Gangliocytoma

Incidence and Sites

Only three such tumors have been reported. All three were in mature dogs and were located in the cerebellum.[1-3] A similar lesion, called a dysplastic gangliocytoma, was described in a horse.[4]

Gross Morphology

The gangliocytoma is described as a solid, soft, grayish mass replacing a segment of the cerebellum. Depending on the tumor size, adjacent cerebellar structures and the fourth ventricle may be compressed.

Histological Features

An almost monomorphic cell population of large cells resembling mature pyramidal cells (fig. 14.18) characterizes gangliocytomas. The cytoplasm is either homogeneously eosinophilic or vacuolated. The large nuclei are round to oval and contain one or two prominent nucleoli. Some tumor cells may be bi- or multinucleated. The cells have multiple processes that can be better visualized by silver impregnation stains. Mitotic figures are rare or absent. The tumor grows by local expansion. In the PNS the ganglioneuroma is the counterpart of the gangliocytoma.

Immunohistochemistry

The tumor cells usually react with one or more neuronal markers such as synaptophysin, triple neurofilament proteins, and/or neuron specific enolase (NSE). GFAP immunoreactivity is seen when astrocytic stromal cells are a constituent of the gangliocytoma.

Ganglioglioma

Incidence and Sites

This is a rare tumor in humans as well as in animals. Only one case has been reported, and that tumor was in the spinal cord of a calf[5]; however, the tumor also occurs in the

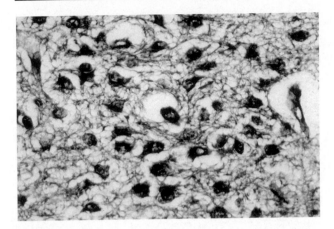

Fig. 14.18. Gangliocytoma in the cerebellum of a 6-year-old German shepherd dog. Consists of a fairly monomorphic population of medium sized neuronal cells. (Courtesy of Dr. Abraham Nyska, Kimron Veterinary Institute, Israel).

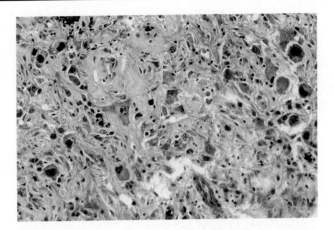

Fig. 14.19. Ganglioglioma showing the mostly astrocytic component.

dog. The two canine cases in our collection were in a 5-year-old female doberman and an 8-year-old miniature poodle. Both had a history of epileptic seizures. Location of the tumors was in the frontal cortex in both cases.

Gross Morphology

Gangliogliomas are well-defined, sometimes lobulated, firm, homogeneous masses compressing the surrounding brain parenchyma. Focal calcification and cyst formation have been described in human gangliogliomas.

Histological Features

Since this is a mixed tumor consisting of neuronal and glial cell elements, the histological appearance varies depending upon the preponderant cellular component. Either neuronal or glial cells may predominate. In both cases in the dog, glial cells predominated (fig. 14.19). Astrocytic and oligodendrocytic cells are mostly intermingled, but clusters of astrocytic or oligodendroglial elements exist. The neuronal cells are well differentiated and form large nerve cells that occur in clusters. Immunohistochemical staining identifies the neuronal and astrocytic cell components. In both canine cases neuronal cells reacted positively with synaptophysin. In addition, neurofilament staining was positive in one case and NSE in the other. GFAP identified the distribution of astrocytic cells.

Olfactory Neuroblastoma (Esthesioneuroblastoma)

Olfactory neuroblastomas are composed of immature neuronal cells derived from a population of precursor neuroblasts of the nasal olfactory epithelium.

Incidence and Sites

These very rare tumors have been reported in dogs, cats, a monkey, horse, and a cow.[6-12] In cats and dogs, they

occupy the caudal nasal cavity unilaterally or bilaterally, are firmly attached to the ethmoid turbinates and nasal bones, and may extend into paranasal sinuses. Penetration through the cribriform plate results in intracranial extension into the frontal lobes. A canine olfactory ganglioneuroblastoma has been described.[13] In the cat, metastases have been found in regional lymph nodes.[7]

Gross Morphology

In the dog and cat, the tumors are usually uniformly soft and granular, pale yellow to gray and may have areas of necrosis and hemorrhage. Some may be divided into lobules by white firm trabeculae. Invasion of the brain can be associated with necrosis and regional edema.

Histological Features

The tumors are comprised of a highly cellular, uniform cell population, sometimes separated into islands or clusters by an arborising fibrovascular stroma. Cells may form pseudorosettes from peritrabecular and perivascular cell palisading (fig. 14.20). Nuclei are densely basophilic with fine, punctate chromatin and a basophilic nucleolus. Rosette formation with central lumens (Flexner-Wintersteiner type) (fig. 14.20) is more common than the neuroblastic rosettes (Homer-Wright type), which have elongate cells aligned radially around a central tangle of cell processes. Similar histological features occur in the metastases of the feline tumors.[7] In some canine tumors, there can be long, branching columns of epithelial-like, cytokeratin positive cells, sometimes forming microcysts, admixed with the typical neuroblastic cell population.

Immunocytochemistry

There can be variably positive immunocytochemical staining for synaptophysin, chromogranin A, and triple neurofilament protein expression. In the cat, tumor cells were also variably positive for NSE, S-100, and cytokeratins.[7, 8] Expression of vimentin and GFAP was consistently negative.

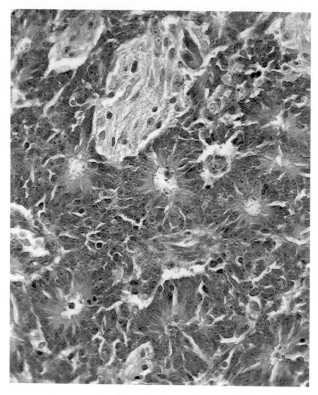

Fig. 14.20. Feline olfactory neuroblastoma (esthesioneuroblastoma) with dense sheets of cells with variable cytoplasm and dark-staining elongate nuclei. Distinctive features are the numerous Flexner-Wintersteiner rosettes and the perivascular pseudorosettes.

Ultrastructure

In the dog and cat, the most helpful diagnostic features were the 9-10 nm diameter intracytoplasmic neurofilaments, with their characteristic side arms, found particularly in cells forming neuroblastic rosettes. Occasional Flexner-Wintersteiner rosettes had intraluminal microvilli, while their cell apices were connected by long, multiple, dense desmosomal-like junctions.[6,7] In the cat, mature type C viral particles were seen both extracellularly and budding from the cisternae of the smooth endoplasmic reticulum. Integrated FeLV was identified by PCR in all feline nasal tumors.[7] These viral particles should not be confused with dense core vesicles.[8,9] There is no causal link established between FeLV and the feline olfactory neuroblastoma.

Differential Diagnosis

In the cat, olfactory neuroblastomas might be confused histologically with ependymomas since both form rosettes and perivascular pseudorosettes. Ependymomas, however, are strongly GFAP positive. Also, the neuroblastic rosettes (Homer-Wright) are distinctive for neuroblastomas; additionally, expression of the neuronal markers synaptophysin and triple neurofilament protein, detected immunocytochemically, also would confirm that diagnosis.[14] Ribbons of epithelial, cytokeratin positive cells, sometimes with microcyst formation, have also been

described in human neuroendocrine carcinoma-like tumors in this region.[14] Such tumors also must be differentiated immunocytochemically from nasal carcinomas.

REFERENCES

1. Nyska, A., et al. (1995) Intracranial gangliocytoma in a dog. *Vet Pathol* 32:190-192.
2. Dahne, E., and Schiefer, B. (1960) Intracranielle Geschwülste bei Tieren. *Zbl Vet Med* 7:341-363.
3. Luginbühl, H. (1962) Geschwülste des Zentralnervensystems bei Tieren (Tumors of the central nervous system in animals). *Acta Neuropathol, Suppl* 1:9-18.
4. Poss, M., and Young, S. (1987) Dysplastic disease of the cerebellum of an adult horse. *Acta Neuropathol (Berlin)* 75:205-211.
5. Roth, L., et al. (1987) Ganglioglioma of the spinal cord in a calf. *Vet Pathol* 24:188-189.
6. Dahme, E., Bilzer, T., and Mannl, A. (1985) Zur Diagnose primaerer Riechschleimhauttumoren, dargestellt an einem ästhesioneuroepitheliom beim Hund. *Tierärzt Prax (Suppl)* 1:112-122.
7. Schrenzel, M.D., Higgins, R.J., Hinrichs, S.H., Smith, M.O., and Torten, M. (1990) Type C retroviral expression in spontaneous feline olfactory neuroblastomas. *Acta Neuropathol* 80:547-553.
8. Cox, N.R., and Powers, R.D. (1989) Olfactory neuroblastomas in two cats. *Vet Pathol* 26:341-343.
9. Popischil, A., and Dahme, E. (1981) Neuroepitheliale Tumoren der Riechschleimhaut bei der Katze. *Zbl Vet Med A* 28:214-225.
10. Correa, P., Dalgard, D.W., and Adamson, R.H. (1975) Olfactory neuroepithelioma in a cynomologous monkey. *J Med Primatol* 4:51-61.
11. Luginbühl, H., Fankhauser, R., and McGrath, J.T. (1968) Spontaneous neoplasms of the nervous system in animals. *Prog Neurol Surg* 2:85-164.
12. Anderson, B.C., and Cordy, D.R. (1981) Olfactory neuroblastoma in a heifer. *Vet Pathol* 18:536-540.
13. Mattix, M.E., Mattix, R.J., Williams, B.H., Ribas, J.L., and Wilhelmsen, C.L. (1994) Olfactory ganglioneuroblastoma in a dog: A light, ultrastructural and immunohistochemical study. *Vet Pathol* 31:262-265.
14. Finkelstein, S.D., Hirose, T., and Vandenberg, S.R. (2000) Olfactory neuroblastoma. In Kliehues, P., and Cavenee, W.K. (eds.) *Pathology and Genetics of Tumours of the Nervous System.* IARC Press, Lyon, France, pp. 150-152.

Embryonal Tumors

The nomenclature of human embryonal neoplasms has been controversial because of the anaplastic nature of these tumors. Therefore it has been decided to consolidate this group of neoplasms under the single term *primitive neuroectodermal tumors* (PNETs).[1,2] This classification is based on the concept that they are all derived from a germinal neuroepithelial cell that has the potential to differentiate along a number of neuroectodermal cell lines, primarily neuronal, ependymal, and glial. There are, in addition, PNETs without specific differentiation and others with multi- or bipotential differentiation. This concept has been applied to a reclassification of domestic animal tumors, in which PNETs that can be specifically identified histogenetically will be specifically designated (e.g., medulloblastoma) and PNET will only be used as a generic term.[3]

Medulloblastoma

Incidence and Sites

While medulloblastomas are common malignant tumors of the cerebellum in children, they are much less frequently observed in young animals. They are chiefly seen in calves and puppies, but have been sporadically observed in pigs and cats.[4] They are currently considered to arise from the matrix cells of the external granular layer of the cerebellum.[4] They are exclusively located in the cerebellum.

Gross Morphology

Medulloblastomas are usually well confined, soft, grayish or pinkish masses unilaterally in the cerebellar cortex or centrally in the vermis, often extending into or compressing the fourth ventricle (fig. 14.21 A). Hydrocephalus is commonly linked to an expanding medulloblastoma.

Histological Features

The neoplasm is usually composed of a fairly uniform and closely packed round to polygonal cell population, often arranged in sheets or bands (fig. 14.21 B). Palisading of cells and complete or incomplete rosette formation are frequently observed. The round to elongated nuclei are hyperchromatic, and mitoses are frequent. There is mostly a scanty vascular stroma. Sometimes there can be paler staining islands of GFAP positive cells interspersed between the predominant medulloblastoma cells.

Immunohistochemistry

Depending upon their degree of differentiation, medulloblastomas may react with one or more neuronal markers. Positive staining for synaptophysin and triple neurofilament protein was more consistent than for NSE in our cases. GFAP reactivity depends upon the presence of astrocytic components that may be found in pale staining islands within the tumor. Some highly anaplastic medulloblastomas may not react with any neuronal or glial markers.

Neuroblastoma

The neuroblastoma is a rare neoplasm in animals. Neuroblastomas are presumably derived from surviving primitive neuroepithelial cells (embryonal remnants), not from dedifferentiation of mature cells. In the PNS these tumors are derived from neuroectodermal cells derived from the neural crest and destined for the adrenal medulla and autonomic nervous system. They show varying degrees of differentiation toward postmitotic neuroblasts.

Incidence and Sites

Neuroblastomas may occur in both the PNS and CNS. Peripheral neuroblastomas (of neural crest origin) have been reported as incidental small and localized lesions in adult slaughter cattle.[5,6] Malignant neuroblastomas have been reported in premature and stillborn calves as well as in dogs of various ages. They are usually located in the

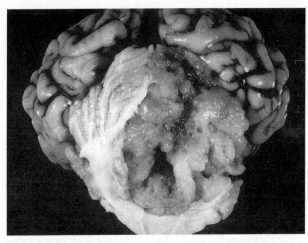

A

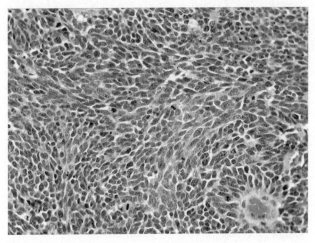

B

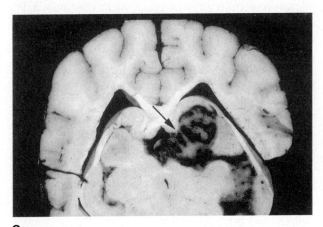

C

Fig. 14.21. **A.** A medulloblastoma in a newborn calf with the midline vermal and intraventricular growth pattern. **B.** Canine medulloblastoma with a dense population of closely packed, hyperchromatic, round to polygonal cells, often arranged in sheets or bands and with numerous mitotic figures. **C.** Canine cerebral neuroblastoma primarily in the thalamus (arrow).

adrenal medulla or in sympathetic gangli, although the primary site is often difficult to determine because of their rapid growth and spread.

Malignant neuroblastomas occur occasionally in the CNS in various locations including the cerebrum, brain stem, and spinal cord. Although mostly young dogs are affected, malignant neuroblastomas may also occur in mature animals. In our collection the youngest dog was 2 months old and the oldest 9 years.

Gross Morphology

Neuroblastomas appear as grayish soft to moderately firm nodules (fig. 14.21 C). Neuroblastomas in supratentorial CNS sites have the same histological appearance as medulloblastomas but are not further differentiated by location.

Histological Features

Neuroblastomas consist of a fairly uniform population of round to oval cells with large hyperchromatic nuclei and a moderate to high mitotic index. Cells often show a tendency toward palisading and neuroblastic (Homer-Wright) rosette formation. The histological similarity to medulloblastomas is often clearly apparent. All neuroblastomas in our series reacted positively to triple neurofilament protein or synaptophysin or both in some areas.

Other Primitive Neuroectodermal Tumors (PNETs)

In addition to the above PNETs specifically characterized by their location, histological features, and immunohistochemical staining (e.g., cerebellar medulloblastoma), there are less well-differentiated supratentorial PNETs that are more difficult to categorize. Some may reveal features of neuronal cells, such as neuroblastic (Homer-Wright) rosette formation, but lack reactivity to neuronal markers. Others are highly anaplastic but possess antigens to diverse types of markers. The latest WHO classification of human brain tumors considers the cerebral neuroblastoma and ependymoblastoma as supratentorial PNETs with neuronal and ependymal differentiation.[2] In some of these poorly differentiated CNS tumors in children or young animals the neuronal, ependymal, or glial origin can neither be confirmed nor excluded.[1] L.P Dehner expressed this dilemma best: "The PNET concept is a useful scheme to organize our understanding and reveal our shortcomings."[7]

REFERENCES

1. Hart, M.N., and Earle, K.M. (1973) Primitive neuroectodermal tumors of the brain in children. *Cancer* 32:890-897.
2. Rorke, L.B., Hart, M.N., and McLendon, R.E. (2000) Supratentorial primitive neuroectodermal tumour (PNET). In Kliehues, P., and Cavenee, W.K. (eds.), *Pathology and Genetics of Tumours of the Nervous System.* 2nd ed. IARC Press, Lyon, France, pp. 141-144.
3. Koestner, A., Bilzer, T., Fatzer, R., Schulmer, F.Y.S., Summers, B,A., and Van Winkle, T.J. (1999) Histological classification of the tumors of the nervous system of domestic animals. In *International Histological classification of Tumors of Domestic Animals.* 2nd series, vol. V. Armed Forces Institute of Pathology, Washington, D.C., pp. 25-26.
4. Fankhauser, R., Luginbühl, A., and McGrath, J.T. (1974) Tumors of the nervous system. *Bull WHO* 50:53-69.
5. Monlux, A.W., et al. (1956) A survey of tumors occurring in cattle, sheep, and swine. *Amer J Vet Res* 17:646-677.
6. Monlux, W.S., and Monlux, A.W. (1972) *Atlas of Meat Inspection Pathology.* Agriculture Handbook No. 367, U.S. Department of Agriculture, Washington, D.C., pp. 70-78.
7. Dehner, L.P. (1986) Peripheral and central primitive neuroectodermal tumors. *Arch Pathol Lab Med* 110:997-1005.

Thoracolumbar Spinal Cord Tumor

Incidence and Sites

This tumor affects young dogs mostly under 1 year of age, but can occur up to 38 months, with an apparent predisposition in the German shepherd and some retriever breeds.[1,2] The tumor is uncommon (about 2.3 percent of all canine primary CNS tumors) but important in the affected age group and breeds. It leads to uni- or bilateral progressive paresis or paralysis. The primary spinal cord tumor occurs at the thoracolumbar segments T10-L2, and an intraspinal tumor metastases or a second site at L4-L6 has also been described.[3] The tumor seems to start and expand either in an intradural-extramedullary or intramedullary location. A clear distinction between an extra- and intramedullary location is, however, not easy to determine because extramedullary tumors mostly invade the spinal cord and those appearing to have started within the cord almost always infiltrate the extramedullary space.

Gross Morphology

A grayish-pinkish discolored soft mass may partially replace the spinal cord at the thoracolumbar segments with intramedullary and extramedullary intradural growth (fig. 14.22 A). Extradural involvement has been reported.

Histological Features

The tumor consists of a mixture of glandular and solid patterns of cells. The former consists of tubules and acinar structures lined by a low columnar to pseudostratified epithelium that sometimes forms a glomeruloid-like component (fig. 14.22 B). In most areas, a clearly defined outer limiting membrane can be identified around these epithelial structures. Nuclei are hyperchromatic with enlarged nucleoli. Mitotic figures can be moderate to numerous. The solid component consists of more ovoid cells, arranged in sheets or interlacing fascicles (fig. 14.22 B). The spindloid cells have ovoid nuclei and small amounts of eosinophilic cytoplasm with indistinct cell borders. Ultrastructural features include the presence of a continuous basal lamina, junctional complexes, microvilli, and occasional cilia.[2]

Differential Diagnosis

The designation of thoracolumbar spinal cord tumor of young dogs is used here because the cell of origin is controversial.[4] Previously this tumor has been labeled as an ependymoma,[5] medulloepithelioma, or neuroepithelioma,[6] all tumors of neuroepithelial origin. However, the histological components of poorly differentiated fusiform cells, together with a stromal and a cytokeratin positive epithelial component that may form tubules or glomeruloid structures is distinctively different from each of those tumors (fig. 14.22 C). The similarity of these features to ectopic renal primordial tissue led to the suggestion that it was a spinal nephroblastoma.[1] Subsequent positive immunocytochemical staining for polysialic acid, and for Wilms' tumor gene product (WT1) in glomeruloid bodies currently supports this hypothesis.[4] There can also be positive staining for vimentin of the spindloid cells and cytokeratin of the epithelial component.[2,3] Staining for neuronal and glial cell markers has been consistently negative.

REFERENCES

1. Bridges, C.H., Storts, R.W., and Read, W.K. (1984) Spinal cord nephroblastoma in a dog. Proceedings of the Annual Meeting of the American College of Veterinary Pathologists, Toronto, p. 97.

2. Summers, B.A., et al. (1988) A novel intradural extramedullary spinal cord tumor in young dogs. *Acta Neuropathol* 75:402-410.

3. Terrell, S.P., Platt, S.R., Chrisman, C.L., Homer, B.L., deLahunta, A., and Summers, B.A. (2000) Possible intraspinal metastasis of a canine spinal cord nephroblastoma. *Vet Pathol* 37:94-97.

4. Pearson, G.R., Gregory, S.P., and Charles, A.K. (1997) Immunohistochemical demonstration of Wilm's tumour gene product WT1 in a canine "neuroepithelioma" providing evidence for its classification as an extrarenal nephroblastoma. *J Comp Pathol* 116:321-327.

5. Luttgen, P.J., and Bratton, C.R. (1976) Spinal cord ependymoma: A case report. *J Amer Anim Hosp Assoc* 12:788-791.

6. Kennedy, F.A., Indrieri, R.J., and Koestner, A. (1984) Spinal cord medulloepithelioma in a dog. *J Amer Vet Med Assoc* 185:902-904.

Meningiomas

Meningiomas are derived from meningothelial (arachnoidal) cells of the arachnoid membrane and pia mater of the nervous system.[1,2] The histological diversity of meningiomas may reflect the mixed mesodermal and neural crest origins of the brain and spinal cord leptomeninges.[1] Human meningiomas have been associated with breast tumors, previous trauma, or cranial irradiation.[2] Such predisposing factors have not been identified in spontaneous meningiomas in animals, but in young cats with mucopolysaccharidosis type 1, meningiomas are claimed to be more frequent.[3] The role of sex steroids, particularly progesterone, in perturbing growth of human meningiomas is controversial and has not been carefully studied in animals.[4,5] In many human meningiomas a variety of genetic abnormalities have been found including deletion of chromosome 22, allelic losses, and mutations in the *NF2* gene.[2] Meningiomas have been experimentally induced in dogs with methylcholanthrene, Rous sarcoma virus, and perinatal X-ray irradiation and in cattle with bovine papilloma virus.[6-9]

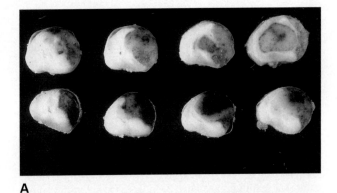

A

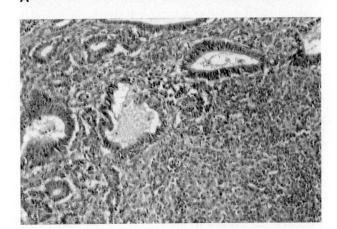

B

C

Fig. 14.22. **A.** Transverse sections of a thoracolumbar spinal tumor in a 13-month-old Great Pyrenees dog. Note the predominant intramedullary location of this tumor with some extramedullary intradural growth. **B.** Higher magnification illustrates the characteristic tubular pattern admixed with more solid cellular areas of this embryonal neoplasm. **C.** Postive cytokeratin staining of some epithelial cells forming the tubules.

Incidence and Sites

Meningiomas are the most common primary nervous system tumor of both dogs and cats but are rare in sheep, horses, and cattle.[10-14] In dogs, meningiomas demonstrate an increasing prevalence with age.[15] Most meningiomas occur in dogs over 7 years of age, with the earliest reported at 16 months. Although there is no obvious gender bias, there is a predilection in the golden retriever breed.[10,16,17] About 82 percent of all canine meningiomas are intracranial, 15 percent intraspinal, and 3 percent retrobulbar.[10] Retrobulbar meningiomas either are extensions of intracranial tumors or arise from the optic nerve.[18] Canine meningiomas occur as solitary, well-demarcated neoplasms that grow either by compression or, less commonly, by infiltration of the adjacent brain. Intracranial canine meningiomas usually occur over the cerebral hemispheres in the falx cerebri, convexities, or basilar areas including the sella turcica.[19] In the caudal fossa they are most common around the brain stem. Canine paranasal meningiomas have been described.[20] In the spinal cord, intradural meningiomas are most common in the cervical segments, often with secondary entrapment of spinal nerve roots or spinal cord and extradural infiltration.[16,21] In female dogs, meningiomas do not exhibit the gender bias reported in human spinal meningiomas.[2] Pulmonary meningiomas have been reported as presumed metastases from primary brain sites.[22] Primary extraneural meningiomas in subcutaneous locations have been described.[23]

Most meningiomas occur in cats over 9 years old, and their prevalence tends to increase with age.[10,11,24] In cats, single or multiple intracranial tumors of varying sizes can either cause neurological deficits or be incidental findings. Although no breed predisposition has been recognized, there is a slightly higher incidence in males. Feline meningiomas are located mainly supratentorially, often within a lateral ventricle. Infratentorial and spinal cord meningiomas are comparatively rare.[24]

Gross Morphology

Meningiomas usually grow as well-demarcated, often lobulated, firm, granular masses that usually have a broad-based or pedunculated attachment to the overlying meninges. Less commonly they can form plaque-like masses over the meninges. In dogs, meningiomas are found commonly in the region of the olfactory bulb (fig. 14.23 A) and frontal lobes, but can occur anywhere over the surface of the cerebral hemispheres (fig. 14.23 A,B,C).[24,25] Supratentorial meningiomas are more common over the meninges of the convexities than in basilar sites and least often involve the midline falx cerebri. In the basilar meninges, meningiomas grow around the optic chiasma and the suprasellar region. Meningiomas can be attached to the brain stem or the tentorium cerebelli. By local compression behind intact meninges, meningiomas generally form depressions into the brain from which they can be easily removed. However, the more invasive types infiltrate deep into the brain parenchyma (fig. 14.23 B). After their exposure by craniotomy, meningiomas appear as very red, fleshy granular masses, but with fixation they become beige to gray or white. Mineralization may impart a gritty feel on sectioning. The plaque form is generally found on the intracranial basilar meninges as a localized velvety villous thickening. Meningiomas can also form large, cyst-like, fluid filled structures in the brain with minimal and periph-

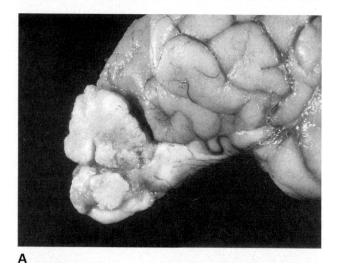

A

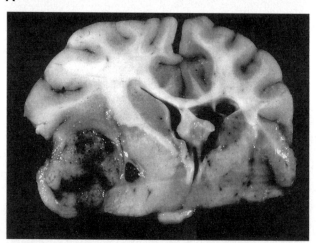

B

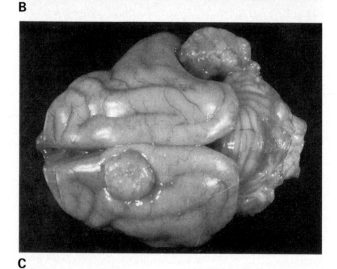

C

Fig. 14.23. Meningioma. **A.** A canine meningioma involving the olfactory bulb and tract. There is associated compression of the frontal lobe. **B.** An invasive canine meningioma. **C.** Multiple meningiomas compressing the brain of a cat.

erally located tumor tissue.[26] Local nodular extension over the periosteum of the cranial vault can occur secondary to meningeal tumor impingement. Invasive types of intracranial meningiomas are especially prone to edema of adjacent white matter, which in turn can exacerbate secondary shifts and brain herniations.

In cats, intracranial meningiomas are globular, well-defined masses with a broad meningeal base of attachment. Generally feline meningiomas can be easily shelled from their intraparenchymal indentation (fig. 14.23 C). Growth usually occurs by local expansion and rarely by parenchymal invasion. Most of the solitary meningiomas occur over the dorsal and lateral hemispheric convexities (fig. 14.23 C). Meningiomas also occur along the falx, base of the brain, or within the third or a lateral ventricle. In about 20 percent of all cats with meningiomas, multiple tumors of smaller size may be found concurrently (fig. 14.23 C). Feline meningiomas tend to be firm to hard, fleshy to yellow gray after fixation, have a granular irregular surface, and are of varying size. Hyperostotic changes in the overlying calvarium are described.[27]

Histological Features

Meningiomas are histologically diverse, with most tumors exhibiting areas of more than one histological subtype. The following classification is based mainly on the WHO classification of human histological subtypes.[2,28]

Meningothelial

This very common pattern is formed by sheets of cells without defined cytoplasmic borders. Cells have elongate to ovoid nuclei and usually solitary prominent nucleoli with delicate heterochromatin. Intranuclear cytoplasmic evaginations can be common. The cytoplasmic borders are indistinct, but the cytoplasm is abundant and homogeneous (fig. 14.24 A). A syncytial variant forms varying sized lobules in which there is a tendency to a whorl-like formation of cells. Larger blood vessels in the canine tumors have a distinct perivascular nuclear-free zone. Mitosis is rare.

Fibroblastic

Cells tend to be more spindle shaped than in the meningothelial subtype and have more elongate nuclei. Cells often form intersecting bundles or streams between which are variably dense collagen fibers. Sometimes a tendency towards whorl formation can be seen in this rare type.

Transitional

There is a mixture of meningotheliomatous and fibrous patterns. There are more syncytial cell clusters or concentric whorls that separate into well-demarcated lobules (fig. 14.24 B), often interspersed with regions of meningothelial cells. Occasional psammoma bodies form, with a core of central hyalinization, necrosis, and mineralization within the whorls.

Psammomatous

There is a background transitional pattern with predominant whorl formation with large numbers of psammoma bodies (fig. 14.24 C).

Papillary

This pattern is formed by meningothelial cells radiating around a central vascular core in papillary formation (fig. 14.24 D). The tapering processes of the meningothelial cells terminating on the central vessels create a prominent perivascular cell-free zone mimicking the formation of pseudorosettes. There are often broad sheets of meningothelial cells interspersed between the papillary areas.

Microcystic

The cells are spindle cell shaped with elongated nuclei, and processes are loosely arranged and intersecting to form empty intracellular cysts, sometimes containing blue-staining mucin-like material (fig. 14.24 E). These areas can be admixed with other foci of more transitional patterns.

Myxoid

The pattern is of papillary structures with a central fibrovascular stroma and ovoid to fusiform cells radiating away from the vessels. The round cells may contain clear vacuoles in an abundant cytoplasm. The cells are embedded individually or in clusters in an amorphous, myxoid matrix that is positive with mucicarmine, alcian blue, and periodic acid-Schiff stains.[29]

Angiomatous

There are numerous prominent dilated blood vessels on a background of a meningioma. This subtype must be differentiated from meningoangiomatosis, which is a vascular malformation within the intracranial leptomeninges with a proliferation of meningothelial cells around blood vessels.[30]

Atypical

This may be a meningothelial subtype with aggressive invasion of the adjacent neuropil (fig. 14.25 A). There are solid sheets of meningothelial cells with multifocal areas of tumor cell necrosis. There can be other intratumoral foci of neutrophils admixed with necrotic tumor cells (fig. 14.25 B). There is a high mitotic index, cellular pleomorphism, and individual cell necrosis.

In the dog the meningothelial, transitional, microcystic, and psammoma types, in descending order, are the most common forms. Each may have multifocal, dense accumulations of T and/or B cell lymphocyte subpopulations scattered throughout the tumor. Areas of chondroid, osseous, myxoid, and xanthomatous-like tissue can be found in the meningothelial and transitional forms. Granular cell differentiation has been described within a canine meningothelial meningioma.[31] The transitional and fibroblastic subtypes appear to be the most common feline subtypes. Feline meningiomas commonly have multiple areas of cholesterol cleft formation, necrosis, and linear mineralization (fig. 14.25 C). Curiously, their incidence appears to be very low in the western compared to the eastern United States.

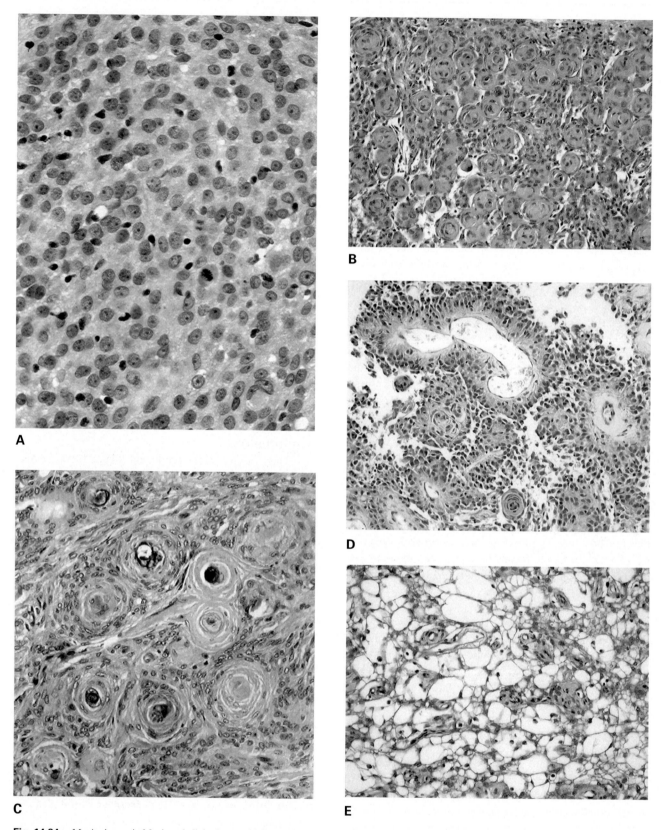

Fig. 14.24. Meningioma. **A.** Meningothelial subtype with broad sheets of cells having elongate to ovoid nuclei, a single nucleolus, abundant cytoplasm, and indistinct cytoplasmic borders. **B.** Transitional meningioma with numerous, concentric whorls in a meningothelial matrix. **C.** Psammomatous meningioma with mineralized psammoma bodies in varying stages and a meningothelial component. **D.** Papillary meningioma with perivascular pseudopapillary pattern. **E.** Microcystic meningioma with varying sized cysts.

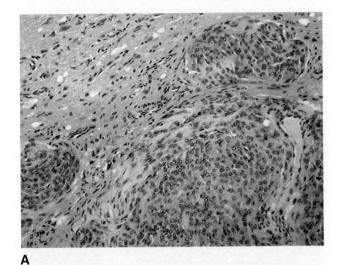

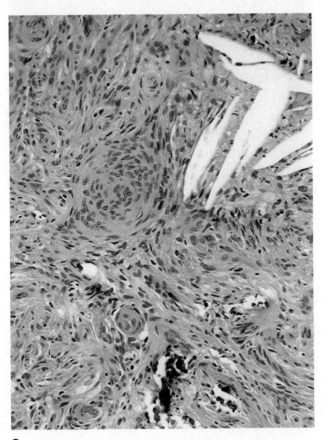

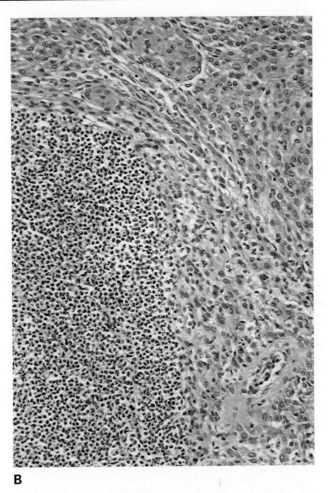

Fig. 14.25. **A.** An atypical canine meningothelial meningioma with aggressive invasion of the brain. **B.** Atypical meningothelial meningioma with focal accumulation of neutrophils. **C.** Feline meningioma with whorl formation, focal mineralization, and cholesterol clefts in a background of spindle shaped tumor cells.

Cytology

Smear preparations can be diagnostically useful, particularly when whorls or psammomatous bodies are present. Meningiomas form characteristic clumps of cells interspersed between blood vessels. Blood vessels are moderately thickened, have a prominent pattern of arborization and peripheral clusters of cells radially oriented away from the vessels. Neutrophils can be a prominent cellular component of some meningiomas.[32]

Immunohistochemistry

Irrespective of their subtype classification, meningiomas are uniformly and strongly positive for vimentin expression. Some tumors have variable, focal expression of low and/or high molecular weight cytokeratins, best demonstrated using fresh-frozen tissue. Epithelial membrane antigen (EMA) is considered the most useful diagnostic marker for human meningiomas, but EMA antibodies do not detect any antigen expression in canine tissue. Positive double labeling of vimentin and desmoplakins is considered distinctive for human meningiomas and also is seen in canine meningiomas.[33] Histochemically, meningiomas generally have strong staining for collagen and reticulin, but these features are not diagnostically useful. Proliferation indices using, for example, MIB-1 have extremely wide variations within individual tumors and between different histological subtypes.[34]

Ultrastructure

Confirmation of a meningioma using ultrastructural criteria is most reliable.[35] Irrespective of their histological subtyping, most meningiomas have very long, interdigitating, parallel layered cytoplasmic processes with endocytotic evaginations of their cytoplasmic membrane (fig. 14.26 A) Their most consistent features are the various types of normal and abnormal desmosomal and gap junctions between their processes (fig. 14.26 B). Tight junctions and hemidesmosomes are almost invariably found, although their numbers can vary widely among the histological subtypes.

Differential Diagnosis

Meningothelial or transitional meningioma subtypes need to be distinguished from metastatic carcinomatosis of the meninges, and this is best done using immunocytochemical staining for positive vimentin detection in meningiomas and cytokeratin expression with carcinomatosis.[36] Some meningiomas, however, can be focally positive for cytokeratins. Angiomatous meningiomas are rare but nevertheless must be differentiated from meningoangiomatosis.[30, 36] Suprasellar germ cell tumors may be confused with meningothelial meningiomas, but the former have positive staining for alpha fetal protein and placental alkaline phosphatase.[37]

REFERENCES

1. Kepes, J.J. (1986) Presidential address: The histopathology of meningiomas. *J Neuropathol Exp Neurol* 45:95-107.
2. Louis, D.N., Scheithauer, B.W., Budka, H., von Deimling, A., and Kepes, J.J. (2000) Meningiomas. In Kliehues, P., and Cavanee, W.K. (eds.), *Pathology and Genetics of Tumours of the Nervous System.* IARC Press, Lyon, France, pp. 176-184.
3. Haskins, M.E., and McGrath, J.T. (1983) Meningiomas in young cats with mucopolysaccharidosis. *J Neuropathol Exp Neurol* 42:664-670.
4. Speciale, J., Koffman, B.M, and Bashirelahi, N. (1990) Identification of gonadal steroid receptors in meningiomas from dogs and cats. *Amer J Vet Res* 51:833-835.
5. Matsuda, Y., Kawamoto, K., Kiya, K., Kurisu, K., Sugiyama, K., and Uozumi, T. (1994) Antitumor effects of antiprogesterones on human meningioma cells *in vitro* and *in vivo. J Neurosurg* 80:527-534.
6. Mulligan, R.M., Neubuerger, K.T., Lucan, J.T., and Lewis, W.B. (1946) Intracranial neoplasms produced in dogs by methylcholanthrene. *Exp Med Surg* 4:7-19.
7. Rabotti, G.F., Bucciarelli, E., and Dalton, A.J. (1966) Presence of particles with the morphology of viruses of the avian leukosis complex in meningeal tumors induced by the Rous sarcoma virus. *Virology* 29:684-686.
8. Benjamin, S.A., Lee, A.C., Angleton, G.M., Saunders, W.J., Miller, G.K., Williams, J.S., Brewster, R.D., and Long, R.I. (1986) Neoplasms in young dogs after perinatal irradiation. *J Natl Cancer Inst* 77:563-571.
9. Gordon, D.E., and Olsen, C. (1968) Meningiomas and fibroblastic neoplasia in calves induced with the bovine papilloma virus. *Cancer Res* 28:2423-2431.
10. McGrath, J.T. (1962) Intracranial pathology of the dog. In Frauchige, E., and Seitelberger, F. (eds.), Symposon uber vergleichende Neuropathologie. *Acta Neuropathol Suppl* 1:3-4.
11. Luginbühl, H. (1961) Studies on meningiomas in cats. *Amer J Vet Res* 22:1030-1040.
12. Zaki, F.A., and Hurvitz, A.I. (1976) Spontaneous neoplasms in the central nervous system of the cat. *J Small Anim Pract* 17:773-782.
13. Luginbuhl, H., Fankhauser, R., and McGrath, J.T. (1968) Spontaneous neoplasms of the nervous system in animals. *Prog Neurol Surg* 2:85-164.

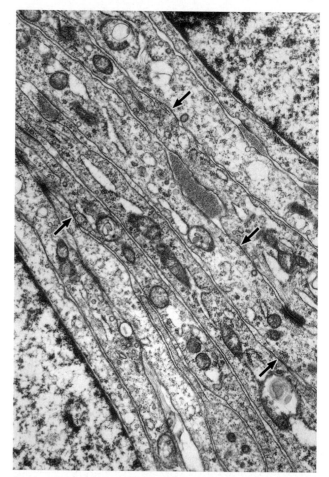

A

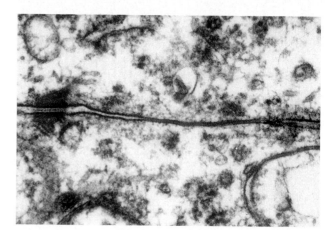

B

Fig. 14.26. **A.** Electronmicrograph of a meningioma with hemidesmosomal and gap junctions (arrows) and cytoplasmic membrane evaginations. **B.** Note the characteristic gap and desmosomal junctions.

14. Josephson, G.K.A., and Little, P.B. (1990) Four bovine meningeal tumors. *Can Vet J* 31:700-703.

15. Patnaik, A.K., Kay, W.J., and Hurvitz, A.I. (1986) Intracranial meningioma: A comparative pathologic study of 28 dogs. *Vet Pathol* 23:369-373.

16. Fingeroth, J.M., Prata, R.G., and Patnaik, A.K. (1987) Spinal meningiomas in dogs: 13 cases. *J Amer Vet Med Assoc* 191:720-726.

17. Andrews, E.J. (1973) Clinicopathological characteristics of meningiomas in dogs. *J Amer Vet Med Assoc* 163:151-157.

18. Paulsen, M.E., Severin, G.A., and LeCouteur, R.A. (1989) Primary optic nerve meningioma in a dog. *J Amer Anim Hosp Assoc* 25:147-152.

19. Schulman, F.Y., Ribas, R.L., and Carpenter, J.L. (1992) Cystic papillary meningioma in the sella turcica of a dog. *J Amer Vet Med Assoc* 200:67-69.

20. Patnaik, A.K., Lieberman, P.H., Erlandson, R.A., Shaker, E., and Hurvitz, A.I. (1986) Paranasal meningiomas in the dog: A clinicopathologic study of ten cases. *Vet Pathol* 23:362-368.

21. Zaki, F.A., Prata, R.G., Hurvitz, A.I., and Kay, W.J. (1975) Primary tumors of the spinal cord and meninges in six dogs. *J Amer Vet Med Assoc* 166:511-517.

22. Schulman, F.Y., Ribas, R.L. and Carpenter, J.L. (1992) Intracranial meningioma with pulmonary metastasis in three dogs. *Vet Pathol* 29:196-202.

23. Herrera, G.A., and Mendoza, A. (1981) Primary canine cutaneous meningioma. *Vet Pathol* 18:127-130.

24. Nafe, L.A. (1979) Meningiomas in cats: A retrospective clinical study of 36 cases. *J Amer Vet Med Assoc* 174:1224-1227.

25. Cordy, D.R. (1990) Tumors of the nervous system and eye. In Moulton, J.E. (ed.), *Tumors of Domestic Animals,* 3rd ed. University of California Press, Berkeley, pp. 650-652.

26. Bagley, R.S., Kornegay, J.N., Lane, S.B., Thrall, D.L., and Page, R.L. (1996) Cystic meningiomas in 2 dogs. *J Vet Int Med* 10:72-75.

27. Lawson, D.C., Burk, R.L., and Prata, R.G. (1984) Cerebral meningioma in the cat; diagnosis and treatment of 10 cases. *J Amer Anim Hosp Assoc* 20:333-342.

28. Kliehues, P., Burger, P.C., and Scheithauer, B.W. (1993) Histological typing of tumors of the central nervous system. In *International Histological Classification of Tumors,* World Health Organization. Springer-Verlag, Berlin, pp. 33-42.

29. Van Winkle, T.J., Steinberg, H.S., DeCarlo, A.J., Dayrell-Hart, B., Steinberg, S.A., Smith, C.A., and Summers, B.A. (1994) Myxoid meningiomas of the rostral cervical spinal cord and caudal fossa in four dogs. *Vet Pathol* 31:468-471.

30. Ribas, J.L., Carpenter, J., and Mena, H. (1990) Comparison of meningoangiomatosis in a man and a dog. *Vet Pathol* 27:369-371.

31. Patnaik, A.K. (1993) Histologic and immunohistochemical studies of granular cell tumors in seven dogs, three cats, one horse and one bird. *Vet Pathol* 30:176-185.

32. Vernau, K.M., Higgins, R.J., Bollen, A.W., Jimenez, D.F., Anderson, J.V., Koblik, P.D., and LeCouteur, R.A. (2001) Primary canine and feline nervous system tumors: Intraoperative diagnosis using the smear technique. *Vet Pathol* 38:47-57.

33. Schwechheimer, K., Kartenbeck, J., Moll, R., Franke, W.W. (1984) Vimentin filament-desmosome cytoskeleton of diverse types of human meningiomas. *Lab Invest* 51:584-591.

34. Higgins, R.J., LeCouteur, R.A., Koblik, P.D., and Fick, J. (1996) Canine meningiomas: Cell to cell communication. *Vet Pathol* 33:598. [Abstract 114]

35. Kepes, J.J. (1982) *Meningiomas: Biology, Pathology and Differential Diagnosis. Masson Monographs in Diagnostic Pathology.* Masson Publishing, New York.

36. Pumarola, M., and Balasch, M. (1996) Meningeal carcinomatosis in a dog. *Vet Rec* 138:523-524.

37. Valentine, B.A., Summers, B.A., deLahunta, A., White, C.L., and Kuhajda, F.P. (1988) Suprasellar germ cell tumors in the dog: A report of five cases and review of the literature. *Acta Neuropathol* 76:94-100.

Granular Cell Tumor

Incidence and Sites

Granular cell tumors (GCTs) of the CNS have been reported most commonly in the rat and occasionally in the brain of the dog and ferret.[1-5] In the rat, the GCT is the most common primary CNS tumor; both histological and ultrastructural evidence suggest that these tumors are of meningeal origin.[1,2] The histogenesis of this tumor in the dog and ferret remains controversial, although one canine meningioma has had a concomitant GCT component.[4] In humans, most GCTs are derived from specialized pituicytes in the neurohypophysis or infundibulum.[6] A granular cell component has also been seen in some human astrocytomas and oligodendrogliomas.

Gross Morphology

In the rat, the tumors may be closely associated with the meninges of the brain and spinal cord.[1,2] In the ferret and dog, the tumors have been reported in supratentorial locations.[3-5] They are granular and congested before fixation and fairly well circumscribed.

Histological Features

The tumors form diffuse sheets of large granular cells interspersed between blood vessels (fig. 14.27 A). The cells have a very large, prominent, cytoplasm formed of large numbers of densely packed eosinophilic granules within a sharp cytoplasmic border (fig. 14.27 B). The granules are diastase resistant, PAS positive. The nuclei have a prominent nucleolus and are displaced toward the cell periphery (fig. 14.27 A,B).[1,3-7] By MIB-1 staining, the proliferative index is up to 2 percent.[5]

Cytology

On smear preparations the large cells are very distinctive, with their granular cytoplasmic content, eccentrically placed nuclei, and sharp cytoplasmic border (fig. 14.27 B).[5,8]

Immunohistochemistry

The cytoplasm is strongly immunopositive for ubiquitin and variably positive with vimentin, S-100, and alpha-1-antichymotrysin and consistently negative for GFAP and canine leucocyte antigens.[5,7]

Ultrastructure

The cytoplasm of the granular cells is packed with autophagosomes including profiles of residual bodies, large dense irregular granules, sheets of membrane bound granules, multivesicular bodies, and sometimes membrane-like whorls.[2,3,5,7]

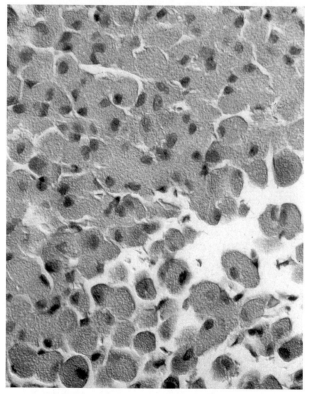

A

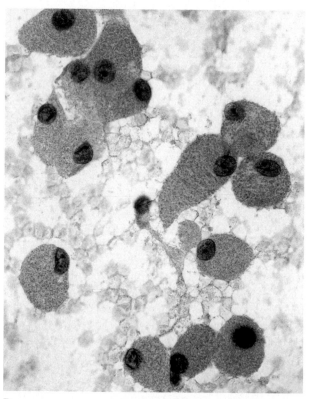

B

Figure 14.27.   Granular cell tumor. **A.** Canine CNS granular cell tumor with sheets of large cells with an eccentric nucleus and granular cytoplasm. **B.** Smear preparation from a CT-guided stereotactic biopsy of a CNS granular cell tumor with typical large, granular, irregularly shaped cells with eccentric nuclei.

Differential Diagnosis

Histologically the features are very distinctive, and only their histogenesis in the dog remains to be determined. The neurohypophyseal site has not been recognized yet in domestic animals.[7]

REFERENCES

1. Krinke, G., Naylor, D.C., Schmid, S., Frolich, E., Schnider, K. (1985) The incidence of naturally occurring tumours in the laboratory rat. *J Comp Pathol* 95:175-192.
2. Yoshida, T., Mitsumori, K., Harada, T,, and Maita, K. (1997) Morphological and ultrastructural study of the histogenesis of meningeal granular cell tumors in rats. *Toxicol Pathol* 25:211-216.
3. Parker, G.A., Botha, W., van Dellen, A., and Casey, H.W. (1978) Cerebral granular cell tumor (myoblastoma) in a dog: Case report and literature review. *Cornell Vet* 68:506-520.
4. Patnaik, A.K. (1993) Histologic and immunohistochemical studies of granular cell tumors in seven dogs, three cats, one horse and one bird. *Vet Pathol* 30:176-185.
5. Higgins, R.J., LeCouteur, R.A., Vernau, K.M., Sturges, B.K., Obradovich, J.E., and Bollen, A.W. (2001) Granular cell tumors of the canine central nervous system. *Vet Pathol* 38:620–627.
6. Sleeman, J.M., Clyde, V.L., and Brenneman, K.A. (1996) Granular cell tumor in the central nervous system of a ferret *(Mustela putorius furo). Vet Rec* 138:65-66.
7. Warzok, R.W., Vogelsang, S., Feiden, W., and Shuangshoti, S. (2000) Granular cell tumor of the neurohypophysis. In Kliehues, P., and Cavanee, W.K. (eds.), *Pathology and Genetics of the Nervous System.* IARC Press, Lyon, France, pp. 247-248.
8. Vernau, K.M., Higgins, R.J., Bollen, A.W., Jimenez, D.F., Anderson, J.V., Koblik, P.D., and LeCouteur, R.A. (2001) Primary canine and feline nervous system tumors: Intraoperative diagnosis using the smear technique. *Vet Pathol* 38:47-57.

Lymphomas and Other Hemopoietic Tumors

There is probably no other group of lesions in veterinary neuropathology that causes more semantic and diagnostic confusion than those classified within the reticulosis complex as originally described in both small and large domestic animals.[1,2] These single or multiple mass lesions were histologically characterized by a perivascular proliferation of "reticulohistiocytic cells" with different patterns of reticulin production and admixed with varying populations of inflammatory cells.[1,2] This morphologically heterogeneous group has included descriptions of inflammatory and neoplastic reticulosis and of microgliomatosis.[2] Inflammatory reticulosis was distinguished from neoplastic reticulosis just using histological criteria for their separation.[2] Currently inflammatory reticulosis in dogs is considered to be part of the spectrum of canine granulomatous meningoencephalitis.[3,4] However, demonstration of immunoglobulin subclass–specific expression within some canine lesions, previously classified as neoplastic reticulosis, first indicated that at least some B cell lymphomas of the CNS were being erroneously included in this group.[5] Subsequently, both canine and porcine T cell lymphomas and feline T and

B cell lymphomas of the CNS have also been identified by immunophenotyping.[6,7] Based on immunocytochemical staining, neoplastic reticulosis is currently considered to be either a neoplastic or an immunoproliferative accumulation of cells expressing various macrophage or histiocyte-like cell markers. Immunocytochemical studies on unfixed tissue from lesions with species and cell specific functional markers will lead most likely to a more accurate classification and understanding of these lesions.[8]

Primary T and B cell Lymphomas of the Central Nervous System

Incidence and Sites

Based on a rigorous necropsy examination and supported by clinical diagnostic information, presumed primary CNS lymphomas have been seen in dogs[5,9] cats[6], cow,[10] and pig as large, deep-seated, single lesions, generally in the cerebrum but also elsewhere in the CNS. Their incidence among all primary CNS tumors is probably less than 3 percent. A canine primary CNS plasma cell tumor in the brain stem expressing IgA has been reported.[11]

Gross Morphology

CNS lymphomas are grayish, soft, poorly defined single masses of varying size, which may extend to the meninges (fig. 14.28).

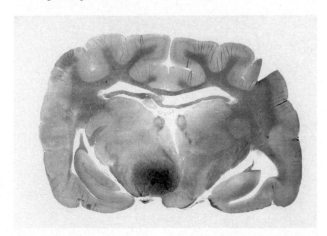

Fig. 14.28. Macrophotograph of a primary canine CNS B cell lymphoma in the hypothalamic area.

Histological Features

The cells form a diffuse infiltration of the neuropil of usually immature lymphoblasts. Their nuclei are densely basophilic, large, and round to sometimes angular with a prominent nucleolus (fig. 14.29 A). There may be a very thin rim of cytoplasm. There are usually both normal and abnormal mitotic figures (2/HP field) and some individual cell necrosis. The cells have an infiltrative pattern of neuropil invasion. At the periphery of the lesion there is often a marked perivascular migration of tumor cells.

Cytology

CNS lymphomas have a characteristic morphological appearance; they form dense sheets with uniform cells that have round basophilic nuclei with prominent nucleoli and minimal cytoplasm. Mitotic figures are uncommon, but individual cell necrosis is striking.

Immunohistochemistry

In the dog, cat, and pig CNS lymphomas, up to 90 percent of tumor cells stain positively for a specific T lymphocyte cell marker antigen (CD3), although there can be admixed smaller populations of macrophages and B cells. In the dog and cat, CNS B cell lymphomas (fig. 14.29 B) have been described based on their uniform expression of an immunoglobulin (Ig) subclass or IgG light chain, respectively.[5,6]

Differential Diagnosis

CNS lymphomas must be carefully differentiated from systemic lymphomas that metastasize to the CNS.[12] Metastatic lymphomas generally target the leptomeninges, choroid plexus, epidural space, or peripheral nerves, but the ultimate diagnosis of a CNS lymphoma depends at the very least on a rigorous clinicopathologic and necropsy examination to exclude any discrete extraneural involvement.

Other Unclassified Tumors

Neoplastic Reticulosis

Incidence and Sites

This lesion occurs mainly in dogs and rarely in cats, cattle, and horses.[1,3,13-16] Based solely on histological criteria, this still unclassified and controversial entity originally termed neoplastic reticulosis has also been variously designated as, for example, reticulum cell sarcoma, histiocytic lymphoma, perithelioma, and adventitial cell sarcoma.[1,2,17] The lesions are most common in older dogs and occur preferentially in white matter of the brain as single or multifocal, well-demarcated masses.[1,2,13,14] A more disseminated form detected microscopically is less common.[14]

Gross Morphology

The masses appear grayish-white, usually sharp bordered, and with granular texture on cut section (fig. 14.30 A). Adjacent parenchyma can also have a granular roughened texture.

Histological Features

Within the mass lesions there is a prominent orientation and concentric perivascular distribution of histiocyte-like cells whose confluence results in solid mass lesions (fig. 14.30 B). Sometimes between these vascularly oriented concentric patterns are areas of acute coagulative necrosis. The perivascular cells are large and elongate with a lobulated vesicular nucleus and prominent nucleoli and a large amount of eosinophilic cytoplasm, often in a bipolar or irregular shape (fig. 14.30 B). Mitoses are infrequent (2/HP field). There can be a few B and T cell positive lymphocytes admixed with these presumably neoplastic cells. Equine reticulosis is composed of a mixture of macrophages, lymphocytes, and some plasma cells and eosinophils and therefore is easily differentiated histologically from a lymphoma.[16]

Immunohistochemistry

Immunocytochemical studies on unfixed tissue with functional species and cell specific markers will best define the lineage of this probable histiocytic or macrophage-like cell population.[18] Whether this entity is an immunoproliferative or neoplastic process also awaits further study.

Differential Diagnosis

Histological examination can readily differentiate between this lesion and lymphoma. Immunohistochemical confirmation of a lymphoma can be done with appropriate antibodies for T lymphocyte or B cell markers (fig. 14.29 A,B).[8] The primary or metastatic CNS lesions of histiocytic sarcoma tend to be somewhat breed specific; have characteristic histological features; often attract an intense inflammatory cell response of T lymphocytes, neu-

trophils, and eosinophils; and stain with canine histiocyte markers.[8]

Microgliomatosis

Canine microgliomatosis is a very questionable entity that was proposed originally as a neoplastic proliferation of endogenous microglial cells and was classified within the reticulosis complex.[2,15,18,19] Currently, we believe that there are insufficient morphological or other criteria to clearly separate this entity from either an astrocytoma or a PNET.

Incidence and Sites

Canine microgliomatosis has been reported in older dogs as a slowly progressive neurological disease.[2,15,19] There are usually no gross lesions.

Histological Features

The lesion is described as a diffuse cellular infiltration within the existing architecture of both white and gray matter in the brain and spinal cord. There are also thick subpial and perivascular cell infiltrates, often separate from the sites of major lesions. In the white matter the cells

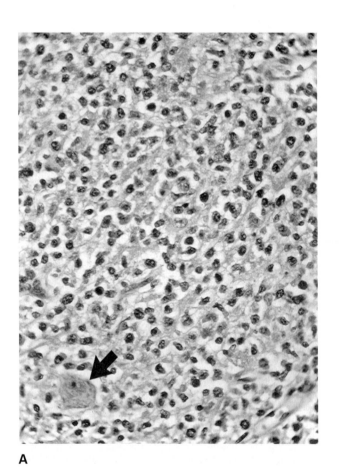

A

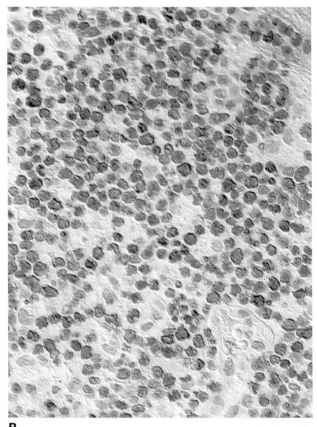

B

Fig. 14.29. **A.** In this primary canine CNS T cell lymphoma there is a diffuse infiltrative pattern within existing neurophil. Lymphoma cells have an angular to round nucleus and minimal cytoplasm. Note the entrapped neuron (arrow). **B.** Immunocytochemical staining in a feline CNS B cell lymphoma.

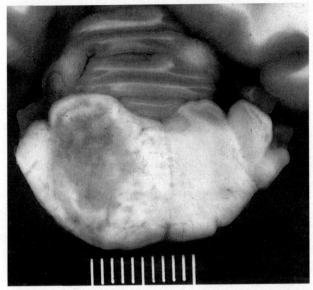

A

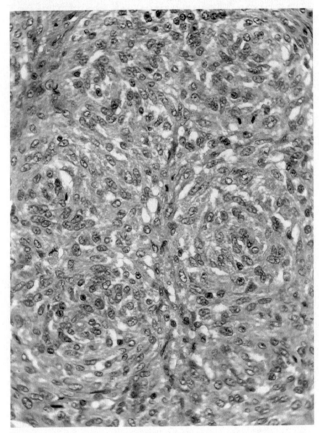

B

Fig. 14.30. **A.** Midbrain section of a dog with a mass lesion of neoplastic reticulosis. (scale = 1 cm). **B.** Canine neoplastic reticulosis with a concentric and confluent angiocentric pattern of histiocyte-like cells.

tend to orient in parallel with existing tracts. Nuclei are uniformly and markedly elongate, ovoid to spiral in shape, with minimal cytoplasm. Mitoses are rare.[18,19]

Immunohistochemistry

Detailed studies have not been reported and the validation of this entity awaits immunocytochemical confirmation using species and defined microglial cell specific antibody markers or possibly lectins. Microgliomatosis may be easily confused histologically with an astrocytoma, but positive immunostaining for GFAP and glutamine synthetase in the latter can be diagnostically useful.

REFERENCES

1. Koestner, A. (1975) Primary lymphoreticuloses of the nervous system in animals. *Acta Neuropathol* 6(Suppl): 85-89.
2. Fankhauser, R., Fatzer, R., Luginbühl, H., and McGrath, J.T. (1972) Reticulosis of the central nervous system (CNS) in dogs. *Adv Vet Sci Comp Sci* 16:35-71.
3. Braund, K.G., Vandevelde, M., Walker, T.L., and Redding, R.W. (1978) Granulomatous meningoencephalomyelitis in six dogs. *J Amer Vet Med Assoc* 172:1195-1200.
4. Cordy, D.R. (1979) Canine granulomatous meningoencephalomyelitis. *Vet Pathol* 16:325-333.
5. Vandevelde, M., Fatzer, R., and Fankhauser, R. (1981) Immunohistological studies on primary reticulosis of the canine brain. *Vet Pathol* 18:577-588.
6. Callanan, J.J., Jones, B.J., Irvine, J., Willett, B.J., McCandlish, I.A.P., and Jarrett, O. (1996) Histologic classification and immunophenotype of lymphosarcomas on cats with naturally and experimentally acquired feline immunodeficiency virus infections. *Vet Pathol* 33:257-367.
7. Fondevila, D., Vilafranca, M., and Pumarola, M. (1998) Primary central nervous system T-cell lymphoma in a cat. *Vet Pathol* 35:550-553.
8. Moore, P.F., Affolter, V.K., Olivry, T., and Schrenzel, M.D. (1998) The use of immunological reagents in defining the pathogenesis of canine skin diseases involving proliferation of leukocytes. In Kwocha, K.W., Willemse, T., von Tscharner, C. (eds.), *Advances in Veterinary Dermatology*. Vol. 3. Butterworth Heinemann, Oxford, pp. 77-94.
9. Couto, C.G.., Cullen, J., Pedroia, V., and Turrel, J.M. (1984) Central nervous system lymphosarcoma in the dog. *J Amer Vet Med Assoc* 184:809-813.
10. mith, B.P., and Anderson, M. (1977) Lymphosarcoma of the brain in a heifer. *J Amer Vet Med Assoc* 170:333.
11. Sheppard, B.J., Chrisman, C.L., Newell, S.M., Raskin, R.E., and Homer, B.L. (1997) Primary encephalic plasma cell tumor in a dog. *Vet Pathol* 34:621-627.
12. Vernau, K.M., Terio, K.A., LeCouteur, R.A., Berry, R.L., Vernau, W., Moore, P.F., and Samii, V.F. (2000) Acute B-cell lymphoblastic leukemia with meningeal metastasis causing primary neurologic dysfunction in a dog. *J Vet Intern Med* 14:110-115.
13. Vandevelde, M., Kristensen, B., and Greene, C.E. (1978) Primary reticulosis of the central nervous system in the dog. *Vet Pathol* 15:673-675.
14. Vandevelde, M. (1980) Primary reticulosis of the central nervous system. *Vet Clin N Amer Small Animal Pract* 10:57-63.
15. Luginbühl, H., Fankhauser, R., and McGrath, J.T. (1968) Spontaneous neoplasms of the nervous system in animals. *Prog Neurol Surg* 2:85-164.
16. Finn, J.P., and Tennant, B.C. (1971) A cerebral and ocular tumor of reticular tissue in a horse. *Vet Pathol* 8:458-466.

17. Cordy, D.R. (1990) Tumors of the nervous system and eye. In Moulton, J.E. (ed.), *Tumors of Domestic Animals,* 3rd ed. University of California Press, Berkeley, pp. 649-650.

18. Fankhauser, R., and Frauchiger, E. (1968) Mikrogliomatose beim Hund. *Dtsch Tierarztl Wschr* 74:142-146.

19. Willard, M.D., and deLahunta, A. (1981) Microgliomatosis in a schnauzer dog. *Cornell Vet* 72:211-219.

Rare Primary Central Nervous System Tumors, Tumor-Like Lesions, Hamartomas, and Cysts

Pineal Tumors

Pineal parenchymal neoplasms are classified as pineocytomas (well-differentiated pineal tumors), pineoblastomas (anaplastic pineal tumors), and mixed pineocytoma-pineoblastomas (a combination of both). Pineal parenchymal tumors are rare in the human population and almost unreported in domestic animals. There are none reported in dogs and cats, the two species in which most intracranial tumor types have been recognized. Among other animal species, pineal tumors have been reported in a single cow, goat, fox, horse, and a zebra.[1-3] There are seven publications on pineal tumors in laboratory rats. A total of 14 pineal tumors occurred in 13,642 rats, for an incidence rate of 0.1 percent.[4] Pineal parenchymal tumors in rats are highly comparable to human pineal tumors, and they have been identically classified. They also react to neuronal markers. As in human pineal tumors, synaptophysin was shown to be the most consistent marker (fig. 14.31). The immunopositivity to other neuronal markers is an additional indicator of their neuroepithelial origin. Not all human pineal tumors are of pineal parenchymal origin. Some are stromal (glial) tumors, but many are germ

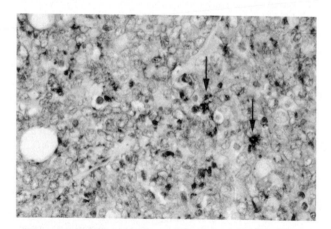

Fig. 14.31. Pineocytoma in a rat. Notice the strongly positive reactivity of the pineal tumor cells for synaptophysin (arrows), indicative of the kinship of pineocytes to neurons. [Reprinted from Koestner, A, and Solleveld, HA (1996) from *Monographs on Pathology of Laboratory Animals,* Springer, pp. 205-213. With permission.]

cell tumors. It is estimated that over 50 percent of the human pineal tumors are of germ cell origin (germinomas). Neither stromal nor germ cell tumors of the pineal gland have been reported in animals, although intracranial germ cell tumors, outside the pineal gland, have been reported in dogs.[5,6]

Germ Cell Tumors (Germinomas)

Intracranial germ cell tumors occur in supra- or intrasellar midline locations in humans and dogs as well as intrapineal locations in humans. They originate from primitive germ cells that migrate to widely separated areas of the embryo during early fetal life.[7] The midline location in the brain is still unexplained. Histologically these tumors resemble testicular seminomas. Identification of intracranial germinomas can be confirmed by detecting alpha-fetoprotein expression.[5,8] The tumors are exceedingly rare in dogs.

Primary Melanomas of the Central Nervous System

Primary melanomas of the CNS are rare in domestic animals, although metastatic melanomas from other regions of the body amount to 5 percent of all secondary tumors in The Ohio State University collection. Primary melanomas of the rat CNS are common in pigmented strains, especially the brown Norwegian rat. One of the two primary CNS melanomas available to us affected the cerebrum and cerebellum of a 42-day-old pig; the other affected the spinal cord of a 3-year-old dog and led to progressive incoordination and paresis. No extraneural melanomas were found in either case.

Chordomas

Chordomas are uncommon in humans and particularly rare in domestic animals. Only a few have been described in dogs, cats, rats, and mink.[9-12] Larger numbers have been reported in ferrets.[13]

Derivation and Sites

Chordomas derive from intraosseous remnants of the notochord. The majority arise in the sacrococcygeal region (fig. 14.32 A), but they may also occur in the sphenooccipital region and rarely in other locations. The chordomas in 20 ferrets were all located on the tip of the tail.[13]

Gross Morphology

Chordomas are usually firm to cystic, slow growing but locally destructive, with a high rate of recurrence following surgical removal (fig. 14.32 A). Up to 30 percent have been reported to metastasize.[13]

Histological Features

The major histological characteristic of chordoma cells is their physaliphorous (bubbly, vacuolated) cytoplasm and

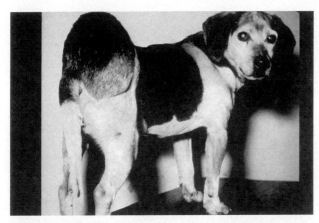

A

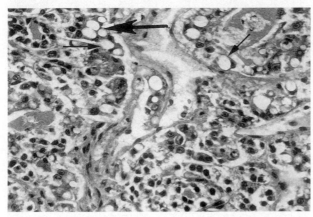

B

Fig. 14.32. A. Large chordoma in the sacrococcygeal region. **B.** Note in the chordoma the typical physaliphorous cytoplasm with eccentric nuclei in many of the cells (arrow).

the eccentrically located dark nucleus (fig. 14.32 B). Immunohistochemically both epithelial (cytokeratin) and mesenchymal (vimentin) markers may be expressed. This duality is also a specific feature possessed by the notochord from which these tumors derive.[14] A special chordoma variant occurs in humans. It is named chondroid chordoma because of its cartilaginous differentiation. It arises primarily in the spheno-occipital region and supposedly has a better prognosis than the physaliphorous type. Among animal species, this variant has only been reported in mink.[13]

Hamartomas

Hamartomas are masses that form by excessive and disorderly growth of local tissue elements. Unlike neoplasms, their growth is limited; once formed, they retain their size with no further expansion. Clinical signs depend upon their size and location; for example, a small (0.4 × 0.4 × 0.3 cm) oval mass on the surface of the left occipital lobe in a 2-year-old cat caused some head tilt and noticeable dementia. This mass was well demarcated and consisted of loose and vacuolated connective tissue with collagen and moderate vascularization. The cellular

elements were heavily pigmented melanocytes, large nerve cells, and cells with astrocytic and oligodendrocytic characteristics (fig. 14.33 A). Vascular hamartomas are less common in animals, but several congenital vascular malformations have been reported.[15-17] In most of the vascular hamartomas in dogs and horses (fig. 14.33 C), there are no clinical signs until later in life even though the hamartomas are congenital malformations. Histologically the vascular malformations comprise various subtypes of arteriovenous anomalies (fig. 14. 33 D). A typical clinical history is of a dog that lived a normal life but at the age of 13 years developed progressive cortical seizures and personality changes. The EEG pointed to a cortical lesion. A vascular hamartoma was diagnosed upon histological examination following necropsy. A vascular rupture triggered the clinical signs. In addition to the intracerebral vascular hamartomas, a few canine cases have been reported to arise within the meninges. They were named meningioangiomatosis.[18-20] Invasion of the cerebral parenchyma may occur in such cases. One case was also described in a horse.[21]

Cysts

A variety of cysts within the CNS have been described in human beings, including Rathke cleft cysts, colloid cysts, epidermoid and dermoid cysts, enterogenous cysts, neuroglial cysts, and arachnoid cysts.[22] Fewer varieties have been reported in animals.[15] The epidermoid cyst is probably the most common cystic lesion in animals. It is also the most frequently encountered CNS cyst in humans. Epidermoid cysts have been reported in dogs and in several rodent species.[23,24] The most common location of such cysts is the cerebellopontine angle. They are considered to result from the inclusion of epithelial elements at the time of closure of the neural groove.[7] They are mostly detected in young dogs following signs of neurological dysfunction. They may, however, be recognized in young or older animals as an incidental finding at necropsy, which is an indication that they may have had a protracted growth rate with no clinical consequences.

Gross Morphology

Epidermoid cysts appear as well-defined, firm, white masses with a smooth and often shiny surface, which suggested the name *pearly tumor.* Upon cutting, cystic structures are filled with a flaky material created by desquamation of keratin from the cyst wall.

Microscopic Features

The cystic character is evident. The cysts are lined by a stratified squamous epithelium that is surrounded by an outer layer of supportive connective tissue (fig. 14.33 B). The illustration is derived from a 2-year-old Boston terrier with a 3 month history of seizures. The epidermoid cyst was located within the aqueduct of Sylvius at its connec-

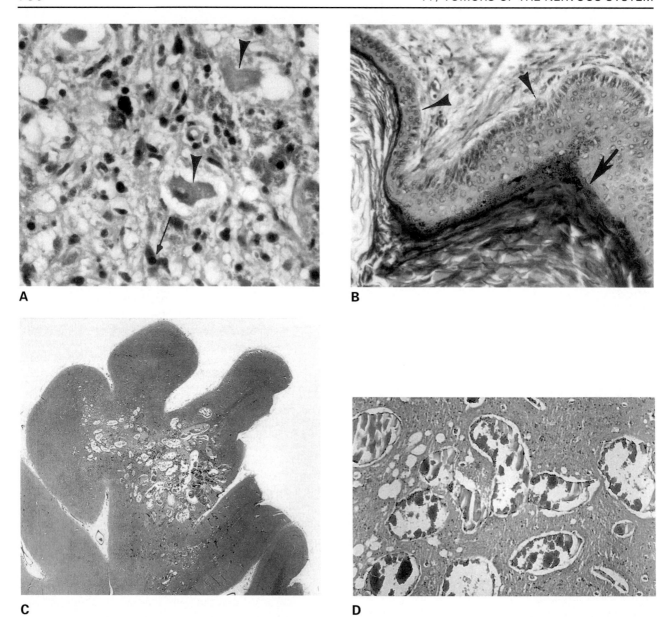

Fig. 14.33. **A.** Hamartoma on the surface of the left occipital lobe in a 2-year-old cat consists of a pleomorphic cell population, including neurons (arrowhead), melanin-containing cells (arrow), and a mixture of mostly unidentifiable cells. **B.** An epidermoid cyst located within the Sylvian aqueduct at its confluence with the fourth ventricle. There is a basal layer (arrowhead) between underlying connective tissue and the metaplastic squamous epithelium with massive keratin production (arrow). [Courtesy of Dr. John Long, The Ohio State University.] **C.** Vascular malformation in the gray and white matter in the frontal lobe of a horse. **D.** Higher magnification illustrating many thin and dilated blood vessels.

tion to the fourth ventricle, occupying most of the aque-ductal lumen. It produced an obstructive hydrocephalus, which was probably the cause of the seizures.

REFERENCES

1. Frauchiger, E. et al. (1966) Pinealome bei Tieren. *Schweiz Arch Tierheilk* 108:368-372.
2. Schlotthauer, G.F., and Keriohan, J.W. (1935) Glioma in a dog and pinealoma in a silver fox (*Vulpus fulvus*). *Amer J Cancer* 24:350-356.
3. Vermeulen, H.A. (1925) Epiphyse und Epiphysentumoren bei Tieren. *Berl Muench Tierärztl Wochenschr* 41:717-719.
4. Koestner, A., and Solleveld, H.A. (1996) Tumors of the pineal gland, rat. In Jones, T.C., Capen, C.C., and Mohr, U. (eds.), *Monographs on Pathology of Laboratory Animals. Endocrine System.* 2nd ed. Springer, Berlin, pp. 205-213.
5. Valentine, B.A., et al. (1988) Suprasellar germ cell tumors in the dog: A report of five cases and review of the literature. *Acta Neuropathol* 76:94-100.
6. Hare, W.R. (1993) Primary suprasellar germ cell tumor in a dog. *J Amer Vet Med Assoc* 203:1432-1433.
7. McClendon, R.E., and Tien, R.D. (1998) Tumors and tumor-like lesions of maldevelopmental origin. In Bigner, D.D., McClendon, R.E., and Bruner, J.M. (eds.), *Russell and Rubinstein's Pathology of Tumors of the Nervous System,* 6th ed. Vol. 2. Oxford University Press, New York, pp. 304-312.

8. Naganuma, H., et al. (1984) Intracranial germ cell tumors. Immunohistochemical study of three autopsy cases. *J Neurosurg* 61:931-937.

9. Luginbuhl, H., Fankhauser, R., and McGrath, J.T. (1968) Spontaneous neoplasms of the nervous system in animals. *Prog Neurol Surg* 2:85-164.

10. Carpenter, J.L., et al. (1990) Chordoma in a cat. *J Amer Vet Med Assoc* 197:240-242.

11. Stefanski, S.A., Elwell, M.R., Mitsumori, K., Yoshitomi, K., Dittrich, K., and Giles, H.D. (1988) Chordoma in Fischer 344 rats. *Vet Pathol* 25:42-47.

12. Hadlow, W.J. (1984) Vertebral chordoma in two ranch mink. *Vet Pathol* 21:533-536.

13. Dunn, D.G., Harris, R.K., Meis, J.M., and Sweet, D.E. (1991) A histomorphological and immunohistochemical study of chordomas in twenty ferrets (*Mustela putorius furo*). *Vet Pathol* 28:467-473.

14. Stosiek, P., Kasper, M., and Karsten, U. (1988) Expression of cytokeratin and vimentin in nucleus pulposus cells. *Differentiation* 39:78-81.

15. Summers, B.A., Cummings, J.F., and de Lahunta, A. (1995) *Veterinary Neuropathology.* Mosby, St. Louis, MO pp. 352-353.

16. Cordy, D.R. (1979) Vascular malformations and hemangiomas of the canine spinal cord. *Vet Pathol* 16:275-282.

17. Fankhauser, R., Luginbuhl, H., and McGrath, J.T. (1965) Cerebrovascular disease in various animal species. *Ann NY Acad Sci* 127:817-819.

18. Ribas, J.L., Carpenter, J., and Mena, H. (1990) Comparison of meningoangiomatosis in a man and a dog. *Vet Pathol* 27:369-371.

19. Stebbins, K.E., and McGrath, J.T. (1988) Meningoangiomatosis in a dog. *Vet Pathol* 25:167-168.

20. Pumarola, M., Martin de las Mulas, J., Vilafranca, M., and Obach, A. (1996) Meningoangiomatosis in the brainstem of a dog. *J Comp Pathol* 115:197-201.

21. McEntee, M., Summers, B.A., and de Lahunta, A. (1987) Meningocerebral hemangiomatosis resembling Sturge-Weber disease in a horse. *Acta Neuropathol* 74:405-410.

22. Kliehues, P., Burger, P.C., and Scheithauer, B.W. (1993) Histological typing of tumors of the nervous system. *WHO International Histological Classification of Tumors,* 2nd ed. Springer-Verlag, Berlin.

23. Kornegay, J.N., and Gorgacz, E.J. (1982) Intracranial epidermoid cysts in three dogs. *Vet Pathol* 19:646-650.

24. Mawdesley-Thomas, L.E., and Hague, P.H. (1970) An intracranial epidermoid cyst in a dog. *Vet Rec* 87:133-134.

PRIMARY TUMORS OF THE PERIPHERAL NERVOUS SYSTEM

Peripheral Nerve Sheath Tumors

This is a heterogeneous group of tumors of peripheral nerves that originate from either Schwann cells or modified Schwann cells, fibroblasts, or perineurial cells.[1] Peripheral nerve sheath tumors (PNSTs) have been subclassified rather confusingly in veterinary literature as neurinomas, neurilemmomas, schwannomas, neurofibromas, and neurofibrosarcomas, depending on their presumed cell of origin.[2] However, it must be pointed out that such classifications in animals are extremely arbitrary and are based more on extrapolation from human tumor studies rather than on any factual basis of their derivation in animals.[2-4] In dogs, cats, and cattle, we prefer to call the benign tumors of presumed Schwann cell origin schwannomas.[2-6] Neurofibromas, similarly to their human counterpart, are rare and have not been convincingly documented in animals.[1] A canine perineurinoma has also been described.[7] We classify the locally invasive and cytologically anaplastic forms as malignant peripheral nerve sheath tumors (MPNST).[1]

Incidence and Sites

In the dog, schwannomas tend to occur in older dogs with a mean age of 8.3 years.[8] The tumors are found most commonly unilaterally in the spinal nerves, with highest frequency in nerves forming the brachial plexus, less in the lumbosacral plexus, and least in subcutaneous sites of distal peripheral nerves.[2,4,8,9] Among the cranial nerves, the trigeminal nerve is most commonly involved. Canine "neurofibrosarcomas" of the brachial plexus and MPNSTs may have presumed pulmonary metastases.[9-11] Both feline schwannomas and MPNST have been observed in dorsal and ventral nerve roots in the lower thoracic and upper lumbar cord segments.[2] In contrast to the dog, brachial and lumbosacral plexus involvement in felines is rare. In cattle, multicentric schwannomas are very common in older animals, although there are usually no associated neurological deficits.[5,6] These tumors have a predilection for the autonomic nervous system including the epicardial plexus, thoracic and cervical sympathetic ganglia, mediastinal nerve plexus, hepatic plexus, tongue, intercostal nerves, and brachial plexus.[5] Intracranial involvement usually affects the vestibulocochlear nerves.[6] A cutaneous plexiform schwannoma in a pig and single or multiple schwannomas in the mediastinum and intestine of horses have been reported.[12-15] A malignant schwannoma of a thoracic spinal nerve in a goat with widespread metastases has been described.[16]

Gross Morphology

In dogs, the gross appearance of schwannomas is distinctive as nodular masses or as varicose or fusiform thickenings of spinal (fig. 14.34 A) or cranial nerves (fig. 14.34 B). The tumors can be very firm or soft and gelatinous, and are white to gray, shiny, and smooth surfaced. Most spread within nerves and are confined by a connective tissue capsule of the epineurium. Centripetal spread in spinal nerve roots from the brachial or lumbar plexus results in extra- or intradural secondary cord compression. Intramedullary infiltration of the spinal cord or pulmonary metastases suggests a more aggressive tumor.[4,8-10,16] Often there is a focal dumbbell shaped swelling of the involved nerve root where it traverses the intervertebral foramen.[2] In schwannomas of the brachial and lumbosacral plexus, there is a varying degree of fusion of individual nerve trunks, but whether this reflects a multicentric origin or spread from a single site is not known. Secondary brain stem compression can occur with schwannomas of the trigeminal or vestibulo-cochlear nerve roots (fig. 14.34 B).

As in dogs, feline MPNST can be locally invasive in vertebral bodies and adjacent musculature and may have pulmonary metastases. Feline schwannomas have also been seen intracranially in the vestibulocochlear nerve with compression of the adjacent brain stem. In cattle, schwannomas also appear as single or multiple nodular or fusiform thickenings of nerve tracts and are whitish-yellow to gray, firm, and glassy.[5,6] On cross section, thickened, separated, and expanded bundles of nerve fibers and a thickened peri- and epineurium can be seen. Affected autonomic ganglia can be enlarged up to 7 cm in diameter. Equine schwannomas have been reported in subcutaneous locations.[17] In the equine intestine multiple schwannomas up to 1 cm in diameter were visible subserosally.[14]

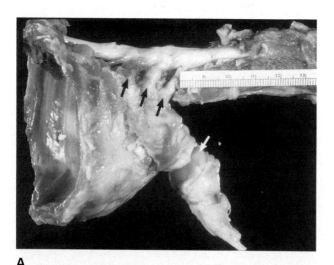

A

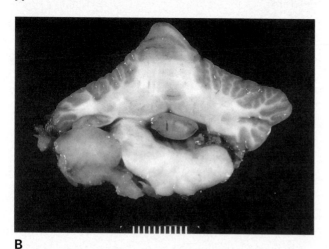

B

Fig. 14.34. Peripheral nerve sheath tumors. **A.** Schwannoma of the brachial plexus in a dog with multiple nerve involvement. (black arrows). On cross section the tumor is still contained by the epineurium (white arrow). **B.** Canine schwannoma in the trigeminal nerve root. (scale = 1 cm).

Histological Features

In dogs, schwannomas consist of densely packed uniform cells, with ovoid to very elongate fusiform shapes, without obvious cytoplasmic borders, and embedded in a variably dense collagen matrix.[2] The tumors are composed of dense cellular sheets arranged in patterns of interwoven bundles, streams, or concentric whorls (fig. 14.35 A). In human schwannomas this form is designated as the Antoni type A pattern. In dogs, palisading or herringbone patterns of nuclear orientation are very uncommon but distinctive (fig. 14.35 B). Verocay bodies formed by stacked parallel rows of palisading nuclei are extremely rare compared to their occurrence in human schwannomas. Mitotic figures are rare. Schwannomas can have areas where cells are low in density, have small dark nuclei, and are embedded in a loose-textured fibrous stroma, designated in human schwannomas as the Antoni type B pattern (fig. 14.35 C). Schwannomas can also have single or multiple foci of osseous, cartilaginous, or mucoid differentiation (fig. 14.35 D).[2] There are often smaller numbers of infiltrating tumor cells within nerve fascicles at some distance from the grossly visible tumor site; these infiltrating tumor cells are visible microscopically and may cause recurrence after surgical intervention. Other types of schwannomas with generalized melanocytic or rhabdomyoblastic differentiation have been described.[18]

The diagnosis of a MPNST rests on macroscopic evidence of local extension and pulmonary metastases and on histological changes including cellular anaplasia, increased mitotic rate, necrosis, and hemosiderin deposition. Multicentric neurofibromas of cranial nerve roots have been reported.[10] A malignant epithelioid canine schwannoma has been described in the trigeminal nerve root.[19] Primary central neurofibromas of uncertain histogenesis have been described in the brains from two dogs.[20]

In cats, schwannomas tend to be overall less cellular, and cells are more spindle shaped and elongate, form streaming patterns, and lie in a more abundant collagenous or mucoid matrix than is seen in the dog. Nuclear palisading is more common than in the dog. Both focal perivascular and more diffuse intratumoral infiltrates of lymphocytes are common. The MPNST has marked cellular pleomorphism with large round or irregular nuclei and prominent nucleoli, bipolar eosinophilic cytoplasm, collagenous stroma, many normal and abnormal mitotic figures, and a propensity for extensive local invasion into adjacent bone and muscle and along fascial planes. In cattle, schwannomas present a variety of admixed cellular patterns and usually have a marked amount of collagenous stroma. The patterns include massive cellular disorganization within nerve tracts, whorls or interlacing bundles, multiple concentric foci of cellular proliferation forming plexiform structures, palisading of nuclei in stacked arrays, and clusters of cells wrapped concentrically in small rings, all embedded within a collagenous and mucoid-like matrix. Myelinated axons may be entrapped within these

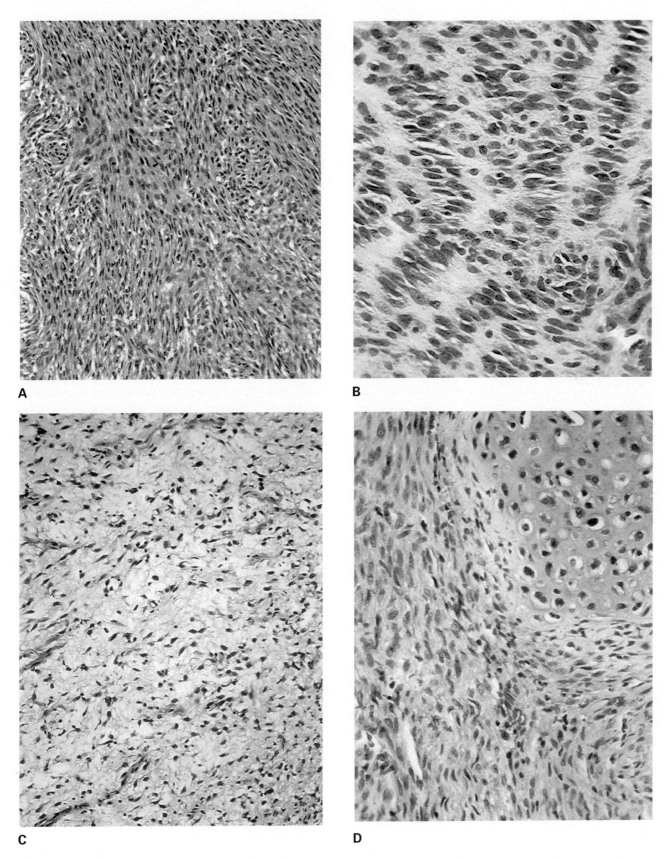

Fig. 14.35. **A.** Canine schwannoma with elongate spindle cells that form interwoven bundles intersecting at various angles. In some areas there is a trend toward whorl formation. Nuclear pleomorphism is not uncommon. **B.** Canine schwannoma with a trend toward cellular palisading. Cell borders are indistinct, and the bipolar processes often are fibrillated. **C.** Canine schwannoma with a mixture of round and spindle shaped cells in a loose cellular arrangement. **D.** Cartilaginous metaplasia in a canine schwannoma.

areas. Affected ganglia have thick, cellular, disorganized nerve fiber tracts with infiltrating spindle cells.[5,6] Neuronal cell bodies appear unaffected. Perivascular cuffing and infiltrates of lymphocytes are common. Although the derivation and morphology of these tumors remains confusing, microscopic and ultrastructural evidence would suggest they are predominantly of Schwann cell origin.[2,3,17,21]

Perineurinomas are extremely rare, and only one, in a dog, has been described.[7] They occur as single or multiple tumors within spinal nerve roots and histologically consist of distinctive concentric whorls of spindle cells in a so-called onion bulb pattern around a central core of a variably myelinated axon (fig. 14.36).

Cytology

In schwannomas, few individual cells detach, so there are usually dense cellular aggregates in which spindle shaped cells may be identified peripherally. Myelinated axons may protrude from the cell masses.

Immunohistochemistry

There are no antigenic markers diagnostically specific for schwannomas. In the dog and cat, schwannomas in formalin fixed, paraffin embedded, tissue sometimes can stain immunocytochemically positive to S-100 protein, GFAP, vimentin, collagen IV, or laminin. The two latter antigens are located extracellularly. With the exception of vimentin, the staining in the dog and the cat is neither consistent between tumors nor uniformly positive within a tumor and is not at all reliable diagnostically. Histochemical staining for reticulin fibrils is usually very dramatic and intense. Presumed tumor metastases to the lungs have been positive for S-100 staining in both dogs and cats. T and B lymphocyte populations are found within schwannomas and MPNST in cats. Two canine cases of possible multiple neurofibromas in cranial nerve roots were negative for S-100 staining.[10]

Ultrastructure

Probably the most definitive evidence of a schwannoma relies on the ultrastructural demonstration of an external basal lamina around neoplastic Schwann cells and their processes (fig. 14.37).[1,3] Compared with normal Schwann cells, the basal lamina of tumor cells can be similar, greatly thickened, often folded into long apparently redundant folds or loops, or in some areas apparently duplicated. In our experience not all tumors contain an exclusive population of such cells, and intermingled fibroblasts and other nonbasal, lamina-forming cells can lead to some diagnostic uncertainty. Desmosomes can be found between closely contiguous cells. Long spacing collagen can also be found extracellularly.[17,21] Perineurinomas have long thin cytoplasmic processes in a perivascular concentric arrangement around intact nerve fibers, bearing pinocytotic vesicles and patchy basal lamina.[7]

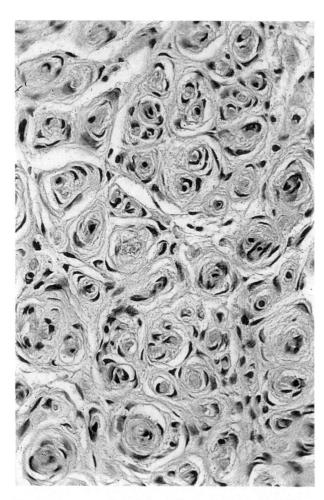

Fig. 14.36. Canine perineurinoma of spinal nerve with the characteristic concentric lamination of spindle cells around a central axonal core.

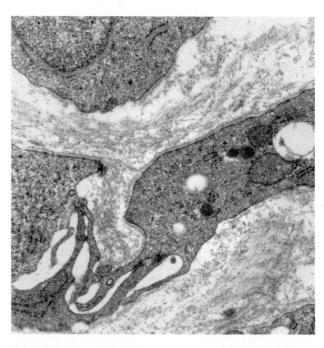

Fig. 14.37. Electronmicrograph from a canine schwannoma, with the basal lamina often thickened or discontinuous around some cells and their processes.

Differential Diagnosis

Canine meningiomas may be a consideration in a differential diagnosis of schwannoma, particularly in intra- or extradural tumors of the spinal cord and in subcutaneous sites. Fibrous meningiomas may resemble schwannomas, and the whorl formation in transitional meningiomas can mimic that of schwannomas. However, meningiomas are S-100 negative and can be distinguished ultrastructurally by their characteristic interdigitating cellular processes, prominent desmosomal and gap junctions, and lack of a basal lamina and positive immunohistochemical staining for desmoplakins. Subcutaneous schwannomas are best differentiated by ultrastructural examination from meningiomas, equine sarcoids, and fibromas.[3,17]

Treatment

Results from surgical intervention in dogs indicate that the overall prognosis is poor with schwannomas and MPNST, with tumors of nerve roots tending to have shorter relapse-free and survival times than those of the brachial or lumbosacral plexus.[4]

REFERENCES

1. Woodruff, J.M., Kourea, H.P., Louis, D.N., and Scheithauer, B.W. (2000) Schwannoma. In Kliehues, P., Cavanee, W.K. (eds.) *Pathology and Genetics of Tumours of the Nervous System.* IARC Press, Lyon, France, pp. 164-166.
2. Cordy, D.R. (1990) Tumors of the nervous system and eye. In Moulton, J.E. (ed.) *Tumors of Domestic Animals,* 3rd ed. University of California Press, Berkeley, pp. 652-654.
3. Summers, B.A., Valentine, B., Van Winkle, T., and Cooper, B. (1992) Divergent differentiation in canine peripheral nerve sheath tumors. *Vet Pathol* 29:447. [Abstract]
4. Brehm, D.M., Vite, C.H., Steinberg, S., Haviland, J., and Van Winkle, T. (1995) A retrospective evaluation of 51 cases of peripheral nerve sheath tumors in the dog. *J Amer Anim Hosp Assoc* 31:349-359.
5. Monlux, A.W., and Davis, C.L. (1953) Multiple schwannomas of cattle (nerve sheath tumors: multiple neurilemmomas, neurofibromatosis). *Amer J Vet Res* 14:499-509.
6. Canfield, P. (1978) A light microscopic study of bovine peripheral nerve sheath tumours. *Vet Pathol* 15:283-291.
7. Cummings, J.F., and deLahunta, A. (1974) Hypertrophic neuropathy in a dog. *Acta Neuropathol* 29:325-336.
8. Bradley, R.L., Withrow, S.J., and Snyder, S.P. (1982) Nerve sheath tumors in the dog. *J Amer Anim Hosp Assoc* 18:915-921.
9. Carmichael, S., and Griffiths, I.R. (1981) Tumors involving the brachial plexus in seven dogs. *Vet Rec* 108:435-437.
10. Zachary, J.F., O'Brien, D.P., Ingles, B.W., et al. (1986) Multicentric nerve sheath fibrosarcomas of multiple cranial nerve roots in two dogs. *J Amer Vet Med Assoc* 188:723-726.
11. Uchida, K., Nakayama, H., Sasaki, N., Tateyama, S., and Goto, N. (1992) Malignant schwannoma in the spinal root of a dog. *J Vet Med Sci* 54:809-811.
12. Tanimoto, T., and Ohtsuki, Y. (1993) Cutaneous plexiform schwannoma in a pig. *J Comp Pathol* 109:231-240.
13. Pascoe, P.J. (1982) Colic in a mare caused by a colonic neurofibroma. *Can Vet J* 23:24-27.
14. Kirchhoff, N., Scheidemann, W., and Baumgartner, W. (1996) Multiple nerve sheath tumors in the small intestine of a horse. *Vet Pathol* 33:727-730.
15. Andreasen, C.B., Hedstrom, A.O., and Allison, P. (1993) Mediastinal schwannoma in a horse. *Vet Clin Pathol* 22:54-57.
16. Veazey, R.S., Angel, K.L., Snider, T.G., Lopez, M.K., and Taylor, H.W. (1993) Malignant schwannoma in a goat. *J Vet Diag Invest* 5:454-458.
17. Fernandez, C.J., Valentine, B.A., Smith, C., and Summers, B.A. (1996) Equine dermal schwannoma. *Vet Pathol* 33:607. [Abstract 152]
18. Patnaik, A.K., Erlandson, R.A., and Lieberman, P.H. (1984) Canine malignant melanotic schwannomas: A light and electron microscopic study of two cases. *Vet Pathol* 21:483-488.
19. Pumarola, M., Anor, S., Borras, D., and Ferrer, I. (1996) Malignant epithelioid schwannoma affecting the trigeminal nerve of a dog. *Vet Pathol* 33:434-436.
20. Vandevelde, M., Braund, K.G., and Hoff, E.J. (1977) Central neurofibromas in two dogs. *Vet Pathol* 14:470-478.
21. Canfield, P. (1978) The ultrastructure of bovine peripheral nerve sheath tumours. *Vet Pathol* 15:292-300.

Paraganglioma

Paragangliomas are rare neuroendocrine neoplasms composed of extra-adrenal paraganglion chief cells associated with segmental or collateral ganglia of the autonomic nervous system.

Incidence and Sites

Paragangliomas involving the spinal cord have been described in a cow and horse, and in a cat in the cauda equina region.[1-3] The feline case also had a pulmonary metastasis. Secondary extension into the spinal cord from paravertebral paragangliomas has been reported in a dog.[4]

Gross Morphology

Paragangliomas are usually soft, well-circumscribed, encapsulated masses but can be locally invasive.

Histological Features

Tumor cells are arranged in packets or lobules of varying size and surrounded by a delicate, well-vascularized, fibrovascular stroma. Cells have distinct borders, eosinophilic granular cytoplasm, and eccentric round to oval nuclei (fig. 14.38 A). The nuclei have finely stippled chromatin and small nucleoli. Binucleate or karyomegalic nuclei may occur. The mitotic index can be high. Mature ganglion cells, when present, may lie in clusters and have prominent Nissl substance.

Immunohistochemistry

Synaptophysin and chromogranin A staining is usually positive, and there is variable expression of NSE. Triple neurofilament staining may be positive when mature ganglionic cells are present.

Ultrastructural Findings

The most consistent features are neurosecretory dense core granules, well-developed Golgi apparatus, and rough endoplasmic reticulum typical of neuroendocrine secretory cells (fig. 14.38 B).

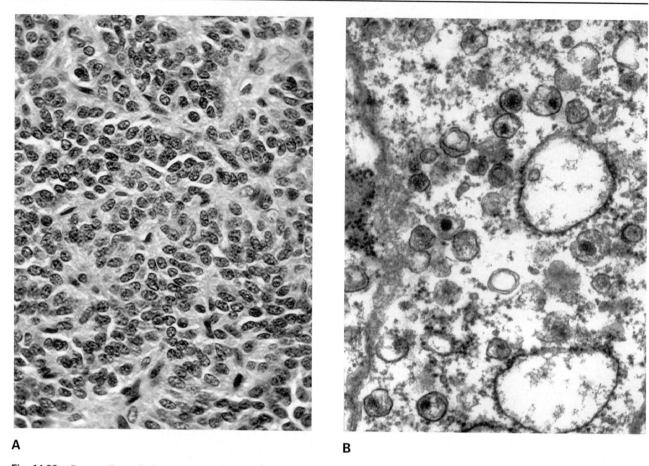

A   **B**

Fig. 14.38.   Paraganglioma. **A.** Canine paraganglioma with clusters of cells in a fibrovascular stroma. **B.** Electronmicrograph illustrating the characteristic dense-core neurosecretory vesicles in a paraganglioma.

REFERENCES

1. Kim, D.Y., Hodgin, C.E., Lopez, M.K., Camus, A.C., and Luther, D.G. (1994) Paraganglioma in the vertebral canal of a cow. *J Vet Diag Invest* 6:389-392.
2. Kim, D.Y., Hodgin, C.E., Lopez, M.K., and Nasarre, C. (1994) Malignant retroperitoneal paraganglioma in a horse. *J Comp Pathol* 110:407-411.
3. Davis, W.P., Watson, G.L., Koehler, L.K., and Brown, C.A. (1997) Malignant cauda equina paraganglioma in a cat. *Vet Pathol* 34:243-246
4. Mascort, J., and Pumarola, M. (1995) Posterior mediastinal paraganglioma involving the spinal cord of a dog. *J Small Anim Pract* 36:274-278.

Ganglioneuroma

Ganglioneuroma and ganglioneuroblastoma are rare neuroblastic tumors of the peripheral nervous system. They originate from the cranial and spinal ganglia and from sympathetic ganglia of the autonomic nervous system.

Incidence and Sites

These can be solitary or multiple tumors in dogs, cats, a pig, a horse, and a steer and are reported from cranial and spinal peripheral nerve ganglia, adrenal medulla, and retro-

pleural, retroperitoneal, mediastinal, and gastrointestinal sites.[1-7] Ganglioneuroblastomas have a mixture of both poorly and well-differentiated ganglion cells.

Gross Morphology

Ganglioneuromas are large, fleshy, gray, firm, poorly defined masses that are locally invasive.

Histological Features

The tumors consist of ganglion cells interspersed between a disproportionate number of nerve fascicles and Schwann cells. The maturation of the ganglion cells varies, and they can be found singly or in clusters. Mature forms have a large, eccentric, vesicular nucleus with a variable amount of Nissl substance, and some may be binucleate (fig. 14.39). Satellite cells are not prominent. The neurons are embedded in a background of tangled, nonmyelinated nerve fibers and fibroblast-like collagen-producing cells.

Immunocytochemistry

Ganglion cells and their processes are strongly immunopositive for triple neurofilament protein expression. The ganglion cells are variably positive for NSE and synaptophysin.

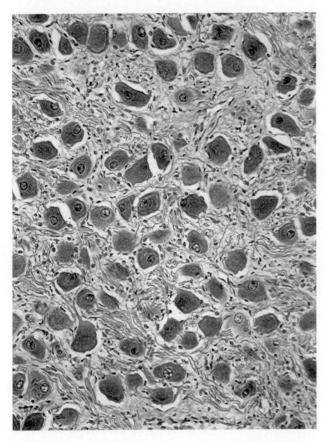

Fig. 14.39. Ganglioneuroma. A well-differentiated perirenal gan-glioneuroma with neoplastic ganglion cells embedded in a stroma of nerve fibers and fibrous tissue.

Ultrastructure

Most ganglion cells have numerous dense core secre-tory vesicles of varying diameter and stacks of rough endoplasmic reticulum.[1,2] Bundles of nonmyelinated nerve fibers identified by their neurofilament content are distrib-uted throughout the mass. There are also some fibroblasts distributed around nerve processes.

Differential Diagnosis

Ganglioneuromas and particularly less well differen-tiated ganglioneuroblastomas need to differentiated from fibromas or schwannomas, which is best done by positive immunocytochemical staining and ultrastructural confir-mation of their neuroblastic origin.[2]

REFERENCES

1. Hawkins, K.L., and Summers, B.A. (1987) Mediastinal ganglioneu-roma in a puppy. *Vet Pathol* 24:283-285.
2. Ribas, J.L., Kwapien, R.P., and Pope, E.R. (1990) Immunocyto-chemistry and ultrastructure of intestinal ganglioneuroma in a dog. *Vet Pathol* 27:376-379.
3. Scheuler, R.O., Rousch, J.K., and Oyster, R.A. (1993) Spinal gan-glioneuroma in a dog. *J Amer Vet Med Assoc* 203:539-541.
4. Patnaik, A.K., Lieberman, P.H., and Johnson, G.F. (1978) Intestinal ganglioneuroma in a kitten. *J Small Anim Pract* 19:735-742.
5. Une, Y., Iwama, K., Yoshida, H., et al. (1984) Multiple ganglioneu-roma derived from the intramural plexus of jejunum in a sow. *Jpn J Vet Sci* 46:247-250.
6. Allen, D., Swayne, D., and Belknap, J.K. (1989) Ganglioneuroma as a cause of small intestinal obstruction in a horse. *Cornell Vet* 79:133-141.
7. Sokale, E.O.A., and Ladds, P.W. (1983) Multicentric ganglioneu-roma in a steer. *Vet Pathol* 20:767-770.

METASTATIC TUMORS OF THE CENTRAL NERVOUS SYSTEM

The incidence of metastases to the CNS from extra-neural primary tumors varies widely within and between species in the few studies reported.[1-3] Most data have been collected from the dog, with only sporadic cases reported in other species. In one series of over 400 canine brain tumors, only 17 percent were from secondary metastases, while in another collection over 60 percent of all tumors were metastatic in origin.[1,3] This seemingly wide disparity, how-ever, may reflect no more than differences in the thorough-ness of the necropsy examination. In an unpublished canine collection of 350 nervous system tumors, the incidence of metastatic tumors was almost 30 percent (A. Koestner). In the latter study, half of these tumors were sarcomas (fibro-, osteo-, chondro-, and hemangiosarcomas), while carcinomas of nasal, pulmonary, mammary, and renal ori-gin comprised the majority of the remaining tumors. Most of these metastatic foci were located in the brain, but the spinal cord was often not examined. In two smaller series of canine spinal cord tumors, over 50 percent were of non-neuroectodermal origin.[4,5] The propensity of specific tumors for metastatic spread into the CNS has been largely ignored, although 14 percent of 85 dogs with disseminated hemangiosarcoma had metastatic tumor foci mainly in the cerebral gray matter.[6]

There are several obvious routes of entry of nonneu-roectodermal tumors into the nervous system that are prob-ably dependent on neurotrophic factors as well as autocrine and paracrine growth factor mechanisms.[7] Hematogenous dissemination within the neuraxis is the most common, with resultant metastatic foci in the neu-ropil, choroid plexus, or the leptomeninges. Such dissemi-nation can occur with carcinomas, sarcomas, and hematopoietic tumors. Within the brain, there appears to be no correlation between the tumor type and site or number of metastases, although detailed studies are not available. There may be a tendency toward more tumors seeding in gray rather than white matter, possibly due to the differ-ences in relative vascularity and blood flow. The massive showering of microscopically detected foci often found in human carcinomas appears to be uncommon in animals. Most carcinomas tend to produce fairly large, multiple masses, while more diffuse showering with smaller sized foci is seen with hemangiosarcomas and melanomas. Hematopoietic tumors (e.g., leukemias) tend to result in small cellular emboli with pinpoint hemorrhages throughout the gray and white matter. A canine myelomonocytic leukemia has selectively involved cranial nerve roots.[8] Diffuse leptomeningeal carcinomatosis is a common secondary manifestation with some human carcinomas but is rarely reported in animals.[9,10] Leptomeningeal involvement has been reported with extraneural malignant lymphomas.[11,12] Angiocentric T cell lymphomas in the dog and cat produce intravascular occlusion leading to hemorrhagic infarcts.[13-15] Peritumoral vasogenic edema can be a secondary manifestation, particularly with mammary carcinomas.

The other major route of entry is by local extension. In the head, infiltration of primary nasal tumors (e.g., adenocarcinomas, chondrosarcomas, and fibrosarcomas) through the cribriform plate into the olfactory bulbs and frontal lobes is most common.[16,17] Primary suprasellar germ cell tumors grow intracranially as compressive extraparenchymal masses.[18] Direct extension through the calvarium, often aided by bony lysis, occurs with squamous cell carcinomas, osteo- and chondrosarcomas, and the multilobular osteochondrosarcoma of bone.[19] In the spinal vertebral bodies, primary osteosarcomas, chondrosarcomas, hemangiosarcomas, as well as metastatic (e.g., multiple myeloma, aortic body tumor) or locally infiltrative tumors (e.g., MPNST, fibrosarcomas) can result in bony lysis with secondary compressive fractures and cord injury.[4,5] Injury to the spinal cord may also result from local infiltration or space-occupying impingement from extradural malignant lymphomas, histiocytic sarcomas, choroid plexus carcinomas, prostatic carcinomas, paravertebral ganglioneuromas, melanomas, and the multilobular osteochondrosarcoma of bone.[20,21]

REFERENCES

1. Luginbühl, H. (1963) Comparative aspects of tumors of the nervous system. *Ann NY Acad Sci* 108:702-721.
2. Luginbühl, H., Fankhauser, R., and McGrath, J.T. (1968) Spontaneous neoplasms of the nervous system in animals. *Prog Neurol Surg* 2:85-164.
3. Fenner, W.R. (1990) Metastatic neoplasms of the central nervous system. *Sem Vet Med Surg* 5:253-261.
4. Lutgen, P.J., Braund, K.G., Brawner, W.R., and Vandevelde, M. (1980) A retrospective study of twenty-nine spinal cord tumors in the dog and cat. *J Small Anim Pract* 21:213-226.
5. Wright, J.A. (1985) The pathological features associated with spinal tumors in 29 dogs. *J Comp Pathol* 95:549-557.
6. Waters, D.J., Hayden, D.W., and Walter, P.A.(1989) Intracranial lesions in dogs with hemangiosarcoma. *J Vet Int Med* 3:222-230.
7. Nicolson, G.L., and Menter, D.G. (1995) Trophic factors and central nervous system metastasis. *Canc Metast Rev* 14:303-321.
8. Christopher, M.M., Metz, A.L., and Klausner, J. (1986) Acute myelomonocytic leukemia with neurologic complications in the dog. *Vet Pathol* 23:140-147.
9. Stampley, A.R., Swayne, D.E., and Prasse, K.W. (1987) Meningeal carcinomatosis secondary to a colonic signet-ring carcinoma in a dog. *J Amer Anim Hosp Assoc* 23:655-658.
10. Pumarola, M., and Balasch, M. (1996) Meningeal carcinomatosis in a dog. *Vet Rec* 138:523-524.
11. Britt, J.O., Simpson, J.G., and Howard, E.B. (1984) Malignant lymphoma of the meninges in two dogs. *J Comp Pathol* 94:45-53.
12. Couto, C.G., Cullen, J., Pedroia, V., and Turrel, J.M. (1984) Central nervous system lymphosarcoma in the dog. *J Amer Vet Med Assoc* 184:809-813.
13. Dargent, F.J., Fox, L.E., and Anderson, W.I. (1988) Neoplastic angioendotheliomatosis in a dog: Angiotropic lymphoma. *Cornell Vet* 78:253-262.
14. Summers, B.A., and deLahunta, A. (1985) Cerebral angioendotheliomatosis in a dog. *Acta Neuropathol* 68:10-14.
15. LaPointe, J.-M., Higgins, R.J., Kortz, G.D., Bailey, C.S., and Moore, P.F. (1997) Feline angiocentric T-cell lymphosarcoma. *Vet Pathol* 34:247-250.
16. Cordy, D.R. (1990) Tumors of the nervous system and eye. In Moulton, J.E. (ed.), *Tumors of Domestic Animals,* 3rd ed. University of California Press, Berkeley.
17. Smith, M.O., Turrel, J.M., Bailey, C.S., and Cain, G.R. (1989) Neurologic abnormalities as the predominant signs of neoplasia of the nasal cavity in dogs and cats: Seven cases (1973-1986). *J Amer Vet Med Assoc* 195:242-245.
18. Valentine, B.A., Summers, B.A., deLahunta, A., White, C.L., and Kuhajda, F.P. (1988) Suprasellar germ cell tumors in the dog: A report of five cases and review of the literature. *Acta Neuropathol* 76:94-100.
19. Straw, R.C., LeCouteur, R.A., Powers, B.E., and Withrow, S.J. (1989) Multilobular osteochondrosarcoma of the canine skull: 16 cases (1978-1988). *J Amer Vet Med Assoc* 195:1764-1769.
20. Spodnick, G.J., Berg, J., and Moore, F.M. (1989) Spinal lymphoma in cats: 21 cases (1976-1989). *J Amer Vet Med Assoc* 200:373-376.
21. Hines, M.E., Newton, J.C., Altman, N.H., Hribernik, T.N., and Casey, H.W. (1993) Metastasizing extra-adrenal paraganglioma with neurologic signs in four dogs. *J Comp Pathol* 108:283-290.

15 Tumors of the Eye

R. R. Dubielzig

GENERAL CONSIDERATIONS

Although tumors of the eye and its supporting tissues in domestic animals are relatively rare, they assume an enhanced importance because of the visibility and effect on function of even small tumors within, or adjacent to, the eyes. Although tumors within the globe may or may not be readily visible, their effect on ocular function can be dramatic, leading to visual defects, discoloration, discomfort, or a change in shape of the globe. These are the consequences of ocular neoplasia that cause an animal owner to seek veterinary attention.

Tumors within the globe present several unique problems to the pathologist. These tumors may be small and are often not apparent from the external surface of the extracted globe. Because the structures of the globe are delicate and the orientation of ocular tissues is important, the globe should be dissected free of extra tissue from the orbit and lids and immersed in fixative without opening the globe. Fixation prior to sectioning will enhance the rigidity of ocular structures and help maintain the ocular structures in their normal anatomic orientation. Table 15.1 summarizes the advantages and disadvantages of commonly used ocular fixatives. It is helpful if information regarding the location of the suspected intraocular tumor can be provided by the attending clinician prior to sectioning of the globe. Without this information, it is useful to have an apparatus that allows the pathologist to candle the globe. In a dark room, a bright light is situated in contact with the posterior sclera, illuminating the globe and revealing intraocular masses as dark shadows. The position of the mass should be recorded, and the section should be made to pass through the largest diameter of the mass. Ideally,

sections of the globe should pass through the optic nerve and pupil; however, oblique sections are often required to assess neoplastic infiltration.

TUMORS OF THE LID AND CONJUNCTIVA

Most of the tumors of the haired skin of the lid are tumors generally found on the skin, and a list of expected tumors of the lid is given in table 15.2.

Tumors of Meibomian Gland Origin

Incidence

Meibomian gland tumors are comparable in frequency to their counterparts in sebaceous glands. They occur in increasing frequency as dogs age, and they invariably occur at the eyelid margin of either the upper or lower lid.[1,2]

Gross Morphology and Histological Features

Meibomian gland adenoma is usually an exophytic, often papillary, protuberance bulging outward from the eyelid margin. Because the tumor contacts the cornea, ocular irritation, pain, and secondary keratitis or conjunctivitis may be a complicating factor. Meibomian gland adenomas are composed of well-differentiated glandular tissue having a sebaceous appearance. Granulomatous or lympho-

TABLE 15.1. **Comparison of fixatives for ocular tissues**

Fixative	Contents	Advantages	Disadvantages
Formalin	Formaldehyde	Cheap, fast, good general fixative	No serious disadvantages
Glutaraldehyde	Glutaraldehyde	Best for electron microscopy	Slow penetration. Must open the globe for surface fixation
Davidson's	Formaldehyde, ethanol, acetic acid	Added rigidity	Shrinkage, not as good as formalin for EM
Bouin's	Picric acid, formaldehyde, acetic acid	Added rigidity plus good for immunohistochemistry	EM impossible, opaque yellow color, dry picric acid explosive
Zenker's	Mercuric chloride, potassium dichromate, acetic acid	Best morphology with paraffin sections	EM impossible. Mercuric chloride is an environmental toxin

TABLE 15.2.   Skin tumors of the eyelids in domestic animals

Tumor	Species
Meibomian gland	Canine, feline
Sebaceous gland	Canine
Squamous papilloma	Canine, feline
Melanocytoma	Canine
Mast cell tumor	Canine, feline
Neurofibroma*	Feline
Trichoblastoma (basal cell tumor)	Canine
Trichoephithelioma	Canine
Basal cell carcinoma	Feline
Sarcoid	Equine

*Peripheral nerve sheath tumor.

cytic inflammation around the exposed adenoma can contribute as much or more to the mass effect as the tumor itself. Unlike sebaceous glands, macrophages surrounding meibomian gland adenoma or simply inflamed meibomian glands often contain intracytoplasmic refractile membranous bodies (fig. 15.1 A,B,C), presumed to be ingested tear-film lipids. *Meibomian gland epithelioma* is analogous to sebaceous epithelioma and is composed of a larger proportion of basal cells, with a smaller proportion that have sebaceous or squamous differentiation. These tumors usually have a coexistent melanocytic component. *Meibomian gland adenocarcinoma* is a rare tumor which is more likely to be invasive and aggressive with local reoccurrence following incomplete excision.[3]

Conjunctival Melanoma

Incidence

Melanomas of the conjunctiva are rare tumors of dogs and cats (fig. 15.2). In 12 cases reported in dogs, there was a predilection for the tumor to arise from the nictitating membrane. Most of these tumors were cytologically malignant; reoccurrence was a problem in over half of the cases, and metastasis occurred in two animals.[4]

Gross Morphology and Histological Features

These are nodular or multinodular masses distorting the conjunctival sac. They are sometimes amelanotic and often multifocal. The histological features of melanoma of the conjunctiva in dogs and cats are similar to those of malignant melanomas in other sites. These tumors have varying pigmentation and features of cytological atypia or anaplasia. The mitotic index is presumed to be the best indicator of prognosis. Tumor cells tend to form tight aggregates, especially subjacent to or within the conjunctival epithelium. Tumors removed by broad excision or enucleation often show aggregates of intraepithelial neoplasm at sites distant from the primary neoplasm. Recurrent tumors often form at different sites in the conjunctiva. Amelanotic melanoma can be confused with anaplastic carcinoma, fibrosarcoma, or lymphoma, and differentia-

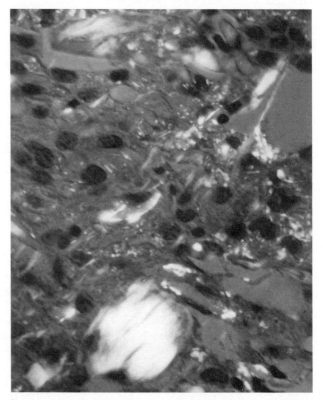

A   **B**

Fig. 15.1.   A. Macrophages surrounding a sebaceous adenoma have dense linear profiles in the cytoplasm. **B.** Same field as A viewed with polarized light, birefringent linear material is in the cytoplasm of the phagocytic cells. (continued)

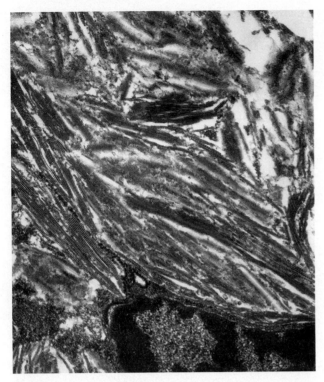

C

Fig. 15.1. **C.** Electron micrograph of phagocytic cells with accumulation of stacked electron dense membranous material in the cytoplasm of cells shown in A. This material is presumed to be tear-film lipid constituted into membranous bodies.

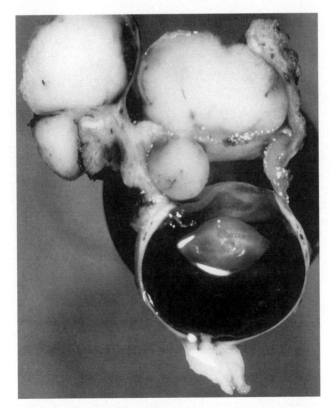

Fig. 15.2. The globe and conjunctiva from a dog with multifocal amelanotic malignant conjunctival melanoma.

tion is best made by immunohistochemical staining with S100, which is reliably positive in melanoma.

Bovine Squamous Cell Carcinoma

Incidence

Ocular squamous cell carcinoma is easily the most common and economically important neoplasm of the eye in cattle. The Department of Agriculture reports a 0.2 percent incidence in cattle from 1950 to 1954.[5]

Geographic Distribution

Squamous cell carcinoma is reported throughout the world. In the United States the tumor is more common in the Southwest, purportedly because of greater exposure to ultraviolet radiation.[6,7]

Age, Breed, and Sex

Squamous cell carcinoma increases in incidence in older animals. Although all breeds are affected, Hereford cattle are the most frequently affected due to the lack of pigmentation around the eyes and the resultant increased dose of penetrating ultraviolet radiation.[8,9]

Gross Morphology and Histological Features

The tumor most commonly begins on the bulbar conjunctiva near the cornea, usually at the limbus (fig. 15.3). Squamous cell carcinoma can be divided into four stages: plaques, 11 percent; papillomas, 7 percent; noninvasive carcinoma, 3 percent; and invasive carcinoma, 79 percent.[5,10] The *plaque lesions* are small and are composed of hyperplastic and dysplastic epithelium. They have smooth margins and a raised surface and are translucent to opaque white. Histologically, there is epithelial hyperplasia with atypia and often hyperkeratosis. A *papilloma* is an exophytic growth which can be multiple and confluent. *Noninvasive carcinoma* is thought to arise from the plaque lesion. This tumor has an exophytic outward irregular growth that distorts the ocular profile and causes pressure on the globe but shows little tendency to invade the scleral tissues. *Invasive carcinoma* shows both exophytic and invasive growth, with invasion of the deep subconjunctival stroma, sclera, and intraocular structures, but metastasis is rare. Microscopically, squamous cell carcinomas exhibit highly anaplastic features, often with a concurrent desmoplastic response.[5,10] In the experience of the author, the presence of a plaque indicates the early stages of a neoplastic process that could progress to papilloma, noninvasive carcinoma, or invasive carcinoma; however, neither papilloma nor noninvasive carcinoma degenerate into invasive carcinoma.

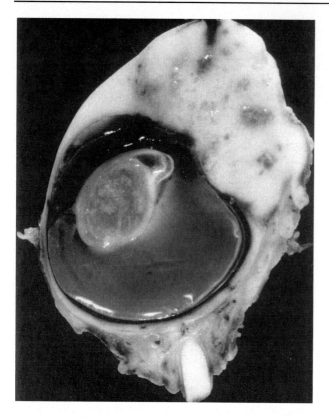

Fig. 15.3. The globe from a bovine with an invasive squamous cell carcinoma infiltrating the limbic sclerocornea and distorting the profile of the intraocular tissues.

Etiology

The cause of ocular squamous cell carcinoma in cattle is definitely multifactorial. Although virus-like particles have been seen in tumors by transmission electron microscopy, their importance in the pathogenesis is unclear.[11,12] Familial lines of cattle with an extremely high incidence of the tumor have been reported.[5,9,13] In most breeds of cattle, a lack of pigmentation around the eyelids is an important predisposing factor to the development of squamous cell carcinoma. The tumor has a higher incidence proportional to the ultraviolet light exposure, and genomic damage related to ultraviolet light undoubtedly plays an important role in the pathogenesis of bovine ocular squamous cell carcinoma.[14] Immunotherapy using phenolized extracts of allogenic carcinomas has been reported to be effective in reducing the size of tumors.[15]

Equine Squamous Cell Carcinoma

Incidence

Squamous cell carcinoma is the most common neoplasm of ocular structures in horses.[16] Although the incidence in horses is less than that in cattle, the biological behavior is similar. Tumors most commonly arise at the limbus as a dysplastic plaque and progress to varying degrees of invasive carcinoma. A hereditary predilection has not been demonstrated in the horse, but exposure to ultraviolet light is thought to be an important predisposing cause.

Gross Morphology and Histological Features

As in cattle, the tumors appear as a plaque progressing to either noninvasive or invasive carcinoma. Histologically the plaque consists of epithelial hyperplasia with or without hyperkeratosis. There is usually an abrupt margin between the intraepithelial neoplasm and the surrounding normal structures. Invasive tumors have features of cytological anaplasia and desmoplastic stromal proliferation. Deep invasion of local tissues is seen, but metastasis is rare. An interesting morphological variant is the stromal invasive carcinoma (fig. 15.4). These tumors show no exophytic growth but directly invade the corneal stromal lamellae, beginning as linear corneal opacities that expand and involve major portions of the corneal tissue without producing tumor-like nodules. Spread beyond the cornea has not been reported.

Canine and Feline Squamous Cell Carcinoma

Squamous cell carcinoma of the conjunctiva, nictitans, and cornea of dogs and cats is rare. These tumors can be multifocal, exophytic papilloma-like lesions, or aggres-

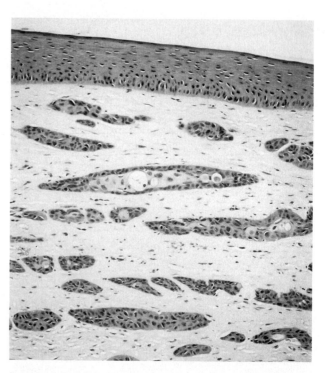

Fig. 15.4. Anterior corneal stroma from a horse with stroma invasive squamous cell carcinoma showing cords of neoplastic cells infiltrating between corneal stromal lamellae.

sive infiltrating carcinomas with destruction of orbital tissue or penetration of the globe. Often squamous cell carcinoma in dogs and cats occurs in conjunction with chronic inflammation of the conjunctiva. In cats, squamous cell carcinoma is often multifocal; the other eye is at risk, as is the ear tip. Because these tumors are irritating and because deep local invasion is possible, enucleation is the treatment of choice.

Carcinoma of the Gland of the Third Eyelid in Dogs

Incidence

Carcinoma of the gland of the third eyelid is a rare, sporadically occurring, invasive, solid neoplasm presenting as a mass lesion at the base of the nictitans on the ventromedial conjunctiva.[17] The tumor displaces the globe, and in large tumors there is invasion of the adjacent orbital tissue.

Histological Features

These tumors are anaplastic, showing solid poorly differentiated epithelial tissue, often mixed with an extensive lymphocytic inflammatory component. Tumor margins are indistinct, with local infiltration that mandates aggressive surgery to remove the mass. Adequately excised tumors have a low recurrence rate, and metastasis is rare or nonexistent. In some cases immunohistochemical markers of epithelial cells such as cytokeratin might be useful in making the distinction between carcinoma of the gland of the third eyelid and granulomatous inflammation.

Hemangioma and Hemangiosarcoma of All Species

Vascular endothelial neoplasms of the conjunctiva, nictitans, and even the avascular cornea are reported in several species, but they are seen most commonly in dogs and horses.[18,19] In dogs these tumors usually present as small, red, raised lesions of the conjunctiva, most commonly on the leading margin of the nictitans. Surgical resection of these tumors with clear margins is curative. Larger invasive lesions of the limbus or cornea can be difficult to resect, and as in subcutaneous tumors, the distinction between hemangioma and hemangiosarcoma depends upon the degree of cellular differentiation and local invasion. Aggressive tumors invade ocular tissues and mandate aggressive or extensive excision including enucleation. In horses there has been speculation that these tumors are of lymphatic vessels,[20] but this interpretation is not clear. Vascular endothelial tumors of the ocular adnexa do not metastasize. Exposure to ultraviolet light may be a risk factor in the pathogenesis of vascular endothelial neoplasms.[20] Differential diagnosis is seldom a problem, but factor VIII is detectable in endothelial cells of both dogs and horses.

Conjunctival Lipogranuloma of Cats

This inflammatory condition causes a tumor-like proliferative mass that may occur at any position in the conjunctiva of cats. Affected cats are usually old animals, and the disease is often bilateral. These lesions can be unilateral or bilateral, and the granuloma lesions have been reported to occur concurrently with invasive neoplasms.[21] Lipogranuloma is refractory to medical therapy, but most cases respond well to surgical excision. Histologically, the lesion is composed of large extracellular pools of lipid surrounded by clusters of large macrophage cells, sometimes with giant cell formation. In most cases, the lesion is purely granulomatous and no birefringent material is seen. The conjunctival epithelium is usually intact, although goblet cell hyperplasia is common. This disease can occur concurrently with conjunctival neoplasia, most often squamous cell carcinoma or spindle cell sarcoma.

REFERENCES

1. Krehbiel, J.D., and Langham, R.F. (1975) Eyelid neoplasms of dogs. *Amer J Vet Res* 36(1): 115-119.
2. Roberts, S.M., Severin, G.A., and La vach, J.D. (1986) Prevalence and treatment of palpebral neoplasms in the dog: 200 cases (1975-1983). *Amer Vet Med Assoc* 189:1355-1359.
3. Case, M.T., Bartz, A.R., Bernstein, M., and Rosen, R.A. (1969) Metastasis of a sebaceous gland carcinoma in the dog. *J Amer Vet Med Assoc* 154:661-664.
4. Collins, B.K., Collier, L.L., Miller, M.A., and Linton, L.L. (1993) Biologic behavior and histologic characteristics of canine conjunctival melanoma. *Prog Vet Comp Ophthalmol* 3:135-140.
5. Russell, W.O., Wynne, E.S., and Loquvam, G.S. (1956) Studies on bovine ocular squamous carcinoma ("cancer eye"). I. Pathobiological anatomy and historical review. *Cancer* 9:1-52.
6. Anderson, D.E., and Skinner, P.E. (1961) Studies on bovine ocular squamous carcinoma ("cancer eye"). XI. Effects of sunlight. *J Anim Sci* 20:474-477.
7. Guilbert, H.R., Wahid, A., Wagnon, K.A., and Gregory, P.W. (1948) Observations on pigmentation of eyelids of Hereford cattle in relation to occurrence of ocular epitheliomas. *J Anim Sci* 7:426-429.
8. Anderson, D.E., and Chambers, D. (1957) Genetic aspects of cancer eye in cattle. In *Oklahoma Agricultural Experiment Station. Miscellaneous Publication.* MP-48, pp. 28-33.
9. Blackwell, R.L., Anderson, D.E., and Knox, J.H. (1956) Age incidence and heritability of cancer eye in Hereford cattle. *J Anim Sci* 15:943-951.
10. Monlux, A.W., Anderson, W.A., and Davis, C.L. (1957) The diagnosis of squamous cell carcinoma of the eye (cancer eye) in cattle. *Amer J Vet Res* 18:5-34.
11. Hod, I., and Perk, K. (1973) Internuclear microspherules in bovine ocular squamous cell carcinoma. *Ref Vet* 30:41-44.
12. Ford, J.N., Jennings, P.A., Spradbrow, P.B., Francis, J. (1982) Evidence for papillomaviruses in ocular lesions in cattle. *Res Vet Sci* 32:257-259.
13. Woodward, R.R., and Knapp, B., Jr. (1950) The hereditary aspect of eye cancer in Hereford cattle. *J Anim Sci* 9:578-581.
14. Kopecky, K.E., Pugh, G.W., Hughes, D.E., Booth, G.D., Cheville, N.F. (1979) Biological effect of ultraviolet radiation on cattle: Bovine ocular squamous cell carcinoma. *Amer J Vet Res* 40:1783-1788.

15. Hoffmann, D., Jennings, P.A. Spradbrow, P.B. (1981) Immunotherapy of bovine ocular squamous cell carcinomas with phenol-saline extracts of allogenic carcinomas. *Aust Vet J* 57:159-162.

16. Blodi, F.C., and Ramsey, F.K. (1967) Ocular tumors in domestic animals. *Amer J Ophthalmol* 64:627-633.

17. Wilcock, B.P., and Peiffer, R.L. (1988) Adenocarcinoma of the gland of the third eyelid in seven dogs. *J Amer Vet Med Assoc* 193:1549-1550.

18. Peiffer, R.L., Duncan, J., and Terrell, T. (1978) Hemangioma of the nictitating membrane in 2 dogs. *J Amer Vet Med Assoc* 172:832-833.

19. Hargis, A.M., Lee, A.C., and Thomassen, R.W. (1978) Tumor and tumor-like lesions of perilimbal conjunctiva in laboratory dogs. *J Amer Vet Med Assoc* 173:1185-1190.

20. Hacker, D.V., Moore, P.F., and Buyukmihci, N.C. (1986) Ocular angiosarcoma in four horses. *J Amer Vet Med Assoc* 189:200-203.

21. Kerlin, R.L., and Dubielzig, R.R. (1997) Lipogranulomatous conjunctivitis in cats. *Vet Comp Ophthalmol* 7:177-179.

TUMORS OF THE GLOBE

The common primary neoplasms of the globe seen in domestic animals are summarized in table 15.3 and Fig. 15.5.

Canine Ocular Melanoma

Incidence

Tumors of melanocytic origin is the most common primary neoplasm of the globe in dogs.[1] Tumors of the scleral limbus have a higher incidence in German shepherd dogs, but other than that, there is no breed or sex predilection for canine ocular melanoma.[2]

Gross Morphology and Histological Features

Melanocytic tumors of the canine globe have been divided into two categories based on histological features. Benign tumors are referred to as melanocytoma (fig. 15.6), and they are composed of two populations of cells. Large, round, heavily pigmented cells occur in clusters within the tumors, often at the peripheral margins, and in some cases, they make up all or nearly all of the tumor mass. Bleached sections are required to evaluate cellular features. These tumors have small, dark, round nuclei and are benign. Since these cells often occur at the periphery of the tumor in large masses extending through the sclera, large round cells can sometimes be left behind by the surgeon, but

there appears to be no risk of recurrence, even if pigmented material is left in the orbit after enucleation. A second population of cells is spindle to stellate cells, often with a small, central, oval-to-round nucleus (fig. 15.7). Mitotic figures are very rare or absent in melanocytoma. More aggressive melanocytomas are composed of a high proportion of spindle cells, and some tumors are composed entirely of spindle cells. Melanocytoma of the globe can occur in several locations, but the most common is the anterior uveal tract, either the iris or the ciliary body stroma. Tumors originating from melanocytes in the limbal sclera (fig. 15.8) (epibulbar melanoma) are always benign. Epibulbar melanocytomas are always composed of heavily pigmented large round cells either alone or mixed with small numbers of heavily pigmented spindle cells. Rare tumors originating in the choroid also tend to be benign, with similar histological features. Although melanocytoma has no metastatic potential, these tumors can be locally aggressive and destructive to the globe. Secondary glaucoma, retinal detachment, intraocular hemorrhage, and ocular pain can lead to clinical disease and visual impairment and can obscure the tumor.[3,4] Even when a small amount of black material remains in the orbit there is seldom recurrence.

Malignant intraocular melanoma (fig. 15.9) comprises about 20 percent of intraocular melanocytic tumors in dogs.[4] These tumors usually arise from the anterior uvea, either the iris or the ciliary body. Histological criteria for anaplasia are useful in distinguishing benign from malignant tumors, and a mitotic profile is probably the single best indicator.[4] More than 1-2 mitotic profiles per high power (HP) field (400×) is evidence of malignancy (fig. 15.10). Malignant ocular melanoma in dogs tends to be less darkly pigmented and is locally aggressive. Occasionally these tumors arise diffusely in the anterior uvea and, very rarely, in the choroid.[5] Even among malignant intraocular melanomas in dogs, systemic metastasis to the extent of changes in the quality of life for the dog have rarely been reported.[3,4] This is in stark contrast to malignant oral melanoma of dogs.

Feline Diffuse Iris Melanoma

Incidence

Tumors of melanocytic origin are the most common primary intraocular neoplasm of cats.[6] There is no known

TABLE 15.3. Primary tumor of the globe

Tumor Type	Cell of Origin	Species	Prognosis
Melanocytoma	Melanocyte	Canine	Good
Malignant melanoma	Melanocyte	Canine	Metastasis possible, rarely fatal
Diffuse iris melanoma	Melanocyte	Feline	Poor unless removal early
Iridociliary epithelial tumor	Pigmented or nonpigmented epithelial cells of iris or ciliary body	Canine/feline	Good
Medulloepithelioma	Primitive neuroectodermal cells	Canine/equine young	Metastasis rare
Posttraumatic sarcoma	Lens: epithelial, fibroblastic, osteoblastic, cells, melanocytes, etc.	Feline	Very poor

PRIMARY TUMORS OF THE GLOBE

	Name of Tumor	Comments
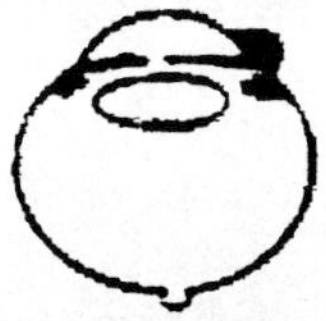	Epibulbar Melanocytoma	Canine, benign, occurs in the limbal sclera by definition, heavily pigmented round cells. Pigmented spindle cells.
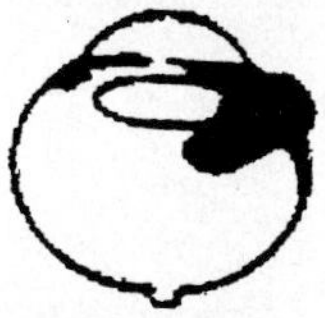	Anterior Uveal Melanocytoma	Canine, benign, occurs in the anterior uveal tissue, a mixture of heavily pigmented round cells and heavily pigmented spindle cells, local invasion, but never metastasizes.
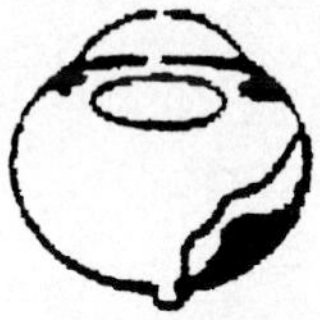	Choroidal Melanocytoma	Canine, benign, occurs in the choroid, a mixture of heavily pigmented round cells and heavily pigmented spindle cells, local invasion but never metastasizes. Retinal detachment common.
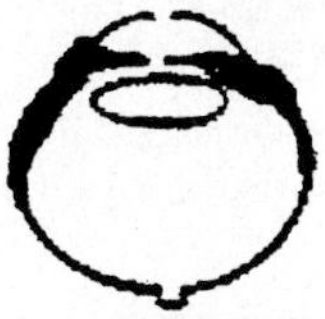	Canine Malignant Ocular Melanoma	Canine, malignant histologically, but slow to cause systemic signs, may occur anywhere in uvea, but anterior uvea is most common. Often diffuse.
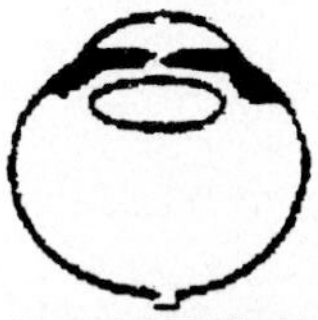	Feline Diffuse Iris Melanoma	Feline, malignant, starts on anterior iris surface and fills iris, then ciliary body, round cell, spindle cell, and balloon cell variants.
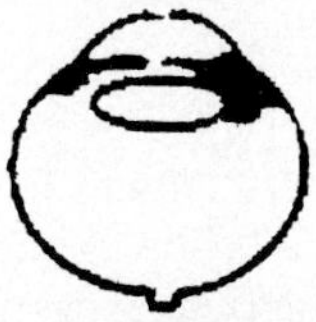	Iridociliary Epithelial Tumor	Canine and rarely feline, may be locally invasive, but never metastasize, tumors of iridociliary epithelial cells, may be pigmented or nonpigmented.
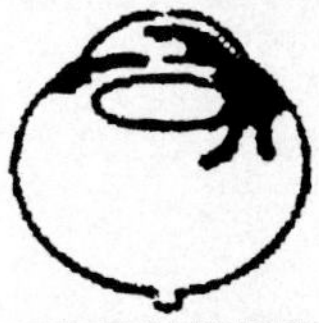	Medulloepithelioma	Canine or equine, usually young, rarely malignant, usually occur in the anterior uvea, tumor of primitive neural tissue which can form rosettes and radiating tubes of tissue.
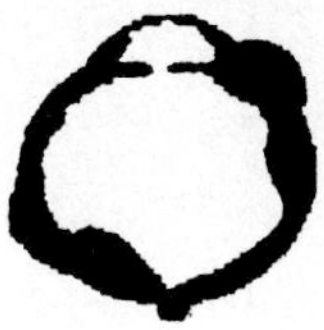	Feline Posttraumatic Sarcoma	Feline, malignant, occurs in damaged eyes with lens rupture. Tumors line the inner globe and invade aggressively. Many different sarcomas possible, including tumors derived from lens cells.

Fig. 15.5. Schematic drawing and comments regarding the distribution and important features of primary tumors of the globe.

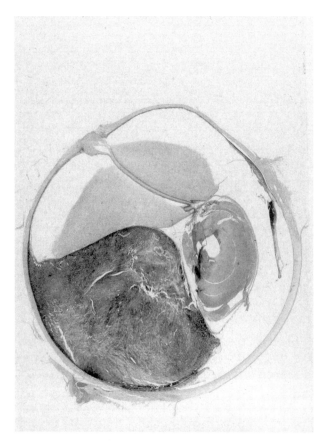

Fig. 15.6. Canine uveal melanocytoma involving the ciliary body and choroid associated with retinal detachment and distortion of the ocular contents.

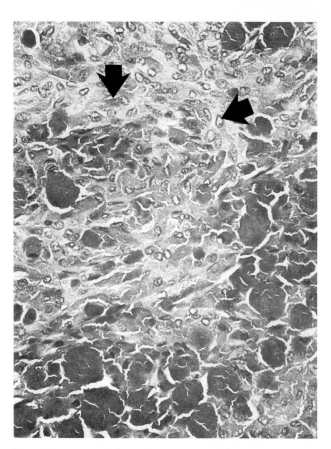

Fig. 15.7. Photomicrograph of canine uveal melanocytoma showing small spindle cells (arrows) mixed with numerous, large, round pigmented cells, H&E bleach.

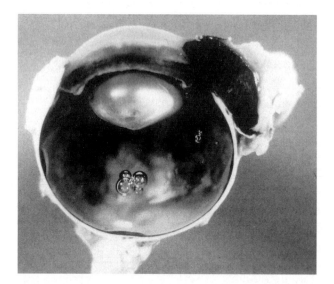

Fig. 15.8. Canine globe with epibulbar melanocytoma extending full thickness through the sclera but not distorting the uvea and lens.

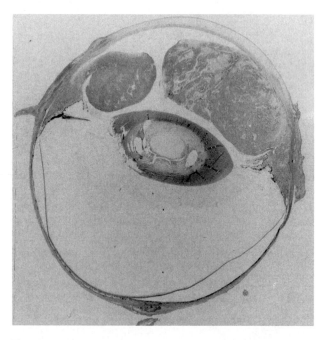

Fig. 15.9. Histological section of canine globe with malignant intraocular melanoma. Arising in the iris vs ciliary body. Tumor was poorly/lightly pigmented, and the mitotic index was high (2/HP field).

breed or sex predilection, and occurrence of melanoma is usually in old cats. Iridal pigmentary changes including localized pigmented foci, expanding or coalescing iridal pigmentation, and diffuse pigmentary changes are often noted prior to the development of melanoma. Pigmentary changes can occur years before neoplasia begins. The most common melanocytic ocular tumor of cats is known as feline diffuse iris melanoma because these tumors tend to

expand diffusely into the iridal stroma, with subsequent invasion of the ciliary body and sclera. Atypical melanomas of the limbus or choroid, or tumors arising multifocally throughout the globe are rarely encountered. I have seen

746

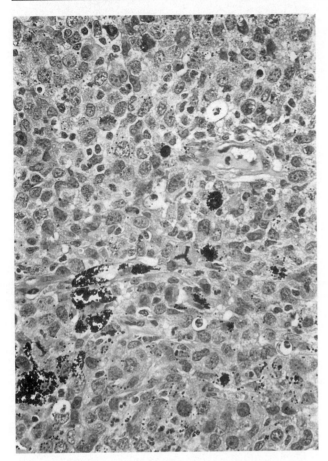

Fig. 15.10. Photomicrograph of malignant intraocular melanoma showing poorly pigmented, anaplastic cells with many mitotic figures.

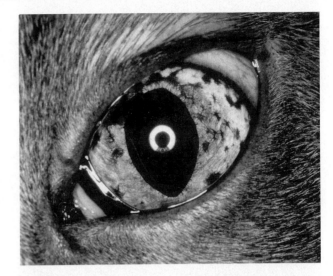

Fig. 15.11. Clinical photograph of a feline eye with multifocal pigmented spots coalescing in some areas. These are the early stages of feline diffuse iris melanoma.

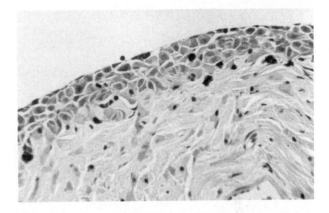

Fig. 15.12. The surface of the anterior iris has angular small pigmented cells with featureless small round nuclei and no tendency to exfoliate into the anterior chamber or infiltrate into the iris stroma. In the absence of infiltrating cells with a larger nucleus, these cells are considered iridal melanosis. This change may be a premalignant change.

two types of atypical melanomas: *multifocal* tumors composed of heavily pigmented round cells that destroy the globe and *anaplastic* poorly pigmented tumors that fill the inner globe and have a history similar to that of posttraumatic sarcoma. These atypical melanomas are rare, and they will not be discussed further because little is known.

Gross Morphology and Histological Features

Feline diffuse iris melanoma appears to begin as abnormal pigmentation of the iris (fig. 15.11). Localized pigmented lesions originate as clusters of small, angular, pigmented cells with small, round nuclei adherent to the iridal surface (fig. 15.12). These pigmented cells have no tendency to exfoliate or invade the iridal stroma. Pigmented lesions can exist locally or expand in the iris for months to several years prior to the development of neoplasia. When pigmented lesions expand, become nodular, or distort the profile of the iris or pupil, neoplasia has replaced the benign pigmented foci. Histologically, malignant transformation is characterized by a change in the histological features of the cell. Although angular cells adherent to the iridal surface may still be visible in early melanoma, the tumor cells have also exfoliated into the anterior chamber, implanted in the iridocorneal angle, and

invaded the iridal stroma (fig. 5.13). Transformed cells tend to be round, with a large round nucleus and a prominent nucleolus. In the early stages of neoplastic transformation, tumor cells seldom show cytological anaplasia. In the later stages of the disease, diffuse iris melanoma is characterized by three distinct cellular profiles.[7] The most common tumor cells are pleomorphic round cells with variable amounts of cytoplasmic pigmentation. Karyomegalic and cytomegalic forms are common, and nuclear pseudoinclusions, secondary to cytoplasmic invagination, are often seen (fig. 15.14). Neoplastic spindle cells are the second most common cell type, and neoplastic balloon cells, characterized by abundant vacuolar-to-granular clear cytoplasm and a small round nucleus are sometimes seen (fig. 15.15). Tumors can be composed of entirely one cell type or mixtures of all three. There is no known prognostic advantage based on the neoplastic cell type.[7]

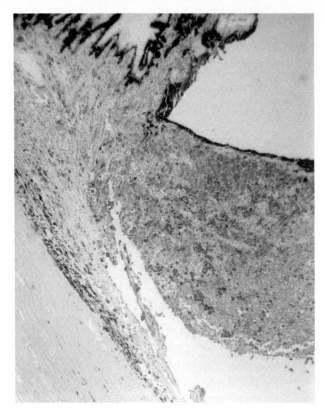

Fig. 15.13. There is distortion of the iris profile due to the diffuse invasion of neoplastic pigmented cells, also seen in the iridocorneal angle and extending into the ciliary body stroma. Notice the posterior iris epithelium is intact. At this stage, diffuse iris melanoma is likely to cause glaucoma, and the possibility of distant metastasis is increased.

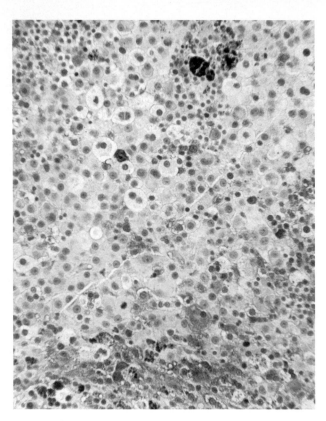

Fig. 15.15. Typical balloon cells sometimes associated with diffuse iris melanoma. Notice the decreased nucleus to cytoplasm ratio and the abundant amount of granular to vacuolated cytoplasm.

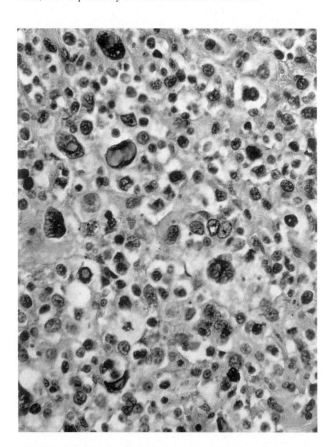

Fig. 15.14. Typical pigmented round cells associated with feline diffuse iris melanoma. Notice the karyomegaly and intranuclear pseudoinclusions caused by cytoplasmic invagination into the nucleus.

Clinical Features

Feline diffuse iris melanoma is a malignant disease, although both its onset and its progression are slow. The stages of development of this tumor are illustrated in table 15.4. Cats in which enucleation was done in the advanced stages of the disease are at risk of life-threatening systemic metastasis to the liver, lung, and kidneys. Cats in which diffuse iris melanoma is removed early in the disease process (abnormal pigmentation of iris) do not have an increased risk of systemic disease over control patients.[6] Tumor progresses slowly from asymmetrical pigmentary changes of the iris to nodular iridal irregularities and, inevitably, to glaucoma before extensive spread into the ciliary body, sclera, and posterior segment occurs.[7,8] Ideally, enucleation should be performed prior to the development of clinical glaucoma; however, alternative modalities of treating early pigmentary lesions are being evaluated.

Equine Melanocytic Tumors

Ocular melanoma in horses is often seen in conjunction with systemic melanomas and rarely is seen as a solitary spontaneous tumor separate from systemic disease. These tumors are usually composed of dense sheets of large, heavily pigmented cells similar to melanomas seen in other parts of the body. Melanomas usually occur anywhere in the uvea, and the risk to the animal depends on the extent of systemic disease. See equine melanoma discussed in chapter 2.

TABLE 15.4. Stages in the development of feline diffuse iris melanoma

Stage	Clinical	Morphological	Prognosis if Globe Removed
Melanosis only	Pigmented spots on iris	Small angular cells	No risk
Early melanoma	Pigmented spots on iris, growing	Rounded cells with large nucleus extending into the iris and in the anterior chamber	No risk
Midstage melanoma	Iris dark and irregular; glaucoma ±	Neoplastic melanocytes in ciliary body	Slightly increased risk
Advanced melanoma	Iris dark and irregular; glaucoma	Neoplastic cells throughout ciliary body	Metastatic disease highly likely

Iridociliary Epithelial Tumors in Dogs and Cats

Incidence

Iridociliary epithelial tumors are rare tumors, but they are the second most common primary intraocular tumor in dogs and cats.[9] They arise from the pigmented or nonpigmented epithelial cells of the iris or ciliary body. These tumors are more frequently diagnosed in dogs than cats. Clinically these tumors can present as white to dark brown or black masses, usually visible through the pupil in the posterior chamber; however, invasion through the iris or protrusion through the pupil can lead to a localized mass visible in the anterior chamber (figs. 15.16 and 15.17).[9,10] Iridociliary epithelial tumors are suspect in cases of glaucoma or intraocular hemorrhage where the media is opaque and direct observation of the tumor is impossible. In these cases, ultrasonographic imaging may prove helpful in delineating a mass lesion in the posterior chamber.

Care must be taken to thoroughly sample the globe histologically before ruling out small iridociliary tumors. Glaucoma is a frequent complication in part owing to the fact that these tumors are associated with the formation of a preiridal fibrovascular membrane, which can lead to peripheral anterior synechia or neovascular membranes that obstruct the iridocorneal angle.[11] Astroid hyalosis is another benign condition seen frequently in association with iridociliary epithelial tumors.

Morphology and Histological Features

Histologically these tumors are pleomorphic, occurring in either the iris or the ciliary body. In dogs, the tumors can be derived from pigmented or nonpigmented epithelium with most tumors containing both elements. Solid, papillary, or cystic tissue organization is possible. Many of these tumors secrete thick, PAS positive, basement membrane-like structures reminiscent of the inner lining of the nonpigmented ciliary body epithelium

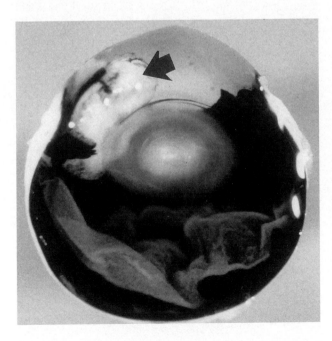

Fig. 15.16. Sectioned canine globe illustrating the typical profile of canine iridociliary adenoma. The nonpigmented tumor is nestled in the posterior chamber between the iris (arrow) and lens, showing extension through the pupillary margin.

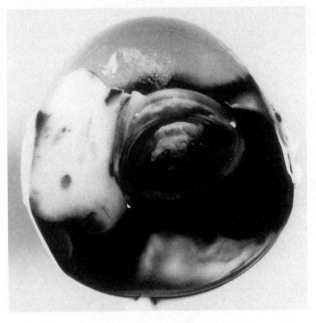

Fig. 15.17. A nonpigmented, feline iridociliary adenoma had invaded into the ciliary body and iris stroma, filling the posterior chamber and distorting the position of the lens.

(fig. 15.18). Secretion of hyaluronic acid is further evidence of iridociliary epithelial differentiation. Hyaluronic acid stains blue with alcian blue stain and resists digestion with hyaluronidase. Iridociliary epithelial tumors also stain positive for S100 and vimentin, as do normal iridociliary epithelial cells. Tumors that are clearly benign show either expansion only into the aqueous filled chambers of the eye, or infiltration of the anterior uvea but not the sclera. Progression into iridociliary carcinoma is recognized by anaplastic features and aggressive infiltration of the scleral stroma.[9] Although the normal iridociliary epithelium and benign tumors stain negative for cytokeratin, carcinomas are often positive. Distant metastasis of infiltrative carcinomas is extremely rare.[12] Differentiation of primary neoplasia from a metastatic tumor can be a problem. The presence of pigmented epithelium, PAS positive membranes, hyaluronic acid secretion, and positive immunohistochemical staining for vimentin or S100 can be useful markers to designate primary iridociliary epithelial tumors.

In cats these tumors are very rare. Histologically they tend to be solid and are composed of fairly monomorphic, usually nonpigmented, small epithelial cells (fig. 15.19). A cystic variant can also occur.

Spindle Cell Tumors in Blue-Eyed Dogs

Spindle Cell tumors of blue-eyed dogs present as nodular nonpigmented masses of the anterior uvea. The iris and ciliary body profile is distorted due to a solid mass composed of pleomorphic spindle cells showing a complex interdigitation with stromal collagen. Cellular aggregating and nuclear palisading are common features and suggest that these tumors are of peripheral nerve origin. Electron microscopy done on one case showed basal lamina around individual cells. All of these tumors, 15 cases, have presented in blue-eyed dogs. Siberian huskies are most commonly affected but several other breeds are represented.

Medulloepithelioma of Dogs and Horses

Gross Morphology and Histological Features

Medulloepithelioma in the eye, as elsewhere, is a neoplasm derived from primitive neuroectodermal tissue and is seen primarily in young animals.[13] These tumors are primary intraocular tumors in dogs and horses. Tumors arise mainly from the ciliary body; however, one tumor from a horse is reported to arise from the optic nerve head.[14] Clinically medulloepitheliomas are recognized by the presence of a fleshy mass seen through the pupillary margin or infiltrating into the anterior chamber. Some tumors are recognized as a white reflection posterior to the lens (leukokoria). Distinctive tubular protrusions are sometimes seen extending from the main mass or floating freely. Histologically these tumors are composed of small, primitive, poorly differentiated, stel-

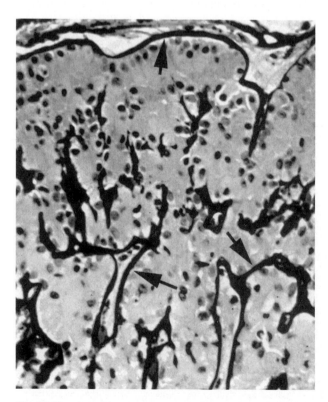

Fig. 15.18. Canine iridociliary adenoma with thick linear extracellular deposits of PAS positive basement membrane material (arrows).

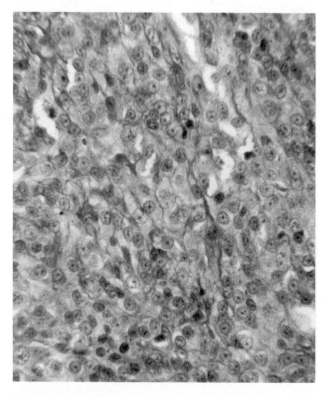

Fig. 15.19. Photomicrograph of feline iridociliary adenoma showing typical solid configuration of tightly packed epithelial cells with indistinct PAS positive extracellular membranes.

late to round cells, and the characteristic histological feature is the formation of rosettes characterized by aggregation of neoplastic cells to form a variably defined tubular structure. The rosettes sometimes have a central lumen (fig. 15.20) (Flexner-Wintersteiner rosettes), or they may be less differentiated, lacking epithelial junctions and a lumen (Homer-Wright rosettes).[13] Distant metastases of medulloepithelioma in dogs and horses are rare, but can occur.

Feline Posttraumatic Sarcoma

General

Cats are at risk of developing malignant sarcomas in eyes that have been traumatized and have rupture of the lens capsule. The onset of neoplastic disease can be as early as several months and as late as 10 years or longer following the traumatic event.[15-17] Tumors are usually first recognized as a change in the shape or color of the blind eye.

Gross Morphology and Histological Features

The posttraumatic sarcoma has a characteristic distribution pattern within the globe. Unless the tumor is detected in its earliest stages, these tumors will be characteristically distributed circumferentially at the peripheral margins within the globe. In many cases the entire globe will be filled with opaque solid tissue, although viable neoplasia may be limited to the periphery, either internal to the uvea and cornea or extending into the sclera depending upon the invasiveness (fig. 15.21). Early invasion into the optic nerve often occurs, and extension through the optic nerve to the brain is a risk for affected animals. The cell of origin of posttraumatic sarcoma is controversial. Some of these tumors form from mesenchymal appearing cells that have intercellular desmosomal attachments and secretion of a thick basement membrane (fig. 15.22) as well as positive immunohistochemical staining for vimentin and smooth muscle actin.[18] All of these features suggest the lens epithelial cell as the cell of origin. Proliferating lens epithelial cells in anterior subcapsular cataract show the same battery of staining reactions as well as desmosomal attachments.[18] Other posttraumatic sarcomas are clearly osteosarcomas, giant cell sarcomas, chondrosarcomas, or anaplastic sarcomas.[19,20] Histological patterns suggesting peripheral nerve differentiation and even melanocytic differentiation have been seen in a similar pattern in traumatized cat eyes. These tumors have a high malignant potential and can cause continued disease because of local reoccurrence, extension into the optic nerve or peripheral nerves and brain, or distant metastases.[17,21] Critical to the diagnosis of posttraumatic sarcoma is the finding of a neoplasm diffusely spread within the globe and evidence of prior lens rupture.

Lymphoma

Although lymphoma is not considered a primary tumor when it occurs in or adjacent to the globe, it is a

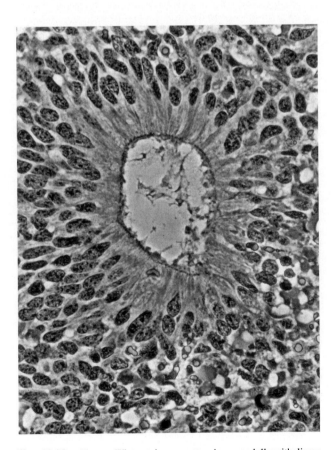

Fig. 15.20. Flexner-Wintersteiner rosettes in a medulloepithelioma from a young horse.

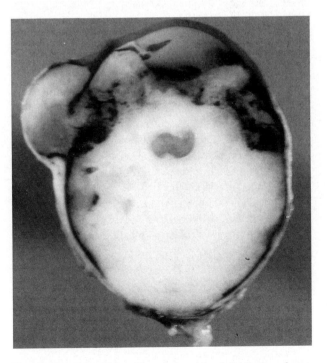

Fig. 15.21. Feline globe with typical peripheral distribution of posttraumatic sarcoma. The nonpigmented tumor fills the globe circumferentially and has aggressive invasion through the sclera.

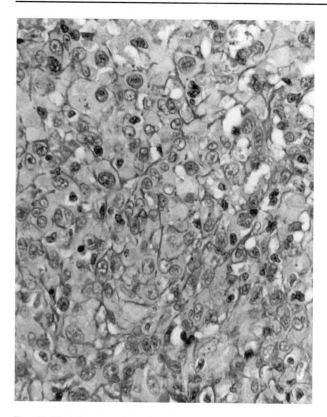

Fig. 15.22. Photomicrograph of posttraumatic sarcoma showing features of lens epithelial differentiation. Pleomorphic angular cells show a thick PAS positive membrane in the extracellular space between sheets of neoplastic cells.

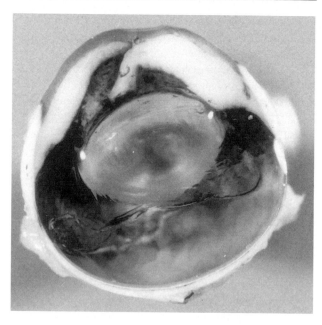

Fig. 15.23. Sectioned feline globe with diffuse thickening of the anterior uvea typical of infiltration with lymphoma.

common ocular tumor in dogs, cats, and cattle.[22-24] The tumors can occur anywhere in the eye, but the anterior uvea is the most frequent site (fig. 15.23). Orbital lymphoma is most commonly seen in cattle and is part of a generalized lymphoma.

Metastatic Ocular Neoplasia

Secondary ocular neoplasia is rare owing to the small size of the ocular tissue, but the clinician and the pathologist should be aware of the potential for clinical ocular disease caused by tumor metastasis. The most common metastatic tumors to the globe in dogs, exclusive of lymphoma, are hemangiosarcoma, mammary adenocarcinoma, and malignant oral melanoma.[25-27] In cats the most common metastatic tumors are pulmonary adenocarcinoma and mammary adenocarcinoma.[28,29] The main differential for these latter tumors is a primary iridociliary epithelial tumor.

REFERENCES

1. Morgan, G. (1969) Ocular tumors in animals. *J Small Anim Pract* 10:563-570.
2. Diters, R.W., and Ryan, A.M. (1983) Canine limbal melanoma. *Vet Med/Sm Anim Clin* 78:1529-1533.
3. Diters, R.W. Dubielzig, R.R., Aguirre, G.D., and Acland, G.M. (1983) Primary ocular melanomas in dogs. *Vet Pathol* 20:379-395.
4. Wilcock, B.P., and Peiffer, R.L. (1986) Morphology and behavior of primary ocular melanomas in 91 dogs. *Vet Pathol* 23:418-424.
5. Collinson, P.N., and Peiffer, R.L. (1993) Clinical presentation, morphology, and behavior of primary choroidal melanomas in eight dogs. *Prog Vet Comp Ophthalmol* 3:158-164.
6. Dubielzig, R.R., Chappell, R.J., Kalishman, J.B., and Flood, L.A. (1997) Survival in cats with diffuse iris melanoma: A matched observational study. Proceedings of the 28th Annual Meeting of the American College of Veterinary Ophthalmology, Santa Fe, NM, p. 5.
7. Patnaik, A.K., and Mooney, S. (1988) Feline melanoma: A comparative study of ocular, oral, and dermal neoplasms. *Vet Pathol* 25:105-112.
8. Duncan, D.E., and Peiffer, R.L. (1991) Morphology and prognostic indicators of anterior uveal melanomas in cats. *Prog Vet Comp Ophthalmol* 1:25-32.
9. Peiffer, R.L. (1983) Ciliary body epithelial tumours in the dog and cat; a report of thirteen cases. *J Small Anim Pract* 24:347-370.
10. Bellhorn, R.W. (1969) Successful removal of ciliary body adenoma. *Mod Vet Pract* 50:47-49.
11. Gelatt, K.N., Henry, J.D., and Strafuss, A.C. (1970) Excision of an adenocarcinoma of the iris and ciliary body in a dog. *J Amer Anim Hosp Assoc* 6:59-70.
12. Bellhorn, R.W., and Henkind, P. (1968) Adenocarcinoma of the ciliary body. *Pathol Vet* 5:122-126.
13. Wilcock, B., and Williams, M.M. (1980) Malignant intraocular medulloepithelium in a dog. *J Amer Anim Hosp Assoc* 16:617-619.
14. Ueda, Y., et al. (1993) Ocular medulloepithelioma in a thoroughbred. *Equine Vet J* 25:558-561.
15. Woog, J., Albert, D.M. (1983) Osteosarcoma in a phthisical feline eye. *Vet Pathol* 20:209-214.
16. Dubielzig, R.R. (1984) Ocular sarcoma following trauma in three cats. *J Amer Vet Med Assoc* 184:578-581.
17. Dubielzig, R.R., Everitt, J.A., Shadduck, J.A., and Albert, D.M. (1990) Clinical and morphologic features of post-traumatic ocular sarcomas in cats. *Vet Pathol* 27:183-189.
18. Dubielzig, R.R., Hawkin, K.L., Toy, K.A., Rosbury, W.S., Mazur, M., and Jasper T.G. (1994) Morphologic features of feline ocular

sarcoma in 10 cats: Light microscopy, ultrastructure, and immuno-histochemistry. *Prog Vet Comp Ophthalmol* 4:7-12.

19. Miller, W.W., and Boosinger, T.R. (1987) Intraocular osteosarcoma in a cat. *J Amer Anim Hosp Assoc* 23:317-320.

20. Hakanson, N., Shively, J.N., Reed, R.E., and Merideth, R.E. (1990) Intraocular spindle cell sarcoma following ocular trauma in a cat: Case report and literature review. *J Amer Anim Hosp Assoc* 26:63-66.

21. Barrett, P.M., Merideth, R.E., and Alarcon, F.L. (1995) Central amaurosis induced by an intraocular posttraumatic fibrosarcoma in a cat. *J Amer Anim Hosp Assoc* 31:242-245.

22. Cello, R., and Hutcherson, B. (1962) Ocular changes in malignant lymphoma of dogs. *Cornell Vet* 52:492-523.

23. Meincke, J.E. (1966) Reticuloendothelial malignancies with intraocular involvement in the cat. *J Amer Vet Med Assoc* 148:157-161.

24. Corcoran, K.A., Peiffer, R.L., and Koch, S.A. (1995) Histologic features of feline ocular lymphosarcoma: 49 cases (1978-1992). *Vet Comp Ophthalmol* 5:35-41.

25. Barron, C.N., and Saunders, L.Z., and Jubb, K.V. (1963) Intraocular tumors in animals. III. Secondary intraocular tumors. *Amer J Vet Res* 24:835-853.

26. Bellhorn, R.W. (1971) Ciliary body adenocarcinoma in the dog. *J Amer Vet Med Assoc* 159:1124-1128.

27. Ladds, P.W., Gelatt, K.N., Strafuss, A.C., and Mosier, J.E. (1967) Canine ocular adenocarcinoma of mammary origin. *J Amer Vet Med Assoc* 156:63-69.

28. Williams, L.W., Gelatt, K.N., and Gwin, R.M. (1981) Ophthalmic neoplasms in the cat. *J Amer Anim Hosp Assoc* 17:999-1008.

29. Gionfridde, J.R., et al. (1990) Ocular manifestations of a metastatic pulmonary adenocarcinoma in a cat. *J Amer Vet Med Assoc* 197:372-374.

TUMORS OF THE OPTIC NERVE

Orbital Meningioma of Dogs

Orbital meningioma is a rare but unique neoplasm occurring by invasion from the optic nerve meninges circumferentially into the connective tissues of the orbit. Characteristically these tumors are conical solid tan masses tightly adherent to the posterior aspect of the globe, tapering as the nerve approaches the brain circumferentially around the optic nerve (fig. 15.24).[1,2] Although the nerve itself may be tightly compressed, invasion of the nerve tissue is usually not prominent.[3] Invasion of adipose and muscular tissue is extensive, and multifocal nodules of myxoid stroma showing both cartilaginous and osseous metaplasia are a feature useful in diagnosis.[4] Osseous foci can sometimes be seen on radiography or orbital ultrasound and are a useful marker of this disease. Neoplastic cells tend to aggregate in invasive clusters (fig. 15.25). The cells are variably sized, but large pleomorphic cells with abundant glassy eosinophilic cytoplasm are often seen in interconnected cords or aggregates. This appearance can mimic the appearance of an invasive epithelial tumor, and an incorrect diagnosis of squamous cell carcinoma or metastatic carcinoma is to be avoided (fig. 15.26). The characteristic tumor distribution, the presence of multifocal mesenchymal differentiation, positive immunohistochemical staining for vimentin, and negative immunohistochemical staining for cytokeratin are morphological features useful in correctly diagnosing this neoplasm.

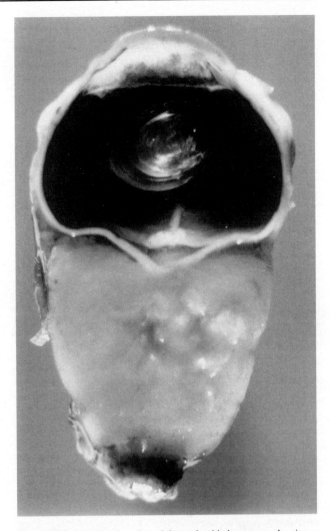

Fig. 15.24. Sectioned canine globe and orbital contents showing a slightly granular mass typical of canine orbital meningioma. The mass distorts the posterior profile of the globe and surrounds the optic nerve.

Astrocytoma

Astrocytomas of the optic nerve and retina have been documented in both dogs and cats as sporadic, very rare neoplasms.[5-7] The morphological and histological appearance are similar to those of astrocytomas seen in the central nervous system (fig. 15.27).

REFERENCES

1. Frith, C.H. (1975) Meningioma in a young dog resulting in blindness and retinal degeneration. *Vet Med/Small Anim Clin* 70:307-312.

2. Karp, L.A., Zimmerman, L.E., Borit, A., and Spencer, W. (1974) Primary intraorbital meningiomas. *Arch Ophthalmol* 91:24-28.

3. Wright, J.E., Maroon, J.C., Malton, M., and Warren, F.A. (1980) Primary optic nerve meningioma. *Brit Ophthalmol* 64:553-558.

4. Dugan, S.J., Schwarz, P.D., Roberts, S.M., and Ching, S.V. (1993) Primary optic nerve meningioma and pulmonary metastasis in a dog. *J Amer Anim Hosp Assoc* 29:11-16.

5. Barnett, K.C. (1972) Retrobulbar tumour and retinal detachment in a dog. *J Small Anim Prac* 13:315-319.
6. Gross, S.L., and Dubielzig, R.R. (1984) Ocular astrocytoma in a dog and a cat. In Proceedings of the Fifteenth Annual Meeting of the American College of Veterinary Ophthalmologists, p. 57.
7. Spiess, B.M., and Wilcock, B.P. (1987) Glioma of the optic nerve with intraocular and intracranial involvement in a dog. *J Comp Pathol* 97:79-84.

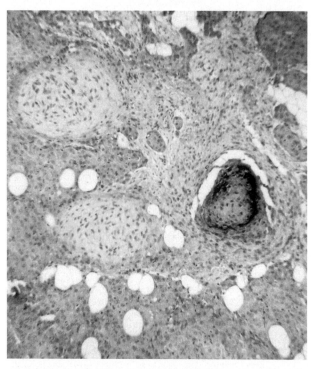

Fig. 15.25. Photomicrograph of canine orbital meningioma with extensive invasion around adipocytes and multiple foci of myxomatous to osseous metaplasia.

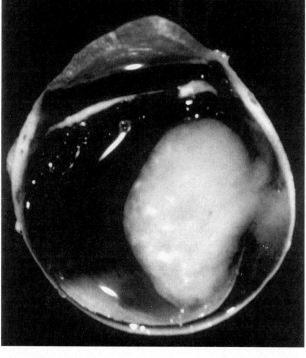

Fig. 15.27. Sectioned feline globe with retinal astrocytoma showing invasion into the choroid.

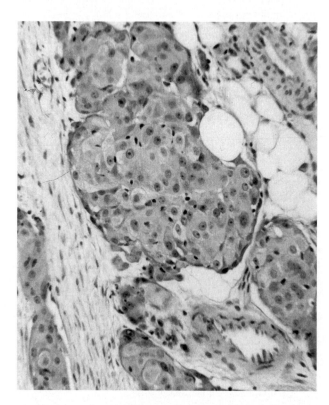

Fig. 15.26. Neoplastic cells from canine orbital meningioma have an epithelial-like appearance yet are tightly aggregated mesenchymal cells infiltrating around adipocytes.

Appendix
Diagnostic Schemes and Algorithms

INTRODUCTION

The diagnostic schemes and/or algorithms that follow this Introduction are used at North Carolina State University in the evaluation of certain tumors in dogs. They were created from information in the literature and have been modified and condensed to make them easier to use. The algorithms and the manuscripts cited are kept in a notebook for the pathologists on duty. Users are encouraged to read the original articles from which the information was drawn and determine if these modifications are suitable for their use. Most of the grading schemes provide prognostic information (survival and/or metastasis), which may also be used to determine therapy. The schemes used most frequently are for connective tissue and mast cell tumors, some are used rarely if requested by the clinician (e.g., lung tumors).

The survival information provided in each figure is derived from the cited articles and based on how the authors gathered the data, not on our modifications. Overall survival time following surgical excision of the tumor is the outcome most often reported in these grading schemes. However, in some studies it is not clear if the patient died as a result of the cancer or from unrelated problems or if euthanasia was elected. These and other confounding problems in retrospective studies may introduce significant inaccuracies associated with survival estimates. Furthermore, the actuarial survival (life span) of age-matched (geriatric) dogs is not known and cannot be compared with the groups being evaluated (e.g., What is the mean, median survival of a 13 year old dog?). Although imprecise, overall survival data can be readily collected, and generally it relates to the severity of a patient's condition.

At our institution, reports contain a description of the tumor, a morphologic diagnosis, an assessment of surgical margins and invasion (of adjacent tissues and vessels), and if applicable, a grade. Margins are evaluated macroscopically and microscopically and are subjective. The number of sites sampled along the margin vary with the size of the specimen, and even with multiple samples the majority of the margin is not assessed. Determination of the presence or absence of neoplastic cells at the surgical margins usually will influence therapy or additional surgery. If neo-plastic cells are present at a surgical margin, that site is reported; if tumor is not present, an estimate of the number of 400× (40× objective) fields from the closest surgical margin to the tumor is provided.

Many of the algorithms use a mitotic index (MI), and there are standardized methods for determining the MI. It is not always clear in some manuscripts how the study pathologist evaluated certain parameters. A recommended approach is to use a 40x objective to count mitoses in 10 contiguous fields in areas of cellular proliferation of the most anaplastic regions, skipping over areas of necrosis. If a tumor has clearly anaplastic areas and well-differentiated areas, start in the anaplastic areas and continue if contiguous fields carry into the more differentiated regions. Formal procedures should be standardized and used.

Grades of tumor, staging, immunohistochemical staining, proliferation indices, etc. are needed on a relatively small percentage of all tumors but are used frequently when treatment is being considered. For the majority of clinical veterinarians and diagnostic pathologists, the morphologic diagnosis and assessment of margins from H&E–stained sections is still the gold standard. Until specialized techniques are standardized, the ancillary aids may be performed best at institutions/centers that have specialists involved in the treatment and microscopic evaluation of tumors. Even immunohistochemical techniques should be standardized because of the many factors that influence immunoreactivity (antibody, concentration of antibody, type and duration of fixative, enzyme digestion, tissue processors, etc.). Our experiences with uterine biopsies, tumor grades, and toxicologic pathology studies have elucidated the variation to seemingly straightforward assessments by different pathologists.

Research correlating morphologic features of cancer with outcome analyses requires a team approach. Histologic criteria should be accurate, reproducible, predictive, and simple. Detailed schemes that evaluate numerous factors are an excellent initial approach to generate data, but subsequently these schemes should be limited to the essential criteria found to separate tumors into biologic categories. These criteria should be sufficiently straightforward so that the variation by pathologists is minimal and of a nature that diagnostic pathologists will have the techniques readily available. Criteria that are difficult to observe consistently will not be used. Diagnostic pathologists want algorithms that are easy to follow, yield reproducible results, and provide important information; for example, correlation with survival, prediction of metastasis, and selection of treatments.

Treatment recommendations are developed from the histopathologic assessment of the tumor and the surrounding tissues. The risk of regional or distant metastasis can be predicted in some tumors using grading schemes. The risk of metastasis is considered against the risk of treatment in order to develop broad treatment recommendations. If the risk of metastasis is high, treatment with an effective protocol is recommended, whereas a low risk of metastasis may not warrant adjuvant chemotherapy or immunotherapy. Such guidelines are imprecise because few studies have confirmed a survival benefit from chemotherapy with comparably graded tumors after surgical excision and no adjuvant therapy. Statistically significant correlation between algorithms and a clinical outcome can be identified best when standardized treatment protocols are followed. Modifying treatment protocols and applying standardized observations generates small groups that are invalid for statistical comparisons. These studies are frustrating because they have limited, if any, value.

The field of veterinary oncology needs prospective studies with rigid protocols and careful correlation of clinicopathologic information. These types of studies can be used to increase the quality of veterinary patient care. As pathologists, we need to standardize the parameters and methods used to evaluate tumors.

The incorporation of presently state-of-the art proliferation indices (AgNOR, Ki67, etc.) and future research techniques need to be compared with light microscopy of H&E-stained sections. Collecting information at research institutes and comparing state-of-the-art indices with basic criteria will determine which techniques are of equal, better, or lesser value in predicting important clinical outcomes. When pathologists generate standardized data and compare them to standardized treatment protocols with large numbers of patients, we will have meaningful information—until then we have some excellent studies to consider. The purpose of these appendixes is to summarize some of the approaches and make them available in one location to diagnostic pathologists.

—Don Meuten

CANINE CUTANEOUS MAST CELL TUMOR

Degree of Differentiation

Differentiation	Grade I	Grade II	Grade III
	Well	**Intermediate**	**Poorly**
Cellularity	Low	Intermediate	High
Cells	Uniform	Anisocytosis moderate	Anisocytosis marked
Giant cells	Zero	Few	Frequent
Pleomorphism	Zero	Moderate	Common
Cytoplasmic granules	Obvious	Visible	Inconspicuous to absent
Nuclei	Uniform, round to oval	Anisokaryosis	Anisokaryosis
Mitoses	None to few	Moderate	Numerous
MI (no. per ten 400 × fields)	<2	≥2–8	>8
% alive (at 200–1500 days postsurgery)	90	50–80	10–40

Comments

Adjuvant treatment is determined by completeness of excision and grade. Irradiation or chemotherapy may be useful for completely excised grade II mast cell tumors (MCT); however, completely excised grade II MCT may not require additional therapy. Chemotherapy is recommended for grade III MCT even with complete excision.

REFERENCES

Patnaik A.K., et al. (1984) Canine cutaneous mast cell tumor: Morphologic grading and survival time in 83 dogs. Vet Pathol 21:469-474.

Abadie J.J., et al. (1999) Immunohistochemical detection of proliferating cell nuclear antigen and Ki-67 in mast cell tumors from dogs. J Amer Vet Med Assoc 215:1629-1634.

Bostock D.E. (1973) The prognosis following surgical removal of mastocytomas in dogs. J Sm Anim Pract 14:27-40.

Simoes J.P.C., et al. (1994) Prognosis of canine mast cell tumors: A comparison of three methods. Vet Pathol 31:637-647.

Sequin B., et al. (2001) Clinical outcome of dogs with grade II mast cell tumors treated with surgery alone: (1996-1999). J Amer Vet Med Assoc 218(7):1120-1123.

CANINE CUTANEOUS SARCOMAS*

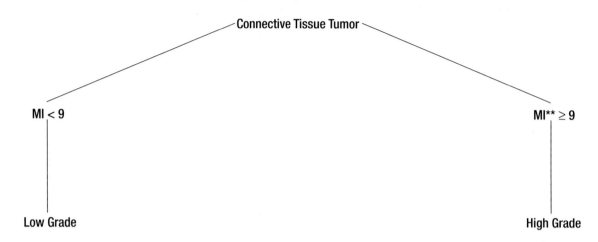

*Fibrosarcoma, hemangiopericytoma, neurofibrosarcoma, schwannoma, peripheral nerve sheath tumors, myxosarcoma, undifferentiated sarcoma: (n = 187 cases)

Mitotic Index: Mitotic figures/ten 400× fields

Low Grade: Recurrence rate of 25% after surgical excision, median survival time of 118 weeks, 2% metastatic rate

High Grade: Recurrence rate of 62% after surgical excision, median survival time of 49 weeks, 15% metastatic rate

REFERENCE

Bostock, D.E., et al. (1980) Prognosis after surgical excision of canine fibrous connective tissue sarcomas. *Vet Pathol* 17:581-588.

Median survival of dogs with soft tissue sarcomas following wide surgical resection as a function of mitotic index (MI = mitotic figures/10-400× fields). Data abstracted from Kuntz, et al; multiple features were evaluated.

Mitotic Index	Survival	% Metastases
< 10	1444 days	13
10-19	532 days	7
>19	236 days	41

Kuntz, C.A., et al. (1997) Prognostic factors for surgical treatment of soft-tissue sarcomas in dogs: 75 cases (1986-1996). *J Amer Vet Med Assoc* 211:1147–1151.

CANINE CUTANEOUS HEMANGIOSARCOMA

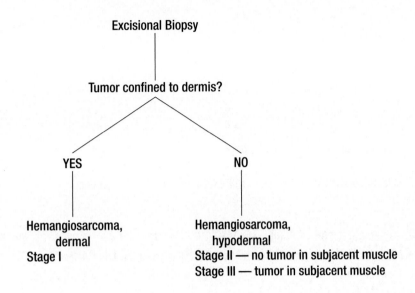

Hemangiosarcoma, dermal: Stage I (n = 10) median survival time 780 days after surgical excision
   3/10 had metastases or multicentric origin in other dermal sites and no distant metastasis

Hemangiosarcoma, hypodermal: Stage II (n = 10) median survival time 172 days
   Stage III (n = 5) median survival time 307 days; adjuvant chemotherapy recommended
   3/15 had additional cutaneous tumors; could not distinguish regrowth, metastases, and multicentric origin; 2 had distant metastasis (1 lung, 1 lymph node)
   Needle, wedge, or punch biopsy = Grading criteria not established—excision recommend

REFERENCE

Ward, H., et al. (1994) Cutaneous hemangiosarcoma in 25 dogs: A retrospective study. *J Vet Intern Med* 8:345-348.

CANINE CUTANEOUS MELANOMA

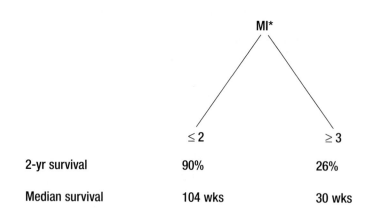

	MI*	
	≤ 2	≥ 3
2-yr survival	90%	26%
Median survival	104 wks	30 wks

*Mitotic Index: Sum of 10 randomly selected high-power fields (400×).
Fields in which nuclei were obscured by pigment were scored a MI of zero.[1]

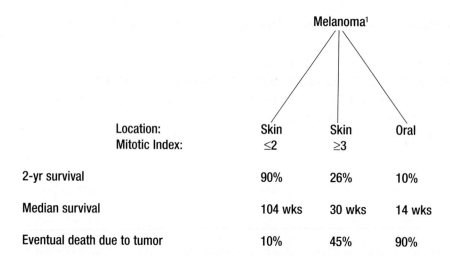

Melanoma[1]			
Location:	Skin	Skin	Oral
Mitotic Index:	≤2	≥3	
2-yr survival	90%	26%	10%
Median survival	104 wks	30 wks	14 wks
Eventual death due to tumor	10%	45%	90%

REFERENCES

1. Bostock, D.E. (1979) Prognosis after surgical excision of canine melanomas. *Vet Pathol* 16:32-40.

Ramos, J.A., et al. (2000) Retrospective study of 338 canine oral melanomas with clinical, histologic, and immunohisto-chemical review of 129 cases. *Vet Pathol* 37:597-608.

DIFFUSE IRIS MELANOMA
(34 cats, 83 age-matched controls)

Cats with melanoma confined to the iris survive at same rate as controls.
Cats with extensive tumors at time of enucleation have lowest survival rates.

Simplified Grades

Early—tumor only in iris and trabecular mesh work (n = 9)

Moderate—tumor in iris and rostral ciliary body but not sclera (n = 12)

Advanced—tumor throughout ciliary body and extending into sclera (n = 13)

Survival Postenucleation (Approximations)

	2 years	4 years
Early	100%	80%
Moderate	90%	70%
Advanced	15%	15%

When enculeation is done early (tumor confined to iris), cats with melanoma survive as long as control cats.

When enucleation is done after invasion of ciliary body or later, there is a progressively shorter survival.

REFERENCES

Kalishman, J.B., et al. (1998) A matched observational study of survival in cats with enucleation due to diffuse iris melanoma. *Vet Ophthalmol* 1:25-29.
Duncan, D.E., et al. (1991) Morphology and prognostic indicators of anterior uveal melanoma in cats. *Prog Vet Comp Ophthalmol* 1:25-32.

CANINE URINARY BLADDER CANCER

Transitional Cell Carcinoma

Features associated with metastases:
  Nonpapillary
  Infiltration
  Concurrent urethral involvement

Features associated with a favorable outcome:
  Tumor size and location such that complete resection is possible
  Females: tumor confined to bladder or urethra
      (spayed females, 358 days survival)
      (castrated males, 145 days survival)

Tumor in bladder **or** urethra—16% survive for 1 year or more

Tumor in bladder **and** urethra—shortest survival

Median survival of dogs with microscopic evidence of lymphatic invasion—145 days

Median survival of dogs without microscopic evidence of lymphatic invasion—349 days

Approximately 85% of dogs with TCC survive less than 6 months

REFERENCES

Norris A.M, et al. (1992) Canine bladder and urethral tumors: A retrospective study of 115 cases (1980-1985). *J Vet Intern Med* 6:145-153.
Valli VE, et al. (1995) Pathology of canine bladder and urethral cancer and correlation with tumor progression and survival. *J Comp Pathol* 113:113-130.
Rocha TA, et al. (2000) Prognostic factors in dogs with urinary bladder carcinoma. *J Vet Intern Med* 14:486-490.

GRADING CANINE SPLENIC SARCOMA

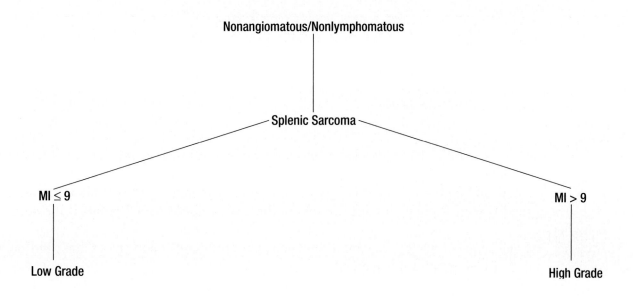

Fibrosarcoma, myxosarcoma, leiomyosarcoma, osteosarcoma, liposarcoma: (n = 87 cases)
Low Grade: Median survival time following splenectomy is 7 to 8 months

High Grade: Median survival time following splenectomy is 1 to 2 months
    80–100% of patients die within 1 year of diagnosis

Comments

The median survival time given for the low grade sarcomas is estimated from a survival rate curve. The median survival time for all splenic sarcomas (excluding lymphoma), regardless of grade, is 5 months following surgery. Both grades are treated similarly.

REFERENCE

Spangler, W.L., et al. (1994) Primary mesenchymal (nonangiomatous/nonlymphomatous) neoplasms occurring in the canine spleen: Anatomic classification, immunohistochemical, and mitotic activity correlated with patient survival. *Vet Pathol* 31:37-47.

CANINE AND FELINE MAMMARY NEOPLASIA

Histologic grading system of canine and feline mammary carcinoma

Characteristic		Score	
1. Tubule formation	1	2	3
2. Hyperchromatism and mitoses	1	2	3
3. Irregular size and shape of nuclei	1	2	3

Scoring

1. Tubule formation: 1 point if the section has well-marked tubule formation and 3 points if there are very few or no tubules.
2. Hyperchromatism and mitoses: 1 point if only an occasional hyperchromatic or mitotic figure per high-power field is seen, 2 points if there are two or three such figures and 3 points if the number is higher.
3. Irregular size and shape of nuclei: 1 point if the nuclei are fairly uniform in size, shape, and staining and 3 points if pleomorphism is marked.

Total Score	Grade of Malignancy
3–5	I
6–7	II
8–9	III

There is no grading system for mammary sarcomas.

Feline Mammary Neoplasia

- Tumor volume < $8cm^3$ — cats have longer disease-free intervals than cats with a tumor volume > $8cm^3$.

- Radical surgical excision of tumor produced significantly longer disease-free intervals than conservative treatment, but survival time was not improved. Cause of death in most cats was metastasis, recurrent tumor, or both.

- Unfavorable prognostic factors: Old age, large tumor volume, numerous mitoses, large amount of necrosis, metastasis to regional lymph nodes, and incomplete surgical excision as assessed by pathologist.

REFERENCE

Misdorp, W. (2002) Chapter 12 of the text.

OTHER REFERENCES

Weyer, K., and Hard, A.A.M. (1983) Prognostic factors in feline mammary carcinoma. *J Natl Cancer Inst* 70:709-716.
McEwen, E.G., Hayes, A.A., et al. (1984) Prognostic factors for feline mammary tumors. *J Amer Vet Med Assoc* 185:201-204.

LYMPHOMA

Our anatomic pathology service provides a morphologic diagnosis and a grade, and indicates if the cell type is <u>immature</u> or <u>mature</u> (a cell type beyond immature/mature must be provided by cytology and/or after immunohistochemistry). More complete schemes and prognostic factors are in Table 3.2 of this book. Our oncologists needs to know if a lymphoma is low or high grade, and they would like to know if it is B or T cell type.

Low grade: Mature cell type — low and medium MI   (any high MI is NOT a low grade)
High grade: Immature cell type — low, medium, and high MI

Mitotic index (MI) is determined from the examination of five to ten 400x fields (40x objective):
—low MI is 0–2/field
—medium is 3–5/field
—high is 6 or more/field
—it may be difficult to recognize mitoses in the lymphoblastic and small cleaved types.
—high MI associated with better initial response to chemotherapy but survival times are not prolonged.

Canine
Grade—High or Low
Grade is based on these criteria:
Low grade: Cell type is mature: lymphocytic and other, less common types.
MI = low or medium (high MI is not a low grade lymphoma)
High grade: The key is to recognize immature lymphoid cells with a medium to high MI.
Immature cell types are: lymphoblastic, immunoblastic, prolymphocytic and small noncleaved. This latter cell type is difficult to identify but they have a high MI which is easy to appreciate and they have "immature" features in nuclei. The MI puts them in the high grade group.
MI = majority (>90%) are medium or high
B vs T: Immunohistochemistry or flow cytometry; decreased survival time with T-cell lymphomas.

Feline
Grade—
Grade is based on these criteria:
Low grade: Cell type is mature:lymphocytic
MI = low to medium
High grade: Cell type is immature: see canine
MI = medium to high
B vs T: There is insufficient data on immunophenotyping B vs T lymphomas in cats to justify including this in our routine service.

REFERENCES

1. Carter, R.F., et al. (1986) The cytology, histology and prevalence of cell types in canine lymphoma classified according to the national cancer institute working formulation. *Can J Vet Res* 50:154-164.
Kiupel, M., et al. (1999) Prognostic factors for treated canine malignant lymphoma. *Vet Pathol* 36:292-300.
Hahn, K.A., Richardson, R.C., Teclaw, R.F., et al. (1992) Is maintenance chemotherapy appropriate for the management of canine malignant lymphoma? *J Vet Int Med* 6:3-10.
Jacobs, R.J., et al. (2002) Tumors of the Hemolymphatic System, chp 3, 4th ed. *Tumors of Domestic Animals,* ed. D.J. Meuten.

(continued)

LYMPHOMA (continued)

Stage and substage: This is assessed by clinician from all the data available; it is not performed by the pathology service. It is a useful indicator of prognosis for lymphoma (see Chapter 3, table 3.2 for complete list of prognostic factors).

   At NCSU immunohistochemistry is CD3 for T cell and BLA36 for B cell. CD3 is fairly reliable in that it identifies most T cells and is specific for T cells. However, BLA36 is less reliable and it will miss some B cells, particularly the more mature B cells and plasma cells, and it cross reacts with macrophages, such as Kupffer cells (see package insert).

   The following table is from reference 1 and it indicates which cell types in dogs are common and which are rare; a similar table is 3.3 in chapter 3 of this text. Note that at NCSU we do not use the "intermediate" grade; most of these lymphomas will fall into the high grade based on MI, and the diffuse, small cleaved lymphomas with a low MI will fall into the low grade.

		MI			Summary		
Grade	**Cell Type**	**Low**	**Med**	**High**	**No.**	**%**	**Total**
Low	Diffuse small lymphocytic	12	2	0	14	4.9	
	Follicular small cleaved	0	0	0	0	0	5.3%
	Follicular mixed	0	1	0	1	0.4	
Intermediate	Follicular large	0	0	1	1	0.4	
	Diffuse small cleaved	15	2	0	17	5.9	
	Diffuse mixed	2	3	1	6	2.1	28.4%
	Diffuse large	3	17	37	57	20	
High	Immunoblastic	2	28	41	71	25	
	Lymphoblastic	2	13	34	49	17.2	66.3%
	Small noncleaved	1	23	45	69	24.2	
	Total no.	37	89	159	285		
	Total %	13	31	56			

Note: "All" large cell types have a medium to high MI; only 7/246 had a low MI.

Note: 62% of 285 canine lymphomas were classified as large cell types and nearly 90% of all types had a medium to high MI.

SCORING SYSTEM AND PROGNOSIS FOR CANINE LUNG TUMORS [1]

Overall Differentiation
  1 Well differentiated (orderly arrangement between cells, basement membrane)
  2 Moderately differentiated (some loss of orderly arrangement)
  3 Poorly differentiated (loss of orderly arrangement)

Nuclear Pleomorphism
  1 Mild (minimal anisokaryosis and anisocytosis)
  2 Moderate (less than twofold difference in nuclear size)
  3 Severe (greater than twofold difference in nuclear size)

Mitotic Rate (per 10 high-power fields— 400×)
  1 1–10
  2 11–20
  3 21–30
  4 > 30

Nucleolar Size
  0.5 = Small (difficult to identify)
  1.   = Medium (identifiable, but not prominent)
  1.5. = Large (at least 1/3 size of the nucleus)

Tumor Necrosis
  0 = None
  1 = 1–20%
  2 = 21–50%
  3 = >50%

Tumor Fibrosis
  0   = None
  0.5 = 1–20%
  1   = 21–50%
  1.5 = >50%

Demarcation
  1 = Well demarcated (unencapsulated but sharp border)
  2 = Moderately demarcated (a few areas of neoplastic cells protrude into adjacent tissue)
  3 = Invasive (borders not distinguishable)

Final Score (Grade): Individual scores added together
  Grade I: <9 (MST: 790 days, MDFI: 493 days); Well differentiated (26 dogs)
  Grade II: 9–14 (MST: 251 days, MDFI: 191 days); Moderately differentiated (32 dogs)
  Grade III: 14.5 or greater (MST: 5 days, MDFI: 0 days); Poorly differentiated (9 dogs)
  MST (Median survival time) = time between surgery and death
  MDFI (Median disease free interval) = time between surgery and clinical evidence of recurrence
  a) Papillary (bronchoalveolar) carcinomas have a better prognosis (MST of 495 days and a MDFI of 365 days) compared with other primary lung tumors (MST of 44 days and a MDFI of 14 days). They were also the most common tumors identified.
  b) Other prognostic indicators that correlated with MST or DFI were presence of clinical signs and lymph node involvement. The MSTs were 26 and 452 days for cases with and without lymph node involvement, respectively.

REFERENCES

1. McNiel EA, et al. (1997) Evaluation of prognostic factors for dogs with primary lung tumors: 67 cases (1985-1992). *J Amer Vet Med Assoc* 211:1422-1427.
Ogilvie GK, et al. (1989) Classification of primary lung tumors in dogs: 210 cases. *J Amer Vet Med Assoc* 195:106-112.

HISTOLOGIC GRADING AND PROGNOSIS FOR FELINE LUNG TUMORS[1]

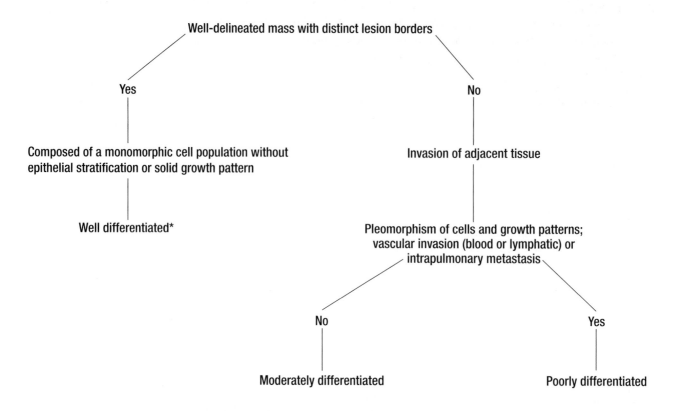

Cats with moderately differentiated tumors had a median survival time of 700 days (range of 19 to 1526 days) (n = 12). (Survival time defined as the time between surgery and death.)

Cats with poorly differentiated tumors had a median survival time of 75 days (range of 13 to 634 days) (n = 9).

*No cats in the study had well-differentiated tumors.

Comments

As with dogs, tracheobronchial lymph node enlargement appears to have prognostic significance in cats, however, further study is needed. Clinical findings (signalment, clinical signs, duration of clinical signs, and radiographic findings) were not significantly associated with survival time. Most tumors were of bronchial origin (n = 65); bronchoalveolar (n = 9); anaplastic carcinoma (n = 10); mesenchymal (n = 2).

REFERENCES

1. Hahn K.A., et al. (1998) Prognosis factors for survival in cats after removal of a primary lung tumor: 21 cases (1979-1994). *Vet Surg* 27:307-311.
Hahn K.A., et al. (1997) Primary lung tumors in cats: 86 cases (1979-1994). *J Amer Vet Med Assoc* 211:1257-1260.

CANINE AND FELINE NASAL TUMORS

The most important diagnostic distinction from a treatment perspective is lymphoma versus carcinoma or sarcoma because oncologists treat nasal lymphoma differently from carcinoma or sarcoma. Nasal carcinoma and sarcoma are treated the "same"; therefore, even though a histologic distinction is attempted, it does not affect treatment choice. It does, however, influence response to treatment (subjective) and survival (sarcomas respond better, also subjective).

Nasal lymphoma is confirmed infrequently in dogs, and it rarely occurs in just the nose. Nasal lymphoma is a relatively common clinical and cytologic diagnosis because many nasal carcinomas and sarcomas exfoliate as poorly differentiated round cells. Most of these tumors are demonstrated to be carcinoma or sarcoma if histology and or immunohistochemistry are used.

Nasal lymphoma occurs in cats more frequently than it does in dogs. It may be confined to the nose at the time of initial diagnosis, but for the majority of cases, if it is truly lymphoma, it will be generalized.

Some nasal tumors will have sarcomatous and carcinomatous areas histologically.

Nasal Adenocarcinoma   (64 dogs)

- Surgical procedure, chemotherapy group, and stage of primary tumor were shown to have no significant association with survival time

- Dogs with radiation therapy—median survival 424 days, which was significantly greater than no radiation therapy

- Dogs without radiation therapy— median survival 126 days

- Dogs with metastasis—median survival 109 days

- Dogs without metastasis—393 days median survival

- 8/64, 12.5% had detectable metastasis at time of initial presentation

REFERENCE

Henry, C.J., et al. (1998) Survival in dogs with nasal adenocarcinoma:64 cases (1981-1995) *J Vet Int Med* 12:436-439.

OTHER REFERENCES

La Due, T.A., et al. (1999) Factors influencing survival after radiotherapy of nasal tumors in 130 dogs. *Vet Radiol Ultrasound* 40:312-317.
McEntee, M.C., et al. (1991) A retrospective of 27 dogs with intranasal neoplasms treated with cobalt radiation. *Vet Radiol* 32:135-139.

Index

ISBN 0-8138-2652-7